Thelma Stoakes
316 Barker Rd.
Michigan City, Ind
482-7879

maternity nursing

maternity nursing

thirteenth edition

Sharon R. Reeder, R.N., Ph.D.

Associate Professor of Nursing, School of Nursing,
University of California, Los Angeles

Luigi Mastroianni, Jr., M.D., F.A.C.S., F.A.C.O.G.

William Goodell Professor and Chairman,
Department of Obstetrics and Gynecology,
University of Pennsylvania School of Medicine

Leonide L. Martin, R.N., M.S.

Family Nurse Practitioner
Assistant Professor, Department of Nursing,
California State College, Sonoma

Elise Fitzpatrick, R.N., M.S.

Professor of Nursing, School of Nursing,
University of Wisconsin, Milwaukee

J. B. LIPPINCOTT COMPANY

Philadelphia

New York   San Jose   Toronto

Thirteenth Edition

Copyright © 1976, 1971, 1966, 1960, 1952, 1948, 1943, 1940, 1937, 1934, 1933, 1931, 1929 by J. B. Lippincott Company

Distributed in Great Britain by
Blackwell Scientific Publications, Oxford
and Edinburgh

ISBN 0-397-54181-3
Library of Congress Catalog Card Number 76-2057
Printed in the United States of America

3 5 7 9 8 6 4

Library of Congress Cataloging in Publication Data

Main entry under title:

Maternity nursing.

    Twelfth ed., 1971, by E. Fitzpatrick, S. R. Reeder, and L. Mastroianni.
    Bibliography: p.
    Includes index.
    1. Obstetrical nursing. I. Reeder, Sharon R.
II. Fitzpatrick, Elise. Maternity nursing. [DNLM:
1. Obstetrical nursing. WY157 M425]
RG951.Z3   1976   610.73'678   76-2057
ISBN 0-397-54181-3

preface

The 13th edition of *Maternity Nursing* reflects extensive revision. Each chapter has been updated, many have been rewritten entirely, and several new chapters have been included.

Today, society is changing at a harrowing pace and the institutions within society, particularly the family, are also undergoing extensive reorganization. As the roles within society change, so, too, must those who occupy the roles alter their thinking and behavior to keep pace with the times. Thus, as clients change their orientations and behavior, providers of care must alter their views and behavior to effect synchrony in their mutual roles.

Of all the institutions in society, perhaps the family has undergone the most innovations in the last decade. The variety of family forms that appear to be emerging, such as single parent families and communal living, as well as the related issues of family planning and abortion, have, of necessity, broadened the scope of obstetrics and maternity nursing. Moreover, the changes and innovations that are occurring within the health care delivery system itself, particularly in nursing, have had an impact on our specialty. Thus, in this edition we have attempted to address these salient issues that affect maternity nursing practice so that students will be aware of their importance and can utilize them as they deliver true family-centered maternity care to their families.

Unit I has been reorganized to provide current concepts and thinking regarding the changing roles in the family, nursing, and parenting. The authors feel that, in order to help students learn to deliver high-quality family-centered nursing care, it is necessary to give them a broad base of knowledge from which to conceptualize the families with which they work. Thus, the concepts of role, the changing family, professional and parental roles in society, and the social factors in society which place the family at risk during their reproductive years are all introduced and explained to provide this broader conceptual base.

Unit II has also been rewritten to reflect the recent advances in knowledge about maternal physiology during reproduction, conception and ovum development, and development and physiology of the embryo and fetus, as well as current clinical aspects of human reproduction. This unit supplies the basic physiology, anatomy, and pathophysiology on which students can base their nursing care.

Dimensions of effective nursing care in each phase of the reproductive cycle have been enlarged, based on recent research and conceptual developments in nursing practice and related disciplines. The areas of antepartal and postpartal care, parent education, the conduct of normal and complicated labor, care of full-term and high-risk infants, and nursing in emergency situations all reflect this current thought and have been expanded accordingly. Of particular interest is the new chapter on the nursing management of pain and discomfort during labor. Basic theories of pain and the response to pain are examined and specific nursing measures to aid the patient who is experiencing pain and discomfort during labor are described in detail.

Current concepts regarding expanded roles for the maternity nurse as well as the role of the nurse-midwife have also been addressed and their implications for maternity nursing practice have been explored.

The subject of fetal medicine which was so new at the beginning of the decade has already advanced beyond fetal diagnosis to include current advances in treatment and genetic assessment. This chapter has been revised to include the most current concepts in this field. Specific fetal problems are examined, and present advances in fetal medicine are reviewed.

The chapters on the care of the preterm infant and the infant with a birth disorder have been extensively rewritten to include recent knowledge and advances in diagnosis and classification of these high-risk infants, as well as the medical and nursing management of infants with such conditions. The material on nursing in crises and emergency situations has been revised, and the chapter on the history of obstetrics has been further enlarged to include the newer developments in present-day maternity nursing in the United States.

Many new illustrations and figures, both photographs and original drawings, have been incorporated into this edition. The suggested reading lists that accompany each chapter have been updated with references from current professional literature. The conference material and study questions at the end of the various study units, as well as the glossary, which are thought to be essential by our readers, have been retained.

Sharon R. Reeder, R.N., Ph.D.
Luigi Mastroianni, Jr., M.D.
Leonide L. Martin, R.N., M.S.
Elise Fitzpatrick, R.N., M.S.

acknowledgments

With the preparation of the 13th edition of this book, we wish to welcome Mrs. Leonide Martin to our list of authors. Her interest and special expertise add a special dimension to the development of this volume.

We wish to express our gratitude for the help and encouragement of our many colleagues and friends in the revision of this text. Specifically, we thank Leo G. Reeder, Ph.D., Elaine Pierson, M.D., Ph.D., and Avner Perry, Ph.D., for their valuable suggestions regarding the content and preparation of the manuscript; Mrs. Shari Deight whose valuable assistance in researching the literature and other editorial services are greatly appreciated; Mrs. Trudy Krohn and Mrs. Debbie Wesley for their expert typing services.

We are also indebted to Mrs. Ruth Lubic, General Director of Maternity Center Association of New York, for permission to publish the exercises taught by Maternity Center Association in its prepared childbirth program. The authors would also like to express their appreciation to colleagues, publishers, and organizations for the use of illustrations, assessment tools, and other forms that are found in the text. We also wish to express our gratitude to the parents and nursing students who granted permission for photographs to appear in this book.

Finally, we take this opportunity to thank the J. B. Lippincott Company, particularly Mr. David T. Miller, Mrs. Mary Morgan, and Miss Val Rementer for their steadfast interest, cooperation, and assistance.

contents

unit I   **Current Issues in Maternity Care 1**

1 Maternity Nursing in Today's Changing
      World 3
      Obstetrics 3
      Maternity Nursing 4
      Maternal and Child Health 6
      Vital Statistics 7
      Natality 9
      Population 10
      Maternal Mortality 11
      Infant Mortality 13
      Current Problems in Maternity Care 14

2 The Family in a Changing World 17
      Roles, Role Theory, and Implications for
         Nursing Practice 18
      What Is the Family? 24
      Theoretical Approaches to the Study of
         the Family 24
      Family Forms of the Seventies 26
      The Nurse and the Changing Family 28
      Ethnic, Social Class, and Cultural
         Variations 35

3 Social Factors in Maternal Care 41
      Leo G. Reeder, Ph.D.
      The Social and Cultural Meaning of
         Pregnancy 42
      Present Societal Trends Affecting
         Childbearing Motivations and
         Maternity Services 42
      Sociocultural Factors Affecting
         Childbearing 44
      Social Class 45
      Sociocultural Patterns in the Use of
         Maternity Health Services 46
      Factors in Utilization 47
      Poverty: Its Relationship to Maternal
         Care 49

4 Selected Risk Factors and Pregnancy
      Outcomes 53
      Sociodemographic Risk Factors 53
      Behavioral Risk Factors 58
      Life Events and Life Crises as Risks 60

unit II   **Human Reproduction 63**

5 Anatomy Related to the Reproductive
      System 65

Pelvis 65
Female Organs of Reproduction 75
Mammary Glands 81
Male Organs of Reproduction 82

6 Maternal Physiology in Relation to Human
      Reproduction 85
      Sexual Maturity 85
      Menstrual Cycle 88
      Bodily Manifestations of Ovarian
         Function 91
      Menopause 93

7 Conception and Ovum Development 95
      Maturation of Ovum and Sperm Cells 95
      Determination of Sex 98
      Fertilization and Changes Following
         Fertilization 103
      Implantation of the Ovum 104

8 Development and Physiology of the Embryo
      and Fetus 107
      Decidua 107
      The Three Germ Layers 108
      Amnion, Chorion and Placenta 108
      Size and Development of the Fetus 110
      Duration of Pregnancy 114
      Calculation of the Expected Date of
         Confinement 115
      Physiology of the Fetus 116
      Periods of Development 118
      Maternal Impressions 119

9 Clinical Aspects of Human
      Reproduction 121
      Contraception 122
      Permanent Means of Sterilization 128
      Pregnancy Termination 129
      Infertility 131

unit III   **Assessment and Management During
               Pregnancy 141**

10 Normal Pregnancy 143
      Physiologic Changes of Pregnancy 144
      Local Changes 144
      Metabolic Changes 148
      Changes in the Various Systems 148
      Effects on the Psyche 150
      Endocrine Changes 150

11 Signs and Symptoms of Pregnancy 153
   Classification of Signs and Symptoms 153
   Presumptive Signs 154
   Probable Signs 155
   Positive Signs 157

12 Antepartal Care 161
   The Importance of Preventive Care 162
   Supervision Within the Health Care
      System 165
   The Nursing Process 170
   Nutrition in Pregnancy 179
   General Hygiene 195
   Minor Discomforts 206
   Preparations for the Baby 212
   Plans for After-Care of Mother and
      Baby 214

13 Patient Teaching and Counseling 217
   Teaching and Learning 218
   Types of Education for Childbearing 220
   Postpartum Teaching 226
   Guide for Preparing Parents for
      Childbirth and the Puerperium 228

unit IV   Assessment and Management During
          Labor and Delivery 241

14 Presentations and Positions 243
   Fetal Habitus 243
   Fetal Head 243
   Presentation 244
   Positions 244
   Diagnosis of Fetal Position 247

15 Phenomena of Labor 251
   Premonitory Signs of Labor 251
   Cause of Onset of Labor 252
   Uterine Contractions 254
   Duration of Labor 254
   The Three Stages of Labor 256

16 The Nurse's Contribution to Pain Relief
      During Labor 265
   Margo McCaffrey, R.N., M.S.
   Nature of the Pain Experience During
      Labor 265
   Assessment of the Patient's Pain and
      Pain Relief Methods 268
   Components of Pain Relief 275
   Pain Relief Measures During Labor 280
   Assistance with Change in Expectations
      and Goals 285
   Aftermath Assimilation 287

17 Analgesia and Anesthesia for Labor 289
   General Principles 289

Methods 290
Special Obstetric Anesthesia
   Problems 298

18 Conduct of Normal Labor 299
   Dimensions of Effective Nursing Care 299
   Prelude to Labor 302
   The Onset of Labor 302
   Continuing Care 307
   Examinations in Labor 310
   Conduct of the First Stage 312
   Conduct of the Second Stage 326
   Conduct of the Third Stage 334
   Conduct of the Fourth Stage 336
   Immediate Care of the Infant 341
   Emergency Delivery by the Nurse 347
   Lacerations of the Birth Canal 348
   Episiotomy and Repair 349

unit V   Assessment and Management of the
         Normal Mother-Infant Dyad 357

19 The Physiology of the Puerperium 359
   Anatomic Changes 359
   Clinical Aspects 362
   Postpartal Examinations 363

20 Nursing Care During the Puerperium 365
   Changes and Reactions During the
      Puerperium 366
   Immediate Care 370
   General Physical Care 371
   Special Physical Care Aspects 375
   The Nursing Couple 379
   Mechanisms in Lactation 379
   Parental Guidance and Instruction 392

21 Care of the Newborn Infant 397
   Physiology of the Newborn 397
   Characteristics of the Newborn 404
   The Environment of the Newborn 408
   Nursing Care of the Newborn 413
   Infant Feeding 420
   Artificial Feeding 423
   The Mother and Her Newborn 428
   Clinical Study: A Nurse and a
      New Mother 431

unit VI   Operative Procedures in Obstetrics 447

22 Operative Obstetrics 449
   Episiotomy and Repair of Lacerations 449
   Version 451
   Cesarean Section 452
   Destructive Operations 456
   Induction of Labor 456

unit VII   Assessment and Management of Disorders Associated with Childbearing 461

23   Complications of Pregnancy 463
        Toxemias of Pregnancy 464
        Hemorrhagic Complications 473
        Hyperemesis Gravidarum 482

24   Coincidental Diseases and Pregnancy 485
        Hematologic Disorders 485
        Heart Disease 486
        Diabetes Mellitus 487
        Disturbances in Thyroid Function 488
        Renal Disease 489
        Ptyalism 489
        Infectious Diseases 489

25   Complications of Labor 493
        Dystocia Due to Abnormalities of Labor
            Mechanics 493
        Hemorrhagic Complications 503
        Prolapse of Umbilical Cord 508
        Amniotic Fluid Embolism 509
        Multiple Pregnancy 510

26   Complications of the Puerperium 515
        Puerperal Infection 515
        Pulmonary Embolism 520
        Subinvolution of the Uterus 521
        Hemorrhage 521
        Vulvar Hematomas 521
        Disorders of the Breast 521
        Bladder Complications 525

27   Fetal Diagnosis and Treatment 529
      Richard H. Schwarz, M.D.
        Determination of Fetal Age 530
        Evaluation of Fetal Well-Being 532
        The Role of the Nurse in Genetic
            Counseling 536
        Intrapartum Evaluation of Fetal
            Well-Being 539
        Specific Fetal Problems 544
        Fetal Treatment 551

28   The High-Risk Infant: Low Birth Weight
        and Premature Classification of
        Infants by Birth Weight and
        Gestational Age 553
        Etiology 555
        Identification of the High-Risk
            Neonate 557
        Prenatal Factors 557
        Intrapartal Factors 557
        Neonatal Factors 558
        Assessment of Gestational Age 558
        Characteristics and Physiology of
            Small-for-Gestational-Age Infants 562

        Characteristics and Physiology of the
            Premature Infant 563
        Physical Care of the Infant 566
        Care of the Mother and Father 575
        Growth and Development 579

29   The High-Risk Infant: Disorders of the
            Newborn 581
        Parental and Staff Reactions to Defects
            and Disorders 581
        Neonatal Respiratory Distress 590
        Injuries 596
        Infections 599
        Malformations (Intrauterine Growth
            Deviations) 603
        Inborn Errors of Metabolism 613
        Miscellaneous Disorders 617

unit VIII   Special Considerations in Maternity Nursing 629

30   Home Delivery 631
        The Home Birth Movement 631
        Nurse-Midwifery 636
        Approach to Home Delivery by Nurse-
            Midwife and Physician Teams 639

31   Obstetrics During Emergency 645
        Commonalities of Disaster Situations 645
        The Organization of Emergency Nursing
            Services in the Hospital
            Environment 646
        Disaster Protection for Mothers and
            Infants 648
        Psychologic Reactions in Emergency
            Situations 651

32   History of Maternity Nursing 657
        Obstetrics over the Centuries 657
        Background and Development of
            Maternal and Infant Care in the
            United States 662
        The Emergence and Development of
            Maternity Nursing 670
        Future Possibilities 674

Appendix 677

    Answer Key for Study Questions 679
    Glossary 681
    Conversion Table for Weights of Newborn 689
    Aid for Visualization of Cervical
        Dilatation 690

Index 693

current issues in maternity care

Maternity Nursing in Today's Changing World
The Family in a Changing World
Social Factors in Maternal Care
Selected Risk Factors and Pregnancy Outcomes

unit I

maternity nursing in today's changing world

1

Obstetrics / Maternity Nursing /
Maternal and Child Health / Vital
Statistics / Natality / Population /
Maternal Mortality / Infant Mortality /
Current Problems in Maternity Care

The study of obstetrics and of the nursing care of women during the various phases of childbearing includes the study of anatomic and physiologic adaptations to human reproduction and, in the full meaning, the study of human growth and development and the many interdependent relationships concerned. The vast importance of professional maternity care to mothers, infants, and families of our country must be fully understood by all who participate in their care.

This chapter is planned to orient the student to maternity nursing. Certain basic terminology will be defined. Basic concepts in care will be introduced, and in the remainder of the unit, concepts relating to childbearing couples, their children, and their interaction with society will be given.

Knowledge of the anatomy and physiology of the reproductive organs and of the development of the unborn child from conception to birth is basic to the understandings required of every maternity nurse. The physiologic mechanism by which conception takes place and a new human being develops is not only a fascinating story in itself, but also one that has far-reaching implications for the mother, the child, and the family. All that a human being be-comes depends on many factors: his heritage, his prenatal environment, his care at birth, and his care thereafter throughout infancy and childhood. Thus, it is all the more important that the safety, health, and well-being of each mother and infant be protected, and, simultaneously, that the highest level of health possible for every childbearing family be achieved in the broader sense of physical, emotional, and social well-being.

In addition, it is important to realize the extent to which the structure and function of the family as it relates to society influence the reproductive behavior and health of the child-bearing family.

Obstetrics

Obstetrics is defined as that branch of medicine which deals with parturition, its antecedents, and its sequels. Therefore, it is concerned principally with the phenomena and the management of pregnancy, labor, and the puerperium under both normal and abnormal circumstances.[1]

The etymology of "obstetrics" is mentioned here to serve as basic information. For many students it will undoubtedly arouse curiosity and interest for further study. Briefly, the word obstetrics is derived from the Latin *obstetricia* or *obstetrix*, meaning *midwife*. The verb form *obsto* (*ob*, before, plus *sto*, stand) means *to stand by*. Thus, in ancient Rome a person who cared for women at childbirth was known as an *obstetrix*, or a person who *stood by* the woman in labor. In both the United States and Great Britain, this branch of medicine was called *midwifery* for several centuries—in fact, until the latter part of the 19th century. The term obstetrics really came into usage little more than a century ago, although reference to a variety of words of common derivation can be found occasionally in earlier writings. With the use of new terminology which has developed over the years, it is not unusual to find that, from the standpoint of semantics, changes have developed also in the present era. Today, in light of the various changes which have evolved in the total care of childbearing women, the usage of the term *obstetric care* is open to question. In the current frame of reference it seems more appropriate to use the term *maternity care*, since this term implies a broader meaning of the care of the mother and her offspring throughout the childbearing experience. Moreover, it focuses attention on the care of a *person*, on the importance of interpersonal relationships—particularly those relationships which are *significant to her*—and the kind of patient care which will assist in promoting the health and the well-being of the expanding family group.

The World Health Organization Expert Committee on Maternity Care has defined maternity care as follows:

> The object of maternity care is to ensure that every expectant and nursing mother maintains good health, learns the art of child care, has a normal delivery, and bears healthy children. Maternity care in the narrower sense consists in the care of the pregnant woman, her safe delivery, her postnatal examination, the care of her newly born infant, and the maintenance of lactation. In the wider sense it begins much earlier in measures aimed to promote the health and well-being of the young people who are potential parents, and to help them develop the right approach to family life and to the place of the family in the community. It should also include guidance in parent-craft and in problems associated with infertility and family planning.[2]

Maternity nursing

Maternity nursing involves direct, personal ministrations to maternity patients and their newborn infants, or related activities on their behalf, during the various phases of the childbearing experience. It differs from the practice of nursing in other areas only in that the clinical focus primarily involves the care of maternity patients (in contrast, for example, with the care of surgical patients or psychiatric patients). How the maternity nurse meets the nursing needs of mothers, fathers, and their newborn infants cannot be spelled out in stereotyped activities any more than it can in any other situation in which individualized nursing care is the underlying objective. In fact, the nurse may be called on at times to perform what superficially appear to be rather elementary nursing tasks, for example, those related to body cleanliness. It is *how* the nurse carries out her care of the patient, the depth of problem-solving ability she employs, that makes the difference between truly professional nursing and nursing on a technical level.

In the practice of nursing, the nurse intervenes to relieve or to reduce the patient's problems due to physical, physiologic, or psychologic stress. A significant aspect of maternity nursing on the professional level is that patient care involves purposeful, sustained interaction between the nurse and the patient, during which the nurse assesses the patient's problems (i.e., makes a nursing assessment concerning the nature of the discomfort or the dysfunction) and takes action to relieve the problem if it can be alleviated properly with nursing measures.

Begetting children is a family affair; thus, the nursing care of maternity patients is properly a family-centered activity. In many situations today the maternity patient is a healthy woman involved in the normal physiologic process of childbearing. However, like individuals facing any other new experience in the family life cycle, maternity patients may begin the experience at various stages of preparation for pregnancy and childbirth, with various kinds of stress and at various levels of contentment. It is safe to say that in almost no other normal physiologic process does one find such individual extremes of reactions within a normal context. These individual reactions may be based on events going back to childhood, to certain experiences shared in growing up, or to later happenings. Certainly, they are influenced by the home environment from which the mother comes and to which, a short time after the delivery, she will return with her newborn infant. The level of satisfaction with which the expectant mother leaves the clinic, or the level of contentment with which the newly delivered mother leaves the hospital environment with her baby will be modified somewhat by the interpersonal relationships of those most significant to her in that environment. Thus, the nurse can provide more continuity in the time spent with patients than other professionals, and by the nature of her position has the ability to make a significant contribution to maternity care.

The authors of this textbook refer to maternal and child health nursing as a philosophy of patient care rather than a special area of nursing. Whether it concerns maternity nursing, pediatric nursing, the nursing of children, or maternal-child health nursing, the patient care involves the nursing of mothers or children. Thus, the crux lies in the care of families. There is a body of knowledge which specifically pertains to maternity nursing, and, likewise, there is a closely related but separate body of knowledge which pertains to the nursing of children, or pediatric nursing. As one develops knowledge, understanding, and skills in these areas, a philosophy of maternal and child health also evolves.

High-level wellness

Good health (i.e., wellness) is not a static condition, but may be manifest in degrees of well-being or overlapping levels of wellness. Providing optimal maternal care requires an explanation of the many facets and factors responsible for the good health of maternity patients. From this point it is then possible to make statements in objective terms about what high-level wellness means for the individual, the family, and others who are significant to the patient.

In maternity nursing, the concept of high-level wellness is particularly appropriate in the promotion of good health for patients, whether the patient is pregnant, is in the course of labor, or is the newly delivered mother with her infant.

"High-level wellness is a term which has been devised to make the person who uses it think about well-being in degrees or levels. High-level wellness for the individual is defined as an integrated method of functioning

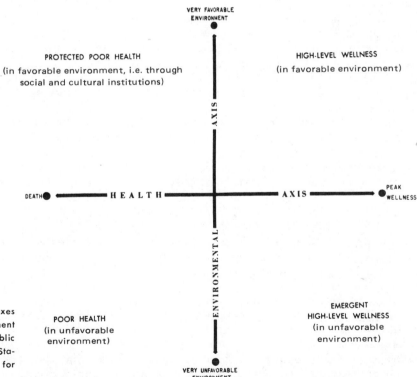

Figure 1-1. The health grid, its axes and quadrants. (Data from U.S. Department of Health, Education and Welfare, Public Health Service, National Office of Vital Statistics) (Dunn, H. L.: High-level wellness for man and society. *Am. J. Public Health*)

which is oriented towards maximizing the potential of which the individual is capable. It requires that the individual maintain a continuum of balance and purposeful direction within the environment where he is functioning."[3] Wellness, then, is a direction in progress toward an even higher potential of functioning for the total individual in all of his uniqueness. Dunn has proposed that, in order to utilize the goal of high-level wellness, it is essential to think in terms of disease and health as a graduated scale.[4] This scale is conceptualized as one axis of the "health grid" (Fig. 1-1). The health grid is made up of 1) the health axis, 2) the environmental axis, and 3) the resulting health and wellness quadrants. The environmental axis includes the physical and biologic factors of the environment, as well as the socioeconomic components affecting the health of the individual. The health axis ranges from death at the left extremity to peak wellness at the right.

As one looks at the health grid, with its health and environmental axes, it seems relatively easy to appreciate the extremes from severe illness and death on one side of the axis to the maximum or peak wellness on the other. Man lives in a very complex environment today which, like progress, tends to become more complicated. Freeman divides the environment into three major areas: the physical, the biologic, and the social.[5] We are in daily interaction with physical factors (or the "elements" in the environment). Temperature and humidity alone can contribute to the comfort or the extreme discomfort of a pregnant woman. For example, considering the various aspects of atmospheric pressure, one might consider the changes in altitude as creating a situation comparable to "Mt. Everest in utero." In the biologic environment, there are forces from the plant and animal kingdoms constantly interacting with man (e.g., microorganisms), some of which contribute to health rather than illness. The biologic area includes the sources which contribute to our food and clothing. Freeman says that the biologic environmental area provides the major source for physiologic growth and development, and that the social segment of the environment provides the major source for psychologic growth and development. As far as the social area of the environment is concerned, we are in constant interaction with people and the culture around us through many avenues of communication, such as the arts, the press, the radio, and television.

When we learn how to diagnose high-level wellness through objective measures, we shall probably find that a substantial amount of creative expression and love of daily life is essential in the approach to a high state of well-being. The goal of high-level wellness for man can be achieved. The needs are for clearcut concepts, for understanding, and for a reassessment of our basic values.

Maternal and child health

Despite the fact that today the use of the term *maternal and child health* seems to imply a relatively new concept of care, it actually was in usage more than 50 years ago. In 1912 the U.S. Children's Bureau was created by an act of Congress for the purpose of promoting maternal and child health "among all classes of people." It was said to be a community health nurse who first conceived the idea of a federal bureau of this kind and originally suggested the plan to President Theodore Roosevelt in 1905. The Children's Bureau has continually stressed the importance of community health nursing in maternal and child welfare. Between the years 1921 and 1929, community health nursing consultants were employed by the Bureau, and their services were offered to the states for maternal and infant hygiene. In rural areas throughout the United States, community health nursing services were greatly extended, and 2,978 centers for prenatal and child health work were established.

Since these early beginnings, the Children's Bureau has continued to make significant contributions to the promotion of maternal and child health in this country (see Suggested Reading).

However, there have been numerous forces arising in the context of society that have had an enormous impact on the delivery of care to childbearing families and children.

Trends in U.S. maternal and child health services were assessed in a recently published report by the late Dr. Edward Schlesinger of the University of Pittsburgh, who has long been active in efforts to upgrade such programs. Writing in *Health and Society*, Dr. Schlesinger cited current and past developments to explain why those in the maternal-child health field feel that they are in the throes of a profound "identity crisis."[6]

These developments are germane to maternity care because they exemplify a broad spectrum of thinking about delivery of health services in general. New systems of personal health services are being developed to serve entire populations regardless of age or categorical needs. Thus, expanding "special purpose" programs in early childhood and adolescence tend to include their own independent health services and have called into question the more traditional types of health services for mothers and children. The latter have tended to be separate and clearly identifiable programs in maternity and newborn care; in health supervisory services for infants, preschoolers, and school-age children; and in rehabilitative services for handicapped children. The new special purpose programs, because of their breadth, often lose specific aspects of care which are badly needed.

However, there have been certain reasons for the development of these newer programs, the most important of which is the unprecedented decline in the U.S. birth and fertility rates. Therefore, further expansion of maternal and child health services can no longer be justified *solely* by the argument of a continuing increase in the number of mothers and children to be served. Moreover, the U.S. infant mortality rate, although poor in relation to the rates of other industrialized nations, has also reached record lows, thus making arguments for broadened services on this point no longer as compelling as they were. Hence, with a much smaller population to serve and a slightly better infant survival rate, what can be the rationale for continued expansion of maternal child services? It appears that the argument must be shifted to the need to provide adequate services in order to maintain and expand the gains of recent years, *especially for those segments of the population that have not shared equally in these gains.*

One other reason for the newer programs deserves mention because it is concerned with basic funding for maternal-child health services. In 1973, there was a drastic reorganization of the federal child development and child health services under the Health Services Administration. While necessary, this reorganization fragmented services and diminished the visibility of mothers' and children's health needs within the federal government. There is no longer a single, clear focus for the expression of concerns for those involved with the health of mothers and children. Before the reorganization, there was firm federal-local cooperation in the provision of special project grants for specific purposes in geographic areas of need—primarily inner-city neighborhoods. However, since the reorganization, the concept of revenue sharing has threatened to reverse this and other salubrious trends that had been growing since 1935 with Title V funding. Inherent in all of this is the hazard that the health needs of the inner-city and other special need populations will receive less emphasis.

In view of these current outside forces and trends, we will summarize in the form of recommendations the major areas of concern in maternal-child health: first, it is necessary to have integration of high-quality maternal-child health services within evolving comprehensive systems of prepaid group health care plans. Moreover, services should include prevention, detection, and maintenance. Second, adequate funding of preventive and ambulatory services, especially during the newborn period, must be included in all the mechanisms for financing maternal-child health services. Third, the present services and special projects must be extended to meet the needs of specific high-risk and disadvantaged groups. Fourth, there is a need to resolve the dilemma of providing health services in settings which do not focus primarily on health, that is, schools. Fifth, there must be a focus on concern for maternal and child health within the federal government and for mechanisms for child advocacy both within and without the federal government. The recent fragmentation has left the federal government without a clear point of entry for those interested in maternal-child health services. Finally, there is a need for continuing, critical evaluative research to explore innovations and alternative methods of delivery of care. For instance, it is necessary to have a much clearer idea about whether increased technology really results in higher quality of care.

Vital statistics

With reference to frequency distribution, an examination of the vital statistics reports gives us quantitative data which have been systematically gathered and collated. These data are presented in this chapter because they relate to statistical changes in the large body of people with whom we are concerned—statistics on births, marriages, population, morbidity, and mortality.

In this country these data are published officially by the U.S. Public Health Service, National Center for Health Statistics, Vital Statistics Division. To understand the significance of the vital statistics quoted in the following discussion, the nurse should be familiar with the following terms, explained according to the definitions of the National Center for Health Statistics. Deaths are classified according to the World Health Organization Manual of International Classification of Diseases, Injuries, and Causes of Death, based on recommendations of the Seventh Revision Conference, 1955, volume 1, Geneva, Switzerland, 1957.

BIRTHRATE. The number of births per 1,000 population.

MARRIAGE RATE. The number of marriages per 1,000 total population.

FERTILITY RATE. The number of birth per 1,000 women aged 15 to 44 years.

NEONATAL. Pertaining to the first four weeks after birth.

NEONATAL DEATH RATE. The number of neonatal deaths per 1,000 live births.

FETAL DEATH, OR STILLBIRTH. One in which the infant of 20 weeks or more gestational age dies in utero prior to birth.

PERINATAL MORTALITY. The sum of deaths of fetuses and infants weighing 1,000 Gm. or over which occur between 28 weeks of gestation and four weeks of age (i.e., to the end of the neonatal period).

INFANT MORTALITY RATE. The number of deaths before the first birthday per 1,000 live births.

MATERNAL MORTALITY RATE. The number of maternal deaths per *100,000* live births.

Table 1-1 Total Fertility Rates and Birthrates by Age of Mother, by Color: United States, 1960-1968

Total fertility rates are the sums of birthrates by age of mother multiplied by five.
Birthrates are live births per 1,000 women in specified group.

Year and Color	Total Fertility Rate	Age of Mother							
		10-14 Years	15-19 Years	20-24 Years	25-29 Years	30-34 Years	35-39 Years	40-44 Years	45-49 Years
Total—Registered Births									
1968	2,476.8	1.0	66.1	167.4	140.3	74.9	35.6	9.6	0.6
1967	2,572.6	0.9	67.9	174.0	142.6	79.3	38.5	10.6	0.7
1966	2,736.1	0.9	70.6	185.9	149.4	85.9	42.2	11.7	0.7
1965	2,928.0	0.8	70.4	196.8	162.5	95.0	46.4	12.8	0.8
1964	3,207.5	0.9	72.8	219.9	179.4	103.9	50.0	13.8	0.8
1963	3,333.2	0.9	76.4	231.2	185.8	106.2	51.3	14.2	0.9
1962	3,473.5	0.8	81.2	243.7	191.7	108.9	52.7	14.8	0.9
1961	3,629.0	0.9	88.0	253.7	197.9	113.3	55.6	15.6	0.9
1960	3,653.6	0.8	89.1	258.1	197.4	112.7	56.2	15.5	0.9
White—Registered Births									
1968	2,368.4	0.4	55.3	162.2	139.7	72.5	33.8	8.9	0.5
1967	2,453.1	0.3	57.3	168.8	140.7	76.5	36.6	9.8	0.6
1966	2,609.2	0.3	60.8	179.9	146.6	82.7	40.0	10.8	0.7
1965	2,790.3	0.3	60.7	189.8	158.8	91.7	44.1	12.0	0.7
1964	3,073.7	0.3	63.2	213.1	176.2	100.5	47.7	13.0	0.7
1963	3,201.2	0.3	68.1	224.7	151.5	102.6	48.9	13.4	0.8
1962	3,347.5	0.4	73.1	238.0	187.7	105.2	50.2	14.1	0.8
1961	3,501.9	0.4	78.8	247.9	194.4	110.1	53.2	14.8	0.9
1960	3,532.9	0.4	79.4	252.8	194.9	109.6	54.0	14.7	0.8
Nonwhite—Registered Births									
1968	3,196.9	4.4	133.3	200.8	144.8	91.2	48.6	15.0	1.2
1967	3,385.3	4.1	135.2	212.1	155.9	99.1	52.4	16.8	1.2
1966	3,614.9	4.0	135.5	228.9	169.3	107.9	57.7	18.4	1.4
1965	3,891.4	4.0	136.1	247.3	188.1	118.3	63.8	19.2	1.5
1964	4,153.4	4.0	138.7	268.6	202.0	127.5	67.5	20.9	1.5
1963	4,268.7	4.0	139.9	277.3	211.8	129.3	68.9	21.0	1.5
1962	4,395.8	3.9	144.6	285.7	217.4	132.4	72.0	21.7	1.5
1961	4,532.6	4.0	152.8	292.9	221.9	136.2	74.9	22.3	1.5
1960	4,522.1	4.0	158.2	294.2	214.6	135.6	74.2	22.0	1.7

Vital Statistics of the United States, 1968, Vol. I—Natality, Table 1-6. Source: U. S. Department of Health, Education, and Welfare, Public Health Service, 1970.

RACE AND COLOR. Births in the United States are classified for vital statistics according to the race of the parents in the categories of white, black, American Indian, Chinese, Japanese, Aleut and Eskimo combined, Hawaiian and part-Hawaiian combined, and "other nonwhite." In most tables a less detailed classification of "white" and "nonwhite" is used (Table 1-1).

The category white includes births to parents classified as white, Mexican, Puerto Rican, or "not stated." If one parent is Hawaiian and the other is not, the birth is classified as part-Hawaiian. If one parent is black, and the other is not Hawaiian, the birth is classified as black. In other cases of mixed parentage in which both parents are nonwhite, the child is assigned the father's race; if the father is white, the child is assigned the mother's race.

Natality

The number of registered births in the United States has decreased appreciably in the last two decades from over 4 million live births in 1957, to 3.5 million in 1968, and to 3.1 million in 1973. In 1947, immediately following World War II, there was a sharp rise in births, reaching a birthrate of 25.8 per 1,000 persons. After this peak, however, the birthrate for the total population declined slightly and remained about 25.0 during the next decade.

The total number of live births in this country began to decline gradually in 1958, and in 1963, the birthrate decreased to 21.7. By 1974, the rate had further declined to 15 per 1,000, and there is some indication that, with the new orientations toward fertility and population controls, there will be further reductions. As in previous years, the birthrate ratios of the white and the nonwhite populations occur in about the same proportion (i.e., about five out of every seven births occur to white couples).

An important consideration which influences the number of children being born annually is the size and the age composition of the female population of childbearing age. Although the fertility rate is computed on the basis of births per 1,000 women between ages 15 and 44, most of the childbearing is concentrated among women in their twenties. In 1973, for example, three out of five births were to women who were in the 20- to 29-age interval. The fertility rate has declined steadily since 1958, dropping from 122.9 births per 1,000 women 15 to 44 years of age to 84.6 in 1973.

Another factor which influences the number of births is the number of marriages. In general, there has been a slight rise in the rate of marriages since 1968. However, more married couples are electing not to have children, and there are children being born more often now from social contract and other nonlegal unions. Thus, marriage is not as accurate a predictor as it was formerly.

Over the years, there has been a decline in the frequency of multiple births in the United States. The frequency of these births is another factor which bears on the natality rate. The rate at present is about ten per 1,000 deliveries. Changes in age and the racial composition of the population, as well as the use of certain ovulation-producing drugs for infertility, contribute to fluctuations in the rate over time. There are differences, for instance, in the occurrence of twins, depending on the number of births the mother has had before delivery of the multiple birth. It should also be mentioned that there are differences between the rate of monozygotic, or identical twins, and dizygotic, or fraternal twins. The relative proportions of monozygotic and dizygotic twins are not the same for all races. The incidence of dizygotic twins is cited: white 60 percent, black 70 percent, Japanese 40 percent. In the United States the twinning rate varies slightly from one region to another (e.g., the region with the highest rate of 10.5 is in the Northeast; the lowest rate, 9.4, is in the West).[7]

The birth certificate

In 1915 the federal government began to collect data on registered births and organized birth registration. At first only ten states and the District of Columbia were included in this method of reporting births, but it gradually expanded so that by 1933 the entire country was included. The dependencies were admitted to the area: the Virgin Islands in 1924, the Territory of Hawaii in 1929, Puerto Rico in 1943, and Alaska in 1950. At the present time all 50 states and the District of Columbia demand that a birth certificate be filled out on every birth, and that it be submitted promptly to the local registrar. After the birth has been registered, the local registrar sends a notification to the parents of the child. Also, a complete report is forwarded from the local registrar to the state authorities, and then to the National Office of Vital Statistics in Washington.

Complete and accurate registration of births

is a legal responsibility (Fig. 1-2). The birth certificate gives evidence of age, citizenship, and family relationships and as such is often required for military service, passports, and even to collect benefits on retirement. On the basis of birth certificates, information which is essential to those agencies concerned with human reproduction is compiled by the National Office of Vital Statistics. The brief reports of statistics presented in this chapter are only a fraction of the volume of such studies compiled by that office.

Population

The population of the United States more than doubled during the first half of this century, and has continued to grow in tremendous proportions as was predicted. Between the time of the 1950 census and 1970, the population of the United States grew from 151 million to over 200 million, the figure indicated by the U.S. Census Bureau projections for 1975. The predominant growth factor in this addition of some 49 million people in 17 years resulted from natural increases rather than international migration. This growth has required huge expenditures, both public and private, for such basic facilities as shelter, schools, and highways. The high birthrates of the 1940s and the early 1950s first produced pressures for expansion of elementary education, then for the expansion of secondary education facilities, and, as we are aware now, for college facilities and jobs.

Three vital factors determine the rate at which population grows: births, deaths, and migration. The decline in the death rate that was so apparent in the first half of this century has fluctuated near the same relatively low level (9.7 deaths per 1,000 population) for the last decade. Control of immigration began in this country about a half century ago, and even with recent modifications it still continues to exert an influence on this factor in our population growth.

One should not be deceived by the falling birthrate, which at first glance gives the impression that there is no need to have any concern about a "population problem" in the United States. The impression left by the tabulation of birthrates is that the number of live births has been relatively stable. However, it must be remembered that the birthrate relates to the number of births *per 1,000 population.*

The decline in the annual number of births is partly related to the age and sex structure of the population. The majority of Americans are young. More than half are under 28 years of age, but the proportion is shifting because

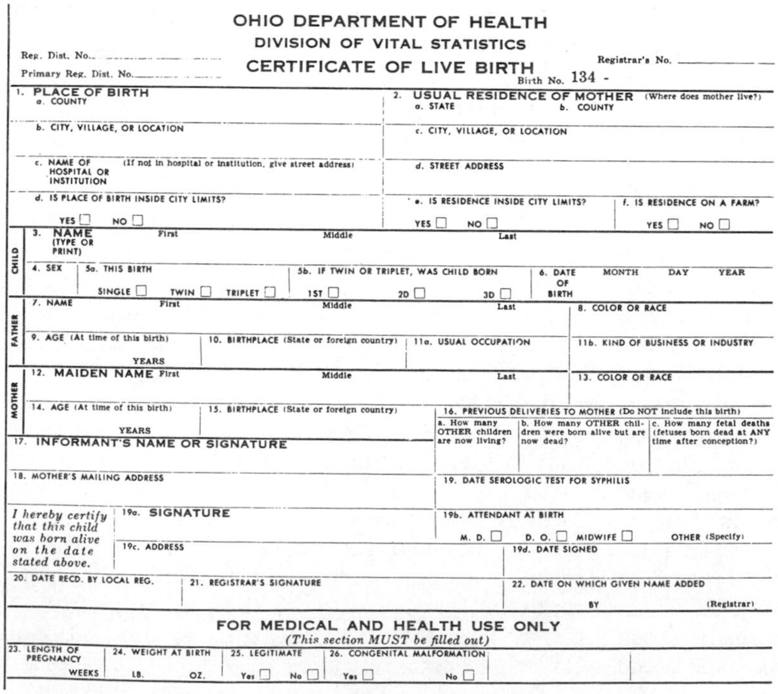
OHIO DEPARTMENT OF HEALTH
DIVISION OF VITAL STATISTICS
CERTIFICATE OF LIVE BIRTH

Reg. Dist. No. ______
Primary Reg. Dist. No. ______
Registrar's No. ______
Birth No. 134 -

1. PLACE OF BIRTH a. COUNTY
b. CITY, VILLAGE, OR LOCATION
c. NAME OF HOSPITAL OR INSTITUTION (If not in hospital or institution, give street address)
d. IS PLACE OF BIRTH INSIDE CITY LIMITS? YES ☐ NO ☐

2. USUAL RESIDENCE OF MOTHER (Where does mother live?) a. STATE b. COUNTY
c. CITY, VILLAGE, OR LOCATION
d. STREET ADDRESS
e. IS RESIDENCE INSIDE CITY LIMITS? YES ☐ NO ☐
f. IS RESIDENCE ON A FARM? YES ☐ NO ☐

CHILD
3. NAME (TYPE OR PRINT) First Middle Last
4. SEX
5a. THIS BIRTH SINGLE ☐ TWIN ☐ TRIPLET ☐
5b. IF TWIN OR TRIPLET, WAS CHILD BORN 1ST ☐ 2D ☐ 3D ☐
6. DATE OF BIRTH MONTH DAY YEAR

FATHER
7. NAME First Middle Last
8. COLOR OR RACE
9. AGE (At time of this birth) YEARS
10. BIRTHPLACE (State or foreign country)
11a. USUAL OCCUPATION
11b. KIND OF BUSINESS OR INDUSTRY

MOTHER
12. MAIDEN NAME First Middle Last
13. COLOR OR RACE
14. AGE (At time of this birth) YEARS
15. BIRTHPLACE (State or foreign country)
16. PREVIOUS DELIVERIES TO MOTHER (Do NOT include this birth)
a. How many OTHER children are now living?
b. How many OTHER children were born alive but are now dead?
c. How many fetal deaths (fetuses born dead at ANY time after conception?)

17. INFORMANT'S NAME OR SIGNATURE
18. MOTHER'S MAILING ADDRESS
19. DATE SEROLOGIC TEST FOR SYPHILIS

I hereby certify that this child was born alive on the date stated above.
19a. SIGNATURE
19b. ATTENDANT AT BIRTH M. D. ☐ D. O. ☐ MIDWIFE ☐ OTHER (Specify)
19c. ADDRESS
19d. DATE SIGNED

20. DATE RECD. BY LOCAL REG.
21. REGISTRAR'S SIGNATURE
22. DATE ON WHICH GIVEN NAME ADDED BY (Registrar)

FOR MEDICAL AND HEALTH USE ONLY
(This section MUST be filled out)

23. LENGTH OF PREGNANCY WEEKS
24. WEIGHT AT BIRTH LB. OZ.
25. LEGITIMATE Yes ☐ No ☐
26. CONGENITAL MALFORMATION Yes ☐ No ☐

Figure 1-2. Certificate of live birth used by Ohio State Department of Health. Similar forms are used by other cities and states.

of the fluctuating birthrates. The young adult group, comprised of those persons between ages 18 and 34, is now the fastest growing portion of the population, reflecting the high birthrates which followed World War II. This group, now 22 percent of the total, will increase to 28.5 percent of the total by 1980. The 40-to-50-year-old segment of the population is not expected to increase proportionately, but moderately large increases are anticipated in the older age groups, that is, those persons 65 years and over.

According to population projections made by the Bureau of the Census, during the next ten years the number of women of childbearing age will probably rise in this country.

The uncertainty as to how much the population will grow rises from the unpredictable number of children who will be born to contemporary young couples. Though their fertility potential is huge, much will depend upon whether they choose to increase or decrease their family size.

Maternal mortality

Maternal mortality refers to the deaths which occur as a direct result of childbearing; in other words, the underlying cause of the woman's death is the result of complications of pregnancy, childbirth, or the puerperium.

In 1968 there were 950 maternal deaths registered in the United States. Over the past decade, there has been a decline so that now complications from pregnancy and childbirth account for about .03 percent of all the deaths per 1,000. The maternal mortality rate in 1972 was about 24 per 100,000 births, and estimated figures for 1974 put the rate at about 15 per 100,000 births.

The reduction in maternal mortality rates has been rather consistent since 1915 (Fig. 1-3). The dramatic decline in these rates began about the mid-30s and continued until 1956. During the succeeding five years, the maternal mortality rate declined more slowly, reaching an all-time minimum in 1962. In 1963 the maternal death rate rose slightly to 35.8 per 100,000 live births, but resumed its decline the following year and reached a record low in 1970.

The risk of maternal death for all mothers is lowest at ages 20 to 24 (15 per 100,000 in 1970). It is slightly higher under age 20, and from age 25 on. Increasing age is associated with a steep rise in maternal mortality. At 40 to 44 years of age, the mortality rate is six times greater than at 20 to 24. At the oldest age in the reproductive age span, 45 years or older, the mortality is about twelve times greater than the low figure.

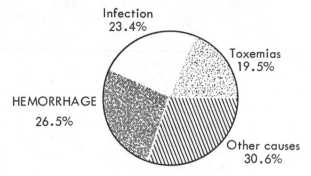

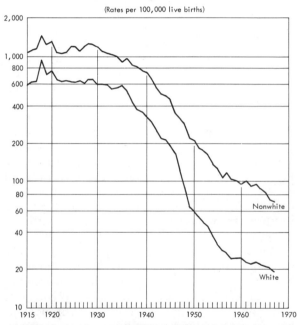

NOTE – Deaths each year are classified according to the International Lists used at that time; for discussion of comparability, see Technical Appendix.

Figure 1-3. *(Top)* Causes of maternal mortality, percentage distribution by cause, 1967. (Data from Vital Statistics of the United States, 1973, Vol. V—Mortality, Part A, Table 1-15, U.S. Department of Health, Education, and Welfare, Public Health Service, 1973) *(Bottom)* Maternal mortality by color: birth registration states, 1915-1967. Deaths from complications of pregnancy, childbirth, and the puerperium per 100,000 live births in the specified groups. (Data from Vital Statistics of the United States, 1973, Vol. V—Mortality, Part A, Table 1-14, U.S. Department of Health, Education, and Welfare, Public Health Service, 1973)

The reduction in maternal mortality from the toxemias of pregnancy was the largest single factor responsible for the reduction in the total maternal mortality rate (from 82.7 per 100,000 live births in 1949-51 to a low of 25 in 1970). Hemorrhage and sepsis (cases other than abortion) were next in importance as conditions affecting the mortality rate. Subsequently, these three conditions will be discussed in detail, but it is important to stress the fact that deaths from these causes are for the most part preventable. Substantial achievements in maternity care have caused the death rate from puerperal infection and toxemias of pregnancy to fall more dramatically than that from hemorrhage. Consequently, hemorrhage has become the predominant cause of death in childbirth. According to the *official classification*, only the direct cause of death is considered, even though the predisposing cause may be an important factor. For example, in a case in which the mother has a massive hemorrhage and then (in her weakened condition) develops a puerperal infection that eventually causes her death, the death is classified as due to puerperal infection. Hemorrhage is often a predisposing factor, and in this manner its toll in maternal mortality probably exceeds all other causes combined.

Puerperal infection is a wound infection of the birth canal after childbirth, which sometimes extends to cause phlebitis or peritonitis. The nurse can play an important role in helping to prevent such infections, not only in terms of flawless technique in performing nursing procedures, but also in protecting the mother from exposure to anyone with an infection.

The toxemias of pregnancy are certain disturbances peculiar to gravid women, characterized mainly by hypertension, edema, albuminuria, and in some severe cases by convulsions and coma. Antepartal care plays an important role in prevention or early detection of symptoms, and with suitable treatment the disturbance often can be allayed.

Many factors are responsible for achieving the overall reduction in maternal mortality in this country during the past 25 years. Most important perhaps is the development of widespread training and educational programs in obstetrics which have provided more and better qualified specialists, professional nurses and other personnel in maternity programs. Better hospital facilities, multiple safeguards provided in the modern maternity hospitals, and advances in therapy have all played major roles.

The distinct change in attitudes of physicians, nurses, and parents also has contributed to this progressive saving of mothers. Childbirth is no longer an event to be awaited helplessly by the expectant mothers with what fortitude she is able to muster; instead, it is the climax of a period of preparation—a true state of preparedness attained through the cooperation of the physician, the nurse, and the expectant mother or parents. As indicated before, this preparation for childbirth, based on careful medical and nursing supervision throughout pregnancy, is called antepartal, or prenatal care.

Antepartal care is one of the most important achievements in maternity care during the present century. It will be of interest to the nurse to know that this salutary contribution to the mother's welfare was initiated by the nursing profession. It had its beginning in 1901, when the Instructive Nursing Association in Boston began to pay antepartal visits to some of the expectant mothers who were to be delivered at the Boston Lying-In Hospital. This work gradually spread until, in 1906, all of these women prior to confinement were paid at least one visit by a nurse from the association. By 1912 this association was making about three antepartal visits to each patient. In 1907 another pioneer effort in prenatal work was instituted when George H. F. Schrader gave the Association for Improving the Condition of the Poor, New York City, funds to pay the salary of two nurses to do this work. In 1909 the Committee on Infant Social Service of the Women's Municipal League, Boston, organized an experiment in antepartal work. The pregnant women were visited every ten days—oftener if necessary. Blood pressure readings and urine tests were made at each visit. This important work was limited because of the effort to make it as nearly self-supporting as possible; therefore, only mothers under the care of physicians and hospitals were accepted. Thus began the movement for antepartal care which has done more than any other single effort to save mothers' lives in our time.

Another important factor in the reduction of maternal mortality has been the development of maternal and child health programs in State Departments of Public Health, particu-

-larly the work of community health nurses in maternal hygiene. These nurses visit a large number of the mothers who otherwise would receive little or no medical care, bringing them much-needed aid in pregnancy, labor, and the puerperium. This service fills a great need not only in rural areas, but also in metropolitan centers.

Still another factor responsible for the decline in maternal mortality is the trend toward hospitalization for childbirth. In the early years of this century, women rarely went to a hospital for such care. In 1935, 37 percent of live births occurred in hospitals, and in 1963, 97.4 percent of the live births were attended by physicians in hospitals. This means that the percentage of hospital births has increased more than two and one-half times during a 25-year period.

Infant mortality

The two groups of problems in infant mortality which are of chief concern in maternity care are 1) those in which the fetus dies in the uterus prior to birth (so-called stillbirth) and 2) those in which it dies within a short period of time after birth (neonatal death). The phrase *perinatal mortality* often is used to designate all deaths in these two categories (Fig. 1-4).

In an effort to end confusion arising from usage of a variety of terms such as stillbirth, abortion, miscarriage, and so on, the World Health Organization recommended the adoption of the following definition of fetal death:

Fetal death is a death prior to complete expulsion or extraction from its mother of a product of conception, irrespective of duration of pregnancy; the death is indicated by the fact

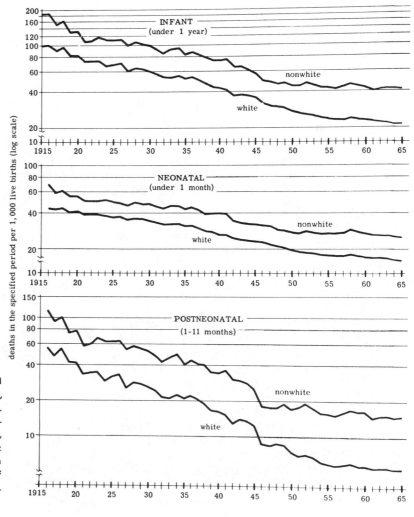

Figure 1-4. Mortality rate of white and nonwhite infants by age, United States, 1915-1965 (birth registration area). (U.S. Department of Health, Education and Welfare, Social and Rehabilitation Service, Children's Bureau. Data from U.S. Public Health Service, National Center for Health Statistics) (Vaughn, McKay, ed: *Textbook of Pediatrics*, ed. 10. Philadelphia, W. B. Saunders, 1975)

that after such separation, the fetus does not breathe or show any other evidence of life such as beating of the heart, pulsation of the umbilical cord, or definite movement of voluntary muscles.[8]

WHO further defined fetal death by indicating four subgroups, according to gestational age in weeks.

A decade ago, there was reported a total of 103,390 infant deaths before the first birthday. By 1970, the infant mortality rate was 20.0 per 1,000 live births, the lowest in U.S. history, and provisional data for 1973 suggests that rate has declined further to 17.6.[9] A falling fertility rate, better contraceptive practices, increasing availability of safe abortion, together with favorable health conditions experienced in the general population, have been suggested as factors in this decline in infant mortality.

However, it has been pointed out that this national figure does not accurately reflect trends in the large urban areas where the rate has declined less. In Philadelphia, for example, the rate decline for the same period was only 14.4 percent, as compared with 20.3 percent nationally. New York's rate declined only 6.2 percent.[10] Moreover, while the national decline in infant mortality may be gratifying, it is not comparable with the fall in maternal mortality in the United States. Also, the United States still ranks about fourteenth in infant mortality, as compared with other nations throughout the world.

Many causes are responsible for this infant mortality. The vast number of infant deaths is the result of several main causes: preterm birth, asphyxia and atelectasis, congenital malformations, and birth injuries.

During the first four weeks of life early gestational age and low birth weight are the most important causes of death. Birth injuries, another of the main causes of infant loss, accounted for almost 7,000 infant deaths in 1970. Almost one-third of these deaths were due to intracranial and spinal injury at birth; for example, cerebral injury as a result of anoxia in utero or traumatic injury to the brain suffered in passing through the birth canal. In the vast majority of these cases death occurred under seven days of life. Subsequently, these conditions will be discussed in detail. It suffices to say that one of the first and most important of them, immaturity, is largely a nursing problem. Indeed, in all the wide range of nursing care there is no area which offers such a challenge to the nurse or such lifesaving possibilities as that of caring for the preterm infant.

The welfare of some 4,000,000 babies born annually in the United States is very much the concern of maternity nurses and obstetricians and one of the main objectives of the entire field of maternity care. To reduce the enormous loss of newborn lives, to protect the infant not only at birth, but also in the prenatal period and during the early days of his life, to lay a solid foundation for his health throughout life—these are the problems and the challenge.

Abortion

The vast number of infants lost by spontaneous abortion, is a matter of grave importance. The abortion rate in this country exceeds stillbirths and neonatal deaths in fetal wastage. About 10 percent of all pregnancies terminate in spontaneous abortion due to such factors as faulty germ plasm; unsatisfactory environmental conditions, hormonal and otherwise; many unknown etiologic causes; and an unknown number of criminal interruptions.

Current problems in maternity care

An orientation to maternity nursing would be incomplete without calling attention briefly to the broad problems in maternity care which reflect on the childbearing potential of families in the United States.

Today the problems for the United States as a whole reflect also a symptom of far-reaching social changes. The tremendous reduction in maternal and infant mortality rates presents concrete evidence of the noteworthy progress that has been achieved in maternity care in this country. Nevertheless, the problems of care which are currently a major cause of concern relate to the care that a large segment of our population is receiving.

The needs resulting from problems of maternal and child health in rural areas continue today, but what is new and alarming is that now there is a parallel situation in the larger cities.

Since World War II, major shifts in population have occurred; urban middle-class families have migrated to suburban areas, whereas large numbers of families from rural areas have moved to the large urban industrial areas.

Despite the increase in employment and in income generally, the population still includes a large segment of disadvantaged, low-income families who recently have concentrated in the major cities. With the increased cost of health services in general and the cost of hospital care in particular, these low-income families are straining the local resources of the communities in which they reside. Also, the number of maternity patients in these areas has greatly increased as a result of migration, producing overcrowding of clinics and hospital maternity in-service divisions. To accommodate such large numbers of patients, many of the hospitals with large maternity services have had to resort to limiting the mother's hospital stay, some women being discharged 24 hours after delivery. The most serious problem by far is that many of these women are receiving poor or, often, no antepartal care, due in part to dissatisfaction with the kind of care provided. Inadequate care during pregnancy has been demonstrated to bear a direct relationship to the rate of immaturity.

It has been mentioned previously that social factors play a role in morbidity and mortality and, in fact, influence the reproduction efficiency of childbearing women.

Much of the difficulty in providing adequate care is due to a shortage of professional personnel. The rapid growth of the population has not been accompanied by a proportionate increase in physicians and nurses. This shortage is compounded by the fact that not enough physicians and nurses are being attracted into this area of specialization. Student nurses might well investigate the reason for this apathy and in good time provide some solution to this problem. These factors will be explored in greater detail in subsequent chapters.

Bibliography

1. Hellman, L. M., and Pritchard, J. A.: *Williams Obstetrics*, ed. 14. New York, Appleton-Century Crofts, 1971.
2. World Health Organization Technical Report Series, No. 51. Geneva, Switzerland, World Health Organization, 1952.
3. Dunn, H. L.: High-level wellness for man and society. *In* J. R. Folta, and E. S. Deck (eds.), *A Sociological Framework for Patient Care.* New York, John Wiley & Sons, 1966, p. 214.
4. *Ibid.*
5. Freeman, B. J.: Human aspects of health and illness: beyond the germ theory. *In* J. R. Folta, and E. S. Deck (eds.), *A Sociological Framework for Patient Care.* New York, John Wiley & Sons, 1966, p. 84.
6. Schlesinger, E.: *Health and Society* 23:16-20, 1974.
7. U.S. Department of Health, Education, and Welfare, National Center for Health Statistics Series 19 and 21, Nos. 12 and 13, 1974.
8. National summaries: fetal deaths, U.S., 1954. National Office of Vital Statistics 44:11, Aug. 1956.
9. Births, deaths, marriages and divorces for 1973. *Monthly Vital Statistics Rep.* 22:12, Feb. 28, 1974.
10. Kendall, N.: The challenge of neonatal mortality in an urban hospital. *Health Services Reports* 89:263, May-June 1974.

Suggested Reading

AUBRY, R., AND PENNINGTON, J.: Identification and evaluation of high-risk pregnancy: the perinatal concept. *Am. J. Ob.-Gyn.* 16:3-27, Mar. 1973.

LAWSON, J.: Avoidable factors in maternal deaths. *Nurs. Mirror* 139, 11:48, Sept. 12, 1974.

NISWANDER, K., AND JACKSON, E.: Physical characteristics of the gravida and their association with birth weight and perinatal death. *Am. J. Ob-Gyn.* 119:3, June 1974.

OSOFSKY, H., AND KENDALL, N.: Poverty as a criterion of risk. *Clin. Ob. and Gyn.* 16:103-119, Mar. 1973.

SCHNEIDER: Changing concepts of prenatal care. *Postgrad. Med.* 53:91-97, June 1973.

the family in a changing world

Roles, Role Theory, and Nursing Practice /
What Is the Family? / Family Forms
of the Seventies / The Nurse and the
Changing Family / Ethnic, Social Class,
and Cultural Variations

Various factors need to be considered when providing high-quality health care for families. It is particularly important that all members of the health team be aware of other theories and experiences regarding human behavior when they work with families. This awareness necessitates using knowledge from other specific disciplines where it is most appropriate in order to deliver optimum health care.

The concept of family-centered care and its logical extension, family nursing, has always been a part of nursing. Some areas of practice, notably that of community health, have traditionally claimed more interest, expertise, and responsibility for total family care than others. Delivering care in the client's home has allowed the nurse more insights into the family and its workings and the implications its structure and function have for the health of its members. Moreover, it has allowed the nurse to assess as a whole the problems and progress of the family members.

However, other nursing specialists, notably those in maternal-child health, have also demonstrated interest in family care, focusing initially on the mother-child dyad and later on parenting. In addition, midwifery has used a family-centered approach to home delivery ser-

vices by utilizing family resources to prepare for care of the mother-infant couple in the home setting.[1] Parents' classes under the auspices of the Maternity Center Association and the Child Study Association in conjunction with the Children's Bureau have also promoted the development, over time, of nursing care of the total family.[2] The philosophy behind this approach has been to meet expressed needs and concerns of parents through the nurse's group leadership role, not necessarily through a course of preplanned instruction. Thus, as nursing has evolved to keep pace with today's health needs, it has become apparent that concepts from other disciplines are badly needed in order to supply a total picture of the family unit for which high-quality care is to be provided.

Probably no force has been so potent or recent in supplying these valuable concepts as the theorists and researchers in the social and behavioral sciences. Efforts to theorize and to conduct research about the family as a social phenomenon have brought together many disciplines and encouraged cooperation and collaboration in the study of that complex social entity. These multidisciplinary contributions have stimulated many teachers and students of nursing to seek advanced preparation and to conduct research about families that have implications for their practice.

The comprehensive overview of family study given by Christensen in his *Handbook of Marriage and the Family*,[3] as well as the identification and classification of conceptual frameworks relating to the family unit done by Hill and Hansen, and Nye and Berardo,[4,5] have been invaluable resources for helping to delineate content in clinical nursing courses and providing conceptual frameworks for the development of assessment tools and the testing of nursing intervention techniques.

Perhaps most significantly, nursing is now joining with other related disciplines whose basic interests and expertise in the family may someday ensure team approaches to research in clinical matters, multidisciplinary educational programs, and, most importantly, team effort in family care.[6] Society's demands, needs, and aspirations are causing rapid changes in all health fields, including nursing practice and educational programs. Tired of fragmentation in service, high costs, barriers to the entry into health services, and the inertia and unresponsiveness of the health care system in general, consumers are taking action in what amounts to a social movement.[7,8]

As a result, health professionals find themselves in the center of a revolution in the health care system. Only by multidisciplinary collaboration will they be able to rise to the occasion and provide adequate health services.

Roles, role theory, and implications for nursing practice

As background for understanding the family, we must deal with another concept that permeates both lay and professional language today. That concept is role, and it is an integral part of the structure and function of the family. As with the concept of family, we have an intuitive sense of what a "role" is, but when attempts are made to systematically study the construct, we find a broad latitude in definitions and understandings of it. Psychologic and sociologic approaches to role are closely interrelated, since an individual's personality develops within a social system which, in our culture, is the family. Hence, roles may be viewed from a psychosocial viewpoint that enables us to focus on the individual and how he integrates his role relationships, and also

from a sociologic viewpoint which guides us in focusing on group or social relationships, primarily those within the family. We must also deal with culture, for the "self" can be viewed as the unit of personality, an individual's "status" or position as the unit of society, and "role" as the unit of culture.[9]

Basic to any discussion of role are the definitions of *role* and *status*. Status, or position, generally refers to a person's location in a system of interaction. On the other hand, role applies to *behavior* that reflects the goals, values, and sentiments operating in a given situation. A further clarification of these definitions can be made by contrasting role as defined by two major theorists, Ralph Linton and George Herbert Mead. According to Linton, roles tend to be defined as constellations of rules or expectations for behavior associated with a given status or position.[10] In the Meadian, or interactionist tradition, however, roles are defined, created, stabilized, or modified as a consequence of interaction between the self and others.[11]

From an interactionist frame of reference, then, role is more than a series of do's and don'ts for the behavior expected of a person occupying a given position. Rather, it is a constellation of behaviors that emerges from interaction between the self and others, that constitutes a meaningful unit, and that is an expression of the values, goals, and/or sentiments that provide direction for that interaction. It is true that these constellations of behaviors become patterned over time and that the actors proceed "as if" there were prescriptions for performance. However, there is much more latitude in the Meadian conception of role, since it allows for innovative, individualistic designing of a person's role performance on the basis of assignment of some sentiment or goal to the behavior of relevant others. This conception of role is particularly salient for nursing practice, since it allows for a broader interpretation of the behavior of all actors than do more traditional concepts. Moreover, it does not limit either the interpretation of the behavior or the nurse's response to the behavior to a prescribed set of do's and don'ts. Hence, it permits creativity and innovation in interaction with clients.

Another basic concept in role theory is that of the *complementarity* of roles or the fact that all roles are learned in pairs. Thus, a role does not exist in isolation but is patterned to mesh with that of a role partner. For instance, the nurse's role meshes with the patient's role, the husband's with the wife's, the child's with the parent's, and so on. Some of these roles which are basic in society, such as husband, wife, child, and so on, have become more patterned in the various cultures than others, and thus firmer expectations have come about. But we need only look at the innovative variation in recent family lifestyles to appreciate how traditional role prescriptions and expectations can, and often must, be modified.

Whether there be firm or loose expectations, this pairing or complementarity of roles provides for reciprocal arrangements in interaction and therefore allows social interaction to proceed in an orderly fashion, since there emerges a predictability in interaction. The actors "know" what they are to do. Without this complementarity, it would be difficult to maintain stable interaction networks such as exist in the family system. Indeed, the family's equilibrium depends on this role pairing.

Roles are learned through the process of socialization. In socialization, individuals learn the ways of social groups so that they can function within these groups. Socialization takes place through both intentional and incidental instruction, that is, by providing specific instruction regarding a certain facet of behavior and by providing examples of desired behavior —in other words, role modeling. All of the various socialization agencies—the family in the beginning and later the church and schools— teach the child certain role behaviors through intentional programs of learning and study. However, operating conjointly may be incidental learning in which the child adopts the ways of others in his environment through play acting, peer-group relations, and observations of adult and peer-role models. Thus, the significant others in the child's world teach him, both by defining the world for him and by serving as models for his attitudes and behavior. The child learns through a system of rewards and punishment and, if he behaves as the significant others desire, he receives positive attention and invitations to continue his participation and interaction. If, on the other hand, he behaves otherwise, he is refused attention, reprimanded, or physically punished. It is important to remember that much of the role learning that takes place in the family is indirect. The child learns by observing and participating in the interpersonal relations patterns established by the family, the examples set by the other family members, and the role that he develops for himself within the family. Hence, he learns and *adopts* basic role skills from family members and concurrently *adapts* to the roles of the other family members.

Another important aspect of role learning is that it is not merely a cognitive process. It comes to be associated with multiple emotional or affective ties that the individual makes with others. These attachments begin with the mother and gradually include increasing numbers of persons with whom the child interacts and comes to identify with. As these attachments grow, the child develops a sense of "self" in that he can take a position from the outside and view his own thoughts, feelings, and actions. In this way, he gradually internalizes the behavior that is expected of him as he figuratively stands back and looks at himself and guides, judges, and reflects on his own behavior according to his perceptions of others' expectations for his behavior. It has been noted that, while individuals learn role behavior in much the same way, there are differences in respective role performances. This differential role performance may be due to differences in the ways persons respond in interpersonal situations, their knowledge of the role in general, their motivation to perform specific roles, their attitude toward themselves, and finally, their response to the behavior of other persons in the interaction.[12]

Another aspect to be considered when considering the concept of role is that of tension and/or discontinuities in role relations. Many terms have been used to illustrate the idea of tension or interruptions in a smooth process of interaction. Terms such as role conflict, role strain, role change, role transition, and the like have been used to convey the various aspects of tension that can occur in a role system. We have made the point that role interaction is dynamic. As theories of the development of human nature change, so do socialization procedures. As these latter change, variant family life systems evolve, which in turn redefine reciprocal role relationships. Tensions and disruptions in smooth and rewarding role interaction may occur at any point. The major determinants of the degree of adjustment an individual makes to a role can be summarized as follows: 1) the clarity with which a specific role and its complementarity is defined and demonstrated; 2) the clarity or definiteness of the transitional procedures in the acquisition of a new role; 3) how well the role is learned and enacted—this is partly dependent on (1) and (2) and the strength of the socialization process to the new role; 4) the consistency of the responses a role evokes; 5) a role's compatibility with the other roles in the individual's set of roles; 6) a role's congruity with the emotional needs of the individual; and 7) the degree of complementarity that exists between reciprocal roles. When there is a high degree of adjustment, the enactment of an individual's set of roles can be rewarding in that they define for him his niche, his self-concept anchorage, a sense of belongingness and purpose. They give him social recognition and support which, in turn, allow him to buy or earn desired conditions or things in the world and to view himself as a worthwhile, contributing member of society.[13]

Family roles and the nurse

Concepts from role theory encompass a body of knowledge that is vital for the nurse who works with families as a group or individuals within families. The application of these concepts can greatly increase the nurse's understanding of the role strains and changes inherent in the phenomenon of family stress that can be precipitated by childbearing, chronic or acute illness in the family, or death of any of the family members. For example, consider the change in the interaction patterns that must be accomplished when a new infant is incorporated into the household—restructuring of all of the members' roles is necessitated, and this is doubly complicated when there are other children present. Sibling rivalry is only one aspect of the impact of a new infant on the family. Or, consider the situational crisis when parents bear a mentally retarded or otherwise defective child. Following the grief reaction and concomitant frustration, conflict, and high anxiety, the family equilibrium can be regained only when parents restructure their roles to either encompass or reject the afflicted member and learn to cope with the situation. Finally, consider acute catastrophic illness in the father of a family with several children. When such an illness occurs, the man is thrust into the role of patient which is, in essence, a dependent role. This necessitates a reorganization of the role behaviors of the other family members. The wife must become more dominant, the children generally must assume more responsibility, and hence, their positions change vis-à-vis other family members. These few examples point up the necessity for the nurse to consider family role relations if she is to intervene in a holistic way.

THE ROLE OF MOTHER. Each society provides many cues and signals that tell individuals how it defines a role and identifies appropriate behavior for the role. These cues may be overt or covert and may be perceived in a subliminal way. In our culture, the ideal mother has been traditionally the nurturer, the one who gave sustenance and unconditional love. A woman's concept of the mother role is based on the norms of the culture, the social class and ethnic group to which she belongs, and the type of socialization she has received from her immediate family. It is important to remember that there is a difference between the role of mother and feelings of motherliness. In a sense, both are learned, but mothering, the enactment of the role of mother, involves skills and a certain understanding of the developmental process of the child. Thus, *motherliness* can be thought of as an emotional feeling that develops over time as the mother has increasing contact with her infant (see Chapter 15). It is a feeling that the child is emotionally hers, and there is a need to identify the infant with the rewarding values and qualities that she considers part of herself and her life. This development of motherliness begins with the maternal claiming process and is evident in the initial and early mother-newborn contact when the mother touches (at first timidly) and later enfolds her infant and exclaims, "Oh, he is finally here! How did I ever produce that?" Our hospital procedures militate against this early claiming behavior, but fortunately we are now beginning to relax many of the restrictions that tend to disrupt the reality testing of this ownership process.

All mothers need reassurance that they are now, indeed, mothers—and adequate if not excellent ones. The disappointment the mother feels when the infant sleeps at the breast instead of nursing is very familiar to everyone. Mothers excoriate themselves with criticism when they are awkward in handling their first-born. They try desperately to "pull themselves together," to assume care of the infant only hours after delivery. Although seemingly small and unimportant, these initial anxieties are the basis of the future relationship between mother and child. Moreover, they are complicated by the many conflicts in modern society where the role of mother has come into increasing competition with other social roles a woman may enact. Paramount among these conflicts are: 1) fantasies of idealized motherhood versus feelings of inadequacy in actual role performance; 2) the need for dependency versus the adult goal of independence and responsibility; 3) love versus resentment for the baby due to fatigue and increased responsibility for such a dependent being; 4) feelings for the baby versus feelings for the husband; and 5) self-actualization versus the demands of motherhood.[14]

If the mother has had problematic relations with her own mother during the early socialization years, these, too, may affect her role enactment. She may project many of these negative feelings onto her own child or, conversely, bend over backwards to avoid socialization techniques her mother used, thereby limiting or missing important features which she might have kept and used. Also, if the normal and increasing dependency needs of pregnancy and the early postpartum are not met, she may not be able to care easily for and give love to her dependent child. One final point deserves mention. For many, children of one age are more appealing than those of another. A mother may be able to respond to the needs of a dependent infant but not adapt readily to the four-year-old's search and insistence on autonomy. Thus, the role of mother and its enactment is shaped by many interacting factors and therefore will have a wide range of behavioral manifestations.

THE ROLE OF FATHER. It has been said that, if the 20th century is proclaimed the "Century of the Child," it certainly will not be remembered as the "Century of the Father."[15] Research on the dynamics of the father role or the development of fatherliness has received much less attention than that of motherhood. Recently, there has been some impetus in research, but it will be some time before there is solid empirical evidence regarding this topic.

As with the mother role and motherliness, there is a difference between the father role or fatherhood and feelings of *fatherliness*. The role of father is learned as is the role of mother —but feeling tones are not initiated physiologically as with the mother. And this may be a very important difference. Moreover, the admission and enactment of fatherliness in our culture is still wrought with conflicts stirred up by discontinuities in cultural conditioning. This is gradually changing with the more modern attitudes toward relaxed sex role structuring. However, we still have a long way to go. By and large, the image of the virile male is still not compatible with the demonstration of tender feelings which have usually been attributed to the female domain. Traditionally, the male-father in our society was supposed to be a leader, hero, disciplinarian, mentor, an authority figure, and the family bulwark against the outside, reality-oriented world. Yet fatherliness must involve feelings of tenderness and gentleness, empathic capacity, the ability to respond emotionally, the valuing of a love object more than the self and, finally, the finding of a gratifying living experience in the experiences of others. Obviously, these feelings are quite different from the simple pride of a man in his child as a symbol of his virility, or his feelings that the child represents a challenge to his own adequacy.[16]

It becomes apparent that, as long as women have an emotional investment in men, they will not be free to express their motherliness wholeheartedly until their relationships with their mates are integrated into the men's fatherliness. It would seem that the coordination of the feelings of motherliness and fatherliness in those who choose to be parents is essential to the mature, creative psychosexual development of both parents and eventually their children's.

It may be that the same basic problems that confront a woman in delineating her role as mother also face the man in defining his father role. Interviews with young fathers indicate that they are immersed in many instrumental problems, such as rearranging work or study schedules, finding or preparing adequate housing, taking on extra jobs to ease the finances, and the like. They also have basic questions and fears about their preparation for the parenting role, as well as changes in their wives during pregnancy and the postpartum periods. In some, the prospect of fatherhood also rekindles thoughts of the less happy aspects of their childhood and their relations with their parents. Their fears and concerns about their rest, quiet, and privacy, their sexual relationships, and their wives' increasing demands for attention all become realities with the advent of childbirth. We can speculate that these developments and problems may be due, at least partly, to our current lack of systematic obstetrical care of the father. It is true that we invite him to childbirth classes (and this has been a big step), and that we are allowing him greater participation in the actual birthing process. However, there is still no systematic attempt (or even acknowledgment of the necessity) to prepare him for his father role. All of these problems are the common components of severe role conflict and how they are resolved becomes the key to ultimate appropriate role transition.[17]

Josselyn has delineated several functions that a father can *creatively* undertake to enrich and maintain a healthy family life. First, a father can be a *true* companion, help-mate, and inspiration for the mother. Second, he can be an awakener of emotional potential for his child as well as a beloved friend and teacher. Third, he can present a role model for masculine love, ethics, and morality. Fourth, he can be a stabilizing influence as the child proceeds through his maturational stages. Fifth, he can be a model and mentor for social and occupational behavior. Sixth, he can provide a model, as mentor and protector for children in general, and finally, he can be a counselor for and friend of the adolescent.[18] While each of these activities will be modified to meet the needs of a rapidly changing society, it is apparent that they provide more of a basis for sound family interaction than does the traditional role of father as sire, disciplinarian, and breadwinner.

THE ROLE OF CHILD. Of all the family roles, the child's role is perhaps the most dynamic, since it is constantly evolving through techniques of socialization. These techniques are essentially future-oriented, since they focus on and emphasize what the child is to become rather than what he is. Helping the child learn his appropriate social roles requires that the parents be emotionally healthy and stable enough to keep the anxiety level under which the child will learn to adapt himself at a point that will allow his self-esteem to be in relative equilibrium with the environmental demands that are made. This does not mean that there be no demand or no anxiety—without these, no learning takes place. However, they must not be excessive or incompatible with reality.

There are many techniques of socialization, and the evidence indicates that no one technique is better than another. Rather, each set of parents must choose and modify what is best for them, and this will depend on the many factors that we have previously alluded to. Spiegel has attempted to delineate the various steps in the maintenance of role complementarity so that the family can balance the demands society's expectations place on it, the family's attitudes, and the child's needs and eventually arrive at a progressively healthier family role equilibrium. He conceives of these steps along the torturous route of socialization as comprising two major groups of five steps each linked by a sixth, or middle step.

The first group consists of *role induction procedures* by which compliance of the child is elicited. These are primarily manipulative and ensure that the child gradually realizes that he must learn and that his parents are his chief source of learning. The first and second steps are *coercion* and *coaxing* in which punishment and rewards are used respectively to focus the child's attention on the fact that there are rules that must be observed and that his parents are the enactors of these rules. The third step is *evaluation* in which a value judgment of good or bad is placed on the behavior and implies or directly gives praise or blame to ensure appropriate behavior. The fourth step is *masking*, or withholding correct information or giving wrong information for the sake of settling a conflict. This can be pernicious and a crisis may occur if the child uncovers the truth—trust can be lost and reality is distorted. Fifth is the technique of *postponing* which can be useful because it puts off dealing with a conflict until a fresher look can be taken at the situation. Of course, if this maneuver is over-utilized, it will intensify and prolong the difficulty.

The sixth is the transitional step and has been called *role reversal* or *role taking*—that is, putting oneself in the role or position of the other and looking at the situation from the point of view of another. Some refer to this as empathic ability. It is the first glimmer of adult thinking and requires a rather well-developed understanding of self and reality. The ability to perform this maneuver early and successfully depends on the degree of masking that goes on in the family. The less the extent of masking, the better the success of role taking.

The second group of procedures has been referred to as *role modification* maneuvers. The basic characteristic here is *communication* and how individuals learn to complement each other in role change. Role modification begins with the seventh step of *joking, or humor*, in which individuals develop the ability to laugh at themselves and each other (but affectionately). It is felt to be an outgrowth of role taking and the first of several tension-relieving mechanisms that families employ. The eighth step employs the *intervention of a third party* (not necessarily a professional) who brings to the situation certain skills, a point of view, or knowledge that is not available to the parents or child within the family unit. *Mutual exploration* is the ninth step, in which each person probes the capacity of the other to come to a solution regarding a conflict or problem. Here, trust and regard are expressed and invested in all members, including the children (to the extent of their capacity). The tenth step, *compromising goals* is an extension of mutual exploration. Here, goals are altered but to no single person's detriment. Similarly, the last step, *consolidation*, is the refined, integrated effort of learning to compromise successfully. It is associated with adjustment, redistribution of rewards, and role clarification. Needless to say, the evolution through these various steps does not necessarily proceed smoothly, nor at times are all accomplished, especially steps 8 through 10. However, the more frequently they can be utilized, the easier each subsequent role adaptation and transition will become.[19]

THE ROLE OF THE NURSE. The understanding and application of role theory in nursing practice provides a conceptual base from which to understand the populations that we serve and gives some anchorage to our therapeutic method. It increases our capacity to view the forces of personality, family interaction, social systems, the health condition, and nursing intervention as a unit. It provides a needed framework for studying motivations for childbearing, reproductive behavior, childrearing techniques, and cultural goals. In addition, it provides a basis for understanding ourselves and our colleagues who provide health care.

Nursing is an applied science. The broad implications of its scientific nature challenge its practitioners to document this aspect with intellectual experimentation, innovations in practice, and constant research. If, indeed, we in maternity nursing, define the family as the unit to be served, we must have a thorough knowledge of its dynamics—and that includes much more than the physiologic and psychologic stages the *mother* passes through during pregnancy, labor, delivery, and the postpartum. The utilization of role theory provides a vehicle to tie all of these disparate aspects of childbearing into related units amenable for study and, hence, practice.

When one is a nurse, one has a role. The professional level at which the nurse functions will depend upon the sophistication of her practice. Inherent in this is the idea of role facets or multiple aspects of the nurse's role. First, the nurse is a practitioner—she assesses, prescribes, and implements nursing regimens for her patients and assists the physician in implementing his medical regimen for his patients. Another facet of her role is that of role model or mother surrogate. Maternity nurses and community health nurses have long been experimenting with providing role models for mothers who are inexperienced or exhibit maladaptive behavior in childrearing and child care. Again, in high-risk situations of child neglect or rejection, techniques of mothering the mother are implemented. Basically, the nurse meets the dependency needs of the mother, and in so doing, allows her to move on to mothering her own children. The nurse may also provide a role model for her peers and other professional colleagues as she initiates newcomers into the institutional or agency routines and practices and demonstrates an interest in delivering high-quality care.

Another facet of the nurse's role is that of teacher and, more recently, that of counselor. Nurses are becoming increasingly involved in parent education on all levels in order to socialize groups of parents expeditiously, thus avoiding the role strain and conflicts that can occur with the assumption of new roles. The counselor aspect has come into the fore with family planning services and abortion and genetic counseling. Similarly, this aspect has become apparent in parental counseling with regard to health problems of the school child, management of sibling rivalry, childhood and maternal nutrition, and the like.

Finally, in her "expanded role" she may bring new physical diagnosis-clinician skills to her basic role. She finds in many instances that her work in an ambulatory care setting provides the bridge between the family in the community and the institution to which they must go from time to time for more severe conditions. The potential for developing these multiple facets of the nursing role is unlimited and will only be fully realized when nursing recognizes its own unique and independent contribution to health.

When delivering care to individuals and families, nurses must observe and analyze the role behaviors of the persons involved, including their own. Cognizance must be taken of the various dimensions of the roles: the behaviors, values, expectations, and attitudes of the actors, as well as their underlying motivations and emotions. Roles are dynamic, continually shaped by the maturational process, developing families, environmental and societal stressors, and the individual's personality. Role conflict and perceptions of inadequacy in role performance have the potential to undermine emotional and physical well-being. On the other hand, satisfactory role performance is a vital self-concept enhancing experience and can promote growth and emotional well-being.[20]

What Is the family?

Most people know intuitively what they mean by "the family." They have known families throughout their lifetime and intuitive definitions are sufficient for everyday conversation and action. However, when we begin to define what constitutes a family, analyze this unit as a social institution, or attempt to deliver comprehensive care to it, it becomes apparent that what we have considered as *the* family is inappropriate for systematic treatment. The characteristics of the families of our own personal experience often do not fit "families" of other segments of society. Family life in different cultures exhibits even greater contrasts.

The family has been defined in a variety of ways. Torbett refers to it as "a group of two or more persons who are united by blood, marriage, or adoption residing in a common household wherein they create and maintain a common culture and interact with each other by way of familial roles."[21] Other authors have referred to the family as a unit of interacting personalities or as a system of roles.[22, 23] Common to all of these definitions is the fact that the members—whether they be a married dyad, a single parent and child, or have anonymous role relationships, or a union unsanctioned by law—relate to each other in some way; that is they *interact* with specified patterns of behavior, and in so doing differentiate or structure roles for themselves.

Theoretical approaches to the study of the family

In attempting to systematically study and delineate patterns of interaction in the family, scholars of the family, primarily sociologists, have developed several interpretive approaches to variations in family life, each one generating unique understanding about family organization while at the same time emphasizing a different aspect. These variations in emphasis result in slightly modified definitions of the family in each approach. For instance, some students of the family try to define the family in terms of a set of ends; others in terms of a kind of social structure organized to gain more general ends in societies; and still others in terms of structure and ends emerging in the unique history of each society.[24] Five different conceptual frameworks have been designated that can be useful to nurses who deal with families. These have been summarized by Hill and Hansen as follows.[25]

1. *The interactional approach* views the family as a unity of interacting personalities. Each person has a position in the family in which he perceives the norms or role expectations held by the other individuals (or by the family as a whole) as the basis for his attitudes and behavior. The individual will define his role expectations primarily in light of their source and his own self-conception. The family is studied through analyzing the interactions of the role-playing members. The primary focus is on the internal structure of the family; this framework, however, neglects the family's relation to the community.

2. *The structure-function approach* views the family as a social system and one of the components of the complete social system—or society. It analyzes the functions which the family performs for society as a whole. The emphasis in this approach has been upon the statics of structure with a concomitant neglect of change and dynamics.

3. *The situational approach* is based on the assumption that all behavior is purposive in relation to the situation that triggered it. The situation itself, or the individual's behavior in the situation, is the focus for the study of families by means of the situational approach.

4. *The institutional approach* takes the perspective that the family must be considered a social unity in which the individual and cultural values are the prime concern. The individual's values and learned needs are transmitted from one generation to the next within the individual family system.

5. *The developmental approach* focuses upon the study of the developmental phases of the family from the wedding to old age, and finally the dissolution of the family through death. The changing developmental tasks and role expectations of parents and children as they go through the family life cycle, as well as the developmental tasks of the family as a whole, are the basis for this approach.

As previously stated, any of these frameworks can be used depending upon the problem under study. It is important to remember that these frameworks are helpful tools and are not to be considered "right" or "wrong." In choosing a framework, an individual must consider the assumptions he makes about the behavior of man, how he views man in relation to the environment, and the problem that he is trying to solve.

The interactional approach

One of the most useful of the above frameworks for those who must deal with the family as a unit is the interactional framework. This conceptual scheme provides a system for viewing the personal relationships between the husband and wife and parents and children, as well as the impact of various health conditions on the family unit. The family is conceived of as a unity of interacting personalities and, as such, is a living, changing, growing thing. This conceptualization, then, does not view the family in a legalistic way or in family contract sense, but rather as it exists by virtue of the interaction of its members. Thus, a single parent with a child would be a family unit, a household with several monogamous couples with children would constitute a family unit, as would an unmarried couple with or without children.

Within the family, each member occupies a position or positions to which a number of roles are assigned or allocated. Through socialization and role differentiation (structuring a role) the individual perceives certain norms (rules) or role expectations that the other members of his family have for his behavior in his role performance. The response of the others in the family reinforces or challenges this conception that he is developing. Thus, a person defines his role expectations in a given situation in terms of a reference group (others who are important to him) and also by means of his own self-conception. Implicit in this formulation is the fact that human beings interpret or define one another's actions instead of merely reacting to them. For instance, a woman's response to her mate is not made merely on the basis of his actions; it also depends upon the meaning which both partners attach to such actions. Thus, the family members act and react by using symbols, and the key concept involved in the use of symbols is *communication*. Interpersonal relations among family members based on communication is one of the major distinguishing aspects of the interactional approach. Foote and Cottrell have pointed out that the emphasis in this framework is on the development of competence in interpersonal relations and as such describes a *process* rather than a *state*.[26]

Several problems for investigation have grown out of these concerns and emphases on family unity, communication, and interpersonal competence. The one that is particularly salient for health practitioners is that of the study of discontinuities in family life, particularly family crises or stress. This includes the impact of the reproductive process and parenthood on the family, stress created by acute or chronic illness of the various family members at any time during the life cycle, and the crisis brought about by death of a family member, particularly during the reproductive years. Using this approach to the family, a practitioner can get inside the family group and analyze its coping as far as it involves interaction among members. Each family member, therefore, can be viewed as a developing member in a changing group. This approach can be particularly useful to the helping professions not only because it provides a practical way of inspecting the family, but also because it allows the professional to isolate and specify the potential sources of difficulty as family members relate to one another and to their society.[27]

Much of the "pregnancy as crisis" literature has developed from this orientation. LeMasters, Dyer, and Hobbs have been contributors in this vein (see Suggested Reading). The extent to which parenthood is a crisis is likely to vary according to definitions (i.e., crisis as a crisis or a critical event), measurements, and the amount of time between the birth of a child and the undertaking of the particular research study. There is little doubt that, when a dyad of a man and woman becomes a triad of a mother, father, and child, a major reorganization of positions, roles, and interaction patterns takes place. The effect of the birth of a child and the preschool years of children on the adjustment of the parents seems fairly well-established. General marital satisfaction of couples tends to decrease after the birth of their children through the preschool and school years, until the children are getting ready to leave the nest. Thus, the experiences of childbearing and childrearing appear to have a rather profound and negative effect on marital satisfaction, particularly for the mother, who may even feel her basic self-worth is affected.[28] All of this has grave implication for maternity health professionals with respect to our family planning counseling, assistance during the reproductive process, and especially in delineating those successful aspects in the parents' coping behavior that can be useful in lessening this "critical" event.

In summary, there are several conceptual frameworks for the study of the family. Of particular use to practitioners is the interactional approach which strives to interpret family phenomena in terms of internal processes. These processes consist of role enactment (role playing) status or position relations, communication problems, decision making, stress reactions, and socialization processes. Little attempt is made to view the overall institutional or cross-cultural relationship of family structure and function, and this has been one of the criticisms of this approach. However, this framework can be used to study the relationship of the family unit to the community, but it is more difficult since one must move from the microlevel of the small cluster of interacting persons to the larger macrolevel sweep of the community. However, where the interface of these units occurs is important for health practitioners.

Other critics feel that the interactional approach fails to recognize the biogenic and psychogenic influences on family behavior. This criticism seems destined to be short-lived since

these influences are recognized by the interactionist as factors that indeed set limits but are not determinants with respect to family interaction patterns. The focus is on the family in process, irrespective of the biologic or personal makeup of its members, not on a static entity. What appears to be needed at this point for this framework to reach its greatest utility is better agreement and more precise definitions of its assumptions and concepts as well as extension of the framework through application and research. In this way, the interactional approach will function more adequately as a frame of reference for the study of the family and eventually will mesh with other frameworks into what could be called a general family theory.[29]

Family forms of the seventies

Ethnic historians and scholars of race relations have long emphasized the pluralistic characteristic of U.S. society. Over the years there has been quibbling over whether a melting pot was cooking an amalgam of ethnic and cultural distillates called "American" or whether this society was persisting as a salad bowl with a variety of shapes, hues, and forms of ethnic, religious and racial identities. The argument continues but the salad bowl adherents are winning in this decade.

It is interesting to note that the idea of pluralism or variability and differentiation has never been strong among those with an interest in the family, including health practitioners. This may be because the family, the bulwark of society, is a sensitive area surrounded by many judgmental and normative statements about what "ought to be." So often the family is still thought of as having some "ideal" form, which is preordained, often religiously sanctioned and adhering to an ideal set of values. Thus, forms that vary from the traditional nuclear family of husband, wife, and children living in their separate residence with the male as breadwinner and female as homemaker have been viewed as deviant. Research in the 1950s and 1960s on single-parent families, working mothers, or dual-work families was, for the most part, concerned with the deleterious effects of the absence of spouses or the effect of gainful employment on the children. The implication was, of course, that the woman should be in the home "where God intended her to be" and if a spouse was alone for any reason, he or she had the obligation to remarry (not just live with someone) as soon as possible.

This preoccupation with ideal types obscured what is rapidly becoming a very obvious phenomenon: a pluralism in family forms existing side by side, with members of each of these forms having different problems to solve and issues to face. It is important to note that not many persons remain in one type of family structure throughout their lifetime, although most have some experience in the traditional nuclear family.[30] Thus, we see along with the traditional family structures, emerging experimental structures which can have an effect on the socialization and health of their members and, hence, on their reproductive motivation and performance.

Traditional Family Structures

There are a variety of forms in traditional family structures. The most prominent among these are:

1. The nuclear family in which husband, wife, and children live in a common household. A single or a dual career may be pursued, and, in the case of the wife, her career may be continuous or interrupted as the children are born.
2. The nuclear dyad in which a husband and wife live alone. They may be childless or not have children living at home. Again, there may be a single or dual career or a "second career" where the wife enters the labor force after the children have left home.
3. The single-parent family in which there is one head as a consequence of death, divorce, abandonment, or separation. Here there are usually preschool or school-age children. There can be a career or noncareer; when financial aid is not forthcoming from the absent spouse, there is usually some form of occupation pursued by the parenting spouse.
4. The single adult living alone.
5. The three-generation family or extended family. These may be characterized by any variant of forms 1, 2, or 3.
6. The kin network in which nuclear households or unmarried members live in close geographical proximity and operate within a reciprocal system of exchange of goods and services.[31]

Each of these will have its problems and resources with respect to health needs and utilization of services. Generally, these traditional households are more favorably looked upon by society in that they are considered stable and provide a legitimating anchorage for the children born of these unions. It has been said that nuclear families suffer from isolation and cannot cope with illness (or repeated pregnancy, reproductive wastage, and the like); hence, they must turn to professionals for sustenance and care. However, current research indicates that the nuclear family probably has less isolation and better coping ability than formerly was thought.[32] This is due to the fact that there appears to be great role adaptability and flexibility in time of stress as well as a greater utilization of kin and other social networks for advice and sustenance during childbearing as well as for other health conditions.

It is apparent that extended family forms can be helpful to counter isolation and to provide help during periods of stress. It must be remembered, however, that kin and friends can also deter family members from appropriately defining themselves in need of care as well as prohibiting or deterring them from prompt and continued utilization of health services.

Emerging experimental structures

1. The commune family. This form can be further divided into:
   a) A household of more than one monogamous couple with children, sharing common facilities, resources, and experiences; socialization of the child is a group activity. Each member is a responsibility of the other members, and there is mutual concern for the various aspects of the members' lives including health matters.
   b) A household of adults and children in which there is "group marriage"; that is, all the individuals are "married" to each other and all parent the children. A status system usually develops with the leader(s) believed to have charisma. These are very small in number.
2. The unmarried parent and child family, often a mother and child for whom marriage is not desired or possible. Children can be natural offspring of the parent or adopted.

3. Unmarried couple and child family. Again, these may be of two varieties:
   a) A social contract marriage in which there is an ideologic commitment to a relationship not sanctioned by law, which must be constantly worked at in order to maintain its vitality and meaningfulness. Common value systems are shared that strongly emphasize humanism and personal relationships. A great deal of time is spent by the members, including the children, in sharing mutual emotional experiences and ideas. The father plays a prominent role in the caretaking and socialization of the children and both parents have intimate, continued, and sustained contact with their children.
   b) The second type of unmarried couple and child family is that usually referred to as common-law marriage with the children either born to the partners or informally adopted. These unions are often found among the poorer strata of society who experience exceptional problems and constraints associated with legal marriage.[33]

The nurse and the changing family

It is with the emerging forms of alternate family styles that today's nurse may have the least experience, and thus we will discuss some of these more specifically so that the health needs during the reproductive cycle can be more sharply defined.

Social contract families or the unmarried marrieds

As stated previously, social contract families are composed of two partners whose structure exists as a social rather than a legal contract. We in maternity nursing become acquainted with these patients when giving family planning counseling and services during pregnancy and childbirth. The literature and current research suggests that in many ways, this group shares the philosophy of the "turned-off" middle-class countercultures. Living together in this form, however, has little similarity to the "shacking-up" of previous generations, or with the large number of common-law marriages found among some of the poor who experience constraints and problems associated with legal marriage, such as no finances to obtain a divorce or inability to manage the bureaucracy to facilitate legal severance. Rather, this form of marriage involves an ideologic commitment to a relationship instead of joint living by virtue of a legal status. Basic to this rejection of a legal marriage is the conviction that the bond of love and trust that binds the partners is more important and stronger than the legal bond authorized by church or state.

In the family setting, parents spend long periods of time with one another and share emotional exchanges of closeness and rejection, desire and repulsion, and all of the certainties and uncertainties involved in living together and bearing and raising children. There is, for the most part, a great deal of frankness and openness about these statuses which include the children. There is little secretiveness about their approach to life, and both names may be displayed on the mailboxes, in financial arrangements, and the like. There are no hang-ups on their part regarding the legitimacy of the children.

Since the possible instability of the relationship can be critical to pregnancy outcomes and the children's development, researchers have explored these facets of alternate family forms. Motivations for this lifestyle are very important. Some partners do not accept the civil contract per se; others do not accept the relevance of the civil marriage contract to their relationship as it exists for them at the moment, wanting no civil constraints on their "splitting" if things change between them. Others seek to avoid the obvious unhappiness in their own family life and upbringing. In general, from the participants' point of view, living together in this family structure is seen as representing true maturity and an acceptance of the faith placed in one another.

The women's liberation movement and the raising of women's consciousness have played a strong philosophical role in determining reproductive behavior and childrearing activities. The choice of having a child appears even more determined than in the traditional nuclear family. Contraception services appear to be utilized and the option of termination of pregnancy is freely available and utilized without the apparent guilt associated with such termination in some of the traditional families. From this point of view, and because of the close interaction and caretaking when the children are born, this family style has been considered a very motivated form of parenting.[34]

The single parent

The single or unmarried mother is far from a new phenomenon in our society. However, there has been a significant change reflecting this alternative way of bearing and raising children in today's society. Available and effective birth control measures have reduced the population for adoption and, more importantly, there has arisen a new perspective on the part of many single parents to keep their children and raise them without the stigma that has previously been associated with unwed pregnancy. There has been a gradual institutionalized acceptance of single parenting, also, with the acceptance of both single men and women as adoptive parents for the older or handicapped "harder to place" children. The women's movement and the counterculture middle-class student were forceful agents in making parenthood a viable option for the woman whether she was married or not. Young women from middle-class families, in increasing numbers, are allowing their pregnancies to continue to term and are electing to keep their children. Older single women are becoming pregnant by choice and keeping their babies or are adopting one or more children. Single men also have chosen adoption as a means of experiencing parenthood without the responsibility of marriage. Under such conditions, a variety of styles of parenting have emerged since different supports are needed by these parents who are alone. The single mother, particularly, must enlarge her social support networks if she is to become economically independent and socially involved.

Among the family styles that have been encountered among the single mother group are small group homes or boarding homes where a small number (four to ten) live together with their children; foster homes for mother and child; and living alone in an apartment.[35] The actual physical arrangements for the child differ among residences, but, in general, there are separate sleeping quarters for the parent and child with common dining and living facilities. The opportunity for the children to eat and play together, share toys and have a shared caretaker is considered one of the advantages for children in groups such as these.

Many communities have developed programs that facilitate a young mother's return to school or work so that she can gain skills that will enable her to be independent. These programs are still in the early stages and are largely experimental but do indicate that society recognizes the complex needs of women who rear children alone. Child care facilities, caretaking arrangements and infant caretakers in the home reflect the kinds of assistance the community has developed, which means that most children of single parents are exposed to multiple caretaking as early as six weeks of life.

Societal recognition has also encouraged single parents to move toward developing organizations and social networks that provide them with tangible supportive contacts. The expansion of such organizations as Parents Without Partners, the Momma League, LaLeche League, and the like into activity programs, information and training centers, and consciousness-raising efforts suggest that the middle-class parent has become more sensitive to his/her needs as a person as well as a parent.

While voluntary single male parents are still much in the minority, they are becoming more numerous. Their living arrangements include group living as well as living alone with the child. Because the male's economic status is generally better than the female's, he has more options for child care and living quarters. Thus, caretakers in the home are found more frequently, although ample use is made of child care centers and children programs. This particular population provides an opportunity for observing an alternative in family style that has voluntarily and proudly rejected the traditional nuclear family.[36]

Communes

The creation of a communal alternate to the isolated nuclear family is not new in this country. Generations of Americans have sought a new start and protested against the status quo. Causes of their dissent and the ways in which they chose to organize their new communal existence varied in the past as they do with today's communards. Some were based upon religious conviction, some on economic idealism, some on rebellion against authority. Some attempted to establish a model of government based upon an absence of central authority; others sought a strict line of hierarchical authority with the rejection of those members who did not adhere to the authority prescribed. Some had relatively long histories, such as the Bruderhof, while others, such as "Brook Farm," an intellectual community in Massachusetts, dissolved rapidly.

Lifestyles displayed by the current commune movement are perhaps even more varied than those of the historical models. This makes attempts to define this alternate lifestyle difficult. Communes vary today in type of membership, organizational structure, and general purpose. Some are involved in agricultural subsistence seeking a closeness to the land characterized by the early close-knit communities reported to have existed in history, while others are composed of middle-class young professionals who do not wish to disengage from the urban scene and its various technologic comforts. Size also varies from 12 or less to hundreds. A significant number is based upon religious commitments of various persuasions. Eastern philosophy is often a guiding force in many of these religiously oriented communes. In others, the "Jesus movement" is central, with the members searching for a new way to live out the traditional Judeo-Christian convictions.

Communes are often formed around common interests, crafts, or some unifying goal. They start with people who like each other and share similar value systems, orientations, and convictions. This aspect is extremely important in these intentional communities, and some see their alternate family arrangement as the beginning of a social revolution that will bring about radical change in society.

Some communes are reported to be group-marriage oriented, but they are in the minority. One such group lives in Taos, New Mexico, and another similar group exists nationally with a sizable base in Los Angeles. Children are shared with the group and there is little concern with respect to knowing or caring which individuals have been biologically responsible for the conception of the child. The rearing of the child is considered more important than who the parents are.

Other groups are oriented as extended families, with couples remaining essentially monogamous in their own private quarters, although partners may change from time to time. Still others live together under a community concept rather than a family unit, sharing those resources which are more effectively achieved in multiple family cooperatives, such as expenses, household chores, and child care responsibilities. The women's consciousness movement has given particular impetus to these groups. As we stated previously, the lifespan of the current communes varies. Such issues as

organization of work and other aspects of living, interpersonal relationships, mutual values, economic feasibility, and ability to cope with outside community harassment have been suggested as important to the stability of communal arrangements.

Living arrangements largely determine parent-child relationships. Great ingenuity is shown—tents, lean-tos, and cabins in the rural areas; apartment houses, motels, and sometimes "single family" dwellings in the city.

The number of children varies from commune to commune. In general, the adults are conscious of the population explosion, and few parents with more than three biologic children are in evidence; however, there are some "families" who have eight to ten children. Birth, pregnancy, and children are esteemed and joyously regarded as an expression of a natural and ecologically appropriate experience.

Adult-child relations are often determined by proximity of living and sleeping quarters. Relations with biologic parents may be infrequent, with children being physically separated from them and assigned to caretakers, as is the case in some instances. In addition, the child's relationship with other adults is related to the extent of the existence of a hierarchical structure. In a family, multiple dwelling arrangements can permit a child to move among households, as when he is in conflict with other members, lonely for playmates or when his family is "splitting" for a time.

Investigators have found a wide range of childrearing practices among the communards.[37,38] Some of the attitudes and value systems that are likely to affect the child's development and, hence, have relevance for health professionals are summarized here:

1. Breast-feeding appears routine and there is usually close tactile contact between mother and child in the first year. Strapped to the mother's back, the baby goes everywhere with her, and is touched frequently.

2. There is often a clear break in the intense mother-infant relationship at around two-and-one-half years, when there is a push in the direction of independence and self-reliance. The mother begins to think of her own needs and returns gradually to activities.

3. Good health, together with a desire for wholesomeness, are revered. Natural foods

are stressed and "junk" foods are restricted. Institutional medical and dental care is limited to emergencies with self-help medical and pharmacologic expertise encouraged. Few preventive measures are sought from organized medicine except prenatal care. The emphasis is on prevention through healthful, natural living.

4. Nonviolence is generally espoused among the counterculture groups, although assertiveness among the children, especially the girls, is sanctioned. Children are often left to work out peer relationships and direct interrelations are fostered. Only the demands of safety take precedence. Children are disciplined, however, and a broad spectrum of this exists from verbal admonition to physical punishment.

5. Humanistic and interpersonal relationships and the direct expression of affectional needs are valued. Artificial repression of sexuality and intimacy are eschewed. Thus, exposure to nudity and observation of adult sexual activity are permitted and there is a permissiveness concerning these sexual drives which may foster opportunities for acting out. There are various degrees of acting out in the latter, but, in general, parents allow more freedom to their children and expect earlier sophistication.

6. Children socialize each other, since, when the child gets into his own groups, he is dependent upon his peers' support. There is a great deal of age specific role peer modeling.

7. Early decision making is encouraged in the child. This is related to the philosophy that the child has individual rights and thus has a role in participatory democracy. This group decision making by parents is often modeled by children as an important mode for solving problems even though their decisions are by necessity immature.

8. The parents experience some difficulty with serving as role models for their children. They appear to be quite reluctant to "lay their trip" on the child. Yet, they admit to value and lifestyle preferences that are consonant with their attitudes, and, because of their verbal admonishings and role modeling, reinforce those behaviors of the child that are consonant with their attitudes. Another problem is that the parents are not willing to serve as sex role models because of their general acceptance of an antisexist philosophy. Yet many of the males are out and out sexists. There is also ambivalence about having the girls identify with the not completely emancipated women.

9. Competency to handle daily life is stressed, while competition and achievement striving is played down; thus, individual potential and creativity are felt to be promoted. Sensory impressions, intuition, and the occult, as opposed to the rational, are data that are considered an enhancement of creativity. Children, because of their competency, are expected to distinguish between what is appropriate behavior within the "family" and the "outside world."

10. The materialistic values are seen as tied in with technologic advances and nonhumanistic goals; thus, dependence on material possessions is minimized whenever possible. Shared objects, toys, and utensils are far in the majority. Some of the children see the adults "ripping off" the outside society and ignoring the social contracts involved in personal ownership (i.e., stealing). There is such great variability in these groups that it is evident that follow-up is indicated to see what the impact is of these childrearing practices.

One of the other findings of the studies that have been done indicates that many of the practices within these lifestyles and relating to childrearing are also practiced in the present-day nuclear family. Much of what appears in the mass media—TV, newspapers, and so on—logically finds expression in many of these alternative lifestyle families. Indeed, the alternates have influenced, if they have not rapidly become, the mainstream.[39]

Working with alternate lifestyle parents
There are several things that the health professional will want to remember when delivering services to almost any who profess an alternate family structure, whether it be a member of a commune, a social contract commitment, or a single parent. There is a certain rejection of "traditional values" and there is the assumption of new beliefs and practices. These beliefs and practices take on aspects of various other cultures, some of which are Eastern; moreover, there is a good deal of change. Therefore, it can become a highly in-

dividualized culture in its own right, in that each takes for his own what he likes and rejects what he does not feel comfortable with. Moreover, there is a strong emphasis on the right of each individual to find the lifestyle that is best for him and the need for acceptance of all of life and other people's beliefs and practices.

This basic viewpoint and value orientation can be most disconcerting when health professionals work with these families. We often find that our theories of cause and prevention of disease, as well as other health matters, are evaluated by the patient with no more assurance of being accepted as true than are other theories about life and living that she may be considering. Thus, opinions of the health professional may be valued no more highly than those of friends, the clerk in the health food store, someone encountered in the street, or a daily column in an underground paper. Most importantly, these patients wish to evaluate new knowledge for themselves and be free from the burden of accepting advice simply because the giver has some assumed expertise or holds a position of authority.

Health professionals often expect patients to accept their information as true because it is drawn from a scientific body of knowledge. However, these thoughtful patients may not necessarily accept Western scientific knowledge. They may, indeed, regard modern science as attempting to bring forth more and more "laws" aimed at finding absolute truth in a relative world and, hence, having little to do with health and, more importantly, happiness. On the other hand, information from other sources, including health information, is also subjected to scrutiny and evaluation before acceptance. Thus, many practices which could be potentially harmful are often rejected. If these patients have any kind of a relationship with a professional to whom they can turn for criteria against which to compare advice, they will usually make appropriate choices.

The tendency to evaluate medical information given by the health professional on an experiential rather than a scientific basis does not preclude an interest in what the health professional has to say. In our experience, particularly in the free clinics, we find that the nurse is respected as a person who has knowledge in her field and *who shares some of the patient's concerns and feelings.* Expectant parents will have many questions and, when the

nurse responds to their inquiries, they may go on to relate information that they have gathered from other sources. It becomes important to discuss this information seriously and with respect since it is valuable to the parent. Health teaching documented with rational explanation and practical experiences is much more readily accepted. The advice and teaching must be practical also. To insist that a vegetarian eat meat, even if she may have anemia, is simply too impractical, especially if there are others in the family to consider.

Moreover, these patients are, for the most part, well educated and, because of this and their value system, expect a fuller and more complete explanation of what is happening than many other patients. If a mother prefers a vegetarian diet and wants to know the food values of the foods she is considering including in her diet, she will not be satisfied with only a suggested menu. Exchanges and equivalents must be discussed. It is not sufficient to tell a mother in an antepartum clinic to return in so many weeks for another blood test without telling her the reason for returning and the purpose of the procedure. If these patients reject some of the advice, this, too, is still to be treated with respect.[40]

Choosing antepartal services

Many factors that affect the alternate lifestyle mother in selecting maternity services are also factors that affect the traditional lifestyle mother. These include past experience with health personnel, geographic location, her feelings about the pregnancy, the influence of significant others, and her physical condition. One major difference, however, is the high priority that is placed on ambience and interpersonal relations by these patients. Modern surroundings and up-to-date equipment are much less important in the value system.

Selection of services is usually made as with any patient: friends are consulted as well as other sources considered reliable. Past experiences are considered. In addition, the free clinics are seen as a source of referral and information if they do not provide prenatal care themselves, and the underground papers may be perused for health services. Since motivation of the personnel is important to these patients, volunteering service in a free clinic is often looked on with high regard, since it is seen as doing something for its own sake and not for monetary reward and is, thus, an indicator of genuine regard for the patient. In these instances, efficiency is not required and the patience of the patient is notable.

Many alternate lifestyle couples feel that they must be on the defensive with the personnel in hospitals and nonfree clinics. They feel very strongly that their freedom to choose be respected and that they and what they represent be treated with respect. It becomes important to assure these patients of their legal rights, including that of signing themselves out of the hospital. Often this information and the regard for the patient that it implies is enough to lessen the apprehension about going to the hospital for delivery or seeking care from a nonfree clinic or private "establishment" physician.

These patients appear to have little difficulty accepting health care from personnel who do not share their lifestyle *provided* that they are treated with respect and their right to choose is clearly articulated AND RESPECTED. An individual's lifestyle is his own affair, and as long as different values are accepted and no imposition of establishment values is attempted, health services are willingly accepted.

Choosing the place and method of delivery

Selection of a hospital for delivery or the choice between hospital and home delivery involves many of the same factors as those involved in the selection of antepartal services. Underlying the process of choice is the fact that childbirth is regarded as a natural process. Thus, prepared childbirth classes, especially LaMaze classes and the "father coached" variety are very popular. The natural food stores and bookstores frequented by alternate lifestyle patients all carry books on this subject. Books on the efficacy and "how to" of home delivery are also popular, and the parents become very knowledgeable and sophisticated about delivery through reading them.

Many mothers wish to deliver without drugs of any kind and feel that it is very important not to have drugs forced upon them, especially anesthetics. The importance of the mother being in a comfortable, efficient position during delivery, that is, legs not strapped down, is often mentioned as a "must." Some mothers wish to help deliver the baby themselves (actually handle the baby as it is expelled) and most want to have the father participate. There is usually a desire to put the baby to breast immediately following delivery and to breast-

feed on demand. Electronic monitoring when there are no complications is considered superfluous.

When the hospital is chosen for delivery, the couple or mother seeks to have as many of the above conditions fulfilled as possible. These parents want to be able to reject professional advice without condemnation and even to leave the hospital without great pressure from hospital staff to remain. Another important consideration is that the father of the child, a friend, a fellow commune member, or a relative be allowed to be present during the labor, delivery, and postpartum stay and that they be active participants during the hospital stay. Family diet preferences are expected to be respected. In addition, rooming-in is often requested as it is felt that it is important to foster close parent-baby relationships.

Hospitals that have the reputation for not permitting fathers or relatives in the labor and delivery areas and/or of having a great deal of "bureaucratic hassle" over money or signing out early are usually avoided irrespective of the quality of care delivered.

The value of the need for control over one's own life has been mentioned previously, and therefore a home delivery is often desired. These types of deliveries remain controversial at this writing because of the fear on the part of professionals that there is a great risk for the mother and infant in the event of complications. There is also the problem of the expeditious use of the health professional's time in that it requires more time for the physician and nurse to come to the patient than for the patient to come to the physician and nurse. However, home delivery is being reconsidered from both a safety and time factor by more physicians (see Suggested Reading), and professional attendance can be obtained more often. Professional attendance notwithstanding, one counterculture writer relates, that, in many cases, the parents have much more control of the situation. They are not in an unfamiliar environment; they are not strapped to a table nor are they separated from the new baby for anywhere from 12 to 24 hours.[41] As providers of care, we know that these are important considerations, and most of them can be carried out in a hospital delivery with help from considerate staff. However, the fear that they cannot is often a factor weighing against the hospital as a place for delivery. In addition to being viewed as a physiologic process, birth has a symbolic meaning. The home represents the cradle of symbolic meaning while the hospital may be seen as a sterile place with little room for symbolism. Expectant mothers who wish to deliver at home but who wish antepartal care often do not inform their physicians of their intentions. They fear that they will be subjected to undue pressure to deliver in the hospital or be refused prenatal care altogether.[42]

Family-centered care

It is with these patients, especially, that the ideal of family-centered care becomes a necessity when providing maternity services. In these families, having a baby is seen as a concern of both parents and the fathers want and expect more active participation in the pregnancy and delivery of a baby than many of the more traditionally oriented fathers. In the case of the single parent, a friend or relative often assumes the "father" role with the intent of providing help, sustenance and support to the mother during this time. The prospective father (or significant other) often plans to be present at the prenatal visits and participate in the expectant mother's conferences with the physician and/or the nurse. Both parents will discuss matters concerning the physical and emotional state of the mother (and often the father), and other matters relating to the infant's arrival. Since such a strong emphasis is placed on the quality of the relationship between the mother and the father, his feelings about the pregnancy and his emotional state are of equal concern. If the mother must make changes in her diet, or daily habits or avoid certain drugs, the father often does the same.

This concern and participation may be extended to others besides the prospective father. If the mother lives with friends, or in a commune, others of the group take responsibility for the mother. They are also concerned about the effect of the infant on the commune or group as a whole and, hence, tend to do whatever they see as necessary to ensure a positive outcome. Some communes, for instance, who generally follow a restricted vegetarian diet, make efforts to ensure that the pregnant member receives an adequate diet for pregnancy and lactation which might include foods not ordinarily eaten by the group. On the other hand, some feel that, since pregnancy is "natural," there is no need to deviate from the group's chosen diet, even though it may be quite restricted in complete protein. Group pressure will also affect seeking prenatal care and the decision as to the place of delivery.

It is important to the couple that the father remain with the mother during her labor and delivery. He will also want to hold and examine the baby after it is born. If the father cannot accompany the mother, she will usually request that a friend or fellow member of the commune be with her. The father will expect to visit frequently during the postpartum period also. If these expectations are not met, it is quite possible that the mother may decide to sign herself out of the hospital early against medical advice.

The importance of nutrition

One of the most important aspects in caring for alternate lifestyle couples is that of nutrition and dietary practices. Although all kinds of foods are eaten and practices vary, nutrition is seen in these groups as a major factor of being healthy and happy (see Chapter 12). Vegetarian diets seem to receive major emphasis, but the type of diet will vary greatly from group to group, individual to individual, and with different periods in the life of any individual. Macrobiotic diets are popular but, again, how they are defined varies greatly. They may include only brown rice and tea, or be varied enough to include fish and vegetables.

There is a strong belief in the superiority of unprocessed foods (this is becoming current in the mainstream culture also) and those grown without chemicals and synthetic fertilizers. Hence, the natural food stores are utilized as food supplies and as a source of nutritional information. Very often a community cooperative food store is arranged that uses the members as buyers and distributors, and this helps defray the cost of the foods. Great attention is given to the quality of the food.

Prices tend to be higher in the commercial natural food stores than in the supermarket, and shopping in these stores often can lead to spending a limited food budget on a few high-priced items, leaving less money for items that ought to be included in the diet during pregnancy and lactation. However, the patient often feels that she eats a more nutritionally balanced diet than the health professional, even though it consists mainly of whole grains and unpeeled vegetables, since the health professional eats many processed and semiprepared foods.

Nutrition is seen as very important in pregnancy and, as stated previously, many mothers and/or the groups with which they live, make special efforts to eat well during pregnancy. This includes modifying the diet to incorporate animal protein. Again, the health food stores provide a source of information with books and pamphlets on diet in pregnancy. It has been our experience and it is documented by others that the nurse is usually regarded as a reliable source of nutritional information. If she imparts information as has been suggested, always allowing the patient the right to disagree, the patient can usually work out a satisfactory diet.[43]

Ethnic, social class, and cultural variations

The recent emphasis on cultural pluralism and ethnic heritage in America seems to contradict the contention that ethnic groups tend to shed their distinctive family patterns as they become socially mobile. It can be seen, however, that the move toward the celebration of national origins represents an extolling of distinctive ethnic art, language, dress, and food patterns for the purpose of promoting a positive identity and ancestral pride in those who have had little of either.

If we examine the contemporary family roles of various ethnic groups, we see illustrated the process of acculturation as this has been accelerated or delayed by the availability of opportunity in the new environment, by the extent of discrimination, and by the degree of cultural and physical similarity or difference of the acculturating group from the dominant society. There are many groups that comprise the "salad bowl" of America and we cannot, unfortunately, include all of them here. However, we will highlight some of the groups to give an indication of the current state of thought on contemporary family roles.

We would like to make clear at the outset that the variations among the different ethnic groups in family styles, health beliefs and practices, utilization of health services, and the like are a function of the socioeconomic status of the individuals far more than their particular ethnicity. Since minority groups in general are often poorer than their white counterparts and because more individuals within each group tend to be poorer than the same proportion of whites, there has been an inability to gain access to education and other resources that money can buy. Thus, behavior and beliefs have come about or been retained which are different from the mainstream white middle-class dominant society. Thus, misconceptions have arisen that have been attributed to ethnicity.

Black families

One of the most significant factors affecting the family roles of the black population of America has been the concentration of a majority of these families at income levels that are grossly inadequate. This has been due largely to discrimination which is more severe for American blacks than for other less visible groups. New opportunities have opened up for the black community in recent years; however, these have benefitted mainly upper-working-class and middle-class families. The poorest strata have not gained proportionally.

Another factor that has been woven into the fabric of what some have called mythology about the black community has been the lack of a strong patriarchal tradition among the black family. The mother is seen as the head of the household and provider, while the father is seen as mostly absent, a nonprovider, and a powerless parent. Research has indicated that, among the middle-class and upper-working-class families, there is no significant difference from whites with respect to family role differentiation and the acceptance of a middle-class value system. In a thoughtful review and evaluation of the empirical research findings regarding lower-class black families, TenHouten concluded that the bulk of the findings do *not* show these fathers and husbands to be powerless in either their conjugal or parental roles. Black wives do appear to be powerful in their parental roles, but there is no indication that this emasculates the black father.[44] Indeed, there is a salubrious effect in that fathers tend to be more expressive in their marital and parental roles and are helpful and willing to share in childrearing and homemaking chores. Moreover, this freedom from patriarchy has enabled the black woman to be more pragmatic, resourceful, and flexible than her counterparts from other cultures where the tradition of authoritarianism and patriarchy is strong.

Since they typically do not have authoritarian fathers, black children do not experience one of the psychologic sources of low-achievement motivation. The increased economic opportunities which will allow black fathers to become economic role models for their children, combined with an early emphasis on independence which is typical among black families, and confident setting of their standards by black mothers should conceivably result in higher levels of achievement motivation among black children than those among children of families where the father plays a more repressive role. There is already evidence that middle-class black children have higher levels of motivation and aspiration than do their white counterparts.

Blacks in the lower socioeconomic strata, especially when confined to the ghetto and/or rural areas and deprived of educational and other acculturating opportunities, tend to hold a traditional value system which includes a strong sense of family (or familism), superstition, religiosity, and fatalism. This is in contrast to the "middle-class" value system generally held by highly industrialized urban societies. These values—rationalism, pragmatism, individualism, equalitarianism, secularism, and achievement—have also become known as the dominant American values. Whether the individual's value system is traditional or middle-class urban, it becomes part of his belief system and is incorporated into the roles of husband, wife, parent, and child.[45] Thus, when dealing with these patients, health professionals often find their values competing with those of the patients. When the basic values are examined, it becomes clearer why there occur certain health beliefs, differential utilization of health services, delay in seeking care and often nonadherence to prescribed regimens.

Mexican-American families
Mexican-Americans have been the forgotten minority in the United States, possibly because the American Southwest has been somewhat neglected by both academicians and writers with the exception of John Steinbeck. There are more than 5 million Mexican-Americans, who are mainly second-generation offspring of peasant immigrants from Mexico. They are concentrated in the border states of Texas, Arizona, New Mexico, and California, and comprise the second largest minority group in the United States.

Since World War II, the isolation of the Mexican-American has been declining; this has been due to the fact that many participated in the war and gradually new perspectives and opportunities have come about which have had an impact on family roles and traditional value and belief systems. Barrios still exist, of course, and in some small rural or isolated urban areas, even the middle-class Mexican-American tends to reside in them.

Familism appears to be the strongest surviving traditional value within the older Mexican-American community, along with patriarchalism and machismo—the cultural ideal of masculinity which equates maleness with sexual prowess.[46] These traditional values and certain folk beliefs persist, particularly because of the isolation of the barrios and the persistence of these values and beliefs make difficult the acceptance of modern health knowledge and practice.

Those Mexican-Americans in the barrios who are educated and have had a positive experience with health services, have accepted the ideas of scientific medicine and health care and allow their children to be immunized, attend clinics and, in some cases, have accepted some kind of family planning. However, there are many others who have their own set of folk beliefs about illness and its treatment which they practice in conjunction with medical care or before seeking scientific health care. These beliefs about diseases and their cures are derived from experience and experimentation and are handed down from generation to generation. Two or more cures may be recognized for one disorder and disorders generally fall into two categories—those of emotional origin and those of magical origin. Folk healers (primarily curanderas [women], or curanderos [men]) are often utilized and some have an important and respected standing in the community. It is felt by the majority of the uneducated that physicians do not know how to treat folk disorders because they lack either faith, knowledge, or understanding of them.

Among those with little education, there is no distinction between the natural and supernatural and many illnesses can be a result of evil forces, witches, spells cast by other persons, or punishment for some sin committed either knowingly or unknowingly. Some of the common conditions that health professionals should be aware of are the following: *mal aire* or bad air, especially night air. It can enter through any of the body cavities under certain circumstances and result in illness of both mother and child. *Mal ojo*, or the evil eye is a culturally defined disease, primarily of children. It is caused when someone looks admiringly or covetously on the child or adult. Its symptoms are restlessness, crying, and headache as well as other nonspecific symptoms. *Susto* or fright can be caused by a frightening experience which can result in excessive nervousness, loss of appetite and loss of sleep. *Mollera calda* or fallen fontanel is a common disorder among infants. It is believed to be due to a fall or from taking the nipple out of the baby's mouth too suddenly, thus causing the fontanel to be sucked in. Symptoms include irritability, crying, diarrhea, sunken eyes, and vomiting. There are other afflictions as well as their home remedies that it is wise for the nurse to know if she will be dealing with these patients. The reader is referred to the books by Hymovich and Barnard, and Reinhardt and Quinn for excellent presentations of these conditions and specific nursing intervention.[47,48]

Japanese-American families

The modernization of the Japanese family in America has proceeded more slowly in some respects than in Japan because the isolation of the Japanese-American from the effects of technologic development and rapid social change has been more pronounced here. However, in California, where the largest concentration of Japanese ancestry occurs, this segment of the population has the highest median levels of income and education of any minority group. Japanese-Americans also have very low rates of crime and delinquency, indicating at the same time the greater persistence of the traditional values of obedience and conformity to parental values and norms. The generational pattern of increasing acculturation is very clearly illustrated in the contemporary Japanese-American community, since other factors such as urban-rural residence do not vary significantly.

A majority of the Issei or first-generation immigrants who were born in Japan arrived here some time between the end of the 19th century and 1924, when immigration from the Orient and Eastern Europe was sharply restricted by the Johnson Act. While the Issei came largely from rural agricultural areas and occupations, they were unusual in that they were relatively literate, compared with peasant immigrants from Europe, and they valued education even before their arrival in this country.

Second-generation Japanese-Americans—the Nisei—born largely before 1940, experienced an unusual push into modernity not only by the parents' preexisting emphasis on education, but by the West Coast evacuations of Japanese-Americans during World War II. Familistic values were weakened by the loss of confiscated family homes and businesses, which removed an important source of Issei control over their second-generation offspring. Thus, after the war, the Issei, who were forced to seek out independent, nonfamily occupational opportunities, were thereby more speedily acculturated into the modern values of individualism and equalitarianism in family relationships, although a cultural lag in this respect is still quite pronounced among many Japanese-Americans.

The third generation—the Sansei—born largely since World War II and now in high school, college, or in the adult occupational world, are the most totally acculturated of all. However, certain subcultural differences remain in family role conceptions, even within the third generation, that are traceable to the survival of traditional ethnic values in marital roles and in childrearing practices.

In the Orient, the patriarchal tradition has been much more crystalized than in the West. The deference and obedience of wife and children toward husband and father, and of the younger generations toward elders, was more intense and more formalized in ritual, ceremony, religion, and law in the Orient than in Western society.

The extended family form, the ancestral clan or house as the basic family unit, was far more salient in the Orient as reality and as cultural ideal, for all social strata. Arranged marriages and emphasis on lineage, important indicators of the value of familism, were common even among the poor in Japan. The values of obedience, deference, duty, and responsibility were constantly reinforced by pervasive mechanisms of control than elicited shame and guilt for the slightest deviation from established convention.[49]

Frequent sources of role conflict in the Sansei generation, especially, are found in the greater prevalence of strict disciplinary measures in childrearing, the greater emphasis on conformity and unconditional obedience, on humility and emotional reserve (particularly the suppression of anger), the continued extensive use of shame and guilt as mechanisms of control, the greater submissiveness of women, even within the higher strata, and the greater strength of extended family pride and intergenerational emotional dependence. These are the residual of traditional values of the parents.

Male dominance is stronger in Oriental American homes, at all class levels, than in any other ethnic group in this country. While the emphasis within Japanese-American homes on achievement and competitiveness has promoted educational and occupational success, the continuing stress of familism and authoritarian values has retarded the flexibility, independence, and the self-reliance that are important attributes of individualistic achievement in highly industrialized society.

While recent studies of the Sansei generation have indicated a shift toward greater independence in this generation, both males and females remain, typically, less assertive, more deferent and conforming, and more emotionally reserved than their Anglo peers. The rigid conformity, status distinctions, and authority relations of traditional Japan that continue to affect family roles of Japanese-Americans in this country are likely to disappear with time, but more quickly in the occupational world than in the world of the family, where they appear less immediately dysfunctional.[50]

There are few folk beliefs and, in general, scientific medicine is accepted especially by the second- and third-generation Japanese-American. Preventive medicine is solicited and, because of the high educational level as well as high achievement aspirations, health and medical regimens are usually followed. Among the older generation there may be some reliance on herbal medicine and some interest in acupuncture.

Bibliography

1. Ford, L.: The development of family nursing. *In* R. D. Hymovich, and M. Barnard (eds.), *Family Health Care.* New York, McGraw-Hill, 1973, pp. 3-17.
2. Corbin, H.: Development of parent classes in the United States. *The Bulletin for Maternal and Child Health, A Symposium: Education for Parenthood.* Am. Assoc. Mat. and Infant Health, Inc., 1960.
3. Christensen, H. T.: *Handbook of Marriage and the Family.* Chicago, Rand McNally, 1964.
4. Hill, R., and Hansen, D.: *Marriage and Family Living* 22:299-311, 1960.
5. Nye, I., and Berardo, F.: *Conceptual Frameworks for the Study of the Family.* New York, Macmillan, 1966.
6. Ford, L., *op. cit.*, p. 9.
7. *Ibid.*
8. Reeder, L. G.: The patient-client as a consumer: some observations on the changing professional-client relationship. *J. Health and Soc. Behav.* 13:400-412, Dec. 1972.
9. Robischon, P., and Scott, D.: Role theory and its application in family nursing. *Nurs. Outlook* 17:52-57, July 1969.
10. Linton, R.: *The Cultural Background of Personality.* New York, Appleton-Century Co., 1945.
11. Mead, G. H.: *Mind, Self and Society from the Standpoint of a Social Behaviorist.* Chicago, U. of Chicago Press, 1934.
12. Robischon, P., and Scott, D., *op. cit.*, p. 53.
13. *Ibid.*
14. *Ibid.*
15. Hines, J. D.: Father—the forgotten man. *Nurs. Forum* 10:177-200, 1971.
16. Josselyn, I.: Cultural forces, motherliness and fatherliness. *Am. J. Orthopsychiatry* 26:264-271, Apr. 1956.
17. Robischon, P., and Scott, D., *op. cit.*, p. 55.
18. Josselyn, I., *op. cit.*
19. Spiegel, J. P.: Resolution of role conflict within the family. *Psychiatry* 20:1-16, Feb. 1957.
20. Robischon, P., and Scott, D., *op. cit.*, p. 56.
21. Torbct, D.: The single-parent family. *In* J. P. Clausen, *et al, Maternity Nursing Today.* New York, McGraw-Hill, 1973.
22. Schvaneveldt, J.: The interactional framework in the study of the family. *In* A. Reinhardt, and M. Quinn, *Family Centered Community Nursing.* St. Louis, Mosby, 1973, 119-138.
23. Turner, R. H.: *Family Interaction.* New York, John Wiley & Sons, 1970.
24. Farber, B.: *Kinship and Family Organization.* New York, John Wiley & Sons, 1966.
25. Hill, R., and Hansen, D., *op. cit.*
26. Foote, N., and Cottrell, L. S.: *Identity and Interpersonal Competence.* Chicago, U. of Chicago Press, 1955.
27. Schvaneveldt, J., *op. cit.*, pp. 119-138.
28. Eshleman, J. H.: *The Family: An Introduction.* Boston, Allyn & Bacon, 1974.
29. Schvaneveldt, J., *op. cit.*, pp. 120-123.
30. Sussman, M. B.: Family systems in the 1970s: analysis policies, and programs. *Annals Am. Academy* 396, July 1971.
31. *Ibid.*
32. Reeder, Sharon J.: The impact of disabling health conditions on family interaction. Unpublished doctoral dissertation, 1974.
33. Sussman, M., *op. cit.*
34. Eiduson, B. T., *et al:* Alternatives in childrearing in the 1970s. *Am. J. Orthopsychiatry* 43:720-731, Oct. 1973.
35. *Ibid.*
36. *Ibid.*
37. *Ibid.*
38. Johnston, C., and Deisher, R.: Contemporary communal childrearing. *Pediatrics* 52:326, Sept. 1973.

39. Eiduson, B., *op. cit.*
40. Bancroft, A. V.: Pregnancy and the counterculture. *Nurs. Clin. North Am.* 8:67-76, Mar. 1973.
41. Maralee: *Our Babies, Our Lives, Our Right to Decide.* Chicago, Chicago Seed, 1972.
42. Bancroft, A. V., *op. cit.*
43. *Ibid.*
44. TenHouten, W.: The black family: myth and reality. *Psychiatry* 33:145-173, 1970.

45. Yorburg, B.: *The Changing Family.* New York, Columbia U. Press, 1973, 141-149.
46. *Ibid.*
47. Hymovich, D. P., and Barnard, M., *op. cit.*, pp. 128-137.
48. Reinhardt, A., and Quinn, M., *op. cit.*, pp. 72-77.
49. Benedict, R.: *The Chrysanthemum and the Sword.* Boston, Houghton-Mifflin, 1946.
50. Yorburg, B., *op. cit.*, pp. 145-149.

Suggested Reading

BERGER, B., *et al*: Child-rearing practices of the communal family. *In* I. Reiss (ed.), *Readings on the Family System.* New York, Holt, Rinehart & Winston, 1972.

DYER, E. D.: Parenthood as crisis: a restudy. *Marriage and Fam. Liv.* 25:196-201, May 1963.

HOBBS, D., JR.: Parenthood as crisis: a third study. *J. Marriage and Fam.* 27:367-372, Aug. 1965.

HOWELL, M. C.: Employed mothers and their families: I. *Pediatrics* 53:252-263, Aug. 1973.

———: Effects of maternal employment on the child: II. *Pediatrics* 52:327-343, Sept. 1973.

LeMASTERS, E. E.: Parenthood as crisis. *Marriage and Fam. Liv.* 19:353-355, Nov. 1957.

NUCKOLLS, *et al*: Psychosocial assets, life crisis and the prognosis of pregnancy. *Am. J. Epidemiology* 95, 2:431-441, 1972.

RAMEY, J. W.: Communes, group marriage, and the upper-middle class. *J. Marriage and Fam.* 647-655, Nov. 1972.

ROSSI, A.: Transition to parenthood. *J. Marriage and Fam.* 30:26-39, Feb. 1968.

TAVEGGIA, T., AND THOMAS, E.: Latchkey children. *Pac. Soc. Rev.* 17:27-34, Jan. 1974.

THORNTON, R., AND NARDI, P.: The dynamics of role acquisition. *Am. J. Sci.* 80, 4:870-885.

social factors in maternal care

Leo G. Reeder, Ph.D.

3

The Social and Cultural Meaning of
Pregnancy / Sociocultural Factors /
Social Class / Sociocultural Patterns
in the Use of Maternity Health Services /
Poverty: Its Relationship to Maternal Care

In most societies, conceptions of health and
well-being reflect the orientations of the person's social class position or group membership. Values, attitudes, perspectives, and the
behavior that we engage in are formed and
conditioned by the social groups in which we
participate from earliest childhood through
adulthood. As a consequence, there are differing
orientations to health and health care among
the various population groups in society that
reflect memberships in differing ethnic, racial,
religious, and social class groups. These varying health orientations become manifest both in
the behavior of individuals and the institutions
that are organized to deliver health services.

In recent years, there has been a heightened
awareness of the importance of social and cultural factors in health status and specifically
maternal care. Although Americans are accustomed to thinking of their health status as
being the best and highest in the world, the
health care of the American people is still far
short of its potential. Large segments of the
population either do not have access to adequate medical care or are deprived of quality
care in the services that they do receive. There
has been a great stimulus to increase efforts to
improve the prenatal care system, in particu-

lar, in order to improve the delivery of services
of maternal care and thus reduce preterm, low
birth weight, and infant deaths (see Chapter
12). Essentially, there has been an expansion
and elaboration of the existing system of maternity services. Whether such an approach to
maternity problems will have the desired effects
depends on a variety of factors, not the least of
which are those concerning the health values,
beliefs, orientations, and ultimately behaviors
of the target populations.

In the present chapter the focus is upon
those forces and features in society that influence the field of maternity services. First, it is
important to examine the social and cultural
meaning of pregnancy; what are the current
social, cultural, and economic forces that influence motivations for childbearing? Second,
we will discuss some of the critical issues in
access and use of maternal services. Relevant
to this issue of use of services, is the problem
of patient satisfaction. This involves the matter of communication between nurses and patients which is a determinant of use of services
by patients.

As discussed in Chapter 2, pregnancy itself
needs to be considered in terms of the social
context in which it occurs, namely, the family

41

and the larger society. Moreover, pregnancy has a different meaning in various societies and even within any given society.

In some societies, pregnancy is typically regarded as a "normal" life process, through which most women at some time pass. In other societies, pregnancy may be regarded as a kind of illness that must be overcome as quickly as possible. The expectations and the prescriptions for behavior surrounding pregnancy in Western society are relatively ill-defined and in some situations they do not exist. Consequently women are often uncertain when and how often they ought to visit the physician, whether they can continue in employment, and what is expected of them in relation to significant others. Part of the answer is related to the lifestyles of population subcultures and part of the answer lies in factors related to social structure (i.e., social class).

The social and cultural meaning of pregnancy

Childbearing motivations

For nurses to function appropriately, to use their talents more creatively than in the past, they must have an understanding of the social and cultural meaning of pregnancy. In the past 15 years, numerous studies have appeared concerned with factors influencing the number of children desired by and born to married couples. Most of these studies have focused on the *number* of children desired rather than on the attitudes held by women regarding *why* they want children. A brief consideration of some of the social and psychologic aspects motivating childbearing will be discussed.

No biologic event has greater significance for society than reproduction and its outcome. Reproduction is important in family dynamics and population dynamics, and in turn, their impact weighs heavily on individual and national welfare. Women begin their preparation for childbearing early in life. In a sense, they begin it at the time of their own conception.

Society is primarily organized for the families with children and the argument for having children can be very persuasive. Couples without children are generally made to feel "out of place," especially if they have been married very long. Many studies have demonstrated that the values of having children are generally accepted by the vast majority of Americans.[1]

In this context it is understandable that all levels of society should be organized in favor of children. Clearly, parenthood, at least in Western society, is still a highly valued phenomenon. As Rossi has noted, the cultural pressure to become parents is great enough that a couple may plan to bear children in spite of a latent desire to the contrary. For the female, the pressure to become a mother may be the equivalent of the cultural insistence that the male assume a productive occupational role.[2]

The availability of acceptable means for preventing conception permits a portion of childbearing today to be a consequence of motivated human action rather than a mere biologic result of sexual behavior. Regardless of when pregnancies occur or the presence or absence of deliberation, the number of children a couple has and the time at which it has them are partially a function of the nature of the couple's childbearing motivations.[3]

Present societal trends affecting childbearing motivations and maternity services

Elsewhere in this book we discuss techniques of contraception and family planning from a more technical perspective. Here we wish to highlight certain social implications of fertility control. A number of important trends is occurring in the United States that has already resulted in low fertility. Indeed, the American birthrate in 1974 reached an all-time low. At the current level, American families are not having enough children to replace themselves. In the opinion of many demographers, a revolution in the fertility regime of American women is taking place that has profound implications for society, including maternity services. At the core of the fertility changes is the apparent change in values associated with fertility control. The rapid diffusion of the pill resulted not only in a quantitative increase in the efficacy of controlling fertility, but also a qualitative leap that seems to have changed the rules under which fertility decisions are made.

First, it must be recognized that the oral contraceptive, diffused throughout the population at an unprecedented rate, not only vastly improved contraceptive protection, but also separated contraception from sexual activity. Now childbearing can be voluntary in a radically different sense than ever before. Under the previous fertility regime, women could not confidently plan a lifetime of childlessness nor the prevention of unwanted fertility. Surely, some women could and did avoid unwanted fertility, but no individual could be sure of the outcome in advance. Not surprisingly, under this regime the adult role expectations of women were structured around motherhood. In fact, cultural values with respect to fertility were, in part, rationalizations of the inevitable. For example, in the early 1960s about one-half of all births were accidental: one-fifth reported by their mothers as unwanted.[4]

The rapid adoption of the pill has facilitated the adoption of other effective means of preventing unwanted births (the IUD, sterilization, and abortion) and has led to reductions in the number of children intended by U.S. women. Contraceptive sterilization had been a relatively infrequent occurrence in the population prior to the introduction of the pill. In recent years there has been a dramatic reversal of this pattern with majority approval and greater use of this procedure. By 1970, for example, among women older than 30, sterilization was the most prevalent contraceptive method.[5]

All of the foregoing processes in contraceptive practice indicate a drastic realignment of values in fertility. These new fertility control values have prepared the way for greater receptivity to the equal opportunity concept by making nonfamilial roles a realistic and viable option for women. Thus the potential for complete fertility control makes childbearing a matter of choice in a sense never before realized. Motherhood itself now becomes a matter of rational evaluation. The costs as well as the virtues can now be weighed. This is, of course, not a new discovery. There has always been a large literature on the psychologic and emotional costs of motherhood. Indeed, we discuss some of these issues later in this chapter. They have, however, become more relevant and salient particularly in the context of increased concern with equality of opportunity for women.

Thus, as nonfamilial opportunities are more equalized, the opportunity costs of childbearing are increased. One of the consequences is to place motherhood more directly in competition with other socially desirable roles. As fertility becomes more a matter for *decision*, greater emphasis is placed on planning. Among the factors that must be taken into account in the decision are the direct social, psychologic,

and economic costs of children themselves, and also the loss of the wife's earnings and intrinsic satisfaction with her job.

This is no small matter. A leading newspaper in the United States featured a story in its Sunday edition written by a young, well-educated couple on the agonizing decision of whether to have a child; this in itself is symbolic of what has been discussed here. That is, the mere fact that such a story is newsworthy is socially significant. Moreover, modern lifestyles are significantly dependent on the wife's earnings. In a majority of the families in which both the husband and wife have incomes, the wife's income represents over one-fifth of the total family income.[6]

The implications of all this are enormous, for fertility statistics influence almost every facet of our lives. Consider the following as examples: 1) elementary school enrollment has been dropping since 1970 and this is soon to have a similar effect on the high schools; 2) a slowdown in the birthrate affects the Social Security system of the country; 3) there will be changes in the consumption patterns that may influence smaller cars and even smaller houses; 4) last, but not least, there is an impact upon maternity services. Two trends in particular are worth mention; first, not only are some hospitals closing their maternity units, but perhaps more importantly, hospitals are merging their obstetrical units. This will hopefully improve the quality of obstetrical care for mothers and newborns, in addition to controlling costs and avoiding duplication of services. In addition, the experience of fertility control may make women more sensitive and aware of the need for better maternal care during the pregnancy period. Indeed, the increased availability of safe abortion after 1970 is temporarily associated with a reduction in pregnancy-associated maternal mortality.[7,8] There is also good reason to connect the trends in fertility control to the recent rapid decline in infant mortality.

It should be recognized that no one knows for certain that the current pattern of fertility control will continue indefinitely, but most demographers concede that it most likely will. Nevertheless, it is important to note that the "baby boom" children of the fifties are now forming their own families. Thus, there will be an increase of approximately 20 percent, within the next few years, in the number of women in the childbearing age groups of 15 to 44 years. This probably means that the absolute number of births will rise even if the birth*rate* does not. This is what happened in 1974, for the first time in four years.

Clearly, the childbearing motivations of women are complex and often interrelated. There is, for example, the social expectation to bear children, previously mentioned. A childless woman may wish to emulate her friends or relatives who already have children, or she may be supported in her desire to postpone childbearing by the fact that her friends are also childless. Some women are confident of their femininity and look forward to childbearing as a further confirmation of their feminine identity. On the other hand, a woman may doubt her femininity and require childbearing as a demonstration of her adequacy as a woman. A woman may desire motherhood as a substitute identity for unachieved career aspirations; or motherhood may be derogated as commonplace in comparison with her identity as a person or as a career woman, and she may postpone childbearing indefinitely. There are various psychologic factors related to feelings with regard to childhood memories and identifications, anticipation of expected relationships with children, that may be involved in childbearing motivations.

Finally, the woman's relationship with her husband, his interest in having children and her appraisal of his potential for fatherhood may also affect childbearing motivations. It is possible that a woman may consider her home incomplete without children. The child may serve as a symbol of the unity of the marriage or perhaps as an expression of her love for her husband. On the other hand, a woman may be reluctant to bear a child by a husband whom she neither loves nor respects. The husband's lack of interest in having children may undermine her childbearing motivations or support her own childbearing reluctance. These and many other factors are involved in the complex problem of childbearing motivations.

Sociocultural factors affecting childbearing

The sick role, illness, and pregnancy

How a society or groups within a society define pregnancy and cope with pregnancy tends to vary considerably. In some societies, pregnancy is regarded as a "normal" situation—a kind of status passage through which most women, at some time or other, will pass. In other societies, pregnancy may be regarded as an illness and is reacted to as other illnesses are. As previously noted in this chapter, there is considerable variation, even within societies, in the way health and illness are perceived by different social classes, ethnic groups, and age categories.

The sick role has been developed as a concept by sociologists to study the role behavior of persons who are considered sick or as having an illness.[9] In brief, the sick role concept refers to the process by which every society ensures that an adequate level of health and normative conformity exists among the majority of its members most of the time. Society has various mechanisms for accomplishing this purpose. Illness as a form of deviance is one method by which society accommodates individuals or groups who are ill, and hence deviating from expected behavior, by placing them in a special position or status. The term "social role" refers to both the regular way of acting expected of persons occupying a given position and the social position itself. Typically there are certain rights or privileges, as well as expectations, associated with given social positions. Parsons has presented an insightful and systematic analysis of the expectations associated with occupancy of the sick role.[9] There are two main rights:

1. The sick person is allowed exemption from the performance of normal social role obligations.
2. The sick person is allowed exemption from the responsibility for his own state.

In addition there are two main obligations:

3. The sick person must be motivated to get well as soon as possible.
4. The sick person should seek technically competent help and cooperate with medical experts.

The sick role is generally conceptualized by sociologists as an ideal type for the purposes of understanding the processes contributing to and the various conditions to be fulfilled in the legitimation of illness conditions. There is an attempt to detect and account for certain uniformities in the behavior of ill persons. Since this is a theoretical model, the concept permits a study of the effects of legitimation on both the individual and on his social milieu. In reality, the concept is not universally applicable to all who claim to be ill; it varies depending on the unique background of the person, the particular illness involved, and the social context within which legitimation is sought.

Sociologists have made a number of criticisms of the sick role including the fact that Parsons has left open the problem of the chronically ill, as well as some illness that is not considered serious enough to warrant more than a slight reduction in normal activities. Furthermore, much illness never reaches the stage of formal consultation with a qualified physician. Individuals who are ill may receive what they consider to be competent help from other than professional medical personnel. Furthermore, Parsons has suggested that his sick role formulation is especially applicable to psychiatric or emotional illnesses. Finally, Parsons's formulation may not be relevant to all societies, and various studies have demonstrated that there are both intercultural and intracultural variations in the definitions of the conditions to which the sick role is thought to be applicable.

The state of pregnancy in its modal or normal situation, where there are no resultant obstetric or delivery complications, must be considered in the discussion of the applicability of the sick role concept. If a woman is experiencing complications of pregnancy, certainly this would make her eligible for the sick role as discussed above. The question that arises is whether pregnancy is in fact a "normal" state.

One may conceivably take the position that illness, or sickness, is statistically normal in most members of the population, at some point in their lives; similarly, pregnancy can likewise be considered statistically normal in that most of the population of possible conceivers at some time are in this state. Pregnancy can also be considered "normal" in the sense that it is a necessary biologic function for the species. Indeed, it can even be considered a desirable state of affairs. In this latter sense, it is not similar to illness at all. In a recent paper, McKinlay has noted that pregnancy differs from illness by "calling forth in both the woman and her significant others a set of responses which are in many ways different from those elicited with the onset of an illness."[10] Considering whether the four sick role expectations noted above apply to pregnancy, McKinlay suggests that for a variety of reasons, the state of pregnancy is in some ways different from

illness and cannot be analyzed in terms of any of the four expectations associated with the sick role.

There is a tendency in the more advanced societies to consider at least some point during pregnancy as illness and to treat it in a manner similar to that in which illness is handled. For example, women are discouraged from home deliveries and are increasingly hospitalized for delivery. Blood pressure, height, weight, and so on are usually taken at several points during the pregnancy. Treating women "as if" they are ill may perhaps encourage the adoption of certain roles because the women perceive this type of treatment as being similar to that for an illness. In sum, the state of pregnancy and the expectations covering it differ from routine illness behavior and the situation is relatively unstructured. This relatively unstructured situation may produce a sense of role ambiguity or strain in pregnant women. Women may take matters into their own hands and reduce such strain or ambiguity by structuring the situation in particular ways.

On the other hand, in the situation where women cannot maintain their homeostatic mechanisms under the physiologic strain of pregnancy, there is a meaningful situation in which the sick role becomes an important role behavior. For women who are at greater risk, either latent or manifest, and who react excessively or unfavorably under the strain of pregnancy, the sick role becomes meaningful and relevant.

Thus, in the "normal" circumstances of pregnancy and under pathologic conditions, the sick role is an important feature of maternal care.

Social class

Social class is an important determinant of maternal reproductive behavior and maternal use of services. Since socioeconomic status or social class has such a pervasive influence upon health and health care, it is well to briefly describe the central features of this concept.

Social class, or socioeconomic status, is a complex concept referring to a theoretical formulation of relationships between subgroups in our society. It is a term frequently used by sociologists and epidemiologists in medical research as an effort to subdivide populations into a few descriptive categories which differ in a variety of social and economic characteristics, background, and behavior.

Typically, in determining socioeconomic status, the usual procedure is to select as indicators of social differences one or several characteristics, each of which are closely related to: income, education, occupation, housing and place of residence, social values, and the general lifestyle of population subgroups. By far the most widely used indicator of socioeconomic status or social class is occupation. It is the best indicator of a person's income, education, standard of living, social values, and a variety of other attributes. Thus, it has a practical property (ease of collection, accuracy, manageability), as well as social significance.

Not all social differences stem from socioeconomic status. Dividing a population along one social dimension does not automatically provide categories which are socially meaningful in other respects. It can be demonstrated that such social variables as age, geographic region, height, parity, and socioeconomic status, each contribute independently to the total picture of social variation in pregnancy outcome. The same may be said of other more complex social influences.

Similarly, other social variables have limitations when studied out of context with other factors. For example, many studies have demonstrated, epidemiologically, that there is a relationship between customs, habits, and general living conditions and a variety of medical disorders and health conditions. But such relationships are meaningful only in the sense that they indicate hypotheses for further study. They become meaningful to the clinician when it is possible to specify more clearly the nature of the linkage between these social background characteristics and biologic consequences such as infant mortality and malnutrition.

Sociocultural patterns in the use of maternity health services

It is generally accepted that adequate medical care during pregnancy, particularly in the early stages of pregnancy, reduces the incidence of neonatal mortality, congenital malformations or other birth defects, maternal mortality, prematurity, and so on. The relationship between low socioeconomic status and failure to receive adequate antenatal care, has been well documented. The data appear to be similar in the United States, Great Britain, and in various other Western nations. Not only do the lower-class women typically comprise the highest proportion of those who have not received antenatal care, they are also the women, as a group, who contribute to the highest proportion of underutilizers of antenatal care.[10]

According to the latest sources of data for the United States, the average American woman made 11.5 visits for medical care during the year before her child was born. On the average, white mothers made 12.2 visits in a 12-month period and nonwhite mothers 7.7. Thus, the average white mother had 60 percent more visits than the average nonwhite mother. This is undoubtedly related to other findings concerning the influence of socioeconomic status and antenatal care. According to these data, as family income increased, the number of visits for medical care also increased. Women living in families below the poverty level made, on the average, 9.3 visits for medical care; women from middle-income families averaged 13.7 visits. Most of the women in the lowest income group visited medical facilities (clinics, hospitals) for their care as contrasted to the women in the highest income group where the majority visited physicians for medical care.

Income appears to be a major factor in the number of visits for prenatal care. There is a large jump in number of visits when the income goes above the poverty line (i.e., $5,000 and over). As would be expected, the average number of visits for medical care was also higher for women who had completed more years of school. Primiparous women made more visits than multiparous women. According to the National Natality Study only 2 percent make no visits at all during the 12 months before childbirth. On the other hand, almost 20 percent of the women made no visits either to a physician or to a medical facility until the third trimester of pregnancy.

The evidence we have to date indicates that white mothers receive care earlier in pregnancy than nonwhite mothers. There is a consistent difference between white and nonwhite mothers in the receipt of medical care during each of the trimesters of pregnancy. There is evidence that women living in metropolitan areas receive care earlier than those outside metropolitan areas; this held true for both white and nonwhite women. Furthermore, more of the nonwhite women in metropolitan areas are known to have received care than nonwhite women residing outside metropolitan areas. It is worth noting, though, that for any given income or educational group the differences between metropolitan and nonmetropolitan areas are insignificant with respect to the time when mothers first receive medical care.

Several factors are worth mentioning with regard to differences in prenatal care patterns. As noted, the lower-socioeconomic-status groups tend to come later in their pregnancy for prenatal care than do the middle- and upper-socioeconomic-status groups. Furthermore, there is a differential by age and parity; the women in the younger age group tend to come later than women in the other age groups. This is probably due to the fact that the highest rates of illegitimacy are in the youngest age groups. Women in the lower-socioeconomic-status groups tend to receive their prenatal care in clinics and other medical facilities; women in the middle- and upper-socioeconomic-status groups tend to receive their prenatal care from private physicians. Similarly, those in the lower-socioeconomic-status groups tend to have higher rates of illegitimacy and, given the stigma attached to this status, they are not likely to be seen by private practitioners but rather in the clinics. The stigma of illegitimacy would probably be a major factor contributing to underutilization of prenatal services by the young primigravidae.

There are crucial differences in the delivery of health services to clinic populations and to private patients. A number of sociomedical factors influence the availability and use of obstetric services. Not only are there variations in the services available, but there are also variations in the quality of antenatal care for obstetric management. Second, there are differential resources available to the lower-socioeconomic-status groups as contrasted to the higher-socioeconomic-status groups. That is to say, there are relatively fewer maternal care facilities, as well as general medical facilities, available to ghetto residents and other low-socioeconomic-status groups than to higher-social-status groups. Thus, the differential distribution of maternity services is influenced by a complex interaction of many factors.

Factors in utilization

Sociocultural patterns

Research into patterns of utilization of health services has begun to establish a theoretical and empirical basis for a number of assumptions that have been made in the past. Typically, the studies of utilization have made comparisons of the use of health services, including prenatal care, by comparing whites with blacks or other racial/ethnic groups, high-income with low-income groups, and upper-social classes with lower-social classes. Mechanic, however, points out that, in considering the factors that influence the utilizations of health services, it is not enough to focus upon availability of services and resources in accounting for entry or nonentry into the medical system.[11] One must also consider the potential *consumer's willingness to seek care*. This characteristic depends on her health attitudes, knowledge about health care, and the social and cultural definitions of health and illness she has learned, specifically those related to pregnancy.

Use of health services for prenatal care cannot be considered independently of the concept of *access to health care*. Thus, this section of the chapter will discuss both of these concepts as they relate to maternal services. Health services utilization research provides a framework to describe those factors that inhibit or facilitate entrance into the maternal care delivery system. Accessibility, as Donabedian observes, is more than the mere "availability" of medical resources.[12] It also, he says, comprises such characteristics of the resource that facilitate or obstruct use by potential clients. Socioorganizational attributes that facilitate or obstruct use by potential patients include such things as: sex of the provider, the specialization or fee scale, and the race or income of the patient. Geographic accessibility refers to the time and physical distance that must be traversed to receive care.

The issues discussed here are also related to the *changing relationships between the client-patient and the providers of maternity services*, physicians and nurses. Walker has succinctly summarized the changes that have taken place in maternity nursing that are due to changing social factors and consumer demands.[13] She notes the usage of different terminology in the profession from "obstetrical nursing" to "maternity nursing" to "family-centered maternity care" to the present situation. Consumers complain that it is becoming more and more difficult to find a primary care physician who will give them the personal attention they want. Regardless of the social class level of the woman, it is very difficult for her to have continuity of care in the personnel who provide maternity services. Regardless of its other merits, group practice sometimes disrupts the relationship between patient and physician; hospital structure requires nursing personnel to change with shift changes; patients have difficulty determining the status of the person in the medical office to whom she is speaking on the telephone. Patients feel that the obstetrician seems to relinquish his responsibility for the neonate during the postpartum period. Similarly, in this period, the pediatrician (from the mother's perspective) does not appear to be centrally involved with the needs of the mother. All of these features of the medical care system are reflected in the concept of "fragmented health care," and consumer dissatisfaction.

Consumer satisfaction, that is, the satisfaction of pregnant women, refers to the attitudes toward the medical care system of those who have experienced a contact with the system. It is different from the medical beliefs of the patient in that it is concerned with the satisfaction of the patient with the quantity or quality of care actually received. There are several dimensions to this concept. These include: 1) accessibility-convenience of services (convenience of care, and emergency care); 2) availability (family physicians, hospitals, specialists, complete facilities); 3) continuity (regular family physician, same physician); 4) physician conduct (consideration for feelings; explanations; prudent risks; quality; regular checkup); 5) financial aspects (cost of services; insurance coverage; payment mechanisms). However, little is known about the relationship of these features of patient satisfaction to other social-psychologic dimensions such as perceived health, values, psychologic well-being, and general sentiments about life.

A crucial feature of this aspect of maternity care is the quality and quantity of patient-provider *communication*. Here we refer not only to the physician, but also to the nurse in communicating with the patient and her needs. One of the more important transactions that occurs in the physician-patient relationship is effective communication from the physician to the patient concerning the nature of the patient's condition and the actions to be taken. The degree to which the patient has understood the physician and can verbalize the physician's advice and instructions depends on the quality of the relationship.[14] Similarly, good medical care results in communication from the patient to the physician. In particular, the degree to which the patient's concerns, worries, and fears about her condition have been perceived by the physician are equally important.

Commentators on the physician-patient relationship frequently have discussed the social class and value differences between physicians and patients as one barrier to communication and ultimately to utilization of medical services. Numerous studies have demonstrated that working-class patients tend to be diffident in questioning physicians about their health or illness condition. These studies indicate that the middle-class patients tend to obtain most of their information about illness by asking their physicians and nurses direct questions. In contrast, working-class patients receive their information from a "passive process in which they were given information without asking; they also tended to receive less information."[15]

Despite their reluctance to request information, working-class maternity patients are not much different from upper-class patients in their *desire* for information.[16] Although upper-class patients may desire more technical details concerning their health condition, there is no general social class difference in patients' desires for as much information as possible presented in nontechnical language.

Part of the issue of better communication between physician and patient results from a reflection of a general social class difference in language use. Working-class patients sense that physicians do not expect them to ask questions; they hold the physicians in awe; and there is a social class distance. But even middle-class patients hesitate to freely communicate with their physician about troublesome problems or symptoms. A virtual legend has been engendered through all of the media about the hard-working, busy physician. It has become generally accepted throughout our society that all physicians are extremely busy professionals. Thus, although there may be some apparent social class differences in the quantity and quality of communication with physicians, it is a matter of degree of communication.

Given this situation, the maternity nurse has a crucial role to play. By and large the nurse is not perceived by the patient in the same manner as the physician. Patients perceive the nurse as filling a substantially different role with accompanying differences in expectations. Thus, the nurse has an opportunity to fulfill a much-needed role in the delivery of health care by seizing the initiative and closing the communications gap in the patient-provider relationship. Such action would be congruent with patient expectations; moreover, several studies have documented that the nurse can perform roles involving the receiving and giving of information to patients far more effectively than physicians.

These problems of communication have been emphasized here because, among other things, there is an influence upon the use of health services as a consequence of the patient's perceived difficulties in communicating with medical providers. That is, the patient encountering difficulties in communication (typically social class linked) and other problems related to their social position in society will tend to delay or not use medical services even when such services are readily available.

Poverty: Its relationship to maternal care

Sociocultural factors

Earlier in this chapter, the concept of socioeconomic status or social class, was briefly discussed. Unlike that concept, the concept "poor" is very ancient, dating back to biblical times (i.e., "The poor always ye have with you," John 12:8). This concept, like socioeconomic status or social class, also expresses social differences between men and has gained general acceptance. It has been used to describe rural tenant farmers, mountain folk in Appalachia, and ethnic and other groups in urban ghettos. The importance of a discussion of poverty and health with particular reference to maternity care is obvious from the foregoing discussion in this chapter which has indicated a close relationship between low socioeconomic status and maternal health care.

Before discussing how the characteristics of lower-income persons influence their behavior in connection with the issues of health, illness, and the utilization of medical services, it is appropriate to briefly discuss some aspects of medical organization and medical care for lower-income groups. The national commitment for equality of medical care for all citizens has led to a variety of important legislative acts. The emphasis is on extending and improving the system of medical organization so that medical care can be offered more rapidly, more effectively, and more efficiently to the poor as well as to those more economically advantaged. For example, the maternal and infant care projects (MIC) supported by the U.S. Children's Bureau has had an important impact on maternity care throughout the United States. These projects are supposed to help reduce the incidence of mental retardation and other handicapping conditions caused by complications associated with childbearing and to help reduce infant and maternal mortality. The projects are concentrated in low-income areas of large and small cities, and the emphasis is on early, comprehensive prenatal care for all patients in the geographic area served. A variety of allied health personnel has been recruited to provide and extend a range of services. As with most of these new programs, there are many problems that have yet to be resolved before they can be called truly successful.

There is a serious question as to whether the inequities in the medical care system can be overcome unless changes are made reflecting greater understanding of lower-income lifestyles. It is well known that when medical facilities are set up in convenient proximity to lower-income housing, they do not automatically draw clientele. No doubt, medical facilities located near the homes of lower-income people are more likely to draw and keep patients, but their mere presence does not solve the problem of delivering effective care to most people in the nearby locale.

There are two factors which contribute to inequities of medical care. The first of these relates to the way in which medical organization facilities are structured; the second factor is concerned with the characteristic lifestyles of lower-income groups. Both factors are obstacles to the delivery and receipt of quality medical care.

What are the features of medical care organization that tend to blunt the effectiveness of medical care for lower-income patients?[17] These negative features of medical organization include the following: first, there is the massiveness of medical organization itself. Most of the lower-income women, as noted earlier in this chapter, tend to visit medical facilities such as hospitals and clinics. These are often large and complex organizations, characterized not only by great specialization of function and specialized clinics, but by a fair degree of impersonality which is felt even by middle-class patients (who register this as one of their chief complaints about hospital care). Lower-class patients are ill-equipped by lack of education and experience to cope with complex bureaucratic organization. Little explanation is provided to the patient of the reasons for diagnostic tests, the necessity of visiting a variety of clinics, and so on.

A second feature of medical organization which tends to decrease the quality of care for lower-income patients is that professionalization with its resultant characteristic set of goals, its perspectives toward work and patients, results in a gap between the patients and the professionals. Lower-income people are less skilled in interviewing matters to get at information that the professionals have but are not yielding. They tend to be less aggressive in demanding explanations. On the other hand, higher-income patients have greater aggressive and interactional skills and can cope more effectively with the professionals' failure to communicate. There are other, more subtle, disadvantages stemming from professional stances, which lower-income patients suffer. These have been discussed by a number of investigators with regard to the field of mental disorders. That is, middle-class patients are preferred by most treatment agents, and are seen as more treatable. In other words, there may be a distinct bias expressed against the lower-income patient, based honestly on professional conceptions. Many regimens are impossible for low-income patients to carry out. Even the simple order that medication is to be taken "with each meal" may not recognize that many lower-income families eat irregularly and may not have three meals a day.

Another characteristic of medical organization that influences the quality of medical care is the middle-class bias of most professional health workers. The staff members, typically, do not understand the perspective, attitudes, customs and lifestyles of the patients. They simply take for granted that the patients have the same attitudes regarding health as they do. Hence, they tend to issue orders that are not understood or cannot be easily followed by lower-income patients. Furthermore, there is a tendency to think of lower-income people in stereotyped terms, "they cannot keep appointments; they have little sense of time or responsibility; they are shiftless, irresponsible;

they have children out of wedlock; they are dirty." Lower-income patients may perceive these class biases and this may affect not only the quality of medical care which the patients receive, but also the underutilization of medical services.

The many hours of waiting, the impersonal routines of institutional care in large hospitals or clinics, particularly in the municipal and county hospitals—and in the larger cities these tend to be massive, complex, crowded, and busy—the real or imagined perceptions of racial and class bias all tend to maximize dissatisfactions of lower-income patients and reduce the possibility of utilization of health facilities. Furthermore, the distances that patients must travel to the medical facilities and the cost of transportation are realistic matters. Customarily, poor people organize their lives so as not to go far for the necessities of living. This is one of the factors in the relative success of the MIC program (i.e., it has reached out into the lower-income communities and brought the clinic facilities into the neighborhood). Similarly, the neighborhood health centers have been relatively successful for this reason.

It is important to briefly take into account the characteristic lifestyles of the poor. The lower-income person's experience of himself and his world is highly distinctive in our country. It is also distinctive for its problems and crisis-dominated character. As S. M. Miller has commented about these people, their "life is a crisis-life constantly trying to make do with string where rope is needed." In other words, health concerns are minor to those who feel they confront much more pressing troubles. Health problems are just one crisis among many that they must try to cope with, control, or just live with.

Indeed, the value orientations of the medical system reflect the values of the middle- and upper-middle classes. These have been characterized as activistic, rational mastery, future-time orientation to life. A large body of empirical research data suggests that the values of the middle class tend to result in a specific outlook on life that gets reflected in health beliefs and behavior. Thus, the lower classes, whose position in the social structure does not support a belief in the rational mastery of the world, tend to have a quite different orientation of the world. There is a feeling of lack of control over events; occurrences are viewed as "luck" or fate rather than as planned by rational design. Planning, education, and involvement in organized activity are less important in this framework; they seek help from those in their social network rather than from "experts" or professionals.[18,19]

The health attitudes and cultural orientations of the poor or lower social class tend to be significantly different from those of the middle classes. Health has narrow, short-range meanings. These orientations provide a frame of reference for the response to the pregnancy; it is what Milio has called a "maternity activities pattern (MAP)," defined as the "characteristic pattern of activities engaged in by women from their awareness of their pregnancy through delivery."[19]

The pattern of activity for maternity cases that is typically prescribed as the ideal is likely to be most closely adhered to by the middle-class women. The maternal services for delivering prenatal care to encourage this pattern is generally based upon middle-class assumptions. Hence, it should not be surprising to discover that since both the ideal pattern of maternity activity and the system of prenatal care are essentially middle-class oriented, the women from the lower social classes are likely to encounter problems of access and utilization. Indeed, Milio substantiated these expected kinds of behaviors in her study of maternal activity in Detroit.[19]

Another problem is that many lower-income households are often much more understaffed than those of higher income. This understaffing of households means that each individual's health receives relatively little attention as far as preventive measures are concerned, and when someone is sick it is more difficult to care for him at home. When the main family member is sick, he or she will be in a disadvantaged position in caring properly for himself or herself. There is a necessity for poor people to learn to live with illness rather than to use their limited financial and psychologic resources to do something about illness. The pressing problems of daily existence tend to minimize the problem of illness so that symptoms that do not incapacitate are often ignored.

Furthermore, self-education is much less advanced among lower-income groups than among people of higher income. Lower-income people do not conform to the expectations of how "good" and "considerate" patients should behave in medical settings. Their behavior is often frustrating and annoying to medical and nursing personnel for a variety of reasons. Finally, lower-income persons do not respond well to the "impersonality" of the professional role; they tend to seek personal rather than professional relationships with staff, as they do in behavior outside of medical settings. As a result there may be considerable anxiety when the lower-income patient is in the medical setting of large hospitals. This pervasive anxiety has been described in Rosengren's study of obstetric patients.[20] Her lack of experience maneuvering within organizational structures makes this a problematic situation, even when she is a paying patient.

In short, the cultural values and the health beliefs that are rooted in these values tend to shape the maternal behavior of pregnant women just as they influence other types of health practices. These values are not easily mutable; thus, in the absence of either powerful attempts to change behavior or the system itself, it is well to recognize the differences in assumptions, values, beliefs and behaviors and attempt to adjust the structure of the maternal health service delivery system. For example, neighborhood-based prenatal and postnatal non-bureaucratic clinics, staffed by low-income personnel and developing programs reflecting the interests and needs of the low-income population, are more appropriate restructuring of medical organization facilities.

When such a situation exists in a lower-social-class community, the maternal activity pattern does indeed begin to resemble the ideal middle-class pattern. For example, in Los Angeles, where there are over one million Spanish-speaking residents in the County, the existence of a major hospital and neighborhood health centers staffed by Spanish-speaking personnel appears to have significant results. In a recent survey of more than one thousand women concerning the adequacy of prenatal care among the residents of East Los Angeles, it was found that 75 percent stated that their first visit to a care facility had occurred in the first trimester. Only 4 percent made their initial visit during the third trimester. Moreover 94 percent made their final visit during the third trimester of pregnancy; only 2 percent of the sample had no care at all. The average number of visits made was 9.5 or approximately one visit per month. More than 80 percent of the sample of these Spanish-speaking women had received at least five prenatal checkups while only 16 percent made only four or less visits. [21]

In this section an effort has been made to depict some of the problems associated with the delivery of services to the poor, even when resources, equipment, and finances are made available, by focusing upon some of the disparities between the assumptions made about lower-income patients by professional staff and the realities of lower-income life, attitudes, and behavior. Yet, such knowledge concerning the poor has not been adequately built into either the training of health professionals, nor has it affected the organization of medical care in hospitals, clinics, and other medical facilities. It is important, therefore, that greater understanding and awareness of the characteristic lifestyles of the poor gain greater currency among health professionals, if we are indeed, to meet the national commitment of good health care for *all* American citizens.

The differential distribution of maternity care services is influenced by a complex interaction of many factors. In this chapter we have attempted to provide some insight into the relevance of social and cultural factors on the delivery of maternal services.

Bibliography

1. Blood, R. O., and Wolfe, D. M.: *Husbands and Wives.* Glencoe, Ill., The Free Press, 1960.
2. Rossi, A.: Transition to parenthood. *J. Marriage and Fam.* 30:33, Feb. 1968.
3. Flapan, M.: A paradigm for the analysis of childbearing motivations of married women prior to birth of the first child. *Am. J. Orthopsychiatry* 39:402-417, Apr. 1969.
4. Bumpass, L. L., and Westoff, C. F.: The 'perfect contraceptive' population. *Science* 169:1177, 1970.
5. Westoff, C. F.: The modernization of U.S. contraceptive practice. *Fam. Plan. Perspect.* 4, 4:9, 1972.
6. Sweet, J. A.: The employment and earnings of married women. *Seminar*, New York, 1973, Chap. 6.
7. Pakter, J., *et al*: Impact of the liberalized abortion law in New York City on pregnancy associated deaths: a two-year experience. *Bull. N.Y. Academy Med.* 49:804-818, 1972.
8. Wright, N. H.: Family planning and infant mortality rate death decline in the United States. *Am. J. Epidemiology* 101:182-187, Mar. 1975.
9. Parsons, T.: Definitions of health and illness in the light of American values and social structure. In *Social Structure and Personality.* Glencoe, Ill., The Free Press, 1964, pp. 257-291, 436-437.
10. McKinlay, J. B.: The new latecomers for antenatal care. *Brit. J. Prev. Soc. Med.* 24:52, Feb. 1970.
11. Mechanic, D.: Public expectations and health care. In *Essays on the Changing Organization of Health Services.* New York, John Wiley & Sons, 1972.
12. Donabedian, A.: Aspects of Medical Care Administration. Cambridge, Harvard U. Press, 1973.
13. Walker, L.: Providing more relevant maternity services. *JOGN, Nursing,* Mar./Apr. 1974, pp. 34-36.
14. Waitzkin, H., and Stoeckle, J. D.: The communication of information about illness. *Adv. Psychosom. Med.* 8:180-215, 1972.
15. Pratt, L., *et al*: Physicians' views on the level of medical information among patients. *Am. J. Public Health* 47:1277-1283, 1975.
16. Jolly, C., *et al*: Research in the delivery of female health care: the recipients' reaction. *Am. J. Ob.-Gyn.* 110, 3:291-294, June 1, 1971.
17. Strauss, A. L.: Medical organization, medical care in lower-income groups. *Soc. Sci. Med.* 3:143-177, 1969.
18. Hyman, H.: The Value Systems of Different Classes. *In* R. Bendix, and S. Lipset (eds.), *Class, Status, and Power.* Glencoe, Ill.: The Free Press, 1953, pp. 426-442.
19. Milio, N.: Values, social class and community health services. *Nurs. Research,* 16, 1, Winter 1967.
20. Rosengren, W. R.: Social class in becoming "ill." *In* A. B. Shostak, and W. Donberg (eds.), *Blue Collar World,* Englewood Cliffs, N.J., Prentice-Hall, 1964.
21. Sabagh, G.: Growth of Mexican-American Families Study. Unpublished, Department of Sociology, U. of California, Los Angeles, 1975.

selected risk factors and pregnancy outcomes

4

Sociodemographic Risk Factors / Behavioral Risk Factors / Life Events and Life Crises as Risks

In this chapter the focus is upon selected risk factors that are associated with such pregnancy outcomes as infant and maternal mortality, low birth weight, and other complications of pregnancy. Elsewhere in this volume, these pregnancy problems will be discussed from a different perspective than is presented here (see Unit VII).

For purposes of convenience, the risk factors to be discussed in this chapter may be grouped as follows: 1) Sociodemographic risk factors—these include maternal age, out-of-wedlock pregnancies, socioeconomic status, and ethnicity or racial factors; 2) behavioral risk factors—these factors include smoking behavior and drug behavior; 3) life events and life crises—this risk factor includes death or other types of significant loss (desertion), economic (job) loss, interpersonal problems, physical illness, and other significant life changes either preceding or occurring during pregnancy.

Although health status of the mother and medical care received are also risk factors for pregnancy outcome, we shall be particularly concerned with only the three risk factors noted above, since we have already discussed the importance of social factors to prenatal care in Chapter 3.

Sociodemographic risk factors

Maternal age

In one of its earliest studies, the U.S. Children's Bureau demonstrated a relationship between age of mother and infant mortality. This relationship has been observed many times in the past—that is, high mortality rates among infants of the youngest mothers and also among those of the older mothers. Moreover, there is a strong correlation between socioeconomic status and age of mother: births to parents with more education and/or higher family income tend to occur to substantially older mothers. The lower the socioeconomic status, the greater the tendency for the mother to be younger. Of course, women age 35 and over account for only about 5 percent of all U.S. births.

First births to older women are of particular interest because they have been viewed as "high risk" and attention has usually been focused on the maternal rather than the fetal results. More recently, however, given careful prenatal care, the emphasis has shifted to fetal risk.

On the other hand, the older *multiparous*

Table 4-1 Illegitimate Births per 1,000 Unmarried Women Age 14, 15-17, 18-19 and 15-19 by Color, United States, 1940-1968

Color and Age	1940	1950	1960	1968
Nonwhite				
14	13	19	20	21
15-17	38	53	56	67
18-19	61	93	114	112
15-19	45.5	65.6	73.9	82.0
White				
14	0.5	0.8	1	1
15-17	2	3	4	6
18-19	5	8	12	17
15-19	3.5	5.1	6.6	9.7
White and Nonwhite				
15-19	8.3	12.8	15.6	19.8

Rates are adjusted for Census undercount of unmarried teenagers and underregistration of births.

Rates to girls 15-19 exclude births to girls age 14 and younger. Age 14 rate relates births to girls younger than 15 to the number unmarried aged 14. Most rates are rounded to the nearest whole number.

Source: P. Cutright, *Illegitimacy in the United States: 1920-1968*, Final Report to the Commission on Population Growth and the American Future, Oct. 1971, Table 1.3 (Washington, D.C., U.S. Government Printing Office), 1972.

woman is also at increased risk for neonatal mortality. In one recently reported Australian study on a relatively large series of cases, women age 40 and over tended to have heavier babies than normal and the perinatal mortality rate was nearly twice that for the hospital.[1] Interestingly, these women were reported to have attended regularly for antenatal and postnatal care. In addition, the older women had a higher rate of miscarriages compared to all other maternity patients.

Age and parity are two biologic categories that have specific social significance. They are associated with perinatal mortality, stillbirths, and more complications of pregnancy and possible risk of brain damage to the baby. The role of the maternity nurse is to counsel women with respect to the problems associated with pregnancy. Thus, patient education is particularly important for this type of patient.

Teenage pregnancy

Of perhaps even greater concern to society is the problem of adolescent pregnancy. Notable among the social and health costs of these pregnancies are the following: 1) About one-half of school-age mothers will have a subsequent unwanted pregnancy within two years of the birth of the first child; 2) the evidence indicates that approximately 60 percent of those who had their first baby at school-age become welfare recipients; 3) young mothers have a disproportionate number of babies of low birth weight, which is associated with mental retardation and other handicapping conditions; 4) problems associated with pregnancy are particularly acute in mothers 15 and younger.[2]

We cannot consider this issue systematically without placing it within a broader social context. The so-called teenage sexual revolution is related to a number of concurrent trends. For example, there is an increased number and proportion of births to women under age 20. One-third of all births are to girls 17 or younger. About two-fifths of these births (about 200,000) were born out-of-wedlock. Thus, we shall consider out-of-wedlock births jointly with the problems associated with teenage or adolescent pregnancy.

There is no question that teenage out-of-wedlock birthrates have been increasing since 1940 for age 19 and younger. As Table 4-1 shows these rates in the 15 to 19 group in the United States increased from 8.3 in 1940 to 19.8 in 1968. Among nonwhite individuals the rates for girls age 14 increased between 1940 and 1950 but have been rather stable since then. Similarly, there are variations for both white and nonwhites in the period 1940 to 1968; the rate for nonwhites seems to be declining recently, but the rate for whites appears to have risen steadily since 1940. The fact that the teenage out-of-wedlock rate continues to increase is considered prima facie proof of increased sexual activity of revolutionary proportions. In a definitive study of the problem, however, Cutright casts doubt on this conclusion.[3]

There are alternative explanations for rising out-of-wedlock births than the simple one of a sexual revolution. In his analytical examination of this issue, Cutright suggests that the extent to which unmarried people are sexually active today may not have increased very much, after all. "Rather, recent health status changes may explain a great deal of the recent increase in teenage out-of-wedlock births, an increase which may be forcing society to acknowledge now what it has refused to acknowledge in the past: that such levels of teenage sexual activity do exist." He presents evidence concerning two such health status changes as possible causes of this phenomenon: those which affect the ability of young girls to conceive (fecundity) and those which affect their capacity to avoid spontaneous abortion.

In a series of analyses, Cutright undertakes to examine the interrelationships of customs, laws, and mean age of menarche. The data for menarche indicates that it has declined in the United States and western European populations. There is general agreement that one major factor responsible for the decline is improved nutrition and health during pre-adolescent years. Recent research suggests that improved nutrition increases the rate of physical growth, which in turn, decreases the age at menarche.

In short, Cutright demonstrates that previous low out-of-wedlock rates in this country, as well as in Sweden, could be explained by biologic factors, as well as social control factors depressing sexual activity. Problems generated by teenage sexuality have probably been with us for many years and society can no longer afford to ignore their existence. Society thus must begin to ask what it can do sensibly and realistically to solve problems that are a consequence of teenage sexuality.

Childbearing at any age is a momentous event for a woman. For the teenager, however, it is often accompanied by a different set of problems than those experienced by older mothers. As indicated above, for very young mothers, at least those under age 17, risks that the baby will be stillborn, or die soon after birth, or be born with a low birth weight, and so on are much higher than those for women in their twenties.

The relationship of infant mortality to maternal age has been noted earlier. In a recently published study matching infants' death certificates to infants' birth certificates, the National Center for Health Statistics reported that although the shape of the curves are similar, at all ages the infant mortality rate is considerably higher among nonwhites than among whites.[4] Moreover, neonatal mortality (in the period when biologic factors related to pregnancy are the primary determinants of survival) risks to infants of young mothers are much higher than those of infants of older mothers in both color groups.

The increased risk of low birth weight may be the most important medical aspect of teenage pregnancy. Increased mortality risk is only one of the dangers facing infants of low birth weight, as will be discussed more fully else-

where. There are apparent linkages to epilepsy, cerebral palsy and mental retardation, and to higher risks of deafness and blindness.

Various studies are not conclusive about the relationship of age of the mother to the intelligence of the child or physical and mental handicaps. Despite this inconclusiveness, these data document that the infant born to a teenage mother has a much higher risk of suffering severe handicaps than infants of somewhat older mothers.

Moreover, there are increased risks of complications of pregnancy for young mothers including toxemia, prolonged labor, and iron-deficiency anemia. Poor diets, inadequate prenatal care, and immaturity (both physical and emotional) are probably all contributing factors. The primary concern would appear to be with social rather than biologic factors.

The sequelae of early childbearing is of special concern to society. Research studies indicate that there is a tendency to have large and closely spaced families with their own set of biologic and social problems. Young mothers are more likely to be disadvantaged in the socioeconomic sense; the family is likely to be unstable.

What is the role of the nurse in prevention of early childbearing? Any action must start with the assumption that these are not inevitable consequences. Many women want to become mothers, but there are data to indicate that a substantial proportion wish that their first child had come later.[5] Moreover, many young women are poorly informed about the reproductive process. By the end of 1973, 43 states and the District of Columbia had affirmed the right of unmarried girls age 18 or older to consent to their own contraceptive care, and in 23 states and the District of Columbia, girls may consent at considerably younger ages, or with no age restriction.

Nurses can be particularly effective in coping with younger women. Concentration on the postpartum approach may be effective for prevention of future unwanted pregnancies, but it does nothing to prevent the initial unwanted pregnancy. Organized family planning programs could reach out to young people who have not yet had babies. If maternity nursing is to continue to expand its role it must participate in this process of outreach. Special teen clinics have been highly successful where they have been organized.[6] Self-help clinics may also be an important factor in the future in preventing early unintended motherhood.

We cannot close this discussion of early childbearing without recognition of the fact that knowledge, accessibility, and contraceptive technology are not the only problems. More than one study has documented that a substantial proportion of young mothers say that they had not used contraception because they did not care whether they became pregnant or not.[7] For some of these women, the motivation is simply not present for them to take advantage of the opportunities to control their fertility. Altering their motivation would be a major undertaking in society.

Socioeconomic and ethnic indicators of risk

In the preceding chapter we have discussed the concept of social class or socioeconomic status as it relates to health and health care. In this section we shall refer to three separate but highly correlated indicators of socioeconomic status—family income, education of father, and education of mother. The discrepancy in pregnancy outcome related to socioeconomic class becomes readily apparent when one analyzes the data which have accrued since 1935 on racial background. Throughout this period marked differences have occurred on the basis of racial background, with nonwhites faring much worse than whites. Indeed, the relative differential has actually risen during this period.

If the data on legitimate live births alone are examined for infant mortality, there are marked differences between white and black infants in the distributions by all three of the socioeconomic variables mentioned above. With respect to family income, for example, exactly one-half of the black but only one-sixth of the white births were in the lowest income category. Indeed, infant mortality rates were substantially higher for black than for white infants at all levels of the three variables of socioeconomic status.[4] Similar trends were observed for the white infants and for both sexes. The most recent government statistics on legitimate births revealed that there was a flattening of the trend of infant mortality in the lower-middle-socioeconomic-status group. Does this imply that, to the extent that infant mortality is preventable in this country, the medical and other resources available to persons with a high school education and/or reported family income levels of $6,000 to $9,000 have attained the minimal rates achievable with existing knowledge?

The racially related differentials in mortality have also been noted beyond the first year of life. It should be stressed that virtually all of the racially related differentials in mortality are socioeconomically associated. In numerous studies, low-income individuals, who are more likely to have early, frequent, and more numerous pregnancies extending into later life, are more likely to have premature deliveries with increased risk of perinatal mortality. Moreover, these individuals are more likely to have medical complications of pregnancy. When one approaches the complications of pregnancy data from a perspective of a spectrum of reproductive casualty, there appears to be a continuum between pregnancy complications and subsequent infant difficulty. Low income individuals are considerably more predisposed to have lowered health status and obstetrical complications during pregnancy. Low birth weight is particularly prevalent in the lowest socioeconomic status groups, especially the black population. Thus it is possible to observe an apparently important relationship to subsequent altered developmental prognosis.[8,9,10,11,12]

One of the most important sequelae of low socioeconomic status is undernutrition. Undernutrition has been identified as one of the causes of low birth weight in infants born to poor urban mothers.[13] (See Chapter 12.)

Recent studies have shown that deficiencies in the diet of a pregnant woman can have profound effects on a number of pregnancy outcomes. For example, it has been shown that nutritional and genetic factors may interact during prenatal development with consequent irreversible results which endure for the lifetime of the individual. Deficiencies in the diet of a pregnant woman can have profound effects on the development of her baby's brain and this is one of the most important recent discoveries in the field of mental retardation. It is estimated that one-tenth of the children born today are seriously affected as a consequence of malnutrition. Recent work at the National Institutes of Health suggests that there is a correlation between the level of the amino acids in the blood of a pregnant woman and the subsequent intelligence of her baby.

The effects of nutritional deficiencies on other outcomes of pregnancy are not so clear. Extremely low birth weights have been reported among poorly fed groups in Asia and

Africa. The relationship between low birth weight and malnourished populations may be more complex than a simple nutritional explanation. Rather than dietary deficiency in pregnancy as the major factor, the small size of the baby may reflect long-term maternal undernutrition dating back to the early childhood of the woman. Conceivably, malnutrition over many generations in the underdeveloped societies may have favored the emergence of genetically different kinds of women with lower dietary requirements. This, however, is highly speculative and needs much carefully designed research to confirm such a possibility.

Recent evidence on the geographic distribution of eclampsia has led Theobald to the "inescapable conclusion that the pregnancy toxemias were inextricably bound up with nutrition. Indeed, no adequate alternative explanation has been advanced." Eclampsia has largely been a condition associated with the very poor and particularly those in towns or urban places rather than rural places. However, this latter situation may be a result of differential diagnosis and the availability and the use of services in urban and rural areas among poverty populations. As a matter of fact, epidemiologic studies of the toxemias of pregnancy are problematical because of differential definition and diagnosis.[14]

The effect of socioenvironmental influences was most dramatically illustrated in World War II in Great Britain. During this period, the mortality from the pregnancy toxemias fell dramatically (Fig. 4-1). The underlying reason for the drop in mortality resulting from this condition in England and Wales, was that large numbers of women were evacuated from their homes in the cities into the country. The antenatal clinics were understaffed and improvisational. The major advantage brought about by this change of social environment was that the rationing system benefited expectant and nursing mothers and children. For the first time, women of the lower-socioeconomic groups were fed as well as other population groups and better than previously. Suffice to say that eclampsia as a syndrome is most commonly seen in poor and badly nourished populations and that there is some evidence that the incidence has been profoundly modified by environmental changes, either situational or behavioral.

The recently completed Ten-State National Nutrition Survey of the federal government revealed that, compared to the more affluent persons, the poor are twice as deficient in four essential diet ingredients. In general, the survey found a greater incidence of malnutrition among blacks than among whites, especially in the rural South, and among children and the elderly than among adults in their working years. Most strikingly, poor persons had about four times as much clear-cut iron deficiency anemia and twice as many borderline cases as had the nonpoor. In three categories of essential diet ingredients—vitamin A, vitamin C, and riboflavin—the poor were found to have about twice the incidence of clear-cut deficiency as the nonpoor. The survey also found a greater percentage of low height and weight measurements for children living below the poverty line than for those who were more affluent.[15]

Obviously, there is a complex interaction between under- or malnutrition, poverty, and other environmental or genetic factors. What can be done to improve the nutritional and other risk factors associated with socioeconomic status and ethnic or racial groups? Clearly, the role of the maternity or family nurse is relatively limited, but not inactive. The nurse can be a force both in the community and in the clinic setting to help improve preventive services to those at highest risk because of situational factors. Better ways can be devised to use the nurse and other health personnel to provide health education to the individuals at risk. This assumes that the nurse herself is equipped with the knowledge concerning nutrition and other precursors of problems of pregnancy to provide the appropriate knowledge to the patient. Moreover, the nurse

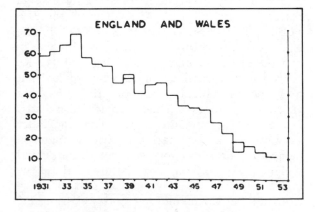

Figure 4-1. The mortality rates per 100,000 live births for eclampsia, preeclampsia, and nephritis. This dramatic fall occurred during World War II. (Theobald, G. W.: The pregnancy toxemias seen in perspective. *J. Reproductive Med.* 3:79, Aug. 1969)

can be a positive force in the community to exert influence on other institutions such as the schools, health departments, government agencies, and voluntary agencies to provide preventive measures to the population at greatest risk.

Behavioral risk factors

Up to now, the discussion has been concerned primarily with factors not easily controllable by the nurse or other health personnel. An individual's social position in society cannot be influenced easily by nursing interventions. In the present section, however, the risk factors of smoking and drug taking are mutable, and, hence, the nurse can have some degree of influence on the patient.

Smoking

Since the interesting paper by Campbell, smoking in pregnancy has received spasmodic but increasing attention.[16] Indeed, in recent years the literature has been growing substantially, reflecting a heightened awareness of the important and substantial effects of smoking on pregnancy outcome. The earlier studies demonstrated that mothers who smoked cigarettes had smaller babies than nonsmoking mothers. Most researchers subscribe to the view that the smaller babies born to smokers are smaller because of a direct effect of the smoking.

Recent evidence, based on prospective studies and other well-designed research has partly substantiated the fact that fetal size, growth, and mortality are related to smoking of cigarettes by the mother. According to the U.S. Public Health Service, some 4600 stillbirths each year in the United States probably can be attributed to women's smoking habits. Research indicates that women who smoked had a 30 percent higher rate of stillbirths than those who did not. These women also had a 26 percent higher rate of perinatal mortality.

A positive association between maternal cigarette smoking and reduced infant birth weight emerges from every study of these two characteristics. The hypothesis that the relationship between smoking and weight reduction in the infant is one of cause and effect is supported by several types of evidence. This relationship has been consistently observed in a wide variety of populations differing by geographic location, race, and social and economic circumstances. Furthermore, there is an inverse relationship between mean birth weights and the number of cigarettes smoked during pregnancy, an evident dose-response effect.

However, there have been a few studies that have not confirmed these findings. Since smoking is a preventable behavior, the focus of concern is to determine whether babies who would otherwise be alive and healthy might die, before or after birth, because their mothers smoked. In an excellent analysis, two epidemiologists have reviewed the problem and proposed suggestions for further work on perinatal mortality.[17] These investigators suggest that the few discrepancies between studies on the effects of smoking and perinatal mortality could be caused by bias in the selection of smokers and nonsmokers, by insufficient numbers to show a significant difference, or by true differences between populations in the effect of maternal smoking on the fetus.

Meyer and her colleagues examined the data from the Ontario Perinatal Mortality Study to look for interactions between maternal smoking and other factors affecting perinatal mortality that could explain why previous studies have not all agreed in their conclusions.[18] They found that perinatal mortality increased significantly with smoking, and was also affected by such factors as maternal age, parity, hospital status, previous pregnancy history, hemoglobin level, and the like. Smoking frequencies also varied by many of these characteristics. Perinatal mortality was analyzed by the amount of cigarettes smoked during pregnancy within subgroups of these antecedent risk factors. Thus, these investigators were able to undertake an analysis of the type not done previously in other studies. They found that in the Ontario population studied, mothers who are young, reasonably healthy, having their first or second child, and smoking less than a pack of cigarettes a day have an increased risk of perinatal loss of less than 10 percent. "At the other extreme, heavy smokers who are high parity, public patients, those who have had previous premature births or whose hemoglobin is under 11 Gm. have an increased risk of perinatal loss of over 70 percent. Other groups are intermediate . . . perinatal mortality increased with maternal smoking, with the magnitude of increase ranging from 4 percent to 97 percent."[18] Thus, their data suggests that maternal smoking may *interact* with other factors in its influence on perinatal mortality.

Meyer and her associates have examined further the contrary evidence from other studies and suggest that these studies were biased in terms of the populations analyzed. That is, they selected study populations that were, in one way or another, not typical of the general population and/or did not impose appropriate statistical controls on the study population. Thus, in conclusion, the weight of evidence indicates that maternal smoking during pregnancy increases the infant's perinatal mortality risk. This risk increases directly with the number of cigarettes smoked. The presence or absence of other risk factors alters the risk.

With such an approach the maternity care service is in a position to estimate the level of increased risk of smoking in a particular pregnancy, and to advise the mother accordingly. There is evidence that smoking depresses fetal growth by depressing caloric intake, reflected by lower maternal weight gain. Moreover, the bulk of research evidence demonstrates that women who stop smoking by the fourth month of pregnancy run no greater risk of incurring fetal loss than do nonsmokers. It thus appears that cigarette smoking, unlike maternal rubella and certain medications, is most dangerous in the last six months, when the central nervous system of the fetus is still forming.

Thus, the implications for prevention are clear. Counseling the patient at the first visit, particularly in the case of mothers with other risk factors, can be done by the maternity nurse. Health education, although it needs to begin early in life, must be an essential part of prenatal care and smoking is one behavior that is preventable. Moreover, the nurse by her own behavior, can provide an appropriate role model for the mother and father.

Drugs

Although there has been considerable interest in the potential genetic and teratogenic effects of a variety of foods and drugs, there needs to be more interest and published research in the maternity literature on the clinical problems of the drug addict. In recent years, the pregnant addict tends to be younger (i.e., the teen and *young* adult) than was evident earlier. Many of these patients will admit to use of drugs or else give some evidence of drug use. Detection of maternal addiction is based on history or physical evidence of administration, particularly puncture marks.

The true prevalence of drug-addicted mothers is unknown. But the indications are that, in large urban centers at least, the ratio of drug-addicted mothers to total deliveries has increased in the past 15 years. This is particularly true for those deliveries that take place in public hospitals.

Most drug-addicted patients are late comers for prenatal care. Indeed, most patients delay until they feel that they are ready for delivery in order to avoid a long labor without drugs and in order to satisfy their need for a last "fix" before submitting to "authority." As a result, there is evidence that a substantial proportion of deliveries to this population occurs at home, in the ambulance, or on the stretcher.[19] This is especially true of the heroin addict. Nevertheless, addicts make considerable efforts to nourish their addiction during enforced periods of confinement in a hospital. Such patients will either hide the drug or obtain it from others in or outside the hospital. A portion of these patients supplement with barbiturates or tranquilizers.

At least insofar as heroin addicts are concerned, there is some difficulty in evaluating the data on total length of labor, but available evidence indicates that labor is not prolonged. Greatest difficulties tend to occur after delivery when withdrawal in the infant and mother is a risk. Symptoms of withdrawal in the mother include nausea, tremors, sweats, abdominal pain, cramps, and yawnings (Chapter 29 discusses withdrawal symptoms in the infant).

The attitude of the medical and nursing staff becomes a critical factor at this stage. The pregnancy outcomes of these heroin-addicted mothers are typical of any nutritionally deprived groups of low-socioeconomic status receiving inadequate prenatal care, with one important exception, congenital addiction of the baby.

There is some suggestion in the literature that narcotic use by the mother may lead to intrauterine growth retardation. The long-term effects on growth and development are now being observed and evaluated in at least one prospective study. As of today, the effects of narcotic addiction on the reproductive process are not clearly reflected in our standard measures of maternal and perinatal mortality rates. Available evidence indicates that the addicted individual, even after withdrawal, detoxification, or rehabilitation remains at risk in that subsequent intake, even years later, may result in the immediate urge for more drugs.

Thus, a pregnant woman who is a user of narcotic drugs of unknown potency and amount, is carrying a potentially addicted fetus, and while detoxification of the newborn infant seems to be initially successful, a detoxified baby is still a problem infant. Even with use of methadone in the management of the pregnant addict, it is possible to magnify the effects on the fetus.

It is important to note that the problem of drug *usage* as distinct from drug addiction, is of considerable magnitude. Although the former is seen more often in private and community hospitals, the addictive patient is a growing problem also. It is increasingly apparent that our *drug-using* population is encompassing greater numbers of individuals from the middle- and upper-socioeconomic segments of our society, in addition to the poor. For these reasons, all maternal service personnel need to be familiar with both the maternal and neonatal aspects of drug use.

Life events and life crises as risks

As we noted in the beginning of this chapter, life events and life crises in the sense used here refer to such events as divorce, illness, death to a significant other, such as a family member, job loss, and the like, rather than to the occurrence of the actual pregnancy itself, although this too may be a factor in pregnancy outcome. Appropriate intervention by nursing staff can be especially effective in meeting the needs and reducing the risks associated with such life crises. The interest in the relationship between the psychologic and social world of the individual and human disorders and disease have a long history. But even the findings of carefully designed and conducted investigations have not always yielded clear-cut and unambiguous results concerning this relationship. This is in sharp contrast to the dramatic results which have been obtained with animal experiments where the various elements in the social environment have been correlated. Nevertheless, there is accumulating evidence of the intimate interaction between the social environment, physiologic reactions and pathologic outcome in the individual. This is particu-

larly true for certain of the chronic diseases such as those of heart and cancer.[20]

With regard to the relationship between disorders of pregnancy and life changes and experiences that may be stressful, the data are relatively scanty. In fact, most of the literature is concerned with the relationship of emotions, psychologic feeling, and attitudes toward the pregnancy and the resulting outcome of pregnancy. This literature and its implications for maternity nursing will be discussed later in this section.

It should be clear that an outcome such as low birth weight is the result of multiple interactions between the human organism and the environment. In a paper published in 1963, Gunter focused on the psychologic and stressful environmental factors operative in the mother *before* conception and during pregnancy. Almost ten years elapsed before another study appeared that was related to the Gunter study, although the importance of the variables had long been recognized and applied in research directed toward other problems.[21] The emphasis in Gunter's research was on critical life events that occurred *before* the onset of pregnancy. Thus, Gunter used a life chart developed by earlier psychologic investigators in medical science, that described such life stressors as: 1) Death within the immediate family of orientation or procreation; 2) desertion by husband or by one or both parents of the subject; 3) economic need; 4) interpersonal problems such as difficulties with husband (including divorce), difficulties with in-laws, family, or neighbors; and 5) physical disability including illness, accident, and bodily harm incidents related to the subject or immediate family. She also had obtained data on events that occurred *during* the gestation period.

Although Gunter found that the "social and life situation of the mother are related to and may, in part, determine the outcome of pregnancy in terms of the birth weight of the infant," the results of her study are perhaps of less importance than the fact that it was not followed up by other investigators until the work of Nuckolls and her associates at North Carolina.[22]

The approach of Nuckolls and her colleagues went beyond an attempt to assess the effects of life experiences on pregnancy outcome. They included, in addition, the supportive or protective psychologic or social elements of the patient, which was termed the adaptive potential for pregnancy (TAPPS). This group of investigators followed the lead of Holmes and his associates in identifying a "stressful" situation through the concept of the magnitude and importance of life changes.[23] In short, Nuckolls and her group were attempting to assess the "balance" between the protective and the deleterious social and psychologic processes and the relationship of this balance to various health parameters of pregnancy and the puerperium.

It is worth noting that other investigators who have examined the relationship of psychosocial factors to pregnancy outcome have focused on either discrete complications or on a total complication score for the whole childbearing episode. The North Carolina group defined the outcome of pregnancy result to be measured as any untoward condition or outcome not related to an anatomical or other known maternal defect.

The results showed that considering the multiple life changes and the psychosocial assets separately, they were not related to complications of pregnancy. When taken together, however, Nuckolls found that in the presence of mounting life change, women with high psychosocial assets had only one-third the complication rate of women whose psychosocial assets were low. In the absence of such life changes, particularly for the period before pregnancy, the level of psychosocial assets was irrelevant.

As these investigators point out, additional research is needed, but their data help to explain some of the discrepant results in the literature. However, in addition to the deficits of life crises, it appears necessary to consider the social supports available to the individual. Moreover, their study lends further support to a theoretical approach that emphasizes general susceptibility to a variety of insults.[24] In short, the research and the approach casts serious doubt on the utility of specificity (as far as current clinical syndromes are concerned) in research concerned with psychosocial factors in disease etiology. Similar psychosocial factors may be related to different disease syndromes. At the present, this research approach is very promising and additional work needs to be done using the approach.

Much has been written in recent years on the role of emotional and attitudinal factors and psychologic stress *during* the pregnancy as these may be related to pregnancy outcomes. The evidence is inconclusive, but more importantly, much of it is based on poorly designed research and inadequate samples of the population-at-risk. Despite this poor state of affairs, there is a general consensus in medical science that psychologic factors are in some way associated with various aspects of the maternity cycle. Indeed, some investigators have asserted that early psychologic assessment of pregnant women holds promise of being predictive of the course and outcome of pregnancy. Most of the literature makes an attempt to measure the attitudes of the woman toward her pregnancy and attempts to measure other psychosocial factors as these may influence the outcome.[25]

Surely there are attitudinal differences among women toward their individual pregnancies. Moreover, findings such as Heinstien's that moodiness, feelings of dullness and indifference, crying easily, and the like, and their association with a "more significant degree of physical complications" may legitimately be suggestive of a relationship to organically stimulated hormonal reactions. There is an intimate interaction between the psychologic stress experienced by the person and physiologic reactions, as Heinstien noted. Complications of pregnancy, labor, and delivery are obscured by this interaction. Thus, physiologic changes and discomfort may trigger psychologically negative attitudes toward the pregnancy and, conversely, life stress may precipitate somatic problems.

There is no doubt that many, perhaps a majority, of women experience some psychologic stress and anxiety during pregnancy. The literature in medical and nursing journals alike tends *to assume* some of these conditions as psychosomatic or emotional in origin. In a paper critical of the cloudy thinking that has characterized such conditions as menstrual pain, nausea of pregnancy, and pain in labor, as caused or aggravated by psychogenic factors, Lennane and Lennane suggest sexual prejudice as the basis for such thinking. Such scientific evidence as exists clearly suggests organic causes for these conditions.[26] The point here is that nurses must not unwittingly and uncritically accept long-established attitudes that are rooted in prejudice rather than in scientific evidence. Stereotypic thinking is not only poor in scientific terms, but, equally important, it tends to influence the course and quality of treatment of women patients.

Nursing staff has a critically important role to play in assisting the pregnant woman to utilize her psychosocial assets to the fullest in coping with the fears, anxieties, somatic complaints, and other problems associated with the pregnancy in the prenatal and hospitalization periods. Emotional and social support during and following the pregnancy can not only be a comfort to the patient, but may also assist in reducing problematic outcomes.

Bibliography

1. Biggs, J. S.: Pregnancy at 40 years and over. *Med. J. Australia* 54:2-5, Mar. 17, 1973.
2. Lesser, A.: Progress in maternal and child health. *Child. Today* 1:7-12, Mar./Apr. 1972.
3. Cutright, P.: Illegitimacy in the United States: 1920-1968. Final Report to the Commission on Population Growth and the American Future. Washington, D.C., U.S. Government Printing Office, 1972.
4. Infant Mortality Rates: Socioeconomic Factors, United States. Series 22, No. 14, Vital and Health Statistics. Washington, D.C., Department of Health, Education and Welfare, 1972.
5. Presser, H.: Early motherhood: ignorance or bliss. *Fam. Plan. Perspect.* 6, 1:8-14, Winter 1974.
6. House, E. A., and Goldsmith, S.: Planned parenthood services for the young teenager. *Fam. Plan. Perspect.* 4, 2:27, 1972.
7. Lindemann, C.: *Birth Control and Unmarried Young Women.* New York, Springer, 1974.
8. Lilienfeld, A. M., and Pasamanick, B.: The association of maternal and fetal factors with the development of cerebral palsy and epilepsy. *Am. J. Ob.-Gyn.* 70:93, 1955.
9. Niswander, K. R., and Gordon, M.: *The Collaborative Perinatal Study of the National Institute of Neurological Diseases and Stroke—The Women and Their Pregnancies.* Philadelphia, W. B. Saunders, 1972.
10. Pasamanick, B., and Knobloch, H.: Brain damage and reproductive casualty. *Am. J. Orthopsychiatry* 30:298, 1960.
11. Pasamanick, B., and Lilienfeld, A. M.: Association of maternal and fetal factors with the development of mental deficiency, I. Abnormalities in the prenatal and paranatal periods. *JAMA* 159:155, 1955.
12. Pasamanick, B., Knobloch, H., and Lilienfeld, A. M.: Socioeconomic status and some precursors of neuropsychiatric disorders. *Am. J. Orthopsychiatry* 26:594, 1956.
13. Naeye, R. L., *et al*: Urban poverty: effects on prenatal nutrition. *Science* 166:1026, Nov. 21, 1969.
14. Theobald, G. W.: The pregnancy toxemias seen in perspective. *J. Reproductive Med.* 3:79, Aug. 1969.
15. Ten-State Nutrition Survey in the United States, 1968-1970. Washington, D.C., Department of Health, Education and Welfare, Pub. No. (HSM) 72-8129 through 72-8134, 1972.
16. Campbell, A. M.: The effects of excessive cigarette smoking on maternal health. *Am. J. Ob.-Gyn.* 31:502-508, 1936.
17. Meyer, M. B., and Comstock, G. W.: Maternal cigarette smoking and perinatal mortality. *Am. J. Epidemiology* 96:1-10, July 1972.
18. Meyer, M. B., *et al*: The interrelationship of maternal smoking and increased perinatal mortality with other risk factors: further analysis of the Ontario perinatal mortality study, 1960-1961. *Am. J. Epidemiology* 100:443-452, Dec. 1974.
19. Stone, M. L., *et al*: Narcotic addiction in pregnancy. *Am. J. Ob.-Gyn.* 109:716-723, Mar. 1971.
20. Syme, S. L., and Reeder, L. G., eds.: Social stress and cardiovascular disease. *The Milbank Memorial Fund Quarterly* Apr. 1967.
21. Gunter, L. M.: Psychopathology and stress in the life experience of mothers of premature infants. *Am. J. Ob.-Gyn.* 86:333-340, June 1963.
22. Nuckolls, K. B., *et al*: Psychosocial assets, life crisis and the prognosis of pregnancy. *Am. J. of Epidemiology* 95:431-441, 1972.
23. Holmes, T. H., and Masuda, M.: 1974, Life Change and Illness Susceptibility. *In* Dohrenwend, B. S., and Dohrenwend, B. P. (eds.), *Stressful Life Events: Their Nature and Effects.* New York, John Wiley & Sons.
24. Thurlow, H. J.: General susceptibility to illness: a selective review. *Canad. Med. Assoc. J.* 97:1397, 1967.
25. Heinstien, M. I.: Expressed attitudes and feelings of pregnant women and their relations to physical complications of pregnancy. *Merril-Palmer Quarterly* 1:217-236, Jan. 1967.
26. Lennane, K. J., and Lennane, R. J.: Alleged psychogenic disorders in women—a possible manifestation of sexual prejudice. *New Eng. J. Med.* 288, 6:288-292, Feb. 8, 1973.

human
reproduction

Anatomy Related to the Reproductive System
Maternal Physiology in Relation to
Human Reproduction
Conception and Ovum Development
Development and Physiology of the
Embryo and Fetus
Clinical Aspects of Human Reproduction

unit **II**

anatomy related to the reproductive system

Pelvis

The pelvis, so called from its resemblance to a basin (*pelvis*, a basin), is a bony ring interposed between the trunk and the thighs. The vertebral column, or backbone, passes into it from above, transmitting to it the weight of the upper part of the body, which the pelvis in turn transmits to the lower limbs. From an obstetric point of view, however, we must consider it as the cavity which contains the generative organs, and particularly as the canal through which the baby must pass during birth.

Structure

The pelvis is made up of four united bones: the two hipbones (*os coxae* or innominate) situated laterally and in front, and the sacrum and the coccyx behind (Figs. 5-1 to 5-3). Anatomically, the hipbones are divided into three parts: the ilium, the ischium, and the pubis. These bones become firmly joined into one by the time the growth of the body is completed (i.e., at about ages 20 to 25), so that on examining them in the prepared pelvis no trace of the original edges or divisions of these three bones

can be discovered. Each of these bones may be roughly described as follows.

The *ilium*, which is the largest portion of the bones, forms the upper and back part of the pelvis. Its upper flaring border forms the prominence of the hip, or crest of the ilium (hipbone). The *ischium* is the lower part below the hip joint; from it projects the tuberosity of

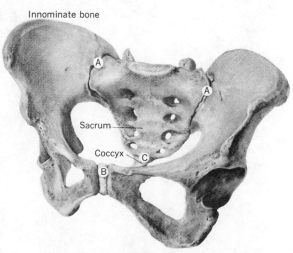

Figure 5-1. Pelvis. (A) Sacroiliac articulations. (B) Symphysis pubis. (C) Sacrococcygeal articulation.

65

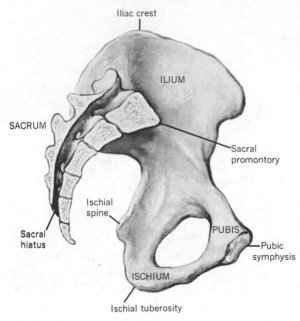

Figure 5-2. Lateral view of left innominate bone showing its three constituent parts (erect position).

ward the ischial tuberosity, thus forming with the bone of the opposite side the arch below the symphysis, the pubic or subpubic arch. This articulation closes anteriorly the cavity of the pelvis.

The *sacrum* and the *coccyx* form the lowest portions of the spinal column. The former is a triangular wedge-shaped bone, consisting of five vertebrae fused together; it serves as the back part of the pelvis. The coccyx forms a tail end to the spine. In the child the coccyx consists of four or five very small, separate vertebrae; in the adult these bones are fused into one. The coccyx is usually movable at its attachment to the sacrum, the sacrococcygeal joint, and may become pressed back during labor to give more room for the passage of the fetal head.

Of special importance is the marked projection which is formed by the junction of the last lumbar vertebra with the sacrum; this is known as the *sacral promontory* and is one of the most important landmarks in obstetric anatomy.

Articulation and surfaces

The *articulations*, or joints of the pelvis, which possess obstetric importance, are four in number. Two are behind, between the sacrum

the ischium on which the body rests when in a sitting posture. The *pubis* is the front part of the hipbone; it extends from the hip joint to the joint in front between the two hipbones, the symphysis pubis, and then turns down to-

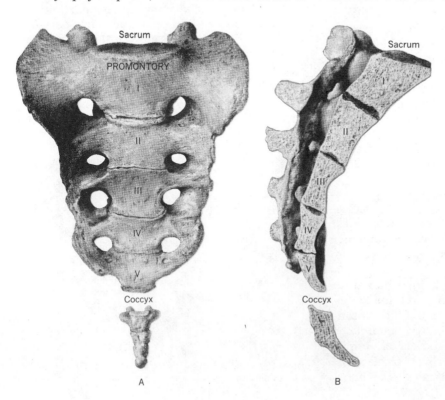

Figure 5-3. Sacrum and coccyx. (A) Front view. (B) Median section. Note how promontory of sacrum juts forward.

and the ilia on either side, and are termed the *sacroiliac articulations* (Fig. 5-1 A); one is in front between the two pubic bones and is called the *symphysis pubis* (Fig. 5-1 B), and the fourth, of little consequence, is between the sacrum and coccyx, the *sacrococcygeal articulation* (Fig. 5-1 C).

All of these articular surfaces are lined with fibrocartilage, which becomes thickened and softened during pregnancy; likewise, the ligaments which bind the pelvic joints together become softened, and as a result greater mobility of the pelvic bones develops. A certain definite though very limited motion in the joints is desirable for a normal labor; however, there is no change in the actual size of the pelvis. From a practical standpoint, one of the most important facts for the nurse to know about these joints is that the increased mobility which they develop in pregnancy produces a slight "wobbliness" in the pelvis and throws greater strain on the surrounding muscles and ligaments. This accounts in large part for the frequency of backache and legache in the latter months of pregnancy.

The pelvis is lined with muscular tissue which provides a smooth, somewhat cushioned surface over which the fetus has to pass during labor; these muscles also help to support the abdominal contents.

Divisions

Regarded as a whole, the pelvis may be described as a two-storied, bony basin that is divided by a natural line of division, the *inlet* or *brim*, into two parts. The upper part is called the false pelvis and the lower part is called the true pelvis (Fig. 5-4).

The *false pelvis*, or upper flaring part, is much less concerned with the problems of labor than is the true pelvis. It supports the uterus during late pregnancy and directs

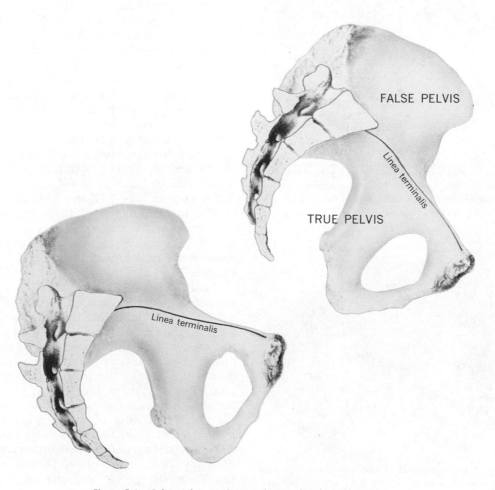

FALSE PELVIS

Linea terminalis

TRUE PELVIS

Linea terminalis

Figure 5-4.   False and true pelves, sagittal section, in erect position.

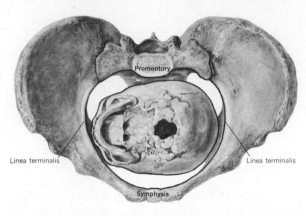

Figure 5-5. Largest diameter of baby's head entering largest diameter of inlet (as viewed from above). Therefore it enters transversely.

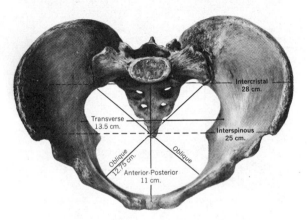

Figure 5-6. Measurements of the inlet of a normal female pelvis, showing the four diameters: the anteroposterior, the transverse, and the two oblique diameters. Broken lines indicate transverse measurements of the false pelvis.

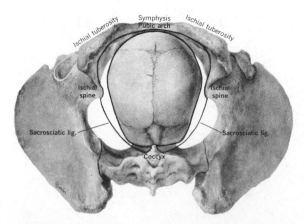

Figure 5-7. Largest diameter of baby's head passing through largest diameter of outlet (as viewed from below). Therefore it passes through outlet anteroposteriorly.

the fetus into the true pelvis at the proper time.

The *true pelvis,* or lower part, forms the bony canal through which the baby must pass during parturition; for convenience in description it is divided into three parts: an inlet or brim, a cavity and an outlet.

PELVIC INLET. Continuous with the sacral promontory and extending along the ilium on each side in circular fashion is a ridge called the *linea terminalis,* or brim (Fig. 5-4). This bounds an area or plane, the *inlet,* so named because it is the entryway or inlet through which the baby's head must pass in order to enter the true pelvis. The pelvic inlet, sometimes called the pelvic brim or superior strait, divides the false from the true pelvis. It is roughly heart-shaped, the promontory of the sacrum forming a slight projection into it from behind (Fig. 5-5). Generally it is widest from side to side, and narrowest from back to front (i.e., from the sacral promontory to the symphysis). It should be noted that the baby's head enters the inlet of the average pelvis with its longest diameter (anteroposterior) in the transverse diameter of the pelvis. In other words, as shown in Figure 5-5, the greatest diameter of the head accommodates itself to the greatest diameter of the inlet. As the inlet is entirely surrounded by bone, it cannot be measured directly with the examining fingers in a living woman. However, the measurements of its anteroposterior diameter can be estimated on the basis of the diagonal conjugate diameter (see Figs. 5-12 and 5-13, pp. 71 to 72).

The measurements of these diameters are very important, since variations from the normal (e.g., smaller in size or flattened) may cause grave difficulty at the time of labor (see Chapter 25.)

PELVIC OUTLET. When viewed from below, the *pelvic outlet* is a space bounded in front by the symphysis pubis and the pubic arch, at the sides by the ischial tuberosities, and behind by the coccyx and the greater sacrosciatic ligaments (Fig. 5-6). It requires only a little imagination to see that the front half of the outlet resembles a triangle, the base of which is the distance between the ischial tuberosities, and the other two sides of which are represented by the pubic arch. From an obstetric point of view, this triangle is of great importance, since the baby's head must utilize this space to gain exit from the pelvis and the mother's body (Fig. 5-6). For this reason Nature has provided a wide pubic arch in females, whereas in males it is narrow (see Fig. 5-11, p. 70). If the pubic arch in women were as narrow as it is in men, natural childbearing would be extremely difficult, since the baby's head, unable to squeeze itself into the narrow anterior triangle of the outlet, would be forced backward against the coccyx and the sacrum, where its progress would be impeded.

In the typical female pelvis, the greatest diameter of the inlet is the transverse (from side to side), whereas the greatest diameter of the outlet is the anteroposterior (from front to back) (Fig. 5-7 and 5-8). Moreover, the baby's head, as it emerges from the pelvis, passes through the outlet in the anteroposterior position, again accommodating its greatest diameter to the greatest diameter of the passage. Since the baby's head enters the pelvis in the transverse position and emerges in the anteroposterior, it is obvious that the head must rotate some 90° as it passes through the pelvis. This process of rotation is one of the most important phases of the mechanism of labor and will be discussed in more detail later (see Chapter 15.)

PELVIC CAVITY. The *pelvic cavity* is the space between the inlet above, the outlet below and the anterior, the posterior, and the lateral walls of the pelvis. The pelvic canal is practically cylindric in shape in its upper portion and curved only in its lower half. It is important to note the axis of the cavity when viewed from the side (Fig. 5-9). It is apparent that during the delivery the head must descend along the downward prolongation of the axis until it nearly reaches the level of the ischial spines and then begins to curve forward. The axis of the cavity determines the direction which the baby takes through the pelvis in the process of delivery. As might be expected, labor is made more complicated by this curvature in the pelvic canal, because the baby has to accommodate itself to the curved path as well as to the variations in the size of the cavity at different levels.

Pelvic variations

The pelvis presents great individual variations—no two pelves are exactly alike. Even patients with normal measurements may present differences in contour and muscular development which influence the actual size of the pelvis. These differences are due in part to heredity, disease, injury, and development.

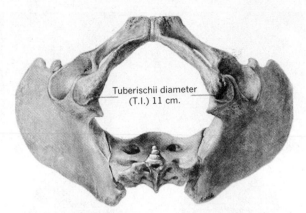

Figure 5-8. Measurement of the outlet, showing transverse diameter in a normal female pelvis.

Heredity may be responsible for passing on many racial and sexual differences. Such diseases as tuberculosis and rickets cause malformations. Accidents and injuries during childhood or at maturity result in deformities of the pelvis or other parts of the body which affect the pelvis. Adequate nutrition and well-formed habits related to posture and exercise have a very definite influence on the development of the pelvis.

It must be remembered also that the pelvis does not mature until between the ages of 20 and 25 years, and that until then complete ossification has not taken place.

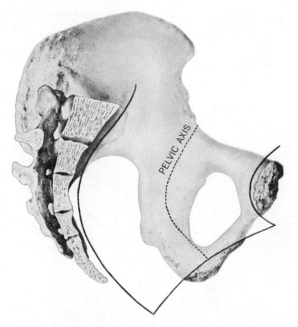

Figure 5-9. Pelvic cavity. Solid line indicates location of soft parts, vagina, and so on.

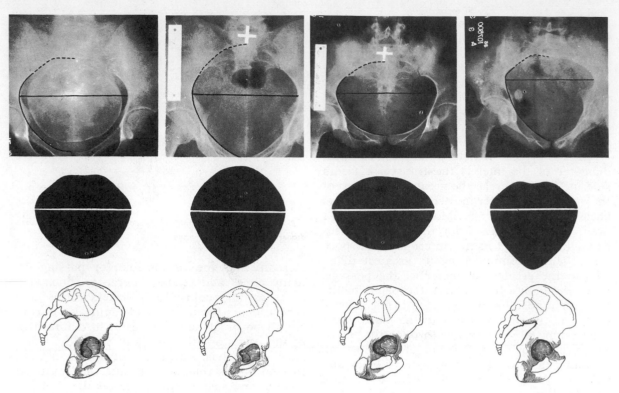

Figure 5-10. (*Left*) Gynecoid (normal female) pelvis. Inlet is well rounded in hind- and fore-pelvis. Sacrosciatic notch is curved, moderate in width and depth. (*Left center*) Anthropoid pelvis. Inlet is deep in hind- and fore-pelvis, increased in anteroposterior diameter. Sacrosciatic notch is broad and shallow. (*Right center*) Platypelloid pelvis. Inlet is a transverse oval, well curved but decreased in anteroposterior diameter. Sacrosciatic notch is curved and small. (*Right*) Android pelvis. Inlet is wedge-shaped with shallow hind-pelvis and pointed fore-pelvis. Sacrosciatic notch is narrow, deep, and pointed. (Roentgenograms from W. E. Caldwell, M.D., and H. C. Moloy, M.D., Sloane Hospital for Women, New York)

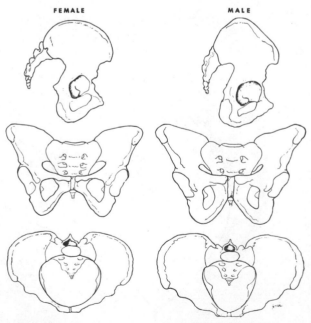

Figure 5-11. Contrast in female and male pelvis, lateral, front, and inlet views.

There are many so-called borderline cases of abnormal pelvic development. Such pregnant patients should be supervised closely. At periodic intervals the size of the fetus is estimated (by palpation of the abdomen), and definite arrangements are made for the type of delivery indicated.

There are several *types of pelves*. Even pelves whose measurements are normal differ greatly in the shape of the inlet, in the proximity of the greatest transverse diameter of the inlet to the sacral promontory, in the size of the sacrosciatic notch, and in their general architecture. These characteristics have been used in establishing a classification of pelves which has been of great interest and value to obstetricians. The four main types according to this classification are shown in Figure 5-10. The manner in which the baby passes through the birth canal and, consequently, the type of labor vary considerably in these pelvic types.

In addition, of course, there are many pelvic types which result from abnormal narrowing of one or the other diameters. These contracted pelves will be described in Chapter 25.

In comparing the male and the female pelves, several differences will be observed (Fig. 5-11). The most conspicuous difference is in the pubic arch, which has a much wider angle in women. The symphysis is shorter in women, and the border of the arch probably is more everted. Although the female pelvis is more shallow, it is more capacious, much lighter in structure, and smoother. The male pelvis is deep, compact, conical, and rougher in texture, particularly at the site of muscle attachments. Both males and females start life with pelves which are identical in type; the major differences observed in adult male and female pelves do not appear until puberty and are therefore due to the influence of the sex hormones. (For the definition and description of the sex hormones, see Chapter 6.)

Pelvic measurements

IMPORTANCE OF PELVIC MEASUREMENTS. The entire problem in childbirth centers on the safe passage of the fully developed fetus through the pelvis of the mother. Slight irregularities in the structure of the pelvis may delay the progress of labor, while any marked deformity may render the delivery by the natural passages impossible. For these reasons, the pelvis of every pregnant woman should be measured accurately in the antepartal period to determine before labor begins whether or not there is anything in the condition of the mother's pelvis that may complicate the delivery. This examination is a part of the antepartal examination. In addition to a general physical examination, the pelvic measurements are made and compared with the dimensions of the normal pelvis.

TYPES OF PELVIC MEASUREMENTS. Internal pelvic measurements, made manually, are an important means of estimating the size of the pelvis. In the past, a number of external pelvic measurements were recorded. Since these are generally of dubious value in evaluating the true pelvis, they are no longer utilized. In the majority of abnormal pelves, the most marked deformity affects the anteroposterior diameter of the inlet. In occasional instances, however, x-ray pelvimetry may be desirable (see pp. 73 to 75).

The internal pelvic measurements are made to determine the actual diameters of the inlet. The chief internal measurement taken is the

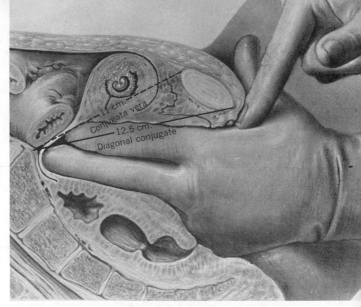

Figure 5-12. Method of obtaining diagonal conjugate diameter (solid line). The broken line represents the conjugata vera.

diagonal conjugate, or the distance between the sacral promontory and the lower margin of the symphysis pubis. The patient should be placed on her back on the examining table, with her knees drawn up and her feet supported by stirrups. Two fingers are introduced into the vagina, and, before measuring the diagonal conjugate, some evaluation of the pelvis is made by palpation: the height of the symphysis pubis and the shape of the pubic arch, the motility of the coccyx, the inclination of the anterior wall of the sacrum and the side walls of the pelvis, and the prominence of the ischial spines.

To obtain the length of the diagonal conjugate, the two fingers passed into the vagina are pressed inward and upward as far as possible until the middle finger rests on the sacral promontory. The point on the back of the hand just under the symphysis is then marked by putting the index finger of the other hand on the exact point (Fig. 5-12), after which the fingers are withdrawn and measured. The distance from the tip of the middle finger to the point marked represents the *diagonal conjugate measurement.* This distance may be measured with a rigid measuring scale attached to the wall or with a pelvimeter, but the former is preferred because there is less chance of error (Fig. 5-13). If the measurement is greater than 11.5 cm., it is justifiable to assume that the pelvic inlet is of adequate size for childbirth. In common medical parlance this measure-

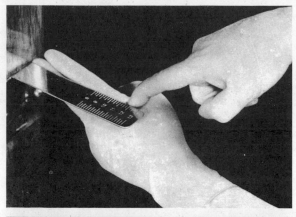

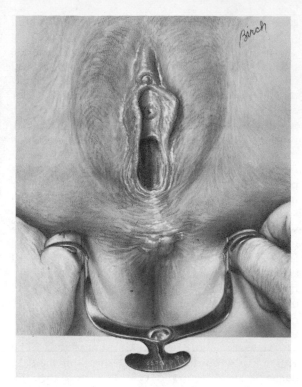

Figure 5-14. Method of measuring tuberischii, or intertuberous, diameter of outlet, using the Williams's pelvimeter. The measurement is made on a line with the lower border of the anus.

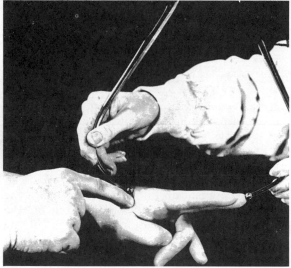

Figure 5-13. Methods of measuring diagonal conjugate diameter. (Top) Wall bracket. (Bottom) Pelvimeter.

ment is often called the "C.D." (conjugata diagonalis).

An extremely important internal diameter is the *true conjugate* or, in Latin, the conjugata vera (C.V.), which is the distance between the posterior aspect of the symphysis pubis and the promontory of the sacrum. However, direct measurement of this diameter cannot be made except by means of a roentgenogram; consequently, it has to be estimated from the diagonal conjugate measurement. It is believed that if 1.5 to 2 cm., according to the height and the inclination of the symphysis pubis, is deducted from the length of the diagonal conjugate, the true conjugate is obtained. For example, if the diagonal conjugate measures 12.5 cm., and the symphysis pubis is considered to be "average," then the conjugata vera may be estimated as

being about 11.0 cm. In this method, the problem consists of estimating the length of one side of a triangle, the conjugata vera; the other two sides, the diagonal conjugate and the height of the symphysis pubis, are known. If the symphysis pubis is high and has a marked inclination, the physician takes this into consideration and may deduct 2 cm. The length of the conjugata vera is of utmost importance, since it is about the smallest diameter of the inlet through which the baby's head must pass. Indeed, the main purpose in measuring the diagonal conjugate is to give an estimate of the size of the conjugata vera.

Students sometimes are confused when they are confronted with the term *obstetric conjugate*. This term identifies a diameter which begins at the sacral promontory and terminates just below the conjugata vera on the inner surface of the symphysis pubis a few millimeters below its upper margin (see Fig. 5-12). The obstetric conjugate is in reality the shortest diameter through which the infant's head must pass as it descends into the true pelvis. A distinction is rarely made between the conjugata vera and the obstetric conjugate, except in x-ray pelvimetry (see below).

Next to the diagonal conjugate measurement, the most important clinical dimension of the pelvis is the transverse diameter of the outlet, the diameter between the ischial tuberosities. This is sometimes called the *tuberischii diameter* (often abbreviated T.I.), or biischial diameter, or intertuberous diameter (see Fig. 5-8, p. 69). This measurement is taken with the patient in the lithotomy position, well down on the table and with the legs widely separated. The measurement is taken from the innermost and lowermost aspect of the ischial tuberosities, on a level with the lower border of the anus. The instruments usually employed are the Williams's pelvimeter (Figs. 5-14 and 5-15) or the Thoms's pelvimeter. The intertuberous diameter may also be estimated by inserting the closed fist between the tuberosities. The known diameter of the hand can then be used as a reference. A diameter in excess of 8 cm. is considered adequate.

X-ray pelvimetry

The most accurate means of determining pelvic size is x-ray pelvimetry. This subjects the maternal ovaries and the fetal gonads to a certain amount of irradiation. Although the amount involved is minimal, exposure of pregnant women to irradiation should be avoided unless this procedure is really necessary. Hence, x-ray pelvimetry is used prior to labor only in cases in which there are sound reasons for suspecting pelvic contraction, such as small manual measurements or a history of difficult labor in the past.

Pelvimetry is also indicated when there has been failure to progress normally in labor, to rule out previously unsuspected cephalopelvic disproportion. It is also important to evaluate pelvic size in term breech presentations, since the head is the largest part of the fetus and the adequacy of the pelvis is not really tested until the body has already been delivered. For this reason, many physicians evaluate pelvic size with pelvimetry routinely in the primigravida at term with a breech presentation.

A variety of techniques have been developed. One which has stood the test of time, with minor modifications, is that devised by Dr. Herbert Thoms, a pioneer in this field. For a complete study, two roentgenograms are made as follows:

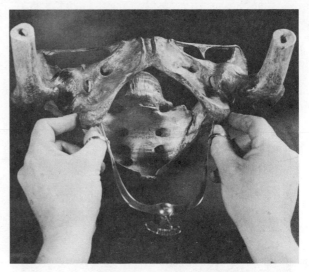

Figure 5-15. Tuberischii, or intertuberous, diameter measured on bony pelvis.

1. The patient is placed on the x-ray table in a semirecumbent position so that her pelvic inlet is horizontal and as nearly parallel as possible with the plate beneath her (Fig. 5-16). The exact plane in which the patient's

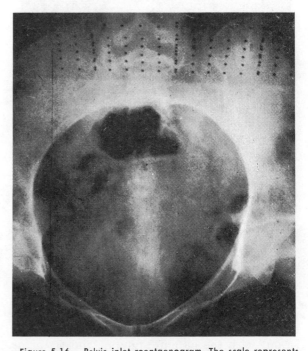

Figure 5-16. Pelvic inlet roentgenogram. The scale represents corrected centimeters for various levels of the pelvic canal. The top line is used for measuring the diameters of the inlet. The other levels are established on the lateral roentgenogram. Pelvic morphology is readily established by viewing both lateral and inlet views. Thoms's technique.

anatomy related to the reproductive system   73

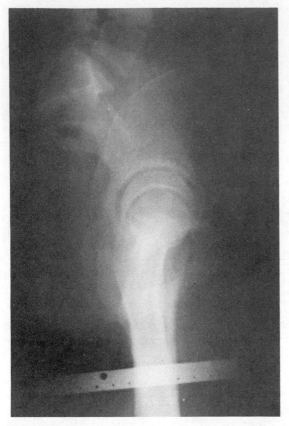

Figure 5-17. Lateral roentgenogram. The scale represents corrected centimeters in the midplane of the body. The various diameters may be measured with calipers. The lateral morphologic aspects are readily visualized.

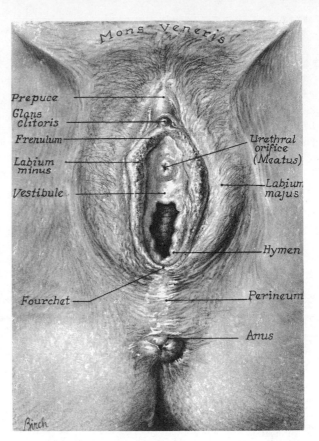

Figure 5-18. External organs of reproduction.

inlet lies, both front and back, is now determined and recorded. After an exposure of the film has been made, the patient is removed from the table, and a lead plate or grid containing perforations a centimeter apart is placed in the plane previously occupied by the inlet of the patient. Another exposure is now made on the same film. When the latter is developed, the outline of the inlet is shown, as are the dots produced by the perforations in the lead plate. Since the projected dots on the film represent centimeters in the plane of the inlet, the diameters of the inlet can be read off directly as centimeters.

2. A somewhat similar procedure is carried out with the patient standing and from the lateral view (Fig. 5-17). Here, however, an upright lead and iron rod, with a centimeter scale notched on its edge, is placed posterior to the patient and close to the gluteal fold. After an exposure has been made, the

developed film will show a lateral view of the symphysis pubis, the sacral promontory, other bony landmarks, as well as, of course, the notched centimeter scale for establishing the distance between important points. Diameters which may be measured by x-ray pelvimetry are the obstetric conjugate, posterior sagittal at the inlet, midpelvis and outlet, and the anteroposterior diameter at the midpelvis and outlet.

Other techniques entail the use of stereoscopic procedures which allow the physician to view the films with three-dimensional vision and thus gain a clear image of all pelvic relationships.

When roentgenograms are made late in pregnancy by any of these methods, it is possible to secure also an impression of the size of the baby's head. When this is considered in relation to the pelvic picture, helpful information may be obtained in forecasting whether or not this particular pelvis is large enough to allow this particular baby to pass through.

PREVENTIVE CARE BASED ON PELVIMETRY. The importance of the knowledge gained through skillful performance of internal pelvimetry cannot be overestimated. Especially it should never be neglected in the case of a woman pregnant for the first time, or in any case in which the patient has suffered previously from difficult or tedious labors.

Female organs of reproduction

The female organs of reproduction are divided into two groups—the external and the internal (Figs. 5-18 to 5-23).

External organs

The external female reproductive organs are called the *vulva,* from the Latin word meaning *covering.* This includes everything which is visible externally from the lower margin of the pubis to the perineum, namely, the mons veneris, the labia majora and minora, the clitoris, the vestibule, the hymen, the urethral opening and various glandular and vascular structures (Fig. 5-18). The term vulva often has been used to refer simply to the labia majora and minora.

The *mons veneris* is a firm, cushionlike formation over the symphysis pubis and is covered with crinkly hair.

The *labia majora* are two prominent longitudinal folds of adipose tissue covered with skin which extend downward and backward from the mons veneris and disappear in forming the anterior border of the perineal body. These two thick folds of skin are covered with hair on their outer surfaces after the age of puberty, but are smooth and moist on their inner surfaces. At the bottom they fade away into the perineum posteriorly, joining together to form a transverse fold, the posterior commissure, situated directly in front of the fourchet. This fatty tissue is supplied with an abundant plexus of veins which may rupture as the result of injury sustained during labor and give rise to an extravasation of blood, or hematoma.

The *labia minora* are two thin folds of reddish tissue covered entirely with thin membrane and situated between the labia majora, with their outer surfaces in contact with the inner surfaces of the labia majora; the labia minora extend from the clitoris downward and

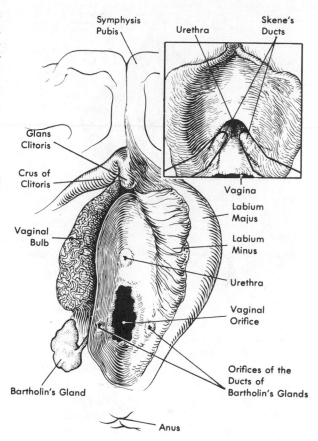

Figure 5-19. The vestibule, showing the urethra, the vaginal orifice and Bartholin's glands. Insert shows the orifices of the ducts of Skene's glands, which open just within the urethral meatus.

backward on either side of the orifice of the vagina. In the upper extremity each labium minus separates into two branches which when united with those of the opposite side enclose the clitoris. The upper fold forms the prepuce and the lower the frenum of the clitoris. At the bottom, the labia minora pass almost imperceptibly into the labia majora or blend together as a thin fold of skin, the fourchet, which forms the anterior edge of the perineum or perineal body.

The *clitoris* is a small, highly sensitive projection composed of erectile tissue, nerves, and blood vessels and is covered with a thin epidermis. It is analogous to the penis in the male and is regarded as the chief seat of voluptuous sensation. The clitoris is so situated that it is partially hidden between the anterior ends of the labia minora.

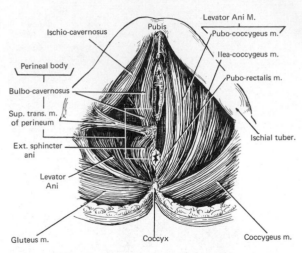

Figure 5-20. Muscles of the pelvic floor viewed from below. (After Dickinson)

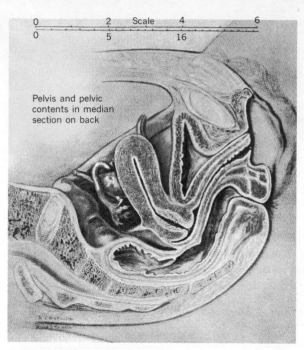

Figure 5-22. Pelvic contents in median section with the subject on her back. (R. L. Dickinson, M.D., New York)

The *vestibule* is the almond-shaped area which is enclosed by the labia minora and extends from the clitoris to the fourchette. It is perforated by four openings: the urethra, the vaginal opening, the ducts of Bartholin's glands and the ducts of Skene's glands. *Bartholin's glands* are two small glands situated beneath the vestibule on either side of the vaginal opening. In women infected with gonorrhea, these ducts sometimes harbor gonococci, which may cause the glands to suppurate, so that the

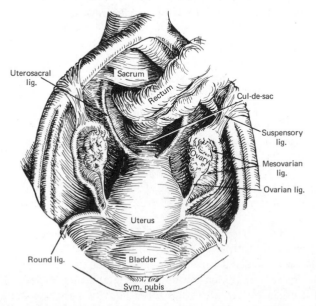

Figure 5-21. Pelvic contents viewed from above, showing position of the pairs of ligaments and their relationship to the uterus, tubes, and ovaries. (After Dickinson)

entire labia become distended by pus. *Skene's ducts* open upon the vestibule on either side of the urethra (Fig. 5-19).

The *hymen* marks the division between the internal and the external organs. It is a thin shelf of mucous membrane situated at the orifice of the vagina. It may be entirely absent, or it may form a complete septum across the lower end of the vagina. The hymen presents marked differences in shape and consistency. In the newborn child it projects beyond the surrounding parts. In adult virgins it is a membrane of varying thickness which closes the vaginal opening more or less completely and presents an aperture which varies in size from a pinpoint to one which will readily admit one or even two fingers. The opening is circular or crescentic in shape. In rare instances, the hymen may be imperforate and cause retention of menstrual discharge if it occludes the vaginal orifice completely.

The *perineum* consists of muscles and fascia of the urogenital diaphragm, which lies across the pubic arch, and the pelvic diaphragm, which consists of the coccygeus and the levator ani muscles. The levator ani is the larger and consists of three portions: the iliococcygeus, the pubococcygeus and puborectalis. These muscles form a slinglike support for the pelvic structure, and between them pass the urethra, the vagina, and the rectum (Fig. 5-20). Between the anus and the vagina the levator ani is reinforced by a central tendon of the perineum to which three pairs of muscles converge: the bulbocavernosus, the superficial transverse muscles of the perineum, and the external sphincter ani. These structures constitute the perineal body and form the main support of the perineal floor. They are often lacerated during delivery.

Internal organs

The internal organs of reproduction are the vagina, the uterus, the fallopian tubes, and the ovaries.

OVARIES. The *ovaries* are two small almond-shaped organs situated in the upper part of the pelvic cavity, one on either side of the uterus. Their chief functions are the development and the expulsion of ova and the provision of certain internal secretions, or hormones. These organs correspond to the testes in the male. They lie embedded in the posterior fold of the broad ligament of the uterus (Fig. 5-21) and are supported by the suspensory, the ovarian and the mesovarian ligaments.

Each ovary contains in its substance at birth a large number of germ cells, or primordial ova (p. 87). This huge store of primordial follicles present at birth more than suffices the woman for life. It is usually believed that no more are formed, and that this large initial store is gradually exhausted during the period of sexual maturity. Beginning at about the time of puberty, one, or possibly two, of the follicles which contain the ova enlarges each month, gradually approaches the surface of the ovary, and ruptures (see Fig. 6-2, p. 87). The ovum and the fluid content of the follicle are liberated on the exterior of the ovary; then they are swept into the tube. The development and the

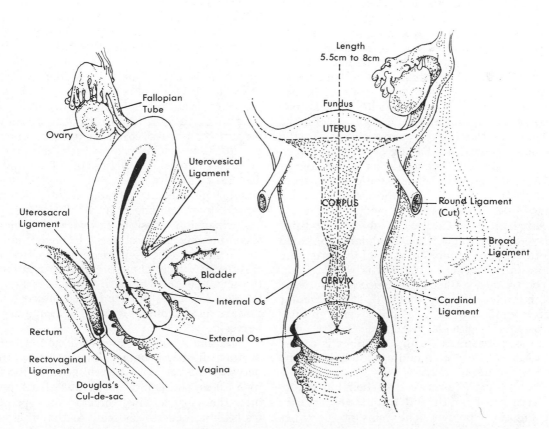

Figure 5-23. Lateral and anterior views of the uterus. The ligaments which support the uterus in the pelvic cavity are two broad ligaments, two round ligaments, and two uterosacral ligaments.

maturation of the follicles containing the ova continues from puberty to menopause.

The arteries which supply the ovary are four or five branches that arise from the anastomosis of the ovarian artery with the ovarian branch of the uterine artery (see Fig. 5-24). The veins proceeding from the ovary become tributary to both the uterine and the ovarian plexus.

The nerves supplying the ovaries are derived from the craniosacral and the thoracolumbar sympathetic systems. The postganglionic and visceral afferent fibers form a plexus surrounding the ovarian artery, which in turn is formed by contributions from the renal and the aortic plexuses and corresponds to the spermatic plexus in the male.

FALLOPIAN TUBES. The fallopian tubes are two trumpet-shaped, thin, flexible, muscular tubes, about 4½ inches long and somewhat thinner than a lead pencil (see Figs. 5-23, 5-24, 5-25, and 7-6). They extend from the upper angles of the uterus, the cornua, in the upper margin of the broad ligament, toward the sides of the pelvis. They have two openings: one into the uterine cavity and the other into the abdominal cavity. The opening into the uterine cavity is minute and will admit only a fine bristle. The abdominal opening is larger and is surrounded by a large number of fine fringes; hence the term *fimbriated end*. The fimbriated extremity lies near the ovary, but it is not necessarily in direct contact with it. It is generally believed that the cilia upon the fimbriated end of the tube create a current in the capillary layer of fluid lying between the various pelvic organs. The fallopian tubes convey the discharged ovum by peristaltic action from the ovaries to the cavity of the uterus; by their tentaclelike processes the fimbriated ends of the tube draw the escaped ovum into the tube. Thus, the function of the fallopian tube is to conduct the ovum along the canal by peristaltic action until it reaches the uterus.

The tubes are lined with mucous membrane containing ciliated epithelium. The muscular layer is made up of longitudinal and circular fibers which provide peristaltic action. The serous membrane covering the tubes is a continuation of the peritoneum, which lines the whole abdominal cavity.

The fallopian tubes receive their blood supply from the ovarian and the uterine arteries (see Fig. 5-24, below). The veins of the tubes follow the course of these arteries and empty into the uterine and the ovarian trunks. The nerves which supply the uterus supply the tubes.

UTERUS. The uterus is a hollow thick-walled, muscular organ (Figs. 5-22 and 5-23). It serves two important functions: 1) it is the organ of menstruation, and 2) during pregnancy it receives the fertilized ovum and retains and nourishes it until it expels the products of conception at the time of labor.

The uterus varies in size and shape according to the age of the individual and whether or not she has borne children. The uterus of the adult nullipara weighs approximately 60 Gm. and measures 5.5 to 8 cm. in length. It resembles a flattened pear in appearance and has two divisions: the upper triangular portion, the *corpus*, and the lower constricted cylindric portion, the *cervix*, which projects into the vagina. The fallopian tubes extend from the *cornu* (the Latin word meaning *horn*) of the uterus at the upper outer margin on either side. The upper rounded portion of the uterus between the points of insertion of the fallopian tubes is the fundus (Fig. 5-23).

The nonpregnant uterus is situated in the pelvic cavity between the bladder and the rectum. Almost the entire posterior wall and the upper portion of the anterior wall is covered by peritoneum. The lower portion of the anterior wall is united to the bladder wall by a thick layer of connective tissue. The lower posterior wall of the uterus and the upper portion of the vagina are separated from the rectum by an area called Douglas's cul-de-sac. Due to its muscular composition, the uterus is capable of enlarging to the size of a pumpkin; at the termination of pregnancy it weighs about 2 pounds. It is made up of involuntary muscle fibers arranged in all directions, making expansion possible in every direction to accommodate the products of conception. Due to the nature of this arrangement of the muscle, the uterus is able to expel its contents at the termination of normal labor (see Fig. 10-6, p. 147). Arranged between these muscular layers are many blood vessels, lymphatics, and nerves.

The cavity of the uterus is somewhat triangular in shape, being widest at the fundus, between the very small openings into the fallopian tubes, and narrowest below at the opening into the cervix. The anterior and posterior walls lie almost in contact, so that if a cross-section of the uterus could be examined, the cavity between them would appear as a mere slit. The uterus is lined with mucous membrane, the endometrium, and is divided into two parts: the cavity of the body of the uterus and the cavity of the cervix.

The cervix is less freely movable than is the body of the uterus. Its muscular wall is not so thick, and its lining is different in that it is much folded and contains crypts, which produce mucus and are the chief source of the mucous secretion during pregnancy. The cervix has an upper opening, the *internal os*, leading from the cavity of the uterine body into the cervical canal, and a lower opening, the *external os*, opening into the vagina. The cervical canal is small in the nonpregnant woman, barely admitting a probe, but at the time of labor it dilates to a size sufficient to permit the passage of the fetus (see Fig. 15-5, p. 256).

Ligaments. The uterus is supported in two ways: by ligaments extending from either half of the uterus (see Fig. 5-23) and by the muscles of the pelvic floor (see Fig. 5-20). The ligaments which support the uterus in the pelvic cavity are the broad ligaments (see Fig. 5-23), the round ligaments, and the uterosacral ligaments. The *broad ligaments* are two winglike structures which extend from the lateral margins of the uterus to the pelvic walls and serve to divide the pelvic cavity into an anterior and a posterior compartment. Each consists of folds of peritoneum which envelop the fallopian tubes, the ovaries, and the round and the ovarian ligaments. Its lower portion, the *cardinal ligament* (see Fig. 5-23), is composed of dense connective tissue which is firmly united to the supravaginal portion of the cervix. The median margin is connected with the lateral margin of the uterus and encloses the uterine vessels. The *round ligaments* are two fibrous cords which are attached on either side of the fundus just below the fallopian tubes. They extend forward through the inguinal canal and terminate in the upper portion of the labia majora. These ligaments aid in holding the fundus forward. The *uterosacral ligaments* are two cordlike structures which extend from the posterior cervical portion of the uterus to the sacrum. These aid in supporting the cervix. The uterovesical ligament is merely a fold of the peritoneum which passes over the fundus and extends over the bladder. The rectovaginal ligament is a fold of the peritoneum which passes over the posterior surface of the uterus and is reflected upon the rectum.

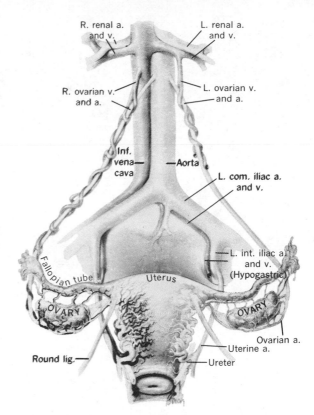

Figure 5-24.   Blood supply of the uterus and the adnexa.

Uterine Blood Supply. The uterus receives its blood supply from the ovarian and the uterine arteries (Fig. 5-24). The uterine artery, the principal source, is the main branch of the hypogastric, which enters the base of the broad ligament and makes its way to the side of the uterus. The ovarian artery is a branch of the aorta. It enters the broad ligament and on reaching the ovary breaks up into smaller branches which enter that organ, while its main stem makes its way to the upper margin of the uterus, where it anastomoses with the ovarian branch of the uterine artery.

The uterovaginal plexus returns the blood from the uterus and the vagina. These veins form a plexus of exceedingly thin-walled vessels which are embedded in the layers of the uterine muscle. Emerging from this plexus, the trunks join the uterine vein, which is a double vein. These veins follow on either side of the uterine artery and eventually form one trunk, emptying into the hypogastric vein, which makes its way into the internal iliac.

Uterine Nerve Supply. The uterus possesses an abundant nerve supply derived principally from the sympathetic nervous system but

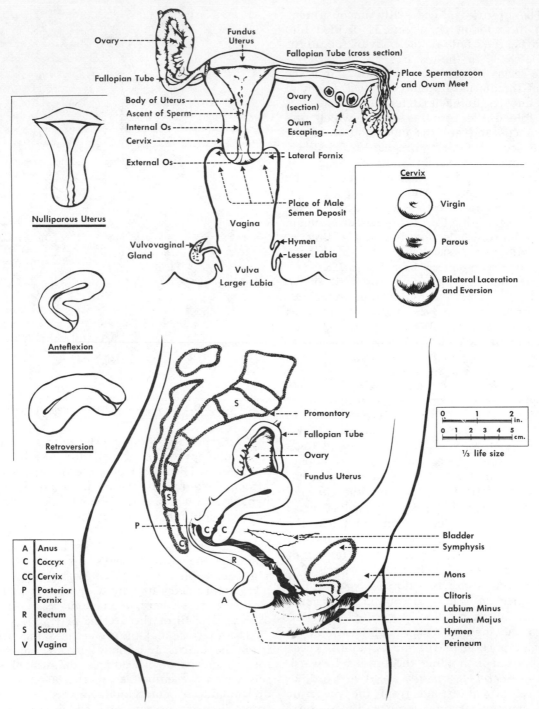

Figure 5-25. Female anatomy. (Dickinson, R. L.: *Human Sex Anatomy*, Baltimore, Williams & Wilkins)

partly from the cerebrospinal and parasympathetic system. Both the sympathetic and the parasympathetic nerve supplies contain motor and a few sensory fibers. The functions of the nerve supply of the two systems are in great part antagonistic. The sympathetic causes muscular contraction and vasoconstriction; the parasympathetic inhibits contraction and leads to vasodilatation.

Since the uterus is a freely movable organ

suspended in the pelvic cavity between the bladder and the rectum, the position of the uterus may be influenced by a full bladder or rectum, which pushes it backward or forward (see Figs. 5-22 and 5-25). The uterus also changes its position when the patient stands, lies flat, or turns on her side. Also, there are variations in position such as anteflexion, in which the fundus is tipped far forward (Fig. 5-25); retroversion, in which it is tipped far backward (Fig. 5-25); and prolapse, due to the relaxation of the muscles of the pelvic floor and the uterine ligaments.

Lymphatic Vessels. The lymphatic vessels drain into the lumbar lymph nodes.

VAGINA. The *vagina* is a dilatable passage lined with mucous membrane situated between the bladder and the rectum. The vaginal opening occupies the lower portion of the vestibule and in the virgin appears almost completely closed by the hymen. The vagina is from 3 to 5 inches in length, and at the upper end is a blind vault, commonly called the *fornix*, into which the lower portion of the cervix projects. The fornices (plural of fornix) are divided into four parts for convenience of description. The lateral fornices are the spaces between the vaginal wall on either side and the cervix; the anterior fornix is between the anterior vaginal wall and the cervix; the posterior fornix is between the posterior vaginal wall and the cervix. The posterior fornix is considerably deeper than the anterior since the vagina is attached higher up on the posterior than the anterior wall of the cervix. The fornices are important because the examiner is usually able to palpate the internal pelvic organs through their thin walls. The vagina serves three important functions: 1) it represents the excretory duct of the uterus through which its secretion and the menstrual flow escape; 2) it is the female organ of copulation; and 3) it forms part of the birth canal during labor. Its walls are arranged into thick folds, the columns of the vagina, and in women who have not borne children, numerous ridges, or *rugae*, extend outward and almost at right angles to the vaginal columns and give the surface a corrugated appearance. Normally, the anterior and the posterior walls of the vagina lie in contact, but they are capable of stretching to allow marked distention of the passage, as in the process of childbirth.

The vagina receives its abundant blood supply from branches of the uterine, the inferior vesical, the median hemorrhoidal, and the internal pudic arteries. The passage is surrounded by a venous plexus; the vessels follow the course of the arteries and eventually empty into the hypogastric veins. The lymphatics empty into the inguinal, the hypogastric, and the iliac glands.

Related pelvic organs

BLADDER. The *bladder* is a muscular sac which serves as a reservoir for the urine. It is situated in front of the uterus and behind the symphysis pubis. When empty or only moderately distended, it remains entirely in the pelvis, but if it becomes greatly distended, it rises into the abdomen. Urine is conducted into the bladder by the ureters, two tubes which extend down from the basin of the kidneys over the brim of the pelvis and open into the bladder at about the level of the cervix. The bladder is emptied through the urethra, a short tube which terminates in the meatus (see Fig. 5-18, p. 74). Lying on either side of the urethra and almost parallel with it are two small glands, less than 1 inch long, known as Skene's glands. Their ducts empty into the urethra just above the meatus. Often in cases of gonorrhea, Skene's glands and ducts are involved (see Fig. 5-19, p. 75).

ANUS. The *anus* is the entrance to the rectal canal. The rectal canal is surrounded at the opening or anus by its sphincter muscle, which binds it to the coccyx behind and to the perineum in front. It is supported by the muscles passing into it (see Fig. 5-20).

The muscles involved are those that aid in supporting the pelvic floor. The rectum is considered here because of the proximity to the field of delivery.

Mammary glands

The *breasts*, or mammary glands, are two highly specialized cutaneous glands located on either side of the anterior wall of the chest between the third and the seventh ribs (Fig. 5-26). Because they are abundantly supplied with nerves, formerly it was believed that direct nervous system connection existed between the uterus and the breasts. But the demonstration that lactation can be established after excluding the spinal nervous mechanism by severing all nerves supplying the breasts clearly indicated that some other factor must be involved in the explanation of mammary

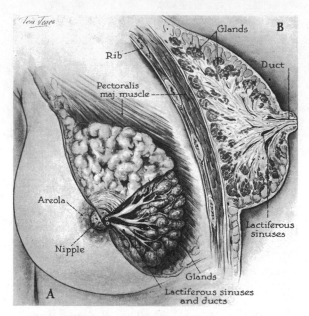

Figure 5-26. (A) Mammary gland showing the lactiferous ducts and sinuses. (B) Cross section of the breast.

with capillaries. By the process of osmosis the products necessary for the milk are filtered from the blood, but the secretion of the milk really begins in the acini cells. As the ducts leading from the lobules to the lobes and from the lobes approach the nipple, they are dilated to form little reservoirs in which the milk is stored; they narrow again as they pass into the nipple. The size of the breast is dependent on the amount of fatty tissue present and in no way denotes the amount of lactation possible.

External structure

The external surface of the breasts is divided into three portions. The first is the white, smooth and soft area of skin extending from the circumference of the gland to the areola. The second is the areola, which surrounds the nipple and is of a delicate pinkish hue in blondes and a darker rose color in brunettes. The surface of the areola is more or less roughened by small fine lumps of papillae, known as the glands of Montgomery (see Plate 3). These enlarged sebaceous glands, white in color and scattered over the areola, become more marked during pregnancy. Under the influence of gestation, the areola becomes darker, and this pigmentation, which is more marked in brunettes than in blondes, in many cases constitutes a helpful sign of pregnancy (see Plate 4). The nipple or third portion is largely composed of sensitive, erectile tissue and forms a large conic papilla projecting from the center of the areola and having at its summit the openings of the milk ducts. These openings may be from 3 to 20 in number. The care of the breasts (see Chapter 12) constitutes one of the important phases of the nursing care of the maternity patient throughout pregnancy and the puerperium.

Male organs of reproduction

The male reproductive system consists of the testes and a system of excretory ducts with their accessory structures (Fig. 5-27).

External organs

The *scrotum* and the *penis* are called the external genitalia. The scrotum contains the testes. In the adult male the testes have descended into the scrotal sac, and the canal connecting the sac with the abdominal cavity has closed, although it is open in the fetus.

changes in pregnancy. It is evident that the stimulation to growth of the mammary gland is hormonal and not nervous in origin.

The internal mammary and the intercostal arteries supply the breast gland, and the mammary veins follow these arteries. Also, there are many cutaneous veins which become dilated during lactation. The lymphatics are abundant, especially toward the axilla. These breast glands are present in the male, but only in the rudimentary state, and are not connected by the sympathetic system to the male generative organs.

Internal structure

The breasts of a woman who never has borne a child are, in general, conic or hemispheric in form, but they vary in size and shape at different ages and in different individuals. In women who have nursed one or more babies they tend to become pendulous. At the termination of lactation, certain exercises aid in restoring the tone of the breast tissue.

The breasts are made up of glandular tissue and fat. Each organ is divided into 15 or 20 lobes, which are separated from each other by fibrous and fatty walls. Each lobe is subdivided into many lobules, and these contain numerous acini cells. The *acini* are composed of a single layer of epithelium, beneath which is a small amount of connective tissue richly supplied

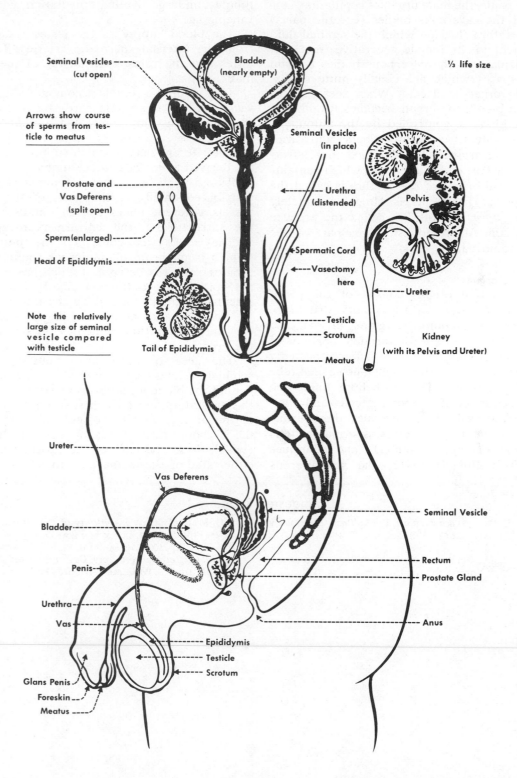

Figure 5-27. Male anatomy. (Dickinson, R. L.: *Human Sex Anatomy*, Baltimore, Williams & Wilkins)

The penis, the male organ of copulation, consists of the cavernous bodies (erectile parts) and a urethra through which the seminal fluid is brought to the female generative tract during ejaculation. The cavernous bodies contain blood spaces which are usually quite empty, and the organ is flaccid. When these spaces fill with blood, the organ becomes turgid. The flow of blood is controlled by the autonomic nervous system (vasodilator fibers) and varies with sexual arousal. The enlarged conic structure at the free end of the penis which contains the external orifice of the urethra is called the glans penis. The glans is almost completely enclosed by a fold of skin called the prepuce or foreskin. At circumcision this part of the skin is removed.

Internal organs

The internal organs consist of the *testes* and a *canal system* with accessory structures. Each testis is a compound gland, divided into lobules. These contain the terminal portions of the seminiferous tubules which join repeatedly and eventually form the single much-coiled tube of the epididymis. The epithelium lining the tubules consists of supporting cells and spermatogenetic cells which produce the spermatozoa. In the human testes, spermatogenesis begins at the age of puberty and continues throughout life. However, the seminiferous tubules undergo gradual involution with advancing age.

The blood supply to the testes is derived from the internal spermatic arteries. The arteries and the veins form a part of the spermatic cords.

The lymphatic vessels accompany the blood vessels in the spermatic cord, and eventually the lymphatics empty into the lumbar lymph nodes.

The efferent nerves which supply the testes are derived from the thoracolumbar and sacral divisions of the autonomic system. They are distributed chiefly to the walls of the blood vessels. Afferent fibers convey impulses from these structures to the central nervous system.

The canal system consists of the epididymis (which is made up of numerous seminiferous tubules), the vas deferens (which passes from the epididymis to the ejaculatory duct), the ejaculatory duct (formed by the union of the vas deferens and the duct of the seminal vesicle) and the urethra, which is surrounded by the prostate gland and terminates in the penis.

The accessory structures consist of the seminal vesicles (sacculated structures located behind the bladder and in front of the rectum), the prostate gland (which surrounds the base of the urethra and the ejaculatory duct) and the bulbourethral glands or Cowper's glands (which lie at the base of the prostate and on either side of the membranous urethra).

Suggested Reading

CHAFFEE, E. C., AND GREISHEIMER, E. M.: *Basic Physiology and Anatomy*, ed. 2. Philadelphia, J. B. Lippincott, 1969.

HELLMAN, L. M., AND PRITCHARD, J. A.: *Williams Obstetrics*, ed. 14. New York, Appleton-Century Crofts, 1971.

GOSS, C. M. (ED.): *Gray's Anatomy of the Human Body*, ed. 28. Philadelphia, Lea & Febiger, 1966.

SMOUT, C. F. V., JACOBY, F., AND LILLIE, E. W.: *Gynecological and Obstetrical Anatomy, Descriptive and Applied*, ed. 4. Baltimore, Williams & Wilkins, 1969.

maternal physiology in relation to human reproduction

6

Sexual Maturity / Menstrual Cycle / Bodily Manifestations of Ovarian Function / Menopause

A general review of reproductive physiology is included here to serve as background material for the more practical aspects of maternity nursing. An understanding of physiology is essential, so that the nurse may recognize the special relation of physiology to the problems in obstetrics.

Sexual maturity

Evidence of sexual maturity in the female begins at the time of puberty, with the onset of dramatic bodily changes. Early in the course of puberty, axillary and pubic hair appears. Shortly thereafter, there is an increase in the size of the external genitalia. The breasts also begin to mature at this time and there is a sudden increase in bodily growth.

These changes usually precede the onset of the first menstruation—the *menarche*. Establishment of the menstrual cycle is the most clearly identifiable sign of puberty and serves as an indication that the internal sex organs are approaching maturity. These physical changes are accompanied by emotional changes, as the young girl recognizes these outward signs that she is now approaching womanhood. The

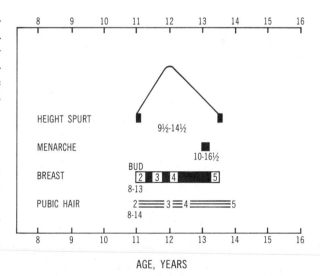

Figure 6-1. Sequence of events at adolescence in girls. An average girl is represented; the range of ages within which some of the events may occur is noted. Breast development progresses from the development of the breast bud (2) through full development (5). There is progression from downy pubic hair (2) through complete development of hair over the mons (5). (Modified for Tanner, J. M.: *Growth at Adolescence*, ed. 2. Oxford, England, Blackwell Science Publication, 1969. Pierson, E. C., and D'Antonio, W. V.: *Female and Male: Dimensions of Human Sexuality*. Philadelphia, J. B. Lippincott, 1974)

85

whole process of puberty spans about five years and is completed with the menarche.

The time-sequence of changes which culminates in the attainment of reproductive potential varies considerably among individuals (Fig. 6-1). Bodily manifestations of puberty, such as the beginning of breast development, the appearance of pubic hair, and a spurt of growth, precede the actual onset of menstruation by a variable amount of time. Throughout puberty there is an interplay of physiologic with sociocultural forces, and often the nurse is called upon to explain the bodily and psychologic changes in puberty to mothers who have daughters approaching their teens. There is often anxiety surrounding the onset of pubertal changes which are thought to be occurring too early or too late. Therefore, it is important to recognize the wide variability from one young woman to the next.

Changes associated with puberty in the male occur somewhat later, on the average, than in the female. These include development of axillary, pubic, and body hair, and maturation and growth of the testes and penis over a two-to-three-year period, accompanied by growth spurt and general muscular development.

Menarche

Menarche usually occurs between the ages of 12 and 16, although heredity, race, state of nutrition, climate, and environment may influence its early or late appearance; for example, maturity tends to occur earlier in warm climates and later in cold regions. The reproductive period spans about 35 years, from some point after the beginning of menstruation until its cessation during the menopause between ages 45 and 50.

Throughout childhood the *gonadotropins*, hormones produced by the pituitary gland which stimulate the ovaries, appear in very low concentrations. Estrogen, produced by the ovaries in the adult, remains undetectable. Puberty is ushered in when there is a rise in the release of gonadotropins from the pituitary gland. These stimulate the ovary to secrete increasing amounts of estrogen, the hormone responsible for many of the bodily changes of puberty. An orderly sequence of endocrinologic events resulting in ovulation may not occur initially. The first few menstrual cycles following the menarche may not, in fact, be associated with ovulation. Once menstruation has occurred, however, it must be assumed that there is ovulation and, therefore, fertility and the potential for pregnancy.

Ovulation and menstruation

Each month, with considerable regularity, a blisterlike structure about 1 cm. in diameter develops on the surface of one or the other ovary. Within this bubble, almost lost in the fluid and cells about it, lies a tiny speck, scarcely visible to the naked eye; a thimble would hold 3 million of these specks. This speck is the human ovum—a truly amazing structure. It not only possesses within its diminutive compass the potential of developing into a human being, but also embodies the mental as well as physical traits of the woman and her forebears: perhaps her own brown eyes or her father's tall stature; possibly her mother's genius at mathematics or her grandfather's love of music. These and a million other potentials are contained in the ovum, which is so small that it is about one-fourth the size of the period at the end of this sentence.

In a process known as ovulation, one blister on one ovary ruptures at a given time each month and discharges an ovum. The precise day on which ovulation occurs is a matter of no small importance. For instance, since the ovum can only be fertilized (impregnated by the spermatozoon, or male germ cell) within hours after its escape from the ovary, the day after ovulation a woman is no longer fertile. However, a person is potentially fertile for a number of days preceding the actual time of ovulation, since spermatozoa survive in the female reproductive tract for hours, even days, awaiting the arrival of the ovum. In a given cycle, the time of ovulation is unpredictable. Even the person who consistently has regular menstrual periods could experience a delayed ovulation, or early ovulation in any one cycle. This possibility of irregularity, combined with the potential for fertility any time prior to ovulation due to the fact that spermatozoa retain their ability for fertilization, makes it difficult to identify accurately the fertile phase of a given cycle. It should be remembered that ovulation can take place any time in a cycle, and that the only really infertile interval is after ovulation has occurred. The time between ovulation and menstruation is standard; the time between menstruation and ovulation is variable enough that ovulation cannot be predicted from one cycle to the next. It should be

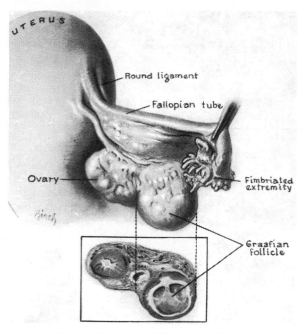

Figure 6-2. Ovary with graafian follicle.

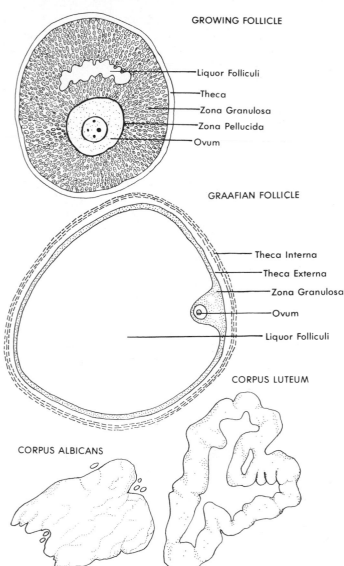

Figure 6-3. Development of the graafian follicle.

assumed that intercourse will result in conception unless some means of contraception is used, or the patient is assured, by the use of the temperature chart described later, that she is past ovulation.

GRAAFIAN FOLLICLE. In delving further into the process of ovulation, we find that at birth each ovary contains a huge number of undeveloped ova, probably more than 400,000. These are rather large, round cells with clear cytoplasm and a good-sized nucleus occupying the center. Each ovum is surrounded by a layer of a few small, flattened or spindle-shaped cells. The whole structure—ovum and surrounding cells—is a *follicle*, while in its underdeveloped state at birth it is a *primordial follicle*. The formation of primordial follicles ceases at birth or shortly after, and the large number contained in the ovaries of the newborn represents a lifetime's supply. The majority disappear before puberty, so that there are then perhaps 30,000 left in each ovary. This disintegration of follicles continues throughout the reproductive period, with the result that usually none is found after the menopause.

Meanwhile, from birth to the menopause a few of these primordial follicles show signs of development. The surrounding granular layers of cells begin to multiply rapidly until they are several layers deep, and at the same time become cuboidal in shape. As this proliferation

of cells continues, a very important fluid develops between them—the *follicular fluid*. After puberty this fluid accumulates in such quantities that the multiplying follicle cells are pushed toward the margin; the ovum itself is almost surrounded by fluid, and is suspended from the periphery of the follicle by only a small neck of cells. The cells within and surrounding the follicle produce estrogenic hormones which in turn act on the reproductive organs and produce cyclic bodily changes. The structure is now known as the *graafian follicle*, after Von Graaf, the famous Dutch physician who, in 1672, first described it (Figs. 6-2 and 6-3).

As it increases in size so enormously, the

graafian follicle naturally pushes aside other follicles, forming each month, as noted previously, a very noticeable, blisterlike projection on the surface of the ovary. At one point the follicular capsule becomes thin, and as the ovum reaches full maturity, it breaks free from the few cells attaching it to the periphery and floats in the follicular fluid. The thinned area of the capsule now ruptures, and the ovum is expelled from the ovary.

CHANGES IN THE CORPUS LUTEUM. After the discharge of the ovum, the ruptured follicle undergoes a change. It becomes filled with large cells containing a special yellow-colored matter. The follicle then is known as the *corpus luteum*, or yellow body. If pregnancy does not occur, the corpus luteum reaches full development in about eight days, then retrogresses and is gradually replaced by fibrous tissue, the *corpus albicans*. If pregnancy occurs, the corpus luteum enlarges somewhat and persists throughout the period of gestation, reaching its maximum size about the fourth or fifth month and retrogressing slowly thereafter. The corpus luteum secretes an extremely important substance, progesterone, which will be discussed later in this chapter.

In the absence of pregnancy, the corpus luteum remains active for about two weeks. The constancy of progesterone production by the corpus luteum accounts for the relatively standard duration of the postovulatory phase of the menstrual cycle.

Menstrual cycle

Menstruation in relation to pregnancy

Menstruation is the periodic discharge of blood, mucus, and epithelial cells from the uterus. It usually occurs at monthly intervals throughout the reproductive period, except during pregnancy and lactation, when it is usually suppressed entirely. Accordingly, the span of years during which childbearing is possible—that is, from about ages 12 to 45—corresponds to the period during which ovulation and, therefore, menstruation occur. In general, a woman who menstruates is able to conceive, whereas one who does not is probably infertile. Ovulation and menstruation are closely interlinked, and since no process of nature is purposeless, menstruation must play some vital and indispensable role in childbearing. What is this role?

If day by day we were privileged to watch the *endometrium*, the lining membrane of the uterus, we would observe some remarkable alterations. Immediately following the termination of a menstrual period, this membrane is very thin, measuring a few millimeters in depth. Each day thereafter it becomes a trifle thicker and harbors an increasing content of blood, while its glands become more and more active, secreting a rich nutritive substance. About a week before the onset of the next expected period, this process reaches its height; the endometrium is now of the thickness of heavy, downy velvet and has become soft and succulent with blood and glandular secretions. At this time the egg, if one has been fertilized, embeds itself into this luxuriant lining.

All these changes have only one purpose: to provide a suitable bed in which the fertilized ovum may rest, secure nourishment, and grow. If an egg is not fertilized, these alterations are unnecessary. Accordingly, through a mechanism which even today is obscure, the swollen endometrium disintegrates, and the encased blood and glandular secretions escape into the uterine cavity; passing through the cervix, they flow out through the vagina, carrying the egg with them. In other words, menstruation represents the abrupt termination of a process designed to prepare board and lodging, as it were, for a fertilized ovum. It forecasts the breakdown of a bed which was not needed because the "boarder" did not materialize. Thus, its purpose is to clear away the old bed so that a new and fresh one may be created the next month.

Hormonal control of menstruation

The menstrual cycle is regulated primarily through the highly coordinated function of the pituitary, the ovaries, and the uterus. If, while watching the changes in the endometrium during the menstrual cycle it were possible to inspect the ovaries from day to day, it would be noted that the uterine alterations are directly related to certain changes that take place in the ovary. If it were possible to look further, it might be seen that the alterations which occur regularly in the ovarian cycle are directly related to certain phenomena which take place in the anterior pituitary gland and the hypothalamus, a portion of the brain which lies above the pituitary. Thus, the whole sequence represents the harmonious, integrated reactions of several processes within the human organism, all of which are necessary to maintain proper relationships in the menstrual cycle.

PROLIFERATIVE PHASE. Immediately following menstruation, it will be recalled, the endometrium is very thin. During the subsequent week or so it proliferates markedly. The cells on the surface become taller, while the glands which dip into the endometrium become longer and wider. As the result of these changes, the thickness of the endometrium increases six- or eight-fold. Each month during this phase of the menstrual cycle (from approximately the fifth to the fourteenth days), a graafian follicle is approaching its greatest development and is manufacturing increasing amounts of follicular fluid. This fluid contains a most important substance, the estrogenic hormone *estrogen*. The word *hormone* comes from a Greek word which means *I bring about*, and in the case of estrogen, it brings about (among other things) the thickening of the endometrium described. Each month, then, after the cessation of menstruation, the cells in and about the developing graafian follicle produce estrogen which acts on the endometrium to cause it to grow (proliferate). For this reason this phase of the menstrual cycle is commonly called the *proliferative phase*, although it is sometimes referred to as the *follicular*, or *estrogenic* phase.

SECRETORY PHASE. Following the release of the ovum from the graafian follicle (ovulation), the cells which form the corpus luteum begin to secrete, in addition to estrogen, another important hormone, *progesterone*. This supplements the action of estrogen on the endometrium in such a way that the glands become very tortuous or corkscrew in appearance and are greatly dilated. This change occurs because the glands are swollen with a secretion. Meanwhile, the blood supply of the endometrium is increased; it becomes vascular and succulent. Since these effects are directed at providing a bed for the fertilized ovum, it is easy to understand why the hormone which brings them about is called progesterone, meaning *for gestation*. It is also clear why this phase of the cycle, occupying the last 14 ± 2 days, is commonly called the *secretory phase* and why occasionally it is referred to as the *progestational, luteal,* or *premenstrual phase*.

MENSTRUAL PHASE. Unless the ovum is fertilized, the corpus luteum is short-lived. Since corpus luteum cells secrete both progesterone and estrogen, cessation of corpus luteum activity means a withdrawal of both of these

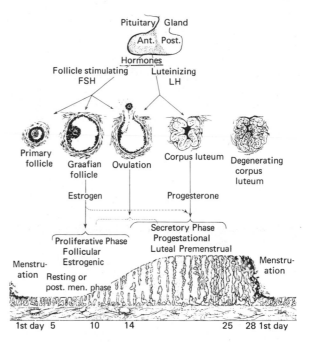

Figure 6-4. Hormonal control of the normal menstrual cycle.

hormones. As a result, the endometrium degenerates. This is associated with rupture of countless small blood vessels in the endometrium with innumerable minute hemorrhages. Along with the blood, superficial fragments of the endometrium, together with mucin from the glands, are cast away, all of which constitutes the menstrual discharge (Fig. 6-4). Naturally, this phase of the cycle (from approximately the first to the fifth days) is called the *menstrual phase*.

ROLE OF THE PITUITARY GLAND. The pituitary gland is of considerable importance in the function of the reproductive system. The anterior lobe of the pituitary, the "master clock," releases, among other hormones, the gonadotropins, whose function is to stimulate the ovary. These hormones produce the ovarian alterations associated with ovulation. There are two principal gonadotropins. One is the *follicle-stimulating hormone*, sometimes abbreviated FSH. As its name implies, FSH stimulates the development of the follicle. The other is the *luteinizing hormone (LH)*, which has its principal activity during ovulation and the luteal phase of the cycle.

The release of the gonadotropic hormones by the pituitary is regulated by the *hypothalamus*—a specialized structure within the brain located just above the pituitary. The hypo-

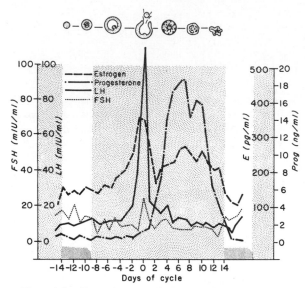

Figure 6-5. Plasma hormones in the normal menstrual cycle.

thalamus has a vascular connection to the pituitary gland, as well as nervous connections with the central nervous system. Indeed, its function can be modified by influences within the central nervous system. Thus, the function of the pituitary gland may be affected by the brain. The cyclic release of gonadotropin is brought about through the influence on the pituitary gland by hormonal agents released by the hypothalamus. These are called releasing factors, since they directly affect the release of both FSH and LH from the pituitary gland.

The *posterior lobe* of the pituitary gland produces *oxytocin*, a hormone that has an important role in obstetrics, but one that differs altogether from the purposes of the present discussion.

OTHER FUNCTIONS OF ESTROGEN AND PROGESTERONE. In addition to their role in controlling menstruation, estrogen and progesterone, have other far-reaching and important functions. Estrogen is responsible for the development of the secondary sex characteristics, that is, all those distinctive sex manifestations which are not directly concerned with the process of reproduction. Thus, the growth of the breasts at puberty, the distribution of body fat, the size of the larynx and its resulting influence on the quality of the voice, as well as mating instincts, are all the results of estrogenic action. Thus, it may almost be said that a woman is a woman because of estrogen.

Aside from its action on the endometrium, progesterone plays a most important role in

preserving the life of the embryo during early pregnancy. It also has a relaxing action on the uterine muscle. For these two reasons, it is sometimes employed therapeutically in cases in which there is a tendency to abort, although its efficacy has not been established.

Sensitive laboratory methods now allow accurate measurement of day-to-day changes in circulating pituitary and ovarian hormones (Fig. 6-5). The interplay between pituitary and ovary, influenced in turn by the central nervous system through the hypothalamus, brings about orderly development of the follicle and ovulation.

In a given cycle (Fig. 6-5) the pituitary gland releases increasing amounts of FSH which, with the help of a small amount of LH, stimulates maturation of several ovarian follicles. These produce modest amounts of the estrogen estradiol. About two days before ovulation, all but the one follicle which is destined to ovulate regress, in a process known as atresia. That one follicle undergoes rapid growth, and estrogen production rises sharply. The increased amount of estrogen produced at this point acts at the central nervous system-hypothalamic-pituitary level to inhibit release of additional FSH, while at the same time stimulating release of LH. There is a dramatic rise in LH level, and associated with this surge, maturation of the follicle is completed. Within 24 hours after the LH surge, ovulation takes place.

The increased levels of preovulatory estrogen prepare the genital tract for sperm migration. The secretions of the cervix, scanty and viscous early in the cycle, become thin and watery and more receptive to spermatozoa. The vaginal wall also reflects the effect of estrogen. A vaginal smear taken at this time reveals a large percentage of mature or "cornified" cells. The endometrium displays maximal proliferation (see Fig. 6-4).

Following ovulation the cyclic pattern continues. The ruptured follicle is transformed into a corpus luteum. LH's second function is the maintenance of the corpus luteum. These endocrine events are associated with further modifications in the cervical mucus, vagina, and endometrium. The mucus becomes thick, "tacky," and viscous, and is no longer as receptive to spermatozoa. The vaginal smear reflects the influence of progesterone with a decreasing "maturation index." The endometrium takes on secretory changes preparatory to implantation.

Progesterone secretion by the corpus luteum reaches its maximum about five to seven days after ovulation (see Fig. 6-5). This is the time when the fertilized egg, now a *blastocyst*, is ready to implant. If pregnancy has occurred another hormone, *human chorionic gonadotropin (HCG)*, appears within two to three days of implantation. HCG acts on the corpus luteum, maintaining its progesterone-providing function, and transforms it into a corpus luteum of pregnancy. If pregnancy has not intervened, the corpus luteum begins its demise at this time. Approximately ten to eleven days after ovulation, progesterone levels decline precipitously, and on about the fourteenth postovulatory day, no longer the beneficiary of hormonal support, the endometrium begins to shed in the process of menstruation.

Bodily manifestations of ovarian function

From what has been said concerning the underlying mechanism of menstruation, it is clear that the monthly flow of blood is only one phase of a marvelous cyclic process which not only makes childbearing possible, but also profoundly influences both body and mind. For this reason the time of the onset of menstruation is a critical period in the life of a young woman.

The average age at which the onset of menstruation occurs is between 12 and 14 years. It may be as early as the ninth year or as late as the eighteenth year and still be within normal limits. Although the interval of the menstrual cycle, counting from the beginning of one period to the onset of the next, averages 28 days, there are wide variations even in the same woman. Indeed, there is scarcely a woman who menstruates exactly every 28 or 30 days. This question has been the subject of several studies on normal young women, chiefly student nurses, who have conscientiously recorded the time and the nature of each period. These investigations show that the majority of women (almost 60 percent) experience variations of at least five days in the length of their menstrual cycles; differences in the same woman of even ten days are not uncommon and may occur without explanation or apparent detriment to health.

The degree and intensity of the outward manifestations of the ovulatory cycle vary from one individual to the next. Some women consistently experience pelvic discomfort during ovulation, or "mittleschmerz," so named be-cause it typically appears in the middle of a 28-day menstrual cycle. Slight staining or, occasionally, bleeding may occur in association with ovulation. In the postovulatory interval there may be breast tenderness and fullness which typically reaches a nadir just before menstruation. Premenstrual "tension" characterized by increased irritability may also occur after ovulation. Cyclic changes in the quality of the cervical mucus may be observed and are often easily detected by the patient when she is made aware of this possibility. In some cases, a clear translucent mucus appears at the labia or may be wiped from the cervix to provide suggestive evidence of impending ovulation. In the postovulatory phase of the cycle, the mucus becomes sticky and less abundant. Daily observations of cervical mucus changes have been suggested as a useful parameter in utilizing the "rhythm" method of contraception.

Normal menstruation should not be accompanied by pain, although quite often there is some general malaise, together with a feeling of weight and discomfort in the pelvis. Painful menstruation is known as *dysmenorrhea* and is usually associated with an ovulatory cycle. If there is a great irregularity or extremely profuse flow or marked pain, a pathologic condition may be present. Absence of menses is known as *amenorrhea*. The most common cause of amenorrhea is pregnancy, but sometimes it is brought about by emotional disturbances, such as fear, worry, or fatigue, which work through the hypothalamus, or by debilitating disease (anemia, tuberculosis).

The cessation of menstrual function usually occurs between the ages of 45 and 50. The time interval over which this alteration takes place is known as the menopause, or climacteric, but generally it is referred to by the laity as the "change of life." About one-half of all women cease menstruating between these years, about one-fourth stop before 45, and another quarter continue to menstruate until past 50.

Variations in basal body temperature

Beginning about the first year of life, slight daily variations in body temperature occur normally in all human beings. These temperature variations have relation to the time of the day and the nature of the circumstances surrounding the individual. For example, the body temperature is lowest in the morning before breakfast, after a good night's rest, and prior to assuming activity. Then after a day of normal activity the body temperature is usually highest toward afternoon and early evening. The fact that physiologic variations in basal body temperature also occur in relation to the menstrual cycle is important here, because it can be useful in assessing ovarian activity and in estimating the time of ovulation. Such an index becomes extremely important in studies of fertility and sterility.

In the woman who is ovulating, there is normally a rhythmic variation in the basal body temperature curve during the course of the

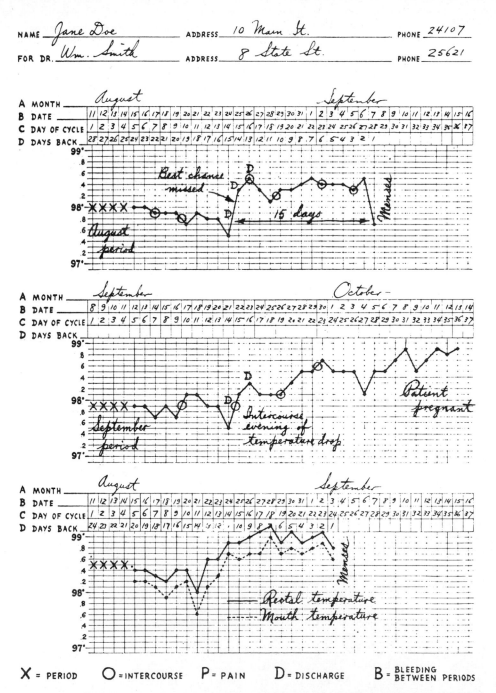

Figure 6-6. Basal temperature chart. Directions for using this chart are given on page 93. (Published under the auspices of the Medical Committee of the Planned Parenthood Federation of America, Inc.)

menstrual cycle (Fig. 6-6). The basal temperature is lower during the first part of the menstrual cycle, the proliferative phase. It rises in association with ovulation and remains relatively higher during the luteal phase of the cycle. The rise in the basal temperature occurs as a result of the influence of progesterone, produced by the corpus luteum following ovulation. Progesterone causes this thermogenic effect through its influence on the central nervous system. The basal temperature rises as much as 0.5 of a degree, and a relatively higher temperature is sustained until just before the onset of the menstrual period. This interval occupies the 14 ± 2 terminal days in the cycle. If pregnancy occurs, the levels of progesterone are maintained, and under its influence the basal temperature remains high past the expected time of the period. In the absence of pregnancy, the basal temperature usually drops a day or so before the menstrual period.

The use of the basal temperature graph

The basal body temperature is one of the most practical means for the diagnosis of ovulation. It is the relative difference in basal body temperature during the course of the cycle which is the important diagnostic criterion for ovulation. It is only useful in the timing of ovulation retrospectively. Thus, when there is infertility, efforts to time intercourse to coincide with changes in the temperature chart have not proved worthwhile. In fact, such regulation of coital habits is not recommended. However, for the diagnosis of ovulation, the temperature chart has proved valuable. The temperature chart is also useful as an adjunct to the rhythm method of family planning. (See Chapter 9.)

DIRECTIONS.

1. The first day of menses is considered to be the first day of the menstrual cycle. The duration of menstrual flow is recorded, beginning on cycle day 1, with X's on the chart (See Fig. 6-6). The date of onset of flow is recorded, and each subsequent date is recorded in the spaces provided. Following cessation of flow, the morning temperature is taken. Oral temperatures are as satisfactory as rectal recordings and are certainly more convenient. The temperature should be taken immediately after waking and before getting out of bed, talking, eating, drinking, or smoking. Ideally, it should be taken at about the same time every morning.

2. The thermometer is read to within 0.1 of a degree, and the reading is recorded on the chart.

3. Any known cause for temperature variation should be noted on the chart, for example, interrupted or shortened sleep, a cold, indigestion, emotional disturbance. If intercourse has occurred, that fact should be recorded with a circle around the recording the following morning.

4. Some women can recognize ovulation by the so-called mittelschmerz; others have vaginal bleeding or clear preovulatory vaginal discharge. Such manifestations should be recorded on the chart.

Menopause

The term *menopause* refers to the cessation of menstruation which usually occurs during a woman's middle years, somewhere between the ages of 45 and 50. The menopause, which is a normal consequence of aging, takes place as a gradual process. The periods first become scanty, then one may be missed, and finally they cease altogether.

The cause of the natural menopause is cessation of ovarian activity. As one considers the normal life cycle of the woman and focuses on the reproductive years, an analogy can be made that as the menarche is associated with puberty, so the menopause is associated with the climacteric. Often the terms menopause and *climacteric* are used synonymously, but one can readily understand that this usage is not accurate. The climacteric, a word derived from the Greek, meaning *rung of ladder, critical point in human life,* is defined as "the syndrome of endocrine, somatic and psychic changes occurring at the termination of the reproductive period in the female. . . ." Consider briefly the implication that these endocrine changes have for the ovaries. Having for some 30 years performed the function of providing a mature ovum each month with some degree of regularity, the ovary now regresses and gradually shrivels up into a small, flat organ composed mostly of scar tissue. As a result, estrogen no longer is produced. This permanent and complete withdrawal of estrogen results in atrophy of the uterus, the fallopian tubes, the vagina, and the vulva. Furthermore, the withdrawal of estrogen is likely to produce other symptoms, such as "hot flashes," vague muscle and joint pains, headache, and manifestations of emotional instability—for example, irritability, sudden outbursts of tears, and so on. Other evidences of the climacteric may be observed in the dryness of the skin and the hair, which makes the fact that she is aging more apparent to the woman.

Hot flashes is a familiar term to most people. Mentioned in association with the menopause down through the years, the expression has been passed along for generations almost like an old wives' tale. But hot flashes are no old wives' tale; they are the result of vasomotor instability, just as sweating or sensations of cold are during this time. The term hot flashes is descriptive; it says what the patient feels—an abrupt sensation of being very hot that seems momentarily to sweep upward from the body to envelop her to the very top of the head, and most particularly about the face and the neck. The face suddenly becomes very flushed, and she may break out in a sweat, manifestations that will be quite apparent to others. The women so affected may have hot flashes at any time and in varying degrees, from very mild to severe.

The menopause may result from other than the natural physiologic alterations of the climacteric. Artificial menopause relates to the cessation of menstruation produced by some artificial means, such as irradiation of the ovaries or surgical operation for the removal of the ovaries (oophorectomy) or the uterus (hysterectomy). Each of these brings about one manifestation in common (i.e., the woman will no longer menstruate). But beyond this the manifestations in the patient are not identical.

Certain misunderstandings based on incorrect interpretation of terminology are rather widespread and should be clarified. The fact that a woman has had a hysterectomy and ceases to menstruate does not mean that her healthy ovaries will now cease to function, because the hysterectomy involves only the removal of the uterus. On the other hand, if the ovaries are removed surgically or are treated by irradiation, the source of estrogen is withdrawn abruptly, and thus the symptoms relating to the sudden withdrawal of this hormone will occur.

When severe symptoms are produced by lack of ovarian function resulting from either the normal climacteric or artificial menopause, the patient may find them intolerable and may require hormone therapy to control the symptoms. Estrogen, either as the pure hormone or as one of the several synthetic estrogens, finds its greatest usefulness in alleviating these menopausal disorders. It can be said that the better the woman's general health is as she approaches her middle years, the better her chances are for an uneventful menopause.

Suggested Reading

GOLDFARB, A. F. (ED.): Dynamics and abnormalities of puberty. *Am. J. Ob.-Gyn.* 11:755-878, 1968.

MASTROIANNI, L. (ED.): Ovulation. *Clin. Ob. and Gyn.* 10: 345-417, 1967.

PIERSON, E. P., AND D'ANTONIO, W.: *Female and Male: Dimensions of Human Sexuality.* Philadelphia, J. B. Lippincott, 1974.

conception and ovum development

In all of Nature's wide universe, there is no process more wondrous, no mechanism more fantastic, than the one by which a tiny speck of tissue, the human egg, develops into a 7-pound baby. So miraculous did primitive peoples consider this phenomenon that they frequently ascribed it to superhuman intervention and even overlooked the fact that sexual intercourse was a necessary precursor. Throughout unremembered ages, our own primitive ancestors doubtless held similar beliefs, but now we know that pregnancy comes about in only one way: from the union of a female germ cell, the egg, or ovum, with a male germ cell, the spermatozoon (Fig. 7-1). These two germ cells, or *gametes* become fused into one cell, or *zygote*, which contains the characteristics of both the female and the male from which these gametes originated.

Maturation of ovum and sperm cells

Until about two days before ovulation, the ovum remains in a resting stage of development. Its nucleus is large and round and has been described as vesicular, because it resembles a bleb or vesicle. While still in the follicle, the ovum undergoes the process of

meiosis, the special method for cell division, through which it is matured and its genetic material (chromosomes) is prepared for fertilization.

The spermatozoon is fully matured before it is discharged from the tubules in the testis. It, too, has undergone a meiotic process preparatory to fertilization.

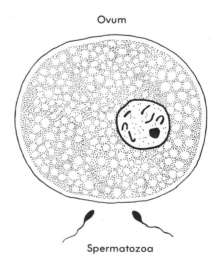

Ovum

Spermatozoa

Figure 7-1. Relative size of spermatozoa and ovum.

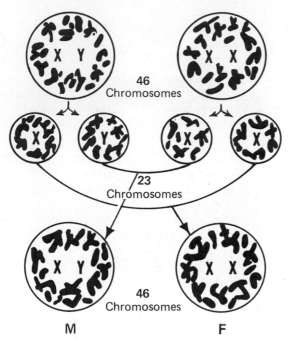

Figure 7-2. The sex of the offspring is determined at the time of fertilization by the combination of the sex chromosome of the spermatozoon (either X or Y) and that of the ovum (X). The ovum fertilized by a sperm cell containing the X chromosome produces a female (44 regular chromosomes + 2 X chromosomes). If it is fertilized by a spermatozoon containing the Y chromosome, the union produces a male (44 regular chromosomes + X + Y).

Note: The structures depicted as chromosomes are diagrammatic only. In this illustration it was not possible to include the total correct number.

In all human cells, with the exception of the mature sex cells, there are normally 46 chromosomes (chroma, color; soma, body). Normally, the chromosomes within each somatic cell are paired. Thus, each cell contains 22 pairs of autosomes (auto, self) and one pair of sex chromosomes. Female cells normally contain two X chromosomes; male cells normally contain one X and one Y chromosome. The sex chromosome of the mature ovum is always of the X type. The mature spermatozoon may have either an X chromosome or a Y chromosome (Fig. 7-2). When fertilization occurs with a spermatozoon containing the X chromosome, the resulting product is genetically female. When an ovum is fertilized by a spermatozoon containing a Y chromosome, the resulting product is genetically male.

Thus, in the human being, age, state of health, and natural physical strength have nothing to do with the determination of the sex of the offspring. The sex is determined at the time of fertilization by the spermatozoon—not by the ovum. At the completion of the fertilization process, the fertilized ovum contains 46 chromosomes, the number normally present in all somatic cells.

Prior to fertilization, each gamete undergoes a reduction in its total number of chromosomes to one-half the usual number, the *haploid number*. This reduction occurs through the process of meiosis. In the meiotic process, each gamete normally receives only one chromosome of each pair. Thus, each mature spermatozoon has 23 chromosomes in its nucleus, and each mature ovum also contains 23 chromosomes, the haploid number. The chromosomes of the ovum have been reduced as a result of extrusion of chromosomal material in the form of a *polar body*, so called because it is observed at one pole of the developing ovum. Altogether, two polar bodies are extruded. The first is released prior to ovulation. Upon penetration by the spermatozoon a second polar body is released from the ovum and, as a result of its release, the number of chromosomes is halved. The final product, the fertilized ovum, once again contains a set of 46 chromosomes. Thus, the chromosomes of the fertilized ovum are derived from both germ cells (i.e., one-half from the ovum and one-half from the spermatozoon that fertilized the ovum).

The chromosomes differ in form and size, ranging from small, spherical masses to long rods. By the use of cell culture techniques, it has been possible to photograph the individual chromosomes in a given cell. The white blood cell has proved to be the most useful cell for this technique. A sample of blood is taken, and the white blood cells are separated and cultured. After a period of culture, cell division, or *mitosis* occurs. This division is arrested by the introduction of the drug colchicine into the culture medium. Colchicine causes arrest of cell division in metaphase, a time when the individual chromosomes are separate from one another. The chromosomes are then photographed and the individual chromosomes are cut out and arranged in pairs according to their relative lengths. *Karyotype* is the technical term for the arrangement of the chromosomes of a single cell in this way. The examples of normal karyotypes are shown in Figure 7-3. The 46 chromosomes (greatly magnified) appear as rod-shaped structures split longitudinally into

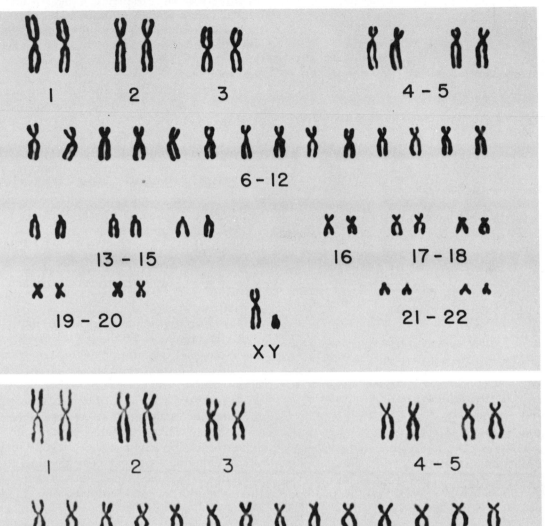

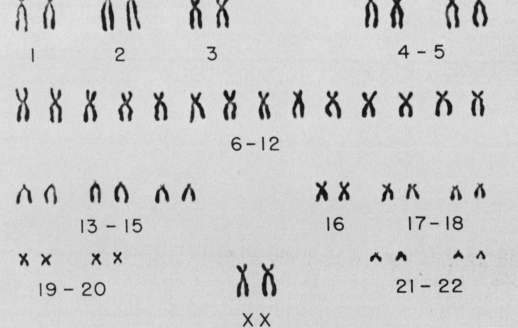

Figure 7-3. (Top) Normal male karyotype. (Bottom) Normal female karyotyping. Total count for each is 46. (Dr. M. Neil Macintyre, Department of Anatomy, Western Reserve University School of Medicine)

sex chromatin

of infant female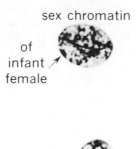

of adult female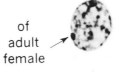

not seen in male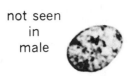

Figure 7-4. Photomicrographs of epithelial cells from the oral mucosa stained with cresylecht violet (× 2,000). The upper two nuclei have Barr bodies, which are indicated by arrows. (Moore, K. L. and Barr, M. L.: Lancet 2:57, July 9, 1955. Ham, A. W.: Histology, ed. 6, p. 72. Philadelphia, J. B. Lippincott, 1969)

two chromatids, lying side by side, and held together at the constricted region, the centromere.

Except for the mature ovum and spermatozoon, which contain the haploid number of chromosomes, each normal cell in the body contains a standard number of chromosomes. After fertilization, the ovum again has its full complement of 46 chromosomes. In every cell division thereafter, throughout the differentiation of all tissues, each cell will have 46 chromosomes. Preparation for the passing on of the requisite number of chromosomes to each of two daughter cells is accomplished by an internal change in the cell before division, the completion of mitosis. Each of the chromosomes replaces itself and splits in half, and each of the two new cells (daughter cells) receives its half of the halved chromosomes. This splitting and halving occurs in all dividing cells until growth ceases.

Within the chromosomes, distributed along the chromosomal threads, are the ultramicroscopic self-perpetuating bodies called genes. When the cell divides into two daughter cells, each daughter cell is an exact duplicate of the other and of the mother cell before division. For the daughter cells to be identical, each must have the same complement of genes in its chromosomes; thus, there must be a duplication of genes before cell division occurs. This is accomplished by mitosis.

As division proceeds, then, the mother cell will have identical sets of 46 chromosomes for each daughter cell.

Now consider briefly what happens when the ovum is fertilized and conception takes place. Each gamete, ovum, and spermatozoon comes from a different person with a different ancestral history—and with different genes in its 23 chromosomes. To these genes are attributed such differences as color of hair and eyes, facial characteristics, and body build. Since a single gene may carry more than one character, there may be numerous variable results in the offspring of any two parents. The hereditary possibilities discarded or retained in the mature gametes is a matter of chance, but the nature of the combination of the germ plasm which occurs in each generation when two gametes fuse in fertilization is of great significance. If either parent brings defective germ plasm, the result may affect the fertilized ovum, or zygote, and later the characteristics of the child.

Biologists have estimated that at the time of the reduction division some 17 million different combinations are possible due to the interchange of genes. Apparently, there is sufficient stability produced during this intricate interchange process to ensure perpetuation of the characteristics of the progenitors.

Determination of sex

Sex chromatin

In females, from 20 to 90 percent of the nuclei of the somatic (body) cells contain a small mass of material, sex chromatin, which stains red with suitable dyes. This is probably formed by an inactive X chromosome, since it is not usually present in the body cells of males. Sex chromatin has proved to be useful in determining the sex of the embryo or fetus in early abortions and under other circumstances in which the generative organs are improperly developed (Fig. 7-4).

Cells may be recovered from the amniotic fluid surrounding the fetus in late pregnancy, and their sex chromatin pattern used to pre-

Table 7-1 Chromosomal Aberrations in Man

I. Anomalies of whole chromosomes (aneuploidy): If present in part of the cells only, a *mosaic* results.
  A. Autosomal trisomy. 47 chromosomes, extra chromosome leads to complex mental retardation—malformation syndrome.
    1. Trisomy 21—mongolism.
    2. Trisomy 18—18 trisomy syndrome.
    3. Trisomy D_1—D_1 trisomy syndrome.
    4. Other autosomal trisomies have been observed in aborted fetuses.
    5. Double trisomies may occur—i.e., mongolism with XXY constitution, etc.
  B. Sex chromosomal abnormalities.
    1. XO condition, females with Turner (Ullrich-Turner) syndrome; commonly associated with mosaicism due to mitotic chromosomal nondisjunction: XO/XX, XO/XXX, XO/XX/XXX, XO/XY are the most common types.
    2. Extra sex chromosomes.
      (*a*) XXX (47, i.e., 44 + XXX constitution) at times associated with mild mental retardation and/or minor anomalies, rarely with serious gonadal dysgenesis.
      (*b*) XXY (47, i.e., 44 + XXY): males with Klinefelter syndrome.
      (*c*) XYY (47, i.e., 44 + XYY): males with unusual height, at times mild mental retardation and/or mental illness, minor somatic abnormalities and aggression.
      (*d*) XXXY, XXYY (48), XXXXY, XXXYY (49): males with gonadal defect and severe retardation—malformation syndromes.

II. Anomalies involving parts of chromosomes (with or without mosaicism in affected individuals).
  A. "Partial trisomy" due to insertions, reciprocal translocations, isochromosomal formation, etc. Chromosome number 46, one altered chromosome may be detectable in the affected individual. In cases of isochromosomes and reciprocal translocations phenotype may also be affected by chromosomal deficiency. Balanced "carrier state" may be transmitted over several generations.
  B. Chromosomal loss due to deletions, ring chromosomal formation, etc. Several "deletion syndromes" are known: the cat-cry syndrome, the 18q- and 18p-syndromes, the Dq-syndrome, etc.

III. Anomalies involving chromosomal sets.
  A. Triploidy (69 XXX or XXY or XYY constitution). Most common chromosomal abnormality in aborted fetuses; compatible with postnatal viability only in presence of normal cells.
  B. Tetraploidy (92 chromosomes) has been observed in aborted fetuses.

Source: Hamilton, W. J., and Mossman, H. W.: *Human Embryology*, ed. 4. Cambridge, England, W. Heffer & Sons, Ltd., 1972.

dict with accuracy the sex of the unborn infant. These fetal cells may then be cultured and karyotyped to determine whether the fetus is male (XY) or female (XX).

CHROMOSOMAL ABERRATIONS. The normal development of the embryo depends on the normal complement of chromosomes in the zygote, as well as the proper genetic balance. When this is not the case, developmental abnormalities occur. Malformations may result from alterations in a single gene, or in a number of genes, and from chromosomal abnormalities involving whole chromosomes. Some of these abnormalities are determined before fertilization takes place (during gametogenesis), and are almost certainly due to failure of separation of chromosomes in the first reduction division in meiosis or nondisjunction. For example, this aberration is now known to be the cause of Down's syndrome (mongolism). Here the zygote has three homologous autosomes, and it is trisomic; thus it is sometimes referred to as "trisomy 21."

A number of chromosomal aberrations have been identified in humans, involving both autosomes and sex chromosomes (Table 7-1). Because this subject is highly specialized, the student is referred to the current literature on genetics for elaboration on it. The role of the nurse in genetic counseling is considered in Chapter 27.

The ovum

As described in Chapter 6, ova normally are discharged from the human ovary at the rate of one a month. Under the influence of the gonadotropins, the graafian follicle that is destined to release an ovum has matured. The ovum itself has been pushed to one side of the fluid-filled cavity of the follicle. It is surrounded by a translucent coat, the *zona pellucida*. Immediately adjacent to the zona pellucida, and connected to it, is a layer of follicular cells, the *corona radiata*, so named because the cells are arranged in a radial pattern. Peripheral to this is a more loosely arranged layer of cells, the *cumulus oophorus*. The ovum, surrounded by this entourage of cells, having matured through release of its first polar body, is released through the process of ovulation. Transfer of

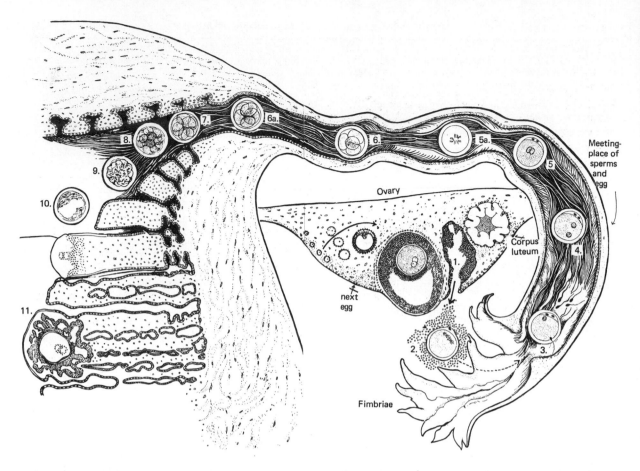

Figure 7-5. Travel of egg from ovary through implantation, with alterations en route: three days in tube, four days in uterus before implantation which occurs midway on rear wall or front of uterus. (1) Follicle ruptures. (2) Ovum with adhering granulosa cells; first polar body; second maturation spindle. (3) Sperm enters egg; second maturation division. (4) Male and female pronuclei. (5) Pronuclei fusing; fertilization accomplished. (5a) First cleavage division. (6-7) Early cleavage. (8) Morula. (9-10) Early and later gastrula. (11) Implanted growing embryo. (R. L. Dickinson, M.D., New York, adapted from Sellheim, with suggestions from Streeter, Frank, Hartman, and Miller)

the ovum into the fallopian tube, the site of fertilization, occurs relatively rapidly and with great efficiency. At this time, the ovum is a relatively large cell, measuring about 0.2 mm. (1/25 of an inch) and is barely visible to the naked eye.

Transport through the fallopian tube

The *fallopian tube* is an important structure which serves a number of functions in reproduction (Fig. 7-5). It is responsible for the transfer of the ovum into its lumen from the rupturing follicle, and for providing a temporary environment for the ovum and the spermatozoon. The fallopian tube also provides the environment in which the fertilization process occurs, and in which the ovum passes through many cell divisions during the early stages of

human life. Finally, the tube is responsible for transport of the fertilized, cleaving ovum into the uterus after a three-day interval.

The tube is uniquely designed anatomically for its various functions. At its ovarian end, it is endowed with specialized structures, the *fimbriae*. These are arranged in fronds and are lined with hairlike projections, the *cilia*, which beat in such a manner as to direct any overlying fluid—as well as any particles that float thereon—in the direction of the uterine cavity. The remainder of the fallopian tube is also lined with cilia, and these are important in the transportation of the newly released ovum along the fallopian tube (Fig. 7-6). The cilia create a current which courses along the fallopian tube, and which is partially responsible for the transportation of particles through it. The anatomical arrangement at the fimbriated end of the tube is important in ovum pickup mechanisms. A separate strand of fimbria, the *fimbria ovarica*, extends from the tube to the ovary to which it is attached. This contains a separate bundle of smooth muscle. At the time of ovulation this muscle contracts, pulling the ovary in the direction of the tubal opening. The remainder of the fimbria are thought to embrace the ovary near the point of ovulation, or over it, and they exercise muscular movement which moves them to and fro over the rupturing follicle. Thus, the cilia lining the fimbriae soon come into contact with the cumulus oophorus surrounding the ovum. Through these mechanisms an efficient process of ovum transfer is arranged, and ovum pickup is practically assured, despite the fact that the ovum itself is miniscule in size. Once the ovum is safely within the tubal ostium, it is transported rapidly to a point well within the fallopian tube. There, fertilization occurs. The fertilizing spermatozoon has previously been conditioned in the female reproductive tract so that it has acquired the ability to fertilize an ovum. After fertilization, the ovum passes through many cell divisions, during which it is retained in the fallopian tube for approximately three days. Eventually it develops into a solid mass of cells, a *morula*, so called because it resembles a mulberry. In the human, the mechanism by which the ovum is retained in the tube is not as yet clear. However, the importance of the three-day residence within the tube can be extrapolated from experiments in other mammals. In the rabbit, for example, if the ovum is removed from the tube and placed in the uterus prematurely, it degenerates and fails to implant. Although for obvious reasons the actual experiment has not been carried out in the human, it is generally accepted that the three-day residence within the human tube is important. Premature expulsion of the ovum from the tube could result in failure of implantation. Prolonged retention could result in ectopic pregnancy, with implantation into the tube itself and consequent tubal rupture and hemorrhage. The latter condition constitutes a serious obstetrical emergency. The importance of the fallopian tube, a once-neglected organ which bridges the space between the ovary and the uterus, is now quite evident.

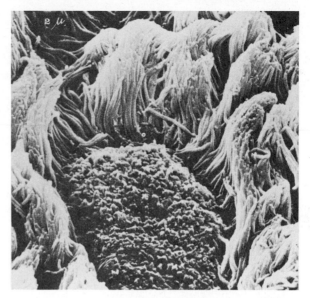

Figure 7-6. Scanning electron micrograph of the human fallopian tube showing ciliated cells surrounding a nonciliated cell in the midproliferative phase of the menstrual cycle. (Patek, E., Nilsson, L., and Johannison, E.: *Fertil. steril.* 23:459, 1972)

Spermatozoa

The minute, wriggling *spermatozoa* are in some respects even more remarkable than the ova which they fertilize. In appearance they resemble microscopic tadpoles, with oval heads and long, lashing tails about ten times the length of the head. The human spermatozoon consists of three parts: the head, the middlepiece (or neck) and the tail (Fig. 7-7). The nucleus, and consequently the chromatin material, is in the head; the tail serves for propulsion. Spermatozoa are much smaller than ova, their overall length measuring about one-quarter the diameter of the egg, and it has been estimated that the heads of 2 billion of them—

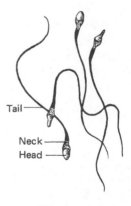

Figure 7-7. Spermatozoa.

enough to regenerate the entire population of the world—could be placed, with room to spare, in the hull of a grain of rice. As a result of the wriggling motion of the tails, spermatozoa swim with a quick vibratory motion and have been "timed" under the microscope at rates as fast as 3 mm. a minute. To ascend the uterus and the fallopian tube, they must swim against the same currents that waft the ovum downward; in their ascent, they are assisted by the muscular action of the uterus, which propels them upward in the direction of the tube. Spermatozoa have been observed in the fallopian tube within minutes of insemination.

The most amazing feature of spermatozoa is their huge number. At each ejaculation, the climax of intercourse in the male, about 300 million are discharged into the vagina. If each of these could be united with an ovum, the babies which would be created would exceed

the total number born in the United States during the past 100 years—all from a single ejaculation. Of the millions of spermatozoa deposited in the vagina during coitus, many are expelled immediately; some remain in the vagina for an interval and are later extruded. Those retained in the vagina lose their motility at the end of about an hour because of the rather hostile acid environment provided by the vagina. Some spermatozoa reach the cervix almost immediately after ejaculation. Those transferred into the secretions of the cervix find a more favorable environment there and may remain motile for as long as several days especially in the preovulatory phase of the cycle. Thousands of spermatozoa find their way into the cavity of the uterus; fewer still reach the lumen of the fallopian tube. Only one is afforded the privilege of continued biologic life through fertilization and, at that, only occasionally. The remainder

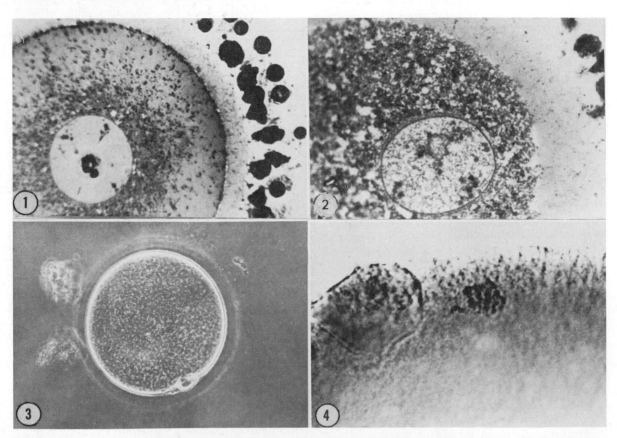

Figure 7-8. (1) Section of a follicular oocyte at the time of recovery. The cytoplasm contains a round, centrally located nucleus with nucleoli. Layers of corona cells are seen outside the zona pellucida. ($\times$ 201.) (2) Section of a human follicular oocyte after 24 hours of culture. A granular nucleus is located near the surface of the cytoplasm. Some altered corona cells surround the zona pellucida. ($\times$ 400.) (3) Human follicular oocyte cultured for 48 hours. The first polar body has been extruded. Phase-contrast microscopy. ($\times$ 102.) (4) Human follicular oocyte displaying metaphase II chromosomes and first polar body. (Lacmoid stained. $\times$ 780.) (Mastroianni, L., and Noriega, C.: Observations on human ova and the fertilization process, Am. J. Ob-Gyn. 107:682-690, 1970)

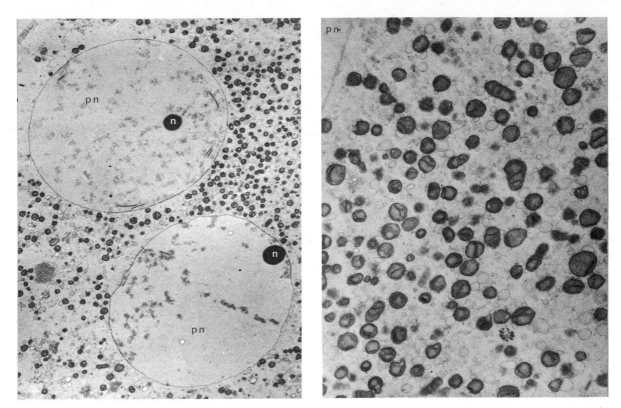

Figure 7-9. (*Left*) Electronmicrograph of a penetrated human ovum showing male and female pronuclei (pn). n = nucleoli. (*Right*) A portion of the penetrating spermatozoon is seen in the cytoplasm of the penetrated human pronuclear ovum. (Zamboni, L., *et al:* Fine structure of the human ovum in the pronuclear stage, *J. Cell Biol.* 30:579, 1966)

are disposed of in the reproductive tract, and as they degenerate they are phagocytized by the white blood cells in that region. However, it should be remembered, that once the spermatozoon is in the female reproductive tract it may retain its motility and, therefore, its potential ability to fertilize for hours, and even for days. Spermatozoa are conditioned to fertilize an egg after they are exposed to the female reproductive tract, a process referred to as *capacitation*. Within the female reproductive tract they "lie in wait" for the ovum (see Fig. 7-5).

Fertilization and changes
following fertilization

After the ovum is well within the fallopian tube, dispersion of the cumulus oophorus occurs (Fig. 7-8). These cells begin to separate, partly as a result of the influence of the enzyme hyaluronidase contained in the head of the spermatozoon. The spermatozoon makes its way through this peripheral layer of cells; meanwhile the densely packed corona radiata

has undergone certain changes. These cells become looser under the influence of tubal fluid, and the spermatozoon then finds its way through this layer to the zona pellucida. It is now thought that the zona pellucida is penetrated by the spermatozoon because of a trypsin-like enzyme which is present in the sperm head. The spermatozoon makes a channel through the zona pellucida. It is then in a position to penetrate the membrane of the ovum itself. As the spermatozoon penetrates the ovum, it brings its tail with it (Fig. 7-9). On penetration the meiotic process is completed with extrusion of the second polar body. Once penetration is complete, a physiologic barrier occurs, and penetration of the ovum by other spermatozoa is somehow prevented. Soon after penetration, the nucleus of the spermatozoon and the nucleus of the ovum undergo characteristic changes. They become pronuclei—distinct, clearly identifiable bodies of chromatin, each contained in a membrane. The male pronucleus and the female pronucleus then fuse, and the process of fertilization is now biologically complete. The new cell presents the full comple-

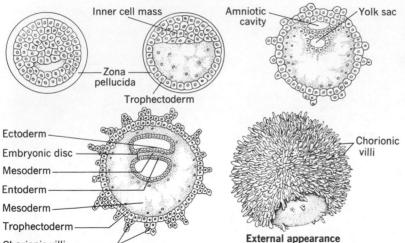

Inner cell mass

Amniotic cavity

Yolk sac

Zona pellucida

Trophectoderm

Ectoderm

Embryonic disc

Mesoderm

Entoderm

Mesoderm

Trophectoderm

Chorionic villi

Chorionic villi

External appearance

Figure 7-10. Early stages of development. (*Top, left and center*) The cells are separated into a peripheral layer and an inner cell mass; the peripheral layer is called the trophoblast, or trophectoderm; the entire structure is called a blastodermic vesicle. (*Top, right*) The formation of the amniotic cavity and yolk sac is indicated. The former is lined with ectoderm, the latter with entoderm. (*Bottom, left*) The location of the embryonic disk and the three germ layers is shown, together with the beginning of the chorionic villi. (*Bottom, right*) The external appearance of the developing mass is shown; the chorionic villi are abundant. (Chaffee, E. E., and Greisheimer, E. M.: *Basic Physiology and Anatomy*, ed. 3. Philadelphia, J. B. Lippincott, 1974)

ment, or *diploid number* of chromosomes, one-half from the spermatozoon and one-half from the ovum. Soon thereafter, the first cell division occurs. In this process, the male and female chromosomes and their genes are mingled and finally split, forming two sets of 46 chromosomes, one set of 46 going to each of the two new cells. This process is repeated again and again until masses containing 8, 16, 32, and 64 cells are produced successively. These early cell divisions produce a morula. At the 8 to 16 cell stage, the dividing ovum is delivered into the uterus (see Fig. 7-5).

Retention in the fallopian tube occupies about three days. The fertilized ovum then spends a period of time, some four days, in the uterine cavity before actual embedding takes place. Thus, a total interval of some seven days elapses between ovulation and implantation. Meanwhile, important changes are taking place in the internal structure of the fertilized ovum. Fluid appears in the center of the mulberry mass which pushes cells to the periphery of the sphere. At the same time it becomes apparent that this external envelope of cells is actually made up of two different layers, an inner and an outer. A specialized portion of the inner layer, after some 260 days, will develop into the long-awaited baby. The outer layer is a sort of foraging unit, called the trophoblast which means "feeding" layer; it is the principal function of these cells to secure food for the embryo (Fig. 7-10).

While the ovum is undergoing these changes, the lining of the uterus, it will be recalled, is making preparations for its reception. Considering that ovulation took place on the fourteenth day of the menstrual cycle and that the tubal journey and the uterine sojourn required 7 days, 21 days of the cycle will have passed before the ovum has developed its trophoblastic layer of cells. This is the period when the lining of the uterus has reached its greatest thickness and succulence. In other words, the timing has been precisely correct; the bed is prepared, and the ovum has so developed that it is now ready to embed itself.

Implantation of the ovum

The embedding of the ovum is the work of the outer foraging layer of cells, the *trophoblast*, which possesses the peculiar property of being able to digest or liquefy the tissues with which it comes into contact. This process

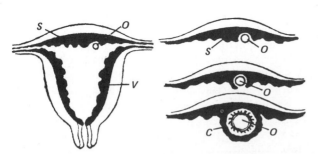

Figure 7-11. Various stages in the process of implantation; the relation of the uterine mucosa to the embryonic vesicle during implantation is shown: (s) decidua basalis, (v) decidua vera, (c) decidua capsularis, and (o) the ovum or embryonic vesicle. (Greisheimer, E. M.: *Physiology and Anatomy*, ed. 8, p. 809, Fig. 421. Philadelphia, J. B. Lippincott, 1963)

is carried out by means of enzymes. In this manner these cells not only burrow into the uterine lining and eat out a nest for the ovum, but also digest the walls of the many small blood vessels that they encounter beneath the surface. The mother's bloodstream is thus tapped, and presently the ovum finds itself deeply sunk in the lining epithelium of the uterus, with tiny pools of blood around it (Fig. 7-11). Sprouting out from the trophoblastic layer, fingerlike projections now develop and extend greedily into the blood-filled spaces. Another name for the trophoblast, and one more commonly employed as pregnancy progresses, is the *chorion*; the fingerlike projections are *chorionic villi*. These chorionic villi contain blood vessels connected with the fetus and are extremely important, because they are the sole means by which oxygen and nourishment are received from the mother. The entire ovum becomes covered with villi, which grow out radially and convert the chorion into a shaggy sac.

The cells of the chorionic villi begin to produce HCG. This hormone maintains progesterone production by the corpus luteum. In turn, progesterone stimulates and supports endometrial growth, providing suitable environment for continued development of the conceptus.

Suggested Reading

HAFEZ, E. S. E., AND BLANDAU, R. J.: *The Mammalian Oviduct*. Chicago, U. of Chicago Press, 1969.

SEITZ, H. M., BRACKETT, B. G., AND MASTROIANNI, L., JR.: Fertilization. *In* Hafez, E. S. E., and Evans, T. N.: *Human Reproduction: Conception and Contraception*. Hagerstown, Md., Harper and Row, 1973, pp. 119-131.

development and physiology of the embryo and fetus

Decidua / The Three Germ Layers / Amnion, Chorion, Placenta / Size and Development of Fetus / Duration of Pregnancy / Expected Date of Confinement / Physiology of the Fetus / Periods of Development

With completion of implantation, the fertilized ovum has survived a series of delicately programmed events. It has been released from its follicle within the ovary, the miotic process having been initiated. Following ovulation the ovum has been transported successfully into the lumen of the fallopian tube. There a single, properly conditioned spermatozoon has traversed the barriers surrounding the ovum to initiate the fertilization process. Ovum miosis is completed, and there is fusion of the male and female genetic components, followed by a series of mitotic divisions. Three days later the ovum, now multicellular, is ushered out of the fallopian tube into the uterus. It lingers free in the uterine cavity, bathed in uterine fluid while it develops further into a blastocyst. Implantation occurs on about the seventh postfertilization day and the conceptus begins to derive its nourishment from the blood and tissue juices of the endometrium. As development continues, the conceptus begins to produce HCG which maintains production of progesterone by the corpus luteum. Thus, the newly formed pregnancy is now essentially self-sufficient and is in control of its own environment. Support of the corpus luteum by HCG results in continued maintenance of the endometrium by progesterone, and the next expected menstrual period is missed. At this point the conceptus is traditionally referred to as an embryo.

Throughout this two-week interval, there is a substantial incidence of pregnancy loss. It is estimated that 35 percent of fertilized ova develop abnormally and fail to progress beyond two weeks. Such a pregnancy loss is not surprising when one considers the complicated series of events which culminate in a successfully implanted pregnancy.

From the second week on, development occurs relatively rapidly. The mechanisms which support pregnancy, as the now nearly self-sufficient embryo develops, will be considered in this chapter.

Decidua

The thickening of the uterine endometrium, which occurs during the premenstrual phase of menstruation, was described in Chapter 6. If pregnancy ensues, this endometrium becomes even more thickened, the cells enlarge, and the structure becomes known as the *decidua*. It is simply a direct continuation in exaggerated

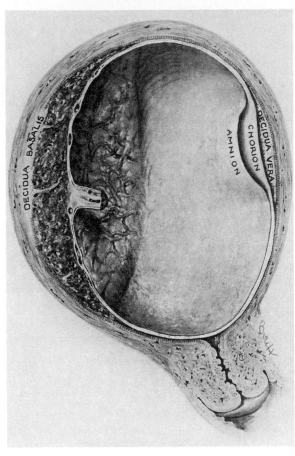

Figure 8-1. Amniotic cavity, placenta, and membranes (amnion and chorion).

three main groups: an outer covering layer (ectoderm), a middle layer (mesoderm), and an internal layer (entoderm).

From the *ectoderm* the following structures are derived: the epithelium of the skin, hair, nails, sebaceous glands and sweat glands; the epithelium of the nasal and oral passages; salivary glands and mucous membranes of the mouth and nose; the enamel of the teeth; and the nervous system. From the *mesoderm* are derived: muscles, bone, cartilage, the dentin of the teeth, ligaments, tendons, areolar tissue, kidneys, ureters, ovaries, testes, the heart, blood, lymph and blood vessels, and the lining of the pericardial, pleural, and peritoneal cavities. From the *entoderm* arise: the epithelium of the digestive tract, and the glands which pour their secretion into this tract; the epithelium of the respiratory tract (except for the nose) and of the bladder; the urethra, the thyroid, and the thymus.

Amnion, chorion and placenta

AMNION. However, even before the above noted structures become evident, a fluid-filled space develops about the embryo, a space which is lined with a smooth, slippery, glistening membrane, the *amnion*. The space is the amniotic cavity. Because it is filled with fluid, it is often called the bag of waters; in this the fetus floats and moves. At full term this cavity normally contains from 500 to 1,000 ml. of liquor amnii, or the "waters." The amniotic fluid has a number of important functions: it keeps the fetus at an even temperature, cushions it against possible injury, and provides a medium in which it can move easily; furthermore, it is known that the fetus drinks this fluid. At the end of the fourth month of pregnancy, the amniotic cavity has enlarged to the size of a large orange and, with the fetus, occupies the entire interior of the uterus.

CHORION. As explained in Chapter 7, the early ovum is covered on all sides by shaggy chorionic villi, but very shortly those villi which invade the decidua basalis enlarge and multiply rapidly. This portion of the trophoblast is the *chorion frondosum* (leafy chorion). Conversely, the chorionic villi covering the remainder of the fetal envelope degenerate and almost disappear, leaving only a slightly roughened membrane, the *chorion laeve* (bald chorion). The chorion laeve lies outside of the amnion, of course, with which it is in contact

form of the already modified premenstrual mucosa.

For purposes of description, the decidua is divided into three portions. The part which lies directly under the embedded ovum is the *decidua basalis* (Fig. 8-1). The portion which is pushed out by the embedded and growing ovum is the *decidua capsularis*. The remaining portion, which is not in immediate contact with the ovum, is the *decidua vera*. As pregnancy advances, the decidua capsularis expands rapidly over the growing embryo and at about the fourth month lies in intimate contact with the decidua vera.

The three germ layers

With nutritional facilities provided, the cells which are destined to form the baby grow rapidly. At first they all look alike, but soon after embedding, certain groups of cells assume distinctive characteristics and differentiate into

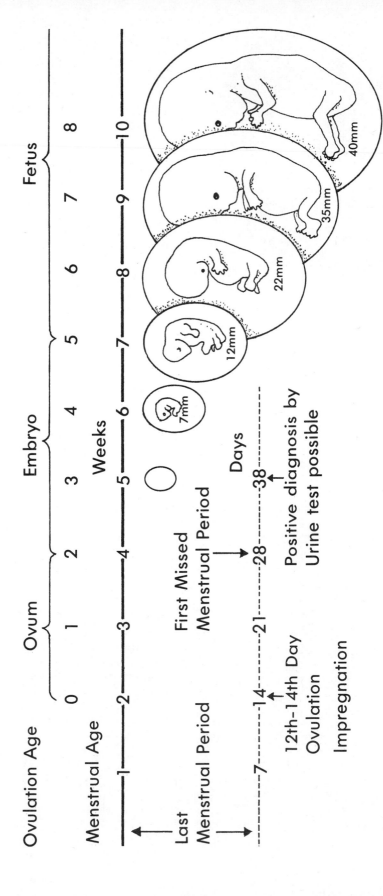

Figure 8-2. Growth of ovum, embryo, and fetus during the early weeks of pregnancy.

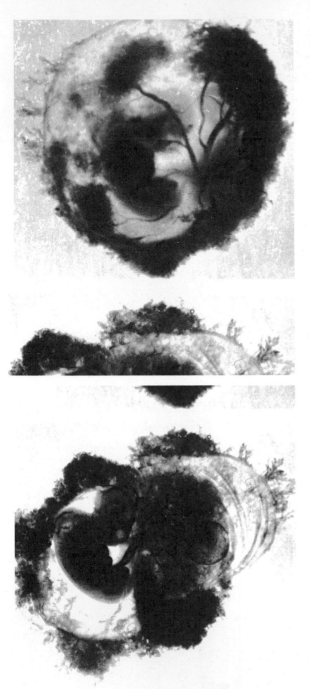

Figure 8-3. Human embryo at approximately 35 days. Length 7 mm. (Top) In the closed sac. (Bottom) In the open sac. (Wesley Kaswell, University Hospitals of Cleveland)

PLACENTA. By the third month, another important structure, the placenta, has formed. This is a fleshy, disklike organ; late in pregnancy it measures about 8 inches in diameter and 1 inch in thickness. It receives its name from the Latin word meaning flat cake, which this structure resembles somewhat in shape. The placenta is formed by the union of the chorionic villi and the decidua basalis. An analogous situation is seen when a tree or a plant sends down its roots into a bed of earth for nourishment; when the plant is removed, a certain amount of the earthy bed clings to the interlocking roots. Similarly, a thin layer of the uterine bed clings to the branching projections of chorionic villi, and together they make up this organ which supplies food to the fetus, as the roots and the earth provide nourishment for a plant. At term the placenta weighs about 500 Gm., or 1 pound. Its fetal surface is smooth and glistening, being covered by amnion, and beneath this membrane may be seen a number of large blood vessels (see Plates 1 and 2). The maternal surface is red and fleshlike in character and is divided into a number of segments, or *cotyledons*, about 1 inch in diameter.

The placenta and the fetus are connected by the *umbilical cord*, or funis, which is usually about 20 inches in length and about ¾ inch in diameter. The cord leaves the placenta near the center and enters the abdominal wall of the fetus at the umbilicus, a trifle below the middle of the median line in front. It contains two arteries and one large vein, which are twisted upon each other and are protected from pressure by a transparent, bluish-white, gelatinous substance called *Wharton's jelly*.

Size and development of the fetus

Size at various months

The physician, as well as the nurse, is sometimes called upon to estimate the intrauterine age of a fetus which has been expelled prematurely.

In general, length affords a more accurate criterion of the age of the fetus than weight. Haase's rule suggests that, for clinical purposes, the length of the embryo in centimeters may be approximated during the first five months by squaring the number of the month to which the pregnancy has advanced; in the second half of pregnancy, by multiplying the month by five. Conversely, the approximate age of the fetus may be obtained by taking the square root of its length in centimeters during

on its inner surface, while its outer surface lies against the decidua vera. The fetus is thus surrounded by two membranes, the amnion and the chorion, and in ordinary clinical discussions these are usually referred to simply as "the membranes."

the first five months, and thereafter by dividing its length in centimeters by five. For instance, a fetus 16 cm. long is about four months old; a 35-cm. fetus is about seven months old.

Development month by month

Most women consider themselves one month pregnant at the time of the first missed menstrual period, two months pregnant at the second missed period, and so on. Since conception does not take place until ovulation, 14 days after the onset of menstruation in a 28-day cycle, it is obvious that an embryo does not attain the age of one month until about a fortnight after the first missed period (assuming a 28-day cycle), and its "birthday" by months regularly falls two weeks or so after any numerically specified missed period. If the cycle is longer than 28 days, or if ovulation was delayed in the conceptive cycle, the duration of actual pregnancy, relative to the last menstrual period, will be shorter. This should be remembered in evaluating the month-by-month development of the fetus. In speaking of the age of a pregnancy in months, physicians use the term *lunar months*, that is, periods of four weeks. Since a lunar month corresponds to the usual length of the menstrual cycle, it's easier to "figure" in this way (Fig. 8-2, p. 109).

Month by month, the fetus develops as follows:

END OF FIRST LUNAR MONTH. The embryo is about ¼ inch long if measured in a straight line from head to tail—for it does have a tail at this early stage—and recognizable traces of all organs have become differentiated. The backbone is apparent but is so bent upon itself that the head almost touches the tip of the tail. At one end of the backbone, the head is extremely prominent, representing almost one-third of the entire embryo. (Throughout intra-uterine life, the head is always very large in proportion to the body, a relationship which is still present, although to a lesser degree, at birth.) The rudiments of the eyes, the ears, and the nose now make their appearance. The tube which will form the future heart has been formed, producing a large, rounded bulge on the body wall; even at this early age this structure is pulsating regularly and propelling blood

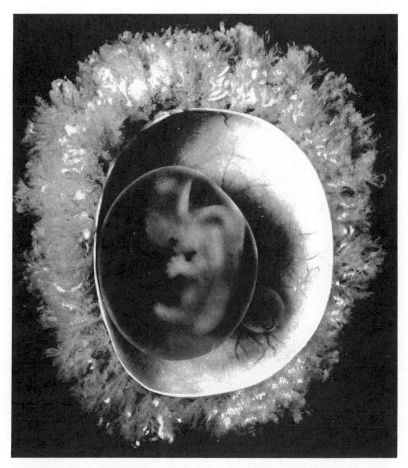

Figure 8-4. Human embryo photographed by Chester F. Reather. This specimen represents about 40 days' development and is shown in the opened chorion. It is reproduced at a magnification of 1.7. (Carnegie Institution, Washington, D.C.)

development and physiology of the embryo and fetus   111

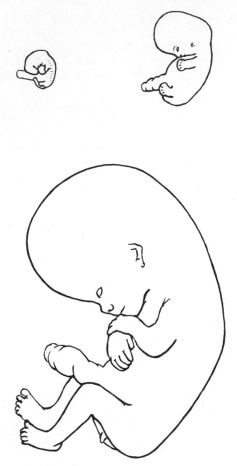

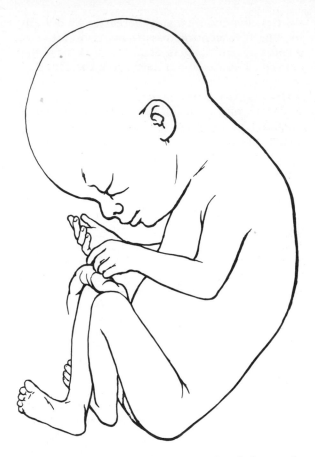

Figure 8-6. Actual size of fetus at approximately four months.

Figure 8-5. Actual size of fetus at approximately one, two, and three months, respectively. (Eastman, N. J., and Russell, K. P.: *Expectant Motherhood*, ed. 5. Boston, Little, Brown, 1970)

through microscopic arteries. The rudiments of the future digestive tract are also discernible—a long, slender tube leading from the mouth to an expansion in the same tube which will become the stomach; connected with the latter the beginnings of the intestines may be seen. The incipient arms and legs are represented by small nubbins that resemble buds (Fig. 8-3, p. 110).

END OF SECOND LUNAR MONTH. The fetus, the term used to refer to the product of conception after the fifth week of gestation, now begins to assume human form (Fig. 8-4). Due to the development of the brain, the head becomes disproportionately large so that the nose, the mouth, and the ears become relatively less prominent. It has an unmistakably human face and also arms and legs, with fingers, toes, elbows, and knees. During the past four weeks it has quadrupled in length and measures about 1 inch from head to buttocks; its weight is approximately 1/30 of an ounce.

The external genitalia become apparent, but it is difficult to distinguish between male and female. During the second month, the human tail reaches its greatest development, but by the end of the month it is less prominent and then undergoes retrogression.

END OF THIRD LUNAR MONTH. The fetus is somewhat over 3 inches long and weighs almost 1 ounce. The sex can now be distinguished because the external genitalia are beginning to show definite signs of sex. Centers of ossification have appeared in most bones; the fingers and the toes have become differentiated, and the fingernails and the toenails appear as fine membranes. Early in this month, buds for all the temporary "baby" teeth are present, and sockets for these develop in the jawbone. Rudimentary kidneys have developed and secrete small amounts of urine into the bladder, which in all probability escape later into the amniotic fluid. Movements of the fetus are known to occur at this time, but they are too weak to be felt by the mother (Fig. 8-5).

END OF FOURTH LUNAR MONTH. The fetus from head to toe is now 6½ inches long and weighs about 4 ounces. The sex, as evidenced by the external genital organs, is now quite obvious (Fig. 8-6).

END OF FIFTH LUNAR MONTH. The length of the fetus now approximates 10 inches, while its weight is about 8 ounces. A fine downy growth of hair, *lanugo*, appears on the skin over the entire body. Usually, about this time the mother becomes conscious of slight fluttering movements in her abdomen, which are due to movements of the fetus. Their first appearance is referred to as *quickening*, or the perception of

life. At this period the physician often is able to hear the fetal heart for the first time. If a fetus is born now, it may make a few efforts to breathe, but its lungs are insufficiently developed to cope with conditions outside the uterus, and it invariably succumbs within a few hours at most (Fig. 8-7).

END OF SIXTH LUNAR MONTH. The length of the fetus is 12 inches, and its weight is 1½ pounds. It now resembles a miniature baby, with the exception of the skin, which is wrinkled and red with practically no fat beneath

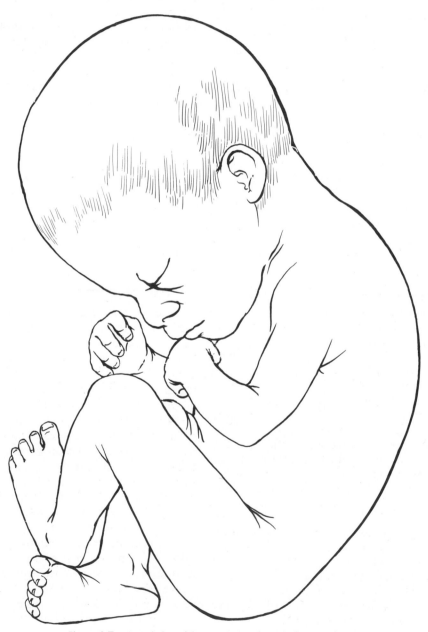

Figure 8-7. Actual size of fetus at approximately five months.

development and physiology of the embryo and fetus   113

Table 8-1 Deviation From Calculated Date of Confinement, According to Naegele's Rule, of 4,656 Births of Mature Infants

Deviation in Days	Early Delivery	Delivery on Calculated Date	Late Delivery
0		189 (4.1)*	—
1–5	860 (18.5)*	—	773 (16.6)*
6–10	610 (13.1)	—	570 (12.2)
11–20	733 (15.7)	—	459 (9.9)
21–30	211 (4.5)	—	134 (2.9)
31 and over	75 (1.6)	—	42 (0.9)

The menstrual cycles of the mothers were 28 ± 5 days. The infants were at least 47 cm. in length and 2,600 Gm. in weight (Burger and Korompai).

* Numbers in parentheses represent percent of cases considered.

Source: Eastman, N. J., and Hellman, L. H.: *Williams Obstetrics*, ed. 13. New York, Appleton-Century Crofts, 1966, p. 220.

it. At this time, however, the skin begins to develop a protective covering, *vernix caseosa*, which means cheesy varnish. This fatty, cheesy substance adheres to the skin of the fetus and at term may be ⅛ inch thick. Although a few cases are on record in which fetuses of this size have survived, the outlook must be regarded as practically hopeless.

END OF SEVENTH LUNAR MONTH. The fetus measures about 15 inches in length and weighs approximately 2½ pounds. If born at this time, it has some chance of survival, at least one in ten. There is a widespread notion, quite incorrect, that infants born at the seventh month are more likely to survive than those born at the eighth month. This is another of those old superstitions which have descended through more than 2,000 years from the time of the ancient Greek physicians. They believed that the fetus is born by means of its own effort; that is, it pushes with its legs against the upper part of the womb and wriggles out into the world. It was their opinion that the fetus first attempts to escape from the uterus at the seventh month and, if strong, it succeeds. If the attempt fails, it is repeated at the eighth month. However, if it now succeeds, it is so exhausted as the result of the previous attempt that it is more likely to die than if it had been successful in the prior attempt a month earlier. We now know, of course, that the fetus is entirely passive, that it is expelled from the mother's body solely through the muscular action of the uterus, and that this old belief is wholly fallacious. The fetus born at the eighth month stands a much better chance of survival than one born at the seventh.

END OF EIGHTH LUNAR MONTH. The fetus measures about 16.5 inches and weighs approximately 4 pounds. Its skin is still red and wrinkled, and vernix caseosa and lanugo are still present. In appearance it resembles a little old man. With proper incubator and good nursing care, infants born at the end of the eighth month have better than even chances of survival, possibly as high as three chances in four.

END OF NINTH LUNAR MONTH. For all practical purposes the fetus is now a mature infant, measures some 19 inches and weighs approximately 6 pounds. Due to the deposition of subcutaneous fat, the body has become more rotund and the skin less wrinkled and red. As though to improve its appearance before making its debut into the world, the fetus devotes the last two months in the uterus to putting on weight; and during this period gains ½ pound a week. Its chances of survival are now as good as though born at full term.

MIDDLE OF TENTH LUNAR MONTH. Full term has now been reached, and the fetus weighs on an average about 7 pounds if a girl and 7½ if a boy; its length approximates 20 inches. Its skin is now white or pink and thickly coated with the cheesy vernix. The fine, downy hair which previously covered its body has largely disappeared. The fingernails are firm and protrude beyond the end of the fingers (Fig. 8-8).

Duration of pregnancy

The length of pregnancy varies greatly; it may range, indeed, between such wide extremes as 240 days and 300 days and yet be entirely normal in every respect. The average duration from the time of conception is 9½ lunar months, that is, 38 weeks or 266 days. From the first day of the last menstrual period its average length is 10 lunar months, that is, 40 weeks or 280 days. That these average figures mean very little, however, is shown by the following facts. Scarcely one pregnancy in ten terminates exactly 280 days after the beginning of the last period. Less than one-half terminate within one week of day 280. In 10 percent of cases, birth occurs a week or more before the theoretical end of pregnancy, and in another 10 percent, it takes place more than two weeks later than we would expect from the average figures cited above. Indeed, it would appear that some fetuses require a longer time, others a shorter time, in the uterus for full development.

Calculation of the expected date of confinement

In view of the wide variation in the length of pregnancy, it is obviously impossible to predict the expected day of confinement (often abbreviated EDC) with any degree of precision. The time-honored method, based on the above "average figures," is simple. Count back three calendar months from the first day of the last menstrual period and add seven days (Naegele's rule). For instance, if the last menstrual period began on June 10, we would count back three months to March and, adding seven days, arrive at the date of March 17. An easier way to calculate this is to substitute numbers for months. Then, this example becomes: $6/10 - 3$ months $= 3/10 + 7$ days $= 3/17$. Although it may be satisfying to the curiosity to have this date in mind, it must be understood that less than 5 percent of all pregnant women go into labor on the estimated date of confinement, and in 35 percent a deviation of from one to five days before or after this date may be expected (Table 8-1).

Yet, whether pregnancy terminates one week before or two weeks later than the day calcu-

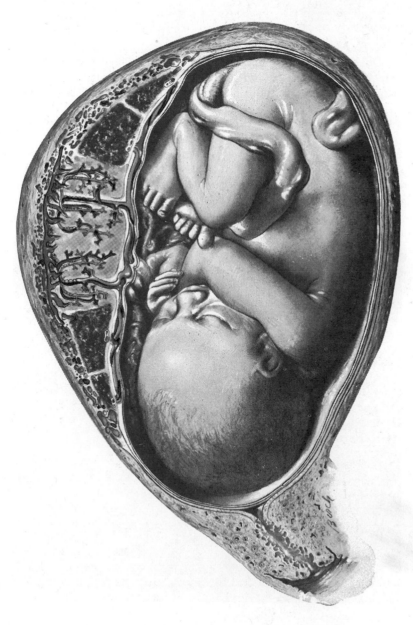

Figure 8-8. Full-term fetus in utero, with placental circulation shown in color.

lated, the outlook for mother and baby is usually as good as though it had ended at "high noon" on the due date. Actually, women seldom go overterm; in most of these cases it is the system of calculation and not Nature which has erred. For example, ovulation and, hence, conception may have occurred some days later than calculated; this error would make the beginning and the end of pregnancy that many days later. If, in addition to this circumstance, we were dealing with a baby which required a slightly longer stay in the uterus for complete development, it would be clear that the apparent delay was quite normal and for the best.

Physiology of the fetus

Nutrition; placental transmission

During the period when the ovum lies unattached in the uterine cavity, its nutriment is provided by an endometrial secretion, often called *uterine milk*, which is rich in glycogen. When burrowing into the endometrium, the ovum lies in a lake of fluid representing the broken-down product of endometrial cells and obtains nourishment from this source.

Very early in pregnancy, certainly by the third or the fourth week, the chorionic villi have blood vessels within them (connected with the fetal bloodstream), and since these villi have already opened up the maternal blood vessels, nourishment is available from the maternal blood by the process of *osmosis*. Such substances as oxygen and glucose in the maternal blood must diffuse through several layers of tissue of the chorionic villi to reach the fetus. These layers are the cellular epithelium covering each villus, the loose connective tissue within it, and finally the endothelium of the capillary blood vessel in the center of the villus. In this manner, oxygen passes into the fetal circulation, while the fetal waste product, carbon dioxide, diffuses in the opposite direction. The placenta thus serves as the lungs of the baby in utero. Simple food substances, such as glucose, salt, calcium, phosphorus, iron, amino acids, and fatty acids, all diffuse through the chorionic villi to the fetus by this process of osmosis.

It is particularly important to note that most drugs pass readily to the fetus and, if given to the mother very shortly before birth, may affect the newborn baby. In addition to this, maternal estrogen is transmitted to the fetus and produces certain effects in the newborn which may be very striking. First, as the result of the action of this hormone, the breasts of both boy and girl babies may become mark-

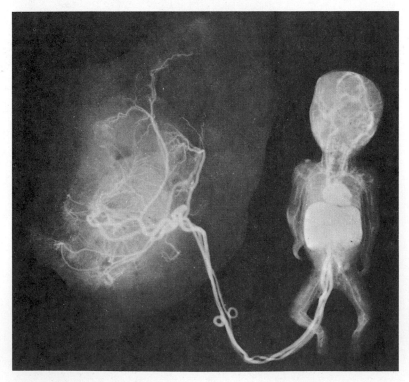

Figure 8-9. Roentgenogram showing fetal and placental circulation at 11 weeks gestation, injected with Thorotrast (a contrast medium) by Charles H. Hendricks, M.D., and Frederick P. Zuspan, M.D. (Department of Obstetrics and Gynecology, Western Reserve University)

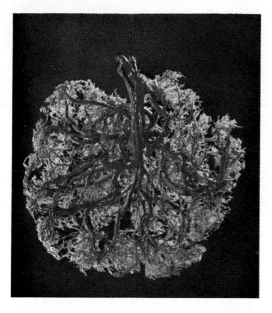

PLATE 1. Placenta stripped to the main vessels. Arteries are red; veins, blue. (Life Magazine. Picture taken by Rudolph Skarda Research Anatomist, University of California, San Francisco, Calif.)

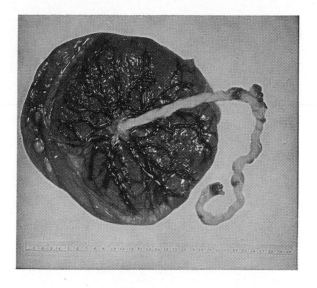

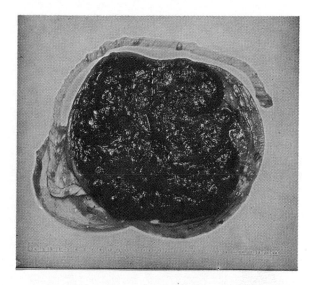

PLATE 2. (*Top*) Fetal surface of placenta. (*Bottom*) Maternal surface of placenta.

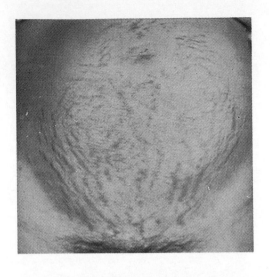

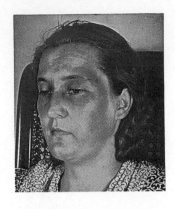

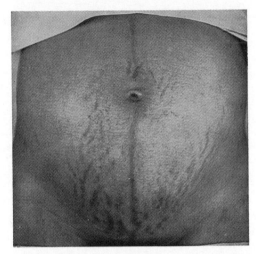

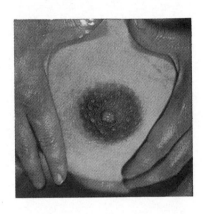

PLATE 3. (*Left, top*) Striae gravidarum.
(*Left, bottom*) Linea nigra and also striae gravidarum.
(*Right, top*) Mask of pregnancy (chloasma).
(*Right, bottom*) Montgomery's tubercles.

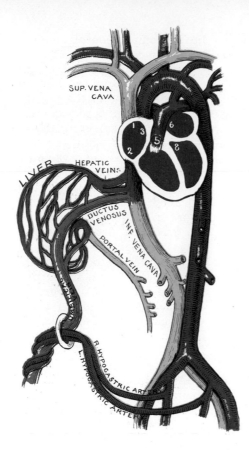

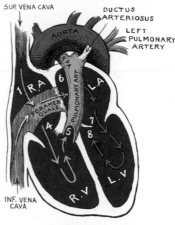

1 OPENING OF SUP. VENA CAVA
2 OPENING OF INF. VENA CAVA
3 FORAMEN OVALE
4 TRICUSPID VALVE TO R. VENTRICLE
5 PULMONARY VALVE
6 OPENING FROM PULMONARY VEINS
7 BICUSPID OR MITRAL VALVES
8 AORTIC VALVE

Figure 8-10. (*Left*) Fetal circulation before birth. The material needed for the nourishment and the development of the fetus is brought to it from the placenta by way of the umbilical vein. Since the lungs do not function in the exchange of gases, the placenta serves as the respiratory organ in supplying oxygen to the fetus and also as an excretory organ for waste products. After the blood is purified in the placenta, it is sent with its nutritive material to the fetus by way of the umbilical vein; this vein divides into two branches after entering the abdominal wall. One of these branches joins directly to the portal vein which empties its blood into the liver, from which it is carried to the inferior vena cava by way of the hepatic veins. The other branch, the ductus venosus, joins directly the inferior vena cava, from which the blood is then carried to the right auricle of the heart. From the right auricle it goes through the foramen ovale to the left auricle and then to the left ventricle to the upper extremity by way of the aorta.

The blood returning from the upper extremity through the superior vena cava enters the right auricle, then the right ventricle, and then goes to the lungs by way of the pulmonary artery. Since the lungs do not function before birth, only a small portion of this blood gains access to them. Most of the blood from the pulmonary artery is diverted through the ductus arteriosus to the aorta and is then carried to the trunk and lower extremities.

(*Right*) Fetal circulation after birth. Pulmonary circulation becomes established with birth. The umbilical cord circulation ceases. The arteries and the vein become obliterated immediately at the body junction. Shortly the hypogastric arteries, which are a continuance of the umbilical arteries after entrance into the body, become obliterated at their distal ends, followed by occlusion and obliteration of the umbilical vein and ductus venosus. The ductus arteriosus and the foramen ovale undergo a slower metamorphosis, finally occluding the circulation through the ductus arteriosus and closure of the foramen ovale. (Philips J. Carter, M.D., Louisiana State University, New Orleans)

edly enlarged during the first few days of life and even secrete milk—the so-called witch's milk (see Chapter 21, Breast Engorgement). Second, estrogen causes the endometrium of the female fetus to hypertrophy, as it does that of an adult woman. After birth, when this hormone is suddenly withdrawn, the endometrium breaks down, and sometimes bleeding occurs. For this reason, perhaps one girl baby in every

fifteen manifests a little spotting on the diaper during the first week of life. This is entirely normal and clears up by itself within a few days.

Fetal circulation

Since the placenta acts as the intermediary organ of transfer between mother and fetus, the fetal circulation differs from that required for extrauterine existence. The fetus receives oxygen through the placenta, since the lungs do not function as organs of respiration in utero. To meet this situation, the fetal circulation contains certain special vessels ("bypasses" or "detours") which shunt the blood around the lungs, with only a small amount circulating through them for nutrition (Fig. 8-9, p. 116).

The oxygenated blood flows up the cord through the umbilical vein and passes into the inferior vena cava; on the way to the inferior vena cava, part of the oxygenated blood has gone through the liver, but most of it has passed through a special fetal structure, the *ductus venosus*, which connects the umbilical vein and the inferior vena cava (Fig. 8-10). The liver is proportionately so large in a newborn infant because it receives a considerable supply of freshly vitalized blood directly from the umbilical vein.

From the inferior vena cava, the current flows into the right auricle and goes directly on to the left auricle through a special fetal structure, the *foramen ovale*, passing thence into the left ventricle and out through the aorta. The blood which circulates up the arms and the head returns through the superior vena cava to the right auricle again, but instead of passing through the foramen ovale, as before, the current is deflected downward into the right ventricle and out through the pulmonary arteries, partly to the lungs (for purposes of nutrition only), but mainly into the aorta through the special fetal structure, the *ductus arteriosus*.

The blood in the aorta, with the exception of that which goes to the head and the upper extremities (this blood has been accounted for), passes downward to supply the trunk and the lower extremities (Fig. 8-10). The greater part of this blood finds its way through the internal iliac, or hypogastric arteries, and so back through the cord to the placenta, where it is again oxygenated; but a small amount passes back into the ascending vena cava to mingle with fresh blood from the umbilical vein and again make the circuit of the entire body.

Circulation change at birth

The fetal circulation is so arranged that the passage of blood to the placenta through the umbilical arteries and back through the umbilical vein is possible up to the time of birth, but it ceases entirely the moment the baby breathes and so begins to take its oxygen directly from its own lungs. During intrauterine life the circulation of blood through the lungs is for the nourishment of the lungs and not for the purpose of securing oxygen (Fig. 8-10).

In order to understand, even in a general way, the course of the blood current and how it differs from the circulation after birth, it must be remembered that in infants after birth, as in the adult, the venous blood passes from the two venae cavae into the right auricle of the heart, thence to the right ventricle and through the pulmonary arteries to the lungs, whence it gives up its waste products and takes up a fresh supply of oxygen. After oxygenation, the so-called arterial blood flows from the lungs, through the pulmonary veins to the left auricle, thence to the left ventricle and out through the aorta, to be distributed through the capillaries to all parts of the body and eventually collected, as venous blood, in the venae cavae and discharged again into the right auricle.

Circulation path after birth

As soon as the baby is born and breathes, the function of the lungs is established, and the placental circulation ceases. This change not only alters the character of the blood in many vessels, but also makes many of these vessels of no use as such: the umbilical arteries within the baby's body become filled with clotted blood and ultimately are converted into fibrous cords, and the umbilical vein within the body, after occlusion of the vessel, becomes the round ligament of the liver. After the umbilical cord is tied and separated, the large amount of blood returned to the heart and the lungs, which are now functioning, causes more or less equal pressure in both of the auricles—this pressure causes the foramen ovale to close. The foramen ovale remains closed and eventually disappears, and the ductus arteriosus and the ductus venosus finally shrivel up and are converted into fibrous cords or ligaments in the course of two or three months. The instantaneous closure of the foramen ovale changes the entire course of the blood current and converts the fetal circulation into the adult type.

The changes in the fetal circulation after birth are shown in Table 8-2.

Periods of development

For the purposes of classification, human life has been divided into periods. The succes-

Table 8-2 Changes in Fetal Circulation After Birth

Structure	Before Birth	After Birth
Umbilical vein	Brings arterial blood to liver and heart.	Obliterated. Becomes the round ligament of liver.
Umbilical arteries	Bring arteriovenous blood to the placenta.	Obliterated. Become vesical ligaments on anterior abdominal wall.
Ductus venosus	Shunts arterial blood into inferior vena cava.	Obliterated. Becomes ligamentum venosum.
Ductus arteriosus	Shunts arterial and some venous blood from the pulmonary artery to the aorta.	Obliterated. Becomes ligamentum arteriosum.
Foramen ovale	Connects right and left auricles (atria).	Obliterated usually. At times open.
Lungs	Contain no air and very little blood.	Filled with air and well supplied with blood.
Pulmonary arteries	Bring little blood to lungs.	Bring much blood to lungs.
Aorta	Receives blood from both ventricles.	Receives blood only from left ventricle.
Inferior vena cava	Brings venous blood from body and arterial blood from placenta.	Brings venous blood only to right auricle.

Source: Williams, J. F.: *Anatomy and Physiology*, ed. 7. Philadelphia, W. B. Saunders.

sive periods, with the duration of each, are indicated below.

THE PERIOD OF THE OVUM extends from fertilization to implantation, about the close of the first week of prenatal life. (The term ovum is used in a strict sense to denote the female germ cell and also to indicate the developing zygote, or fertilized ovum, prior to implantation.)

THE PERIOD OF THE EMBRYO extends from the second to the fifth weeks of gestation, during which time the various organs are developed, and a definite form is assumed.

THE PERIOD OF THE FETUS extends from after the fifth week to the time of birth.

THE PERIOD OF THE NEWBORN (NEONATAL) extends from birth to the close of the first month of postnatal life.

THE PERIOD OF INFANCY extends from the close of the first month to the close of the second year of life (Nelson's Textbook of Pediatrics, Saunders, 1959).

THE PERIOD OF CHILDHOOD extends from the close of the second year to about the fourteeth year in females and to about the sixteenth year in males. Puberty ends the period of childhood.

THE PERIOD OF ADOLESCENCE extends from puberty to the last years of the second decade (late teens) in females and to the first years of the third decade (early 20s) in males.

THE PERIOD OF MATURITY extends from the end of the adolescent period to senility (old age).

Development goes on throughout life; during senility, retrogressive or degenerative changes occur.

Maternal impressions

One of the commonest superstitions relating to childbearing is the old belief that the mental condition of the mother may modify the development of the unborn infant or, as people used to say, "mark it." For instance, if a pregnant woman were frightened by some ugly beast, it used to be thought that when the baby was born, it might be "marked" or distorted in the likeness of the animal. Very often the marking took the form of reddish blotches on the skin of the infant, which in the mother's imagination seemed to resemble the beast. Or, sometimes it was thought that the blotch resembled some article of food that the pregnant woman particularly craved.

This belief, like most obstetric superstitions, is of hoary antiquity. The Biblical story of Jacob and the "speckled and spotted" cattle and goats and the "brown" sheep reflects it, and dramatists and novelists from Shakespeare to Dickens have perpetuated the idea in stirring plots. The facts are these: There is no nervous connection between mother and fetus —in other words, no possible pathways along which any such impulses, pleasant or otherwise, could travel. Furthermore, the anlagen for the various organs of the fetus are developed by the sixth week of pregnancy, that is,

development and physiology of the embryo and fetus   119

at a period when most women scarcely realize that they are pregnant; and, almost without exception, the causative mental shock or experience which is alleged to have brought about the marking occurred much later, long after the organ in question was in its final state of formation. Finally, all modern experience refutes the belief. Obstetricians of vast experience, as well as maternity hospitals with thousands of deliveries annually, never have reported an authentic case.

How, then, is this age-old superstition to be explained? A number of factors probably contribute to it, chiefly coincidence. Approximately one baby in every two hundred is born with some kind of blemish. In the event that such a blemish is present—perhaps a reddish blotch on the buttocks of the baby—would it not be easy for an introspective mother, who had been told of this legend, to think finally of some object, some animal, or possibly some article of diet that she craved during pregnancy and, in her imagination, correlate it with the little red blotch?

Suggested Reading

BARNES, A. C.: *Intrauterine Development.* Philadelphia, Lea & Febiger, 1968.

MOORE, K. L.: *The Developing Human.* Philadelphia, W. B. Saunders, 1973.

TORPIN, RICHARD: *The Human Placenta: Its Shape, Form, Origin and Development.* Springfield, Ill., Charles C Thomas, 1969.

clinical aspects of human reproduction

9

Contraception / Permanent Means of Sterilization / Pregnancy Termination / Infertility

Increased levels of technology have introduced an element of choice in reproduction. Yet, during the course of nursing practice, one will surely encounter patients who are pregnant when they do not wish to be or are infertile when pregnancy is consummately desired.

Regulation of fertility is most often expressed in demographic terms. Indeed, population pressures represent a major social force. For the practicing nurse or physician, however, the importance of understanding and controlling reproductive potential is perhaps more cogently expressed in individual terms. The right of choice of the individual has recently been emphasized by international bodies. In 1966, the General Assembly of the United Nations declared that, "The size of the family should be the free choice of each individual family." Three years later, the concept had evolved to include the right to the means to space and limit births.

At the behavioral level, we have witnessed what has been euphemistically termed the "sexual revolution." Sexual intercourse—with its attendant risk of pregnancy—has increasingly supplanted the nonvaginal variations of sexual communication used by earlier generations. Availability of more reliable methods of contraception may have provided some of the impetus for changing sexual attitudes. Be that as it may, as a result of attitudinal changes, contraceptive advice has become all the more important. The alternative choices are formidable. Abortion is not a benign procedure, even when done under ideal conditions. Neither is a hasty marriage, nor carrying pregnancy to term and delivering the child to its adopting parents.

At the other end of the spectrum, fertility is not always a matter of choice. The generally accepted estimate is that about 10 percent of couples are infertile. One can realistically project a rise in the incidence of infertility due to social causes. The increase in the prevalence of gonorrheal salpingitis, and recent changes in women's social orientation—with the concomitant trend toward postponement of childbearing until the late reproductive years—will materially influence reproductive potential. A shortage of children for adoption has created additional pressures. Often the nurse is called upon to act as counselor in what inevitably is an emotionally charged situation—as a couple faces the prospect of a barren marriage. Ideally the nurse should be equipped to schedule and interpret the various tests used in an infertility investigation and to understand, in order to be

Table 9-1   Methods of Contraception Currently Available

Male and Female	Male	Female

ABSTINENCE
  Total
  Periodic
    Rhythm
    Basal Body
       Temperature (BBT)
  Nonvaginal Variations
    Masturbation
      Solitary
      Mutual
    Oralgenital
    Anal Intercourse
	WITHDRAWAL
	CONDOMS
	VASECTOMY
		SPERMICIDES*
		  Foam, Cream, Gels
		  Diaphragm with Gel or Cream
		OVULATION PREVENTION†
		  Oral
		  Injectable
		  Implanted
		UNKNOWN ACTION
		  Minipill
		  Morning-After Pill
		  Intrauterine Device
		    Mechanical
		    Chemical
		    Hormonal
		    Heavy Metals (Copper)
		TUBAL STERILIZATION**

   * Douching is not a contraceptive method.
   † Breast-feeding is not a contraceptive method.
 ** Abortion is not a contraceptive method.
Source: Pierson, E. C.: *Sex Is Never an Emergency*, ed. 3. Philadelphia, J. B. Lippincott, 1973, p. 5.

able to explain to the patient, the physiologic basis for treatment.

The purpose of this chapter is to review the various available methods of family planning—contraception on the one hand and means for promoting fertility on the other. In preceding chapters, basic reproductive mechanisms were discussed and events beginning with spermatogenesis and oogenesis and ending in the development of the term fetus were explored. This information will now serve as a basis for understanding the clinical approach to problems of human reproduction.

Contraception

The role of the nurse

Both the maternity and the community health nurse play an important role in the care of the patient seeking contraceptive advice. The nurse need not advocate a particular method, but the professional nurse has a responsibility to see that help, understanding, and guidance in family planning are available to all parents.

The parents' cultural and religious beliefs must be taken into account. It might be added in this connection that at least one method of contraception has the approval of all religions. Those who are committed to the moral teachings of the Roman Catholic Church realize that the only method which has official sanction is the rhythm method, or variations of rhythm using basal body temperature and/or observations of cervical mucus. The nurse who, in conscience, finds that she cannot give general contraceptive advice should state this to her patients. This will allow them to go elsewhere for the information which they may wish to have.

Certainly, every nurse who will give contraceptive advice needs to be aware of all of the available methods of birth control, and she should be conversant with the advantages and disadvantages of each method, both at the mechanical and psychologic levels. The choice of a suitable contraceptive depends on many factors which vary even from year to year in any couple's contraceptive life span. These factors include expense, bathroom facilities, frequency of intercourse, number of children, the risk of pregnancy the couple wishes to accept, illness, and physical problems.

The nurse should also be acquainted with the increasing availability and acceptability of vasectomy and tubal ligation. Studies have shown that one-fourth to one-third of all couples look to this permanent method of contraception when their families are completed. Currently available methods of contraception are listed in Table 9-1.

General approach to the patient

A number of important principles should be observed as the nurse assists the couple to select a suitable means of contraception. Unlike other health measures, pregnancy prevention ideally involves the participation of both male and female partners. Good family planning programs should encourage participation of the male and provide an opportunity for him to share responsibility for fertility control. A discussion of some of the male methods of contraception, such as withdrawal, the use of condoms, or even vasectomy, then becomes possible, as well as education on rhythm when it is the method of choice. Since family planning deals with the patient's sexuality, a private setting should be arranged whenever possible. The patient's feelings about contraception should be explored in a nonjudgmental way and the variety of choices summarized to allow selection of a method which fits the individual circumstance of the couple. There is no "best method" of contraception, but there is always a method which can work best in the circumstances at hand. It should also be recognized that some patients appearing in a family planning clinic may be there because they may have an infertility problem, or because they wish to have a Pap smear, a breast examination, or an evaluation for venereal disease. Family planning clinics often serve as a patient's initial introduction into the health care system and offer opportunities for general health maintenance.

One of the optimal times for exploring methods of family planning is in the postpartal period. During hospitalization after delivery, the opportunity for patient education is great. Choices can conveniently be reviewed with the patient at that time so that knowledgeable selection of a method can be made. It is general experience that availability of contraceptive advice has resulted in a marked increase in the number of patients returning for postpartal care.

Oral contraception

Oral contraceptives ("the pill") are hormonal agents. The commonly used preparations contain a combination of estrogen and a synthetic progestational agent. They act principally at the central nervous system level to inhibit ovulation. There are secondary effects on uterine and tubal motility and cervical mucus. Under the influence of the progestational agent, the cervical mucus becomes thick, viscous, and unreceptive to spermatozoa. These effects are of minor importance, however, inasmuch as inhibition of ovulation results in the lack of availability of ova. In the standard approach, the pill is administered daily beginning on the fifth day of the menstrual cycle through cycle day 25. Two to three days after the last pill there is usually a "withdrawal" menstrual flow. Since it is possible to control the menstrual cycle with these agents, they are also used extensively in patients with menstrual abnormalities.

In some cases, the amount of menstrual flow decreases markedly and occasionally there is amenorrhea. In such instances, the patient is advised to reinstitute pill taking seven days after administration of the last pill, to obviate the possibility of unexpected ovulation which could occur during a more prolonged period of nonpill taking. When amenorrhea occurs and menstruation is desired, a pill containing a greater amount of estrogen may be tried. If this is ineffective in producing withdrawal flow, one may wish to consider switching to a sequential form of oral contraception. The sequential regimen involves the use of estrogen initially followed, in the last five to six days, with estrogen and a progestational agent in combination. Estrogen stimulates growth of the endometrium, and the estrogen and progestogen together produce changes in the endometrium which are followed by bleeding two to four days after cessation of treatment. The sequential approach has the disadvantage of higher doses of unoppressed estrogen. The estrogen in the pill is thought to be responsible for some of the complications which have been reported with oral contraception.

The theoretical effectiveness of the combined formulation pill approaches 100 percent. In fact, the method failure rate—failure when properly used—is negligible. When patient error is included—and this involves failure to take the pill for one or more days during the cycle—use effectiveness falls to approximately 95 to 98 percent. The discontinuation rate has been reported to be from 20 percent to as high as 50 percent. The reasons for discontinuation include appearance of side effects and untoward symptoms, as well as variations in motivational factors in the populations studied.

Generally accepted, absolute contraindications to oral contraception include thrombophlebitis, thromboembolic disorders, cerebral vascular accident, or a history of any of the three. Other contraindications include marked impairment of liver function, malignancy of the breast or of the reproductive tract, and, of course, pregnancy. Common side effects of the pill include accentuation of premenstrual symptoms, such as mastalgia, irritability, and edema. The most untoward side effect of any contraceptive modality—pregnancy—occurs very rarely and it is generally related to failure to take the pill.

Upon discontinuing the pill, many patients have immediate return of ovulation and menstrual periods. Some, however, may experience a delay in ovulation and, therefore, of menstruation for several months. There is no evidence that future pregnancies are affected by the prior use of oral contraceptives.

Patients on the pill should be seen regularly, ideally at intervals of six months. The initial visit should include assessment of the patient for contraindications to the pill, a blood pressure determination, Pap smear, hematocrit or hemoglobin, urinalysis, and when circumstances dictate, a culture for gonorrhea and a serologic test for syphilis. An alternate method of birth control should be reviewed thoroughly, against the possibility that the patient would discontinue the pill without prior consultation. In many family planning centers, an early follow-up visit at six to twelve weeks is suggested. On that occasion, evidence of side effects and the patient's general attitude are reviewed with specific questions about headaches, blurred vision, chest pain, leg pain, as well as a blood pressure check and an evaluation to be sure the pills are being taken correctly.

Intrauterine device (IUD)

This technique (actually an ancient practice but only recently validated scientifically) involves the insertion into the uterine cavity of a small, usually flexible appliance (Fig. 9-1). This foreign object is allowed to remain in the uterus for as long as contraception is desired. Devices have been made in various shapes (spirals, loops, rings) and of various materials (plastic tubing, nylon thread, stainless steel). Although the mechanism by which these appliances prevent conception is not completely understood, they are about 97 percent effective (three pregnancies in one hundred users with the IUD in place). They rank second only to the oral progestogens and probably equal the properly used diaphragm in the protection they afford. The advantages of intrauterine devices are that they are inexpensive and, once inserted, require no further attention, provided they remain in place. The main drawback of these appliances is that they are frequently expelled, and some have to be removed because of bleeding or cramps. Spontaneous expulsion or necessary removal occurs in from 15 to 20 percent of patients.

Many commonly used IUDs have a nylon string attached. This serves two purposes: 1) it aids in removal, and 2) it allows the patient to check for its presence by palpating the strings at the cervix. The nurse should emphasize to the patient that it is important to check for the presence of the IUD before each sexual exposure during the first several months of use. Beyond this time the chance of spontaneous expulsion without the patient's knowledge is much less, and it is at this time that the quoted 97 percent rate of effectiveness is valid.

The rate of expulsion and removal is greater than 20 percent in patients who have never been pregnant. For this reason many physicians reserve the method for the multiparous patient. There are probably two factors operating here: 1) the irritability of the nulliparous uterus, and 2) lack of sufficient motivation among women who have never been pregnant to tolerate the initial two to three months of cramping and spotting. The severity of these

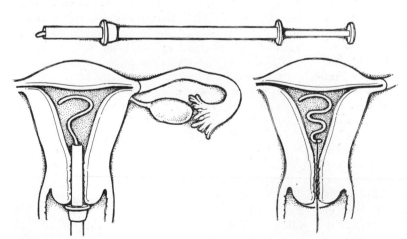

Figure 9-1. (Left) Method of insertion of a Lippes loop. Note location of head which protrudes beyond the cervix.

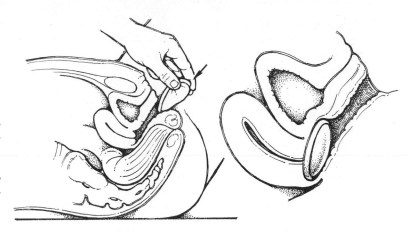

Figure 9-2. *(Left)* Method of manual insertion of diaphragm. Prior to insertion, contraceptive cream or jelly is placed over the dome around the edges of the diaphragm. Plastic inserters are also available for ease of insertion of the diaphragm. *(Right)* Diaphragm in place.

symptoms varies from none to quite severe or intolerable. The IUD is being widely used throughout the world, especially in developing countries, where its low cost and lack of need for continuing motivation constitute particular advantages.

Recently metallic copper has been incorporated in intrauterine devices. These copper-containing devices, shaped like a "T" or "L," appear to be associated with a lower expulsion rate and an increased effectiveness. The copper is slowly delivered from the device into the uterine fluid. For this reason, it is recommended that the copper device be replaced every two to four years. Experimental intra-uterine devices which contain progesterone, slowly released from the device to provide a local effect on the endometrium, may soon become available for general use. These will have to be replaced at intervals because the progesterone is gradually dispersed.

Commonly reported side effects of the IUD include increased menstrual flow, dysmenorrhea, and intermenstrual spotting. Since flow is sometimes excessive, patients should be checked routinely for anemia. They should be instructed to report any fever, pelvic pain or tenderness, or unusual vaginal bleeding, since these may be signs of pelvic infection. If pregnancy occurs when the IUD is in place, removal is recommended. An increased danger of intra-partum infection and deaths from sepsis has been reported among patients whose IUD was allowed to remain in place in pregnancy. The risk of spontaneous abortion is somewhat higher when the IUD remains in place (about 50 percent) than if it is removed when the pregnancy is discovered (25 percent). Another major complication is uterine perforation. This usually occurs at the time the IUD is inserted.

When perforation through the uterine wall into the abdomen occurs, it is generally recommended that the IUD be removed. This can be done with the use of a laparoscope, avoiding an exploratory laparotomy.

Occasionally on insertion, the IUD may produce enough pain and stimulation to result in syncope. The nurse should be aware of this complication and should be ready to place the patient in a recumbent position if there are any signs of lightheadedness, sweating, or nausea.

The diaphragm

The diaphragm is a dome-shaped rubber cup, which may range in diameter from 7 to 10 cm. and is inserted into the vagina and over the anterior vaginal wall and cervix prior to intercourse (Fig. 9-2). The diaphragm, by itself, is not a contraceptive device; it must be used with a spermicidal jelly or cream which is placed in the diaphragm between it and the cervix. The use of the diaphragm insures the placement of spermicidal jelly over the cervix.

A common objection to the diaphragm is the vaginal manipulation necessary to insert it, a procedure which is repugnant to some women. This problem is easily solved if the patient is fitted with a flat or coil-spring diaphragm (in contrast to the arc flex diaphragm). These diaphragms may be used with an "inserter" which allows the patient to insert it like a tampon, without touching the genital area. The arc flex diaphragm cannot be used with an inserter. It was designed for ease of manual insertion and may, in some cases, give a better fit in the presence of a mild cystocele. Some women, after one or more pregnancies cannot be fitted with a diaphragm. The nurse may assure the patient that neither she nor her husband will be aware of the presence of a well-fitted diaphragm.

When the diaphragm is properly used—each time intercourse occurs without exception—it is associated with a failure rate of three pregnancies per one hundred women years, a very acceptable rate. In practice, however, the overall failure rate varies from twenty to twenty-five pregnancies per one hundred women years of use, possibly because of inconsistent use. A diaphragm requires motivation and premeditation, but despite these drawbacks has again gained favor, as some of the disadvantages of the pill and IUD are weighed.

One of the stated disadvantages of prescribing a diaphragm is the office time consumed during fitting and instruction on its use. Increasingly the nurse is called upon to play an active role in both. Sample diaphragms or rings of known size are inserted until a size is found which will cover the cervix and fit snugly behind the symphysis pubis. The patient is then asked to remove the diaphragm by hooking a finger over it just beneath the symphysis and then to reinsert it. Before the patient leaves the office, one should be satisfied that she is able to insert and remove the diaphragm with ease. She should be instructed always to use a spermicidal cream or jelly with the diaphragm, placing some around the rim and in the dome. If intercourse occurs a second or third time, additional spermicidal agent should be inserted for added protection. The diaphragm should be left in place for at least six hours following intercourse. A douche is recommended after removal to remove the remaining jelly or cream.

The condom

If used properly, the condom is an effective contraceptive modality. The patient will probably tell the nurse that she knows this, but that there is really a decrease in "sensation" and that her partner will not use one for the same reason. The nurse might point out that no method of contraception is perfect (i.e., all have some disadvantages for one or both partners and have some anxiety-producing aspects). If used before any penetration, condoms are safe, and they rarely break. This information will help those couples who have anxiety over other forms of contraception.

The condom is applied over the shaft of the penis after erection. Before withdrawal of the penis from the vagina, the condom should be held in place on the penis so that it does not slip off into the vagina. Some condoms are packaged with a lubricant. In some cases, this causes an irritation at the introitus and an unpleasant "stinging" sensation. In general, a lubricant should not be necessary if there is sufficient foreplay to produce the natural lubrication associated with female sexual arousal.

The safe period or rhythm method

The rationale of the safe period or the rhythm method is that when there are regular periods, ovulation occurs at approximately the same time in each cycle (i.e., 14 days prior to the beginning of the next cycle). The ovum is capable of being fertilized only for a period of 48 hours, at the most, after ovulation. Theoretically, therefore, abstinence from sexual intercourse on that day and for the two days before and after (a total of five days) should forestall conception.

In actual experience, however, even normal, regular cycles are often one to two days in either direction (e.g., 28 ± 2 days). This puts the day of ovulation in the same four day range $\pm$ two days, and the period of abstinence must then be, realistically, about eight days. For more accuracy the basal body temperature should be used.

The most important point about the rhythm method and its repeated failures really has more to do with the longevity of the sperm than with the day of ovulation. Sperm are found in the cervical mucus as soon as 20 seconds after ejaculation and as late as seven days after ejaculation. Any motile sperm must be regarded as capable of fertilizing an egg. There are many "day six and day seven" pregnancies that attest to this fact (i.e., that intercourse on day six or seven of a 28-day cycle resulted in pregnancy).

If rhythm is to work, there must be regular cycles and abstinence for at least 14 days out of each 28-day cycle. Intercourse during the first days of a cycle (menses) is not contraindicated, except on an aesthetic basis by some couples nor is it contraindicated during the last five or six days of a cycle, if these can be determined accurately.

ANCILLARY AIDS TO RHYTHM. Use of the basal body temperature provides variation of the rhythm method. Oral temperatures are recorded on a chart daily for three cycles and submitted to the physician or nurse for analysis (see Fig. 6-6 and Chapter 6). Special thermometers are sold at most drugstores for this purpose. An increase in basal body temperature which is sustained indicates that ovulation has occurred.

Temperature chart variation of rhythm is all the more useful if periods are irregular. In general, when a temperature rise of a degree or more is sustained for three days, it can be assumed that ovulation has occurred and that intercourse is safe. Since the time of ovulation cannot accurately be forecast in a given cycle and since the longevity of spermatozoa may occupy several days, abstinence should begin shortly after the end of menses. When cycle length is prolonged the method requires a long period of abstinence.

Self-observed changes in the quality of the cervical mucus are also recommended to time ovulation. When daily observations of cervical mucus are combined with the basal body temperature chart, the approach is called the *symptothermal method*. Characteristically, in the ovulatory cycle there is a rapid increase in the quantity of cervical mucus just prior to ovulation. At that time, the mucus becomes clear and stringy. The patient may observe the presence of such mucus at the introitus or may wipe the cervix to obtain a sample for observation. Subsequent to ovulation, mucus becomes more viscous. When this change is associated with a rise in temperature, it is assumed that ovulation has occurred. Many workers in rhythm clinics have been successful in teaching patients to observe bodily signs associated with ovulation by encouraging increased awareness of such changes. For the couple who has developed a degree of mutual understanding such that prolonged abstinence can be accepted and, especially, when an accidental pregnancy would not be a tragedy or constitute a health hazard, rhythm can be recommended, provided the drawbacks are recognized and accepted.

Douches
Not a method of contraception.

Jellies, creams, suppositories, foams
These contraceptives are inexpensive and available without consulting a physician. They are relatively ineffective, however, because the woman cannot be sure of the placement or

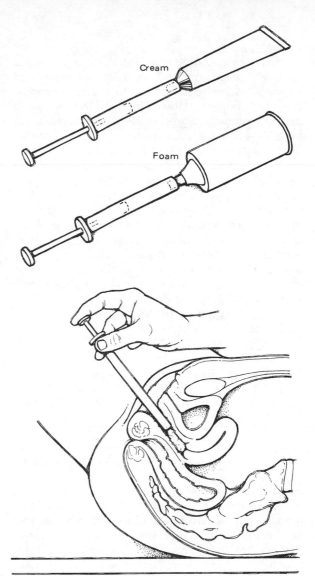

Figure 9-3. Insertion of foam or cream near the cervix.

the retention of the spermicidal agent. These are especially useful for the patient who is contemplating another pregnancy and has been on the pill. She could stop the pill a few months earlier than the time she planned for conception and use a contraceptive (foams, jellies, creams, and the like) that is less effective until her periods are reestablished (Fig. 9-3). Points to be remembered are: 1) The foam or cream should be placed in the vagina no more than one-half hour before intercourse; 2) the agent should be inserted before each intercourse; and 3) the patient should not douche for at least eight hours after intercourse.

Withdrawal

Withdrawal, or *coitus interruptus* is an extensively used method of contraception and appears to be satisfactory to a large proportion of couples. However, withdrawal, as a method of contraception, is a compromise at best. It requires concentration and willpower on the part of the male and trust on the part of the female. This trust is not always well founded and creates anxiety. Neither of these factors is conducive to relaxation and pleasure and may leave the couple with a distorted idea of what sexual pleasure is or can be. Also, there is a preejaculatory secretion which may contain motile spermatozoa. This is especially true when there has been prolonged erection. Despite these drawbacks, many couples are able to develop sufficient expertise so that there is mutual satisfaction while avoiding intravaginal ejaculation.

Contraceptive advice for the postpartal patient

Patients may be reluctant to discuss methods of contraception to be used prior to the postpartal visit because they may have been told by the physician to abstain until the six-week visit. The patient is often more realistic, especially the multiparous patient, and she will discuss this matter with the nurse if given an opportunity. Of all of the methods available, the condom is the most practical for use during this period. Insertion of an IUD and the use of the diaphragm or foams and other spermicidal agents are generally postponed until involution of the uterus is complete. Withdrawal might be suggested if the couple has used this method previously. Some physicians will put their patients on the pill immediately after delivery, whether or not the mother is nursing. Others will not prescribe the pill for use during the nursing period because of the possibility that it suppresses lactation.

Permanent means of sterilization

Increasingly, vasectomy in the male and tubal ligation in the female have gained popularity and acceptability as a means of limiting family size. Both are permanent methods and, therefore, the decision in favor of either must be very carefully considered. In many settings, the role of the nurse in the decision-making process is pivotal. It is the responsibility of the counselor to be sure that both husband and wife are aware that these methods are considered irreversible. Total family circumstances which could influence the decision should be reviewed in depth and such factors as the number of children, stability of the marriage, age of marital partners, and ability to use nonpermanent methods should be considered.

Vasectomy

The *vas deferens* is a tube leading from the testis to the urethra in the male, carrying spermatozoa from the testis to the urethra. It is a firm structure somewhat less than .5 cm. in diameter which can be felt bilaterally in the scrotum, lateral to the base of the penis. *Vasectomy*, which involves surgical interruption and ligation of the vas, is a relatively minor operation. It can be carried out under local anesthesia. It is associated with minimal risk and only slight morbidity. The procedure itself is simple, requires about 15 minutes, and can be done on an outpatient basis. Its major disadvantage is that it is permanent. Although surgical methods have been developed to reanastomose the ligated vas, the success rate is low. Even when a channel is recreated, the spermatozoa which subsequently appear in the ejaculate are not always normal, as they are affected by sperm antibodies which sometimes are produced after ligation. Vasectomy failure is the result of recannulization of the ends of the ligated vas, and occurs in 0.15 per 100 cases. Additional pregnancies occur when unprotected intercourse takes place following vasectomy before the male reproductive tract is cleared of spermatozoa. The first few postvasectomy ejaculates contain active spermatozoa. Except for the absence of spermatozoa, vas ligation does not affect the ejaculate itself, nor does it affect the ejaculatory process.

Tubal ligation

Tubal ligation is, of course, designed to eliminate the passage along which spermatozoa and ova pass. A number of approaches have been used to interrupt the continuity of the fallopian tubes. The procedure may be carried out via an abdominal incision and is commonly done along with cesarean section or in the first few postpartal hours. Many workers in the family planning field now feel that patients should be encouraged not to accept a permanent form of contraception during emotionally charged intervals in their lives. An "on the spot" decision to have a tubal sterilization following an abortion or delivery should be explored with great care.

Coagulation and interruption of the fallopian tubes can be carried out using a *laparoscopic approach* (Fig. 9-4). In some centers this procedure is carried out under local anesthesia, but generally a general anesthetic is utilized. After the abdomen is distended with carbon dioxide, the laparoscopic trocar is introduced through a small incision in the umbilicus. The laparoscope is then passed into the peritoneal cavity. Visualization of the adnexae is usually complete. Using a coagulating instrument the fallopian tubes are grasped, coagulated, and severed. The procedure can be carried out on an outpatient basis. Although it is associated with a relatively low morbidity, the morbidity is considerably higher than for vas ligation.

Although tubal ligation must be considered a permanent method, surgical techniques have been developed to reunite the fallopian tubes. These are difficult procedures at best. The success rate is variable, depending upon the experience of the surgeon and the extent of the segment of tube which was damaged or removed. A decision to attempt reanastomosis is usually based on social circumstances—the death of a child, divorce and remarriage, or an agonizing reappraisal of an earlier decision which was made in haste.

Pregnancy termination

In 1973 there was a substantive change in the legal status of pregnancy termination in the United States. The Supreme Court announced a decision which legalized abortion. Before the end of the first trimester, the decision is left to the judgment of the pregnant woman and her physician. The Court allows regulation of abortion procedures by states when pregnancy is advanced beyond the first trimester, and states can regulate and even proscribe abortion subsequent to viability, defined to be between 24 and 26 weeks gestation, except when necessary for the preservation of the life or health of the mother. As the result of the changed legal status, pregnancy terminations are now being sought and obtained in large numbers throughout the United States.

Availability of legal abortion has dramatically decreased the maternal mortality and morbidity previously associated with illegal,

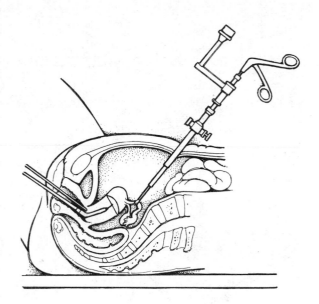

Figure 9-4. One-incision technique using the operating laparoscope.

criminal abortion (see Chapter 23). Although abortion is now legal, it is still associated with misgivings on the part of many, based mainly on religious and personal attitudes toward pregnancy termination. Most agree that abortion is not a happy substitute for pregnancy prevention and that the procedures necessary for bringing about termination, though generally safe, are associated with a higher morbidity than are most contraceptive modalities. The nurse must recognize that attitudes toward abortion are varied and personal and that there are strong religious and moral influences in these attitudes. One is entitled to one's own conclusions on this matter but should respect those of others. Personal convictions in this area are generally respected, and those who do not feel that abortion is ethically acceptable should make their views known so that arrangements can be made well in advance for substitute medical personnel.

The approach to pregnancy termination varies according to gestational age. Prior to the twelfth week, abortion is generally a relatively uncomplicated vaginal procedure. Beyond the eleventh to twelfth week, termination should not be carried out vaginally and other techniques must be used.

First trimester abortion may be carried out as an outpatient procedure. Extra-hospital fa-

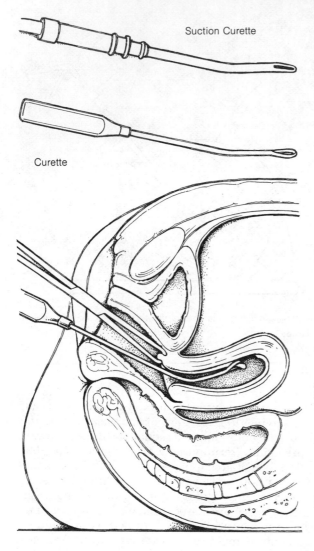

Suction Curette

Curette

Figure 9-5. Curettage, or vacuum aspiration for first trimester abortion.

used. The cervix is dilated with graduated dilators (see Chapter 23) and a suction curette is placed into the endometrial cavity to the fundus. Suction is applied, usually by electric pump, and the products of conception are evacuated into a container. These are usually sent to the pathology laboratory for confirmation of the pregnancy and to rule out unusual conditions such as hydatidiform mole (see Chapter 23). Generally, recovery takes from two to three hours, during which time the patient is observed for excessive bleeding.

When pregnancy has progressed beyond the twelfth week, termination is usually carried out by instillation of *hypertonic saline* into the amniotic cavity. This procedure is most easily carried out beyond the fourteenth week, when there is sufficient fluid in the amniotic cavity to be identified and aspirated. The bladder is emptied, and the patient is placed in the supine position. The skin is prepped and draped with sterile towels, and infiltrated with a local anesthetic over the injection site. An 18-gauge spinal needle is then inserted through the uterus into the amniotic cavity. When properly placed, clear amniotic fluid flows into the syringe attached to the needle. After a small amount of fluid is removed to verify proper placement of the needle, hypertonic saline is injected into the amniotic cavity. Initially a small amount is placed, and if there is no reaction, the remainder is delivered over approximately 15 minutes.

Following a latent period of several hours, labor usually ensues and the fetus with part or all of the placenta is delivered. If the placenta cannot be extracted completely after delivery, a curettage must be carried out to complete the abortion. During the course of labor, the contractions can cause considerable discomfort. As the cervix dilates, the patient should be medicated at intervals and generally a substantial amount of emotional support is needed during this process. The previable fetus is usually dead at the time of delivery, but at this late stage of gestation it has human form.

In cases where the hypertonic saline fails to induce contractions, a repeat dose must be administered. In some cases, there is failure to respond to the second attempt and a *hysterotomy*, a mini-cesarean section, must be resorted to. In some circumstances, infusion of hypertonic saline is contraindicated, for example, severe hypertension, and abortion is

cilities have been established, and many hospitals have designed facilities for outpatient procedures. Personnel in such units should include counselors. Their role is to help the patient to evaluate the decision to terminate pregnancy, to review alternate possibilities—having the baby and placing it for adoption—and to provide contraception advice. Termination of a pregnancy is often an emotionally charged situation and must be handled with the greatest skill and delicacy.

Increasingly the procedure of choice for the termination of early pregnancy is *suction curettage* (Fig. 9-5). A local anesthetic (paracervical block) or a light general anesthetic may be carried out by hysterotomy. Hysterotomy, being a cesarean section in principle, has the obvious disadvantage of requiring a major intra-abdominal procedure.

In some circumstances, the cervix is prepared for the abortion by the use of *laminaria.* These are lengths of sterile hydroscopic material, derived from seaweed, which absorb moisture at a rapid rate. When placed in the cervical canal, they expand in three to six hours and cause cervical dilatation. Insertion of laminaria several hours prior to a first trimester abortion can reduce the need for mechanical cervical dilatation. Some feel their use decreases the incidence of cervical lacerations.

Oxytocin infusion is often used as an adjunct to saline abortion, to decrease the time needed for completion of the process. Oxytocin is used in a manner similar to that employed for induction of labor (see Chapter 23) except that a more concentrated solution is used. The oxytocin drip is begun six to twelve hours after amnio infusion of saline. Maximum time of oxytocin use should be limited to 24 hours. When used longer, there is an increased incidence of water retention which could lead to water intoxication.

Recently some naturally occurring chemical agents, prostoglandins, have been used to induce labor. These powerful agents are capable of initiating smooth muscle contractions. They have been used intravenously, intravaginally, and intraamniotically. They may produce nausea, vomiting, and diarrhea as they stimulate the smooth muscle of the gastrointestinal tract, as well as the uterus.

Pregnancy termination in either the first or second trimester involves operative procedures and is, therefore, associated with some morbidity and a low mortality rate. In combined figures obtained from California and New York, there was a case mortality ratio of 2.6 per 100,000 abortions in patients treated by suction curettage. The mortality increased to 18.3 per 100,000 when pregnancy interruption was carried out by amniotic infusion. Causes of death included hemorrhage, infection, anesthesia, and complications of the hypertonic saline itself. As a point of reference, maternal mortality in the state of California in 1972 was 17 per 100,000 live births. Thus, morbidity and mortality rates in the first trimester are lower when compared to either second trimester abortions or carrying a pregnancy to term.

These figures speak for an early decision and availability of facilities so that the patient can have her decision implemented without delay.

Infertility

It is generally felt that infertility should be explored after a year's exposure without contraception. When one considers the complexity of reproductive processes, it is not surprising that unprotected coitus at about the time of ovulation does not always result in a pregnancy. In fact, under normal circumstances an average of three cycles of exposure is required. On the other hand, it is unwise to insist on an interval of one year before investigation is initiated in each case. A reassuring consultation is often helpful, if only to dispel doubts concerning the existence of major abnormalities. Since fertility declines with age, it would seem justifiable for couples in their thirties to seek advice somewhat earlier. Even among younger couples when the nurse or physician senses that there is anxiety over failure to conceive or when on cursory exploration there is an obvious reason for infertility, for example, amenorrhea, or a history of acute salpingitis or postabortal infection, early evaluation is in order.

Standard for infertility studies

Before selecting a method of treatment, efforts should be made to identify the underlying cause for the infertility. Minimal standards which are suggested for a complete infertility investigation include evaluation of seminal, cervical, ovarian, tubal, peritoneal, and uterine factors. In addition, the frequency and technique of intercourse should be explored.

The infertile couple

Since infertility is usually caused by abnormalities in the anatomy or physiology of the male and/or female reproductive tracts, management of the problem involves both marital partners. In the initial interview, sexual habits should be reviewed with both the husband and wife. Certainly, when intercourse occurs infrequently, the sexual adjustment in the marriage should be explored. Patients who have made it a habit to arise from bed immediately after intercourse, spilling much of the ejaculate shortly after it is placed in the vagina, should be advised to remain in bed. Occasionally couples admit to the use of lubricants during intercourse which may interfere with sperm migration, and even to douching postcoitally. These factors may not cause infertility when the husband's fertility potential is normal but may play a role when sperm production is marginal. In the occasional patient, there is even anatomical evidence that normal intercourse has not, in fact, occurred. Other sexual problems, such as premature ejaculation, may have resulted in failure of proper placement of sperm. Sympathetic and knowledgeable advice in these areas is often useful not only in the treatment of infertility, but also in bringing about a better marital adjustment in the sexual sphere.

Seminal factor

Because evaluation of the male is much less complicated than the series of tests required to explore female infertility, his reproductive potential should always be assessed initially. The postcoital test—evaluation of cervical mucus for the presence of spermatozoa—is useful in this regard. When adequate numbers of spermatozoa are not seen in cervical mucus following coitus, the husband should be evaluated with a semen analysis. This involves analysis of the fresh ejaculate obtained by masturbation after at least three days of abstinence. The volume of the specimen, sperm density, percentage of motile forms, quality of the motility of the spermatozoa, and the percentage of abnormal spermatozoa are determined. The volume of the normal ejaculate ranges from 2 to 5 ml. A sperm count of more than 20 million per ml. is considered normal, provided the quality and percentage of motility in the specimen are also normal. The single, most useful criterion is the actual quality of motility—the ability of spermatozoa to progress.

The postcoital test— evaluation of insemination

The couple is instructed to have intercourse during the preceding 12 hours. The test is timed to coincide with a day or two before expected ovulation, for example, day 12 to 13 in a presumed 28-day menstrual cycle. At that time the cervical mucus, under the influence of estrogen, is normally clear and abundant and most receptive to spermatozoa. A sample of mucus is removed from the endocervical canal, the quality of the mucus evaluated, and the specimen examined microscopically for spermatozoa. The test is normal when there are more than 20 spermatozoa per HPF in areas of clear, abundant cervical mucus. In addition to allowing assessment of proper placement of spermatozoa during coitus, the postcoital test permits evaluation of the quality of cervical secretions and their ability to support the life of the spermatozoon—the cervical factor.

When either the semen analysis or the postcoital test is abnormal, the male partner should be evaluated further for anatomical, genetic, or endocrine abnormalities. These evaluations are usually carried out by a urologist with special interest in fertility. Recently a subspecialty, *andrology*—devoted to the study of male fertility problems—has emerged which will place major emphasis on the diagnosis and treatment of the infertile male.

Artificial insemination

When semen is deficient, and especially in cases of *azoospermia*, the absence of spermatozoa in the ejaculate, insemination with the use of a specimen from a donor has gained increasing popularity and acceptability. Because of the serious ethical implications involved, such an approach should not be taken lightly. Certainly those advising patients on this matter should be aware of the social and ethical implications of the procedure and should allow adequate time to explore matters with the couple in depth before proceeding. On the positive side, when donor insemination is accepted by informed consenting partners, the end result is usually satisfactory, and there is a remarkable marriage stability among properly selected couples. Recently freeze-stored semen has been used to increase the ready availability of specimens for donor insemination.

The ovarian factor

Clearly conception does not occur when there is failure of ovulation, and fertility is impaired when ovulation is infrequent. Thus, ovulation detection is an integral part of the infertility investigation. Clues as to the occurrence of ovulation are derived from menstrual history (see p. 88), evaluation of characteristic changes in cervical mucus, and by the basal body temperature chart (see p. 92). Additional parameters used to assess ovulation include histologic evaluation of a sample of endometrium obtained by biopsy and the plasma progesterone determination obtained late in the cycle.

Endometrial biopsy is a simple office procedure and offers the additional advantage of ruling out a chronic inflammatory condition in the endometrium. A number of specially designed biopsy curettes may be used. After the position of the uterus is determined, a curette is gently introduced through the cervical canal to the level of the fundus and one or two samples of tissue removed. The endometrial sample is then sent to the pathologist's laboratory for evaluation. Following ovulation, the endometrium takes on "secretory" changes under the influence of progesterone. The changes in the endometrium after ovulation are progressive and predictable and timing of ovulation can be established retrospectively. Additional evidence of corpus luteum function and, therefore, indirect evidence of ovulation is obtained when plasma progesterone levels are greater than 3 ng. per ml.

Treatment of ovulatory failure

Treatment of anovulatory infertility depends on the underlying cause. When failure of ovulation is suspected, a thorough endocrine evaluation is in order. The defect may occur at the level of the hypothalamus, the pituitary, or the ovaries themselves. Ovulation is also influenced by the patient's general state of health and thyroid and adrenal abnormalities. Recent availability of effective agents for the induction of ovulation has made careful evaluation of patients suspected of anovulatory infertility all the more important. In properly selected cases,

the use of an estrogen antagonist, *clomiphene citrate*, is associated with a success rate above 50 percent. In patients whose ovulatory failure is the result of a defect at the hypothalamic-pituitary level, the use of *human menopausal gonadotropin* (*HMG*), derived from the urine of postmenopausal women, is associated with some success. Multiple pregnancies, which have received considerable attention in the press, are usually the result of HMG treatment. Even in expert hands, it is difficult to avoid overstimulation of the ovary with HMG and induction of more than one ovulation in a given cycle.

Tubal factors

The clinical approach to tubal disease involves assessment of tubal and peritubal anatomy. Since the human tube is a conduit which provides a passage between the ovary and uterus, tubal obstruction, of course, results in infertility. In addition, since the fimbriated end of the tube is important in transferring the ovum from the rupturing follicle to the tubal lumen, when the relationship between it and the ovum is distorted by pelvic adhesions, fertility is diminished. Anatomic defects in and about the fallopian tubes are generally a result of a past infection or pelvic irritation. Acute gonorrheal salpingitis, seen with increasing frequency, is a common offender. A ruptured appendix associated with pelvic peritonitis may also cause peritubal and periovarian adhesions (Fig. 9-6). *Endometriosis*, a condition in which the endometrium has been displaced into the peritoneal cavity around the tube and

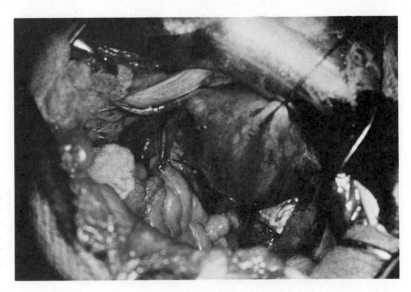

Figure 9-6. Pelvic (peritubal and periovarian) adhesions associated with infertility. Ruptured appendix occurred at age eight. (Mastroianni, L., Jr.: Variations of fertility. *In* S. Romney, et al (eds.): *Gynecology and Obstetrics: The Health Care of Women.* New York, McGraw-Hill, 1975)

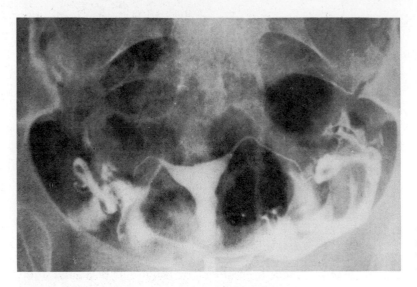

Figure 9-7. A normal hysterosalpingogram revealing bilateral tubal patency with spill of radiopaque material into the peritoneal cavity. (Mastroianni, Variations of fertility)

ovaries, may also result in pelvic adhesions and distortion of pelvic architecture. Treatment of anatomic tubal disease is surgical, involving lysis and excision of the adhesions and special techniques to reestablish the patency of the fallopian tubes.

The commonly used tests for evaluation of tubal function include uterotubal insufflation (the Rubin's test), hysterosalpingography, and finally endoscopy. *Uterotubal insufflation* involves the introduction of carbon dioxide into the uterus via a cannula. If one or both of the tubes are patent, the carbon dioxide flows along the uterus and tubes into the peritoneal cavity. When the patient sits up, the carbon dioxide rises to the diaphragm, causing pain in the shoulder referred there via the phrenic nerve. This test is useful only as a screening measure and, increasingly, physicians have substituted other methods for it.

Hysterosalpingography involves introduction of radiopaque material into the uterus and fallopian tubes (Figs. 9-7 and 9-8). This is usually done under fluoroscopic visualization, and x-rays are taken at intervals to provide a permanent record. When the tubes are patent, the radiopaque material enters the peritoneal cavity and is evenly distributed there. When the tubes are closed, the peritoneal egress is prevented by the obstruction, and a diagnosis of tubal occlusion can be made without further delay.

Peritoneoscopy involves direct visualization of the tubes and ovaries with an endoscope.

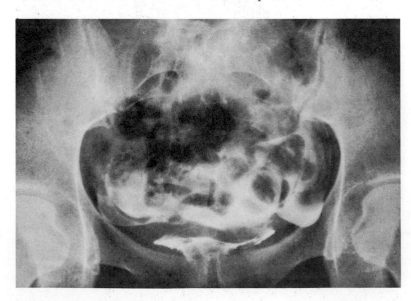

Figure 9-8. Delayed follow-up film revealing distribution of radiopaque material throughout the pelvis, continuing tubal patency. (Mastroianni, Variations of infertility)

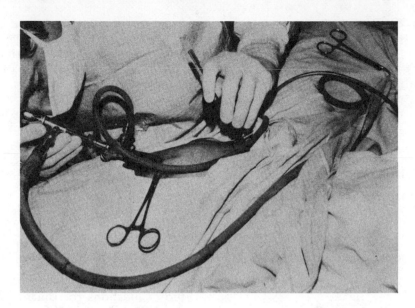

Figure 9-9. The double-puncture laparoscopic technique utilizing the probe to position the pelvic structures for optimum visualization. (Seitz, H. M., Jr., and Rosenfeld, R. L.: *Clin. Ob. and Gyn.* 17:86, 1974)

This may be carried out either through the cul-de-sac (*culdoscopy*) or through the umbilicus (*laparoscopy*). The former is carried out under local anesthesia with the patient in the knee-chest position. In expert hands, visualization is usually satisfactory. It is a more difficult procedure, however, than laparoscopy. Diagnostic laparoscopy is generally carried out under general anesthesia (Fig. 9-9). This is the same procedure as that used for tubal sterilization. In this case, however, tubal patency is evaluated by the introduction of a dilute solution of dye while the ends of the tubes are under visualization. Dye can be seen spilling from the ends of patent tubes. In addition, the area in and about the fallopian tubes can be evaluated directly for the presence of adhesions. When the latter are present, the condition is called the peritoneal factor in infertility. The treatment of adhesions is surgical.

The uterine factor

Pathologic conditions of the uterus associated with decreased fertility include uterine fibroids, congenital malformations, and intrauterine adhesions. Inflammatory lesions of the endometrium also occur. Pelvic tuberculosis is usually first detected at the time of endometrial biopsy.

Congenital defects of the uterus and uterine fibroids are more often related to habitual abortion than to infertility. Fibroids may distort the endometrial cavity and if strategically located and large enough, presumably could interfere with implantation. If located adjacent to the tube, they may cause tubal obstruction. When a causal relationship is thought to exist, *myomectomies* (removal of the fibroids) with preservation of the uterus are usually technically possible. Treatment of congenital abnormalities, more commonly associated with habitual abortion than infertility, is also surgical.

Asherman's syndrome, or adhesions within the uterine cavity are usually the result of a postpartal or postabortal infection or pelvic tuberculosis. There is often a history of a previous dilatation and curettage followed by a stormy postoperative course. Increasing use of abortion as a backup for contraceptive failure may be associated with an increased incidence of this uncommon but potential fertility-impairing lesion. Treatment of intrauterine adhesions is surgical, in association with the use of steroids and estrogens to decrease the incidence of repeat formation of adhesions.

Some patients, for reasons that are not understood, conceive during the course of the diagnostic evaluation for infertility. Occasionally conception occurs after not more than a preliminary examination and discussion of the diagnostic approach to follow. It is tempting to conjecture that, in some cases, the decision to seek aid for infertility is associated with a release of emotional tension followed, somehow, by improved reproductive performance. With the exception of ovulatory failure, which may have a psychologic basis, and decreased frequency of intercourse which certainly has a psychologic basis, there is as yet no proved somatic basis for psychologically induced infertility. The general impression that adoption is often followed by conception has not been substantiated. Nevertheless, throughout the infertility investigation, the emotional support provided by those involved in patient management is especially important. Infertility is threatening, and both husband and wife inevitably display anxiety. The role of the nurse in such situations is to understand the purpose of the various diagnostic procedures for infertility and to provide the couple with information so that both partners can cope with the problem knowledgeably.

Suggested Reading

BEHRMAN, S. J., AND KISTNER, R.: *Progress in Infertility,* Vol. 2. Boston, Little, Brown, 1968.

HAFEZ, E. S. E., AND EVANS, T. N.: *Human Reproduction: Conception and Contraception.* Hagerstown, Md., Harper & Row, 1973.

HOLZMAN, G. B.: Implementation of legal abortion: a national problem. *Clin. Ob. and Gyn.* 14, 1971.

KLEIN, S., AND GARCIA, C. R.: Asherman's syndrome, a critique and current review. *Fertil. Steril.* 24:722, 1973.

MASTROIANNI, L., JR. (ED.): Current concepts in infertility. *Clin. Ob. and Gyn.* 17, 1974.

PIERSON, E. C.: *Sex Is Never an Emergency,* ed. 3. Philadelphia, J. B. Lippincott, 1973.

WALLACH, E. W.: The uterine factor in infertility. *Fertil. Steril.* 23:138, 1972.

Study Questions for Unit II

Read through the entire question and place your answer on the line to the right.

1. In each of the following write the term or the phrase by which the pelvic measurement described is commonly called.

   A. From the lower margin of the symphysis pubis to the sacral promontory. A. _____

   B. The posterior portion of the symphysis pubis to the promontory of the sacrum. B. _____

   C. From the inner aspects of the ischial tuberosities. C. _____

2. By using the letter or letters of the measurements described in Question 1 indicate:

   A. The one which must be estimated rather than measured directly. A. _____

   B. The one which represents the most important clinically measured diameter. B. _____

   C. The most important externally measured diameter of the pelvis. C. _____

3. A patient's chart shows pelvic measurements of 9.5 cm. for the diagonal conjugate and 7.0 cm. for the true conjugate; therefore, the nurse caring for the patient in the labor room should anticipate that the patient might have:

   A. An easy, rapid delivery.

   B. A delivery of reasonable duration.

   C. A protracted labor with difficult delivery. _____

4. To give adequate care to the patient during and after delivery, the nurse should fully understand the structure of the uterus. Which of the following are true of the uterus?

   A. Its muscular tissue is:
      1. Chiefly striated.
      2. Chiefly nonstriated.
      3. Entirely striated.
      4. Entirely nonstriated. _____

   B. Its muscle fibers are arranged to run:
      1. Circularly.
      2. Longitudinally.

3. In all directions.
4. In three layers, the inner and the outer circularly, the other longitudinally. _____

C. Its blood is supplied directly from:
1. Ovarian and uterine arteries.
2. Abdominal aorta and uterine arteries.
3. Internal iliac and ovarian arteries.
4. Internal iliac and uterine arteries. _____

D. Normally, it is:
1. Attached anteriorly to the bladder wall.
2. Suspended freely movable in the pelvic cavity.
3. Suspended between the bladder and the rectum.
4. Attached posteriorly to the anterior wall of the sacrum. _____

5. The perineum lies between the vagina and the rectum. This structure has:
A. A single, strong elastic muscle.
B. A strong elastic tendon.
C. A tendon to which five muscles are attached.
D. Two strong muscles, the anal and the transverse perineal. _____

6. The hymen, which marks the division between the internal and external organs is characterized by the following description:
A. A rigid structure which ruptures during delivery.
B. Variation in shape and consistency from one patient to the next.
C. Often imperforate, preventing menstrual discharge. _____

7. Every effort is made to prevent the tearing of the perineum during childbirth. The chief hazard to the patient from laceration of the perineum would likely be:
A. Incontinence.
B. Postpartal hemorrhage.
C. Perineal abscess.
D. Prolapsed uterus. _____

8. A patient with small breasts in her first pregnancy was worried about her ability to feed her baby.
A. The nurse could respond correctly to the patient by telling her that:
1. She probably would be unable to feed her baby.
2. The size of the breasts does not influence the amount of lactation possible.
3. Mothers with small breasts usually have less difficulty feeding their babies.
4. Her baby would be fed better by means of a formula. _____

B. Milk is produced by the process of:
1. Dialysis.
2. Osmosis.
3. Secretion. _____

C. The structures most directly involved in the production of milk are:
1. Papillae.
2. Glands of Montgomery.
3. Acini cells.
4. Lactiferous sinuses.
5. Areola.
6. Lactiferous ducts. _____

9. What are the ovarian hormones produced by the graafian follicle and the cells of the corpus luteum?
   A. Progesterone and gonadotropin.
   B. Estrogen and progesterone.
   C. Gonadotropin and FSH.
   D. FSH and estrogen. _____

10. Ovulation characteristically precedes menstruation in the normal menstrual cycle by:
    A. 14 ± 2 days.
    B. 18 ± 2 days.
    C. 26 ± 2 days. _____

11. In a given menstrual cycle, the pituitary gland releases:
    A. FSH only.
    B. LH only.
    C. FSH and LH.
    D. FSH, LH, and HCG. _____

12. During the ovulatory menstrual cycle there is an increase in the basal body temperature which occurs:
    A. In association with ovulation.
    B. Four days after ovulation.
    C. Three days before ovulation. _____

13. A young mother-to-be told a nurse that she was sure that she would have a boy because her husband was such a strong, physically well-developed man. The nurse could respond correctly by saying:
    A. "It is the female cell which determines the sex of the child."
    B. "It is unlikely because there are more girls born than boys."
    C. "Physical strength does not influence the sex of the child."
    D. "You are probably right." _____

14. Fertilization normally occurs:
    A. In the ovarian follicle.
    B. In the fallopian tube.
    C. In the uterus. _____

15. Spermatozoa remain motile in the female reproductive tract for:
    A. 30 minutes.
    B. Several days.
    C. Up to three weeks. _____

16. The first polar body is released from the ovum:
    A. At the time of fertilization.
    B. Prior to its release from the ovarian follicle.
    C. During the first cell division. _____

17. The hormone human chorionic gonadotropin (HCG) is produced:
    A. By the placenta.
    B. By the pituitary gland.
    C. By the corpus luteum. _____

18. The only direct connection between the fetus and any other structure is through the umbilical cord. The umbilical cord contains which of these important structures?
    A. Umbilical artery.
    B. Umbilical arteries.
    C. Umbilical vein.
    D. Umbilical veins.
    E. Umbilical nerves.
    F. Umbilical lymphatic duct.
    G. Wharton's jelly.

    Select the number corresponding to the correct letters.
    1. A, D and F
    2. B, C and G
    3. C, E and G
    4. All of them   _____

19. Oral contraception, the "pill," generally exerts its contraceptive action by:
    A. Inhibition of ovulation.
    B. Modifying progesterone production by the corpus luteum.
    C. Altering sperm migration and motility.
    D. Regulating the menstrual cycle.   _____

20. Generally accepted absolute contraindications to oral contraception include:
    A. Thrombophlebitis.
    B. Cerebral vascular accident.
    C. Recurrent urinary tract infections.
    D. Obesity.
    E. A history of venereal disease.   _____

    Select the number corresponding to the correct letters.
    1. A and D
    2. C and E
    3. B and C
    4. A and B   _____

21. Commonly reported side effects of the IUD include:
    A. Dysmenorrhea.
    B. Intermenstrual spotting.
    C. Increased menstrual flow.
    D. All of the above.   _____

22. For maximal protection the diaphragm should be left in place:
    A. Until immediately after intercourse.
    B. For at least six hours following intercourse.
    C. For 24 hours after intercourse.
    D. None of the above.   _____

23. In considering a decision to have a tubal ligation the patient should understand that:
    A. This is a permanent form of pregnancy prevention.
    B. It is easily reversed.
    C. It is associated with a 0 percent failure rate.
    D. It can delay the menopause.   _____

24. Postabortion complications are least when the abortion is performed:
  A. In the first trimester of pregnancy.
  B. After the twelfth week of pregnancy.
  C. Beyond the sixteenth week.   _____

25. In the infertile patient, the postcoital test is best timed:
  A. Immediately after menstruation.
  B. Within one or two days of presumed ovulation.
  C. In the postovulatory phase of the menstrual cycle.
  D. Just prior to the expected onset of the next menstrual period. _____

26. Complete occlusion of the fallopian tubes results in:
  A. Failure of ovulation.
  B. Failure of union of sperm with egg.
  C. Pituitary abnormalities.
  D. Defective implantation of the fertilized ovum.   _____

assessment and management during pregnancy

Normal Pregnancy
Signs and Symptoms of Pregnancy
Antepartal Care
Patient Teaching and Counseling

unit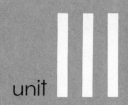

normal pregnancy

10

Physiologic Changes of Pregnancy / Local Changes / Metabolic Changes / Changes in the Various Systems / Effects on the Psyche / Endocrine Changes

This chapter is concerned with the anatomic and the physiologic adaptations of the human organism to pregnancy. Knowledge of human reproduction, presented in the previous unit, is essential to the understanding of this phase of the reproductive process. From a biologic point of view, pregnancy and labor represent the primary function of the female reproductive system and should be considered as a normal process.

The length of human pregnancy varies greatly, but the average duration, if counted from the time of conception, is approximately 267 days or 38 weeks (see Chapter 8).

Many changes in maternal physiology occur during pregnancy. These adaptations to pregnancy, although most apparent in the reproductive organs, involve other body systems as well. Concomitant with these changes, the expectant mother usually has many emotional adjustments to make: sometimes fear, apprehension, worries (financial as well as physical), and family problems are present. The fact that delivery must be "faced," that there is no turning back or "changing the mind," can in itself sometimes create an overwhelming crisis (see Chapters 12 and 13). However, these are all temporary alterations. Usually they regress after the birth of the baby (see Chapter 19).

IMPORTANT DEFINITIONS

Gravida   A pregnant woman.

Primigravida   A woman pregnant for the first time.

Primipara   A woman who has given birth to her first child. Usage is not uniform.

Multipara   A woman who has had two or more children.

Para I   A Primipara.

Para II   A woman who has had two children (and so on up numerically, Para III, Para IV, etc.).

(The plural of these words is usually formed by adding "e," as "primigravidae.")

The term *gravida* refers to a pregnant woman, regardless of the duration of pregnancy. In reference it includes the present pregnancy. The term *para* refers to past pregnancies which have produced an infant which has been of viable age, whether or not the infant is dead or alive at birth. The terms *gravida* and *para* refer to pregnancies, not to fetuses.)

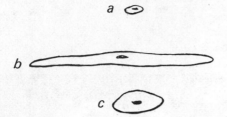

Figure 10-1. Illustration of the size of the muscle cells of the uterus (a) before pregnancy, (b) during pregnancy, showing the change in the size of these cells, and (c) in the puerperium. (After Stieve)

Physiologic changes of pregnancy

The physiologic changes of pregnancy are those alterations, both local and general, which affect the maternal organism as the result of pregnancy, but subside at or before the end of the puerperium. Such changes are to be re-

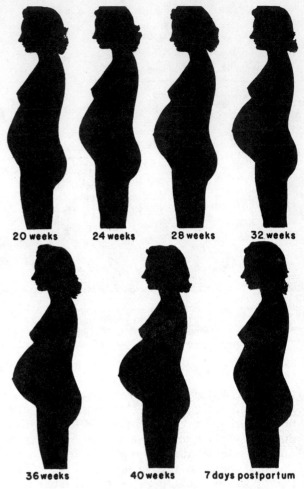

Figure 10-3. Changes in abdominal contour in pregnancy. Photographic study of actual patient.

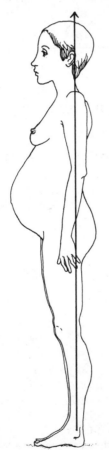

Figure 10-2. Pregnancy should and usually does improve posture. This diagram illustrates the correct standing posture showing that a straight line may be drawn from the ear to the ankle. During pregnancy "walk tall, stand tall, and sit tall."

garded as normal, inevitable, and purely temporary. They are present in varying degrees in every instance, and in the case of a physically healthy woman there should be no significant traces of them after convalescence is complete. However, it must be remembered that after pregnancy the uterus does not return to its normal nulliparous size, though it does return to a normal nonpregnant state. The adult parous uterus is slightly larger and weighs more than that of a woman who has never borne children.

Local changes

Uterus

The uterus increases in size to make room for the growing fetus. Naturally, the enlargement of the uterus is the most striking change in pregnancy. Moreover, it is directly responsible for other important alterations. The growth of this organ in gestation is phenomenal. It increases in size from approximately 6.5 cm. long, 4 cm. wide, and 2.5 cm. deep to about 32 cm. long, 24 cm. wide, and 22 cm. deep. Its weight increases from 50 to 1,000 Gm. The small, almost solid organ which has a capacity of about 2 cc. increases to become a thin-walled muscular sac capable of containing the fetus, the placenta, and over 1,000 ml. of amniotic fluid. The tremendous growth is due partly to the formation of new muscle fibers during the early months of pregnancy, but principally to the enlargement of preexistent muscle fibers which are seven to eleven times longer and two to seven times wider than those observed in the nonpregnant uterus (Fig. 10-1). Simultaneously, fibroelastic tissue develops between the muscle bands and forms a network around the various muscle bundles. This is of great importance in view of the function of the uterus in pregnancy and labor, because it strengthens the uterine walls. During early pregnancy, the hypertrophy of the uterus is probably due to the stimulating action of estrogen on muscle fibers. The uterine wall thickens during the first few months of pregnancy from about 1

cm. to almost 2 cm., but thereafter it thins to about 0.5 cm. or less. By the end of pregnancy, the uterus becomes a thin, soft-walled muscular sac which yields to the movements of the fetal extremities and permits the examiner to palpate the fetus easily.

The muscle fibers are arranged in three layers: the external hoodlike layer which arches over the fundus; the internal layer of circular fibers around the orifices of the fallopian tubes and the internal os; and the figure-8 fibers in the middle layer which make an interlacing network through which the blood vessels pass. This last group plays an important role in childbearing and will be referred to particularly in the care of the mother during labor and after delivery; for when these muscle fibers contract, they constrict the blood vessels.

Between the third and the fourth months of pregnancy, the growing uterus rises out of the pelvis and can be palpated above the symphysis pubis, rising progressively to reach the umbilicus at approximately the sixth month and almost impinging on the xiphoid process at the ninth month (Figs. 10-2 to 10-4).

In the majority of pregnancies the uterus is rotated to the right as it rises out of the pelvis. This dextrorotation is probably caused by the presence of the rectosigmoid on the left.

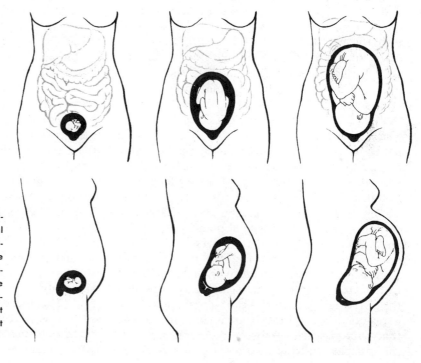

Figure 10-4. Relative size of the growing uterus, (top) front views, (bottom) lateral views, showing the fetus at four, six-and-a-half, and nine months of gestation. The fundus reaches a height between the symphysis pubis and the umbilicus by the fourth month, is about the level of the umbilicus at six-and-a-half months, and almost impinges on the xiphoid process at about the ninth month of gestation.

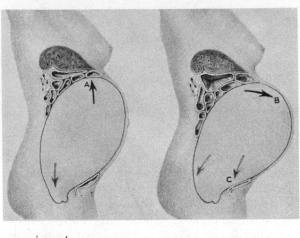

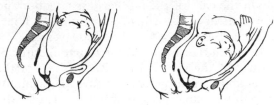

Figure 10-5. The changes which take place in "lightening." (A) Pressure exerted on diaphragm before lightening. (B) Pressure relieved by falling forward of uterus. (C) Descent of head causes pressure on pelvic structures, particularly bladder.

As the uterus becomes larger, it comes in contact with the anterior abdominal wall and displaces the intestines to the sides of the abdomen. About two weeks before term, in most primigravidae, the fetal head descends into the pelvic cavity. As a result, the uterus sinks to a lower level and at the same time falls forward. Since this relieves the upward pressure on the diaphragm and makes breathing easier, this phenomenon of the descent of the head has been called *lightening* (Fig. 10-5). These changes usually do not occur in multiparas until the onset of labor. By palpating the height of the fundus, experienced examiners can determine the approximate length of gestation.

Since the full-term pregnant uterus and its contents weigh about 12 pounds, a gravid woman may be likened to a person carrying a heavy basket pressed against the abdomen. Such a person will instinctively lean backward to maintain equilibrium. This backward tilt of the torso is characteristic of pregnancy. From a practical viewpoint it is important to note that this posture imposes increased strain on the muscles and the ligaments of the back and the thighs, and in this way is responsible for many of the skeletomuscular aches and cramps so often experienced in late pregnancy.

An additional contributing factor is a relaxation of the ligaments which support the joints of the spinal column and pelvis. This feature is increasingly prominent as. pregnancy progresses. Relaxation of the sacroiliac joints and the pubic symphysis creates a certain amount of pelvic instability, producing additional strain on the back muscles and thighs. These changes account for the waddling gait observed in late pregnancy and in the early postpartal period.

The cervix undergoes certain remarkable changes during pregnancy. One of the first physical signs of pregnancy, softening of the cervix, may be apparent as early as a month after conception (see p. 156). The softening of the cervix in pregnancy is due to increased vascularity, edema, and hyperplasia of the cervical glands. As shown in Figures 10-6 and 10-7, the glands of the cervical mucosa undergo marked proliferation and distend with mucus. As a result they form a structure resembling honeycomb and make up about one-half of the entire structure of the cervix. This is the so-called mucous plug and is of practical importance for a number of reasons. First, it seals the uterus from contamination by bacteria in the vagina. Second, it is expelled at the onset of labor and along with it a small amount of blood; this gives rise to the discharge of a small amount of blood-stained mucus, or *show*. Frequently, the onset of labor is heralded by the appearance of show. While these changes in the uterus and the cervix are taking place, the vagina and the external genital organs are being prepared for the passage of the fetus at the time of labor. These parts become thickened and softened, and their vascularity is greatly increased. This increase in the blood supply of the genital canal gives a dark violet hue to the tissues (Chadwick's sign), in contrast with the ordinary pink color of the parts, and is often described as a valuable sign of pregnancy. As the result of the succulence of the parts, the vaginal secretions may be considerably increased toward the end of gestation. The increased vascularity extends to the various structures in the vicinity (i.e., tissues in the perineal region, skin, and muscle) and effects changes in preparation for labor.

As pregnancy advances, there is a marked change in the position of the ovaries. Ovulation ceases during pregnancy. New follicles do not ripen, and only the single large corpus luteum can be found on one of the ovaries. The large size of the corpus luteum of pregnancy is due mainly to the increased vascularity of the organ.

Abdominal wall

The abdomen naturally enlarges to accommodate the increase in size of the uterus. The mechanical effect of this distention of the abdominal wall causes in the later months of pregnancy the formation of certain pink or slightly reddish streaks, or *striations* in the skin covering the sides of the abdomen and the anterior and the outer aspects of the thighs. These streaks, or *striae gravidarum*, are due to the stretching, rupture, and atrophy of the deep connective tissue of the skin (see Plate 3, *left*, *top and bottom*). They grow lighter after labor has taken place and finally take on the silvery whiteness of scar or cicatricial tissue. In subsequent pregnancies new pink or reddish lines may be found mingled with old silvery-white striae. The number, size, and distribution of striae gravidarum vary exceedingly in different women, and patients occasionally are seen in whom there are no such markings whatever, even after repeated pregnancies. Striae are not peculiar to pregnancy but may be found in other conditions which cause great abdominal distention, such as the accumulation of fat in the abdominal wall or the development of large tumors of rapid growth.

Coincident with the uterine and the abdominal enlargement, the umbilicus is pushed outward until at about the seventh month its depression is completely obliterated, and it forms merely a darkened area in the smooth and tense abdominal wall. Later, it is raised above the surrounding integument and may project, becoming about the size of a hickory nut.

When the abdominal wall is unable to withstand the tension created by the enlarging uterus, the recti muscles become separated in the median line—so-called *diastasis recti*.

Breasts

Slight temporary enlargement of the breasts, causing sensations of weight and fullness, is noted by most women prior to their menstrual periods. The earliest breast changes of pregnancy are merely exaggerations of these changes. After the second month, the breasts

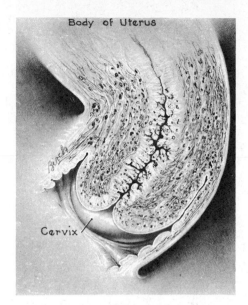

Figure 10-6. Normal pregnant cervix.

begin to become larger, firmer, and more tender; a sensation of stretching fullness, accompanied by tingling both in the breasts and in the nipples, often develops, and in many instances a feeling of throbbing also is experienced. As time goes on, the nipple and the elevated, pigmented area immediately around it—the *areola*—become darker in color. The areola tends to become puffy, and its diameter, which in the nulligravida rarely exceeds 1½ inches, gradually widens to reach 2 or 3 inches. Embedded in this areola lie tiny sebaceous glands

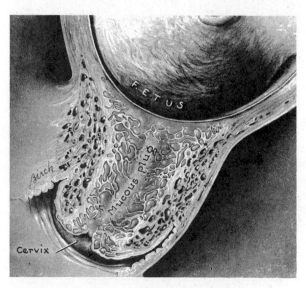

Figure 10-7. Cervix at full term, showing mucous plug.

which take on new growth with the advent of pregnancy and appear as little protuberances or follicles.

(See Plate 3, *bottom, right*). In a few cases, patches of brownish discoloration appear on the normal skin immediately surrounding the areola. This discoloration is known as the secondary areola and is a sign of pregnancy, provided the woman has never nursed an infant previously (see Plate 4, *center, right*). With the increasing growth and activity of the breasts, it is not surprising that a richer blood supply is needed; consequently, the blood vessels supplying the area enlarge. As a result, the veins beneath the skin of the breast, which previously may have been scarcely visible, now become more prominent and occasionally exhibit intertwining patterns over the whole chest wall.

The alterations in the breasts during pregnancy are directed ultimately to the preparation for breast-feeding the baby. After the first few months, a thin viscous yellowish fluid may be expressed by gentle massage, or appears spontaneously, from the nipples. This is a watery precursor of breast milk, *colostrum.*

Metabolic changes

Weight gain

A desirable total weight gain in pregnancy for the average woman is about 20 pounds. During the first three months there may be a slight weight loss, or if weight is gained, it is perhaps only a small percentage. About one-half of the increment is gained in the second trimester and a similar amount in the last trimester. However, there are wide individual variations observed, even in completely normal patients. The greater part of this 20-pound increment is quite understandable, as shown by the following figures:

Baby	7	pounds
Placenta	1	"
Amniotic fluid	1½	"
Increase in weight of uterus	2	"
Increase in blood volume	1	"
Increase in weight of breasts	1½	"
	14	pounds

The remaining 6 pounds gained by the pregnant woman represent, in part, general accumulation of fat and, in part, the increased amount of fluid that tissues tend to retain at this time. As pregnancy progresses, there is an increasing tendency toward salt retention. The salt holds water with it, and the net result is an accumulation of body fluid. This contributes to the total weight gain in pregnancy. A sudden increase in weight, especially in the last trimester of pregnancy, suggests excessive fluid retention. Recognition of this possibility is especially important, since abnormal water retention may presage the onset of toxemia (see Chapter 23). Normally, there is a diuresis, a rapid elimination of the accumulated salt and water, during the first 24 hours after delivery.

Gains between 15 and 20 pounds are natural and in keeping with good health; usually they are lost after the baby is born.

Carbohydrate metabolism

Pregnancy has a decided influence on carbohydrate metabolism. In general, the levels of fasting blood sugar are lower, and the secretion of insulin by the pancreas is increased. The stress of pregnancy may actually bring to light subclinical diabetes (see Chapter 24). In fact, diabetes is often detected for the first time during the course of prenatal care.

Changes in the various systems

Blood

The total volume of blood in the body increases approximately 30 percent during pregnancy. The minimal hematologic values for nonpregnant women apply to pregnant women, namely, 12 Gm. of hemoglobin, 3.75 million erythrocytes, 35 percent hematocrit. If there are adequate iron reserves in the body, or if sufficient iron is supplied from the diet, the hemoglobin, the erythrocyte count, and the hematocrit values remain within normal limits during pregnancy.

During pregnancy, there is an increased production of red blood cells by the bone marrow. At the same time, the maternal blood volume, the total amount of fluid circulating in the vessels, increases. Thus, under normal conditions, the actual concentration of red blood cells is relatively the same, and the normal values cited above apply.

The marked increase in production of red blood cells places an inordinate demand on bodily iron stores. Iron stores in the female are often marginal anyway because of the normal loss at menstruation. Iron deficiency anemia is often present prior to pregnancy, especially

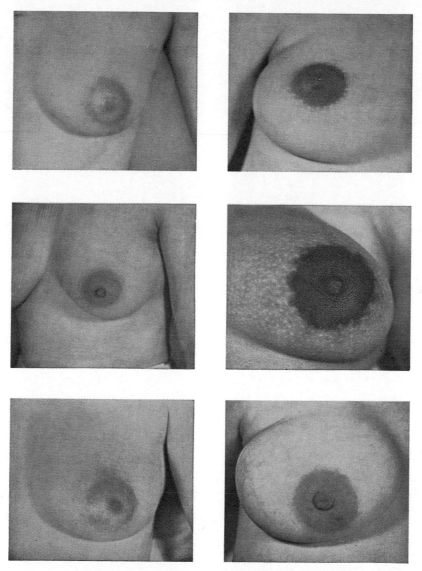

PLATE 4. (*Left, top*) Breast in nonpregnant blonde.
(*Right, top*) Breast in pregnant blonde, showing pigmentary changes.
(*Left, center*) Breast in nonpregnant brunette.
(*Right, center*) Breast in pregnant brunette, showing pigmentary changes
and marked secondary areola.
(*Left, bottom*) Breast in nonpregnant red-haired woman.
(*Right, bottom*) Breast in pregnant red-haired woman.

when there has been inadequate dietary intake of iron, frequently the case among patients in poor socioeconomic circumstances. Iron deficiency is markedly aggravated by pregnancy because of the heavy demand for iron by the growing fetus, especially late in gestation. The increased demand for iron as a result of the changes associated with pregnancy should be kept in mind during the course of prenatal care, and the use of supplementary iron should be seriously considered.

Heart

An important aspect of this increase in blood volume relates to its effect on the heart. As a natural result of this change, the heart has more blood to pump through the aorta—about 50 percent more blood per minute than it did prior to pregnancy. This augmented cardiac output attains a peak at the end of the second trimester, then declines to the nonpregnant level during the last weeks of gestation. Immediately following delivery there is a sharp rise again. In women with normal hearts this is of no particular concern. However, in women with heart disease this increase in the work that the heart has to do may add to the seriousness of the complication (see Chapter 24).

Palpitation of the heart is not uncommon; in the early months of pregnancy this is due to sympathetic nervous disturbance, and toward the end of gestation to the intraabdominal pressure of the enlarged uterus.

Respiration

In the later months of pregnancy the lungs are subjected to pressure from the underlying uterus, and the diaphragm may be displaced upward as much as 1 inch. As a consequence, shortness of breath at that period is common. It might seem that this upward displacement of the diaphragm would decrease the capacity of the lungs, but a concomitant widening of the thoracic cage occurs which more than compensates for the other change. Actually, indeed, the pregnant woman breathes in much more air than the nonpregnant woman. This is necessary, since the mother is called upon to oxygenate not only her own blood, but, by osmosis, that of her baby as well.

Digestion

The function of the digestive organs may be somewhat altered during pregnancy. During the early months the appetite may be diminished, particularly if nausea exists. Since the nutritional requirements to meet the needs of the mother's body and the growing fetus demand quality of the diet rather than an appreciable increase in the quantity of food ingested, this temporary manifestation should not produce injurious effects. As pregnancy advances, and the digestive apparatus seems to become accustomed to its new conditions, the appetite is increased and may be voracious. Heartburn and flatulence may occur at this time. Also, the pressure from the diaphragm and the diminished tone may delay the emptying time of the stomach. Constipation is exceedingly common in pregnancy; at least one-half of all gravid women suffer from this disorder. This suggests that the entire gastrointestinal tract is limited by diminished tone and pressure of the growing uterus during gestation.

Skin

Striae gravidarum, which have already been discussed in relation to changes in the abdominal wall, often develop in the breasts, the buttocks, and the thighs, presumably as the result of deposition of fat in those areas with consequent stretching of the skin. Certain pigmentary changes also are common, particularly the development of a black line running from the umbilicus to the mons veneris, the so-called *linea nigra* (see Plate 3, *bottom*, *left*).

The external genitalia and any pigmented nevi also darken. In certain cases irregular spots or blotches of a muddy brown color appear on the face. This condition is *chloasma*, or the "mask of pregnancy" (see Plate 3, *top*, *right*). Oral contraceptives may also cause chloasma in some women. These facial deposits of pigment often cause the patient considerable mental distress, but her mind may be relieved by the assurance that they will often disappear after delivery. However, the increased pigmentation of the breasts and the abdomen never disappears entirely, although it usually becomes much less pronounced. All these pigmentary deposits vary exceedingly in size, shape, and distribution and usually are more marked in brunettes than in blondes. Vascular spiders are minute, fiery-red blemishes in the skin with branching legs coming out from a central body. They develop more often in white women; however, they are of no clinical significance and will disappear. The skin changes may be associated with hypertrophy of the cortex of the adrenals.

In addition to the above skin changes, there is a great increase in the activity of the sebaceous and the sweat glands and of the hair follicles. The augmented activity of the sweat glands produces an increase in perspiration, an alteration which is helpful in the elimination of waste material.

Urinary system

The urine in pregnancy usually is increased in amount and has a lower specific gravity. Pregnant women show a tendency to excrete dextrose in the urine. Although a reduction in the renal threshold for sugar is often associated with pregnancy, the presence of any sugar in the urine should always be reported to the physician. Lactosuria may be observed at times, especially during the latter part of pregnancy and the puerperium. It is of no significance, being due to the presence of milk sugar which is supposed to be absorbed from the mammary glands.

The ureters become markedly dilated in pregnancy, particularly the right ureter. This change apparently is due in part to the pressure of the gravid uterus on the ureters as they cross the pelvic brim and in part to a certain softening which the ureteral walls undergo as the result of endocrine influences. These dilated ureters, the walls of which have now lost much of their muscular tone, are unable to propel the urine as satisfactorily as previously; consequently, stasis of urine is common. Following delivery, the ureters return to normal within four to six weeks. The stretching and the dilatation do not continue long enough to impair the ureter premanently unless infection has developed, or pregnancies are repeated so rapidly that a subsequent pregnancy begins before the ureters can return to normal.

The bladder functions efficiently during pregnancy. The urinary frequency experienced in the first few months of pregnancy is caused by pressure exerted on the bladder by the enlarging uterus. This is observed again when lightening occurs prior to the onset of labor.

Effects on the psyche

The effect of pregnancy on the psyche varies greatly. Although many women escape nervous manifestations entirely, some patients present more or less altered mental and emotional characteristics, varying all the way from cravings for unusual foods, fretfulness, and peevishness to rare instances of true psychoses. In exceptional cases the change is to the opposite extreme, and a woman who is ordinarily of an irritable disposition becomes exceedingly amiable and agreeable. The more unstable emotionally the patient is, the more likely is her mental status to be affected by the strain of pregnancy.

Endocrine changes

Placenta

In Chapter 8 the placenta was considered simply as an organ designed to transmit nutritive substances from mother to fetus and waste products in the reverse direction. The placenta has another highly important function; it is one of the most important organs of internal secretion. As discussed previously, the early chorionic villi of the implanted ovum secrete a hormone, human chorionic gonadotropin (HCG), which prolongs the life of the corpus luteum. The result is the continued production of estrogen and progesterone, which are so necessary for the maintenance of the endometrium. During pregnancy this hormone is excreted in the mother's urine and makes possible the standard tests for pregnancy (see p. 157).

The chorionic cells of the placenta produce yet another unique protein hormone—*chorionic somatomammotropin*, or human placental lactogen. This hormone is detectable in placental cells as early as the third week after ovulation and is found in maternal serum by the sixth week. Its name suggests its actions. It influences somatic cell growth of the fetus and facilitates preparation of the breasts for lactation.

In addition to its function in the formation of HCG and chorionic somatomammotropin, the placenta takes over the production of estrogen and progesterone from the ovaries, and after the first two months of gestation becomes the major source of these two hormones. The increase in these hormones in the maternal organism is thought to be responsible for many important changes that take place during pregnancy, such as the growth of the uterus and the development of the breasts. In the breasts, the development of the duct system is promoted by estrogen, and the development of the lobule-alveolar system by progesterone.

Pituitary body

The pituitary gland enlarges somewhat during pregnancy, but, as such, is not essential for the maintenance of pregnancy. The *anterior lobe* of this small gland, located at the base of the brain, has already been referred to as the "master clock," which, under the influence of the hypothalamus, controls the menstrual cycle (see Chapter 6). In addition to gonadotropins, it secretes hormones which act on the thyroid and adrenal glands, and yet another hormone which influences the growth process. Production of these hormones continues during the course of pregnancy. Gonadotropins, on the other hand, are no longer released. The estrogen and progesterone produced by the placenta inhibit their release from the pituitary gland.

The *posterior lobe* of the pituitary secretes an oxytocic hormone, *oxytocin*, which has a very strong stimulating effect on the uterine muscle. That portion of extracts of the pituitary gland which contains oxytocin, is widely employed in obstetrics to cause the uterus to contract after delivery, thereby diminishing postpartal hemorrhage. It is sometimes used also to initiate labor and to stimulate contractions during labor when they are of poor quality. Oxytocin also has an influence on the breasts. It causes *milk let-down*, or ejection of milk from the nipples. This effect is of clinical usefulness in the care of the nursing mother. Oxytocin is marketed under the names Pitocin and Syntocinon, the latter a synthetic product, and is administered either parenterally or, for milk let-down, by a nasal spray.

Other endocrine glands

It is quite clear that the placenta is the major endocrine gland in pregnancy. Other endocrine glands display alterations during normal pregnancy. During the course of pregnancy, there is slight to moderate enlargement of the thyroid. It is now known that this hypertrophy of thyroid tissue is not associated with increased thyroid activity, although there is an elevation in the basal metabolic rate which increases throughout the course of pregnancy. This is merely a reflection of the increased oxygen consumption as a result of the metabolic activity of the products of conception. Other parameters for the measurement of thyroid function also display changes. The serum protein-bound iodine (PBI), butyl extractable iodine (BEI) and thyroxine (T_4) levels increase, and the elevated levels are maintained until shortly after delivery. The increase is due not to increased thyroid activity as such but, rather, to an elevation in the level of thyroid-binding protein normally present in the blood. Thus, although there is an increase in the amount of circulating thyroid hormones and, therefore, the total concentration of hormone is elevated, the actual amount of unbound or available hormone remains within normal limits. The triiodothyronine (T_3) uptake test displays decreased values in pregnancy. This, again, is the result of an increase in the binding of circulating triiodothyronine. A similar increase in the level of thyroid-binding proteins is seen in the nonpregnant patient following the administration of estrogen, and it is likely that in pregnancy the increase is a reflection of the high level of circulating estrogen.

The *adrenal cortex* hypertrophies during pregnancy, and it is believed that its activity increases. The actual secretion of cortisol by the adrenals is unchanged, although there are alterations in the metabolism of cortisol as a result of the influence of estrogen. There is clearly an increase in the production by the adrenal glands of aldosterone, the hormone responsible for the retention of sodium by the kidneys. This increase begins early in pregnancy and continues throughout. The net result of the increase is a decreased ability of the kidneys to handle salt during pregnancy. In the absence of proper dietary control of salt intake, there is often fluid retention, and either occult or overt edema.

The *ovary*, except for the activity of the corpus luteum of pregnancy, remains relatively quiescent. Gonadotropin levels are low, inasmuch as their release is inhibited by the estrogen and progesterone produced by the placenta. Thus, follicular activity in the ovary remains in abeyance, and there is no further ovulation until after delivery.

Suggested Reading

EASTMAN, N. J., AND RUSSELL, K. P.: *Expectant Motherhood*, ed. 5. Boston, Little, Brown, 1970.

HELLMAN, L. M., AND PRITCHARD, J. A.: *Williams Obstetrics*, ed. 14. New York, Appleton-Century Crofts, 1971.

signs and symptoms of pregnancy

Classification of signs and symptoms

The first visit of the expectant mother to her physician is usually prompted by the query, "Am I really pregnant?" Oddly enough, this is the one question which the physician may answer equivocally, because even the most careful of examinations will rarely reveal clear-cut evidence of pregnancy until two menstrual periods have been missed, and occasionally the diagnosis may remain uncertain for a longer time. Some of the signs and symptoms of pregnancy can be recognized readily by the nurse, whereas others can be determined accurately only by one who has had some additional medical or technical training. The availability of rapid, accurate, and easy-to-perform pregnancy tests, thought not 100 percent accurate, has markedly improved our ability to substantiate the diagnosis.

Certain signs are absolutely indicative of pregnancy, but even these may be absent or lacking if the fetus has died in the uterus. Some so-called positive signs are not present until about the middle of gestation, and at that time the physician usually can make a diagnosis without them by the "circumstantial evidence" of a combination of earlier and less significant symptoms.

The signs of pregnancy are usually divided into three groups, as indicated in the following classification:

A. Presumptive signs
  1. Menstrual suppression
  2. Nausea, vomiting, "morning sickness"
  3. Frequency of micturition
  4. Tenderness and fullness of the breasts, pigmentation, and so on
  5. "Quickening"
  6. Dark blue discoloration of the vaginal mucous membrane (Chadwick's sign)
  7. Pigmentation of the skin and abdominal striae
  8. Fatigue

B. Probable signs
  1. Enlargement of the abdomen
  2. Fetal outline, distinguished by abdominal palpation
  3. Changes in the uterus—size and shape and consistency (Hegar's sign)
  4. Changes in the cervix
  5. Braxton Hicks contractions
  6. Positive pregnancy test

C. Positive signs
 1. Fetal heart sounds
 2. Fetal movements felt by examiner
 3. Roentgenogram—outline of fetal skeleton

Presumptive signs

Menstrual suppression

In a healthy married woman who previously has menstruated regularly, cessation of menstruation strongly suggests that impregnation has occurred. However, not until the date of the expected period has been passed by ten days or more can any reliance be put on this symptom. When the second period is also missed, the probability naturally becomes stronger.

Although cessation of menstruation is the earliest and one of the most important symptoms of pregnancy, it should be noted that pregnancy may occur without prior menstruation and that occasionally menstruations may continue after conception. An example of the former circumstance is noted in certain cultures where girls marry at a very early age; here pregnancy may occur before the menstrual periods are established. Again, nursing mothers, who usually do not menstruate during the period of lactation, often conceive at this time; more rarely, women who think they have passed the menopause are startled to find themselves pregnant. Conversely, it is not uncommon for a woman to have one or two periods after conception; but almost without exception these are brief in duration and scant in amount. In such cases the first period ordinarily lasts two days instead of the usual five, and the next only a few hours. Although there are instances in which women are said to have menstruated every month throughout pregnancy, these are of questionable authenticity and are probably ascribable to some abnormality of the reproductive organs. Indeed, vaginal bleeding at any time during pregnancy should be regarded as abnormal and reported to the physician at once.

Absence of menstruation may result from a number of conditions other than pregnancy. Probably one of the most common causes of delay in the onset of the period is psychic influence. Change of climate, exposure to cold, as well as certain chronic diseases, such as anemia, may also suppress the menstrual flow.

Nausea and vomiting

About one-half of pregnant women suffer no nausea whatsoever during the early part of pregnancy. About 50 percent experience waves of nausea; of these perhaps one-third experience some vomiting. *Morning sickness* usually occurs in the early part of the day and subsides in a few hours, although it may persist longer or may occur at other times. When morning sickness occurs, it usually makes its appearance about two weeks after the first missed menstrual period and subsides spontaneously six or eight weeks later. Since this symptom is present in many other conditions, such as ordinary indigestion, it is of no diagnostic value unless associated with other evidence of pregnancy. When the vomiting is excessive, when it lasts beyond the fourth month, when it begins in the later months, or when it affects the general health, it must be regarded as pathologic. Such conditions are termed *hyperemesis gravidarum*, or pernicious vomiting, and will be discussed with complications of pregnancy in Chapter 23.

Frequent micturition

Irritability of the bladder with resultant frequency of urination may be one of the earliest symptoms of pregnancy. It is attributed to the fact that the growing uterus stretches the base of the bladder, so that a sensation results identical with that felt when the bladder wall is stretched with urine. As pregnancy progresses, the uterus rises out of the pelvis, and the frequent desire to urinate subsides. Later on, however, the symptom is likely to return, for during the last weeks the head of the fetus may press against the bladder and give rise to a similar condition. Although frequency of urination may be somewhat bothersome, both at the beginning and at the end of pregnancy, it never should constitute a reason for reducing the quantity of fluid consumed.

Breast changes

The breast changes of pregnancy have already been described (p. 147). In primigravidae these alterations are helpful adjuncts in the diagnosis of pregnancy, but in women who have already borne children, particularly if they have nursed an infant within the past year, they naturally are of much less significance.

"Quickening"

Quickening is an old term derived from an idea prevalent many years ago that at some particular moment of pregnancy life is suddenly infused into the infant. At the time this notion was in vogue, the first tangible evidence of intrauterine life lay in the mother's feeling the baby move, and the conclusion was only natural that the infant "became alive" at the moment these movements were first felt. As is reflected in the Biblical reference to "the quick and the dead," the word quick used to mean alive, and the word quickening meant becoming alive. Hence, our forebears were accustomed to say that when fetal movements were first felt, quickening or coming to life of the baby had occurred. We now know that the infant is a living organism from the moment of conception, but the old term quickening is still used in obstetric terminology, whereas among the laity feeling life is the common synonym. As used today, quickening refers only, of course, to the active movements of the fetus as first perceived by the mother.

Quickening is usually felt toward the end of the fifth month as a tremulous fluttering low in the abdomen. The first impulses caused by the stirring of the fetus may be so faint as to raise some doubt as to their cause; later on, however, they grow stronger and often become disturbingly active.

Many fetuses, although alive and healthy, seem to move about very little in the uterus, and, not infrequently, a day or so may pass without a movement being felt. Inability to feel the baby move does not mean that it is dead or in any way a weakling but, in all probability, that it has assumed a position in which its movements are not felt so readily by the mother. Should three or four days pass without movements, the nurse or physician should listen for the fetal heart sounds. If these are heard, it means beyond doubt that the fetus is alive and presumably in good condition. It might seem that the sensations produced by the baby's movements would be so characteristic as to make this a positive sign of pregnancy, but, oddly enough, women occasionally misinterpret movements of gas in the intestines as motions of a baby and on this basis

imagine themselves to be pregnant. Therefore, the patient's statement that she feels the baby move cannot be regarded as absolute proof of pregnancy.

Vaginal changes

On inspection of the vagina, one is able to observe discoloration of the vaginal mucous membrane due to the influence of pregnancy. The mucosa about the vaginal opening and the lower portion of the anterior wall frequently becomes thickened and of a dark bluish or purplish congested appearance instead of its customary pinkish tint in the nonpregnant state. This sign, *Chadwick's sign*, is of no special value in women who have borne children; and, as it may be due to any condition leading to the congestion of the pelvic organs, it can be considered only as a presumptive sign of pregnancy.

Skin changes

The changes in the skin which may accompany pregnancy (i.e., striae gravidarum, linea nigra, chloasma, pigmentation of the breasts, and so on) have been described in Chapter 10. These manifestations often are observed in pregnant women but vary exceedingly in different persons, often being entirely absent. The pigmentation changes in particular are frequently absent in decided blondes and exceptionally well marked in pronounced brunettes. As already mentioned, this pigmentation may remain from former pregnancies and cannot be depended on as a diagnostic sign in women who have borne children previously.

Fatigue

During the early months of pregnancy the expectant mother becomes easily fatigued and experiences periods of lassitude and drowsiness. This condition frequently accompanies pregnancy and usually disappears after the first few months of gestation.

Probable signs

Abdominal changes

The size of the abdomen in pregnancy corresponds to the gradual increase in the size of the uterus, which at the end of the third month is at the level of the symphysis pubis. At the end of the fifth month it is at the level of the umbilicus, and toward the end of the ninth

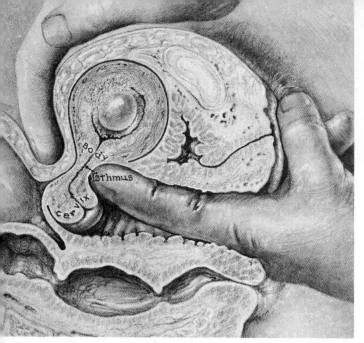

Figure 11-1. Hegar's sign.

week, the so-called Hegar's sign, named for the man who first described it, is perceptible (**Fig. 11-1**). At this time, the lower uterine segment, or lower part of the body of the uterus, becomes much softer than the cervix. So soft does it become, that in its empty state (for it has not yet become encroached upon by the growing embryo) it can be compressed almost to the thinness of paper. This is one of the most valuable signs in early pregnancy. Another valuable sign found on vaginal examination is ballottement (from the French *balloter*, to toss up like a ball). During the fourth and the fifth months of pregnancy, the fetus is small in relation to the amount of amniotic fluid present; a sudden tap on the presenting part makes it rise in the amniotic fluid and then rebound to its original position and, in turn, tap the examining finger. When elicited by an experienced examiner, this response is the most certain of the probable signs.

month, at the ensiform cartilage (see Figs. 10-3 and 10-4, pp. 144 and 145). Mere abdominal enlargement may be due to a number of causes, such as accumulation of fat in the abdominal wall, edema, or uterine or ovarian tumors. However, if the uterus can be distinctly felt to have enlarged progressively in the proportions stated above, pregnancy may properly be suspected.

Fetal outline

After the sixth month, the outline of the fetus (head, back, knees, elbows, and so on) usually may be identified sufficiently well by abdominal palpation to justify a diagnosis of pregnancy. As pregnancy progresses, the outline of the fetus becomes more and more clearly defined. The ability to outline the fetus makes pregnancy extremely probable. In rare instances, however, tumors of the uterus may so mimic the fetal outline as to make this sign fallible.

Changes in the uterus

Changes in shape, size, and consistency of the uterus which take place during the first three months of pregnancy are very important indications. These are noted in the bimanual examination which shows the uterus to be more anteflexed than normal, enlarged, and of a soft, spongy consistency. About the sixth

Cervical changes

Softening of the cervix usually occurs about the time of the second missed menstrual period. In comparison with the usual firmness of the nonpregnant cervix (which has a consistency approximate to that of the cartilaginous tip of the nose), the pregnant cervix becomes softened, and on digital examination the external os feels like the lips or like the lobe of the ear (Goodell's sign).

Braxton Hicks contractions

Uterine contractions begin during the early weeks of pregnancy and occur at intervals of from 5 to 10 minutes throughout. These contractions are painless, and the patient may or may not be conscious of them. They may be observed during the later months by placing the hand on the abdomen and during the bimanual examination. By means of these contractions, the uterine muscles contract and relax, thereby enlarging in size to accommodate the growing fetus. These contractions are referred to as the Braxton Hicks sign, after a famous London obstetrician of the last century who first described them. They often account for false labor.

Pregnancy tests

Since the dawn of civilization efforts have been made to devise a satisfactory test for pregnancy. The priest-physicians of ancient

Egypt, in the earliest writings handed down to us, tell of a test then in vogue based on the seeming ability of pregnancy urine to stimulate the growth of wheat and barley seeds. The itinerant physicians of classical Greece employed similar tests, and during the Middle Ages the omniscient physician merely gazed at the urine and claimed in this way to be able to diagnose not only pregnancy, but also many other conditions.

Today, interestingly enough, as in the tests of old, urine is used in a large number of tests for pregnancy. The tests are based on the fact that the early chorionic villi of the implanted ovum secrete HCG, which is excreted in the maternal urine. The method of its detection depends on the fact that this hormone may be detected in urine by biologic or immunologic methods. Some of the biologic tests which were used extensively in the past include: 1) the Aschheim-Zondek test (immature female mouse), 2) the Friedman test (female rabbit), 3) the Hogben test (South African toad), and 4) the American male frog test.

Recently, numerous systems for immunologic pregnancy testing have been devised. These have largely supplanted those which require the use of animals. Since HCG is an antigen capable of producing specific antibodies when injected into an animal, such as the rabbit, the serum of the animal so injected will contain an antibody or antihormone specific for HCG. This serum then can be used by reliable immunologic methods to establish the presence or absence of HCG in pregnancy urine.

Kits for immunologic pregnancy testing are available and have been simplified so that with a little practice the test can be carried out by the nurse, within minutes. Immunologic tests have two main advantages over the older biologic ones: 1) They provide an answer within a few minutes rather than many hours; 2) they eliminate the need for maintaining an animal colony. These tests are at least as accurate as the older biologic methods.

The great value of the endocrine tests lies in the fact that they become positive very early in pregnancy, usually about ten days after the first missed menstrual period, sometimes even a few days earlier than this. If any of the tests has been carried out properly, the results are accurate in more than 95 percent of cases. They are not, therefore, absolutely positive signs of pregnancy, but very nearly so.

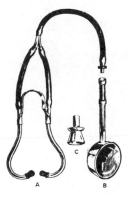

Figure 11-2. Left stethoscope for use with interchangeable bells (A). Weighted bell used for auscultation of fetal heart sounds (B). Small bell used to determine mother's blood pressure (C). (J. Sklar Manufacturing Co., Long Island City, N.Y.)

Positive signs

Although certain of the signs mentioned above—notably, the hormone tests, ballottement, and palpating the fetal outline—are nearly positive evidences of pregnancy, they are not 100 percent certain; errors in technique occasionally invalidate the hormone tests, and on rare occasions the other signs may be simulated by nonpregnant pathologic states. If the term "positive" is used in the strict sense, there are only three positive signs of pregnancy, namely, the presence of fetal heart sounds, fetal movements felt by the examiner, and the x-ray outline of the fetal skeleton.

Fetal heart sounds

When heard distinctly by an experienced examiner, the fetal heart sounds can leave no doubt about the existence of pregnancy. Ordinarily, they become audible at about the middle of pregnancy, or approximately the twentieth week. If the abdominal wall is thin, and conditions are favorable, they may become audible as early as the eighteenth week, but obesity or an excessive quantity of amniotic fluid may render them inaudible until a much later date. Although the usual rate of the fetal heart is approximately 140 beats per minute, it may vary under normal conditions between 120 and 160. The use of the ordinary bell stethoscope, steadied by rubber bands, is entirely satisfactory, but in doubtful cases the head stethoscope is superior, since the listener receives bone conduction of sound through the headpiece in addition to that transmitted to the eardrum.

The nurse will find it advantageous to determine the fetal position by abdominal palpation before attempting to listen to the fetal

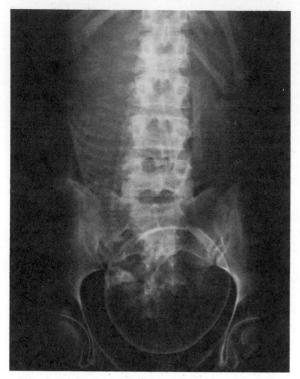

Figure 11-3. Normal vertex position. (Bonner, K. P.: Radiography and Clinical Photography, Eastman Kodak Company, Rochester, N.Y.)

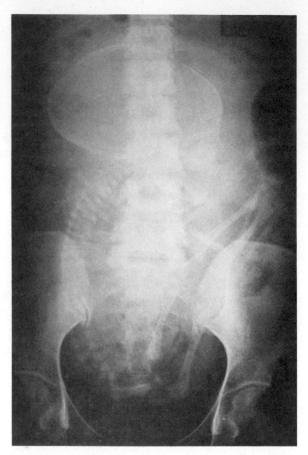

Figure 11-4. Normal breech position. (Bonner, K. P.: Radiography and Clinical Photography)

heart tones, since ordinarily the heart sounds are best heard through the infant's back (see Chapter 14). Also, she will do well, while learning the characteristics of the fetal heart sounds, to accustom herself to place one hand on the maternal pulse and feel its rate at the same time that she hears the fetal heart tones through the stethoscope. Occasionally, the inexperienced attendant, particularly when listening high in the abdomen, may mistake the mother's heart sounds for those of the baby. Since the two are not synchronous (fetal, 140; maternal, 80), the method suggested above will obviate this mistake; in other words, if the rate that comes to the ear through the stethoscope is the same as that of the maternal pulse, it is probably the mother's heartbeat; on the other hand, if the rates are different, it is undoubtedly the sound of the fetal heart.

Two additional sounds may be heard in listening over the pregnant uterus: the funic souffle and the uterine souffle. Since the word *souffle* means a blowing murmur, or whizzing sound, the nature of these two sounds is simi-lar, but their timing and causation are quite different. The word *funis* is Latin for umbilical cord, and, accordingly, the term *funic souffle* refers to a soft blowing murmur caused by blood rushing through the umbilical cord. Since this blood is propelled by the fetal heart, the rate of funic souffle is synchronous with that of the fetal heart. It is heard only occasionally, perhaps in one case out of every six. The funic souffle is a positive sign of pregnancy, but it is not usually so listed, because it is almost always heard in close association with the fetal heart sounds. The *uterine souffle* is produced by blood rushing through the large vessels of the uterus. Since this is maternal blood, propelled by the maternal heart, it is synchronous with the rate of her heartbeat. In other words, the rate of the funic souffle is ordinarily around 140 per minute (or the same as that of the fetal heart rate); the rate of the uterine souffle, near 80 (that of the maternal heart rate). The fetal heart may also be detected electronically or with ultrasound techniques described in detail in Chapter 27 (Fetal Diagnosis and Treatment).

Fetal movements felt by examiner

As already noted, fetal movements supposedly felt by the patient may be very misleading in the diagnosis of pregnancy. However, when an experienced examiner feels the characteristic thrust or kick of the baby against his hand, this is positive evidence of pregnancy.

Often this can be felt after the end of the fifth month.

Roentgenogram

A roentgenogram showing the outline of the fetal skeleton is, of course, undeniable proof of pregnancy. How early the fetal skeleton will show in the roentgenogram depends on the thickness of the abdominal wall, the x-ray equipment and other factors. It has been demonstrated as early as the fourteenth week and is quite easily demonstrated as a rule after the twentieth week (Figs. 11-3 and 11-4).

Suggested Reading

HELLMAN, L. M., AND PRITCHARD, J. A.: *Williams Obstetrics,* ed. 14. New York, Appleton-Century Crofts, 1971.

antepartal care

12

The Importance of Preventive Care /
Health Care Supervision / Nutrition /
General Hygiene / Minor Discomforts /
Preparations for the Baby / After-Care

Within the last decade, there has appeared a rising tide of comment about what constitutes "adequate antepartal care" as well as whether or not antepartal supervision does, in fact, accomplish the goal of better reproductive outcomes for all members of society. It has been documented that the presence of antepartal care does have a positive relationship to more successful outcomes for both mother and infant. However, exactly what factors within the total complex of "antepartal care" are crucial to these successful outcomes remains to be determined. There has been a disparity in successful outcomes dependent on the economic status of the patient. This indicates that the delivery of care has been based largely on a middle-class model; that is, the delivery and utilization of care depends on the assumptions of middle-class persons—that the individual has the knowledge, incentive, and resources to seek and to follow through with care. It has been evident that this model is ineffective for many of our reproductive population.

In the literal sense, antepartal care refers to the medical and nursing supervision and care given to the pregnant woman during the period. between conception and the onset of labor. Opinions vary, but, generally in current prac-

tice, adequate antepartal care is that care which considers the physical, emotional, and social needs of the woman and her unborn baby, her mate, and their other children. It attempts to provide the best of medical and nursing science to protect the life and the health of the mother and fetus. In addition, it takes into consideration the social conditions under which the family lives (i.e., its economic status, educational level, housing, nutrition, and so on; see Chapter 3) so that the mother and fetus may pass through pregnancy, labor, and the puerperium with a maximum of mental and physical fitness. It is this former aspect, in particular, that is now being given more attention than formerly. Innovative styles in delivery of care, together with the utilization of personnel who have a better understanding of the lifestyles of the clients they serve, are gradually but surely improving utilization of health services. It becomes evident, then, that the goals of adequate antepartal care are accomplished through the combined efforts of the expectant parents, the physician, the nurse, and the various other members of the health team.

Adequate antepartal care also aims to increase the knowledge of the mother-to-be and her family, so that she and her infant may be kept healthy and happy after delivery.

Antepartal care may be considered the foundation for the normal development, adequate growth, and good health of the baby. During this formative period, the teeth, bones, and various systems of the body have their beginnings, as well as the foundations for the infant's future health. Adequate antepartal care also aids in stabilizing the daily health of the mother. As pregnancy advances, the demands of the fetus increase. Since individuals react differently to pregnancy, this supervision is of the utmost importance in detecting these reactions; for it not only helps to relieve discomforts and to prevent accidents and complications, but also aids in ensuring a more rapid convalescence and continued good health.

The importance of preventive care

Prior to the rise of present-day obstetrics, the physician usually had only one interview with his patient before he saw her in labor, and often at this interview he merely sought to compute the expected date of confinement. When he next saw her, she might be in the throes of an eclamptic convulsion or striving vainly to overcome the resistance offered by a contracted pelvis. It is in the prevention of such calamities that care and supervision of the pregnant mother have been of value. Indeed, antepartal care is an absolute necessity if a substantial number of women are to avoid disaster; and it is helpful to all.

From a biologic point of view, pregnancy and labor represent the highest function of the female reproductive system. As mentioned previously, this should be considered a normal process. But the numerous physiologic changes which occur in the mother's body during pregnancy (see Chapter 10) demonstrate that the borderline between health and illness is less distinctly marked during pregnancy than during the nonpregnant state. A slight variation in bodily function, which might be of little significance in the nonpregnant woman, may be a warning signal of a potentially pathologic condition in pregnancy which could seriously threaten the health of the mother, the child, or both. Examples of such symptoms might be a weight gain of several pounds during one week or a persistent headache. Health supervision and teaching begun early in pregnancy often help to avoid complications of pregnancy; and if symptoms do occur, their early detection and prompt treatment may avert serious problems.

The importance of early and continued medical supervision during pregnancy cannot be overemphasized. If possible, care should begin when the patient conceives, or perhaps even earlier—at the very beginning of her pregnant period, or ideally with her own mother's antepartal state, which likewise greatly affected the patient's health. In recent years, much has been accomplished through premarital and prepregnancy examinations to determine the patient's fitness for pregnancy. This type of preventive medicine greatly enhances the general well-being and good health of our childbearing population.

However, it must be noted that there are several forces in society today that militate against the ultimate goal of high-quality maternity care for all. These have been designated as the crisis of quality, the crisis of logistics, the crisis of community agencies, and the crisis of medical economics.

The first of these, the crisis of quality, concerns the differential quality and delivery of medical services that often exist for the different socioeconomic groups in our society. Those in greatest need of good maternity care, who generally have the highest death and sickness rates, often lack confidence in the community facilities for their care. They believe that adequate health care is a right of citizenship; however, when they seek it, they often find that two kinds of care exist: one for those who can pay and another for those who cannot. Since so many people now feel that proper health care is a right of citizenship, the provision of adequate health services for all requires a restructuring of present national priorities and an escalation of the public's social consciousness. Most health professionals agree that any worthwhile program should provide financial support, and in addition, should maintain the mother's dignity. The establishment of area health education centers based on or affiliated with university hospitals, neighborhood free clinics, and innovative programs in hospital clinics have been attempts to provide a better calibre of care for all segments of society.

Within the last ten years, the focus of service in many outpatient departments and clinics of hospitals has changed from dispensing first aid to giving ambulatory care. As a result, the ambulatory care department is now one of the most dynamic, change-oriented departments in many hospitals.

As part of this change, nursing service in these ambulatory care settings has discarded the managerial role and replaced it with a care-centered, more independent role in which nurses are expanding their functions of educating patients, providing supportive guidance, and making observations. In this role, the professional nurse becomes the health professional who is primarily responsible for maintaining continuity of health care for a specific patient population.

The second crisis, that of logistics, refers to the current problem of the shortage of maternity personnel at various levels. It is now becoming more and more accepted that quality maternity care in the future will be provided by a closely integrated team of physicians, professional nurses, nurse-midwives or nurse practitioners, laboratory technicians, social workers, nutritionists, health educators, and homemakers. None of these are available in sufficient numbers at the present. However, the development of expanded roles for nurses, together with training programs for the education of paraprofessionals, are proving to be viable efforts to ease this aspect of the present crisis. Research has indicated that when nurses utilize expanded roles and are integral members of the health care team, there are considerably fewer broken antepartal appointments, better postpartal clinic attendance, better utilization of family planning services and techniques, and reduction of infant mortality.[1,2] Utilization of indigenous populations to improve the quality of care has also been effective. Their familiarity with the lifestyles of childbearing families, their knowledge of the socioeconomic factors to be considered and their willingness to provide whatever service is needed, be it transportation or referral for counseling, are salient factors in the improvement of reproductive outcomes. There is a very important message in the majority of the current research on the delivery of antepartal services to the various segments of society. Programs that are planned by outsiders and that do not consider the involvement of those whom they serve are doomed to failure and will in no way deliver the quality of care that they ostensibly were designed to give.

The third crisis arises in community agencies. Many agencies still remain competitive and repetitive in some areas and entirely lacking in others. For example, there may be several community health nursing services in one area, such as the health department, a voluntary nursing agency, and school nursing services. Many times they all serve one family, but seldom communicate with one another regarding the total needs of the family. Similarly, some hospitals may be overcrowded, while others have empty beds. Nothing is done to relieve the shortage because the first hospital may be governed by economic considerations to the exclusion of the comfort and safety of its patients. There are ways to circumvent these problems which use innovation in building hospitals and planning patient care. Light unit-type buildings with interchangeable walls and rooms have been proposed. In some places, motel-type "half-way" houses staffed by nurse-midwives under medical supervision could provide adequate care. Unfortunately, many of these innovations are blocked by long entrenched rules and regulations of local building codes, mortgage companies, and the like which require the massive stereotyped construction found in traditional hospitals. Thus, in many cases, we see vested interests of existing social and health agencies, professional and individual competition, politics, regulations, and false community pride standing in the way of services which can promote the health and life of future generations.

One of the most interesting and innovative phenomena of recent years, the development of the free clinic, is a move to counteract this bureaucratic obstruction. Free clinics have had an important impact, not only on maternity care, but health care in general. The first clinic was opened in the Haight-Ashbury district in San Francisco in 1967. Subsequent clinics were developed in many of the major cities in the United States and Canada. The total number is now more than 135 throughout the country. The derivation of the name of the clinic indicates the reaction against the highly bureaucratic structure of American society. Free does not necessarily mean no charge for services. Rather, a free clinic is "free" of eligibility requirements, questions, and "bureaucratic hassle."[3] It must be noted, however, that the typical client usually does not have many resources to pay for care.

There have been problems with delivery of care, since not all of the types of clinics are able to deliver maternity care to the populations they serve. For instance, in clinics where the clients are mostly adolescent, and where antepartal care is needed the most, there are often too few or no maternity services offered. Moreover, while referrals may be made for obstetric care in the neighborhood family clinics, few can follow through to make arrangements for delivery and hospitalization. It is hoped that as free clinics continue and their benefits are more appreciated they will be able to attract the personnel to provide for these gaps in service.

The final crisis is that of medical economics. The chief protection for the medical needs of most of America's young parents is voluntary and commercial prepayment insurance. Unfortunately, the maternity benefits traditionally have been distressingly low. Young people with low incomes are frequently saddled with a large medical and hospital bill at a time when they can least afford to pay. Many professionals feel that maternity care should be entirely covered, but the actuarians believe that the rates for this kind of coverage would be prohibitive. However, it might be noted that insurance companies have had this opinion about other forms of coverage and under public pressure have increased benefits. Many community health leaders feel that the resources of this country are so vast that full coverage is feasible if there is a public mandate to provide it. However, if this mandate does not come, these leaders foresee only increased costs to future parents.

While the above comments are perhaps unsettling, it is hoped that they give food for thought for tomorrow's nursing practitioners. Our society is undergoing a time of great social change and the commensurate stress that accompanies such change. The nurse, as she becomes better educated and increasingly knowledgeable regarding the forces in society that impinge on the health needs of her patients, is in an advantageous position to help her patients learn what forces and pressures they can bring to bear to help achieve their right of citizenship—adequate health care.

Mothers and infants at risk

In recent years, the term *high risk* has been applied to groups of mothers and babies who have an actual or potentially higher incidence and prevalence of morbidity and mortality than the general population of mothers and infants. Unfortunately, there has developed a stereotype of these mothers as being chiefly un-

married, nonwhite, unemployed, and from broken families. However, recent research indicates that this stereotype, as with most stereotypes, is not altogether useful in assessing whether or not the situation is truly high risk. Many, if not most, of these mothers have children born in wedlock and are now members of intact families headed by males, and in most cases, almost all the males have full-time employment of some kind. However, the crucial factor is that the remuneration for this employment is often very low—which makes the total economic picture precarious. Furthermore, many of these mothers come from low-economic-status homes and, hence, have experienced many deprivations during their formative years (see Chapter 3). While it is wise to beware of stereotyping these families, there are some commonalities that tend to appear. Many have inadequate pre- or postnatal care; some are teenagers and/or do not want their babies; the mothers may have metabolic or chronic diseases, take drugs, or have chronic cervical or vaginal infections or disease; finally the babies may sustain damage at birth or be one of a multiple birth. Early and continued prenatal care is a "must" for these patients to ensure both maternal and fetal salvage. However, case finding and motivating these patients to seek prenatal care present formidable problems.

Although maternity clinics across the country have been improved by federal funding, and satellite clinics have been opened in many cities, many mothers, particularly those in the poverty group, are not seeking the care that is offered. Having been brought up in poverty and having known deprivation or medical indigence all their lives, they simply have never become accustomed to using medical care except in emergencies, and not surprisingly, they will not start when they become pregnant. These findings only reinforce the necessity of extending prenatal and preconceptual care back to childhood, through adolescence and adulthood. It must be remembered that this is not only a problem of prenatal care, but rather a problem of the ill-health and poverty of the total community. Similarly, it is not just a question of dietary supplements during pregnancy, but of life nutrition; nor is it simply a problem of the organization of maternal and child health services, but a question of the organization of family health services. What is even more important is that it is not just a question of a considered referral to a prenatal clinic, but rather the way in which social agencies concern themselves with all the issues of health, and whether they encourage use of medical services preventively or curatively. Most expectant mothers who need motivation to seek prenatal care would go to the clinic if they could see some concrete benefits that accrue to them. Family planning services, for instance, are being found to more than double the attendance at postpartum clinics. In some programs, they also seem to exert a positive influence in attracting women to prenatal clinics early, when they hear by word of mouth that family planning services are available.

Today's climate seems to call for innovation in thought and practice. Ryan, for example, has suggested that regionalization of antepartal care is one method of providing quality care both prenatally and perinatally and avoiding overlap in services. He points out that 60 percent of perinatal mortality will occur in the high-risk group which we are now better able to identify. Moreover, with new techniques of fetal evaluation, both antepartally and intrapartally, and the ability to monitor the mother more exactly during pregnancy and labor, we are in a much better position to define and follow closely the high-risk group. Regionalization has three basic components: First is the development of a system of neonatal intensive care with appropriate transport system; second is the development of a high-risk maternity center in conjunction with the neonatal intensive care unit. Patients identified as high risk could then be delivered at a site where the infant could receive intensive care services if necessary. This would lower the admittedly high costs of these sophisticated services and prevent overlap and/or discontinuity of services. Third is the aspect of consolidation of services. Every patient should be delivered in a setting with the highest *practical* capability for managing her problems and those of her infant. Operationally, this means that we can no longer justify the numerous small maternity units within minutes of each other, all lacking the resources and personnel to provide modern obstetric care for complicated patients in particular.[4] While regionalization is not the only answer to providing quality care to both our high-risk and normal populations, it is one example of innovative practice that appears necessary.

In addition to these types of innovations, there is the likelihood that some form of national health insurance or prepayment scheme will be developed in the near future to help cover some of the crises mentioned previously.

Supervision within the health care system

In present-day maternity care, the physician, nurse, nurse-midwife, nurse clinician, and other specialized health personnel all collaborate to provide services to the family. While many of these roles are still evolving, especially with respect to nursing, there is a beginning clarification as the various programs become established and activities are assigned and carried out by the members of the health team. In general, the physician is the diagnostician of normal and abnormal conditions associated with the childbearing cycle. He is also a technical specialist in the sense that he carries through the technical medical procedures associated with the childbearing cycle, including, of course, delivery of the infant. The nurse-midwife also shares some of these activities. However, she works under the supervision of the physician and is not responsible for the complicated or abnormal patients. She can also be teacher, counselor, and coordinator for the patient. The role of the nurse as clinician, practitioner, or associate, as she is variously known, is somewhat newer in the health care spectrum. This nurse can be responsible for physical assessment of the patient as well as the teaching, counseling, and coordination aspects of care. The nurse is primarily the teacher, counselor, developer, and implementer of teaching programs, coordinator and general factotum for assuring continuity of care in the total patient experience. It is apparent that all of these health professionals have some similar skills, but may differ somewhat in their orientations as to their primary responsibilities.

Several variables interact to determine who provides which services to the family. The number and availability of health professionals, for instance, is a crucial factor. In some rural areas, both physicians and allied health personnel are in short supply; hence, the nurse-midwives and nurses must truly fulfill every aspect of their roles. Usually a minimum of time is available and patients with the greatest need are seen in triage. This emphasizes the necessity for accurate and thorough patient assessments so that appropriate referrals can be made to other professional services. In some of the larger metropolitan clinics, there may be a surfeit of various personnel, but a large patient population, and the nurse will find that providing continuity of care and the coordination aspect of her role must be emphasized. Another variable influencing who provides what services is the orientation of the nurse herself to her role. If she perceives it as being technically oriented, she will concentrate on the technical aspects of the care. If she is interested and skilled in the interpersonal and teaching aspect, she will spend time in supportive, interpretative, and counseling activities. The nurse's strong preparation in interpersonal communication and supportive techniques as well as formal and informal teaching techniques places her in an ideal position to work with total families as they move through the reproductive cycle.

In the last five years, there have been more programs developed where the maternity nurse may manage the normal pregnancy of the mother in consultation with the obstetrician after the initial medical assessment.[5] This trend in expanded role means more responsibility in establishing long-term relationships which have often been absent for the nurse in the maternity setting. As this new trend continues, the nurse will need to rely even more

UCLA HOSPITAL & CLINICS
PRENATAL RECORD

PATIENT NO.: ____________________
NAME: ____________________
ADDRESS: ____________________
____
TELEPHONE:

MARITAL STATUS (CIRCLE) M S W D	AGE	EDC
RACE: ☐ Cauc ☐ Oriental ☐ Negro ☐ Others:		TYPE RH

PRIOR PREGNANCIES

TERM	PREMATURE	ABORTIONS	LIVING

	YEAR	PLACE OF CONFINEMENT	DURATION OF GESTATION	CHARACTER OF DELIVERY	LABOR DURATION	COMPLICATIONS	INFANT WEIGHT	INFANT COND	REMARKS
1	19								
2	19								
3	19								
4	19								
5	19								
6	19								
7	19								
8	19								
9	19								

FAMILY HISTORY
(Especially diabetes, hypertension, tuberculosis, renal disease, hemorrhagic tendencies, allergy)

FATHER'S HISTORY
AGE:
HEIGHT ft. in. WEIGHT lbs.
OCCUPATION AND MEDICAL HISTORY

PATIENT'S HISTORY
MEDICAL HISTORY
SURGICAL HISTORY

ALLERGIES
TRANSFUSIONS

MENARCHE	DURATION	INTERVAL	FLOW	RECENT IRREGULARITY:
PMP	LMP	EDC	QUICKENING	INFERTILITY OR CONTRACEPTION

CURRENT PREGNANCY — COMPLAINTS
EARLY PREGNANCY ILLNESS
FIRST TRIMESTER MEDICATIONS
PELVIC PAIN BLEEDING
OTHERS

SUGGESTED ANESTHESIA:
RECOMMENDATIONS

FORM 232 (REV APR 74) (PREV USABLE)

PRENATAL RECORD

Figure 12-1. Prenatal record.

on her interpersonal communication skill background in interpreting the reproductive process and the various roles of the health providers to today's knowledgeable client.

With today's emphasis on positive health, ideally every patient ought to be under the care of obstetric personnel during the entire period of her pregnancy. This supervision aids greatly in determining the health status of those anticipating parenthood. The mother-to-be should be seen as early as possible and at least every four weeks thereafter until the seventh month. Then her visits can be made every two weeks until the last month of pregnancy, during which time it is most important that she be seen every week. The therapy of all patients should be individualized. In the case of an expectant mother who has an abnormal condition, the visits can be spaced according to the demands of the situation.

When a woman thinks that she may be pregnant, she will contact her physician or clinic. She is generally asked preliminary questions regarding why she thinks she may be pregnant and is given an appointment for a pregnancy test. If the test is positive, an appointment is made for her to see the physician and nurse. At the initial visit, a general history of the patient is taken, and a general medical examination is performed, followed by an obstetric examination

■ PHYSICAL EXAMINATION ■		By ▶		Consultant		DATE	
AREA CHECKED	NORM √	BP	PRESENT WEIGHT LBS	NON-PREGNANT WEIGHT LBS	HEIGHT FT INS		
EYES		IF ABNORMAL, EXPLAIN					
ENT							
NECK							
BREASTS							
HEART							
ABDOMEN							
EXTREMITIES							
NEUROLOGICAL							
BACK/SPINE							
PSYCHIATRIC							
CONGENITAL ANOMALIES							
SKIN/HAIR DISTRIBUTION							

PELVIC

RECTAL

PELVIC MEASUREMENTS	DIAGONAL CONJ.	SIDE WALLS	PUBIC ARCH
	SACROSCIATIC NOTCH	ISCHIAL SPINES	TRANSISCHIAL
PELVIC MORPHOLOGY	SACRUM	POST SAGITTAL	

DIAGNOSIS

■ LABORATORY DATA ■					TITERS ▶	D A T E S		R H	
STS	DATE	CHEST X-RAY	DATE	URINALYSIS	DATE				
TUBERCULIN TEST	DATE	VAGINAL SMEAR	DATE	HEMOGLOBIN	DATE				
BLOOD TYPE	RHO	HUSBAND'S BLOOD TYPE		HUSBAND'S RHO					
OTHER LABORATORY DETERMINATIONS	2 HR. B.S.								
HCT	DATE								
UA	DATE								

■ IMMUNIZATIONS ■				DATE
		DATE		DATE
		DATE		DATE

antepartal care   167

which includes a vaginal examination. It is important to note that, with the modern collaborative efforts of the various health personnel, a variety of persons may be responsible in varying degrees for the following activities. For instance, an admissions clerk or nurse may initiate the information on the history. The physician together with the nurse-midwife or nurse practitioner may perform the general physical and obstetric examination. Laboratory tests may be done by laboratory technicians. Some aspects of dietary instruction may be given by a nutritionist or all aspects of patient instruction may be handled by the nurse. Whatever the participation of the various personnel, the initial visit usually proceeds as follows.

The history

The name and address of the patient, her age and parity, and the date of the latest menstrual period are recorded, and the date of delivery is estimated. Inquiries are made into the family history, with special reference to any condition likely to affect childbearing, such as hereditary disease, tuberculosis, or multiple pregnancy. The personal history of the patient then is reviewed not only with regard to previous diseases and operations, but particularly in relation to any difficulties experienced in previous pregnancies and labors, such as miscarriages, prolonged labor, death of infant, hemorrhage, and other complications. Inquiry is made into the history of the present pregnancy, especially in relation to nausea, edema of the feet or the face, headache, visual disturbance, vaginal bleeding, constipation, breathlessness, sleeplessness, cramps, heartburn, lower abdominal pain, vaginal discharge, and varicose veins. Usually a suitable form for recording these particulars is employed. As a rule, obstetricians, hospital clinics and other community health agencies have their own forms for recording these details (Fig. 12-1).

General medical examination

The general medical examination includes weighing the patient, taking the blood pressure, inspecting the teeth and the throat, and making an examination by auscultation and percussion of the heart and the lungs. Opportunity is taken at this time to inspect the breasts and the nipples, particularly in relation to their suitability for subsequent nursing. From an obstetric viewpoint, one of the important details of the general medical ex-

amination is the measurement of the blood pressure (Fig. 12-2). This is usually carried out first and is also done when the patient is seen on subsequent visits. As will be explained later, any substantial increase in blood pressure indicates one of the most serious complications in pregnancy—toxemia. A fact for the nurse to keep in mind is that any sudden or gradual rise in the systolic or the diastolic blood pressure is significant and may be alarming.

Obstetric examination

The obstetric examination is comprised of three parts: 1) palpation and auscultation of the abdomen; 2) estimation of pelvic measurements; and 3) vaginal examination. Palpation and auscultation of the abdomen yield valuable information concerning the size and position of the fetus and the rate of the fetal heart. The importance of careful pelvic measurements has already been emphasized, and the purpose of the vaginal examination (aside from its use in the diagnosis of pregnancy) is to rule out abnormalities of the birth canal (particularly those which might impede labor) and to take the diagonal conjugate measurement (Fig. 12-3).

Laboratory tests

The laboratory tests carried out in antepartal care are the urine examination, the blood test for syphilis, the estimation of the hemoglobin, and tests for the Rh factor and blood type. Recently, more institutions are instituting tests for the mother's status to rubella immunity. At the first and subsequent examinations, the urine is tested for albumin and sugar. The patient is instructed to collect a part of the first urine voided in the morning before breakfast. The reason for this is that glucose may spill into the urine of a normal pregnant woman due to a decreased kidney threshold for glucose. Hence, it is more likely to appear in the urine after a meal. The test for sugar is the same as that used to test a diabetic's urine; several simple tests are available today and may be completed quickly and accurately in a matter of minutes. Any positive reaction to sugar is reported to the physician so that the possibility of diabetes or a prediabetic condition can be ruled out.

The test for albumin also is simple. The principle involved here is the application of heat in chemical form, which solidifies any albumin present and causes a whitish precipitate. The presence of albumin in the urine is another symptom of possible toxemia and should be reported immediately. The sudden appearance of albuminuria is regarded as a symptom of preeclampsia.

The blood for the Wassermann or other serologic test for syphilis is usually obtained by venipuncture. A sufficient quantity of blood is drawn at this time so that a portion may be employed for the Rh factor and hemoglobin estimation. Since many pregnant women develop anemia, the latter examination is highly important. A metabolism test is routine in the practice of some obstetricians.

If the test for the Rh factor shows the patient to be Rh negative, it may be necessary to check the father. It is also a wise precaution for the physician to have the father's blood type (see Chapter 27).

In many antepartal and postpartal clinics, the secretions in the cervix and the vagina are examined microscopically to ascertain whether the cells contained therein exhibit certain changes suggestive of incipient uterine cancer. A drop of the cervical or the vaginal fluid is placed on a glass slide, and after this has been spread out in a very thin layer, it is stained for microscopic study. This is called a Papanicolaou smear or Papanicolaou spread. According to the cellular picture seen, it is classified by number from Class 1 to Class 5. Smears in Classes 1 and 2 are characterized by the complete absence of malignant or "suspicious" cells. They are regarded as normal. Smears in Classes 3, 4 and 5 contain cells that either are suggestive of malignancy or actually malignant. These call for further investigation and, in some cases, intensive treatment. The rationale of this procedure is that it provides a method whereby incipient cervical cancer can be detected in its earliest stages. Since the success of treatment in any form of cancer depends on early diagnosis and early treatment, the use of the Papanicolaou smear promises to prevent many fatalities from uterine cancer, one of the most common causes of death in women.

Weight

The routine estimation of weight at regular intervals during pregnancy is an important detail of antepartal care. Any *marked gain* or *loss* in weight will be discussed by the obstetrician. At first the average gain in weight of the fetus is 1 Gm. daily; nine-tenths of the

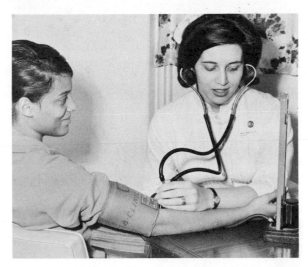

Figure 12-2. Clinic nurse taking blood pressure of pregnant patient.

weight is gained after the fifth month, and one-half of the weight of the fetus is acquired during the last eight weeks. Most physicians agree that a weight gain of about 25 to 30 pounds is desirable for a woman who is average or "normal" in her prepregnant weight. However, there is increasing evidence among investigators that the weight gain for pregnancy needs to be individualized for every patient, particularly those of under and over average prepregnant weights. In the former

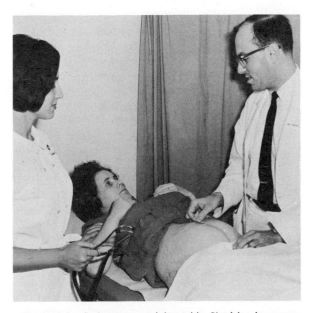

Figure 12-3. Patient on examining table. Physician is measuring the height of the fundus.

case, a gain of 30 pounds or more has had no deleterious effects on the mother and has resulted in a healthy normal weight infant. For all patients the emphasis is becoming less centered on gain per se, but rather on a balanced nutritional status related to the patient's general physical condition.

Return visits

At return visits careful inquiry is made into the general well-being of the patient, and questions are asked concerning any untoward signs and symptoms, such as edema of the fingers or the face, bleeding, constipation, and headache. The patient then is weighed, her blood pressure is taken, and the urine is analyzed for albumin and sugar. An abdominal examination is usually carried out at this time. Abdominal, vaginal, and rectal examinations should be done at regular intervals to determine that pregnancy is progressing at the expected rate and, following quickening, that the fetus is living. During these visits the patient should be encouraged and given ample opportunity to ask the physician and nurse any questions that may be of concern to her.

Instructions to patients

After the routine examination the physician or the nurse may instruct the patient regarding diet, rest and sleep, daily intestinal elimination, proper exercise, fresh air and sunshine, bathing, clothing, recreation, and dental care.

It is usually possible and always desirable to assure the patient that the findings on examination were normal, and that barring complications, she may anticipate an uneventful pregnancy followed by an uncomplicated delivery. However, at the same time, she is tactfully instructed regarding certain danger signals which demand immediate report to the physician. These symptoms are as follows:

1. Vaginal bleeding, no matter how slight
2. Swelling of the face or the fingers
3. Severe continuous headache
4. Dimness or blurring of vision
5. Flashes of light or dots before the eyes
6. Pain in the abdomen
7. Persistent vomiting
8. Chills and fever
9. Sudden escape of fluid from the vagina

In addition to this detailed supervision the patient needs an explanation of the changes that are taking place within her body. This point cannot be stressed enough. Intelligent exploration with the patient regarding her concerns about these changes and appropriate instruction will give her greater reassurance and self-confidence. An understanding and empathic attitude on the part of the physician and the nurse will do much to buoy the patient's morale and to diminish unnecessary anxiety.

As the patient approaches full term, she can be instructed also about the signs and symptoms of oncoming labor, so that she may know when the process is beginning and when to notify the physician. At this time the physician will want to know the frequency of contractions and any other pertinent symptoms.

Most hospitals conduct routine tours of the maternity division for the expectant parents. It is advisable to encourage them to take advantage of this opportunity sometime during the pregnancy. Becoming familiar ahead of time with the surroundings where the mother-to-be will be delivered reduces the anxiety that may be experienced in going to a strange hospital for the first time after labor has begun. The details of the hospital admission routine are explained, so that she is familiar with this procedure before being admitted for delivery.

The nursing process

Although adequate antepartal care is becoming more readily available throughout the nation, health workers find that because of one or several factors in the previously mentioned crises, many women who want this care often do not utilize available services, or they may discontinue their care at some point in the pregnancy. This is particularly true of those who attend clinics. There are several reasons that have been cited by patients as deterrents: 1) extremely long periods of waiting, 2) impersonal treatment by staff, 3) complicated procedures for clinic registration, 4) different physicians at each visit, 5) inadequate comfort facilities, such as toilets and sitting rooms, 6) no evening or weekend clinic, and 7) lack of personnel who understand the problems that the patient faces in her daily life.

If those who provide care merely focus on a maintenance type of physical care and make no attempt to discover and help the expectant mother to satisfy her needs as she perceives them, the patient does not really receive good nursing care. Those who attend her must recognize that the pregnant woman is an individual involved in one of life's most important experiences. When the atmosphere of the hospital, the clinic or the physician's office is such that a patient encounters regard for her human dignity and worth, and her concerns are listened to with interest and respect, she returns for care and profits by it. Therefore, one of the most important activities of the nurse who attends antepartal patients is to establish a relationship with the patient that conveys regard for her as a human being and permits free and frank discussion. This type of relationship not only will enable the nurse to instruct and counsel the mother more effectively about the various aspects of her pregnancy, but also will allow the patient to express the more covert concerns and nuances of the pregnancy that trouble her. The nurse then will be in a better position to deal with these herself or to refer them, as the occasion warrants, to the other members of the health team.

The nurse involved in antepartal care will find herself in one of three settings: a private physician's office, a clinic, or the community. Whatever the setting, the nurse should be skilled in communication techniques, since these are basic to establishing a productive nurse-patient relationship. The nurse must be able to notice what goes on in the interaction between herself and the patient, to interpret what she observes, and to determine appropriate nursing intervention accordingly. In conferring with patients, the nurse needs not only to teach and give information, but also to be able to get it as well. Hence, she must be able *to listen* to what the patient is saying, to make nonjudgmental responses, to question, and to elicit significant information from the patient when it is appropriate in order to increase her own understanding.

The nurse who *listens actively* to what the patient is saying will discern the covert as well as the overt cues. In conversation she can reflect the gist of the patient's remarks so that both patient and nurse may gain insight into the topic under discussion. The skilled nurse can also probe gently but effectively to get at the crux of the problem or the concern. In helping the patient to separate fact from fiction in the situation and eventually to see what alternatives she has for action, the nurse helps the patient to confront her problems more realistically.

The nurse's understanding of human behavior will guide her in choosing the appropriate time and circumstances to help the

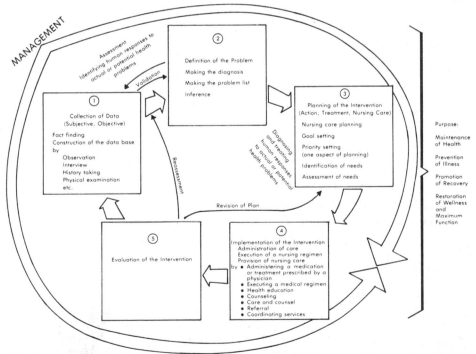

Figure 12-4. Contextual scheme for some currently used terms in the conceptualization of nursing practice. (Block, D.: Some crucial terms in nursing: what do they really mean? *Am. J. Nurs.* 22:11, Nov. 1974)

patient in this way. The skillful nurse focuses her attention on the mother and listens, reflects, and questions to learn more about the mother-to-be as an individual, her usual methods or ways of coping with problems, whether she needs help, and how she reacts to advice.

Nursing assessment

From the time of initial contact with the patient, the nurse will be gathering data about the patient so that she can formulate a plan of nursing care and pass on information needed by other members of the health team. These data tell the nurse what needs or problems the patient has, and the type and extent of intervention that is required. Over the years, new terminology has evolved, and as nursing science develops, other terminology no doubt will be employed. Figure 12-4 presents a model for a contextual scheme of some current terms used in the conceptualization of nursing practice.

In general, nursing assessment provides data from which a total picture of the patient will be drawn. Each facility generally has some form on which to note information obtained in the various assessments, and this form often accompanies the patient to the labor and delivery area. Figure 12-5 illustrates a form developed by one hospital in the northwest.

Alternatively, the nurse may develop her own tool. Whatever the format, the following general areas are to be included, as well as a description of the plan of care:

1. Social and personal characteristics of the patient: age, marital status, occupation, ethnicity, religion, height, weight, number of children in the home.
2. Information summary of spouse (father of baby): name, address, age, height, weight, ethnicity.
3. Characteristics influencing the course of pregnancy: EDC, LMP, blood type and Rh, pertinent medical conditions and/or hospitalizations, current medications and medication habits, usual bowel patterns, usual sleep patterns, resumé of dietary habits.
4. Attitudes toward the pregnancy: Was this child planned? What are the patient's goals and values regarding this pregnancy (and life in general)? Does she view this pregnancy as a boon or interference in her life? What is her knowledge about health in general and pregnancy and childrearing in particular? Does she have any previous ex-

perience with pregnancy and/or childrearing? What are her expectations and concerns about this pregnancy, birth, and care of the infant? What is her apparent willingness or disinclination to prepare herself in the areas that need attention?
5. Resources: What appears to be her general level of intelligence and/or education? What is the level of economic stability? Is the family intact? Is there family available to her? Does she have sufficient friends from which she can get tangible help and emotional support if necessary?
6. Resumé of antenatal classes and instruction: antenatal classes and films attended, individual and group instruction and counseling.
7. Nursing care plan: nursing prescriptions, interventions, and evaluations.

The office and clinic settings

THE PROBLEM OF LIMITED TIME. The nurse accustomed to caring for patients on the inpatient hospital service, where she has continuous contacts with the same patient for days or weeks at a time, often finds the initial adjustment to an office, or especially a clinic service, difficult because of the limited time that the schedule usually permits for contacts with each patient. During the patient's brief appointment period in these last two settings, the nurse must evaluate the present and continuing nursing needs of the individual and plan to meet these needs effectively. The nurse who recognizes and understands this problem of limited time will find the orientation period less frustrating, and as she becomes more skilled in communication and observation of nonverbal as well as verbal behavior, she will enjoy the satisfactions of giving patient care and guidance in these types of settings.

TEACHING THE PATIENT. In addition to assisting the physician with examinations and performing various procedures, the nurse in the office or the clinic can devote much of her nursing care to health teaching and anticipatory guidance (i.e., informing mothers about what to expect regarding their pregnancy, delivery, postpartal and childrearing periods before they begin to worry or to make mistakes). Therefore, the nurse needs to have broad knowledge and understanding about the physiology of pregnancy and childbearing, general hygiene, nutrition, the emotional, psychologic, and socioeconomic aspects of family living, and the part

University of Oregon Medical School
Hospitals & Clinics

MATERNAL–CHILD NURSING ASSESSMENT CARE PLAN

Date   Bldg.   Fl.   Rm.

Unit No.

Name

Birthdate

Age   Marital Status Religion   Ht   EDC   LMP

    M S W D Sep

G   P   AB   CIRC   Blood Type   Rh   No. of Children

           if boy   at home

           Y   N

Labor & Delivery Progress, Problems, Behavior

Spouse (baby's father) Name   Address Age   Ht   Wt   Race

Allergies   Previous Hospitalization   Medications on now

Baby   Weight   Status

Describe Usual Bowel Routine   Describe Usual Sleep Patterns

Self-Care Instructions & Observations
(check when instructed)

☐ Breast self-exam   ☐ clean catch
☐ Breast care for   ☐ peri care
    breast-feeding   ☐ heat lamp

Future Plans (outcome of preg, home situ, job, lifestyle)

Has patient been observed doing these completely?
Y   N   Explain.

PRENATAL CLASSES attended:

☐ Anatomy, physiology,   ☐ family planning,
    hygiene   baby care
☐ Nutrition, breast- &   ☐ labor, delivery PP,
    bottle-feeding   Anesthesia
☐ Exercises, Group   ☐ other

Will pt. need follow-up help with any of above?

Individual Prenatal Instruction—check when pt. instructed

☐ warning signs of pregnancy   ☐ prenatal Lit given
    20-28 weeks   ☐ bottle-feeding
☐ Breast-feeding   ☐ bottle sterilization
☐ Breast care
☐ Method of Prepared
    Childbirth Referral_____

Mothering Tasks:
☐ Mother has looked over baby completely.
    If no, why?

☐ Doing breathing & relaxation   ☐ Room for infant
    exercises   ☐ Clothing for infant
☐ Sibling preparation
    36-40 weeks   Referrals Made
☐ signs of labor and what to do   _____
☐ someone at home to help   _____
☐ family planning   _____
☐ postpartum & well baby care   _____

Mother observed doing tasks:
    + correct   — needs help
☐ diapering   ☐ holding
☐ feeding   ☐ burping
☐ other
Does this mother or family need help in
any above area?

NURSING CARE PLAN

(General Observations, Concerns of Patient or Family/and/or problems observed by staff, knowledge and attitudes concerning childbirth and care, restrictions to visitors, etc.)

Date	Area of Concern/Problem list	Intervention (Plan of action)	Progress	Signature

---

Figure 12-5. Front side of the Maternal-Child Nursing Assessment Care Plan. The reverse of this form continues the Nursing Care Plan chart and under the heading "Discharge Planning" asks the following questions: 1) Has the baby's father come to visit the baby and/or mother? 2) Who is at home to help this mother? 3) Which of the following have been discussed: Bathing baby; Sibling rivalry; Baby's crying; Circumcision care; Navel care; New routine at home; Other. 4) Where will she take baby for well baby care and PKU test? 5) Are any problems anticipated when she goes home? 6) What consults or referrals were planned while in hospital or upon discharge? 7) Date of discharge? There is also a place for the nurse's signature. (Nunnaly, D. M.: A nurse establishes prenatal program with med-school clinic, JOGN, Jan.-Feb., 1974)

played by a family in the larger community. Her teachings are individualized for each patient, and should include instruction in ways of maintaining good health habits in daily living, interpretation of the reasons that these practices are important, and suggestions of ways in which undesirable habits may be changed or modified. It is important to remember that health teaching and anticipatory guidance in any setting involve motivating the patient—and consequently influencing the degree of her interest and her desire to change or to continue present patterns of behavior. To accomplish the desired end, the nurse first identifies the level of knowledge and understanding of the patient through exploration of what the patient knows and feels about the topic in question. Second, the nurse clarifies any misinformation or misconceptions. Finally, she adds to the base of knowledge and understanding through reinterpretation, clarification, reemphasis, and reinforcement.

The problem of motivating patients is complex, and unfortunately no simple steps or methods exist to explain how to accomplish this. Generally, it seems that valid information about the subject, reference groups, and the patient's personal values are key *preconditions* to motivation. Another key precondition is the selection of a goal or "request" which the patient can reasonably achieve. If, for instance, a patient is well informed on a subject and can identify in some way with the group from which the request comes, and if the subject or the request is not at too much variance with the patient's values, she can comply without an enormous degree of change or effort; then the stage is set to "motivate."

The initial contact with the patient is particularly important. By her pleasant greeting and professional manner the nurse can initiate a productive relationship that conveys her interest and concern for the patient. In making a patient comfortable who is waiting for her appointment with the physician, the nurse can utilize the opportunity to find out any questions, symptoms, or problems that the mother may have and deal with them or report them to the proper person. This is an example of one way that the nurse can utilize limited contacts with the patient constructively.

Referrals. The problems that come to light are not always of a physical nature; emotional and social problems also may interfere with the patient's ability to derive full benefit from health services. It is the responsibility of the nurse to find out in what ways the patient needs help and to make appropriate referrals when they are indicated (e.g., to the nurse in the community, to allied community services or to other members of the extended health team). This is one of her most important nursing activities, since through the use of referrals she can keep lines of communication open between her particular health agency, the community, and the members of the health team. Thus comprehensive care for the patient is assured.

Visual Aids; Teaching Groups. In hospitals and offices where the appointment system is used, the waiting time for the patient is minimized. In others the patient may have to wait longer periods. Waiting time in any setting may be utilized advantageously by providing reading material that will contribute to the patient's knowledge of her condition. Visual aids such as posters and charts may be both instructive and diverting. Flannelboard posters are excellent in this respect, since they can be changed frequently. These visual aids also provide an outlet for the creative ideas of the staff. Some offices and more and more clinics are using a group approach for discussion, teaching, and guidance. These groups are usually under the leadership of the nurse and provide a maximum amount of instruction for a large number of patients in a short period of time. In addition, in the large, busy clinic, this group discussion technique provides patients with a feeling of continuity of care since the nurse leader remains a stable figure (Fig. 12-6).

THE PHYSICAL EXAMINATION. When the nurse assists the physician with the physical examination, she has an opportunity to learn more about the patient's condition. She should be alert to the cues and the events that transpire during this time, since she may be questioned afterward by the patient regarding her condition, or she may have to interpret the physician's instructions to make certain that they are understood. Often a patient is hesitant to discuss some matter with the physician, because she considers it too trivial, but she may feel comfortable in talking about it with the nurse. In turn, the nurse may consider this a problem of some importance, and on reporting it to the physician, she may find that it has a bearing on the course of treatment that he prescribes.

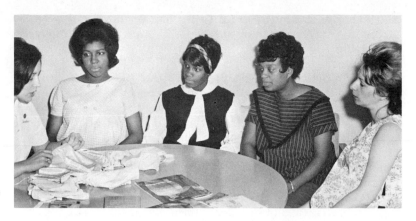

Figure 12-6. Group counseling by the nurse in the clinic.

Another of the nurse's responsibilities is to prepare the patient for the physical examination. Since the initial examination is thorough, it is desirable that the patient disrobe completely and wear a gown that opens easily. In addition, the expectant mother should be covered with a small sheet to prevent unnecessary exposure and chilling. The nurse will want to instruct the patient to empty her bladder, since a full bladder is uncomfortable and may interfere with the physician's manipulations. A good footstool is imperative if the patient is to mount the table in safety and comfort. Many patients move somewhat awkwardly, especially as they near term, and the nurse can contribute a great deal to their safety and also help alleviate embarrassment by assisting the mother, as she changes her position, to move slowly but steadily. For the patient's physical and emotional comfort and for the physician's protection, the nurse should be present during the entire examination.

The Pelvic Examination. One aspect of the physical examination, the vaginal or pelvic examination, deserves special consideration, because often it is the most stressful part of the experience for the patient. This examination is carried out with the patient in the dorsal recumbent position. In this position the patient lies on her back with the lower extremities flexed and rotated outward. Her heels are supported in stirrups, which are level with the table, perhaps a foot in front of her buttocks. In this position the anxious patient, already under stress during the physical examination, is likely to tense her abdominal, pelvic and thigh muscles, attempting to adduct her thighs. Moreover, if the patient arches her back as her tension increases, her pelvis will be tilted downward, a position that makes the pelvic examination almost impossible to achieve.

The nurse can be most effective in assisting the patient to relax if she encourages her to keep breathing naturally, reminds her to breathe if she holds her breath, and helps her to let the small of her back press down on the table. Merely telling the anxious patient to relax is of no avail; thus the nurse needs to give the patient rather direct guidance, often step by step. For example, if the patient is clenching her fists, the nurse may say, "See, your wrists and hands are tense. Try to let them go limp—very limp—like a rag doll's. That's it—very limp." And a moment later, "Keep breathing naturally." Such short, explicit requests and instruction give the mother a simple task that she can do with guidance. This diverts her attention from the anticipated discomfort and promotes relaxation.

Since the examiner must see the cervix clearly, he will need a stool to sit on and a good light to focus into the vagina. Any equipment that he may need, such as vaginal speculum, swabs, cotton balls, slides, lubricating jelly, and the like should be close at hand, so that he can reach them readily.

The pelvic examination will begin with an examination of the external genitalia and will include the urethra, Skene's and Bartholin's glands. If any unusual discharge is present, a specimen may be obtained for culture or microscopic examination. Usually, the physician will next insert a speculum into the vagina to distend the folds so that he may observe the cervix. If a Papanicolaou smear is to be taken, no lubricating jelly will be used; instead, the speculum may be rinsed under *tepid* running water to facilitate the ease of insertion. Occasionally, the dilatation of the vagina by the speculum may cause an unpleasant sensation of stretching. Unfortunately, the patient already may be tense from the effect of strange surroundings and experiences, and the intrusion of this instrument may contribute to her discomfort, increasing her tenseness.

The fear, tension, pain syndrome in labor, first described by Dr. Grantly Dick-Read (see Suggested Reading), can affect the expectant mother under these circumstances as well. Her fear of the examination increases her tenseness, which enhances the discomfort; hence a vicious circle is established. The nurse can do much to break this circle by encouraging the mother to breathe naturally while she is being examined. Allowing the patient to squeeze or to hold her hand is often very helpful, although the nurse should recognize that not all patients want or need this physical contact. It is wise to be readily available to the patient but to let her initiate the contact. In our culture, it is important that people "control themselves"; this is difficult to do when a person's privacy is invaded, as it is by these intrusive procedures. It becomes especially important, then, to help the patient to preserve a positive concept of herself in this obstetric situation, since these early encounters all help to form an integral part of the mosaic that determines her self-concept as a mother.

As the examination proceeds, the cervix is visualized, and the examiner will note its color and character. Normally, the cervix of the primigravida is pink or bluish and smooth, with a dimple for the os. The cervix of a multigravida may have an irregular os due to lacerations from previous deliveries. If erosions of the cervix are present, they may be treated with silver nitrate swabs. Any discharge, such as a purulent, a greenish or a frothy discharge, is considered to be abnormal, and a specimen may be secured for microscopic examination or culture.

After the cervix has been examined, the examiner will withdraw the speculum and proceed with the bimanual examination to evaluate the uterus and the adnexa. He will determine the size, the consistency and the contour of these organs as well as the relationship of the uterus to the pelvis. At this time he will take the internal measurements to determine the diameters of the pelvic inlet (see Chapter 5). The physician usually completes the pelvic examination with an examination of the rectum to ascertain the presence of hemorrhoids, polyps, or other abnormalities.

At the completion of this examination, disposable tissues should be offered the patient so that she may wipe the perineum adequately. Optimally, further activity and demands should be kept at a minimum, so that the mother may recoup the energy which has been dissipated through trying to absorb all the new experiences and information. Further specific health teaching and counseling is better postponed until a subsequent visit, when the patient is not so overloaded with new stimuli and fatigue.

THE PATIENT AND HER FAMILY. In a program which emphasizes family-centered service, the health problems of the individual patient and their relationship to other members of the family are of major importance. An example of a situation might be the case of Mrs. Brown, the wife of a laborer and the mother of a small toddler and a four-year-old boy. Her physician has advised her that she needs more rest in the course of the day. Her husband is at work, and the older boy is in nursery school until noon. In order to get more rest, she needs help to make plans for the safety and the care of the children during these rest periods; otherwise the physical rest would not accomplish its purpose. Even the consideration of meeting the nutritional needs for this family with a limited income may require guidance. To give real help at this point requires some knowledge of nutrition and entails extra planning so that the meals supply the nutritional requirements for a pregnant woman, a father who performs hard physical labor, and two small children. Wherever facilities and personnel permit, more clinics are utilizing the services of a "resident" nutritionist for guidance and counseling regarding nutritional aspects and planning. Depending on the clinic's procedure, the nurse may then have the responsibility of referring the patient to the nutritionist or arranging for the patient to join a group of mothers who meet with the nutritionist for planning. In the case where a nutritionist is not available, the responsibility for this counseling falls to the nurse.

The nurse in the office or the clinic who is alert to such actual or potential health problems that affect both the patient and her family recognizes that a home visit by a community health nurse often is very helpful. If such a situation arises, she can tell the patient about available community health services and explain what this nurse might do while making a home visit and how such a visit could benefit the patient. With the physician's knowledge and the patient's permission, she can institute a referral through the proper channels. Each institution or agency will have its particular method and procedure. Real value may be derived from a visit in which the nurse is able to see the patient in her usual surroundings. For instance, if the patient has the problem of excessive weight gain and is not responding to clinic therapy, the community health nurse, visiting the patient in her home, may gain some insight into the basis of the problem during her visit. In her report to the clinic or the office staff, she would relate information that would contribute to both the medical and the nursing management of this pregnancy. In situations in which the clinic program is limited in educational opportunities, such as parents' classes and/or individual guidance, the community health nurse's visit to the home may be necessary to supplement the health care teaching and anticipatory guidance done in the clinic.

The community setting

The extensive adoption of early antepartal care by various institutions, both lay and medical, is doing much to improve obstetric standards; and, in connection with this movement, the community health nurse has been an invaluable asset. During the period before antepartal care was fully accepted, a case-finding program was a part of the work done by some organizations (i.e., the nurse would canvass the district for pregnant mothers). In recent decades the demand for hospital deliveries has increased rapidly; thus the present trend is toward hospital care. This has resulted in an increased demand for hospital beds, and some hospitals, especially those in congested areas or those with limited facilities, have requested that patients register early in their pregnancy to be assured of adequate accommodations for their deliveries. This early registration has resulted in more mothers getting adequate antepartal supervision early in pregnancy. In some isolated rural areas the community health nurse does case finding in the course of her usual activities and can assist the local practitioner in the antepartal care of maternity patients in the community.

IDEAL ROLE OF THE COMMUNITY HEALTH NURSE SERVING IN AN AGENCY. The nurse in the community is "home-based" in either an official or a voluntary agency. The official health agency may have an antepartal clinic offering complete antepartal services for those families who are having financial crises that may or may not be a result of the pregnancy. Many agencies have recognized that the community health nurse is not being utilized to her fullest potential when she is responsible for the administrative aspects of the clinic. When the professional nurse is caught up in the mechanics of record work, room preparation, directing traffic, and assisting with procedures, she can barely reinforce the physician's orders and perhaps clarify information relative to the obstetric condition. To utilize the time of the professional nurse more efficiently, so that she is free to counsel patients in depth in any matters relative to health, many agencies are employing registered nurses for clinic management who do not have the community health credential (i.e., formal preparation in community health and community health certification). In addition, to maximize patient care, various types of other auxiliary personnel may be utilized (e.g., lay volunteers, licensed vocational nurses, nursing aides, and so on). The clinic managers together with other nonprofessional personnel may be responsible for all of the clinic activities with the exception of patient counseling. Similarly, more hospital clinics throughout the nation are beginning to utilize a community health nurse for the health teaching and the anticipatory guidance aspects of patient care. As has been described already, most clinic schedules are very full, and the distribution of activities in such a manner results in more comprehensive patient care.

If the patient and/or her family has a problem that the community health nurse in the clinic thinks needs follow-up in the home (between clinic visits), she will contact her district counterpart and communicate the necessary information. In turn, the district nurse will inform the clinic personnel of any pertinent findings. If complete comprehensive care is to be given to patients, open lines of communication and an expeditious interagency referral system are basic to the best service of all members of the health team, whatever their level of responsibility.

HOME VISITS. The district community health nurse does not follow a stereotyped routine when she makes her home visits, since each visit involves an individual patient in her own home setting. She does not have the "captive audience" that the hospital nurse does; rather she is a guest in her patient's home, and this involves a somewhat different approach and orientation. In such a situation, it is especially important to orient the visit to what the patient wants and needs to know. Repeated visits based on the *nurse's* needs (to impart certain information, instruction, and so on) may very well result in a firmly closed door and a consequent severing of the nurse-patient relationship. Astute assessment of the situation at each visit includes, first of all, finding out what the patient needs to know. Communication and observation skills (previously mentioned) are, of course, of paramount importance here. It is the wise nurse who takes her cues from the mother and handles each need as it arises without feeling compelled to "teach" a certain amount of material each visit. If the visits are managed in this way, topics may include basic information about pregnancy, hygiene, and nutrition, specific preparations for the baby, how to handle sibling rivalry, and so on. These subjects may come up naturally in the course of the visits, or the nurse can guide conversation around to them as she explores with the mother certain areas of need. By the end of the antepartal supervision period, all necessary counseling usually can be accomplished.

Opportunities for Family Health Supervision. During the course of antepartal care, the nurse has many opportunities for family health supervision. In her observation of other children in the home, she may be the first person to notice a neglected orthopedic condition, to suspect a need for a chest roentgenogram, or to observe a possible vision or hearing difficulty. In addition, observation of the mother's interaction with her children may give valuable clues to the patient's mothering patterns. This will aid the nurse in planning more effective anticipatory guidance and health teaching.

COMPREHENSIVE ANTEPARTAL CARE, then, is a quality of patient care that is goal-directed toward the total health and the well-being of the pregnant woman. With this as the central objective, the combined efforts of several disciplines, in addition to those of medicine and nursing, may be required in the cooperative plan to achieve the ultimate goals. The practitioner-patient relationship is reciprocal, involving one giving and the other receiving care, and, to be meaningful, it must be a positive interaction. This type of interaction can be achieved only if the patient and her problems are understood and viewed with respect. The patient, in turn, must be helped to understand the goals of the health practitioners. A positive effort on the part of the health team becomes possible if each member has a clear under-

standing of his own role, appreciates and understands the contribution of the other professions represented on the team, knows something of the processes involved in the differing approaches, recognizes commonality of interest and skill, and has the intellectual and the emotional capacity to enter into a team relationship.

The medical social worker

Although nursing care is the primary consideration in this section, one member of the extended health team will be mentioned specifically since she works so closely with the nurse in the care of the pregnant woman. Most hospitals today have a substantial Social Service Department; it is hoped that more community health agencies will be able to take advantage of this service as more funds and personnel make this possible.

THE FUNCTION of Social Service workers is to help people to meet and to cope with problems that interfere with social functioning. These problems may include unmarried parenthood, divorce, desertion, placing older children during the mother's hospital stay, arranging for a working housekeeper, planning convalescent care for the mother, or arranging financial or material assistance. In their professional role, social workers are called on to evaluate these problems. Then, with the patient's cooperation they help her to mobilize her resources and assist her, when necessary, through referral and counseling to alleviate the condition. They may make home visits and interview the patient, and perhaps other family members, to aid them in diagnosing the extent of the problems. Social problems may seem overwhelming if the patient's physical condition is affected, and these concerns, in turn, may interfere with the benefit that the patient may derive from medical services. The social worker may act as an understanding counselor between the family and the patient during her hospital stay. In many hospitals the need for a social service referral is apparent when the patient is registered early in pregnancy. In that event, the patient is interviewed after the initial medical examination, and from both the physical and the social findings, plans are made with the patient to mobilize her resources.

By her observation, counseling, and liaison work, the social worker combines her efforts with the other members of the health team to see the patient not only as an individual mater-

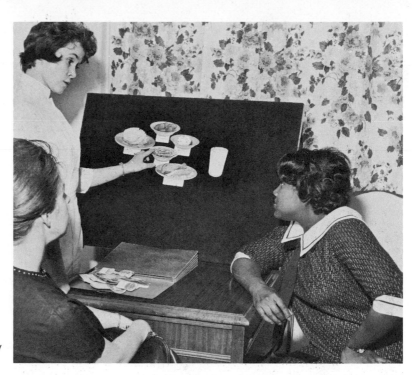

Figure 12-7. Nutritional counseling by the dietitian in the clinic.

nity patient, but also as an important member of the family, and the family as an integral part of the community.

Nutrition in pregnancy

As previously mentioned, present day antepartal clinics are utilizing the services of nutritionists for dietary counseling and planning whenever possible (Fig. 12-7). When nutritionists are available, the nurse will find that she can work in conjunction with them to provide adequate guidance. Her role in these cases may be to explore with the mother the extent of her need to have nutritional counseling and/or arrange for the mother to participate in some form of counseling under the auspices of the nutritionist. However, many areas do not have the services of a nutritionist, and in these instances, a very important activity of the nurse is that of nutritional counseling. Attention has been focused on the diet of the pregnant mother in recent studies, and it has been demonstrated that the improved nutritional status of the mother promotes not only her wellbeing, but also her baby's. For instance, a significant relationship has been found between the protein intake of the mother and the physical condition of the infant. Moreover, research has demonstrated an association between in-

adequate protein intake during pregnancy and mental deficiency in the fetus, as well as low birth weight (see Suggested Reading). Thus, an appropriate diet promotes building materials for the growth and the development of the mother's offspring. The student is advised to study the recommended dietary allowances so that she can compare necessary increases in pregnancy (see Table 12-1).

General factors in planning the diet

CALORIC INTAKE. Calories provide the energy requirements for the body. They are needed to maintain bodily processes, thermal balance, and physical activity. Caloric allowances are established to provide for adequate energy requirements and to support growth and body weight levels for the fetus and mother which are commensurate with health and well-being.

In the past, it was generally recommended that weight gain be limited by caloric restriction with the purpose of preventing and controlling toxemia and eclampsia. This idea goes back to some observations that were made after World War I. It was noted that pregnant women in Germany and Austria-Hungary gained less because of protein and fat scarcity and seemed to have a lower incidence of toxemia. Subsequent studies were not done and from these unsystematic observations

Table 12-1 Recommended Daily Dietary Allowances

Designed for the maintenance of good nutrition of practically all healthy people in the United States[a]

	Age (years)	Weight (kg.)	Weight (lbs.)	Height (cm.)	Height (in.)	Energy (kcal.)[b]	Protein (g.)	Vitamin A Activity (RE)[c]	Vitamin A (IU)	Vitamin D (IU)	Vitamin E Activity[e] (IU)	Ascorbic Acid (mg.)	Folacin[f] (µg.)	Niacin[g] (mg.)	Riboflavin (mg.)	Thiamin (mg.)	Vitamin B6 (mg.)	Vitamin B12 (µg.)	Calcium (mg.)	Phosphorus (mg.)	Iodine (µg.)	Iron (mg.)	Magnesium (mg.)	Zinc (mg.)
Infants	0.0–0.5	6	14	60	24	kg. × 117	kg. × 2.2	420[d]	1,400	400	4	35	50	5	0.4	0.3	0.3	0.3	360	240	35	10	60	3
	0.5–1.0	9	20	71	28	kg. × 108	kg. × 2.0	400	2,000	400	5	35	50	8	0.6	0.5	0.4	0.3	540	400	45	15	70	5
Children	1–3	13	28	86	34	1,300	23	400	2,000	400	7	40	100	9	0.8	0.7	0.6	1.0	800	800	60	15	150	10
	4–6	20	44	110	44	1,800	30	500	2,500	400	9	40	200	12	1.1	0.9	0.9	1.5	800	800	80	10	200	10
	7–10	30	66	135	54	2,400	36	700	3,300	400	10	40	300	16	1.2	1.2	1.2	2.0	800	800	110	10	250	10
Males	11–14	44	97	158	63	2,800	44	1,000	5,000	400	12	45	400	18	1.5	1.4	1.6	3.0	1,200	1,200	130	18	350	15
	15–18	61	134	172	69	3,000	54	1,000	5,000	400	15	45	400	20	1.8	1.5	2.0	3.0	1,200	1,200	150	18	400	15
	19–22	67	147	172	69	3,000	54	1,000	5,000	400	15	45	400	20	1.8	1.5	2.0	3.0	800	800	140	10	350	15
	23–50	70	154	172	69	2,700	56	1,000	5,000		15	45	400	18	1.6	1.4	2.0	3.0	800	800	130	10	350	15
	51+	70	154	172	69	2,400	56	1,000	5,000		15	45	400	16	1.5	1.2	2.0	3.0	800	800	110	10	350	15
Females	11–14	44	97	155	62	2,400	44	800	4,000	400	12	45	400	16	1.3	1.2	1.6	3.0	1,200	1,200	115	18	300	15
	15–18	54	119	162	65	2,100	48	800	4,000	400	12	45	400	14	1.4	1.1	2.0	3.0	1,200	1,200	115	18	300	15
	19–22	58	128	162	65	2,100	46	800	4,000	400	12	45	400	14	1.4	1.1	2.0	3.0	800	800	100	18	300	15
	23–50	58	128	162	65	2,000	46	800	4,000		12	45	400	13	1.2	1.0	2.0	3.0	800	800	100	18	300	15
	51+	58	128	162	65	1,800	46	800	4,000		12	45	400	12	1.1	1.0	2.0	3.0	800	800	80	10	300	15
Pregnant						+300	+30	1,000	5,000	400	15	60	800	+2	+0.3	+0.3	2.5	4.0	1,200	1,200	125	18+[h]	450	20
Lactating						+500	+20	1,200	6,000	400	15	80	600	+4	+0.5	+0.3	2.5	4.0	1,200	1,200	150	18	450	25

[a] The allowances are intended to provide for individual variations among most normal persons as they live in the United States under usual environmental stresses. Diets should be based on a variety of common foods in order to provide other nutrients for which human requirements have been less well defined.

[b] Kilojoules (kJ) = 4.2 × kcal.

[c] Retinol equivalents.

[d] Assumed to be all as retinol in milk during the first six months of life. All subsequent intakes are assumed to be half as retinol and half as β-carotene when calculated from international units. As retinol equivalents, three fourths are as retinol and one fourth as β-carotene.

[e] Total vitamin E activity, estimated to be 80 percent as α-tocopherol and 20 percent other tocopherols.

[f] The folacin allowances refer to dietary sources as determined by *Lactobacillus casei* assay. Pure forms of folacin may be effective in doses less than one-fourth of the recommended dietary allowance.

[g] Although allowances are expressed as niacin, it is recognized that on the average 1 mg. of niacin is derived from each 60 mg. of dietary tryptophan.

[h] This increased requirement cannot be met by ordinary diets; therefore, the use of supplemental iron is recommended.

Source: Adapted from Food and Nutrition Board, National Academy of Sciences—National Research Council Recommended Daily Dietary Allowances, Rev., 1974.

came the notion that caloric restriction to limit weight gain protected women from toxemia and other pregnancy complications. We now have evidence to indicate that the incidence of toxemia can be significantly higher in women who are markedly underweight as compared to those who are extremely overweight. Moreover, it has been found that even an excessive weight gain of from 9 to 10 pounds at the end of pregnancy for very *underweight* women is still compatible with *minimum* risk for developing toxemia symptoms![6]

In pregnancy there is an increased need for calories to provide for energy requirements necessary for building the fetal and placental tissue and for maintaining the mother's tissue requirements. An additional 200 calories above the mother's usual caloric intake are recommended during pregnancy. This caloric consumption is consistent with the average 24-pound weight gain that is recommended by the Committee on Maternal Nutrition. We now have evidence that a strong positive association exists between the weight gain of the mother and the birth weight of the infant. Among *healthy* women who have a *well-balanced* diet and eat "to appetite," the range in weight gains can be very wide. The Committee on Maternal Nutrition suggests that a range of from 20 to 25 pounds is a reasonable target and is most consistent with favorable outcomes in pregnancy.

However, as Cross and Walsh[7] point out, weight gain above the recommended range, if *proceeding at a regular rate*, should not be criticized *without consideration of cause*. Because of limited incomes, many women have to purchase a major portion of their protein and other nutrients in combination with large quantities of fats and carbohydrates. For instance, pinto beans cost about seven cents per serving of 30 Gms. of protein, while ground meat costs 23 cents for the same amount of protein, and roast beef costs 53 cents. In these days of soaring and fluctuating prices, to restrict this woman's caloric intake would also restrict her intake of protein and other needed nutrients.

In addition, the Committee on Maternal Nutrition recommends that weight reduction programs should not be imposed during pregnancy as distortions in normal pregnancy weight gains are apt to occur. The focus should be on the birth weight of healthy infants and not on a social norm of figure maintenance for

Table 12-2 Food and Nutrition Board National Academy of Sciences National Research Council Recommended Daily Dietary Allowances, 1968

Nutrients	Moderately Active Healthy Female 18-35 yrs. Wt. 128 lb. Ht. 64 in.	Moderately Active Healthy Girls 16-18 y.	14-16 y.	12-14 y.
Calories	2,200	2,500	2,600	2,500
Protein Gm.	65	65	65	60
Calcium Gm.	1.2	1.7	1.7	1.7
Iron mg.	18	18	18	18
Vitamin A (I.U.)	6,000	6,000	6,000	6,000
Vitamin D (I.U.)	400	400	400	400
Ascorbic Acid mg.	60	55	55	50
Folacin mg.	0.8	0.8	0.8	0.8
Niacin mg. equivalent	15	17	18	17
Riboflavin mg.	1.8	1.8	1.7	1.7
Thiamin mg.	1.1	1.3	1.3	1.3
Vitamin B_6 mg.	2.5	2.5	2.3	2.1
Vitamin B_{12} mg.	8	8	8	8
Iodine mg.	125	140	145	140

Source: Adapted from Cross, A. T., and Walsh, H. E.: Prenatal diet counseling, *J. Reproductive Med.* 7:266, Dec. 1971.

the mother. The recommendation of 1.5 to 3.0 pound gain during the first trimester and a 0.8 pound per week during the reminder of the pregnancy is commensurate with good health for both the mother and fetus *even if the mother is overweight at the beginning of pregnancy.*

A more positive approach to the problem of caloric intake would be to advise the mother that "every calorie should count"; that is, calories eaten during pregnancy should provide an abundance of other nutrients as well. Table 12-2 lists the nutrient need of pregnancy for the various childbearing age groups recommended by the Food and Nutrition Board of the National Academy of Sciences, National Research Council, 1968.

There are some women who need particular attention to their nutritional needs during pregnancy. They can be grouped for purposes of discussion as follows:

1. Biologically immature mothers. These are women who are pregnant and are under the age of 17. The stresses of pregnancy are

added to the nutritional needs for body growth and maturation at a time when existing poor or marginal nutritional status may further contribute to poor pregnancy outcome.

2. Mothers who are experiencing rapid, successive pregnancies which often deplete maternal nutrient stores.

3. Women who have low prepregnancy weight for their height—a greater-than-average incidence of toxemia and a strikingly increased incidence of prematurity occurs in this group.

4. Mothers who have a limited weight gain during pregnancy which may result in low birth weight infants.

5. Overweight expectant mothers. While weight per se is not an indication of nutritional status, food selections of some obese women are likely to emphasize "empty calorie" foods—rich in fat and carbohydrates—which are low in essential proteins, minerals, and vitamins.

6. Mothers who have low incomes. Inability to purchase needed foods during pregnancy coupled with a history of poor diet and suboptimal health makes pregnancy outcome experience in this group exceptionally poor. High rates of maternal and infant mortality and prematurity exist for these mothers and infants.

7. Mothers who because of religious, philosophical, or other reasons have limited their food intake to certain groups of foods, such as vegetarian diets, macrobiotic diets, fruitarian diets, and the like.

8. "Healthy" mothers who are besieged with confusing, conflicting and misleading nutrition information. These mothers also need guidance in selecting a high-quality diet.

During the early months the appetite may be affected, and there may be phases of dislike for certain foods and beverages. Later, there may be an increase in the desire for all food or certain types of food. The mother may need help to discipline her appetite in accord with the amount of food needed. Thoughtful and cooperative meal planning with the patient, with specific and thorough direction as to quantity and quality of nutrients, does much to help the mother to maintain motivation and discipline during these times.

Also, it is well to counsel the mother early in her pregnancy to avoid sweets and high caloric desserts, as well as the habit of frequent nibbling, since these interfere with appetite for the more essential foods. Early pregnancy is a good time to institute health teaching of this sort, since many mothers are motivated to attain good health for themselves and their impending child at this time and hence are very receptive to anything that will bring this about. Appetite tends to be diminished, and therefore appropriate choosing of the quantity of food may be easier; later, when the "newness" of the pregnancy has worn off, and the appetite is unleashed, self-discipline is much harder, especially without previous reinforcement. Occasional "cravings" for unusual types of food may occur. These sometimes indicate the lack of a certain element in the diet that the body demands. Any desires of this nature may be granted with safety, if they agree with the patient and are not exceptional in amount or content. If the diet supplies all the needs of the patient and the growing fetus, such cravings may not occur.

There is one other consideration in planning the diet for the pregnant woman. That is the *deemphasis* in sodium restriction during pregnancy. Like the former calorie restriction, restriction of salt was thought to be an important factor in the prevention of toxemia. Clinical and laboratory data now indicate that this restriction is not necessary for all pregnant women and can, indeed, be harmful when imposed indiscriminately. Flowers[8] has noted that there is a mechanism present in pregnancy that increases sodium reabsorption and retention when there is a reduction in sodium intake during pregnancy. An adequate renal and placental blood flow demands an adequate circulating blood volume. When there is a stringent reduction in sodium intake, there is a reduction in circulating blood volume which is intolerable during pregnancy and causes damage to both the mother and fetus. Thus, the routine restriction of salt for the healthy woman is being questioned, as well as the indiscriminate use of diuretics for reduction of edema that was heretofore thought to have been associated with sodium retention caused by excessive salt in the diet. Many physicians now advise their patients early in the pregnancy to simply "salt their food to taste" and not to cut down inordinately on their sodium intake.

There are some specific suggestions that the nurse can make to help the mother attain the philosophy of "every calorie should count." In so doing, a high-quality diet can be maintained and an adequate weight gain can be achieved without excessive poundage due to "empty calories."

1. The patient can be acquainted with the amazing fattening potentials of certain common *nonessential* foods—foods which, in many people's minds, scarcely deserve that term at all, because most of them are likely to be regarded as mere snacks without perceptible effects on total caloric intake. Actually, these little extras taken between meals or at bedtime constitute one of the most common causes for excessive weight gain in pregnancy and at other times. A glass of ginger ale or cola drink averages 100 calories. A chocolate bar approximates more than 300 calories. A single cocktail or highball has 200 calories. A doughnut without icing plus a cup of cocoa yields 400 calories, and the average malted milk served at soda fountains contains some 500 calories. Pie à la mode approximates 600 calories. When it is recalled that 2,200 to 2,600 calories per day generally is recognized as a satisfactory allowance for pregnancy, it is plain that these "little snacks" loom tremendously large in relation to the total caloric allotment. If she is hungry between meals, the patient may take the glass of milk scheduled for dinner, omitting it from her evening meal. Raw vegetables and fruit also are helpful in assuaging hunger pangs.

2. The patient should be reminded that the way in which a food is prepared may affect its caloric value almost as much as the nature of the food itself. Perhaps the simplest way to show how the preparation of a food affects its caloric value is to be found in fried foods. Although the caloric content of a poached or boiled egg is about 80 calories and is so calculated in dietary lists, once that egg is fried, its caloric value jumps to around 120 calories because of the fat absorbed by the egg in cooking. A level tablespoon of fat, let it be emphasized, yields approximately 120 calories. With regard to soups and desserts, it is common knowledge that those made with milk are of much less caloric content than those made with cream, and that those made with skim milk are still lower. When flour or cheese in addition to cream is used, as in escalloped or au gratin dishes, the calories soar to unbelievable heights; in general, for this group of foods, the smoother and the more delicious the taste, the higher is the caloric value.

The intrinsic caloric value of foods of the same type varies widely. Fruits show considerable variation according to their degree of sweetness. For instance, canned fruit can be very high in calories because of the sugar in the syrup. Therefore, the mother can be reminded to use fresh fruits regularly, and if for some important reason canned fruit must be served, the unsweetened varieties or those packed in light syrup are the only ones that should be taken. It might be added that these varieties are more economical than those packed in the rich heavy syrups. Likewise, meats vary greatly in their caloric contents; lean meats being low and those with much fat in their substance being high. As as example of the latter, an average serving of linked country sausage may exceed 600 calories. To summarize this aspect of caloric intake, the patient should be reminded that fried foods invariably possess a high caloric content; that milk, preferably skim milk, should be substituted for cream in preparing soups and desserts; and that lean meat rather than fatty meat must be chosen, and fresh fruit rather than canned.

The balanced diet

The physician will regulate the patient's diet according to her needs and condition, and the nurse will follow through, planning with the mother to how best meet her nutritional requirements. If the patient's previous diet has been nourishing and well balanced, few changes will be necessary except to provide for the adjustment in protein, mineral, and vitamin intake.

DELIVERING NUTRITIONAL COUNSELING. Each mother is an individual whose attitudes and beliefs toward emotional response to food, cultural meaning of food, and knowledge of nutrition are unique. Creating a positive attitude toward nutrition during pregnancy requires patience, understanding, and respect for her particular nutritional patterns of behavior.

To deal with each patient's individuality, the physician and nurse must provide an opportunity and atmosphere for the mother to discuss her concerns about food and diet and to give information about her current dietary patterns. Nutritional evaluation requires information on not only what is eaten, but also the quantities and the method of preparation. Information will also be needed regarding purchasing practices as certain foods may not be purchased because of cost and more economi-

Table 12-3 Diet History and Evaluation Form

Name_____ Date_____

_____ Due Date_____

Patient's childhood home_____ Height_____

  (State or country)_____ Present weight_____

Patient's occupation_____ Pregravid weight_____

Last year school completed_____

Husband's occupation_____ Birth date_____

Money available for food weekly_____ Number in household_____

Food currently bought by_____

Meals currently prepared by_____

Foods liked especially, including cravings_____

_____

_____

Foods never eaten and why (storage problems, equipment, and so on)_____

_____

_____

Nutritional supplements currently used during pregnancy (kind and amount used)_____

_____

_____

_____

Diet modified previously or currently (type of diet and date)_____

_____

_____

Meals and snacks often eaten at these times:

Morning: _____

_____

_____

Midmorning: _____

_____

Midday: _____

_____

_____

_____

Afternoon: _____

_____

Evening: _____

_____

_____

_____

Before bedtime: _____

_____

Prenatal diet prescribed and date_____

Instruction received on prenatal diet including materials given_____

_____

_____

Additional information_____

_____

Followup remarks_____

_____

Prenatal dietary history recorded by: _____

_____

It is desirable to obtain a dietary history as early as possible in pregnancy and before recommending a specific diet for an individual mother. This history should include: information concerning the expectant mother's usual food practices, meals often omitted, typical menu patterns, food likes and dislikes, cultural factors, methods of food preparation, financial situation, and so on. Nutritional gaps will be obvious from an evaluation of this information. During the process of taking a diet history, useful information is obtained concerning the patient's level of nutrition knowledge and clues to methods of counseling. Explaining any recommended changes will help the expectant mother understand her present needs. (If history is kept in patient's chart and information is recorded elsewhere, interviewer may prefer to omit some questions. Sample form may be changed to fit situation).

Source: Cross, A. T., and Walsh, H. E.: Prenatal diet counseling, *J. Reproductive Med.* 7:269-270, Dec. 1971. From *Nutrition—During Pregnancy and Lactation*, Berkeley, Calif., California State Dept. of Public Health, 1971.

cal substitutions may be needed. Table 12-3 illustrates the type of nutritional assessment form that can be used to obtain adequate dietary information.

To provide appropriate guidance for the mother and to better assess her level of understanding and knowledge about her diet, a brief diet history can be taken to find out her present eating patterns. The nurse may ask the mother to write down her usual daily and/or weekly meal pattern and any "extras" that she is likely to consume. These menus then are checked for an adequate intake of those foods that provide a substantial amount of the essen-

Table 12-4 Sample Menus*

	Regular	Mexican	Black	Oriental	American Indian	Lacto-Ovo
Breakfast						
2 Energy Foods	1 Cup Cream of Wheat / 1 Tbsp. Sugar	2 Corn Tortillas / 2 Tbsp. Jelly	1 Cup Grits / 1 Tbsp. Sugar	1 Cup Rice / 1 Tsp. Sugar (in Tea)	1 Cup Corn Mush / 1 Tbsp. Sugar	1 Cup Brown Rice / 1 Tbsp. Honey
1 Calcium/Protein Food	1 Cup Milk	½ Cup Evaporated Milk in Coffee	1 Cup Milk	1 Cup Milk	1 Cup Milk	1 Cup Milk
1 Vitamin C Food	1 Cup Orange Juice	1 Cup Orange Juice	1 Cup Orange Juice	1 Cup Orange Juice	1 Cup Orange Juice	1 Cup Orange Juice
Lunch						
1 Energy Food	1 Slice Bread	1 Tortilla	1 2" Square Corn Bread	½ Cup Rice	1 Slice Indian Fried Bread	1 Slice Whole Wheat Bread
2 Protein Foods	2-1 oz. Slice Cheese	1 Cup Beans	1 Cup Pork and Beans	3½ oz. Tofu / 1 Egg	1 Cup Pinto Beans	1 Cup Lentils
1 Calcium/Protein Food	1 Cup Milk	½ Cup Evaporated Milk and Chocolate	1 Cup Milk	1 Cup Milk	1 Cup Milk	1 Cup Milk
1 Vitamin A Food	½ Cup Spinach	½ Cup Spinach / 1 Green Pepper	½ Cup Collard Greens	3/5 Bok Choy	½ Cup Spinach	½ Cup Spinach
1 Vitamin/Mineral Food	1 Banana	1 Banana	1 Banana	1 Banana	1 Apple	1 Banana
Dinner						
1 Energy Food	1 Small Baked Potato	½ Cup Spanish Rice	2 Halves Candied Yams	½ Cup Rice	½ Cup Fried Potatoes	1 Small Baked Potato
3 Protein Foods	3 oz. Beef Roast	1 Cup Beans / 1 Cup Caldo	3½ oz. Fried Pork Chops	Okazu (Stewing Beef 3 oz. ½ Cup Broccoli) and 2 oz. Tofu)	3½ oz. Fish	3½ oz. Cheese (Cheddar)
1 Calcium/Protein Food	1 Cup Milk	½ Cup Evaporated Milk and Coffee	1 Cup Milk	1 Cup Milk	1 Cup Milk	1 Cup Milk
2 Vitamin/Mineral Foods	1 Stalk Broccoli / 1 Cup Fruited Jello	1 Cup Fruited Jello	1 Cup Peas / 1 Cup Fruited Jello	1 Cup Fruited Jello	1 Stalk Broccoli / 1 Cup Fruited Jello	1 Stalk Broccoli / ½ Cup Fruited Jello
Snacks						
1 Calcium/Protein Food	1 Cup Custard	1 Cup Flan	1 Cup Custard	1 Cup Custard	1 Cup Custard	1 Cup Custard
1 Vitamin/Mineral Food	1 Pear	1 Pear	1 Pear	1 Pear	1 Pear	1 Pear
1 Energy Food	2 Oatmeal-Raisin Cookies	2 Oatmeal-Raisin Cookies	2 Oatmeal-Raisin Cookies	2 Oatmeal-Raisin Cookies	2 Oatmeal-Raisin Cookies	2 Oatmeal-Raisin Cookies

* The menus above show the cultural variations possible when planning a nutritionally adequate prenatal diet. All meet the Recommended Dietary Allowances for calories, provide a minimum of 90 Gm. of protein, and exceed the Recommended Dietary Allowances for vitamins A and C and calcium. Only the black and Mexican dietary pattern meets the Recommended Dietary Allowances for iron, providing 21.9 mg. and 23.1 mg. The regular, American-Indian, and the Oriental pattern provide 15.3 mg., 15.8, and 15.3 respectively. The lacto-ovo plan provides only 12.0 mg.

Source: Cross, A. T., and Walsh, H. E.: Prenatal diet counseling, *J. Reproductive Med.* 7:274, Dec. 1971.

tial nutrients. As the nurse and the mother plan together, the patient's likes and dislikes are recognized, and those foods that provide the essential nutrients are encouraged. Suggestions may be given for the addition of certain foods or the modification of existing methods of selection and/or preparation. During these planning sessions, it is important to remember that the mother is a member of a family, and although she plans the meals, many of her choices are dictated by the likes and dislikes of her family. The young teenage bride who has just learned to fry cheeseburgers and french fries for her spouse may not be persuaded easily to broil and to bake instead; furthermore, she deserves recognition for accomplishing something as important as preparing a meal that is pleasing to her husband.

The religious, racial, and ethnic background of the patient and her family is another important consideration with respect to nutritional counseling and other aspects of care. Many families are fond of their regional or national diet and prefer it to the American "meat and potatoes" regimen. Whenever possible, the preferred diet should be considered and planned through the use of "exchanges" for food groups (see Suggested Reading). Many nutrition books give a "basic national" diet for the various countries, which provide a springboard for planning. Table 12-4 gives sample menus that illustrate the common variations in diet found in this country.

In considering the diet of persons of a different ethnicity, the nurse also will consider the degree of *acculturation* of the patient. This term refers to the acquisition by a group or an individual of the traits of another culture. For instance, in the case of a bilingual patient with the name of Munoz, it should not be assumed that beans and tortillas are staple in the diet. Mrs. Munoz may be a third-generation American and very familiar with and accepting of North American nutrition and eating patterns (i.e., she is acculturated).

The young "counter culture" has stimulated a new interest in a lifestyle and dietary pattern which is "natural" and emphasizes an ecologic system of living. Many positive attitudes toward nutrition exist in this group. There is the rejection of highly processed foods which contain little nutritive value, that is, cake-type snack food made from refined sugar and flour, processed and fried items such as potato chips, and foods which have many additives. There is

also a general return to foods that are in their more natural forms (rice and flour, particularly) and that are prepared in wholesome ways—little frying and overcooking. However, a good deal of guidance often is needed to avoid food faddism and to meet nutritional needs. Those who choose alternate lifestyles for various philosophical, religious, and/or health reasons often follow vegetarian diets also, either pure or lacto-ovo. It is possible to meet the protein and mineral requirements of pregnancy on many of these various diets, but to do so requires considerable knowledge of the protein content of foods and continual attention to including these foods in the diet. However, some of the patients who subscribe to these diets do not have the requisite knowledge and/or resources to procure the appropriate amount of protein. Moreover, they may be swayed more by philosophical and religious considerations than by those which are nutritional.

Several of the vegetarian diets have certain inherent deficiencies.[9] They can be adequate only if they are supplemented with dairy and poultry products, which are necessary to meet the nutritional requirements of all age groups. If the majority of the calories are obtained from unrefined grains, legumes, nuts, and nut-like seeds, accompanied by a wide variety of vegetables including the green leafy variety, the result is a diet rich in bulk and many vitamins. This is very helpful in alleviating constipation, but is sparse in providing the complete proteins and minerals essential for adequate nutrition.

Those who exclude all animal products, including dairy products and eggs, run the risk of developing a vitamin B_{12} deficiency. The diets prescribed by the Vegan group contain adequate amounts of folic acid which masks the symptoms of B_{12} deficiency, so one who strictly follows such a diet may be totally unaware of the deficiency until irreversible degeneration of the spinal cord has occurred. This condition has occurred often enough to become known as "Vegan back." The symptoms are soreness of the tongue, anemia of the pernicious type, menstrual irregularity, and paresthesia. Vitamin B_{12} alleviates the symptoms dramatically if they are detected early enough.

Those who adhere to the Krishna group, who eat neither meat nor eggs but do consume dairy products, encounter few nutritional problems other than iron-deficiency anemia. However, this can be important during pregnancy. Those who do exclude dairy products increase the risks inherent in lowered intake of protein, riboflavin, and calcium. An exaggerated cereal consumption enhances zinc deficiency. It is important to remember that, while most of the vegetarian diets contain an adequate *amount* of protein, the quality of the amino acids is not the best; that is, they are incomplete proteins. Thus, some form of complete protein (eggs, dairy products, fish, or fowl) must be taken with the incomplete proteins (legumes, nuts, cereals) at the *same meal*. Patients also need to be advised to keep their calorie intake from fats and carbohydrates high enough so as not to deplete their protein as a calorie source.

Individuals who *strictly* subscribe to the macrobiotic diet can suffer from a combination of all the nutritional afflictions that are seen in the other vegetarian groups who have stringent anti-dairy, poultry, and fish proscriptions. The deaths and debilitation in recent years that were attributed to the *extreme* adherence to the macrobiotic diet prompted the Council on Foods and Nutrition of the American Medical Association to warn health professionals that these diets can produce major health problems by inducing scurvy, hypoproteinemia, anemia, hypocalcemia, and the emaciation of starvation with the accompanying loss of kidney function.

Pregnant and lactating women and their infants appear to be especially vulnerable to the defects of the strict macrobiotic diet. Pediatricians in the San Francisco Bay area have reported a high incidence of low birth weight babies (less than 5 pounds), many of whom gained little or no weight during breast-feeding. Young women who adhere to a *stringent* macrobiotic regimen during pregnancy may have a heavy discharge and experience fatigue, muscle cramps, and a variety of infectious diseases. They can lose fat and muscle tissue and, not infrequently, have severe anemia in addition to showing all the signs of hypoproteinemia.

Any health professional who tries to counsel those who adhere to a strict vegetarian group must try to understand each group in the context of its own terms and must appreciate the influences that govern food selection if he or she hopes to effect a stable and effective nutritional status (see Suggested Reading). Reinforcement of the positive aspects of the dietary practices helps to modify the more negative aspects in the context of the vegetarian's belief system. In making attempts at education, there must be tolerance and a nonjudgmental attitude and respect for the client's rejections of dietary information if she chooses. These may be difficult as providers of care traditionally expect their advice to be followed. However, more may be gained in the long run by accepting the "client's right to choose" since she will be more likely to seek care from those whom she feels respect her views even if they differ considerably from the provider's views.

Psychological Aspects of Nutrition. Other aspects to be considered are the stage of growth and development of the patient and the psychologic factors involved in nutrition (e.g., the meaning that food has for the mother). We are aware, for instance, that foods enjoyed by adolescents are different from the foods enjoyed by older people; the hamburger-soda-french fry "typical" teenage diet has received wide publicity. It seems to meet some need in much the same way as peanut butter sandwiches do for the preschooler. Many persons are marrying younger and becoming parents at an earlier age, and, of course, they carry their eating patterns into marriage with them. In addition, adolescence is a time for developing independence, and this is healthy. However, many foods are rejected (milk, vegetables, cereal, and the like), because they are associated with "home" and a dependency period. The desire to be free and to select the "forbidden" foods is very strong. Permitting assertion of independence is important if the overall developmental task is to be accomplished, and the patient is to make a healthy adjustment in roles from that of the child to that of the adult; yet limits often must be set if the health of the mother and the health of the baby are to be safeguarded. Therefore, incorporating the mother into the planning and allowing her choices whenever possible, helping her to increase her knowledge of nutrients, encouraging and reinforcing correct choices or willing adaptations, and giving firm guidance when indicated, all help the patient and the nurse to achieve their respective goals.

The psychologic aspects of nutrition lend themselves less well to clear-cut analysis. It has been said that people can survive a state of celibacy, however uncomfortably, but no one has been able to survive without food. Food is a basic need, according to the survival criterion, more basic even than the need for sex. We know that hunger is the most fundamental of all sensations. Related to hunger, but of a very different origin, is appetite. Appetite is Nature's primary defense for the prevention of hunger. Based on the anticipation of eating, the impulse is determined by the person's previous experience. Only by coincidence and training does appetite become associated with health-giving foods. Factors affecting food-seeking behavior are the main determinants of eating (i.e., hunger, appetite, and custom). The great deterrents to normal appetite are worry, fear, and preoccupation with troublesome or difficult problems—and these may be reflected in either an increase or a decrease of appetite. Some of the positive emotional stimulants include a situation of calm contentedness, a feeling of mild elation, or a condition of ego-stimulation.

Present-day cuisine is a potpourri of heritage, superstition, custom, knowledge, and opportunity. Subtle cravings are passed along from one generation to the next by the process of training and imitation. Unique methods of food preparation as well as food selection, combinations, and prejudices are embodied in this training. Congeniality and hospitality among normal people are enhanced by the serving of good food; and it has become the custom to serve food at practically all functions, business as well as social.

From infancy onward, food and closeness are associated with love and security. Food and eating, in and of themselves, are looked upon as symbolizing interpersonal acceptance, warmth, and sociability. Throughout all societies this symbolic undertone is unmistakable; from the "breaking of bread" in antiquity to the modern banquet the serving of food is a vehicle for expressing honor, joy or mutual bonds. It is easy to see why food has become associated with the symbolism of motherliness. Feeding is not only kindly and warm in its emotional meaning to those who receive food, but it is also essential to growth and well-being; hence it has become bound up with the idea of the mother, the one who originally nurtured, loved, and supported.

The pregnant woman makes a close identification with the concept of the mother, and selections and choices may be influenced profoundly by these symbolic meanings of food. She may respond to worry, frustration, or anxiety by overeating—either by nibbling or gorging. Conversely, another patient may develop anorexia. Or she may crave certain foods and reject others, and not because of physiologic factors. For instance, she may feel that certain foods will "mark" her baby or will give him strength. It is crucial that the meaning which food has for the patient be explored, and that her feelings and attitudes be respected. Care must be taken not to make her feel deprecated or deprived while she is helped to understand the dynamics involved in hunger and appetite.

In summary, if counseling is to be effective and the results lasting, the nurse should strive to elicit wholehearted cooperation from the patient through involving her in the planning; considering her and her family's needs, background, preferences, and attitude; encouraging and reinforcing appropriate choices and preparation; providing gentle but firm limit setting, when indicated, and careful, thorough explanation regarding the rationale behind the advice.

The following discussion might provide some guidelines in helping patients to plan their diet. Foods have been grouped according to four general classifications: dairy foods, meat group, vegetables and fruits, and breads and cereals. This type of classification is a useful one to employ with the patient as most individuals have an understanding of dairy foods, meat groups, and so on, but may be less familiar with the more basic terminology of protein, carbohydrates, and the like. However, an effort should be made to incorporate these latter terms into the mother's vocabulary since she will encounter this language in everyday life. Table 12-5 presents a summary of the sources and functions of the major nutrients needed during pregnancy and lactation.

DAIRY FOODS. The expectant mother needs a quart of milk or its equivalent daily. Milk is nature's most nearly perfect food and is invaluable as a nutrient. It contains all the different kinds of mineral elements that are needed for fetal development. The high content of calcium and phosphorus in milk makes it almost indispensable for good growth of bone and teeth; it provides these minerals in the correct proportions and in a digestible form which permits optimum utilization by both mother and fetus. It is not only an excellent source of protein or tissue-building material, but also the most readily digested and easily absorbed of all food proteins. Milk is also rich in energy-providing values, so that one quart a day alone furnishes almost one-fourth of the total energy requirements. Finally, milk contains some of the most important vitamins, particularly vitamin A, which increases resistance to infection and safeguards the development of the fetus.

Unfortunately, many persons are not able to tolerate milk well and/or decidedly do not like it. If the mother is able to tolerate it, and if she can overcome her aversions, an effort should be made to have her drink two glasses a day; the remainder may be taken in some other form, such as soups, custards, and so on. Evaporated milk and instant dried milk are acceptable and may be substituted if fresh cow's milk is not available or desired. Other dairy products, such as cottage cheese, ricotta cheese, farmer's cheese, hoop cheese, yogurt, and the hard cheeses are also adequate substitutes. Hard cheeses, such as cheddar, jack, swiss, and the like, are higher in calories than the soft cheeses—cottage, ricotta, hoop; two exceptions are mozzarella and the Armenian string cheeses. Both of these are often made from skim milk. One ounce of cheese contains approximately the same amount of minerals and vitamins as a large glass of whole milk. However, the total protein and fat content will vary and must be considered when making substitutions.

For some individuals, milk may cause distressing gastrointestinal symptoms, such as nausea and diarrhea. These symptoms indicate a milk allergy and intolerance and the product should not be encouraged. Substitutes can be found in other protein sources. For other patients, milk may be constipating, and, if amenable to treatment, an effort should be made to treat the constipation other than by omitting the milk. If the milk is merely distasteful without causing physical symptoms, it may be disguised in other foods as mentioned previously.

The instant nonfat and whole dry milks may be used in a quantity that provides an adequate intake. Approximately five tablespoons of dried skim milk will equal one pint of fluid milk. The milk may be used dry and worked into meatloaf, mashed potatoes, cereals, sandwich spreads, baked articles, and so on. Reconstituted with less than the usual amount of water, it has a richer taste than the regular liquid skim milk. Certain condiments and flavorings (vanilla, nutmeg, instant coffee,

Table 12-5 Summary of Major Functions and Sources of Nutrients

	Function	Source	

Protein	Growth of fetus and accessory tissues
	Production of breast milk
		Animal Protein
		  meat
		  fish
		  poultry
		  eggs
		  milk
		  cheese
			Vegetable Protein
			  dried beans
			  dried peas
			  lentils
			  nuts
			  peanut butter

Iron	Maintain hemoglobin level of mother
	Maintain mother's stores of iron
	Furnish iron for fetal development
	Furnish infant with iron stores needed for blood formation during neonatal period before food sources of iron are added to diet
		Good Sources
		  pork liver
		  kidney
		  beef liver
		  oysters
		  clams
		  canned dried beans
		  prune juice
		  liverwurst
		  heart
		  lean pork
		  lean beef
		  raisins
		  cooked dried beans
		  cooked dried peaches
		  cooked dried apricots
		  cooked dried prunes
		  canned green peas
			Fair Sources
			  enriched pastes
			  spinach
			  canned mackerel
			  enriched white bread
			  kale
			  mustard greens
			  whole wheat bread
			  canned string beans
			  eggs
			  brussels sprouts
			  broccoli

Calcium	Skeletal structures of the fetus
	Production of breast milk
	Blood coagulation, neuromuscular irritability and muscle contractility
		Good Sources
		  skim milk
		  buttermilk
		  whole milk
		  nonfat dry milk
		  cheese
		  ice milk
		  ice cream
			Fair Sources
			  dark green
			    leafy vegetables
			  dried beans
			  broccoli
			  cottage cheese
			  canned fish—
			    including bones
			  oranges

Vitamin A	Tooth formation
	Normal bone growth
	Healthy skin
	Vision—light/dark adaptation
		Vitamin A
		  butter
		  egg yolk
		  fortified margarine
		  kidney
		  liver
		  whole milk
		  cream
			Carotenes
			  dark green and deep
			    yellow vegetables
			    and a few fruits
			  apricots
			  broccoli
			  cantaloupe
			  carrots
			  chard
			  collards
			  kale
			  mustard greens
			  persimmons
			  spinach
			  pumpkin
			  sweet potatoes
			  turnip greens
			  winter squash

Riboflavin	Functions in number of enzyme systems in tissue respiration
	Metabolism of amino acids and carbohydrates
		Good Sources
		  heart
		  kidney
		  liver
		  milk
		  ice milk
			Fair Sources
			  broccoli
			  cheese
			  dark green leafy
			    vegetables
			  eggs
			  ice cream
			  lean meat
			  poultry

Thiamine	Appetite and digestion normal
	Nervous system health
	Completion of carbohydrates
		Good Sources
		  whole grain and
		    enriched bread
		  whole grain and
		    enriched cereals
		  dried peas
		  dried beans
		  oranges
		  liver
		  heart
		  kidney
		  lean pork
		  nuts
		  potatoes
		  peas
		  wheat germ
			Fair Sources
			  eggs
			  fish
			  meat
			  poultry
			  milk
			  many vegetables

Niacin	Helps translate sources of energy into useable form	Good Sources
		  fish
		  heart
		  lean meat
		  liver
		  peanuts
		  peanut butter
		  poultry
			Fair Sources
			  milk
			  potatoes
			  whole grain and
			    enriched bread
			  whole grain and
			    enriched cereal

Ascorbic Acid	Production of inter-cellular substances necessary for the development and maintenance of normal connective tissue in bones, cartilage and muscles
	Improves health of bones and teeth
	Increases absorption of iron
		Good Sources
		  citrus fruits or juice
		  broccoli
		  brussels sprouts
		  cantaloupe
		  greens—collards,
		    mustard, turnip
		  peppers
			Fair Sources
			  asparagus
			  cabbage, raw
			  cauliflower
			  chile fresh or canned
			    fresh chile
			  kale
			  liver
			  other melons
			  potatoes or sweet
			    potatoes in jackets
			  spinach
			  tomatoes or prunes

Vitamin D	Promotes absorption and retention of calcium and phosphorus necessary for growth and formation of bones and teeth	butter egg yolk fish oils liver milk fortified with vitamin D other foods may contain added vitamin D— check labels	

Source: Cross, A. T., and Walsh, H. E.: Prenatal diet counseling, *J. Reproductive Med.* 7:271-272, Dec. 1971.

cinnamon), when mixed with the milk, will enhance the flavor.

Some patients complain that milk is "fattening." In most instances the weight gain is due to the consumption of more food than is needed or an excess of such foods as bread, potatoes, and desserts. These should be the articles that are restricted, and not the milk. Occasionally, however, it will be necessary to substitute skim milk or churned buttermilk for whole milk. This is acceptable and will reduce calories. Most dairies nowadays reinforce skim milk with vitamins A and D, which otherwise would be deficient. Many companies now have another variety of skim milk, one that is fortified by the addition of nonfat milk solids, 400 USP units of vitamin D and 4,000 USP units of vitamin A per quart. It has a standardized 2 percent butterfat, so that the butterfat content in general is 1½ percent less than that of whole milk.

If the mother can be helped to realize the importance of this one article of food in relation to the development of her baby, the sacrifices or modifications that may be involved may be made more willingly.

MEAT GROUP. This is a rich source of one of the most essential nutrients, protein. Three or more servings of beef, pork, lamb, veal, organ meats, fish, poultry, eggs, or cheese are recommended daily. Legumes (dried beans, peas) or nuts may be used occasionally as alternates. In addition, these foods contain vitamins and valuable minerals, but their main value is in their amino acids or "building stones," as they sometimes are called. These are the elements that are needed not only by the mother, but also by the fetus for the development of all the delicate and intricate systems of his body. Meat, eggs, and fish contain complete proteins, with all the ten amino acids that are necessary to maintain life and support growth. Often the family's budget restricts the quantity and the variety of these proteins, especially with respect to meat. The substitution of cheese, peanut butter, poultry, fish, or legumes then may be suggested. The mother may also need advice regarding the preparation and the utilization of the organ meats that are so rich in protein, vitamins, and minerals. Because some of these are relatively inexpensive, many women do not realize their nutritional worth and further avoid them because of the aesthetics that may be involved in the preparation—skinning, soaking, and so on. Taste also is sometimes a factor.

Nevertheless, with a little ingenuity and suggestions from a good nutrition and/or cookbook, the nurse can do much to help the family to utilize this valuable and inexpensive source of protein. Liver, for instance, can be *lightly* broiled, ground, and incorporated into a meatloaf or ground meat patties. The taste and looks are disguised, the nutritional value is retained, and the meat goes further.

VEGETABLES AND FRUITS. Four or more servings should be included from this group, especially the leaf, stem, green, and yellow varieties of vegetables, as well as the citrus fruits and tomatoes. It is desirable to serve at least one portion of each vegetable and fruit raw.

Vegetables, particularly, are rich sources of iron, calcium and several vitamins. At mealtimes there is no reasonable limit to the amount of lettuce, tomatoes, celery, string beans, carrots, beets, and asparagus which may be eaten, provided that they are not heavily salted, sauced, buttered, or served with a rich dressing. By increasing the quantity of such foods to several times the amount ordinarily taken, it is usually possible to satisfy the appetite without gaining abnormally in weight.

Fresh frozen vegetables are a good alternate. Canned vegetables may be used if fresh are not available. If a good brand is obtained, the vitamin content often is higher than that of vegetables cooked at home. Careful preparation and cooking of vegetables will help to retain the maximum vitamin and mineral content. Some vegetables contain several incomplete proteins which add to the total protein intake.

In addition to their value as nutrient agents, these vegetables deserve an important place in the diet as laxative agents, since their fibrous framework increases the bulk of the intestinal content and thereby stimulates the muscular, eliminative action of the intestines.

Fruits. Citrus fruits—oranges, lemons, and grapefruit—are the best sources of vitamin C. Most of these fruits also supply vitamins A and B. Tomatoes are also an excellent source of vitamin C; the amount, however, must be twice that of the citrus fruits to supply the same amount of vitamin. Other fruits, raw and cooked, such as prunes, raisins, apricots, contain important minerals (iron and copper) as well as vitamins. Fruits may stimulate a lagging appetite and counteract constipation. They may be used in many ways: as juices, combined in salads, additions to cereals or in-between meal refreshments and in desserts, such as gelatins and puddings. Fruits contain some incomplete proteins but only supplement the other proteins.

BREAD AND CEREALS. Four or more servings should be included from this group. In the past it has been the practice to counsel patients to eliminate white bread and cereals and to substitute the darker and whole wheat varieties. This is no longer necessary, since almost all breads and cereals are enriched with vitamins, minerals, and protein. A careful perusal of the label is usually all that is necessary. However, the darker varieties do provide a welcome change and, of course, are nutritious. When cereals are supplemented by milk, they become adequate for growth, as well as for maintaining life. Bread that is buttered increases the vitamin A intake. The coarse cereals and the dark breads add roughage to the diet. Vitamin B and roughage both help to counteract constipation.

In addition to the four basic food groups, special attention should be given to the following:

FLUIDS. Fluids should be taken freely, averaging six to eight glasses daily. Water aids in the circulation of the blood, body fluids, and the distribution of mineral salts, as well as in stimulating the digestion and the assimilation of foods. Fluids help to increase perspiration and to regulate elimination from intestines and kidneys. Tea and coffee may be included in the daily fluid quota if not found to be diarrhetic or sleep disturbing. Alcohol is to be used sparingly, particularly if the mother must watch her weight, since alcoholic beverages have a high "empty calorie" content. The use of a small amount of alcohol by the pregnant woman has not shown a tendency to produce any pathologic changes in the mother or fetus.

VITAMINS. Vitamins are the *live* elements in food and are essential to life. The best sources are the natural foods. To retain the vitamin value in foods, they must be fresh, carefully prepared, and not overcooked. During pregnancy and lactation the vitamin needs are increased, and so it is apparent that a well-balanced diet containing all the vitamins is of first importance. Some physicians add vitamin preparations to the diet to be sure that an adequate requirement has been met.

Vitamin A is essential in the diet for the maintenance of body resistance to infection. Foods which are good sources of this vitamin include whole milk, fortified skim milk, dairy products containing butterfat, eggs, green leafy and yellow vegetables, and liver.

The vitamin B complex is essential to good nutrition. During pregnancy, thiamine (B_1) is necessary in increased amounts, as the fetus readily depletes the mother's reserve. Milk, eggs, lean meat, and whole grain or enriched bread and cereal are good sources of thiamine. Riboflavin and nicotinic acid, absolute essentials in the diet, are found in such foods as meat, milk, eggs, and green vegetables.

Vitamin C is necessary for the proper development of the fetus. Since an adequate reserve of this water-soluble vitamin is not stored in the body, an abundant supply of this vitamin is needed daily throughout pregnancy and lactation. Fresh citrus fruits, berries, and green leafy vegetables (with the exception of lettuce) are foods which are a good source of vitamin C. These foods should be eaten raw as often as possible, since cooking destroys about half of their vitamin content.

Vitamin D is of great importance in safeguarding the mother and the fetus during pregnancy, since it bears some relationship to calcium and phosphorus metabolism. Liver, eggs, fortified sweet milk, and fish (particularly Atlantic herring and mackerel) are food sources of vitamin D. The National Research Council recommends a daily intake of 400 IU for the pregnant and lactating woman. This amount, the Council says, will protect all normal growing individuals from deficiency with an adequate margin of safety. In evaluating vitamin D intake, all fortified foods in the diet should be taken into account, since large doses of either vitamin A or D may be toxic.

MINERALS. Studies indicate that 13 or more mineral elements are essential for good nutrition. It is believed that if calcium, phosphorus, iron, and iodine are provided in adequate amounts, the others also will be present in sufficient quantities.

Calcium. Although two-thirds of the calcium in the fetus is deposited during the last month of pregnancy, the mother's daily requirement of calcium is increased during the entire course of pregnancy to prepare adequate storage for this demand. The principal foods from which calcium is obtained are cheese, eggs, oatmeal, vegetables, and milk. A quart of milk alone supplies 1.2 Gm. of calcium.

Phosphorus. This element is an essential constituent of all the cells and the tissues of the body. Milk provides an abundant source of

Table 12-6 Basic Daily Pregnancy Diet

Predominant Nutrient	Foods	Number of Servings*
Protein and Iron	Lean meats, fish, poultry, lentils, dried beans and peas, eggs, nuts	3 or more (7 ounces)
Protein and Calcium	All milks, cheese, cottage cheese	4 or more
Vitamin C	Citrus fruits and juices, broccoli, brussels sprouts, greens, peppers	1 or more
Vitamin A	Fortified margarine, kidney, dark green and deep yellow vegetables	1 or more
Energy and B Vitamins	Whole grain or enriched breads and cereals	5
Other Vitamins and Minerals	All fruits and vegetables	2 or more
Energy	Fats and sugars	Only as needed for energy

*A serving is:

A two to three ounce serving of lean cooked meat, fish, or poultry without bones is—

¼ pound of hamburger after it is cooked
½ cup cooked diced lean meat, fish or poultry
One medium meat or fish patty
One slice roast meat or poultry, 5 inches by 2¼ by ¼ inch
Two frankfurters
Two slices of liver
Two slices meatloaf
Two medium chicken drumsticks (fryer)
One chicken leg including thigh
One medium sized fish steak

A substitute for a two to three ounce serving of lean cooked meat, fish or poultry without bone is—

½ cup cottage cheese	½ cup shelled peanuts
3 ounces cheddar or jack cheese	4 tablespoons peanut butter
1 cup cooked dried peas, beans, or lentils	3 eggs

A serving of vegetable or fruit is—

½ to ¾ cup or a portion as ordinarily served such as

1 medium apple	1 medium potato
1 medium banana	½ medium grapefruit
1 medium orange	½ medium cantaloupe

A serving of whole grain or enriched breads and cereals is—

1 slice enriched or whole grain bread
½ to ¾ cup cooked whole grain cereal such as cracked wheat, oatmeal, brown rice, rolled wheat
½ to ¾ cup cooked enriched cereal such as grits, cornmeal
½ to ¾ cup enriched noodles, macaroni, spaghetti
¾ cup enriched ready-to-eat cereal
½ to ¾ cup rice, enriched or converted
1 large enriched flour tortilla
2 small corn tortillas

Source: Cross, A. T., and Walsh, H. E.: Prenatal diet counseling, *J. Reproductive Med.* 7:273, Dec. 1971.

phosphorus. Actually, since phosphorus is an almost invariable constituent of protein, a diet which includes sufficient protein-rich foods, such as eggs, meat, cheese, oatmeal, and green vegetables, will provide also an adequate amount of phosphorus.

Iron. During the first two trimesters of pregnancy, iron is transferred to the fetus in moderate amounts, but during the last trimester, when the fetus builds up its reserve, the amount transferred is accelerated about ten times. Therefore, the diet should be balanced and nutritious as well as rich in iron-containing foods. It is believed that certain amino acids, vitamin C, and folic acid may be essential to normal iron absorption. If the daily diet contains egg yolk, lean meat (particularly liver), vegetables, fruit, and whole grain cereals, the problem of anemia is less likely to occur. Recent studies indicate that expectant mothers who were in good health prior to pregnancy can maintain their hemoglobin concentration at known levels of health by eating a balanced diet (see Suggested Reading). However, some physicians prescribe additional iron in the form of such preparations as ferrous sulfate and ferrous gluconate. These preparations are administered three times a day, following meals, to allow for maximum absorption and to eliminate much of the intolerance for iron which would occur if the daily prescription for iron were administered in one dose.

Iodine. Only very small amounts of iodine are needed for the health of the mother and the fetus. This mineral is obtained very readily from seafoods; cod liver oil is another good source. In certain localities around the Great Lakes and in parts of the Northwest the water supply and the vegetables grown are poor in iodine. Hence, daily use of iodized salt ensures an adequate intake and prevents deficiency.

Table 12-6 illustrates a basic daily pregnancy diet from which various daily menus can be constructed.

OTHER INFORMATION ON NUTRITION. When consultation with a nutritionist is advisable and one is not available on the clinic or hospital staff, one may be found in the area through the local community health department or a home economist's office. Publications and visual aids, charts, and so on, may be secured from city, county, and state health departments. The U.S. Government Printing Office is another invaluable source of publications. Certain professional organizations offer additional resources: Food and Nutrition Board, National Research Council, Council on Foods and Nutrition, American Medical Association, American Home Economics Association, American Public Health Association. The above associations serve to illustrate only a few of the resources that the nurse and the physician have to assist their patients in planning for adequate nutrition.

General hygiene

The remainder of the counseling that the physician and nurse will want to give the mother falls under the heading of general hygiene. Pregnancy ought to be a normal, happy, healthy experience for a woman. During the months preceding labor, the physician and the nurse will advise her about her mode of life. She will be encouraged to continue her usual habits with very little change, unless, of course, it is found that she has been leading an existence not conducive to healthy living.

Rest, relaxation and sleep

Because rest and sleep are so essential to health, it is well to emphasize this detail in the nurse's teaching during the antepartal period. Pregnant women become tired more readily; therefore, the prevention of fatigue must be stressed emphatically. The body is made up of various types of cells, each of which has a specific function. Depletion of nerve-cell energy results in fatigue, and fatigue causes certain reactions in the body that are injurious. For all body processes, such as digestion, metabolism, working, playing, and studying, nerve-cell energy is utilized. Nature has made provision for some reduction in normal energy without injury to health. Beyond this limit the symptoms of fatigue are evidenced in irritability, apprehension, a tendency to worry, and restlessness. These symptoms are sometimes very subtle and misleading, but, in contrast, human beings are very conscious of tired muscles. It is more important to avoid fatigue than to have to recover from overfatigue. The pregnant woman should rest to prevent this fatigue. Rest and sleep replenish the cell energy. As Dr. Jastrow says of this code of rest and sleep, they "must be shaped according to the individual's nervous disposition, habits of life, age, and circumstances."

If patients cannot sleep, they can attempt to rest. Rest is the ability to relax. Patients often need to learn how to relax. There is no code so variable, so necessarily adapted to the individual, as that of rest and sleep. The final test is whether the day's work is done with zest and energy to spare. The expectant mother ought to get as much sleep as she feels she needs. Some people need more than others. In addition to a good night's sleep, it is advisable that the mother take a nap or at least rest for a half hour every morning and afternoon. If this is not possible, shorter rest periods, preferably taken lying down (several times a day) are beneficial.

The nurse must recognize that all mothers are not able to follow the recommended rest periods to the letter. Both the woman who works throughout her pregnancy, and the mother of several preschool children need special attention with respect to planning for adequate rest. Rigid recommendations are to be avoided, and the nurse can search with the mother for minutes in her busy day that can be utilized for rest; again, counseling the family may be necessary to maximize the mother's free moments. Although the nurse strives for flexibility, she also needs to emphasize the necessity of this aspect of general hygiene. It can be explained that rest means not only to lie down and perhaps to sleep, but also to lie down or to sit comfortably—to rest the body, mind, abdominal muscles, legs and back, and to stretch out whenever possible, and so make it easier for the heart to pump the blood to the extremities. During the last months of pregnancy, a small pillow used for support of the abdomen while the patient lies on her side does much to relieve the discomfort common during this period and adds materially to the degree of rest that the patient gets in a given time.

It should be suggested that the patient sit whenever possible, even while doing her housework. Sitting to rest for other brief periods during the course of the day can be beneficial if the feet and the legs are elevated.

Often the so-called minor discomforts of pregnancy can be overcome by rest. Rest and the right-angle position (see Fig. 12-11, p. 209) are advised for swelling, edema, and varicosities of the lower extremities. Rest and Sims's position (see Fig. 12-13, p. 211) are advised for varicosities of the vulva and the rectum. Even for the more serious abnormalities, the simple aids included in "diet and rest" may help measurably until more specific orders from the obstetrician can be obtained. In such instances, the nurse must be aware of the mother's interpretation of "rest," and, if indicated, she can provide the necessary guidance to help the mother to understand and to plan for it.

Exercise

Outdoor exercise during pregnancy is usually very beneficial, because it affords diversion in the sunshine and fresh air. However, for each patient the obstetrician usually decides whether the customary exercise should be increased or diminished. There are differences in the amount of exercise for the early and late periods of pregnancy. When pregnancy is advanced, exercise may be limited in comparison with the amount advised previously. Exercise usually means diversion, and, of course, this phase is most important. Exercise also steadies the nerves, quiets the mind, promotes sleep, and stimulates the appetite, all of which are valuable aids to the pregnant mother.

Walking in the fresh air is quite generally preferred to every other form of exercise during pregnancy, because it stimulates the muscular activity of the entire body, strengthens some of the muscles used during labor, and is available to all women. Exercise of any kind should not be fatiguing; to secure the most beneficial results, it should be combined with fresh air and sunlight, as well as periods of rest.

The woman who does her own housework needs little or no planned exercise from the physical viewpoint. However, she does need fresh air, sunshine, and diversion. It is far better for the patient to be occupied than to sit idly, but standing for long periods of time should be avoided. Lifting heavy objects, moving furniture, reaching to hang curtains, any activity which might involve sudden jolts, sudden changes in balance which might result in a fall or the likelihood of physical trauma should be avoided. The more strenuous sports (i.e., horseback riding, skiing, hikes involving long climbs, rough water swimming) are subjects to be discussed with the obstetrician for his guidance. The pregnant woman who is accustomed to participating in certain sports and finds this participation an enjoyable form of recreation usually will be permitted to continue in moderation and at a mild pace, if it proves harmless.

Employment

The same attitude of moderation can be maintained whether for work or play. Ideally, no work or play should be continued to the extent of even moderate fatigue; however, it is not realistic to expect the mother to willingly discontinue her job because it is tiring, especially if it is essential to the family sustenance. If her employment is influencing her health adversely, the matter needs conscientious exploration by the health team to see what realistic adjustments can be made. A referral to a social worker may be indicated to better ascertain the economic situation of the family and/or the resources in the community that might be helpful. Different job opportunities can be discussed, and the patient's skills, satisfactions and preparation can be considered.

In general, jobs requiring moderate manual labor should be avoided if they must be continued over long hours, or if they require delicate balance, constant standing, or constant working on night shifts. Actually, the woman who has a "desk job" in an office often does less strenuous work than the average homemaker who does not go out to work. Nevertheless, positions which require the worker to sit constantly can be extremely tiring. Adequate rest periods should be provided for all pregnant women employed in such positions.

In some countries the time of discontinuing routine jobs has been regulated by law, and the limits, although arbitrary, are generally from six to eight weeks prior to the expected date of confinement.

Many women are employed in industry, and the problem of pregnancy for the working mother in this type of employment is a most important one. To safeguard the interests of expectant mothers so engaged, the following Standards for Maternity Care and Employment of Mothers in Industry have been recommended by the U.S. Children's Bureau.

1. Facilities for adequate prenatal medical care should be readily available for all employed pregnant women; and arrangements should be made by those responsible for providing prenatal care, so that every woman would have access to such care. Local health departments should make available to industrial plants the services of prenatal clinics; and the personnel management or physicians and nurses within the plant should make available to employees information about the importance of such services and where they can be obtained.

2. Pregnant women should not be employed on a shift including the hours between 12 midnight and 6 A.M. Pregnant women should not be employed more than 8 hours a day nor more than 48 hours per week, and it is desirable that their hours of work be limited to not more than 40 hours per week.

3. Every woman, especially a pregnant woman, should have at least two 10-minute rest periods during her work shift, for which adequate facilities for resting and an opportunity for securing nourishing food should be provided.

4. It is not considered desirable for pregnant women to be employed in the following types of occupations, and they should, if possible, be transferred to lighter and more sedentary work:

   a. Occupations that involve heavy lifting or other heavy work.

   b. Occupations involving continuous standing and moving about.

5. Pregnant women should not be employed in the following types of work during any period of pregnancy, but should be transferred to less hazardous types of work.

   a. Occupations that require a good sense of bodily balance, such as work performed on scaffolds or stepladders and occupations in which the accident risk is characterized by accidents causing severe injury, such as operation of punch presses, power-driven woodworking machines, or other machines having a point-of-operation hazard.

   b. Occupations involving exposure to toxic substances considered to be extrahazardous during pregnancy, such as:

   Aniline
   Benzene and toluene
   Carbon disulfide
   Carbon monoxide
   Chlorinated hydrocarbons
   Lead and its compounds
   Mercury and its compounds
   Nitrobenzol and other nitro compounds of benzol and its homologs
   Phosphorus
   Radioactive substances and x-rays
   Turpentine

Other toxic substances that exert an injurious effect upon the blood-forming organs, the liver, or the kidneys.

Because these substances may exert a harmful influence upon the course of pregnancy, may lead to its premature termination, or may injure the fetus, the maintenance of air concentrations within the so-called "maximum permissible limits" of state codes, is not, in itself, sufficient assurance of a safe working condition for the pregnant woman. Pregnant women should be transferred from workrooms in which any of these substances are used or produced in any significant quantity.

6. A minimum of six weeks' leave *before* delivery should be granted, on presentation of a medical certificate of the expected date of confinement.

7. At any time during pregnancy a woman should be granted a reasonable amount of additional leave on presentation of a certificate from the attending physician to the effect that complications of pregnancy

have made continuing employment prejudicial to her health or to the health of the child.

To safeguard the mother's health she should be granted sufficient time off after delivery to return to normal and to regain her strength. The infant needs her care, especially during the first year of life. If it is essential that she return to work, the following recommendations are made:

a. All women should be granted an extension of at least two months' leave of absence after delivery.

b. Should complications of delivery or of the postpartum period develop, a woman should be granted a reasonable amount of additional leave beyond two months following delivery, on presentation of a certificate to this effect from the attending physician.

Diversion

Recreation is as necessary during pregnancy as it is at any other time in life. The patient is preparing for one of the most important role changes that she will undergo during life, and concomitant with any such change is the production of anxiety. It is to be expected that a certain amount of concern about the impending labor will be present; the additional responsibility of having a helpless new baby in the household, plus caring for and integrating him into the family unit, is also anxiety-provoking. The parents will have occasion to wonder whether they are equal to the enormous responsibility of rearing children, and whether or not they will be "good" parents. Therefore, activities which are diverting, healthful, and relaxing help the patient and the family to keep things in their proper perspective. Hence, it is beneficial to discuss with the mother some types of recreation that are most relaxing and pleasing for her and her family. Family group activities still can be enjoyed, even though the mother's energy and dexterity may be somewhat curtailed.

Consideration and understanding on the part of the father, the family, the physician, and the nurse can do much to relieve any uncertainties or concerns that the mother may have. When the father, in particular, understands more about the processes involved in the pregnancy (see Suggested Reading), his helpfulness can be increased. If a "blue" day comes, the father can make it his particular responsibility to provide a means of counteracting it. On a home visit the nurse might discuss with the family ways in which they might help to diminish the strain in this period. This may necessitate changes in attitudes, understanding and habits; certainly it will mean increased tolerance and forbearance on the part of those involved; yet this is one of the ways that others can make their contribution to a successful pregnancy. The father's gentleness and tenderness are especially appreciated and therapeutic at this time; the mother, for her part, can help him to maintain his supportive attitude and behavior by letting him know when his actions are helpful and gratifying. This type of "feedback" conveys her appreciation to the father and leads to reinforcement of his positive behavior. He is perhaps the key person in helping the mother to secure the kind of social relaxation that she enjoys most.

With respect to the activities themselves, books, radio, music, movies, sporting events, television, sewing clubs, church functions, visiting, drives, walks, and entertaining friends are some of the means of providing relaxation and diversion. However, the mother should avoid crowds, chances of infection and all conditions likely to cause a sense of discomfort. Amusements, exercise, rest, and recreation at proper intervals help to keep the pregnant mother well and happy in an environment conducive to her well-being and happy anticipation of the baby.

Traveling

This is perhaps a detail of antepartal care which most patients think very little about, unless they have a tendency to become nauseated or have had a previous miscarriage.

The restriction of travel to short trips had been a rule for maternity patients until World War II, when many women found it necessary to follow their husbands regardless of distance or modes of travel. It is now possible to apply the data compiled during that era to show that travel, almost regardless of distance and type of conveyance, has no deleterious effect on pregnancy.

Even though there is little restriction on travel from a medical point of view, this topic is to be discussed with the mother, so that any of her concerns or misinformation may come to light. The general information usually given to a pregnant woman is to avoid any trip which will cause undue fatigue, since she is prone to tire easily. For traveling long distances the railway or airplane is safer and provides greater comfort. If travel is by private automobile, rest periods of 10 to 15 minutes ought to be planned at least every two hours. This not only avoids fatigue, but the chance to stretch and walk about also benefits the general circulation.

If there are questions about the safety of wearing seat belts by the pregnant woman, it is advisable that they be recommended. Seat belts have been found to decrease the maternal mortality in severe car accidents. They should be worn low and comfortably under the abdomen and in conjunction with the shoulder strap if one is available. Both belts can be adjusted so that they are not too tight or pressing tightly against the neck and abdomen.

Thus, while traveling in general is not usually contraindicated during pregnancy, the expectant mother can consult her physician concerning the advisability of extensive travel at any time during the period of pregnancy.

Immunizations and vaccinations

Another important topic that is interrelated with travel is that of immunization and vaccination protection for the pregnant woman. The diseases that she will be exposed to during her travels, as well as in the course of her daily life, must be considered. In *The Medical Letter on Drugs and Therapeutics*, the Advisory Committee on Immunization of Infectious Diseases of the American Academy of Pediatrics[10] reviewed the following vaccinations and made these recommendations:

1. Cholera. This is a killed bacterial vaccine and should be given only if there is danger of infection. As yet there is no definitive evidence of abortogenic effect.
2. Mumps and measles (rubeola). These are live viruses and should never be given to pregnant patients.
3. Poliomyelitis. Immunization during pregnancy is rarely indicated since this disease has been almost irradicated in *the United States.*
4. Rubella. Pregnancy is a contraindication for administration of the live rubella vaccine. This virus has been shown on occasion to infect both the placenta and the fetus and for this reason is to be avoided.
5. Smallpox. Vaccinia virus administered during pregnancy occasionally infects the fetus. This fetal vaccinia has almost always been associated with primary vaccination. Hence, primary vaccination should only be given in those cases where exposure in an endemic area has occurred.
6. Yellow fever. Since this is a live virus, it should be given to pregnant women only if there has been an exposure or if there is a great risk of exposure.
7. Other vaccines and immunizations. There were no recommendations made by the Committee regarding vaccination against influenza, epidemic typhus, and typhoid. Tetanus and diphtheria toxoids are considered safe and the tuberculin and histoplasmin tests are also permitted.

Since there is at least somewhat of a risk with many of these vaccinations, it is well for the nurse to counsel her patients regarding the spacing of conception well after receiving these injections. The patient can be counseled also to plan vacations and travels during pregnancy to minimize the opportunity for disease exposure and the consequent need for post hoc vaccination. In addition, all patients should be advised to report any illness, no matter how trivial, to their physician so that appropriate follow-up can be done.

Care of the skin

The glands of skin may be more active during pregnancy, and there may be increased or decreased perspiration, resulting in irritation or dryness. Since the skin is one of the organs of elimination, bathing is obviously important, and baths should be taken daily because they are stimulating, refreshing, and relaxing. They not only act as a tonic and a general invigorator, but also favor elimination through the skin as well. Elimination through the skin is thought to lessen the strain of elimination by the kidneys.

During pregnancy, showers or sponge baths may be taken at any time. The old idea that tub baths should be avoided because the wash water enters the vagina and thereby carries infection to the uterus now is believed to have little validity. There is only one objection to tub baths during the last trimester of pregnancy. At this period the heavy weight of the large abdomen may put pregnant women off balance and make climbing in and out of the tub awkward. Therefore, the likelihood of slipping or falling in the bathtub is increased. Chilling the body should be avoided; thus, cold baths, sponges, or showers should be avoided if they produce this sensation.

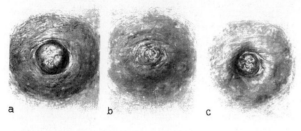

Figure 12-8.   Types of nipples. (a) Normal. (b) Flat. (c) Inverted.

Care of the breasts

Special care of the breasts during pregnancy is one of the important preparations for breast-feeding. During the antepartal period the breasts often have a feeling of fullness and weight and in fact do become larger, heavier, and more pendulous. A well-fitted supporting brassière which holds the breasts up and in may relieve these discomforts. It may also help to prevent the subsequent tissue sagging so often noticeable after pregnancy due to the increased weight of the breasts during pregnancy and lactation.

There may be sufficient secretion of colostrum from the nipples to necessitate wearing a pad to protect the clothing. The daily care of the nipples and the reason for it, as well as the actual procedure, should be explained to the patient. Early in pregnancy the breasts begin to secrete, and this secretion often oozes out on the surface of the nipple and in drying forms fine imperceptible crusts. If these crusts are allowed to remain, the skin underneath becomes tender; if left until the baby arrives and nurses, this tender skin area is likely to crack. With this condition there is always a possibility of infection. Nipples that are kept clean and dry do not have a tendency to become sore or cracked.

The breasts are to be bathed daily; this may be done at the beginning of the tub, shower, or the sponge bath. The patient ought to use a clean washcloth and warm water. Some studies have demonstrated that the use of soap, alcohol, and other such materials during the antepartal period and puerperium tends to be detrimental to the integrity of the nipple tissue, since they remove the protective skin oils and leave the nipple more prone to damage (see Suggested Reading). Therefore, the patient can discuss the use of these with the physician. She begins cleansing each breast by washing the nipple thoroughly with a circular motion, making sure that any dried material

has been removed, then gradually continues working away from the nipple in this fashion until the entire breast is washed. She rinses the breast in this manner and dries with a clean towel. Rubbing the nipples with a rough towel during the last trimester of pregnancy may be helpful in attempting to toughen them. The physician may advise the use of nipple cream, a hydrous lanolin preparation, to prepare the nipples for nursing. This can be applied after the breasts are bathed. First, a small quantity of cream is placed on the thumb and the first finger; then the nipple is grasped gently between the thumb and this finger and, with a rolling motion, the cream is worked into the tiny creases found on the surface of the nipple. The position of the thumb and finger should be gradually shifted around the circumference of the nipple until a complete circuit has been made. This procedure is limited to about 30 seconds on each breast.

A nipple which is flat or even slightly inverted in early pregnancy (Fig. 12-8) very probably will become protractile by delivery. If the nipples are inverted, some physicians prefer to start special care in the fifth or sixth month of pregnancy or earlier. Dr. J. B. Hoffman has suggested a treatment which has proved helpful. With the thumbs placed close to the inverted nipple, press firmly into the breast tissue and gradually push the thumbs away from the areola. The strokes should follow an imaginary cross drawn on the breast and be done four or five times in succession on awakening each morning (Fig. 12-9). The nipple will assume an erect, projected position and then can be grasped as a unit and gently teased out a bit further. This is done daily, so that the nipples may be made more prominent for the baby to grasp. In extreme cases in which the nipples are badly inverted, the obstetrician will give instructions concerning the care needed.

Clothing

During pregnancy the clothes should be given the same or perhaps even a little more attention than at other times. The young mother who feels that she is dressed attractively and is well groomed will reflect this in her manner. Her clothing should be practical, attractive, and nonconstricting. Most women are able to dress in the manner to which they are accustomed in the nonpregnant state until the enlargement of the abdomen becomes apparent. Maternity specialty shops and department stores have made maternity fashions available, which has settled the problem of suitable clothing during pregnancy. Today designers and stylists are giving consideration to the pregnant mother's clothing, so that she may dress attractively and feel self-confident about her appearance. The clothes are designed to be comfortable and "hang from the shoulders," thus avoiding any constriction; they are made in a variety of materials. The expectant mother can dress according to the climate and the temperature for her comfort.

ABDOMINAL SUPPORT. Women who have been unaccustomed to wearing a girdle will scarcely feel the need of abdominal support, especially during the early months of pregnancy. Later, however, a properly fitted maternity girdle often gives the needed support to keep the mother from becoming fatigued. The natural softening of the pelvic joints which accompanies pregnancy and the increasing weight of the abdomen may encourage a change in posture to such a degree that severe backache results.

If the mother's abdomen is large, or if previous pregnancies have caused her abdomen to become lax or pendulous, a properly made and well-fitting maternity girdle will give support and comfort. The purpose of the garment is support, not constriction of the abdomen.

BREAST SUPPORT. It is advisable that every pregnant woman wear a well-fitted brassière to support the breasts in a normal uplift position. Proper support of the breasts is conducive to good posture and thus helps to prevent backache.

The selection of a brassière is determined by individual fitting and influenced by the size of the breasts and the need for support. It is important to see that the cup is large enough, and that the underarm is built high enough to cover all the breast tissue. Wide shoulder straps will afford more comfort for the woman who has large and pendulous breasts. The size of the brassière is, again, determined by the size of the individual being fitted, but in most instances the brassière is approximately two sizes larger than that usually worn. The mother who is planning to breast-feed will find it practical to purchase nursing brassières which can be worn during the latter months of pregnancy, as well as during the postpartal period for as long as she is nursing her baby.

GARTERS. Round garters or any tight bands (rolled stockings, elastic tops on stockings)

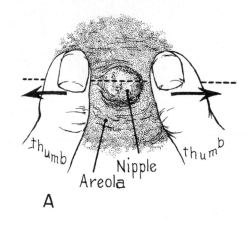

A

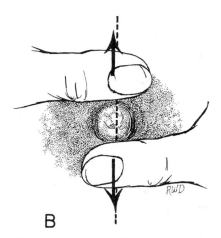

B

Figure 12-9. A suggested treatment for inverted nipples. The thumbs are placed close to the inverted nipple, pressed firmly into the breast tissue, then gradually pushed away from the areola. The strokes should be directed horizontally (A) and vertically (B) and be done four or five times in succession.

that encircle the leg tend to aggravate varicose veins and edema of the lower extremities and should be discarded in favor of suspender garters or some form of stocking supporters attached to an abdominal support. If pantyhose do not aggravate any discharge that the mother may have, she may use these. It will be remembered that arteries have muscular tissue in their walls, whereas veins have little or none, so that arteries are able to resist pressure. The external veins lie close to the surface, but the arteries are embedded deeper in the tissues. Hence, any constriction of any extremity affects the veins far more than the arteries. Blood which apparently meets no obstruction whatever in its flow down the extremity through an artery may on its return through the vein find at the point of constriction sufficient closure

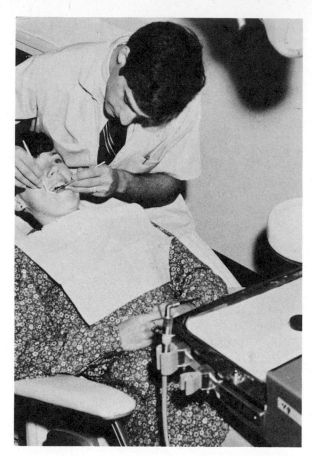

Figure 12-10. Dental care as part of obstetric health service. Because of the importance of good dental care, some hospitals have dental clinic facilities available as part of antepartal supervision. (School of Dentistry, Case Western Reserve University, Cleveland)

fatigue. It is advisable that low-heeled shoes be worn during working hours and for busy daytime activities. For evening or more fashionable afternoon attire, a 2-inch heel is permissible if the patient does not develop backache from the increased lordosis induced by the heels, and if she can maintain adequate balance.

The nurse will want to remember that the height of the heel is but one consideration here, and that the support which the shoe gives the foot adds materially to the mother's comfort. Many flat-heeled shoes give little or no support to the feet and thus may cause fatigue and aching legs and backs. A simple method to check the support of a shoe is to place the shoe flat on the floor, and press the thumb down on the inner sole against the shank (the part that would come under the arch of the foot). If the shoe gives under this pressure, it will give weak support to the foot.

Care of the teeth

Good dental care is necessary because the teeth are important for adequate mastication of food. This care need be little different during pregnancy from what is considered good, general mouth hygiene in any person who is not pregnant. The teeth should be brushed carefully on arising, after each meal, and before retiring at night. An alkaline mouthwash may be used, if desired. It is advisable for the expectant mother to visit her dentist at the very beginning of pregnancy and to follow his recommendations (Fig. 12-10). Any extensive elective work is better postponed until after the pregnancy. The most favorable period for routine, minor procedures is from the fourth to the seventh month. The mother is usually less nauseated, not as yet very large and, in general, feeling well. Diagnostic dental x-rays ought to be postponed until the latter half of pregnancy. A lead apron over the abdomen will give sufficient protection.

The old saying, "For every child a tooth," based on a belief that the fetus takes calcium from the mother's teeth, has no real scientific basis. It should be carefully explained to the mother that an adequate diet during pregnancy will supply the baby with lime salts and other necessities in sufficient amounts to build his bones and teeth. Therefore, this old adage need not be true if proper attention is given to the care of the teeth and nutrition during pregnancy.

of the vessel to "dam it back" and so stretch the vein wall that a varicosity is formed. There is already a marked tendency toward this condition, because the enlarged and constantly enlarging uterus tends to impede the return circulation from the lower extremities by compression of the great abdominal vessels; round garters definitely tend to aggravate the condition. Garters that encircle the leg should never be worn, even by growing children, for the tendency to varicosities is always present; and when once formed, they never entirely disappear and later may lead to great discomfort.

SHOES. A comfortable, well-fitting shoe is essential for the expectant mother. The postural changes which occur as the mother's abdomen enlarges may be aggravated by wearing high-heeled shoes, with resulting backache and

Bowel habits

The pregnant woman who heretofore has adhered to regular habits of elimination usually experiences little or no change in the daily routine. Those who have a tendency toward constipation become noticeably more irregular during pregnancy due to 1) decreased physical exertion, 2) relaxation of the bowel in association with the relaxation of smooth-muscle systems all over the body, and 3) pressure of the enlarging uterus. Particularly during the latter part of pregnancy, the presenting part of the fetus exerts pressure on the lower bowel.

Personal habits of intelligent, daily hygiene are the best resource that the expectant mother has to prevent constipation. The alleviation of this problem in modern society may be attributed to education, more reasonable bowel habits, and greater latitude in physical exercise. During pregnancy, the mother should pay close attention to bowel habits, drink sufficient quantities of fluid, eat fruits and other foods which add roughage to the diet, and get reasonable amounts of daily exercise.

If these simple measures are not effective, the physician should be consulted about the problem. Harsh laxatives and enemas should be avoided unless the physician orders them specifically. He probably will prescribe some mild bulk-producing laxative and/or stool softener. If the mother has been taking a non-absorbable oil preparation, such as mineral oil, she should be advised to take the medication at bedtime, since it has the ability to dissolve and to excrete the oil-soluble vitamins if taken at mealtime, thus depriving her of the vitamins so necessary for good nutrition.

Constipation is conducive to the development of hemorrhoids and may be associated with the incidence of pyelitis. Aside from the discomfort associated with the passage of hard fecal material, this may injure the rectal mucosa and cause bleeding.

Douches

Vaginal douching, long considered a requisite of feminine hygiene by some women, should be kept at a reasonable minimum during pregnancy. If it is indicated because of excessive vaginal secretion or infection, the physician will prescribe the kind of douche and the frequency with which it is to be taken. In the absence of excessive secretions or infec-

tion, the nurse might reassure the patient that a washcloth and soap and water are quite adequate for general cleanliness, with emphasis on washing anteriorly first, and the rectal area last. The use of moist towelettes that are sold in foil packages is not contraindicated.

Deodorant, "feminine hygiene" sprays are contraindicated as they have been found to cause severe perineal irritation in many women, as well as urethritis and cystitis in the more severe cases. During pregnancy, the sebaceous glands in the genital area are quite active and there may be a characteristic odor that some women find quite unpleasant. Plain soap and water is a very effective agent to keep this odor under control. Any suggestions that the nurse might give for general cleanliness will usually be appreciated. Mothers may find that the genital area is a little more sensitive to heat and cold and pressure during pregnancy, but they should be reassured that there is nothing they can harm with the use of the above methods.

Specific instructions about douching are to be given, and the physician usually gives this responsibility to the nurse. This instruction can be very time-consuming, and, if she has permission, the nurse might consider writing out and having copies of instructions for douching that would agree with the philosophy of the office or clinic in which she is working. Women who avoid douching or douche infrequently have usually been instructed to do this in the bathtub, which is very awkward and time-consuming. The instructions should be clear enough for the patient who has never douched and knows nothing about it, and perhaps has never heard the word or seen it in print.

The nurse can include the following points in her instructions, making sure that the language and the vocabulary is understandable to the group of patients with whom she is working:

1. It is a four-minute procedure (after the initial few times).
2. It can be done while sitting on the toilet.
3. A gravity bag must be used (never a hand-bulb syringe).
4. During pregnancy, the douche tip should not be inserted more than 3 inches.
5. The frequency and the solution are prescribed by the physician.

6. The douche bag may be placed (hung or held) no higher than 2 feet above the level of the vagina.

7. The douche tip should be held at about the 3-inch length and inserted in the vagina, and the labial tissue in that area should be held around the douche tip with the same hand.

8. The solution is allowed to run in until there is a slight feeling of fullness, then it is expelled (the douche bag will hold enough solution to do this four or five times).

9. The bag and the tube should be rinsed and hung to dry with a towel underneath.

10. The solution, for comfort, should only be barely warm to the hand. Holding the labial tissue around the douche tip allows the water to flow in without flowing out immediately, and this, along with rapid expelling, enables the solution to get into the folds of the wall of the vagina. In the nonpregnant woman there is no contra-indication to inserting the entire douche tip or as much of it as the vagina will accommodate.

If douching is made a simple procedure, more women will use it both as a voluntary hygienic measure and, more important, as frequently as the physician requests it for medicinal reasons. There is no need to get undressed and get into a bathtub (which many patients do not have) and spend a half an hour with a procedure that requires only four or five minutes.

Sexual relations

From the standpoint of all parties involved —patient, nurse, and physician—the area of sexual relations, because of its intimate nature, often becomes one of the most difficult in which to give appropriate guidance. Many patients are reluctant to discuss sex in general, especially when the patient-physician-nurse relationship is new; yet they are disturbed because of the changes which may be taking place in their bodies and emotions, with consequent influences on their sexual relationship. Because of this reluctance, nurses (and physicians) often avoid exploring with the patient the possibility of an existing problem, and the counseling then consists mostly of prohibitions regarding the time and frequency of intercourse. However, when there is a need, most patients will discuss the subject with a little help, especially when the physician or the nurse conveys the idea that these are "expected" changes, and that there is nothing "shameful" or unique about them. Some patients prefer to speak only to the physician about this matter, but some turn to the nurse at this time, because she is a woman and is also likely to have experienced similar feelings and concerns. Since she may be utilized as a resource person, the nurse can prepare herself as she would for any other counseling activity.

She needs to know about the anatomical, physiologic, and psychologic aspects involved; she can ascertain the physician's wishes regarding any particular advice relating to sex for this patient. She should be aware that her approach here is extremely important and requires adroit use of communication skills, especially those of listening, reflecting, and gentle probing. Finally, she can examine her own feelings and attitudes about sexuality, pregnancy, and motherhood so that she can understand and better empathize with the patient's situation.

Early pregnancy has an almost unpredictable effect on the sexual desire of the expectant mother. Some women feel a sense of pleasant release from pregnancy fears, which enhances their desire; others find their ardor distinctly curbed. If this is a gross change from what is usual, concern may be generated in the couple, especially if sexual activity is refused, and misunderstandings ensue. Sudden unexplained aversion to the man also may occur, which is quite traumatic for both partners. Fortunately, these idiosyncrasies are temporary, and desire and responsiveness soon return. It is important that the couple become aware of this fact before misunderstanding and hurt lead to the establishment of unhealthy and negative patterns of interaction. It is especially gratifying for the man to realize that these apparent caprices are only a temporary accompaniment of the new condition of pregnancy and do not signify any real change in the woman's basic attitude or love for him.

During the first trimester, the pregnant woman is very aware of her pelvis. The feeling of fullness, the sharpened sensations, and the round ligament twinges that may occur deep in the groin with sudden movement all give rise to some anxiety. Even though she may have had previous successful pregnancies and enjoyed sexual relations, she still tends to view these symptoms as possible threats to the pregnancy. If there is occasional (common) spotting, there is all the more reason for her to believe (however mistakenly) that the pregnancy is in danger. Very different sensations from those usually experienced occur with deep penile penetration with an enlarging soft uterus, although the uterus is still entirely in the pelvis. This does not imply that intercourse should not take place or that thrusting or movement need be curtailed. However, it does have implications for the woman's immersing herself in the pleasures of sexual stimulation, since she may be preoccupied with these other thoughts and sensations. Hence, she may not be orgasmic on all occasions or as often as is usual for her. This preoccupation may also give rise to the unpredictableness in her general sexual desire. If there appear to be large changes from what is usual, concern may be generated in both partners. It is important for them to understand that the time of pregnancy can be one of the most anxiety-free, spontaneous sexual interludes of a couple's life. They can be counseled that intercourse poses no threat to pregnancy under normal circumstances. If they have been reasonably comfortable with their sexuality before the pregnancy, and there are no unusual problems, there is no reason to anticipate that their sexual *activity* need be curtailed.

If there are times when intercourse should wait for a few days because of the psychic factor, there need not be a limitation of any of the other variations of sexual stimulation and orgasmic release for either the man or the woman. Sexual techniques may need modification due to the breasts' and genitals' increased sensitivity. As the secretions increase and change in character, there may be an accompanying odor which need not be unpleasant if standards of hygiene are maintained daily. Medication and/or douching may be required if there is the yeast overgrowth common to pregnancy. The physician will prescribe these as needed and the nurse can be helpful in eliciting the needed information about the existence of any of these problems in the patient.[11]

In the second trimester, early in the fourth month, the uterus enlarges rather rapidly and becomes an abdominal organ rather than a pelvic organ. The expectant mother has usually adapted to the pelvic awareness and does not approach intercourse so gingerly. However, with the rapidly enlarging abdomen, new concerns are engendered regarding crushing the fetus. While these are not valid concerns, they are very real to both partners. The fetus is very well protected by the uterus and the abdominal wall, but the enlarging uterus can get in the way about the fifth month if the partners assume the top and bottom position for intercourse. Hence, modifications in positioning may be needed. Since the uterus is not pressing down in the vagina, there is not the feeling of hitting an immovable object with penetration.

Vaginal bleeding during the second trimester is very unusual. Even abortions and premature deliveries during this period are not generally preceded by bleeding, but by cramping and a gush of amniotic fluid. Stress incontinence of urine (losing urine with coughing, sneezing, or orgasm) may continue into this trimester, since the uterus is pressing on the bladder, although it is out of the pelvis. This incontinence is sometimes confused with a gush of amniotic fluid and can be frightening during intercourse.

Intercourse using the side position can be successful, and from a purely mechanical point of view, is necessarily gentle. As the uterus grows larger, the expectant mother is usually much more comfortable lying on her side, with her uterus supported by a pillow. If she is on her back for any length of time, with the enlarged uterus pressing on the great blood vessels in the abdomen, there may be problems with hypotension and lightheadedness. Using a pillow under the hips during intercourse can be helpful in avoiding hypotension.

It is often difficult for a thoughtful, caring man to initiate sexual overtures to a woman who is lying on her side with a pillow under her uterus and two pillows under her head to enable her to breathe without difficulty. But the warmth that comes from physical closeness is always desired, even though it may not be defined in terms of sexual activity. However, some women may push away well-meaning attempts to physical closeness if they have found by experience that these overtures usually terminate in intercourse—as bulkiness grows, the desire for intercourse per se may be variable, and the male needs to be able to understand this. Just as important, the woman should know and remember that it is difficult for males *only* to be physically close constantly without eventually needing some kind of physiologic and psychic orgasmic release. The presence of constant, unreleased sexual desire results in aching pelvic congestion, particularly for the male, and this is especially true if there has been frequent regularity in the couple's sexual life prior to pregnancy.

In contrast to previous thinking and counseling about sexual activity in the last trimester and particularly in the last weeks of pregnancy, many physicians are no longer discouraging maintenance of sexual relations during this period when the pregnancy has been normal. The threat of possible infection from penile penetration or of stimulating vaginal bleeding does not seem to warrant abstinence. Moreover, any contractions associated with orgasm do not warrant adherence to types of sexual stimulation that stop short of orgasm for the female. Caution about deep penetration is often in order but for comfort and ease reasons.

It is well to remember that the maintenance of sexual activity does not have to include intercourse per se, and often the female genitalia are so sensitive that the woman is not interested in intercourse and many prefer alternate practices or caressing. The contractions that accompany orgasm and the postcoital spotting may cause concern in both partners. Many of the vague transient signs and symptoms, all within the range of normal, may now be interpreted in the light of their possible effects on the child. The father shares some of this same concern and does not want to endanger the child; hence, abstinence from intercourse often becomes a mutual unspoken decision. This commonly occurring mutual concern is the rationale for allowing sexual activity during this period, and saying nothing to discourage it unless medically indicated. A really demanding man will continue to require sexual access; telling the expectant mother to abstain will only put her in an even more difficult position in relation to him and will cause her undue worry and guilt about what effects this might have on the fetus. Frequently, she can control the vigor of the act and this point can be explored. Most couples, however, modify their activity by mutual consent.[12]

Smoking

The Surgeon General's report, as well as other recent studies, has indicated that cigarette smoking is a health hazard of sufficient importance in this country to warrant remedial action. Lung cancer and heart disease have been linked significantly with cigarette smoking. With respect to pregnancy, several studies have found a relationship between smoking and lower birthrates, higher rates of prematurity, and higher neonatal mortality. The mechanism is somewhat obscure, but it is thought that the nicotine in the cigarettes causes peripheral vasoconstriction, with subsequent changes in the heart rate, the blood pressure, and the cardiac output that appear to have a detrimental effect on the development and the health of the fetus. Carbon monoxide also is found in higher concentrations in smokers, with a consequent decrease of oxygen; this apparently also affects the fetus.

The subject of smoking should be discussed thoroughly with the physician, and his recommendations followed. Several "smoking clinics" have been developed around the country, and books and articles have been published on the topic of "how to stop smoking." No one claims to have a sure answer. A combination of motivation, education in the destructive effects of smoking for both mother and infant, and support seem to be the basic ingredients. The health team certainly can supply the last two and help the patient to achieve the first.

Minor discomforts

The so-called minor discomforts of pregnancy are the common complaints experienced by most expectant mothers, to some degree, in the course of a normal pregnancy. However, all mothers do not experience all of them, and, indeed, some mothers pass through the entire antepartal period without any of these discomforts. They are not serious in themselves, but their presence detracts from the mother's feeling of comfort and well-being. In many instances they can be avoided by preventive measures, or entirely overcome by common sense in daily living, once they do occur.

Frequent urination

One of the first signs the young woman may notice to make her suspect she might be pregnant is the frequent desire to empty her bladder. This is caused by the pressure of the growing uterus against the bladder and will subside about the second or the third month, when the uterus expands upward into the abdominal cavity. Later, during the last weeks of pregnancy the symptoms will reoccur.

Nausea

Nausea and vomiting of mild degree, the so-called morning sickness, constitute the most common disorder of the first trimester of pregnancy. For many years it has been thought that this condition has an emotional basis. In all life's encounters, there are probably few experiences which are so anxiety provoking as the realization by a woman that she is pregnant. At first there is the anxious uncertainty before she can be sure of the diagnosis. Then, there are numerous adjustments that have to be made and responsibilities that may seem to be overwhelming. Emotionally, the implications of pregnancy extend far back into her childhood, long before she met her husband. It is understandable that women who cannot adjust themselves to all these new circumstances could have problems. Moreover, whether causative or not, the stress of pregnancy and all its ramifications can contribute to the symptoms caused by the metabolic changes associated with pregnancy. Thus, a neurotic factor cannot be posited as the sole cause of nausea and vomiting. Symptoms are now thought to be due to the invasion nature of the pregnancy-implantation and the change in the carbohydrate metabolism.

Symptoms usually appear about the end of the fourth or sixth week and last until about the twelfth week. Nausea occurs in about 50 percent of all pregnancies; of these, about one-third experience some vomiting. Usually, it occurs in the morning only, but a small percentage of patients may have nausea and vomiting throughout the entire day.

THE TYPICAL PICTURE of morning sickness starts with the patient's experiencing a feeling of nausea on arising in the morning. The mother is unable to retain her breakfast, but by noon she has completely recovered and has no further episodes until the next morning. This does not always occur in the morning, but may happen in the afternoon or in the evening. In a small percentage of patients the nausea and the vomiting may persist throughout the day and even be worse in the afternoon. With the majority of patients this problem lasts from one to three weeks and then suddenly ceases. There may be a slight loss of body weight but no other signs or symptoms.

TREATMENT. Often this condition can be controlled, and frequently it may be greatly relieved. Various before breakfast remedies often are used. If a half hour before rising the patient takes a dry piece of toast or a cracker, relief may be obtained. In some instances sips of hot water (plain or with lemon juice), hot tea, clear coffee, or hot milk have been tried, with successful results. However, the dry carbohydrate foods seem to be more effective. After taking any one of these remedies, the patient remains in bed for about a half hour; then she gets up and dresses slowly (meanwhile sitting as much of the time as possible). After this she is usually ready for her breakfast.

Greasy foods, and those known to disagree with the patient, should be avoided in the diet. Other suggested remedies include eating an increased amount of carbohydrate foods during this period of disturbance or eating simple and light food five or six times a day instead of the three regular full meals. Unsweetened popcorn during the morning is sometimes advised. The patient may be helped by drinking sweet lemonade, about half of a lemon to a pint of water sweetened with milk sugar. Usually, after vomiting, the patient is quite thirsty, and it is not difficult for her to drink lemonade. Small amounts of ginger ale or cola drink also are often helpful.

Nausea and vomiting, if once established, are difficult to overcome; and so it is especially desirable to prevent the first attack, or at least to control this condition as soon as possible after it develops. It must be remembered that if the patient is unable to retain most of her food, her system is being depleted when daily health should be maintained. Pregnancies may differ, and what may help one person may not benefit another. The trial-and-error method often is necessary to obtain results. If persistent vomiting develops, as it does with a small number of these patients, the condition is no longer considered to be a minor discomfort but then may develop into a serious complication. (See Chapter 23, Complications of Pregnancy.)

Heartburn

This is a neuromuscular phenomenon which may occur any time throughout gestation. As a result of the diminished gastric motility which normally accompanies pregnancy, reverse peristaltic waves cause regurgitation of the stomach contents into the esophagus. It is this irritation of the esophageal mucosa which causes heartburn. It may be described as a burning discomfort diffusely localized behind the lower part of the sternum, often radiating upward along the course of the esophagus. Although referred to as heartburn, it really has nothing to do with the heart. Often it is associated with other gastrointestinal symptoms, of which acid regurgitation, belching, nausea, and epigastric pressure are most troublesome. Nervous tension and emotional disturbances may be a precipitating cause. Worry, fatigue, and improper diet may contribute to its intensity.

Very little fat should be included generally in the diet. Although fatty foods are especially aggravating in this disturbance, strangely enough, the taking of some form of fat, such as a pat of butter or a tablespoon of cream, a short time before meals acts as a preventive, because fat inhibits the secretion of acid in the stomach. However, this will not help if the heartburn is already present.

Home remedies are not to be used to relieve this condition. The physician usually will prescribe some alkaline preparation, because it gives the best results. However, *sodium bicarbonate is not to be used*, because the sodium ion tends to promote water retention. It is important to make sure that the patient understands this point. Equally effective medications are aluminum compounds, such as aluminum hydroxide gel, or this medication in tablet form with magnesium trisilicate.

Flatulence

This is a somewhat common and very disagreeable discomfort. Usually it is due to undesirable bacterial action in the intestines, which results in the formation of gas. Eating only small amounts of food which are well masticated may prevent this feeling of distress after eating. Regular daily elimination is of prime importance, as is the avoidance of foods that form gas. Such foods as beans, parsnips, corn, sweet desserts, fried foods, cake, and candy ought to be avoided. If these measures fail to relieve the condition, the physician should be consulted.

Constipation

This is not unusual during pregnancy. It is due largely to impaired peristaltic motion of the intestine caused by pressure from the gravid uterus. The patient should understand the importance of good bowel habits (see General Hygiene, p. 195), the influence of drinking adequate fluids and the appropriate diet in avoiding or alleviating this problem. Proper elimination cannot be emphasized too much, and daily regularity of habit aids in preventing constipation. In mild cases of constipation a diet of fruits, vegetables, dark breads, and coarse foods, with several glasses of water daily, may relieve the condition.

Enemas, laxatives, or cathartics are not to be used unless prescribed by the physician. Some obstetricians advise milk of magnesia or cascara for their patients. Cascara is easier to take in the pill form, but it seems to be less effective; when the fluid extract is given, the size of the dose and the frequency of its administration must be determined according to the individual patient's reactions. When the proper dosage has been determined, this drug is generally very satisfactory. The salines are usually reserved for the cases in which they are distinctly indicated, such as certain types of toxemia.

Simple measures, combined with adequate diet, are ordinarily all that is necessary.

Backache

Most pregnant women experience some degree of backache. As pregnancy advances, the woman's posture changes to compensate for the weight of the growing uterus. The shoulders are thrown back as the enlarging abdomen protrudes, and, in order to maintain the body balance, the inward curve of the spine is exaggerated. The relaxation of the sacroiliac joints, in addition to the postural change, causes varying degrees of backache following excessive strain, fatigue, bending, or lifting. The mother can be advised early in pregnancy how to prevent such strain through measures such as good posture and body mechanics in everyday living and avoidance of fatigue. Appropriate shoes worn during periods of activity and a supporting girdle may be helpful (see Clothing, in General Hygiene, p. 200).

A woman who has a pendulous abdomen, with a weak abdominal wall which allows the uterus to fall forward, will experience severe back pain, in addition to a "drawing sensation" in the abdomen and general discomfort in walking or standing. The physician will prescribe measures to be taken here or for any persistent complaint.

Dyspnea

Difficult breathing or shortness of breath occasionally results from pressure on the diaphragm by the enlarged uterus and may be sufficient in the last weeks of pregnancy to interfere considerably with the patient's sleep and general comfort. Usually it is not a serious condition, but unfortunately it cannot be wholly relieved until after "lightening" (p. 146) (the settling of the fetus into the pelvic cavity with relief of the upper abdominal pressure) or after the birth of the baby, when it will disappear spontaneously. It is most troublesome when the patient attempts to lie down, so that her comfort may be greatly enhanced by propping her well up in bed with pillows. In this semisitting posture she at least will sleep better and longer than with her head low. It is well for the nurse to demonstrate how these pillows may be arranged comfortably so that the patient's back is well supported.

In patients with known heart disease, shortness of breath, especially of rather sudden onset, may be a sign of oncoming heart failure and should be reported at once to the physician.

Varicose Veins

Varicose veins or varices may occur in the lower extremities and, at times, extend up as high as the external genitalia or even into the pelvis itself. A varicosity is an enlargement in the diameter of a vein due to a thinning and stretching of its walls. Such distended areas may occur at short intervals along the course of the blood vessel; they give it a knotted appearance. Varicosities generally are associated with hereditary tendencies and are enhanced by advancing age, multiple pregnancy, and activities which require prolonged standing. During pregnancy the pressure in the pelvis due to the enlarged uterus, which presses on the great abdominal veins, interferes with the return of the blood from the lower extremities. Added to this, any debilitated condition of the patient favors the formation of varicosities in the veins because of the general flabbiness and lack of tone in the tissues.

Naturally, the greater the pressure in the abdomen, the greater will be the tendency to varicose veins of the lower extremities and the vulva. Therefore, any occupation which keeps a patient constantly on her feet, particularly in the latter part of pregnancy, causes an increase in abdominal pressure and so acts as an exacerbating factor.

SYMPTOMS. The first symptom of the development of varicose veins is a dull aching pain in the legs due to distention of the deep vessels. Inspection may show a fine purple network of superficial veins covering the skin in a lacelike pattern, although this does not always appear.

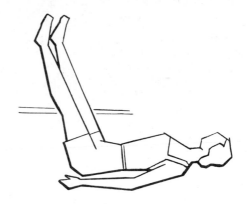

Figure 12-11. Right-angle position for swelling, edema and varicosities of legs.

Later, the true varicosities appear, usually first under the bend of the knee, in a tangled mass of bluish or purplish veins, often as large as a lead pencil. As the condition advances, the varicosities extend up and down the leg along the course of the vessels, and in severe cases they may affect the veins of the labia majora, the vagina, and the uterus.

THE TREATMENT consists in promptly abandoning any constricting garters, stockings, or other clothing that will cause pressure, particularly on the legs or thighs. If varicosities persist in spite of this precaution, the patient can be taught to take the right-angle position, that is, to lie on the bed with her legs extended straight into the air at right angles to her body, with her buttocks and heels resting against the wall (Figure 12-11). At first, this position is taken for two to five minutes several times a day, and that will soon demonstrate what can be accomplished. For some patients this position is very uncomfortable at first; but if it is explained, and the discomfort is therefore anticipated, the patient is less likely to discontinue the exercise. Late in pregnancy this position may be too difficult to assume because of pressure against the diaphragm.

To give support to the weak-walled veins, either an elastic stocking or elastic bandage often is recommended. The initial cost of elastic stockings is somewhat more than that of bandages, but they are easier to put on, more effective, have a neater appearance and a longer usefulness than bandages. A regular nylon stocking put on over the elastic hose further improves the appearance. Many hosiery companies are manufacturing "support" hose which do not have the strength of the elastic stockings but are very effective in giving a

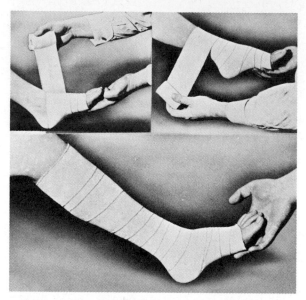

Figure 12-12. Application of bandages for varicosities or edema of the legs. (*Top*) The Ace bandage (Becton, Dickinson and Company). (*Bottom*) The Elastoplast bandage (Duke Laboratories) is applied firmly, adjusting the stretch to produce the amount of compression desired, each turn overlapping to avoid gaps.

moderate amount of support. This type of stocking is useful in cases in which the varicosities are very mild or may not even be apparent peripherally, but may be suspected because of the ache they produce. Many women who must be on their feet a great deal, and do not have the opportunity to rest frequently, wear these stockings during working hours as a "prophylactic" measure. The nurse can be very helpful in apprising mothers of the varieties of hose now available and which will meet the needs of individual patients.

If bandages are used, they should be applied spirally with firm, even pressure, beginning at the foot and continuing up the leg above the varicosities (Fig. 12-12). The nurse can demonstrate the technique of wrapping to the mother and let the patient practice in her presence; this will ensure that the mother understands and is able to wrap the bandages effectively. The patient also must be told that the stocking or the bandage should be removed at night for greater comfort and reapplied in the morning after the legs have been elevated so that the vessels will be less dilated. The longer stocking or bandage is more satisfactory when the varicosities are above the knee. Either the elastic stocking or bandage is washable; indeed, washing helps to maintain the original elasticity of these appliances. However,

mild soap rather than detergent should be used.

Varicosities of the vulva may be relieved by placing a pillow under the buttocks and elevating the hips for frequent rest periods or by taking the elevated Sims's position for a few moments several times a day (Fig. 12-13). Patients suffering from this condition should not stand when they can sit, and they should not sit when they can lie down.

More important than the treatment of this condition is its prevention. Every pregnant woman should be advised to sit with her legs elevated whenever possible. And when the legs are elevated, care should be taken to see that there are no pressure points against the legs to interfere with the circulation, particularly in the popliteal space. Tight constricting garments, round garters, constipation, standing for long periods of time and an improper amount of rest, all tend to aggravate this condition.

A varicose vein in the vagina may rupture during the antepartal or intrapartal period, but this is rare. The hemorrhage is venous and can be controlled readily by pressure. The foot of the bed can be markedly elevated.

Hemorrhoids

Hemorrhoids, varicosities of the veins about the lower end of the rectum and the anus, may develop during the antepartal period and may cause rectal bleeding. On the other hand, they may become thrombosed or protrude through the anus. The little bumps and nodules seen in a mass of hemorrhoids are the distended portions of the affected vessels. Like varicosities in other areas, they are due to pressure interfering with return venous circulation and are aggravated by constipation. They often cause great distress to the pregnant patient and, due to pressure at the time of delivery, may cause great distress during the postpartal period.

The first step is the prevention and the treatment of constipation. The guidance that the nurse gives the mother in this respect cannot be stressed enough. In addition, when internal hemorrhoids protrude through the rectum, the mother can be instructed to replace them carefully by pushing them gently back into the rectum. Usually the patient can manage this quite well, after a thorough explanation and/or demonstration. She lubricates her finger with petrolatum or mineral oil to aid ease of insertion and to avoid trauma to the veins. If the patient wishes, a finger cot can be used to cover her finger. Also, taking either the knee-chest position or elevating her buttocks (see Fig. 12-13) on a pillow facilitates replacement through gravity.

The application of an icebag, or cold compresses wet with witch hazel or Epsom salts solution, gives great relief. The physician may order tannic acid in suppositories, or compresses of witch hazel and glycerin. If the hemorrhoids are aggravated the first few days after labor, the same medications usually give relief. Surgery is seldom resorted to during pregnancy.

Cramps

Cramps are painful spasmodic muscular contractions in the legs. They may occur at any time during the pregnancy, but more generally during the later months due to pressure of the enlarged uterus on the nerves supplying the lower extremities. Other causes have been attributed to fatigue, chilling, tense body posture and insufficient calcium in the diet. They are commonly noted after the use of diuretics. A quart of milk in the daily diet has been generally recommended to meet the calcium needs during pregnancy. However, studies show that large quantities of milk or dicalcium phosphate predispose to muscular tetany and leg cramps as the result of the excessive amount of phosphorus absorbed from these products. Some authorities suggest that small quantities of aluminum hydroxide gel be taken with the quart of milk as it removes some of the dietary phosphorus from the intestinal tract. Immediate relief may be obtained by forcing the toes upward and by making pressure on the knee to straighten the leg (Fig. 12-14). Elevating the feet and keeping the extremities warm are preventives. Cramps, while not a serious condition, are excruciatingly painful for the duration of the seizure. If the husband has been taught the procedure for immediate relief, much pain will be prevented.

Edema

Swelling of the lower extremities is very common during pregnancy and is sometimes very uncomfortable. It is especially prone to occur in hot weather. Often it may be relieved by a proper abdominal support or by resting frequently during the day. Elevating the feet or taking the right-angle position often gives relief (see Fig. 12-11, p. 209). If the swelling is persistent, the patient may have to stay in bed, but ordinarily this condition proves to be no more

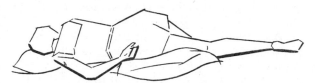

Figure 12-13. Sims's position for varicosities of vulva and rectum.

than a discomfort. However, edema is one of the symptoms of toxemia, and it must never be overlooked.

When edema of the lower extremities is observed, careful investigation should be made to see if other parts are affected—the hands or the face, and so on. The condition should be reported to the physician at once.

Vaginal discharge

In pregnancy there is increased vaginal secretion so that a moderately profuse discharge at this time usually has no particular significance. However, it is wise to instruct the patient to call any copious and/or yellow or greenish foul-smelling or irritating discharge to the attention of the physician. For instance, a profuse yellow discharge may be regarded as a possible evidence of gonorrhea (see Chapter 25), especially when it is accompanied by such urinary manifestations as burning and frequency. A smear may be taken, and the microscopic result will indicate whether or not definite treatment is necessary. If any discharge becomes irritating, the patient may be advised to bathe the vulva with a solution of sodium bicarbonate or boric acid. The application of KY jelly after bathing often relieves the condition entirely. Instructing a patient to wear a perineal pad is sometimes all the advice that

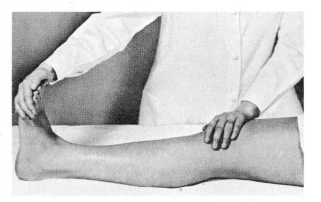

Figure 12-14. The nurse helping the patient during a leg cramp, forcing the toes upward while making pressure on the knee to straighten the leg.

is needed. A douche never should be taken unless the obstetrician orders it.

A particularly stubborn form of leukorrhea in pregnancy is caused by the parasitic protozoan known as the *Trichomonas vaginalis*. It is characterized not only by a profuse frothy discharge (white or yellowish in color), but also by irritation and itching of the vulva and the vagina. The diagnosis is easily made by the physician by taking a small quantity of the fresh secretion and putting it under the microscope in a hanging-drop. Here the spindle-shaped organisms, somewhat larger than leukocytes, with whiplike processes attached, can be seen in active motion.

A highly effective specific agent of very low toxicity, metronidazole, is available for this infection. It is given orally and the usual course is 21 tablets of 200 mg., one tablet three times a day. Simultaneous treatment of the sexual partner with the same regimen is highly advisable, otherwise the mother will only become reinfected. Other topical preparations are available, but are usually necessary only when the infection is extremely resistant or when the patient cannot tolerate metronidazole. The physician will evaluate this aspect.[13]

Candidiasis, a yeast infection caused by the *Candida albicans*, is another common cause of profuse vaginal discharge. The organism is frequently present in the vaginal canal without producing symptoms, but during pregnancy the physical changes in the vagina produce conditions that foster its development. It is characterized by white patches on the vaginal mucosa and a thick cottage-cheeselike discharge which is extremely irritating, so that burning or pruritus is present. Even the external genitalia often become inflamed, and occasionally extensive edema is observed. Bleeding may accompany the other symptoms if the patches on the mucosa are removed in any way.

It is not necessary to treat patients in whom *Candida* are found if signs and symptoms are not present. Specific fungicidal suppositories are used to treat this condition. Although this treatment is effective, the infection is stubborn and likely to recur and require repeated treatment during the pregnancy. The *pruritus*, or itching of the skin, may be relieved to a marked degree if proper hygienic measures are employed to keep the area free of the irritating material being deposited on the skin surface. The mother who has this infection may transmit it to her infant during the process of delivery. *Thrush* develops when the organisms attack the mucous membrane of the mouth.

Preparations for the baby

Layette

The baby's layette and equipment are of real interest to all parents—in fact, they are interesting to almost everyone. The cost of the layette should be in keeping with the individual economic circumstances. The entire layette can be purchased ready-made or can be made at home quite inexpensively. Much or little may be spent in its preparation, but nurses who are teaching parents should know why certain types of clothes and equipment are preferable. In the selection of clothing the following points should be considered: comfort, ease in laundering, ease in putting on and taking off, and that it be very light in weight. The new baby's skin is easily irritated by wool. Any clothing which comes in contact with the infant's skin should be made of soft cotton material. Knitted materials have the advantage of ease in laundering and sufficient stretch quality to allow for more freedom in dressing the baby. Garments that open down the full length and fasten with ties or grippers are easier to put on. Ties or grippers are not only less difficult to fasten than buttons, but also are more desirable from the standpoint of safety. The geographic location and climate will greatly influence the selection of the infant's clothing. Size 1 shirts and gowns are recommended, since the infant grows rapidly in the first six months and quickly outgrows his garments. It is well to remember that his clothing should not inhibit his normal activities. The complete outfit of clothes that the baby wears need not weigh more than 12 to 16 ounces.

The mother can be advised to prepare a very simple layette. As she sees how fast her baby grows, and what he will need, the additional items can be secured. The complete layettes which can be purchased often contain unnecessary items and are often costly. Also, many articles may be received as baby gifts. Therefore, it is wise to choose only those things which are necessary for immediate use.

Layette necessities include:
Five or six shirts
Three to four dozen diapers (if diaper service is not used)

Four to six receiving blankets (These are very versatile items and can be used in various ways. For instance, they can be rolled firmly and used to support the infant's back when he is on his side; in emergencies, they can be used as bathtowels, diaper pads, sheets)

Three to six nightgowns, kiminos, or sacques

Six cotton covered waterproof diaper pads (11" x 16")

Two waterproof protectors for under diaper pads

Two afghans or blankets ⎫
One bunting ⎬ (if climate is cold)
⎭

Two to four soft towels (40" x 40")

Two to four soft washcloths

Nursery equipment should consist of:

basket, bassinet or crib
mattress (firm, flat and smooth)
mattress protector (waterproof)
sheets or pillowcases for mattress
chest or separate drawer
cotton crib blankets
bathtub
diaper pail
toilet tray—equipped
absorbent cotton—or cotton balls
baby soap (bland, white, unscented)
rustproof safety pins
soapdish
bath apron (for mother)
table, for bath or dressing
chair (for mother)

Additional suggestions for layette and equipment are:

sweaters	footstool
crib spreads	diaper bag (for traveling)
bibs	disposable diapers
clothes drier	nursery light
chest of drawers	carriage
nursery stand	

Some further suggestions in relation to the selection of specific items are as follows:

SHIRTS, GOWNS, AND THE LIKE. The sleeves should have roomy armholes, such as the raglan-type sleeve. If the pullover-type garments are used, the neck openings should be so constructed that they are large enough to be put on easily from over the feet or the head.

DIAPERS. Of the several varieties of diapers available, bird's-eye or gauze diapers are the most popular. The selection of diapers should be considered from the standpoint of their comfort (soft and light in weight), absorbency and washing and drying qualities. The mother who plans to use a commercial diaper service may either use the company's diapers or her own. Disposable diapers are also available, but they are generally more expensive in the long run than cloth diapers or a diaper service.

RECEIVING BLANKETS. These should be made of cotton flannelette 1 yard square. This square is used to fold loosely about the baby. If properly secured, the baby may lie and kick and at the same time keep covered and warm. In the early weeks these squares take the brunt of the service and in this way save the finer covers from becoming soiled so quickly.

AFGHANS OR BLANKETS. These can be of very lightweight cotton or polyester material. The temperature and the weather will determine the amount of covering needed.

SHEETS. Crib sheets are usually 45" x 72" and are available in muslin, percale, and knitted cotton materials. The knit sheets are practical for bottom sheets and do not need to be ironed. Pillowcases are very usable for the carriage or the basket mattress. Receiving blankets may be used for top sheets.

WATERPROOF SHEETING. Various waterproof materials are suitable to protect the mattress and to be used under the pads. Even though the mattress may have a protective covering, it it necessary to have a waterproof cover large enough to cover the mattress completely—something that can be removed and washed.

WATERPROOF PANTS. These offer protection for special occasions. If the plastic variety is used, they should not be tight at the leg or the waist. For general use, a square of protective material such as Sanisheeting or a cotton quilted pad can be used under the baby next to the diaper.

BATH APRON. This is a protection for both mother and baby and may be made of plastic material covered with terry cloth.

Nursery equipment

In choosing the equipment, again the individual circumstances should be considered. Expense, space, and future plans all influence the selection. Most nurseries are planned for the satisfaction of the parents. Eventually the baby's room becomes the child's room; and if economy must be considered, furniture should be selected that will appeal to the child as he grows and develops.

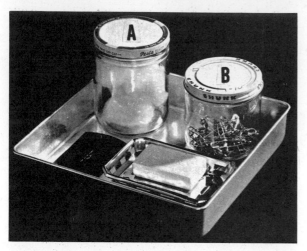

Figure. 12-15. Improvised toilet tray for infant. A household tray or baking pan and miscellaneous jars may be utilized. Comb has fine teeth with smooth rounded edges. Soap dish contains mild, white, unscented soap. (A) Jar for clean absorbent cotton. (B) Jar for safety pins.

THE BABY'S ROOM. Preferably, the baby should have his own room. If this is not feasible, a quiet airy place, out of drafts, may be selected.

BED. The baby needs to have his own bed. This may be a basket, a bassinet, or a crib. The trimming on the basket or the bassinet should be such that it can be removed easily and laundered. A bed may be improvised from a box or a bureau drawer, placed securely on a sturdy table or on chairs which are held together with rope. Many parents may have a carriage that may be used as a bed. However, after about the first two months, the baby will need a crib. The crib should be constructed so that the bars are close enough together to prevent the baby's head from being caught between them. If it is painted, a paint "safe for babies" should be used, that is, nonleaded.

MATTRESS. The mattress is to be firm (not hard) and flat. All mattresses, including the waterproof-covered, can be protected by a waterproof sheeting to prevent the mattress from becoming stained and from absorbing odors. The waterproof sheet is easily washed and dries quickly.

NETTING. This will be needed for the carriage, the basket, or the crib during the insect season. If a Kiddie-Koop is used, it is screened to protect the baby from insects and animals.

BATHTUB. The plastic tub is safe and easy to keep clean.

BATHTUB TABLE. The table on which the tub is placed for the baby's bath should be of convenient height. A kitchen table, or other sturdy table without wheels, may be used for this purpose.

MOTHER'S CHAIR. The chair also should be a convenient height and comfortable for the individual mother.

DIAPER PAIL. This should be large enough for at least the day's supply of soiled diapers. It may be used also for boiling the diapers.

TOILET TRAY. This tray can be prepared and ready for use immediately after the delivery of the baby (Fig. 12-15).

Plans for after-care of mother and baby

It is always a relief to the mother and the father when the plans for delivery and the arrangements for the period following have been completed. The parents should make some provision for the mother to be free from other responsibilities until she has regained, in part at least, her physical strength, and until lactation has been established.

The nurse should make an effort to include the father when discussing the details of the mother's care. Often it is only with his help that the mother gets the full care she needs, care that the physician and the nurse wish her to have (see Chapter 13).

Return to employment

The expectant mother who is employed may desire to know how early she may return to work after the baby is born. Following delivery, six weeks is the recommended time that is needed for the physician to determine whether or not the reproductive organs are returning to their approximate normal size and position. This is an important time also for the mother to regain her general strength and begin to establish the important role transition to parenthood. A role relationship must be established with her infant and adjustments in the role relationship(s) must begin to be made with the father and/or other children in the household. Accordingly, it is advisable that no commitments should be made until at least six to eight weeks after the baby's birth. There are, of course, certain unavoidable circumstances within some family units which leave the mother no alternative but to return to work.

In these situations, the mother may require special guidance from the health team to insure that adequate care and attention be given to herself as well as her infant and family. In the long run, research has demonstrated that the employment of the mother has *no deleterious* effects on the personalities and general well-being of the children and family. However, during these weeks following delivery, attention must be given so that the mother may attain adequate rest and nutrition and the infant and family receive appropriate care and attention.

Bibliography

1. Grimm, L. M.: Changed patterns of obstetric care: maternity continuity clinic. *Am. J. Nurs.* 73:1723-1725, Oct. 1973.
2. Thompson, H. E., *et al*: Factors contributing to improved maternal care and fetal outcome in a medium-sized city-county hospital. *Am. Ob-Gyn.* 116: 229-238, May 15, 1973.
3. Schwartz, J. L.: First national survey of free medical clinics 1967-69. *HSMHA Health Reports* 86:788, 1971.
4. Ryan, G. M.: Improving pregnancy outcome via regionalization of prenatal care. *JOGN Nursing* 38-40, July/Aug. 1974.
5. Grimm, L. M., *op. cit.*
6. Tompkins, W. T., *et al*: The underweight patient as an increased obstetric hazard. *Am. J. Ob-Gyn.* 69: 898-919, 1955. Winich, M., *et al*: Effects of prenatal nutrition upon pregnancy risk. *Clin. Ob. and Gyn.* 16: 184-198, March 1973.
7. Cross, A. T., and Walsh, H. E.: Prenatal diet counseling. *J. Reproductive Med.* 7:265-274, Dec. 1971.
8. Flowers, C. E.: Editorial: Nutrition in pregnancy. *J. Reproductive Med.* 7:198-204, Nov. 1971.
9. Erhard, D.: The new vegetarians. *Nutrition Today,* 4-12, Nov.-Dec. 1973.
10. Drugs and therapeutic information. *In* Safety of Immunizing Agents in Pregnancy. *Medical Letter of Drugs and Therapeutics* 18:5, March 6, 1970, issue 291.
11. Pierson, E., and D'Antonio, W. V.: *Female and Male: Dimensions of Human Sexuality.* Philadelphia, J. B. Lippincott, 1974, pp. 153-163.
12. *Ibid.*
13. Dennerstein, G. J.: Vaginitis: diagnosis and treatment. *Drugs* 4:419-425, 1972.

Suggested Reading

BANCROFT, A. V.: Pregnancy and the counterculture. *Nurs. Clin. North Am.* 8:67-76, March, 1973.

BLOCK, D.: Some crucial terms in nursing: What do they really mean? *Nurs. Outlook* 22, 11:689-694, Nov. 1974.

BOLTON, J. H.: Dietary protein in pregnancy, its importance. *Australian and New Zealand J. Ob-Gyn.* 8:20-21, Feb. 1968.

BRANDL, E.: Cigarette smoking and pregnancy. *Nurs. Sci.* 3:71-76, Feb. 1965.

BROOK, M.: The use of artificial sweeteners in food products. *Roy. Soc. Health J.* 89:140-142, May/June 1969.

BRUSER, M.: Sporting activities during pregnancy. *Am. J. Ob-Gyn.* 32:721, Nov. 1968.

CHOW, B. F., *et al*: Maternal nutrition and metabolism of the offspring: studies in rats and man. *Am. J. Public Health* 58:668-677, April 1968.

CLARK, L.: Introducing mother and baby. *Am. J. Nurs.* 74, 8:1483-1848, Aug. 1974.

CLARK, A. L., AND HALE, R. W.: Sex during and after pregnancy. *Am. J. Nurs.* 74, 3:1430, Aug. 1974.

CROSS, E. T., *et al*: Prenatal diet counseling. *J. Reproductive Med.* 7:265-274, Dec. 1971.

DANSFORTH, D. N.: Pregnancy and labor—from the vantage point of the physical therapist. *Am. J. Phys. Med.* 46:653-658, Feb. 1967.

DICK-READ, G.: *Childbirth Without Fear.* New York: Harper & Row, 1972.

EASTMAN, N. J., AND JACKSON, E.: Weight relationships in pregnancy. *Ob-Gyn. Survey* 28:1003-1025, Nov. 1968.

———: Iron and folic acid in pregnancy. *Drug Ther. Bull.* 5:21-23, Mar. 17, 1967.

———: Moving iron to the mother. *JAMA* 205:33 and 36, Sept. 1968.

ERHARD, D.: The new vegetarians, Part one—Vegetarianism and its medical consequences. *Nutrition Today* 4-12, Nov./Dec. 1973.

———: The new vegetarians, Part two—The zen macrobiotic movement and other cults based on vegetarianism. *Nutrition Today* 20-27, Jan./Feb. 1974.

ESTEY, G. P.: Word from a mother. *Am. J. Nurs.* 69:1453-1454, July 1969.

FLOWERS, C. E.: Editorial: Nutrition in pregnancy. *J. Reproductive Med.* 7:199-204, Nov. 1971.

FRAZER, A.: Health aspects of artificial sweeteners. *Roy. Soc. Health J.* 89:133-136, May/June 1969.

GAGE, M. A.: Educational aspects of prenatal care. *Med. Serv. J. Canad.* 23:527-531, April 1967.

GOLDMAN, J. A., AND SCHECHTER, A.: Effect of cigarette smoking on glucose tolerance in pregnant women. *Israel J. Med. Sci.* 3:561-564, Aug. 1967.

HAMMEL, F.: Nurses in private practice as montrices. *Am. J. Nurs.* 69:1446-1450, July 1969.

HARDING, E. H., *et al*: The Berkeley free clinic. *Nurs. Outlook* 21, 1:40-43, Jan. 1973.

HASSALL, D.: A home visit program for students. *Nurs. Outlook* 22:522-524, Aug. 1974.

INZER, L. C.: A study of nutrition in pregnancy. *J. School Health* 40:392-396, Oct. 1970.

IYENGER, L.: Effects of dietary supplements late in pregnancy on the expectant mother and her newborn. *Indian J. Med. Res.* 55:85-89, Jan. 1967.

JACHE, M. C.: Nursing goals in working with families under multiple stress. *Nurs. Clin. North Am.* 4:69-75, Mar. 1969.

JONAT, L. V.: Continuing maternal health care. *Med. Serv. J. Canad.* 23:531-534, April 1967.

JORDAN, A. D.: Evaluation of a family-centered maternity care hospital program. *JOGN Nursing* 2, 1:13-35, Jan./Feb. 1973.

KELLER, N. S.: Care without coordination: a true story. *Nurs. Forum* 6:280-323, 1967.

KENNELL, J. H., *et al*: Attachments begin in fixed period after birth. *Ob. Gyn. News* 9, 20:37, Oct. 15, 1974.

KOWALSKI, K. E.: Changed patterns of obstetric care on call staffing. *Am. J. Nurs.* 73, 10:1725-1727, Oct. 1973.

LEVINE, M. M., *et al*: Live-virus vaccines in pregnancy: risks and recommendations. *Lancet* 2:7871, July 6, 1974.

LEVY, B. S., *et al*: Reducing neonatal mortality rate with nurse-midwives. *Am. J. Ob-Gyn.* 109:50-58, Jan. 1, 1971.

LIPKIN, G. B.: *Psychosocial Aspects of Maternal-Child Nursing.* St. Louis, Mosby, 1974, 160 pp.

LUBIC, R. W.: What the lay person expects of maternity care. *JOGN Nursing* 1:25-31, June 1972.

MANN, V. R.: Food practices of the Mexican-American in Los Angeles County. Los Angeles County Health Dept., 1963.

MANNING, M. L.: The psychodynamics of dietetics. *Nurs. Outlook* 13:57-59, April 1965.

McCLURE, W.: National health insurance and HMOs. *Nurs. Outlook* 21, 1:44-48, Jan. 1973.

MOORE, M. L.: The importance of culture in childbearing. *JOGN Nursing* 1:29-32, July/Aug. 1972.

NATIONAL INSTITUTE OF CHILD HEALTH AND HUMAN DEVELOPMENT: *Optimal Health Care for Mothers and Children: A National Priority.* Bethesda, Md., National Institutes of Health, 1967.

NEWTON, M. E., *et al*: Nutritional aspects of nursing care. *Nurs. Res.* 16:46-49, Winter 1967.

NISWANDER, K., *et al*: Physical characteristics of the gravida and their association with birth weight and perinatal death. *Am. J. Ob-Gyn.* 119, 3, June 1, 1974.

OSOFSKY, H. J.: Psychological and sociological aspects of normal pregnancy. *Med. Serv. J. Canad.* Proceedings of the National Conference on Maternal and Child Health 23, 4:512-521, April 1967.

OTTE, M. J.: Correcting inverted nipples. *Am. J. Nurs.* 75:454-456, Mar. 1975.

PIKE, R. L., *et al*: Juxtaglomerular degranulation and zona glomerulosa exhaustion in pregnant rats induced by low sodium intakes and reversed by sodium load. *Am. J. Ob-Gyn.* 95:604-614, July 1, 1966.

PION, R. P., *et al*: Prenatal care, a group psychotherapeutic approach. *Calif. Med.* 97:281-285, Nov. 1962.

RECOMMENDED DIETARY ALLOWANCES, rev. ed., Publication No. 1146, Washington, D.C., National Academy of Sciences, National Research Council, 1963.

REEDER, S. R., AND REEDER, L. G.: Some correlates of prenatal care among low income wed and unwed women. *Am. J. Ob-Gyn.* 90:1304-1314, Dec. 15, 1964.

REEDER, S. R., AND DECK, E.: Nurses' participation in a group psychotherapeutic approach to antepartal management. *Nurs. Forum* 2:82-93, 1963.

RICHIE, J.: Using an interpreter effectively. *Nurs. Outlook* 12:27-29, Dec. 1964.

ROSE, P. A.: The high risk mother-infant dyad—a challenge for nursing. *Nurs. Forum* 6:94-102, 1967.

ROSENGREN, W. R.: Social instability and attitudes toward pregnancy as a social role. *Soc. Prob.* 9:371-378, Spring 1962.

RUBIN, R.: Behavioral definitions in nursing therapy. Conference on Maternal and Child Nursing. Columbus, Ohio, Ross Laboratories, 1964.

———: Food and feeding: a matrix of relationships. *Nurs. Forum* 6:195-205, 1967.

SCHNEIDER, J.: Changing concepts in prenatal care. *Postgrad. Med.* 53:91-97, June 1973.

SCHULKIND, M. L., *et al*: Neonatal health insurance. *Ob-Gyn. Survey* 29, 10:714, Oct. 1974.

SCOTT, J. N.: The changing health care environment: its implications for nursing. *Am. J. Public Health* 64:364-369, April 1974.

SILVER, G. A.: National health insurance, national health policy, and the national health. *Am. J. Nurs.* 71, 9:1730-1735, Sept. 1971.

TAYLOR, E. S.: Four crises in maternity care. *Ob-Gyn. Survey* 24:253, Mar. 1969.

THOMPSON, H. E., *et al*: Factors contributing to improved maternal care and fetal outcome in a medium-sized city-county hospital. *Am. J. Ob-Gyn.* 116:229-238, May 15, 1973.

TOKUHATA, G. K.: Smoking in relation to infertility and fetal loss. *Arch. Environ. Health* 17:353-359, Sept. 1968.

ULIN, P. R.: Changing techniques in psychoprophylactic preparation for childbirth. *Am. J. Nurs.* 68:2586-2591, Dec. 1968.

VELLAY, P.: *Childbirth Without Pain.* New York, Dutton, 1960.

WATTS, W.: Social class, ethnic background and patient care. *Nurs. Forum* 6:155-162, 1967.

WHITESIDE, M. G., *et al*: Iron, folic acid and vitamin B_{12} levels in normal pregnancy, and their influence on birth-weight and the duration of pregnancy. *Med. J. Aust.* 1:338-342, Mar. 2, 1968.

WINICH, M., *et al*: Effects of prenatal nutrition upon pregnancy risk. *Clin. Ob. and Gyn.* 16:184-198, Mar. 1973.

YOUNG, E. W.: Prepared childbirth: its impact on nursing. *Canad. Nurse* 64:39-43, Jan. 1968.

YOUNOSZAI, M. K., AND HAWORTH, J. C.: Cigarette smoking during pregnancy: the effect upon the hematocrit and acid-base balance of the newborn infant. *Canad. Med. Assoc. J.* 99:197-200, Aug. 3, 1968.

patient teaching and counseling

13

Teaching and Learning / Types of Education for Childbearing / Postpartum Teaching / Guide for Preparing Parents for Childbirth and the Puerperium

Education of the patient is a major component of the professional nurse's role. In this era of the consumer movement, enabling the patient and family to fully understand the body processes and rationale for medical and nursing management of their health problems assumes even greater significance. Particularly in the area of maternity, patients and families are not only very interested in learning, but have come to view such knowledge as their right. They expect the nurse to be willing and able to assist in their acquisition of knowledge, and to take their individual wants and needs into consideration.

The increased involvement of childbearing couples in all phases of the reproductive cycle is beneficial for them as receivers of care and for nurses as givers of care. A concerned and knowledgeable woman will follow a more healthful regimen during pregnancy, including nutrition, exercise and rest, physical care and psychological processes. A prepared woman and an involved partner can cope positively with the stresses of labor, enriching their relationship and promoting psychological maturation. Parents who are informed and actively seek understanding of their child's numerous needs concerning comfort, security, and stimulation during the early formative years can attain a happier, more satisfying parent-child relationship and foster optimal growth and development of the child.

When the childbearing couple desires to learn, and the health professional is ready to teach, their shared experiences can be most satisfying to all involved. The roles of teacher and learner are not rigid, however, for often the nurse learns much of value from the parents, and gains deeper understanding of the reproductive experience through appreciating their perspectives. The cornerstone of patient education is recognition and respect of the learning needs of patients. The nurse may design content, but if it does not meet the patient's learning needs, it is pointless and ineffective. A responsibility of the nurse is developing the skill to assess these learning needs accurately.

Patient teaching encompasses an enormous body of knowledge, only a portion of which is included in this chapter. Throughout the text additional information about teaching as a part of nursing intervention for specific patient needs or problems will be found. Concepts related to the teaching-learning process, some approaches to group and individual teaching, and programs providing preparation for childbirth and parenting are discussed here.

Teaching and learning

"Teaching is an interactive process between a teacher and one or more learners."[1] The teaching-learning process is a complex entity composed of various interrelated parts. These parts might be summarized as: 1) identifying the need or needs of the learner, 2) determining the motivation of the learner, 3) establishing the objectives of learning, and 4) evaluation in terms of desired learning. Learning may be defined as a (desired) change in behavior. Teaching is accomplished only when the learner learns, retains new knowledge, and is able to use it at the present or in the future. Many factors affect the teaching-learning process, and the nurse must be aware of those which might either enhance or interfere with learning. The following concepts about learning illustrate some of these influences:

1. Learners (and teachers) bring with them to the classroom a cluster of understandings, skills, appreciations, attitudes, and feelings that have personal meaning to them and are in effect the sum of their reactions to previous stimuli.
2. Learners (and teachers) are individually different in many ways even when ability grouped.
3. Learners (and teachers) have developed concepts of self, which directly affect their behavior.
4. Learning may be defined as a change in behavior.
5. Learning requires activity on the part of the learner. The learner should not be passive.
6. Learners ultimately learn what *they* actively desire to learn; they do not learn what they do not accept or come to accept.
7. Learning is enhanced when learners accept responsibility for their own learning.
8. Learning is directly influenced by physical and social environment.
9. Learning occurs on successively deeper levels.
10. Learning is deepened when the learning situation provides opportunity for applying learnings in as realistic a situation as is feasible.
11. Learners are motivated when they understand and accept the purposes of the learning situation.
12. Learners are motivated by success experiences.
13. Learners are motivated by teacher acceptance.
14. Learners are motivated when they can associate new learnings with previous learnings.
15. Learners are motivated when they can see the usefulness of the learning in their own personal terms.[2]

The idea of educating mothers during pregnancy is probably very ancient. In Manchester, England, during the 18th century, Dr. Charles White wrote a book on instructions for the supervision of mothers during pregnancy, and how to help them in labor and make them more comfortable. During the last few decades of this century, increased understanding of the psychodynamics of pregnancy and the puerperium has established a scientific basis for the content and structure of antepartal and postpartal education.

Psychologic tasks of pregnancy and mothers' interests

Nurses have long observed that pregnant women ask different kinds of questions and express different concerns in early pregnancy as compared to later periods in gestation. The widely recognized receptiveness of women in the third trimester toward information about baby care and behavior led to the common practice of scheduling prenatal classes at this time. Women in the first or second trimester did not exhibit the same level of interest in "mothercraft" classes; thus they were largely omitted from prenatal education.

Professional interest in the many behavior changes characteristic of pregnant women led to identification of the specific and unique psychologic tasks which appear to be a universal phenomenon of pregnancy. Viewing pregnancy as a developmental process, involving profound endocrine and general somatic as well as psychologic changes, it can be understood as a period of disequilibrium and a significant turning point in the woman's (and probably her partner's) life.[3] Certain specific psychologic tasks are necessary to cope with the numerous changes, and these seem to occur at characteristic times during gestation. The first, incorporation and integration of the fetus, occurs during the first trimester and is not evident during later stages of pregnancy. The second, perception of the fetus as a separate object, seems to begin in the second trimester and to be quite well established by the third trimester. Readiness to assume the care-taking relationship with the baby, the third task, increases from the second to the third trimester and is not apparent in early pregnancy. The highest level of anxiety about labor is manifest during the second trimester, while women in the third trimester express more confidence about undergoing labor.[4]

This "time schedule" of involvement with different psychologic tasks suggests that pregnant women's interests and needs for information will vary according to stage of gestation. While research has not yet identified exactly what periods of time are involved in each psychologic task, nurses can utilize these data to plan appropriate antepartal education. During early pregnancy, when the woman is working through the idea of being pregnant, informational needs center around validation of pregnancy, understanding physical changes, and recognition of normal emotions and feelings. In midpregnancy, women begin to identify the baby as a unique individual, and are receptive to information about fetal growth and development and about maintaining their own and the baby's health. As pregnancy draws to an end, women become concerned about preparing for the baby's arrival, thus the interest in preparation for childbirth, infant behavior, and care-taking activities including feeding, handling, bathing, and so on. By tailoring the information presented to the different interests of each group and providing mothers with the opportunity to express their own learning needs, nurses can conduct meaningful antepartal educational programs.

Postpartum processes and the mother-child relationship

Although the experience of labor is undoubtedly significant for the woman's self-concept, maternal-infant bonding, and possibly the couple's relationship, few data are available to substantiate what impact nursing intervention during labor might have on these. Advocates of prepared childbirth believe women move more rapidly into the care-taking role when they are awake and actively participating in their labor. There is some empirical evidence that fathers who act as labor coaches develop paternal feelings toward the babies of these labors which are stronger and more recognizable than toward their other children. The work of some neonatologists in the area of high-risk infants strongly suggests that early and prolonged contact between mother and baby following labor and delivery enhances the bonding process (see Chapter 18). As with other mammals, humans seem to have a critical time for optimal mother-infant bonding, and this time probably is the first several hours after delivery. There also appear to be certain species-specific maternal behaviors which initiate and carry out the attachment process.[5]

On first contact with their babies, mothers seek an "en face" position in which their eyes are in the same vertical plane as the baby's. It has been suggested that this eye-to-eye contact may initiate or release maternal care-taking responses. Mothers then begin to explore the infant, first with fingertips touching the infant's extremities, then within a few minutes proceeding to massage, with encompassing palm contact, the infant's trunk. Some fathers have been observed going through these same steps. Kennell and Klaus[6] described this process as taking only a few minutes. Rubin, writing many years earlier, observed very similar behavior patterns in mothers as they moved from fingertip to palm touch, then encompassed their infants in their arms. However, this process took about three days according to Rubin's observations.[7]

Other physiologic and psychologic changes occur during the puerperium which are part of the process of regeneration undergone by the mother. There is a "taking-in" period which lasts for the first day or two, possibly three. During this restorative period the mother has a great need for sleep, may indeed have "sleep-hunger" for several days. Among other normal reactions associated with this taking-in phase is the mother's passive and dependent behavior. However, when the "taking-hold" phase follows, the mother is physically and psychologically ready to assume active care of her infant, and seeks information and support to facilitate her mothering behaviors. Once her dependency needs have been met in the taking-in phase, she needs to move toward greater independence.[8] For further details of nursing care during the puerperium, refer to Chapter 20.

Effective patient teaching must take into account what is known about the processes occurring during labor and the puerperium, as well as individual variation and specific need. If the labor experience is as important as we suspect, health professionals have an obligation to assist parents to prepare for it and support them during this stressful time. When labor has started, a certain amount of teaching is possible, and sensitive care can be helpful, but this is not as effective as antenatal preparation. While parents have long recognized the significance of being together with their new baby in the hours right after birth, health professionals have largely been oblivious to this in their concern for asepsis, technology, and immediate dangers to the newborn. Perhaps it is time to rethink delivery and recovery routines, and educate both parents and professionals in the new data concerning mother-infant attachment. During the few days the postpartal woman spends in the hospital, her needs may conflict with the nursing staff's needs to maintain the routine or provide the teaching they believe necessary. Mothers will progress at different speeds in their assumption of the care-taking role, and will have individualized concerns. Finding a way to respond to individual needs yet conduct an efficient postpartal educational program is a major challenge to postpartal nurses. Patient teaching activities must also extend into the community, to respond to the needs of families integrating a new member during the early years of childrearing.

The learning process will vary according to culture and socioeconomic situation. Mothering practices in lower income groups are influenced by economic circumstances which limit equipment, supplies and mobility; by the organization of the family group and the authority structure; and by the accumulated folk knowledge which establishes specific practices for many common activities and problems of childrearing. Standard educational programs about formula preparation, clothing and supplies for the baby, integration of the baby into the family, and the mother's nutritional and rest needs are often meaningless to low income mothers because of a lack of resources and a different value system. Family and friends are generally viewed as more reliable consultants for health concerns than professionals, whose assistance is sought only when community knowledge cannot solve the problem. Sometimes the use of language itself precludes useful exchange of information, as differences in terms used,

accent and speed of delivery vary substantially between middle-class nurses and low income mothers. In lower socioeconomic levels, the grandmother's word is often law in terms of baby care, and she may be the major caretaker of the baby. Teaching given solely to the mother may thus have little consequence for the actual care given to the baby. Different cultural groups also have their unique approaches to childrearing and patterns of assistance to new mothers. Values, language, style, and knowledge will exert influences within other cultural groups in a manner similar to that discussed above.

The nurse must come to understand different cultural and low income lifestyles if effective antepartal and postpartal teaching is to occur. The approach to teaching utilized with these groups will probably need to shift from the giving of information to assessing present practices, then supplementing these practices when necessary with information presented in a form that can be understood and accepted.[9]

Types of education for childbearing

Preparation for motherhood actually begins with the mother's own birth or earlier (as was stated in the last chapter), and its development is influenced by an accumulation of her experiences through infancy, childhood, adolescence and maturity. The father's feelings and attitudes are influenced in a like manner by his previous experiences. There is an increasing tendency for schools to incorporate information about childbearing and parenthood into "health education" and "family life" courses. Classes about pregnancy, sexuality and parenthood are becoming more common in college and university curricula, as well as more widely available in continuing education and private adult educational programs. Couples thus bring a wealth of previous learning to their experience of childbearing, some of it useful and positive and some frightening and inaccurate. With the advent of pregnancy, preparation for parenthood begins in earnest as the immediacy of the event escalates the need for information.

Individual teaching and counseling

One-to-one teaching is widely used in all nursing settings, and is frequently a most effective means of assisting patients to understand and adapt to a variety of health problems. In most nurse-patient contacts, some individual teaching occurs. During pregnancy numerous opportunities are present in which nurses can enhance the effectiveness of medical care through explanations of treatments and procedures, interpretations of what the physician tells parents, and specific instructions for carrying out the regimen of care. When the patient asks questions about symptoms or feelings or seeks general information, an on-the-spot response by the nurse meets that particular learning need. Some clinics and offices have pamphlets or audiovisual material intended to provide individualized instruction to antepartal patients. The amount of actual structure necessary to ensure that these materials are used varies widely. The effectiveness of written or media information without reinforcement through discussion is questionable.

Counseling, an interchange of opinions or giving of advice to help direct the judgment or conduct of others, is often hard to separate from teaching. While counseling is more personal and feeling oriented, its use in combination with presentation of facts usually results in enhanced learning. Individualized nursing care in which the mother is assisted to recognize her feelings and fears, reassured that such feelings are normal, and given certain facts to dispel myths or anticipate and prepare for coming events is a common example of how teaching and counseling are combined in antepartal care. Mothers frequently seek the nurse's advice about their own care during pregnancy, family conflicts, problems with children, diet and nutrition, and many specifics about care of the newborn baby. They want not just information, but the nurse's opinion about the subject or practice. The wise nurse will elicit the mother's opinion and the unspoken concerns behind the question before proceeding to answer. Provided the nurse is well informed on the subject, has a well reasoned approach to the practices that are recommended, and is sensitive to the mother's reactions, offering advice can often be very helpful. What must be avoided, however, is discrediting or dismissing the mother's practices or philosophy, for this only serves to alienate her. Appropriate use of counseling takes into consideration the patient's viewpoint and works within an acceptable framework to bring about increased understanding, leading to a change in behavior in the desired direction through the patient's internalization of the new goals.

Although individual teaching and counseling will continue to be a major mode of nursing intervention, concerns for more efficient utilization of the health professional's time have led to increased use of groups for antepartal education. Groups are also beneficial because the exchange of experiences among patients with common concerns provides support and encouragement, and expertise and knowledge of the group members combined often exceeds that of the professional alone.

Groups and classes

Most institutions providing maternity care also offer some type of antepartal group instruction, but the goals and purposes of these groups vary widely. Many private organizations also offer programs in antepartal education, preparation for childbirth, and preparation for parenthood. Classes may be affiliated with continuing education programs in colleges and universities, or with national health care organizations such as the Red Cross. The teachers in these groups or classes usually have some type of preparation or certification. They may represent one or, less commonly, several disciplines.

These educational programs can enhance, strengthen, and broaden the care and services provided by the physician and maternity nurse. Programs in parent education should be related segments in the total constellation of services provided to families. In order to make these sessions truly a preparation for parenthood and family-centered nursing, special attention has to be given to timing and availability of these courses. Sometimes hospitals and institutions arrange classes at times which are not feasible for the parents attending, especially for the father and often for the mother (e.g., in the middle of a busy day). Therefore, attendance is sparse and limited and many valuable aims of the programs may be thwarted.

INFORMATIONAL GROUPS. The most widely used type of program in this country, these groups are planned to serve everyone in the community and place emphasis on a general type of "education for childbirth." Courses usually include the physiology of childbearing, general hygiene, including nutrition during pregnancy and lactation, preparations for the baby, and the care of the mother and baby after delivery. In this type of program a multidisciplinary approach may be used in the teaching, or the nurse may be responsible for teaching all of the content.

In general, the material is usually covered in a lecture-type format with time allowed for questions and discussion. At times a semi-structured approach may be used, with certain topics being suggested by the participants and additional relevant information introduced by the nurse-discussion leader as it seems appropriate. Audiovisual materials such as films and slides are often used, with a film depicting actual childbirth a standard component. Tours of the hospital labor unit, postpartum floor and nursery are usually included.

Some of these classes are given for expectant mothers or fathers alone; in others the parents attend classes together. In the latter group the classes aid the parents in their mutual appreciation of the value of antepartal preparation and tend to promote the idea of sharing parenthood. The goals set for the parents in any of these classes are similar, namely, to gain increased knowledge about childbearing and increased understanding of ways to promote and to maintain optimum health through the practice of good health habits in daily living.

These classes are included as a part of the programs of private "public health" agencies such as the Visiting Nurse Association, official public health agencies such as the local and state departments of health, private organizations such as the Maternity Center Association in New York City, and many hospitals throughout the states.

DISCUSSION OR COUNSELING GROUPS. In this format no structured curriculum is set in advance. Group discussion is developed from the contributions of the group members. The leader is responsible for guiding the discussion and for opening essential areas not probed by the group members. The various areas described in the informational type programs (i.e., physiology of childbearing, general hygiene, etc.) are covered as the nurse-leader introduces these topics when they fit with the areas brought up by the participants. The group situation demands that the nurse develop a new concept of self as a leader and acquire new skills. Knowledge and understanding of what material is relevant is essential so that it can be drawn upon as the group needs it. Hence, the nurse must be totally prepared each time that the group meets since the discussion may range from nutrition in the first trimester of pregnancy to the physiology of labor. In addition, she must be skilled in communication techniques with the ability to listen, to probe, and to reflect so that the group can be helped to elaborate on germaine comments and statements. The nurse must recognize the importance and the implication of "iceberg questions," sometimes spoken of as "the question behind the question," knowing that such questions may indicate an underlying concern of the questioner. For example, an expectant mother in the last trimester of pregnancy asks, "How common is going crazy after having a baby?" In such instances the professional nurse should be able to explore and to sift alternatives until the real question can be asked and appropriate action may be taken. In this instance the patient really was not concerned with how often people became psychotic after childbirth but rather she wanted to know whether she was likely to experience this malady. Because of a history of mental illness in her family and her own extreme emotional lability during this pregnancy she was afraid that she might become psychotic after delivery.

Since training group leaders is a costly and time-consuming business (and it is essential that those who manage parents in this way be trained in the techniques), group education is not a commitment to be undertaken lightly by either the participating nurses or the sponsoring agencies. Unfortunately, many of these agencies rate the success of a program by the numbers attending; and in the group situation, by definition, only *small groups* can be served at one time.

Group discussion programs are usually well received by those who become involved on a continuing basis, with high levels of professional and patient satisfaction. Small groups are also quite effective in bringing about behavior change. Moreover, group education has the advantage of not limiting the discussion to certain topics usually discussed by particular class groups, and it can focus upon any of the aspects of pregnancy or childbearing which are of interest to the group.

Whatever the approach, the nurse who participates in parent classes is in a favorable position to help the patients and families to develop a better understanding of their immediate situations, together with a balanced view of the sociology of pregnancy and parturition, growth and development, and the psychologic and emotional aspects of family life.

PREPARED CHILDBIRTH GROUPS. The interpretation of "labor" as "pain" has been held by women from time immemorial, with the result that many women approached childbirth in dread of a fearful ordeal. Orthodox Christian teaching considered pain the natural accompaniment of childbirth in partial reparation for Eve's enticing Adam into the original sin. As most body processes are free from discomfort, the question of labor pain as a social phenomenon is frequently raised. Whatever the basic causes and mechanisms of childbirth pain (see Chapter 16), concern developed gradually over finding a means to help relieve the suffering of women during labor.

The influence of the attitude of a woman toward her confinement upon the ease of labor was stressed for many years by the British obstetrician, the late Grantly Dick-Read. He emphasized certain psychological aspects of labor—that "fear is in some way the chief pain-producing agent in otherwise normal labor." The neuromuscular mechanism by which fear exerts a deleterious effect on labor is obscure, but the general validity of Dick-Read's contention is in keeping with common clinical knowledge. The mother builds up a state of tensions because she is frightened, and these tensions create an antagonistic effect on the muscular activity of normal labor, with resulting pain. The pain causes more fear, which further increases the tensions, and so on, until a vicious circle is established.

Dick-Read's approach included an educational component so the women could comprehend the physiologic processes of labor, exercises to improve muscle tone, and techniques to assist in relaxation so the fear-tension-pain mechanism would not be instituted. These three components are included in most childbirth preparation programs which developed after Dick-Read's work became well known.

The educational component during pregnancy is designed to eliminate fear. Facts which concern the anatomy and the physiology of childbearing and the appropriate care of the mother are taught. The mother not only learns how labor progresses but also is helped to gain an understanding of the sensations likely to accompany labor and methods of working cooperatively with them. The exercises which are included are designed for the muscles which will be used in labor, as well as those which will promote the general well-being of the body. In the performance of any skill the individual is more efficient if the muscles involved are in the best condition. The exercises are not strenuous and, for the most part, are ones that will contribute to improved posture, body balance, agility and increased strength and endurance.

The mother learns breathing techniques that will aid her ability to relax in the first stage of labor, and techniques that will help her to work effectively with muscles used in the delivery. To enable the parents to better meet the needs of their baby after birth, information about growth and development also is included in these classes.

An important consideration throughout such programs is "to help the mother help herself," so that her pregnancy will be a healthy, happy experience, and at the time of labor she will be better able to participate actively in having her baby. In former days when mothers often were given heavy sedation, they were unable to have this satisfying experience.

Currently most prepared childbirth programs include the father as an active participant, with a role in helping the woman cope with labor. In this way fathers are made to feel involved and useful, and through learning the physiologic and emotional processes of pregnancy, gain an appreciation of the woman's experience. They are also able to explore their feelings and role as parents, and prepare psychologically for fatherhood.

Prepared childbirth is variously called *natural childbirth*, *participant childbirth*, or by the particular program's founder as with Lamaze and Bradley. Early in the movement in the United States, prepared childbirth earned a bad name through publicity about its more overzealous advocates. "Painless childbirth" was held up as a goal by some extremist groups, and the woman who did experience pain and resorted to pain medication during labor was made to feel a failure. This can be extremely destructive to the woman's self-concept at a time when she needs positive reinforcement in her abilities to achieve and perform competently. Fortunately, current thinking recognizes the variability in individual responses to stress and the differing character of individual labors, and teaches that pain medication used judiciously may serve to enhance the woman's ability to use relaxation techniques, thus helping her cope better with labor and achieve a satisfying outcome.

For some years there was resistance on the part of many obstetricians and labor room nurses toward prepared childbirth. Couples who had been trained in a particular method often had to buck staff pressures in their attempt to practice the relaxation techniques they had learned. Medication was at times forced upon the laboring woman on the premise that the physician felt it would be best for her, even when she protested that it was not necessary. Such practices as laboring in a semi-upright position instead of lying flat, having ice chips or sips of water, eliminating the perineal shave, holding and putting the baby to breast immediately after delivery, and constant presence of the father throughout labor and delivery cause much staff consternation and were often vetoed. Although prepared childbirth advocates had long been reporting the increased satisfaction the couple experienced, and the reduction of depressed babies which resulted when these methods were used, it took economic consumer pressure to bring about widespread acceptance of prepared childbirth. When childbearing couples began avoiding physicians and hospitals not allowing them to practice their method, the recalcitrants began to see the benefits of involvement and participation of the parents.

The *psychoprophylactic*, or *Lamaze, method* is the most widely used prepared childbirth method in the United States today. It was first propounded by two Russian doctors, Nicolaiev and Velvovskiy. The rationale of the program was based on Pavlov's concept of pain perception and his theory of conditioned reflexes (i.e., the substitution of favorable conditioned reflexes for unfavorable ones). The theory intrigued a Paris obstetrician, Fernand Lamaze, who studied Russian-trained mothers-to-be in a Leningrad clinic. Lamaze returned to France and began to prepare his patients in *psychoprophylaxis* or *mental prevention* of pain in childbirth. He gradually introduced certain adaptations, the most important of which was the rapid shallow breathing which came to characterize the Lamaze method. As the technique spread throughout Europe and Latin America the *Lamaze method* and psychoprophylaxis became synonymous. The late Marjorie Karmel was perhaps the most responsible for introducing this technique to America. There are now programs in psychoprophylaxis throughout this country. Many are under the auspices of the American Society for Prophylaxis in Obstetrics (ASPO) which was founded through joint efforts of Mrs. Karmel and a physical therapist, Elizabeth Bing, and others. In general, the teaching in the program consists of combating the fears associated with pregnancy and childbirth by instructing the pregnant woman in the anatomy and the neuromuscular

activity of the reproductive system and the mechanism of labor. The underlying theory of these programs remains firmly based on the neurophysiology of cortical excitation and conditioned response. That is, the mother is taught to replace responses of restlessness, fear and the loss of control with more useful activity. Its usefulness lies in the fact that a high level of activity can excite the cerebral cortex efficiently to inhibit other stimuli, in this case, the pain usually associated with labor. In some programs nutrition and general hygiene are included. Exercises which strengthen the abdominal muscles and relax the perineum are taught, and breathing techniques to help the process of labor are practiced. Thus, the mother is conditioned to respond with respiratory activity and dissociation (or relaxation) of the uninvolved muscles. She then controls her perception of the stimuli associated with labor and learns to work more effectively with the obstetric team.

Several changes have occurred in the Lamaze method as a result of experiences gained over many years of use. Exercises, breathing techniques, theories of learning and motivation, and emphasis on the childbirth team constitute the major changes. Exercises in the Lamaze method are intended to promote physical fitness, good posture, comfort, and controlled relaxation. One exercise which was found to be associated with sciatic nerve irritation, the straight leg raise-abduction exercise, has been eliminated. The "tailor-press" exercise has been modified from applying downward pressure on the knees while sitting in the tailor position to placing hands under knees and using thigh muscles to exert downward pressure against the hands. This modification results in less jerking of the muscles and is more effective for strengthening.

The main modification in breathing technique has been to use shallow breathing rather than rapid panting. Shallow effortless breathing, moderate in pace and high in the chest, is now taught in combination with the slower chest breathing to be used as labor intensifies and slow chest breathing is no longer effective by itself. Using this combined pattern, the woman begins her contraction with slow chest breathing, switches to shallow chest breathing for the peak of the contraction, and returns to slow chest breathing as the contraction declines. The shallow breathing itself has several variations, and an acceleration-deceleration pattern is used as transition nears. In the second stage of labor, the woman prefers to assume a 35° angle, grasp legs and pull them up and out, take several deep breaths, and then hold her breath, tighten abdominal muscles, relax the perineum, and push out through the vagina. This pushing effort is repeated about every 15 seconds throughout the contraction, timed and coached by the partner.

In the area of learning and motivation, Lamaze has progressed to a more individualized approach. The original psychoprophylactic training was rather rigid, with goals set by the teacher. Now, the couple set their own goals for labor and delivery, and the teacher assists them to learn ways in which these goals can be realized. This approach removes any set criterion for the success of the labor experience, avoiding the disappointment of externally imposed goals which may be unrealistic for the particular couple. The childbirth team also receives greater emphasis, in which the couple, obstetrician, nurse and Lamaze teacher are perceived as working together toward a satisfying labor experience. Rather than anticipating thwarting of their goals, the couple are encouraged to discuss these with their physician so he can understand what they hope to do. They also gain appreciation of some of the physician's responsibilities and alternate plans should labor not progress normally. Labor room nurses tend to be better informed about methods of prepared childbirth, and more committed to helping couples achieve their goals. Discussion of these goals with the nurses early in labor helps them understand and work more effectively with the couple. The theme of cooperation with the childbirth team has led to improved relations between prepared childbirth couples and health professionals.[10]

Other approaches to prepared childbirth, such as the *Bradley* method, also called *husband-coached childbirth*, the programs of the American Institute of Family Relations and the Maternity Center Association of New York, and others, utilize the same general approach of education, exercise, and relaxation. Although these programs may derive from different theories, and specific techniques vary, there are many points in common including the basic beliefs that 1) fear enhances the perception of pain but may diminish or disappear when the parturient knows about the physiology of labor, 2) psychic tension enhances the perception of pain but the parturient may relax more easily if childbirth takes place in a calm and agreeable atmosphere, and if good human contacts have been established between her and the personnel attending her, 3) muscular relaxation and a specific type of breathing diminish the pains of labor.

Nurses are often concerned about hyperventilation during labor when prepared childbirth breathing techniques are used. Undue fatigue, hyperventilation, and subsequent carpopedal spasm have been observed when breathing techniques are improperly used. Maternal respiratory alkalosis and a paradoxical acidosis in the fetus are also possibilities if hyperventilation is prolonged. It has been reported that a comparative physiologic study carried out with four groups of mothers in labor demonstrated that under certain circumstances hyperventilation did occur. Each group of mothers in the study had different preparation during pregnancy: 1) no antepartal training, 2) training in psychoprophylaxis, 3) training in psychophysical technique, 4) autohypnosis. Breathing patterns, alveolar gas samples and acid-base balance of maternal and umbilical cord blood were compared for the four groups of mothers. Hyperventilation was observed in all four groups of women, but the mothers prepared by the psychophysical method were more relaxed and overbreathed less than any other group.[11]

Hyperventilation and its complications can occur in any labor when the woman breathes improperly. Correct use of prepared childbirth breathing techniques can help prevent hyperventilation from occurring, which is another benefit of these programs.

Hypnosis

This technique is an induced state of extreme suggestibility in which the patient is insensible to outside impressions, except the suggestions of her attendant. There is no particular "program" associated with the use of this technique; rather, training in achieving a hypnotic state or autohypnosis is usually given by an obstetrician who himself is especially trained in this area. While there is no general regimen for learning this technique the conditioning required is usually presented in several individual sessions at the time of the antepartal visits, usually in the latter half of pregnancy. The modus operandi of hypnotically induced relaxation has been explained by suggesting that whenever all the voluntary muscles are completely relaxed during labor, the uterus has a monopoly on available energy and hence can work more efficiently. In addition, it is likely that when fears are abolished or diminished efficient uterine action is promoted. The utilization of comfort measures, such as low back massage, has also been suggested as enhancing the hypnotic state. The major drawback to this technique lies in the difficulty in securing adequately prepared physicians.

Postpartum teaching

Parenthood often constitutes a crisis in the developmental processes of both mothers and fathers. The postpartum period is particularly stressful due to the numerous physical changes the mother undergoes, the incomplete integration of her pregnancy and labor experiences, the changing roles which must occur within the family complex, and the uncertainty of the nature of the early mother-child relationship. Fatigue, confusion, feelings of helplessness and inadequacy, and depression often complicate this period. Isolation from the extended family, lack of community resources, economic strains, and pressures upon the mother to resume her full previous role within the family as rapidly as possible create additional stresses.

The nurse on the postpartum unit has a unique opportunity to intervene early in the developing mother-child relationship, and assist the parents to anticipate and plan for the first few critical weeks at home. If the mother can attain a level of confidence in her ability to perform care-taking tasks, and begin to recognize her baby's behavioral messages, a good foundation can be laid and perhaps later difficulties minimized. Sources for continuing care and counseling need to be available to parents during the baby's first few months at home, and the postpartum nurse can direct them to such sources in the particular community.

Individual teaching

Part of the postpartum nurse's daily responsibility is to provide individual instruction and support to those mothers to whom she provides care. This can range from information about infant sleep and activity patterns, growth and development, and how to dress the baby for different types of weather to sibling rivalry, contraception and organizing the household to get the necessary tasks done. Mothers' concerns may be small and particular, such as getting the baby to stay awake and suck well, or they may be larger and more general, such as the changes in her own and the father's lifestyle after the advent of the baby. The nurse needs to be informed about a wide variety of topics including contraception, sexuality, and family dynamics as well as infant care and involutional physiology.

Individual teaching allows the nurse to respond to the personal questions and concerns of mothers, and relate information to that particular situation. Reinforcement of mothering skills is particularly effective on an individual basis, as is counseling regarding family problems or emotions. However, the nurse may not have the time to give each mother the amount of individual teaching and counseling needed. Certain types of teaching can be effectively done in groups, and the use of postpartum groups has increased on hospital postpartum units. Baby care classes seem well suited to group methods, because the more experienced mothers can add their wisdom and practices to the pooled knowledge available.

Postpartum classes

The organization of classes for postpartum mothers, and sometimes for fathers as well, differs considerably from one institution to another. Each unit must work out the most convenient time for both staff and patients, and a method of communicating with patients to ensure maximum attendance. At times a conference room on the unit is utilized, or a large patient room can be adapted and extra chairs brought in. The teachers may be postpartum nurses only, or nursery nurses, physicians, social workers, nutritionists, and public health nurses may be involved. A variety of media aids can be used, ranging from films to flip charts, books, or other printed material. Closed-channel television which can be viewed by each mother in her room has also been explored as a method of postpartum group instruction.

The content of postpartum teaching varies, but generally contains a section about the mother and one about the baby. Personal care of the mother includes information about pericare, breast care, involutional physiology, bathing and hair washing, medication and its effects, contraception, fatigue and depression. In relation to the baby, mothers are instructed in the bath, breast- or bottle-feeding, holding and handling, dressing, care of the cord, the

PKU test, care of the circumcision, sleep patterns, crying, individual behavior of babies, and sibling rivalry. During most classes, mothers have their babies with them, and can practice what they have just been taught with the nurse available for assistance and clarification.[12]

SPECIAL CLASSES. Some postpartum units organize special classes for mothers with particular needs. Breast-feeding classes in which only breast-feeding mothers participate, are examples. They are instructed in techniques of nursing and assisted to have successful nursing experiences, and possible problems and their prevention are discussed. Mothers whose babies are in the intensive care nursery, but who plan to nurse, are also invited to these classes. More experienced mothers can be encouraged to attend, as they are most helpful to new mothers who have never breast-fed before. Common situations which breast-feeding mothers might encounter are brought up, and group solutions developed. Questions the mothers have are elicited, such as what foods should be avoided, whether breast-feeding ruins the breasts, and what to do when the mother plans to be away for several hours. Answers to these questions can be provided by the nurse or other mothers in the group. Having the telephone number of the nurse for consultation if problems arise after discharge is very helpful to mothers, and promotes continued success with breast-feeding.[13]

If the hospital is large enough to have a regular census of diabetic mothers, postpartum classes to address their particular needs and concerns are helpful. A group of adolescent mothers would also present a different set of needs, and require a special teaching approach to address their unique attitudes and problems. As discussed previously in this chapter, low income mothers constitute another distinct group whose perceptions of parenting differ, and who face particular types of problems to which postpartum teaching would have to be tailored. Perhaps mothers who delivered by cesarean section could make up another group, as their physiologic problems often affect accomplishment of mothering tasks. If, however, the maternity service is relatively small and could not support many different types of postpartum groups, the commonalities of baby care could be taught to a group of varied composition, with particular needs for information handled on an individual basis.

Outpatient groups

Increasingly nurses and other health professionals are aware of the need to extend services to parents after discharge from the hospital. This care may be provided through the public health department, hospital-affiliated clinics, the private sector, or possibly a community liaison nurse from the postpartum unit. The importance of the first year of life in the child's development, both behaviorally and physically, has led to establishment of "mother's groups" in a variety of settings. The goals of such groups generally include increasing the parents' knowledge of child development and methods of childrearing, helping parents to understand the child's nutritional needs and plan the family's diet wisely, providing role models and social contacts to the participating mothers and a supportive atmosphere in which the parents can explore their feelings about themselves as parents. One outcome noted for such groups was that as the mothers gained confidence in themselves as parents and felt more relaxed and in control, their children showed fewer behavioral problems.[14]

Parents' groups provided by local facilities can be helpful to low income mothers and fathers. Particularly if mothers receive little or no instruction in the hospital before discharge, these groups can offer answers to many common concerns about care of small babies and support in mothering abilities. Cultural differences must be respected and the structure informal and friendly if such groups are to be effective. The content of each class would vary, but information about infant nutritional needs and feeding methods is important and should be covered in detail, as inadequate nutrition and protein deprivation are common problems among this group, posing serious implications for the baby. General care of the infant, particularly bathing, diaper care, and causes of simple skin rashes is another standard topic. Sharing among the mothers can also enhance learning. If the atmosphere is comfortable, these mothers can be encouraged to examine practices that might be contributing to the baby's health problems, and possibly modify these. The nurse has the opportunity to observe the infants for signs of illness and refer them to the pediatrician if needed, as well as to identify serious emotional problems and make appropriate referrals.[15]

CLUSTER VISITS constitute a new approach to pediatric care which utilizes the group approach. A small number of mothers and their babies, usually four pairs, are scheduled for a joint visit with the pediatric nurse practitioner or pediatrician. Each baby is examined with the mother standing by, findings explained and instructions given for minor illness or problems. Subjects of general interest are postponed until discussion time which follows the examinations. While one mother and baby are involved in the examination, the others are getting acquainted and comparing notes. During the discussion period, the nurse and mothers talk about childrearing, feelings related to motherhood and baby care, changes in the family structure, or other topics relevant to the baby's age or the mother's needs. The groups are formed to include mothers with babies of about the same age. The mothers generally take the lead in the discussion, and often provide specific information and teaching for one another. During the last ten minutes, the next cluster visit is planned and immunizations given to the babies as needed.

These cluster visits are usually alternated with individual visits. They permit more care to be provided to mothers and babies using less professional time. The mothers involved tend to respond very positively, as they enjoy the camaraderie, sharing problems and anxieties, the chance to observe other babies, and the knowledge and support gained through the discussion. Increased confidence as parents, and recognition that babies are individuals whose weights and development vary were also outcomes of the experience. There appears to be no increased cross-contamination. Cluster visits thus are one way to provide improved health care at a lower cost to parents.[16]

Guide for preparing parents for childbirth and the puerperium

Whether or not the maternity nurse is involved in offering classes for parents or group preparation, it is important that education for childbirth and the puerperium be part of the professional repertoire. This information can be used for individual teaching or to reinforce what has been learned from other sources. The guide for preparing parents presented here aims at helping the mother to manage her body well in activity and rest, to use her natural resources effectively during labor, and to achieve optimal postpartal restoration. Inclusion of the father in this instruction, when possible, will assist him to understand his partner's needs during the childbearing process and offer support.*

Comfort during pregnancy

The majority of women can maintain their usual work and play activities. However, changes do occur in weight and weight distribution. Comfort in pregnancy can be significantly improved by good posture and body mechanics in everyday activities. It is often possible to reduce or overcome discomfort by correct positions, body movements and exercises (Table 13-1). Since the major postural changes begin in the second trimester of pregnancy, this is the logical time for learning. Correct posture for standing, sitting, and stair climbing, and good body mechanics for carrying packages or lifting objects must be reinforced. The spinal muscles and joints should be protected from undue strain; thus the mother needs to know how the feet can be used efficiently for balance and for movement.

Certain principles are applicable to activities in everyday living. For instance, activities need to be varied (e.g., walking, standing, sitting), and they may need to be of shorter duration. Walking back and forth is preferable to standing still. When the mother does housework which requires standing (e.g., using equipment such as a mop), she should stand with one leg forward to enable her to shift her weight easily and efficiently from foot to foot and turn her body comfortably.

As she walks, she should keep her head erect, back upright and chin up and forward.

When the mother climbs stairs she should place her entire foot on the stair and use leg muscles to lift herself up each step, without leaning forward.

Whenever possible, it is better for the expectant mother to avoid stooping and lifting. When it becomes necessary to stoop, she should squat down in front of an object she wants to reach or lift, keeping her feet wide apart and her back straight. A good axiom to remember

*The illustrative material and much of the information in the following section were provided through the courtesy of the Maternity Center Association, based upon their publication *Preparation for Childbearing*, ed. 2, New York, 1969.

is "use the legs to spare the back." As an alternate method of squatting, have the mother place one foot in front and to the side of the other, as when taking a step forward; then she is ready to squat. In carrying bulky packages such as groceries, the load should be divided and carried in two hands if it seems heavy. Better still, the mother should let someone else do the lifting for her. Whenever possible a cart that rolls easily should be employed to carry heavy loads. Work surfaces in the home can be adjusted for the individual mother to minimize stooping and stretching. A footstool is often an invaluable aid for the mother when she is sitting.

For rest and comfort during pregnancy, the mother can learn the position for lying on her side, on her back, in the side relaxation position, and equally important, how to get up and out of bed without strain.

Backache is one of the most common complaints, and *pelvic rocking* performed daily will help to relieve abdominal pressure and low back pain during pregnancy and early labor. This exercise is useful also to firm the abdominal muscles following the birth of the baby.

Other exercises to promote comfort and give relief from some of the common discomforts of pregnancy include *rib cage lifting*, *shoulder circling*, *leg elevating*, *hip elevating*, *and calf stretching*.

Muscle control

Two muscle groups undergo great changes during pregnancy, the abdominals and the muscles of the pelvic floor. The abdominal muscles stretch from the pressure of the enlarged uterus, and the pelvic floor muscles soften to prepare for the vaginal delivery. Loss of muscle tone can be minimized during pregnancy and can be regained after delivery through proper exercise.

Abdominal contraction is an exercise which increases muscle tone and thus helps to strengthen the abdominal wall during pregnancy and the postpartal period. The mother assumes any comfortable position, even standing or walking, and tightens her abdominal muscles as much as she can, holds them for a few seconds, then relaxes. This should be repeated frequently throughout the day, and may be performed simultaneously with *pelvic floor*

Table 13-1 Relief of Common Discomforts that May Occur During Pregnancy

Discomfort	Exercise or Position
Leaking urine when coughing, laughing	Pelvic floor contraction
Abdominal pain when coughing	Abdominal contraction
Heaviness in pelvis	Knee-chest; pelvic floor contraction
Hemorrhoids and swelling around vagina	Knee-chest; resting with hips elevated; pelvic floor contraction
Low back pain—one side	Knee-chest
Cramps in thighs, buttocks	Knee-chest
Cramps in legs	Leg elevating; calf stretching
Tired legs	Leg elevating; calf stretching
Varicose veins in legs	Leg elevating; calf stretching
Shortness of breath	Good posture; good body mechanics; rib cage lifting
Low backache	Pelvic rocking; good posture; pushing posture; squatting
Middle backache	Pushing position
Upper backache	Shoulder circling; good posture
Numbness in arms and fingers	Shoulder circling; lying on side
Abdominal muscle spasm (stitch)	Squatting; pushing posture

contraction. The latter exercise reduces congestion and general discomfort in the pelvic region and increases ability to control the muscles surrounding the orifice of the vagina, bowel, and bladder. It also improves muscle tone, thereby providing better support for the pelvic organs. Whenever exercises are taught to the patient with instructions to "repeat frequently throughout the day," the patient should understand about muscle fatigue and its consequences which may result from overdoing.

Conscious relaxation

Relaxation is one of the most natural activities known to humans. However, human beings living in a civilized society, unlike their feline pets, seem to have forgotten how to relax naturally.

Relaxation enables a person to obtain maximum benefit from any rest period, it relieves bodily tensions that cramp muscles, producing fatigue, and promotes a feeling of physical and mental well-being.

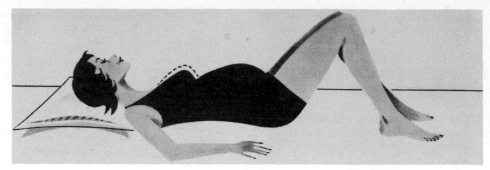

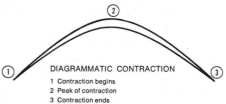

DIAGRAMMATIC CONTRACTION

1 Contraction begins
2 Peak of contraction
3 Contraction ends

DIAGRAMMATIC BREATH PATTERN

1 Complete breath
2 Slow rhythmic breathing

Figure 13-1.   Complete breath and breath control.

Physical relaxation may reduce the pain of labor and equally important, can put the mother in a calm frame of mind which permits her to cope more effectively with the demands of her situation.

The key to relaxation may be found in two principles—*correct posture* and *proper breathing*. Correct posture minimizes muscular stress, and coupled with this, controlled breathing makes it easier to relax.

Once the mother has developed the art of relaxing by using the following techniques, she is advised to practice regularly and at other times when she is under pressure or excited. The mother may need to be reminded that her ultimate purpose in this preparation is to be able to relax during labor, when feelings of excitement and tension are apt to run high.

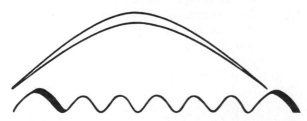

Figure 13-2.   Application of complete breathing to labor.

Complete breath and breath control— technique 1

A complete breath is one in which the chest wall expands and the diaphragm descends to its maximum extent. The breath is let out slowly under pressure so that a more complete exchange of oxygen and carbon dioxide can take place. It is used periodically during relaxation and should be followed by slow, quiet, easy respiration (Fig. 13-1).

1. Breathe in once as deeply as possible.
2. Hiss or blow the air out slowly, letting your whole body go limp.
3. Continue breathing quietly, easily and rhythmically.
4. Let yourself go completely loose.
5. Soon your body will begin to feel very heavy and any exertion will be difficult. You can test this out:
   a. Gradually bend an elbow bringing your hand toward your chin. Notice how much effort this requires.
   b. Slowly lower your arm to its resting position. Again you will find yourself actually working to prevent its falling too quickly.

Breath control in the first stage of labor

Application of complete breathing to labor:

1. Pretend that you are having a contraction lasting 30 to 45 seconds.
2. At the beginning of each contraction take a complete breath and hiss or blow it out.
3. Breathe deeply, slowly and rhythmically throughout the remainder of the contraction.
4. When the contraction has ended, take another complete breath and hiss or blow it out slowly.
5. Return to normal breathing between contractions.
6. During labor, you will continue to use this pattern of breathing with contractions as long as it continues to be helpful (Fig. 13-2).

Modified complete breathing

As labor advances and contractions increase in strength, there is often a desire on the mother's part to keep the diaphragm as still as possible. Yet, the uterus continues to need a good supply of oxygen. For this reason the mother should breathe deeply as the contraction begins and ends, and modify her breathing so that it is quiet and shallow at the peak of each contraction. To practice this:

1. Pretend that you are having stronger contractions, lasting almost a minute.
2. Breathe in deeply as the contraction starts. Then slowly hiss or blow out, letting yourself go completely limp.
3. Make each of the next four or five breaths a little shallower than the previous one. Soon you will notice that you are breathing very lightly.
4. Light breathing is quiet and effortless, almost like a throat breath. Experiment to find your own comfortable rate and continue for 15 to 45 seconds. If you become dizzy or lightheaded, your breathing is too vigorous. If you have trouble getting enough air or difficulty maintaining the rhythm, try taking a quick, deep breath, and return to light breathing.
5. Make each of the next four or five breaths a little deeper than the previous one.
6. End the breath pattern with one complete breath (Fig. 13-3).

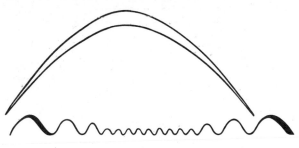

Figure 13-3. Modified complete breathing.

Further adaptation for transition

For the latter part of the first stage of labor (if you feel a tendency to hold your breath or to push during strong contractions) do the modified complete breath, but with one important change:

During light breathing, puff out gently as you exhale on every third or fourth breath (Fig. 13-4).

Pushing position with pushing breath for second stage

During the second stage of labor, the mother pushes, actively helping in the delivery of her baby. Contractions at this time last 60 to 65 seconds and generally are accompanied by a strong urge to push. To practice for this (Fig. 13-5):

1. Lie on your back with head and shoulders elevated. Pillows may be used for practice at home. In the labor room the head of the bed may be elevated.
2. Bend your knees and separate your legs.
3. Take a deep breath and hiss or blow out.
4. Breathe in as quickly and deeply as you can; then hold your breath. (In labor, this "held" breath will help to fix your diaphragm so that your abdominal wall will make more effective downward pressure on the uterus and baby, aiding the baby's birth.)

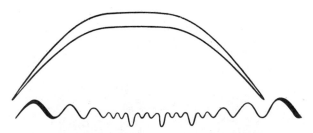

Figure 13-4. Modified complete breathing with adaptation for transition.

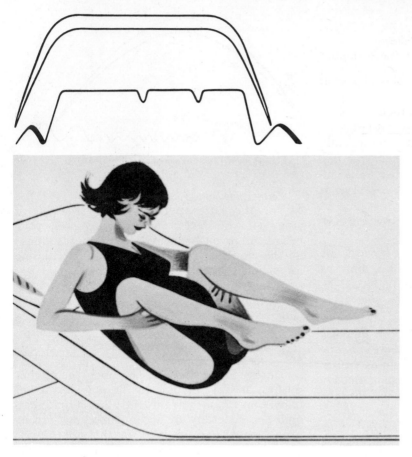

Figure 13-5. Pushing position.

5. Draw up your legs against your abdomen, in a squatting position, holding your legs or feet with your hands. (On the delivery table your feet and legs will be supported in stirrups so that you won't have to hold them, and there will be handles on which to pull.) Raise head.

6. During practice, do *not* actually push. You will be able to do so in labor.

7. Take *catch breaths* as needed. A catch breath is a short breath that may be taken when-ever you can no longer hold your breath comfortably. Try to take no more than two or three catch breaths in each 60- to 65-second breath pattern.

a. Maintain the pushing position.

b. Exhale, moving your head back.

c. Take in a quick, deep breath.

d. Tilt your head forward again and hold your breath.

8. When the contraction is over, relax completely, take a deep breath and sigh it out.

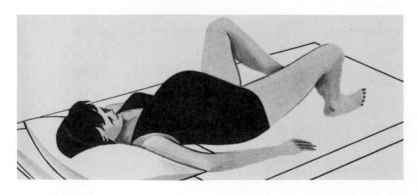

Figure 13-6. Practice position for the delivery table.

Note: *You may wish to practice breath holding and catch breaths without assuming the pushing position. You may do this while sitting in a chair by following the instructions relating to breathing described above.*

Practice position for the delivery table

On the delivery table the mother's legs and feet are supported in stirrups, adjusted to the mother's comfort. It is important that the inner thigh and pelvic floor muscles be relaxed so that they offer no resistance to the baby's oncoming head (Fig. 13-6). Practice relaxation of these muscles as follows:

1. Lie flat on your back.
2. Draw up your knees and place your feet flat on the bed.
3. Tense your inner thigh and pelvic floor muscles.
4. Relax these muscles, allowing your knees to drop apart gradually.
5. Have your partner apply gentle pressure to your knees and outer thighs so that he is supporting them in a widely separated position and you do not experience a pulling sensation.
6. Remain in this relaxed position for a few minutes.

Panting

Your physician may tell you to pant or to stop pushing in the middle of a contraction. If so, begin panting immediately. This will make your diaphragm move up and down. Although this will not decrease the desire to push, it will physically prevent you from doing so. To practice panting:

1. Start doing the exercise described in the section on Pushing Position with Pushing Breath.
2. All at once, drop your head and shoulders, allowing your arms and hands to relax.
3. Breathe in and out very quickly, keeping your mouth open—like a panting dog.

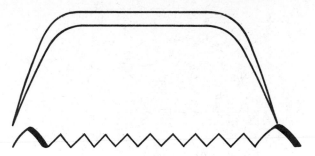

Figure 13-7. Diagrammatic breath pattern for panting.

4. Continue breathing this way until the contraction ends (Fig. 13-7).

Postpartum

During the puerperium, the six weeks following childbirth, the body undergoes major changes. The organs that had adjusted during pregnancy to make room for the growing baby gradually return to their original positions in the mother's body. The uterus, cervix, and vagina slowly return to the nonpregnant state. Important hormonal changes also occur. In effect, a bodily transformation that took nine months to complete is being reversed in the course of a few weeks.

Good nutrition and adequate rest are essential during this period. A new mother needs at least one rest period each day. Lying on the abdomen may help her uterus to return to good position (Fig. 13-8). A pillow under the hips when she is lying this way prevents back strain.

Postpartum exercises are important in restoring muscle tone and the mother's figure. In an uncomplicated delivery, these may be begun during the first few postpartal days, starting with the simpler exercises and progressing to the more strenuous ones. If the mother had an abnormal delivery or extensive perineal repair, exercises may need to be delayed. Practiced properly, the exercises should not be tiring, as they are done slowly and rhythmically, only

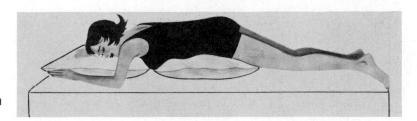

Figure 13-8. Prone position for rest and relaxation postpartally.

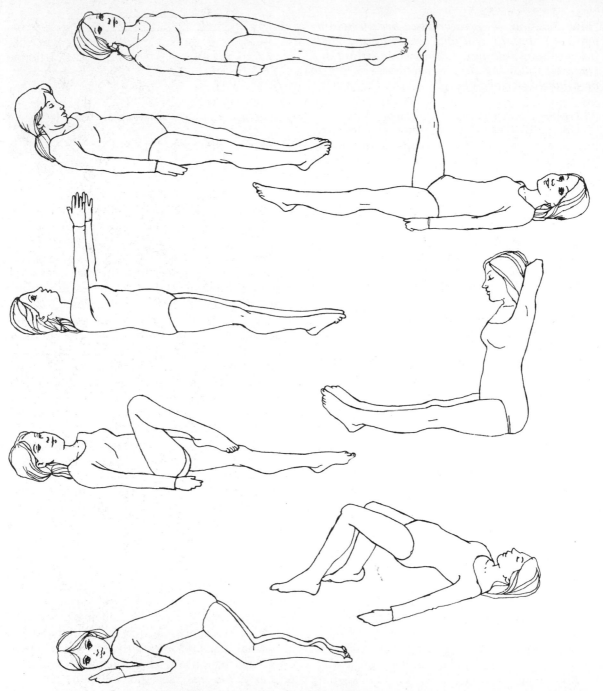

Figure 13-9.   Postpartum exercises. First day: lie on your back with your body and legs straight. Inhale slowly, expanding your chest. Pull your abdominal muscles in and press the lower part of your back to the floor. Hold, then relax. Repeat 5 to 10 times. Second day: raise your head from the floor, bringing it as close to your chest as possible. Try not to move any other part of your body. Repeat 5 to 10 times. Third day: put your arms straight out at your sides, then raise them over your head until your hands meet. Keeping your arms stiff, lower them again until they rest at your sides. Repeat 10 to 15 times. Seventh day: bring one leg up over your body until your foot touches your buttocks. Straighten and lower it, then repeat the exercise with your other leg. Repeat one more time each day. Fourteenth day: lying on your back, cross your arms on your chest and raise your body upright, keeping your legs close together on the floor. Later, when you are stronger, sit up while clasping your hands behind your head. Repeat one more time each day. Next, bend your legs almost to a right angle and raise your body, supporting it on your shoulders. Press your knees together, but keep your feet apart. Contract the muscles of your buttocks at the same time. Repeat one more time each day. Seventh to tenth day: without using your hands, raise one leg at a right angle to your body. Repeat using the other leg. Later when you are stronger, raise both legs at once. Repeat 5 to 10 times. If ordered by your physician: turn on your stomach and raise your body so that your knees and chest are close together. Your chest should be against the floor, and your legs about a foot apart. Hold this position for two minutes.

a few times at first, and gradually increased (Fig. 13-9).

The Kegal exercise, used to strengthen and tone the muscles of the pelvic floor, can be started a few days postpartum and continued daily for the rest of the woman's life. The exercise can be done in almost any position, and no one need know it is being done. The woman tightens the muscles around the anus as if to control a bowel movement, and then tightens the muscles around the vagina and urethra as if to stop urine in midstream. She holds these muscles tight to the count of three or four, then relaxes. This should be repeated 50 to 100 times at least once a day. This exercise is widely used for women with sexual dysfunction to increase their capacity for orgasm, and is also helpful for minor degrees of cystocele. It is an excellent exercise to maintain lifelong pelvic tone and enhance sexual enjoyment.

Bibliography

1. Redman, B. K.: *The Process of Patient Teaching in Nursing.* St. Louis, Mosby, 1968, p. 11.
2. Gorman, A. H.: *Teachers and Learners in the Interactive Process of Education.* Boston, Allyn and Bacon, Inc., 1969, p. 12.
3. Bibring, G. F., Huntington, D. S., and Valenstein, A. F.: A study of the psychological processes in pregnancy and of the earliest mother-child relationship. *Psychoanal. Stud. Child* 16: 9-71, 1961.
4. Tanner, L. M.: Developmental tasks of pregnancy. *In* B. S. Bergersen (ed.): *Current Concepts in Clinical Nursing,* Vol. II. St. Louis, Mosby, 1969, pp. 292-297.
5. Klaus, M., and Kennell, J.: Care of the mother. *In* Klaus and Fanaroff (eds.): *Care of the High-Risk Neonate.* Philadelphia, W. B. Saunders, 1973, pp. 98-118.
6. Kennell, J., and Klaus, M.: Care of the mother of the high-risk infant. *Clin. Ob. and Gyn.* 14: 926, 1971.
7. Rubin, R.: Maternal touch. *Nurs. Outlook* 11: 829-831, Nov. 1963.
8. Rubin, R.: Puerperal change. *Nurs. Outlook* 9: 753-755, Dec. 1961.
9. Spaulding, M. R.: Adapting postpartum teaching to mothers' low-income lifestyles. *In* B. S. Bergersen (ed.): *Current Concepts in Clinical Nursing,* Vol. II. St. Louis, Mosby, 1969, pp. 280-291.
10. Sasmor, J. L., Castor, C. R., and Hassid, P.: The childbirth team during labor. *Am. J. Nurs.* 73: 444-447, Mar. 1973.
11. Buxton, R. St. J.: Maternal respiration in labor. The Obstet. Assoc. of Chartered Physiotherapists. Herefordshire, England, St. Albans, 1969.
12. Walker, E. G.: Concerns, conflicts, and confidence of postpartum mothers. *In* E. H. Anderson (ed.): *Current Concepts in Clinical Nursing,* Vol. IV, St. Louis, Mosby, 1973, pp. 230-236.
13. Bird, I. S.: Breast-feeding classes on the postpartum unit. *Am. J. Nurs.* 75: 456, Mar. 1975.
14. Shaw, N. R.: Teaching young mothers their role. *Nurs. Outlook* 22: 695-698, Nov. 1974.
15. Cooper, I.: Group sessions for new mothers. *Nurs. Outlook* 22: 251, Apr. 1974.
16. Feldman, M.: Cluster visits. *Am. J. Nurs.* 74: 1485-1488, Aug. 1974.

Suggested Reading

BING, E.: *Six Practical Lessons for an Easier Childbirth.* New York, Grosset and Dunlap, 1967.
DICK-READ, G.: *Childbirth Without Fear.* New York, Harper & Row, 1972.
GOODWIN, B.: Psychoprophylaxis in childbirth. *In* M. Duffy (ed.): *Current Concepts in Clinical Nursing,* Vol. III. St. Louis, Mosby, 1971, pp. 194-203.
HASSALL, D.: A home visit program for students. *Nurs. Outlook* 22: 522-524, Aug. 1974.
KARMEL, M.: *Thank You, Dr. Lamaze.* Philadelphia, J. B. Lippincott, 1959.

Read through the entire question and place your answer on the line to the right.

1. Below are some signs, symptoms and conditions commonly associated with pregnancy. Those which the patient might notice and describe in the first trimester of pregnancy are:

   A. Amenorrhea.
   B. Enlargement and tenderness of breasts.
   C. Enlargement of uterus.
   D. Frequent micturition.
   E. Goodell's sign.

   Select the number corresponding to the correct letters.
   1. A and C
   2. A, B and D
   3. B, D and E
   4. All of them   _____

2. **A.** In pregnancy, morning sickness is most common during which of the following periods?
   1. First month
   2. First six weeks
   3. Sixth to twelfth week
   4. First four months
   5. Eighth to sixteenth week   _____

   B. A patient complains of morning sickness. Which of the following measures should the nurse suggest as a possible means of overcoming this discomfort?
   1. Keep the stomach empty when nausea is present.
   2. Drink plenty of water upon arising.
   3. Eat six small meals instead of three per day.
   4. Increase daily intake of whole milk.   _____

3. A pregnant woman seen for the first time in the antepartal clinic has a hemoglobin of 70 percent. The nurse should understand that this condition is:

   A. A true anemia.
   B. Caused by increased blood volume.
   C. Dangerous to baby's development.
   D. Predisposing to postpartal hemorrhage.   _____

4. The nurse in the obstetrician's office should instruct the patient regarding the collection of the specimen for the Aschheim-Zondek test by telling the patient to:

   A. Save the first voided specimen in the morning.
   B. Withhold fluid intake during the night and collect the first voided specimen in the morning.
   C. Report to the laboratory in the morning for a blood specimen.
   D. Take a warm voided specimen to the laboratory.   _____

5. Though the pregnant woman is usually advised to include a quart of milk in her diet daily, which of the following, if any, would justify the omission of milk?

   A. Milk makes her constipated.
   B. She is gaining weight too rapidly.
   C. She is not gaining fast enough and needs more concentrated foods.
   D. Milk causes a feeling of fullness, decreasing her appetite for other foods.
   E. Milk causes heartburn.
   F. None of the above; milk should not be omitted for these reasons. _____

6. The most essential foods in a 2,500-calorie diet for a pregnant woman are:
   A. High in carbohydrate, low in protein.
   B. High in protein, low in carbohydrate.
   C. High in protein, low in fat.
   D. High in fat, low in protein. _____

7. The nurse in the antepartal clinic will encourage the pregnant woman to see her dentist at the earliest convenience because:
   A. Each baby causes the mother to lose one tooth.
   B. Bone development of the baby requires calcium.
   C. Foci of infection should be removed early in pregnancy.
   D. The increased carbohydrate needed in pregnancy is detrimental to sound teeth. _____

8. What instruction should the clinic patient be given concerning the care of her breasts during pregnancy?
   A. A brassière should:
      1. Not be worn.
      2. Be worn snugly enough to support and lift up the breasts.
      3. Be worn snugly enough to press the breasts flat against the chest wall.
      4. Be worn snugly enough to apply constant firm pressure toward the midline. _____

   B. Special care of the nipples should begin:
      1. As early as pregnancy is confirmed.
      2. Between the third and fourth months.
      3. Between the sixth and seventh months.
      4. At the beginning of the ninth month. _____

9. "Preparation for Childbearing" is a term applied to a maternity center's program in antepartal education.
   A. The program includes certain "exercises" as one aspect of preparation. Which of the following are these exercises intended to accomplish?
      1. Promote control of muscle tension for coordination and economy of effort in all the mother's activities.
      2. Develop intraabdominal space for uterine enlargement.
      3. Obviate the need for pharmaceutical analgesics. _____

   B. Prepared childbirth programs prepare the pregnant patient for some of the experiences of labor. In addition to muscular control, which of the following measures will be most helpful to her during labor?
      1. Sympathetic care
      2. Moderately heavy sedation
      3. Understanding the progress of labor _____

   C. Which of the following best explains the purpose of conscious control of respiration during the first stage of labor?
      1. Gives mechanical relief of pressure by depression of the diaphragm to expand the abdominal wall.
      2. Limits the downward movement of the diaphragm through restriction of breathing to the upper chest.
      3. Gives the patient a calming rhythmic activity upon which to concentrate. _____

10. A. If the pregnant woman complained of painful, swollen veins in the legs, the nurse would understand that the condition would be likely to be due to:
      1. Infection of the blood-vessel wall.
      2. Toxins accumulating in the blood.

    3. Pressure against the veins in the pelvis.
    4. Pressure directly against the walls of the arteries.
    5. Force of gravity. _____

B. To remedy this condition, the nurse would expect that the patient would be advised that she should:

1. Refrain from wearing restricting clothing around the legs or the abdomen.
2. Refrain from wearing a girdle.
3. Lie down each day for an hour's rest.
4. Apply an Ace bandage, starting above the source of obstruction. _____

11. The nurse teaching parents' classes will stress the importance of which one of the following?

    A. Fathers doing the housework for mothers during the period of pregnancy
    B. The idea of sharing responsibility in parenthood
    C. The causes of invalidism during pregnancy
    D. The moral responsibility of being parents _____

12. If a woman six months pregnant asked if she should or should not wear a girdle, in your opinion the patient should be advised to:

    A. Avoid wearing any girdle.
    B. Adjust her regular girdle loosely.
    C. Wear a girdle that will keep the uterus from rising too high in the abdomen.
    D. Wear a girdle that will firmly support the lower portion of the abdomen and the back.
    E. Wear a girdle that will not disclose her condition. _____

13. The reason that pregnant women are warned against wearing high-heeled shoes from the seventh to the ninth months is:

    A. To avoid additional backstrain.
    B. To increase venous pressure in the legs.
    C. To allow freer movement in taking daily exercises.
    D. To dress themselves according to current styles. _____

14. The expectant mother who is employed as a stenographer can be advised that:

    A. Rest periods are unnecessary if the job requires only "desk work."
    B. Part-time employment should be requested after the fourth month of pregnancy.
    C. A position which requires moderate manual labor would be more advantageous because it affords physical exercise.
    D. Employment should be discontinued if the work causes moderate fatigue. _____

15. The clinic nurse would expect the pregnant patient to be advised to get in touch with her physician *immediately* as soon as she observed which of the following?

    A. Abdominal pain
    B. Bleeding with bright blood
    C. Blood-streaked mucus
    D. Chills and fever
    E. Constipation

Select the number corresponding to the correct letters.

    1. A, B and D
    2. B, C and E
    3. C, D and E
    4. All of them _____

16. In teaching the pregnant woman how to take a vaginal douche prescribed by the physician, the following is to be emphasized:

   A. A handbulb syringe is satisfactory if the mother is accustomed to using it.
   B. The medicated solution must be prepared according to the physician's instructions.
   C. The external genitalia should be cleansed with soap and water before taking a douche.
   D. The douche may be taken while sitting on the toilet if the douche bag is placed no higher than 2 feet above the level of the hips.
   E. The douche nozzle should be inserted gently into the vagina as far as it will go.

   Select the number corresponding to the correct letters.
   1. A and B
   2. B and D
   3. B, D and E
   4. All of them   _____

17. During her first visit to the clinic the mother confides to the nurse that she is afraid to have a baby. The most appropriate response of the nurse might be:

   A. "Modern obstetrics makes having a baby so safe that you have absolutely nothing to fear."
   B. "Perhaps if you discussed this with a psychiatrist he would help you to overcome this feeling."
   C. "Many women feel this way, so I wouldn't be concerned about it if I were you."
   D. "I can understand that you might feel this way. What is it in particular that you are worried about?"   _____

assessment and management during labor and delivery

Presentations and Positions
Phenomena of Labor
The Nurse's Contribution to Pain Relief During Labor
Analgesia and Anesthesia for Labor
Conduct of Normal Labor

unit IV

presentations and positions

Fetal Habitus / Fetal Head /
Presentation / Positions /
Diagnosis of Fetal Position

Fetal habitus

Habitus, or attitude, of the fetus means the relation of the fetal parts to one another. The most striking characteristic of the fetal habitus is flexion. The spinal column is bowed forward, the head is flexed with the chin against the sternum, and the arms are flexed and folded against the chest. The lower extremities also are flexed, the thighs on the abdomen and the calves of the lower legs against the posterior aspect of the thighs. In this state of flexion the fetus assumes a roughly ovoid shape, occupies the smallest possible space and conforms to the shape of the uterus. In this attitude it is about half as long as if it were completely stretched out. However, there are times when the fetus assumes many other positions.

Fetal head

From an obstetric viewpoint the head of the fetus is the most important part. If it can pass through the pelvic canal safely, there is usually no difficulty in delivering the rest of the body, although occasionally the shoulders may cause trouble.

The cranium, or skull, is made up of eight bones. Four of the bones—the sphenoid, the ethmoid and the two temporal bones—lie at the base of the cranium, are closely united and are of little obstetric interest. On the other hand, the four bones forming the upper part of the cranium are of great importance; these are the frontal, the occipital and the two parietal bones. These bones are not knit closely together at the time of birth but are separated by membranous interspaces called *sutures*. The intersections of these sutures are known as *fontanels* (Fig. 14-1).

By means of this formation of the fetal skull the bones can overlap each other somewhat during labor and so diminish materially the size of the head during its passage through the pelvis. This process of overlapping is called "molding," and after a long labor with a large baby and a snug pelvis, the head often is so definitely molded that several days may elapse before it returns to its normal shape.

The most important sutures are: the sagittal, between the two parietal bones; the frontal, between the two frontal bones; the coronal, between the frontal and the parietal bones; and the lambdoid, between the posterior margins of the parietal bones and the upper margin of

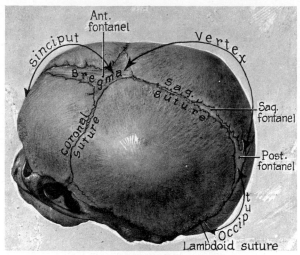

Figure 14-1. Fetal skull, showing sutures and fontanels.

the occipital bone. The temporal sutures, which separate the parietal and the temporal bones on either side, are unimportant in obstetrics because they are covered by fat parts and cannot be felt on the living baby.

The fontanels of importance are the anterior and the posterior. The anterior fontanel, large and diamond-shaped, is at the intersection of the sagittal and the coronal sutures, while the small triangular posterior fontanel lies at the junction of the sagittal and the lambdoid suture. The sutures and the posterior fontanel ossify shortly after birth, but the anterior fontanel remains open until the child is over a year old, constituting the familiar "soft spot" just above the forehead of an infant. By feeling or identifying one or another of the sutures or fontanels, and considering its relative position in the pelvis, one is able to determine accurately the position of the head in relation to the pelvis.

Presentation

The term *presentation* or *presenting part* is used to designate that portion of the infant's body which lies nearest the internal os, or, in other words, that portion which is felt by the examining fingers when they are introduced into the cervix. When the presenting part is known, by abdominal palpation, it is possible to determine the relation between the long axis of the baby's body and that of the mother.

Head or *cephalic presentations* are the most common, being present in about 97 percent of all cases at term. Cephalic presentations are divided into groups, according to the relation

which the infant's head bears to its body. The most common is the *vertex presentation*, in which the head is sharply flexed so that the chin is in contact with the thorax; then the vertex is the presenting part. The *face presentation*, in which the neck is sharply extended so that the occiput and the back come in contact, is more rarely observed.

Next to the cephalic presentation, *the breech presentation* is the most common, being present, however, in only about 3 percent of cases. In breech presentations the thighs may be flexed and the legs extended over the anterior surface of the body (*frank breech presentation*), or the thighs may be flexed on the abdomen and the legs on the thighs (*full breech presentation*), or one or both feet may be the lowest part (*foot or footling presentation*).

When the fetus lies crosswise in the uterus, it is in a "transverse lie," and the shoulder is the presenting part—*shoulder presentation*. The common causes of a "transverse lie" are: 1) abnormal relaxation of the abdominal walls due to great multiparity, 2) pelvic contraction, and 3) placenta previa. Shoulder presentations are relatively uncommon, and, with very rare exceptions, the spontaneous birth of a fully developed child is impossible in a "persistent transverse lie."

Positions

In addition to knowing the presenting part of the baby, it is important to know the exact position of this presenting part in relation to the pelvis. This relationship is determined by finding the position of certain points on the presenting surface and relating these to the four imaginary divisions or regions of the pelvis. For this purpose the pelvis is considered to be divided into quadrants: left anterior, left posterior, right anterior and right posterior. These divisions aid in indicating whether the presenting part is directed toward the right or the left side and toward the front or the back of the pelvis. Certain points on the presenting surface of the baby have been arbitrarily chosen as points of direction in determining the exact relation of the presenting part to the quadrants of the pelvis. In vertex presentations the occiput is the guiding point; in face presentations, the chin (mentum); in breech presentations, the sacrum; and in shoulder presentations, the scapula (acromion process).

Position, then, has to do with the relation of some arbitrarily chosen portion of the fetus

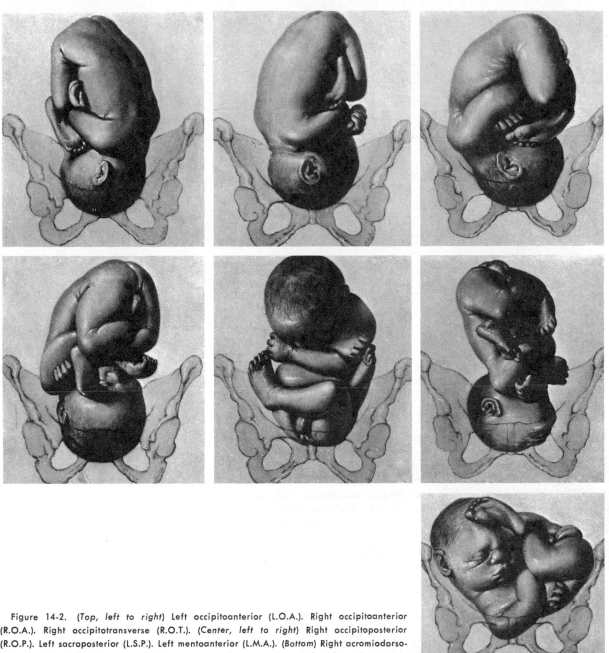

Figure 14-2. *(Top, left to right)* Left occipitoanterior (L.O.A.). Right occipitoanterior (R.O.A.). Right occipitotransverse (R.O.T.). *(Center, left to right)* Right occipitoposterior (R.O.P.). Left sacroposterior (L.S.P.). Left mentoanterior (L.M.A.). *(Bottom)* Right acromiodorso-posterior (R.A.D.P.). This means that the *acromium* lies toward the *right* side of the mother and the back of the infant lies toward the *posterior* part of the pelvis.

to the right or the left side of the mother's pelvis. Thus, in a vertex presentation, the back of the head (occiput) may point to the front or to the back of the pelvis. The occiput rarely points directly forward or backward in the median line until the second stage of labor, but usually is directed to one side or the other.

The various positions are usually expressed by abbreviations made up of the first letter of each word which describes the position. Thus,

left occipitoanterior is abbreviated L.O.A. This means that the head is presenting with the occiput directed toward the left side of the mother and toward the front part of the pelvis. If the occiput were directed straight to the left with no deviation toward front or back of the pelvis, it would be termed left occipitotransverse, or L.O.T. The occiput might also be directed toward the back or posterior quadrant of the pelvis, in which case the position would

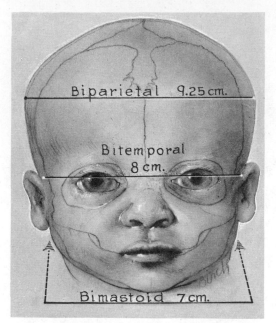

Figure 14-3. Fetal head, showing transverse diameters.

be left occipitoposterior, or L.O.P. There are also three corresponding positions on the right side: R.O.A., R.O.T. and R.O.P. (Fig. 14-2).

The occipital positions are considered the most favorable for both mother and baby, and of these, the L.O.A. position is preferred. The same system of terminology is used for face, breech and shoulder presentations, as indicated in the following list of abbreviations (S indicating breech; M, chin or face; and A, shoulder).

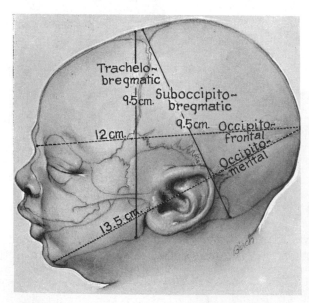

Figure 14-4. Fetal skull, showing anteroposterior diameters.

Although it is customary to speak of all "transverse lies" of the fetus simply as shoulder presentations, the examples of terminology sometimes used to express position in the shoulder presentation are listed. Left acromiodorso-anterior (L.A.D.A.) means that the acromion is to the mother's left and the back is anterior (Fig. 14-2).

POSITIONS—VERTEX PRESENTATION

L.O.A.—Left occipitoanterior
L.O.T.—Left occipitotransverse
L.O.P.—Left occipitoposterior
R.O.A.—Right occipitoanterior
R.O.T.—Right occipitotransverse
R.O.P.—Right occipitoposterior

POSITIONS—BREECH PRESENTATION

L.S.A.—Left sacroanterior
L.S.T.—Left sacrotransverse
L.S.P.—Left sacroposterior
R.S.A.—Right sacroanterior
R.S.T.—Right sacrotransverse
R.S.P.—Right sacroposterior

POSITIONS—FACE PRESENTATION

L.M.A.—Left mentoanterior
L.M.T.—Left mentotransverse
L.M.P.—Left mentoposterior
R.M.A.—Right mentoanterior
R.M.T.—Right mentotransverse
R.M.P.—Right mentoposterior

POSITIONS—SHOULDER PRESENTATION

L.A.D.A.—Left acromiodorso-anterior
L.A.D.P.—Left acromiodorso-posterior
R.A.D.A.—Right acromiodorso-anterior
R.A.D.P.—Right acromiodorso-posterior

Figures 14-3 and 14-4 show the principal measurements of the fetal skull. The most important transverse diameter is the biparietal; it is the distance between the biparietal protuberances and represents the greatest width of the head. It measures, on an average, 9.25 cm. There are three important anteroposterior diameters: the suboccipitobregmatic, which extends from the undersurface of the occiput to the center of the anterior fontanel and measures about 9.5 cm.; the occipitofrontal, which extends from the root of the nose to the occipital prominence and measures about 12.0 cm.; and the occipitomental, which extends from the chin to the posterior fontanel and averages about 13.5 cm.

In considering these three anteroposterior

diameters of the fetal skull, it is important to note that with the head in complete flexion and the chin resting on the thorax, the smallest of these, the suboccipitobregmatic, enters the pelvis, whereas if the head is extended or bent back (with no flexion whatsoever), the greatest anteroposterior diameter presents itself to the pelvic inlet. Herein lies the great importance of flexion; the more the head is flexed, the smaller is the anteroposterior diameter which enters the pelvis. Figure 14-5 shows this basic principle in diagrammatic form.

Diagnosis of fetal position

Diagnosis of fetal position is made in four ways: 1) abdominal palpation; 2) vaginal or rectal examination; 3) combined auscultation and examination; 4) in certain doubtful cases, the roentgenogram.

Inspection

Nurses thus should be able to determine whether a presentation is normal or otherwise, as work in rural, sparsely settled localities often may require knowledge not demanded of her in her hospital experience.

Palpation

The nurse should become thoroughly familiar with this method. It is extremely helpful to palpate the abdomen before listening to the fetal heart tones. The region of the abdomen in which the fetal heart is heard most plainly varies according to the presentation and the extent to which the presenting part has descended. The location of the fetal heart sounds by itself does not give very important information as to the presentation and the position of the child, but it sometimes reinforces the results obtained by palpation. To obtain satisfactory information by abdominal palpation for the determination of fetal position, the examination should be made systematically by following the four maneuvers suggested by Leopold, often called the *Leopold maneuvers*.

The nurse should make certain that the patient has emptied her bladder before the procedure is begun. This will not only contribute to the patient's comfort but also will aid the nurse to gain more accurate results in the latter part of the examination. During the first three maneuvers the nurse stands at the side of the bed facing the patient; during the last one

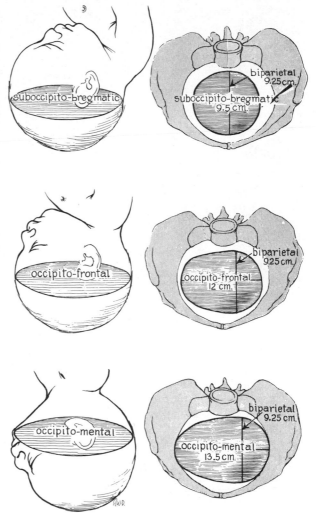

Figure 14-5. (Top) Complete flexion allows smallest diameter of head to enter pelvis. (Center) moderate extension causes larger diameter to enter pelvis. (Bottom) Marked extension forces largest diameter against pelvic brim, but head is too large to enter pelvis.

the nurse faces the patient's feet. Although a diagnosis should not be made on the basis of inspection, actual observation of the patient's abdomen should precede palpation. For the examination the patient should lie flat on her back, with her knees flexed, to relax the abdominal muscles; the nurse should lay both hands gently and, at first, flat upon the abdomen. If done in any other manner than this, or if the hands are not warm, the stimulation of the fingers will cause the abdominal muscles to contract. One should accustom oneself to palpating the uterus in a definite, methodical way, and it will be found best to carry out the following four maneuvers.

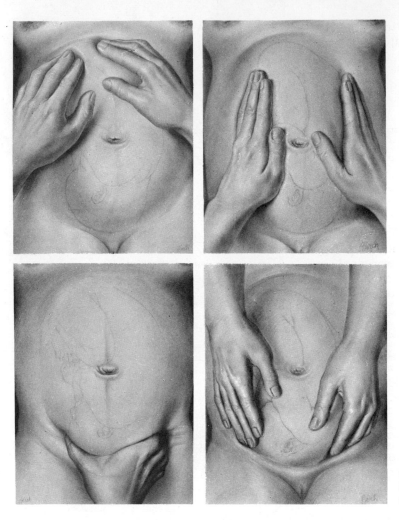

Figure 14-6. Palpation. (*Top, left*) First maneuver; (*top, right*) second maneuver; (*bottom, left*) third maneuver; (*bottom, right*) fourth maneuver.

FIRST MANEUVER. The nurse should ascertain, facing the patient, what is lying at the fundus of the uterus by feeling the upper abdomen with both hands; generally one will find there a mass, which is either the head or the buttocks (breech) of the fetus. The nurse must decide which pole of the fetus this is by observing three points (Fig. 14-6):

1. Its relative consistency: the head is harder than the breech.
2. Its shape: if the head, it will be round and hard, and the transverse groove of the neck may be felt. The breech has no groove and usually feels more angular.
3. Mobility: the head will move independently of the trunk, but the breech moves only with the trunk. The ability of the head to be moved back and forth against the examining fingers is spoken of as ballottement.

SECOND MANEUVER. Having determined whether the head or the breech is in the fun-dus, the next step is to locate the back of the fetus in relation to the right and the left sides of the mother. Still facing the patient, the nurse places the palmar surfaces of both hands on either side of the abdomen and applies gentle but deep pressure. If the hand on one side of the abdomen remains still to steady the uterus, a slightly circular motion with the flat surface of the fingers on the other hand can gradually palpate the opposite side from the top to the lower segment of the uterus to feel the fetal outline. Then, to palpate the other side, the functions of the hands are reversed (i.e., the hand which was used to palpate now remains steady), and the other hand palpates the opposite side of the uterus. On one side is felt a smooth, hard, resistant plane, the back, while on the other, numerous angular nodulations are palpated, the small parts; these latter represent the knees and the elbows of the fetus.

THIRD MANEUVER. This maneuver consists of an effort to find the head at the pelvic inlet and to determine its mobility. It should be conducted by gently grasping the lower portion of the abdomen, just above the symphysis pubis, between the thumb and the fingers of one hand and then pressing together. If the presenting part is not engaged, a movable body will be felt, which is usually the head.

FOURTH MANEUVER. In this maneuver the nurse faces the feet of the patient and places the tips of her first three fingers on both sides of the midline about 2 inches above Poupart's ligament. Pressure is now made downward and in the direction of the birth canal, the movable skin of the abdomen being carried downward along with the fingers. It will be found that the fingers of one hand meet no obstruction and can be carried downward well under Poupart's ligament; these fingers glide over the nape of the baby's neck. The other hand, however, usually meets an obstruction an inch or so above Poupart's ligament; this is the brow of the baby and is usually spoken of as the "cephalic prominence." This maneuver gives information of several kinds:

1. If the findings are as described above, it means that the baby's head is well flexed.
2. Confirmatory information is obtained about the location of the back, as naturally the back is on the opposite side from the brow of the baby, except in the uncommon cases of face presentation, in which the cephalic prominence and the back are on the same side.
3. If the cephalic prominence is very easily palpated, as if it were just under the skin, a posterior position of the occiput is suggested.
4. The location of the cephalic prominence tells how far the head has descended into the pelvis. This maneuver is of most value if the head has engaged and may yield no information with a floating, poorly flexed head.

Vaginal examination

Vaginal examination is done by the physician and consists of identifying the fontanels and the suture lines of the fetal skull. During pregnancy the vaginal examination gives limited information concerning the position of the fetus because the cervix is closed. However, during labor, after more or less complete dilatation of the cervix, important information about the position of the baby and the degree of flexion of its head can be obtained.

Auscultation

The location of the fetal heart sounds, as heard through the stethoscope, yields helpful confirmatory information about fetal position but is not wholly dependable. Certainly, it never should be relied on as the sole means of diagnosing fetal position. Ordinarily, the heart sounds are transmitted through the convex portion of the fetus, which lies in intimate contact with the uterine wall, so that they are heard best through the infant's back in vertex and breech presentations, and through the thorax in face presentation. In cephalic presentations the fetal heart sounds are heard loudest midway between the umbilicus and the anterior superior spine of the ilium. In general, in L.O.A. and L.O.P. positions the fetal heart sounds are heard loudest in the left lower quadrant. A similar situation applies to the R.O.A. and R.O.P. positions. In posterior positions of the occiput (L.O.P. and R.O.P.) often the sounds are heard loudest well down in the flank toward the anterosuperior spine. In breech presentation the fetal heart sounds usually are heard loudest at the level of the umbilicus or above.

Roentgenograms

Roentgenograms are of particular value in diagnosis of fetal position in doubtful cases, particularly in obese women or in those with abdominal walls so rigid that abdominal palpation is difficult. In such situations the roentgenogram enables the physician to recognize the existence of conditions which might otherwise have escaped detection until late in labor. They give accurate information concerning position, presentation, flexion and descent of the fetal head (see Fig. 11-4, p. 158).

Suggested Reading

DANFORTH, D. N.: *Textbook of Obstetrics and Gynecology*, ed. 2. New York, Hoeber Medical Division, Harper & Row, 1971.

GREENHILL, J. P., AND FRIEDMAN, E. A.: *Biological Principles and Modern Practice of Obstetrics*. Philadelphia, W. B. Saunders, 1974.

HELLMAN, L. H., AND PRITCHARD, J. A.: *Williams Obstetrics*, ed. 14. New York, Appleton-Century Crofts, 1971.

WILSON, J. R., BEECHAM, C. T., AND CARRINGTON, E. R.: *Obstetrics and Gynecology*, ed. 4. St. Louis, Mosby, 1971.

phenomena
of labor

15

Premonitory Signs of Labor / Cause of
Onset of Labor / Uterine Contractions /
Duration of Labor / The Three Stages
of Labor

Labor refers to the series of processes by which the products of conception are expelled by the mother (Fig. 15-1). Childbirth, parturition, accouchement, and confinement are also terms for these processes. The actual birth of the baby is called delivery.

Premonitory signs of labor

During the last few weeks of pregnancy a number of changes indicate that the time of labor is approaching. Particularly in primigravidas, "lightening" occurs about 10 to 14 days before delivery. This alteration is brought about by a settling of the fetal head into the pelvis (Fig. 15-2). This may occur at any time during the last four weeks, but occasionally does not occur until labor actually has begun. Lightening may take place suddenly, so that the expectant mother arises one morning entirely relieved of the abdominal tightness and diaphragmatic pressure that she had experienced previously (Fig. 10-5). But the relief in one direction often is followed by signs of greater pressure below, such as shooting pains down the legs from pressure on the sciatic nerves, an increase in the amount of vaginal discharge and greater frequency of urination

due to pressure on the bladder. In mothers who have had previous children, lightening is more likely to occur after labor begins.

For a varying period before the establishment of true labor, women often experience "false labor." The nurse can distinguish between this and effective uterine contractions, as true labor contractions will produce a demonstrable degree of dilatation of the cervix in the course of a few hours, while false labor contractions do not affect the cervix. The crux of the matter, then, between true and false labor is whether or not the uterine contractions effect cervical effacement and dilatation.

False contractions may begin as early as three or four weeks before the termination of pregnancy. They are merely an exaggeration of the intermittent uterine contractions which have occurred throughout the entire period of gestation but now may be accompanied by discomfort. They are confined chiefly to the lower part of the abdomen and the groin and do not increase in intensity, frequency and duration. The discomfort is rarely intensified if the mother walks about and may even be relieved if she is on her feet. Examination will reveal no changes in the cervix. The signs that accompany true labor contractions present a contrast-

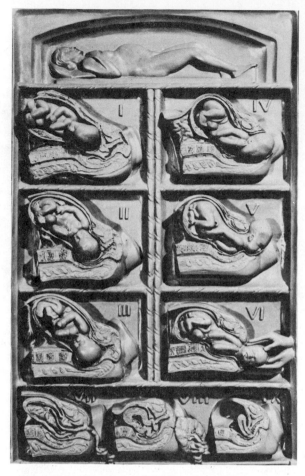

Figure 15-1. "The Birth Relief." This distinguished sculptured relief depicts the nine stages of birth with vertex presentation from before labor through the delivery of the placenta. (Dickinson-Belskie models, Cleveland Health Museum, Cleveland)

Occasionally, rupture of the membranes is the first indication of approaching labor. It used to be thought that this was a grave sign, heralding a long and difficult dry labor, but present-day statistics show that this is not true. Nevertheless, the physician must be notified at once; under these circumstances, he may advise the patient to enter the hospital immediately. After the rupture of the membranes there is always the possibility of a prolapsed cord if the presenting part does not adequately fill the pelvic inlet. This is more likely if the infant presents as a footling breech, or by the shoulder, or in the vertex presentation when the fetal head has not descended far enough into the true pelvis prior to the rupture of the membranes (see Fig. 25-6, p. 508).

Cause of onset of labor

In mammalian species, whether the fetus weighs 2 Gm. at the end of a 21-day pregnancy, as in the mouse, or whether it weighs 200 pounds at the end of a 640-day pregnancy, as in the elephant, labor usually begins at the right time for that particular species, namely, when the fetus is mature enough to cope with extra-uterine conditions but not yet large enough to cause mechanical difficulties in labor. The process responsible for this beautifully synchronized and salutary achievement has not yet been clearly identified.

The uterus during pregnancy consists of a large number of greatly hypertrophied smooth muscle cells. Each cell is activated by a series of chemical reactions to begin rhythmic contractions in a highly coordinated way, and with such force that the cervix is dilated and the baby expelled. The fundamental question is what stimulates these uterine cells, at a precise time in most pregnancies, to begin labor contractions. Various theories have been advanced to explain the onset of labor. It appears that several mechanisms are involved in initiating and maintaining labor, each having varying importance depending upon individual circumstances.

Progesterone deprivation theory

Progesterone, secreted first by the corpus luteum, and then by the placenta, is essential in maintaining pregnancy. Since the uterus is composed of smooth muscle, and most smooth muscle organs will contract when stretched, it is significant that the uterus remains quiescent

ing picture. True labor contractions usually are felt in the lower back and extend in girdle-like fashion from the back to the front of the abdomen. They have a definite rhythm and gradually increase in frequency, intensity and duration. In the course of a few hours of true labor contractions a progressive effacement and dilatation of the cervix is apparent.

Another sign of impending labor is pink "show." After the discharge of the mucous plug that has filled the cervical canal during pregnancy, the pressure of the descending presenting part of the fetus causes the minute capillaries in the cervix to rupture. This blood is mixed with mucus and therefore has the pink tinge. It must be differentiated from substantial discharge of blood, which would indicate a medical complication.

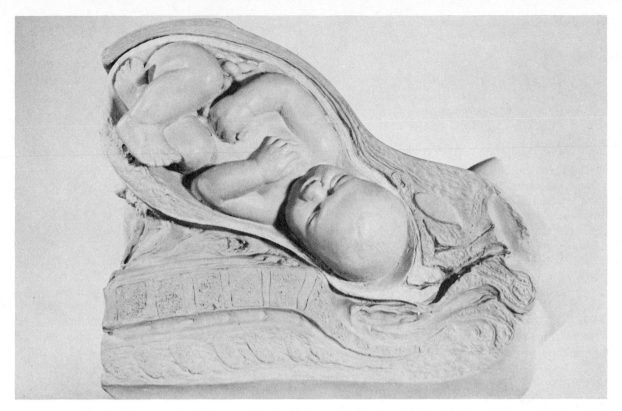

Figure 15-2. Before labor, showing the uterus relaxed with the cervix closed and thick pelvic floor. (Dickinson-Belskie models, Cleveland Health Museum, Cleveland)

throughout the greater part of pregnancy. This suggests that some substance is acting to inhibit uterine contractility. Progesterone is the most likely substance, and the role of a "progesterone block" in the maintenance and termination of pregnancy has been upheld by some investigators for many years. In several animal species, this theory is well supported by studies showing a drop in maternal progesterone with a rise in estrogen, which has opposite effects on uterine musculature, before labor begins. This could not be documented in humans until recently, when new methodology was able to identify a fall in circulating progesterone with a continuing increase of estrogen in a study population of women during the five weeks preceding labor. The onset of labor in humans is felt to result, then, from withdrawal of progesterone at a time of relative estrogen dominance.[1]

Oxytocin theory

It has been clearly demonstrated that the human uterus is increasingly sensitive to oxytocin as pregnancy advances. Oxytocin is an effective stimulant of uterine contractions in late pregnancy, and is commonly used to induce or augment labor. While oxytocin-like activity in the blood has been found in women during labor, with the highest concentration during the second stage, it is also present in both males and females having surgery. It is possible that any stress may release this hypophyseal hormone. Also, blood contains an enzyme which promptly inactivates oxytocin. Humans, as well as several other mammals, still go into labor normally when the hypophysis has been removed or destroyed. While oxytocin alone seems unlikely as initiator of the labor process, it may well be significant in combination with other substances.

Fetal endocrine control theory

At the appropriate time of fetal maturity, it appears that the fetal hypothalamus secretes cortical steroids which are felt to trigger the mechanisms leading to labor. Destruction of the fetal pituitary or hypothalamus in sheep leads to prolonged pregnancy, while administration of corticotropin or cortisol directly to the fetus leads to premature labor.[2] Cortical steroids are released during periods of stress, which suggests one cause of premature labor in the instance when the fetus is compromised. Conditions which cause decreased blood flow to the uterus, such as toxemia or uterine overdistention due to multiple pregnancy or polyhydramnios, are known to be related to premature labor. These conditions also compromise the fetus, and thus could be implicated in fetal release of cortical steroids. The suggested mechanism of action is that fetal steroids stimulate the release of precursors to prostaglandins which in turn produce uterine labor contractions.

Prostaglandin theory

Recent research has shown prostaglandins to be very effective in inducing uterine contractions at any stage of gestation.[3] Prostaglandins are formed by the uterine decidua, and their concentration in the amniotic fluid and blood of women increases during labor. Study of the mechanisms of prostaglandin synthesis has shown that arachidonic acid, the obligatory precursor to prostaglandin, increases markedly in comparison to the other fatty acids in the amniotic fluid of women in labor. Arachidonic acid injected into the amniotic sac during the second trimester is highly effective in producing abortion, while other fatty acids do not induce labor. It is hypothesized that initiation of human labor results from a sequence of events including the release of lipid precursors possibly triggered by steroid action, release of arachidonic acid from these precursors perhaps at the site of the fetal membranes, increased prostaglandin synthesis from the arachidonic acid, and increased uterine contractions as a consequence of prostaglandin action on the uterine muscle.[4]

Uterine contractions

In all languages the word for the uterine contractions of labor has been interpreted the same, namely, "pain." The degree of discomfort during labor varies considerably from patient to patient. The patient who anticipates a painful experience generally will have more pain than the patient who is properly prepared for what can be a good experience. To allay preexisting fear, one should refer to uterine contractions as *contractions*, not *pains*. The duration of these contractions ranges from 45 to 90 seconds, averaging about one minute. Each contraction presents three phases: a period during which the intensity of the contraction increases (increment), a period during which the contraction is at its height (acme), and a period of diminishing intensity (decrement). The increment, or crescendo phase, is longer than the other two combined. The contractions of the uterus during labor are intermittent, with periods of relaxation between, resembling, in this respect, the systole and the diastole of the heart. The interval between contractions diminishes gradually from about ten minutes early in labor to about two or three minutes in the second stage. These periods of relaxation not only provide rest for the uterine muscles and for the mother, but also are essential to the welfare of the fetus, since unremitting contractions may so interfere with placental functions that the resulting lack of oxygen produces fetal distress. Another characteristic of labor contractions is that they are quite involuntary, their action being not only independent of the mother's will, but also of extrauterine nervous control.

During labor, the uterus is soon differentiated into two identifiable portions—the upper and lower uterine segments. The upper segment is the active, contractile portion of the uterus. Its function is to expel the uterine contents. It displays a decreasing gradient of intensity of contractions from the fundus downward. As labor progresses, a passive lower segment is developed. With each contraction, the muscle fibers of the upper segment retract, becoming shorter as the fetus descends. The upper segment, therefore, becomes thicker. Fibers of the lower segment stretch and, consequently, it becomes thinner. The distinct boundary between the upper and lower uterine segments is referred to as a physiologic retraction ring.

Duration of labor

Although there is usually some degree of variation in all labors, an estimate of the average length of labor can be based on studies of records of some several thousand primigravidas and multiparas.

The average duration of first labors is about 14 hours, approximately 12½ hours in the first stage, 1 hour and 20 minutes in the second stage, and 10 minutes in the third stage.

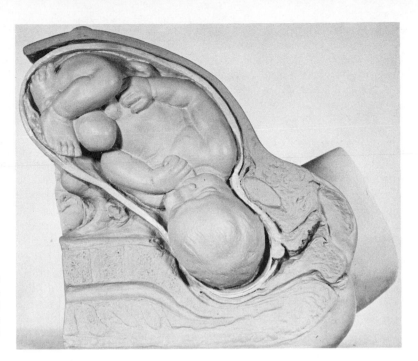

Figure 15-3. First stage of labor. The rhythmic contractions of the uterus aid the progressive effacement and dilatation of the cervix, as well as the descent of the infant. (Dickinson-Belskie models, Cleveland Health Museum, Cleveland)

The average duration of multiparous labors is approximately six hours shorter than for first labors; for example, seven hours and 20 minutes in the first stage, a half hour in the second stage, and ten minutes in the third stage.

During the first stage of labor full dilatation of the cervix (10 cm.) is accomplished, but for the greater part of this time the progress of cervical dilatation is slow. This has been clearly demonstrated in Friedman's study of 500 labors of primigravidous women. From his study labor is divided into the latent phase and the active phase. The *latent phase*, from the onset of uterine contractions, takes many hours and accomplishes little cervical dilatation. But with the beginning of the *active phase*, cervical dilatation proceeds at an accelerated rate and then reaches a deceleration phase shortly before the second stage of labor.

The first 4 cm. of cervical dilatation occurs during the slow, latent phase. The remainder

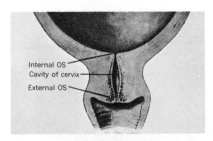
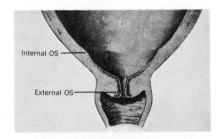
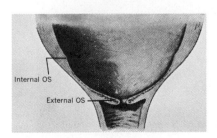
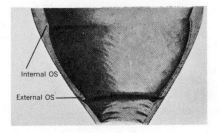

Figure 15-4. Cervix in primigravida. (*Top, left*) At beginning of labor; no effacement or dilatation. (*Top, right*) About one half effaced, but no dilatation. (*Bottom, left*) Completely effaced, but no dilatation. (*Bottom, right*) Complete dilatation.

of cervical dilatation is accomplished much more rapidly in the active phase. Hence, 5 cm. of dilatation has taken the patient well past the halfway point in labor, even though 10 cm. represents full dilatation. In fact, at that point the average labor is more than two-thirds over.

The three stages of labor

The process of labor is divided, for convenience of description, into three distinct stages.

The first stage of labor, or the dilating stage, begins with the first true labor contraction and ends with the complete dilatation of the cervix. This stage may be further subdivided into the latent phase and the active phase.

The second stage of labor, or the stage of expulsion, begins with the complete dilatation of the cervix and ends with the delivery of the baby.

The third stage of labor, or the placental stage, begins with the delivery of the baby and terminates with the birth of the placenta.

The first stage of labor

At the beginning of the first stage the contractions are short, slight, 10 or 15 minutes or more apart and may not cause the woman any particular discomfort. She may be walking about and is generally quite comfortable between contractions. Early in the first stage the sensation is usually located in the small of the back, but, as time goes on, it sweeps around, girdlelike, to the anterior part of the abdomen. The contractions recur at shortening intervals, every three to five minutes, and become stronger and last longer. When labor has progressed to the active phase, the woman usually prefers to remain in bed as ambulation is no longer comfortable. She becomes intensely involved in the sensations within her body and tends to withdraw from the surrounding environment. As cervical dilatation progresses to 8 to 9 cm., the contractions reach peak intensity. This phase, between 8 to 10 cm. dilatation, is called *transition,* and is frequently the most difficult and painful time for the woman. At this time, there is usually a marked increase in the amount of show due to rupture of capillary vessels in the cervix and the lower uterine segment.

As the result of the uterine contractions, two important changes occur in the cervix during the first stage of labor—*effacement* and *dilatation* (Fig. 15-3, p. 255).

EFFACEMENT is the shortening of the cervical canal from a structure 1 or 2 cm. in length to one in which no canal at all exists, but merely a circular orifice with almost paper-thin edges. As may be seen in Figure 15-4, the edges of the

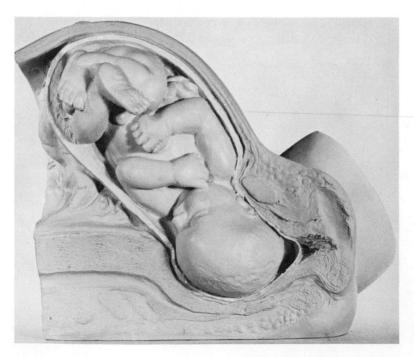

Figure 15-5. Full dilatation: cervix high, head deep in birth canal, membranes intact. (Dickinson-Belskie models, Cleveland Health Museum, Cleveland)

internal os are drawn several centimeters upward, so that the former endocervical canal becomes part of the lower uterine segment. In primigravidas, effacement is usually complete before dilatation begins, but in multiparas it is rarely complete, dilatation proceeding, as a rule, with rather thick cervical edges. The terms *obliteration* and *taking up* of the cervix are synonymous with effacement. Effacement is measured during pelvic examination by estimating the percentage by which the cervical canal has shortened. For example, in a cervix 2 cm. long before labor, 50 percent effacement has occurred when the cervix measures 1 cm. in length.

DILATATION OF THE CERVIX. This means the enlargement of the cervical os from an orifice a few millimeters in size to an aperture large enough to permit the passage of the fetus—that is, to a diameter of about 10 cm. When the cervix can no longer be felt, dilatation is said to be complete. Although the forces concerned in dilatation are not well understood, several factors appear to be involved. The muscle fibers about the cervix are so arranged that they pull upon its edges and tend to draw it open. The uterine contractions cause pressure on the amniotic sac and this, in turn, burrows into the cervix in pouchlike fashion exerting a dilating action (Fig. 15-5). In the absence of the membranes, the pressure of the presenting part against the cervix and the lower uterine segment has a similar effect.

Measurement of cervical dilatation is done during pelvic examination through digital estimation of the diameter of the cervical opening. It is expressed in centimeters, and often tactile charts are available in labor rooms to help the examiner translate into centimeters the mental picture obtained during this "blind" examination.

Dilatation of the cervix in the first stage of labor is solely the result of uterine contractions which are involuntary. In other words, there is nothing that the mother can do, such as bearing down, which will help the slightest in expediting this period of labor. Indeed, bearing-down efforts at this stage serve only to exhaust the mother and cause the cervix to become edematous.

The second stage of labor

The contractions are now strong and long, lasting 50 to 70 seconds and occurring at inter-

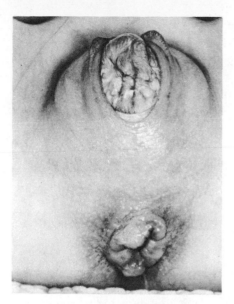

Figure 15-6. Extreme bulging of perineum showing patulous and everted anus.

vals of 2 or 3 minutes. Rupture of the membranes usually occurs during the early part of this stage of labor, with a gush of amniotic fluid from the vagina. Sometimes, however, membranes rupture during the first stage and occasionally before labor begins. In rare cases the baby is born in a "caul," which is a piece of the amnion that sometimes envelops the baby's head. Superstitious parents consider this to be a good omen.

During this stage, as if by reflex action, the muscles of the abdomen are brought into play; and when the contractions are in progress the woman will strain, or "bear down," with all her strength so that her face becomes flushed and the large vessels in her neck distended. As a result of this exertion she may perspire profusely. During this stage the mother directs all her energy toward expelling the contents of the uterus. There is a marked pressure in the area of the perineum and rectum, and the urge to bear down is usually beyond her control.

Toward the end of the second stage, when the head is well down in the vagina, its pressure causes the anus to become patulous and everted (Fig. 15-6), and often small particles of fecal material may be expelled from the rectum with each contraction. This should receive careful attention to avoid contamination. As the head descends still further, the perineal region begins to bulge, and the skin over it becomes tense and glistening. At this time the scalp of

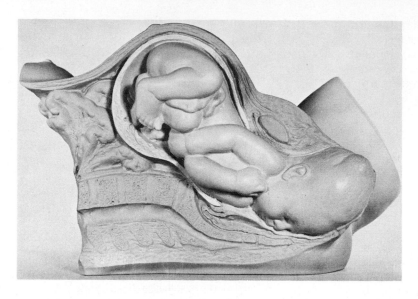

Figure 15-7. Second stage of labor. "Caput," or top of infant's head, begins to appear through the vulvar opening. (Dickinson-Belskie models, Cleveland Health Museum, Cleveland)

the fetus may be detected through a slitlike vulvar opening (Fig. 15-7). With each subsequent contraction the perineum bulges more and more, and the vulva becomes more dilated and distended by the head, so that the opening is gradually converted into an ovoid and at last into a circle. With the cessation of each contraction the opening becomes smaller, and the head recedes from it until it advances again with the next contraction.

The contractions now occur very rapidly, with scarcely any interval between. As the head becomes increasingly visible, the vulva is stretched further and finally encircles the largest diameter of the baby's head. This encirclement of the largest diameter of the baby's head by the vulvar ring is known as "crowning." The physician usually does an episiotomy at this time, supports the tissues surrounding the perineum and delivers the head. One or two more contractions are normally enough to effect the birth of the baby.

Whereas in the first stage of labor the forces are limited to uterine action, during the second stage two forces are essential, namely, uterine contractions and intraabdominal pressure, the latter being brought about by the bearing-down efforts of the mother. (The force exerted by the mother's bearing down can be likened to that used in forcing an evacuation of the bowels.) Both forces are essential to the successful spontaneous outcome of the second stage of labor, for uterine contractions without bearing-down efforts are of little avail in expelling the infant, while, conversely, bearing-down efforts

in the absence of uterine contractions are futile. As explained in Chapter 18, Conduct of Normal Labor, these facts have most important practical implications.

THE MECHANISM OF LABOR. In its passage through the birth canal, the presenting part of the fetus undergoes certain positional changes which constitute the mechanism of labor. These movements are designed to present the smallest possible diameters of the presenting part to the irregular shape of the pelvic canal, so that it will encounter as little resistance as possible. The mechanism of labor consists of a combination of movements, several of which may be going on at the same time. As they occur, the uterine contractions bring about important modifications in the attitude or habitus of the fetus, especially after the head has descended into the pelvis. This adaptation of the baby to the birth canal, as descent takes place, involves four processes, flexion, internal rotation, extension and external rotation (Fig. 15-8).

For purposes of instruction, the various movements will be described as if they occurred independently.

DESCENT. The first requisite for the birth of the infant is descent. When the fetal head has descended such that its greatest biparietal diameter is at, or has passed, the pelvic inlet, the head is said to be *engaged*. This provides a clear indication that the pelvic inlet is large enough to accommodate the widest portion of the fetal head and is, therefore, of adequate size. For the average fetal head, the linear dis-

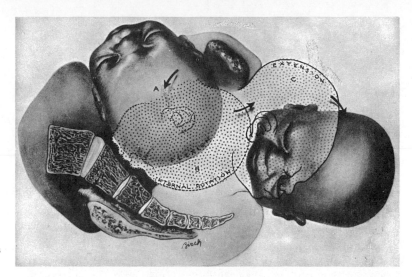

Figure 15-8. L.O.A. Positional changes of head in passing through birth canal.

tance between the occiput and the plane of the biparietal diameter is less than the distance between the pelvic inlet and the ischial spines. Thus, when the occiput is at the level of the spines, its biparietal diameter has usually passed the pelvic inlet, and the vertex is therefore engaged. However, one cannot assume that engagement has occurred simply because the vertex is at the spines. When the fetal head has been molded markedly, with consequent increase in the distance between the occiput and the biparietal diameter, the vertex may be felt at the spines, but its longest diameter may still be above the pelvic inlet.

The ischial spines are used as a landmark to describe the relative position of the fetal head in the pelvis. When the vertex is at the level of the spines, it is at 0 station. If 1 cm. below, it is a +1 station; 2 cm. below, +2 station; 3 cm. below, +3 station. When the vertex is 1 cm. above the spines, it is a −1 station; 2 cm. above, −2 station; 3 cm. above, −3 station. This relationship is evaluated during the course of each pelvic examination and recorded, along with the assessment of cervical dilatation and effacement.

In primigravidas, engagement often precedes the onset of labor. This is the process of

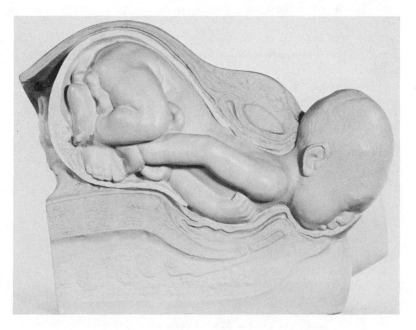

Figure 15-9. Head extends upward: pelvic floor retreats. (Dickinson-Belskie models, Cleveland Health Museum, Cleveland)

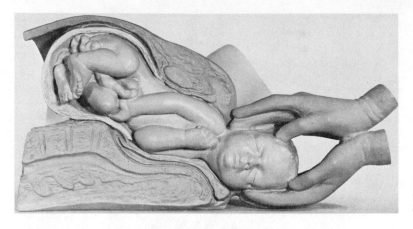

Figure 15-10. Birth of shoulders: rotating to accommodate to birth passage. (Dickinson-Belskie models, Cleveland Health Museum, Cleveland)

"lightening." Because the vertex is frequently deep in the pelvis at the onset of labor, further descent does not necessarily begin until the second stage of labor. In multiparas, on the other hand, descent often begins with engagement. Once having been inaugurated, descent is inevitably associated with the various movements of the mechanism of labor.

FLEXION. Very early in the process of descent the head becomes so flexed that the chin is in contact with the sternum, and, as a consequence, the very smallest anteroposterior diameter (the suboccipitobregmatic plane) is presented to the pelvis.

INTERNAL ROTATION. As seen in Chapter 5, the head enters the pelvis in the transverse or diagonal position. When it reaches the pelvic floor, the occiput is rotated and comes to lie beneath the symphysis pubis. In other words, the sagittal suture is now in the anteroposterior

diameter of the outlet (see Fig. 5-7, p. 68). Although the occiput usually rotates to the front, on occasion it may turn toward the hollow of the sacrum. If anterior rotation does not take place at all, the occiput usually rotates to the direct occiput posterior position, a condition known as persistent occiput posterior. Since this represents a deviation from the normal mechanism of labor, it will be considered in Chapter 25, under Abnormal Fetal Positions.

EXTENSION. After the occiput emerges from the pelvis, the nape of the neck becomes arrested beneath the pubic arch and acts as a pivotal point for the rest of the head. Extension of the head now ensues, and with it the frontal portion of the head, the face and the chin are born (Fig. 15-9, p. 259).

EXTERNAL ROTATION. After the birth of the head, it remains in the anteroposterior position only a very short time and shortly will be seen

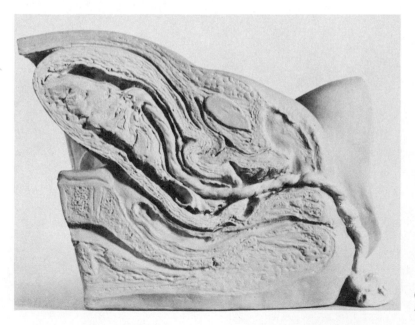

Figure 15-11. Separation of placenta. (Dickinson-Belskie models, Cleveland Health Museum, Cleveland)

to turn to one or another side of its own accord —*restitution*. When the occiput originally has been directed toward the left of the mother's pelvis, it then rotates toward the left, and to the right when it originally has been toward the right. This is known as external rotation and is due to the fact that the shoulders of the baby, having entered the pelvis in the transverse position, undergo internal rotation to the anteroposterior position, as did the head; this brings about a corresponding rotation of the head, which is now on the outside. The shoulders are born in a manner somewhat similar to that of the head. Almost immediately after the occurrence of external rotation, the anterior shoulder appears under the symphysis pubis and becomes arrested temporarily beneath the pubic arch, to act as a pivotal point for the other shoulder (Fig. 15-10). As the anterior margin of the perineum becomes distended, the posterior shoulder is born, assisted by an upward lateral flexion of the infant's body. Once the shoulders are delivered, the infant's body is quickly extruded (expulsion).

The third stage of labor

The third stage of labor is made up of two phases: *the phase of placental separation* and *the phase of placental expulsion*.

Immediately following the birth of the infant, the remainder of the amniotic fluid escapes, after which there is usually a slight flow of blood. The uterus can be felt as a firm globular mass just below the level of the umbilicus. Shortly thereafter, the uterus relaxes and assumes a discoid shape. With each subsequent contraction or relaxation the uterus changes from globular to discoid shape until the placenta has separated, after which time the globular shape persists.

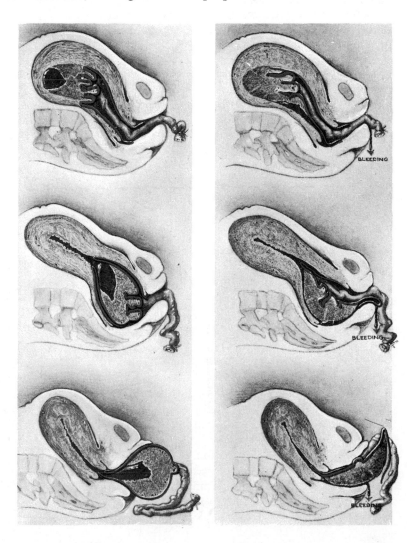

Figure 15-12. Successive stages of extrusion of placenta: (*left*) by Schultze's mechanism; (*right*) by the Duncan mechanism.

PLACENTAL SEPARATION. As the uterus contracts down at regular intervals on its diminishing content, the area of placental attachment is greatly reduced. The great disproportion between the reduced size of the placental site and that of the placenta brings about a folding or festooning of the maternal surface of the placenta (Fig. 15-11, p. 260); with this process separation takes place. Meanwhile, bleeding takes place within these placental folds, and this expedites separation of the organ. The placenta now sinks into the lower uterine segment or upper vagina as an unattached body.

The signs which suggest that the placenta has separated are: 1) the uterus becomes globular in shape and, as a rule, firmer; 2) it rises upward in the abdomen; 3) the umbilical cord descends 3 or more inches farther out of the vagina; and 4) a sudden gush of blood often occurs. These signs usually occur within five minutes after the delivery of the infant.

PLACENTAL EXPULSION. Actual expulsion of the placenta may be brought about by bearing-down efforts on the part of the mother if she is not anesthetized. If this cannot be accomplished, it is usually effected through gentle pressure on the uterine fundus by the physician after he has first made certain that the uterus is hard. Excessive pressure should be avoided to obviate the rare possibility of "inversion" of the uterus (see Chapter 25).

The extrusion of the placenta may take place by one of two mechanisms. First, it may become turned inside-out within the vagina and be born like an inverted umbrella with the glistening fetal surfaces presenting. This is known as Schultze's mechanism and occurs in about 80 percent of cases. Second, it may become somewhat rolled up in the vagina, with the maternal surface outermost, and be born edgewise. The latter is known as the Duncan mechanism and is seen in about 20 percent of deliveries (Fig. 15-12, p. 261). It is believed that Schultze's mechanism signifies that the placenta has become detached first at its center, and usually a collection of blood and clots is found in the sac of membranes. The Duncan mechanism, on the other hand, suggests that the placenta has separated first at its edges, and it is in this type that bleeding usually occurs at the time of separation.

The contraction of the uterus following delivery serves not only to produce placental separation but also to control uterine hemorrhage. As the result of this contraction of the uterine muscle fibers, the countless blood vessels within their interstices are clamped shut. Even then, a certain amount of blood loss in the third stage is unavoidable, commonly amounting to 500 cc. or more. It is one of the aims of the conduct of labor to reduce this bleeding to a very minimum.

SUMMARY OF MECHANISM OF LABOR

First Stage—Dilating Stage

Definition Period from first true labor contraction to complete dilatation of cervix.

What Is Accomplished Effacement and dilatation of cervix.

Forces Involved Uterine contractions.

Second Stage—Expulsive Stage

Definition Period from complete dilatation of cervix to birth of baby.

What Is Accomplished Expulsion of baby from birth canal—facilitated by certain positional changes of fetus: descent, flexion, internal rotation, extension, external rotation and expulsion.

Forces Involved Uterine contractions plus intraabdominal pressure.

Third Stage—Placental Stage

Definition Period from birth of baby through birth of placenta.

What Is Accomplished (A) Separation of placenta; (B) expulsion of placenta.

Forces Involved (A) Uterine contractions; (B) intraabdominal pressure.

The fourth stage of labor

The first hour postpartum is sometimes referred to as the fourth stage of labor. During this time *restoration of physiologic stability occurs*, following the tumultuous events of labor. It is a period of potential crisis, with increased incidence of hemorrhage, urinary retention, hypotension, and side effects of anesthesia; it requires careful monitoring of uterine contraction, vital signs, and other physiologic indices.

The first hour after the baby's birth is also considered critical for initial formation of the mother-child relationship and consolidation of the family unit.[5] The process of maternal-child attachment is still under study, but it is possible that early parental interactions with the new baby and each other set the tone for the later quality of their relationships. If so, this is a key time for nursing care which includes assessment of potential problems and support of satisfying interactions for the new family.

Bibliography

1. Turnbull, A. C., *et al*: Significant fall in progesterone and rise in oestradial levels in human peripheral plasma before onset of labour. *Lancet* 1:101-103, Jan. 26, 1974.
2. Liggens, G. C., *et al*: The mechanism of initiation of parturition in the ewe. *Recent Prog. Horm. Res.* 29:111-159, 1973.
3. Karim, S. M. M.: *The Prostaglandins.* New York, Wiley-Interscience, 1972, pp. 73-164.
4. MacDonald, P. C., *et al*: Initiation of human parturition. I. Mechanism of action of arachidonic acid. *Am. J. Ob-Gyn.* 44:629-636, Nov. 1974.
5. Rising, S. S.: The fourth stage of labor: Family integration. *Am. J. Nurs.* 74:870-874, May 1974.

Suggested Reading

HELLMAN, L. M., AND PRITCHARD, J. A.: *Williams Obstetrics,* ed. 14. New York, Appleton-Century Crofts, 1971.

QUILLIGAN, E. J. (ED.): Symposium on physiology of labor. *Clin. Ob. and Gyn.* 11:13-191, 1968.

the nurse's contribution to pain relief during labor

Margo McCaffery, R.N., M.S.

Nature of the Pain Experience During Labor / Assessment of the Patient's Pain; Pain Relief Methods / Components of Pain Relief / Pain Relief Measures During Labor / Aftermath Assimilation

Nature of the pain experience during labor

Beliefs about pain during labor

Is childbirth painful or painless? Most laypeople have learned to expect pain to occur during childbirth. This expectation may evolve from a variety of sources, such as television, movies, books, comments from one's own parents, and reports from friends who have had babies. However, sexual activities, including reproduction, have not been discussed openly in the United States until the last few years. As a result information about childbirth may be incomplete, if not inaccurate. Hence fear is also likely to be felt by the expectant parents both of whom expect pain during labor but know little about labor.

The fear of pain is second only to the fear of death. Understandably, then, some expectant parents are eager to examine and accept any information suggesting that childbirth need not be associated with pain. Information convincing to laypeople is available in several forms.

Reports of how childbirth is handled in some other cultures, especially the more primitive ones, often emphasize the lack of expression of pain. In other words, there is an absence of the overt behavioral responses usually associated with pain, such as crying and moaning, inactivity or fatigue following pain, or requests for pain relief. Some women are noted to have their babies in the fields and to resume work immediately following delivery. Other women are observed to remain quiet with relaxed facial expressions during childbirth.

From this information some people erroneously conclude that these women experience no pain, and therefore, that pain results *only* from cultural conditioning. However, lack of expression of pain does not mean that pain is absent. Indeed, a recent study of Samoan women has revealed that while their expressions of pain were minimal during labor, they admitted afterward in interviews that they did experience pain or discomfort.[1]

Some methods of prepared childbirth may also suggest that labor is painless. One paperback book about a method of childbirth states "painless childbirth" in bold, large print on the cover. Currently most methods of prepared childbirth do not purport to be painless, but they seem inadvertently to insinuate lack of pain in their films of childbirth and in the written narratives of couples utilizing their particular method of childbirth. Expectant parents exposed to this information may be left with the impression of painless childbirth because these films and reports do not focus on pain. They focus on the techniques of a particular method and on the "peak experience" or ecstasy of giving birth fully conscious.

In answer to the question of whether childbirth is painful or painless, one must simply conclude that there are a number of very different ways to respond to the event of childbirth. Some responses entail minimal expression of pain, but this does not mean pain is absent. Certainly there are reports of painless labors, but these are infrequent. Most labors are accompanied by some degree of pain, ranging from minor discomforts and feelings of pressure to intense pain with suffering.

Importance of pain control during labor

The relief of pain and suffering is traditionally a humane and moral act. But, the health-care professional is also aware of the physiologic and emotional benefits of freedom from pain.

EMOTIONAL ADVANTAGES. In the instance of childbirth, control or relief of pain potentially enables the mother and father to have a positive experience during this significant step toward becoming parents. Ultimately one or both parents may be able to witness that moment which remains miraculous and awesome even to many obstetricians—a new human being emerging into the world. Even when the delivery is not observed, there are other desirable outcomes. If the mother and father can handle the discomforts during childbirth, they can feel they are active participants in the actual birth of their own child.

The parent who is willing and able to participate in labor probably more easily comprehends the transition from expecting a baby to having a baby. This may facilitate the parent's ability to perform in the new role of mother or father to this particular child.

In any event, relief or control of pain at a tolerable level helps to make it possible for parents to participate in childbirth in the ways they have chosen, whether or not this involves their active participation. When people jointly plan for an event such as childbirth and are then able to carry through with these plans, the event probably fosters growth in the relationship between them. In the case of childbirth, a satisfying labor experience for both parents probably also fosters their relationship with their baby.

At least a childbirth experience where pain is adequately controlled will not impede these relationships. Pain has the potential for eliciting angry and aggressive responses, often referred to as the fight or flight response. Such feelings resulting from a miserably painful childbirth experience sometimes are projected onto the infant or the father. The mother temporarily may express hatred toward the infant or father, and she may withdraw from these relationships for a while. During and following very painful labors mothers have been quoted as saying they despise their partners. Fathers have been known to say they felt angry toward the baby because its birth caused the mother pain. One mother even commented that her labor was so painful it took her a year to forgive her child and establish a warm relationship with him.

It does not seem likely, however, that pain and suffering during labor could be the sole reason for permanent or prolonged impairment of mother-father-child relationships. Labor may be a convenient scapegoat. Other more significant factors operating over a long period of time have probably affected the relationships.

PHYSIOLOGIC ADVANTAGES. The adequate relief of pain also results in physiologic benefits. The mother who experiences tolerable discomforts in labor is able to be cooperative with examinations and to work with her contractions. Consequently she facilitates efforts of the health team members to obtain information and she avoids prolongation of labor. After childbirth she is less fatigued. If she is able to utilize pain relief measures other than medication, she may eliminate the need for medication or reduce the amount necessary. This is of enormous physiologic benefit to the infant since many analgesics and anesthesics, including regional anesthesia, have untoward effects upon the fetus, such as respiratory depression and bradycardia.

Definitions

PAIN. Pain defies definition. It is always a personal and subjective experience, differing from one person to another and varying within the same person from one time to the next. Quite simply pain is a localized sensation of hurt. But, for both the nurse and patient who work together to relieve pain, it seems more productive for the nurse to adopt the patient's definition of pain. The nursing definition of pain may then be stated as whatever the experiencing person says it is, existing whenever he or she says it does.[2] A crucial aspect of this definition is that the nurse believes what the patient tells her. And, of course, the patient may communicate the pain experience in any number of ways besides verbalization. For example, in some patients a marked increase in rate and depth of respirations may alert the nurse to the intensification of discomfort.

PAIN EXPERIENCE. The phrase "pain experience" has been used repeatedly thus far in this chapter and deserves some explanation. The pain experience encompasses all the patient's sensations, feelings, and behavioral responses, including physiologic activities such as blood pressure changes. The pain experience may also refer to any or all of the three phases of pain—anticipation, presence, aftermath. And it may include not only the patient's actions, but also the impact upon the patient of the actions of others while the patient is in one of the phases of pain.

PAIN EXPRESSIONS. Several examples have already been given of ways patients may express pain. "Pain expressions" refer to the many different ways people respond, voluntarily and involuntarily, to pain. The manner in which an individual responds to pain is dependent upon numerous and varied factors such as the culture in which the person lives, the personal meaning of the pain, and the intensity of the pain. Hence pain expressions may be absent or minimal, i.e., none, very few, or not easily observed. For example, a slight and momentary frown may be the only sign that the patient is experiencing pain. Or, the patient may be more expressive. Prolonged moaning is one example. Expressions of pain are usually observed in one or more of the following categories of behavioral response: physiologic, verbal, vocal, facial, body movement, physical contact with others, and general response to the environment.[3]

PAIN TOLERANCE. In caring for the patient with pain it is very important to differentiate between the presence of a pain sensation and the patient's tolerance for that pain. Pain tolerance may be defined as the intensity and duration of pain that the patient is willing to endure at that time without pain relief or without additional relief.

Pain tolerance differs markedly from one person to another. Some patients will state that the pain sensation is severe, yet they willingly tolerate the pain and do not want anything done for them. Other patients will utilize or request pain relief measures when they rate their pain as mild. The latter group may be said to have a low tolerance for pain. While a high pain tolerance is valued by many people, the nurse realizes that a patient's tolerance for pain is not a matter of good or bad, or right or wrong. Indeed, none of the patient's responses to pain are to be judged in this way.

SUFFERING. Suffering is an affective state that may accompany pain. Copp, a nurse-researcher in the field of pain, pointedly uses the term suffering in reference to pain and defines it as "the state of anguish of one who bears pain, injury, or loss."[4] When pain cannot be eliminated, it is imperative that the patient receive whatever assistance is necessary to prevent or diminish feelings of suffering. While a painful experience is at best only unpleasant, in most cases it need not be unrelenting agony.

Descriptions of painful sensations of normal labor

UTERINE CONTRACTIONS. During the first stage of normal labor one source of pain or discomfort is usually the involuntary contraction of the uterine muscle. The contraction tends to be felt in the lower back at the beginning of labor. As labor progresses the sensation of a contraction encircles the lower torso, covering both back and abdomen.

Contractions are frequently referred to as wavelike in character: they rhythmically come and go, each one increasing to a certain height or intensity and then decreasing, finally disappearing. Contractions last from about 45 to 90 seconds. In early labor the contractions are not necessarily uncomfortable. As labor progresses the intensity of each contraction increases, resulting in a greater possibility or intensity of discomfort.

The quality of the discomfort is difficult to describe and certainly is varied. Basically there appear to be three possible qualities to any painful sensation—burning, pricking, aching. And, quite simply, pain can be either deep or superficial. Consequently one may say that a labor contraction is felt as deep aching, as opposed to being localized superficially on the skin and as opposed to being felt as burning or pricking sensations.

The intervals between contractions shorten

Table 16-1 Tools for Assessing the Pain Experience During Labor

I. **Contractions**
  Onset
  Frequency
  Duration
  Intensity
  Description of sensation
  Attitude toward contractions

II. **Pain Relief Methods Employed by Parent(s) for Labor**
  Person(s) to assist or be present during labor
  Positioning
  Relaxation techniques
  Distraction (or concentration) methods
  Breathing patterns
  Physical activities
  Medication
  Usage and effectiveness of above

III. **Current Discomforts of Mother Other than Labor**
  Pregnancy
  Chronic illness
  Recent illness or injury
  Methods of handling above; effectiveness of methods

IV. **Parents' Current Concerns Other than Labor**
  Activities or plans interrupted by labor
  Care of children at home
  Financial arrangements
  Condition of mother or unborn child
  Plans for care of infant
  Unexpected change in childbirth plans
  Plans and needs for assistance regarding above

V. **Parents' Goals and Expectations Regarding Labor**
  Presence and intensity of pain
  Provisions for pain relief (if any)
  Father's (coach's) presence
  Opportunity to observe, especially delivery
  Photographs
  Episiotomy
  Contact with baby immediately after delivery
  Differences between mother and father regarding above
  Which of above not possible or not discussed with physician

as labor proceeds. Early labor contractions are about 20 minutes apart. Then for several hours they are three to five minutes apart. During about the last hour prior to delivery the intervals between contractions may be only a few seconds long. This period, when the cervix is dilating from about 7 cm. to 10 cm., is referred to as transition.

Uterine contractions are at their highest intensity and greatest frequency during transition. This is usually when the mother will experience the most discomfort and will have the most difficulty handling her discomfort.

BACK LABOR. In addition to uterine contractions, approximately 25 percent of women in labor will also have to cope with the discomfort of *back labor*. This occurs when the fetus is in an occipitoposterior position (see discussion of persistent occipitoposterior positions in Chapter 25). With each contraction the occiput presses on the mother's sacrum, causing extreme discomfort as the intensity of contractions increases. Back labor is considerably more painful for the mother than labor in which there is an anterior occipital position.

DELIVERY. A common but false assumption about labor is that the most painful part is the expulsive stage. Of course, the mother certainly may experience discomfort during delivery but it is generally much less intense than what she felt during transition. The predominant sensations during delivery occur in the vaginal and perineal area and can be described as pressure, stretching, or splitting, and sometimes burning. Most of the time the mother has an overwhelming desire to push. Pushing may relieve whatever discomfort is felt. Also, the pressure of the baby's head causes a degree of numbness in the perineum. If desired, the physician can take advantage of this numbness during a contraction and perform a painless episiotomy.

The foregoing is a description of the painful or uncomfortable sensations often felt during normal labor. Considerably more pain may be experienced with certain complications of labor, such as hypertonic uterine dysfunction, delivery of an oversized baby, or a contracted pelvis.

Assessment of the patient's pain and pain relief methods

When the laboring mother is admitted to the hospital, the nurse identifies several factors important to the management of pain. Table 16-1 summarizes those items which are usually the more pertinent. Since a thorough assessment is inextricably related to intervention, some pain relief measures will be mentioned in the discussion of assessment. Actually, the manner in which the nurse assesses the patient often contributes to pain relief. When the nurse conveys to the mother that she believes her and that she desires to understand the mother's experience as completely as possible, this can reduce anxiety and thereby relieve pain.

Items for assessment

CONTRACTIONS. Any time the nurse discusses labor contractions with the patient she refers to them as contractions, not as pains. Although many laypeople continue to use the term pains, the nurse should attempt to help the parents substitute the word contractions. One reason for this is that the word pain tends to suggest not just discomfort but an unbearable sensation. The initial contractions are not necessarily uncomfortable, and it is usually a misnomer to refer to them as pains. Later in labor the contractions may be uncomfortable but not unbearable. Most mothers probably are not so suggestible that they would actually feel unbearable pain during contractions simply because the nurse used the term pains rather than contractions. But the use of the term pains may generate needless anxiety about the sensations of labor.

With regard to assessment of the characteristics of uterine contractions (see Table 16-1, I), the onset of labor is important to note since prolonged labor intensifies the painful experience. Not only is there simply a longer time spent in discomfort, but a lengthy labor often fatigues and discourages the parents. Thus they have more difficulty coping with labor.

Regularity and increasing frequency of contractions along with increasing intensity of contractions assist in determining the normality of labor. Such information can be used to assure the parents that progress is being made. To obtain more detailed and useful information about intensity of contractions, the nurse may ask the mother to use a scale for rating. The scale may be composed, for example, of the following terms: mild, moderate, intense (strong), very intense (strong).

In addition to asking the mother about the intensity of contractions, it is important to encourage her to describe other characteristics of the contraction, such as where the sensation begins and where it is felt the most intensely. This information often suggests the need for specific pain relief measures. For example, if the contraction begins in the lower back and is felt most intensely there, rubbing that area and applying pressure may provide considerable comfort.

During the mother's discussion of her contractions she may reveal her attitude toward them or toward labor in general. If not, the nurse may ask her how she feels about her labor. Of special importance is the degree of fear or anxiety experienced by the mother. These feelings have a profound effect upon pain. They decrease pain tolerance and increase the perceived intensity of pain. Anxiety or fear also increases muscle tension, and in labor this may increase painful stimuli by interfering with contractions.

There are innumerable potential sources of anxiety or fear during labor. In relation to the contractions themselves some common sources of anxiety appear to be how pain will be managed and how labor is progressing. Considerable anxiety may be alleviated by discussing with the mother the various pain relief measures that may be employed. Concern over the progression of labor, or the effectiveness of the contractions, may be partially diminished if the nurse keeps the mother informed of signs of progress such as increasing cervical dilatation or regularity of contractions. It is sometimes helpful to assure the mother that it is possible to stop or correct ineffective or dysfunctional uterine contractions.

PAIN RELIEF METHODS EMPLOYED BY PARENT(S) FOR LABOR (Table 16-1, II). Whether or not the parents have any special or well-defined method of handling childbirth (e.g., Lamaze method), the nurse questions them about how they have handled the discomforts of labor thus far and what their plans are for the remainder of labor. In the United States there are many methods of preparation for childbirth. These methods not only employ different techniques and philosophies but within each method variations may be encountered. Techniques may be developed, deleted or added by the individual instructor or by many instructors in a particular geographical area. Some childbirth education classes combine two or more methods. And, of course, some mothers do not inquire about these methods, but they intuitively devise their own special way of handling childbirth.

The following alphabetized list at least introduces the nurse to some of the existing methods of preparation for childbirth. Other ways of referring to the methods are mentioned in parentheses.

GAMPER METHOD (Margaret Gamper)
HUSBAND-COACHED CHILDBIRTH
    (Robert A. Bradley)
MATERNITY CENTER ASSOCIATION
PSYCHOPROPHYLACTIC METHOD
    (PPM, Lamaze method)
PSYCHOSEXUAL METHOD (Sheila Kitzinger)
READ METHOD (Grantly Dick-Read)
WRIGHT METHOD (Erna Wright)

Part II of Table 16-1 lists aspects that are common to methods of childbirth taught to expectant parents as well as those unique styles sometimes developed by the parents themselves. For example, regardless of the type of formal or informal preparation for childbirth, some attention is almost always directed at comfortable positioning, efforts to relax, and the persons who will be in attendance during labor.

It is difficult to list all the variations in methods of childbirth and to keep abreast of the constant changes taking place within each method, but the nurse can be reassured by the fact that in any single hospital labor suite she is likely to observe only one or two methods being used. This is partially because physicians using one particular method of childbirth tend to congregate at the same hospital where they can share ideas and know that the nursing staff is reasonably familiar with the method. Also, certain methods tend to be popular only in certain geographical areas. Thus the nurse is likely to be able to identify quickly which methods are most common where she is employed, and she can then study them in greater depth.

With regard to the *person or persons to assist or be present during labor*, the father is almost always included if the couple has attended classes on one of the methods of prepared childbirth. Sometimes the couple's children are allowed an occasional and brief visit to the labor room. When the father is absent or does not want to attend labor or when the mother is unwed, the person in attendance may be a childbirth educator or the mother's friend or relative.

After identifying this person the nurse finds out if that person has been with the mother prior to hospital admission and if the mother wants that person to remain with her in the labor and delivery rooms. She also assesses the attending person's attitudes and desires. It is possible, for instance, that the mother might want the father to remain with her, but the father may be quite reluctant and fearful. (For the sake of convenience the person the mother brings to the hospital to be with her during labor henceforth will be referred to as the father.)

In addition the nurse determines what the father has done for the mother prior to admission, what is planned for the remainder of labor, what (if any) preparation the mother and father have had, and whether they have practiced what they plan to do. Sometimes the father simply stays near the mother, touching her gently and offering verbal encouragement. In other cases the father is expected to take a very active role in the following pain relief measures.

Some of the techniques and pain relief methods employed by methods of prepared childbirth initially appear, in all fairness and at the very least, simply odd. Not uncommonly mothers feel foolish doing them and nurses are shocked to see them. Hopefully the following examples will be sufficiently informative to encourage the nurse to investigate the situation rather than automatically suspect that a laboring mother is mentally unbalanced.

A variety of *positions* may be assumed during normal labor, in particular during a contraction. At the beginning of labor the mother may walk between contractions, and during a contraction she may remain standing but lean forward with her husband's arms or back as support. As labor progresses she may be more comfortable sitting or lying in bed. Ordinarily the mother is encouraged to assume any position that is comfortable, with the possible exception of lying flat on her back. Some mothers may be more comfortable "on all fours" with gentle pelvic rocking during a contraction.

When the mother is admitted the nurse asks her which positions have been comfortable and which have not. The nurse also inquires about positions the mother may wish to consider later in labor. Some positions require additional pillows which the nurse can then obtain before they are needed. For pushing during delivery most childbirth educators teach the father to stand behind the mother and to prop her up with pillows at a 35° to 45° angle.

Numerous techniques are utilized to achieve and maintain total skeletal muscle *relaxation*. Usually the mother needs adequate support of her limbs, such as a pillow between her legs if she is on her side. Beyond that she may employ regular intervals of smiling, yawning, or taking a deep breath. One mother may visualize the contractions as soothing ocean waves and another may try to simulate sleeping. The father may give tactile or verbal cues to induce relaxation. Again, the nurse finds out what techniques are used for relaxation. Knowing that the mother intends to keep her eyes closed, for example, will prevent the nurse from mistakenly concluding that this laboring mother is sleeping most of the time.

Methods of *distraction* and concentration are probably the most individualized and therefore varied of all the techniques a mother may employ during childbirth. Some patients will bring with them to the hospital their personal choice for a "concentration point," an object the mother stares at during a contraction. Hence the nurse may find a mobile hanging from the ceiling, a seashell on the bed, a drawing pinned to the drapes or a brilliant circle taped to the wall. Combined with other techniques this concentration point helps the mother distract her thoughts from discomfort. Toward the end of labor the mother may distract herself from discomfort by emphatically mouthing the words to a song and tapping her finger to the rhythm or slapping her thigh in rhythm. Some mothers may close their eyes and utilize mental relaxation as a distracter. This may be accomplished by the father's whispering "sweet nothings" in the mother's ear during a contraction and/or by the mother's closing her eyes and visualizing previously selected, pleasant childhood experiences.

The nurse asks the parents if they will be employing any special objects or techniques to facilitate concentration or distraction. In addition to the examples given here it is well to remember that the mother's efforts to achieve relaxation and to perform certain breathing patterns and other activities also serve as profound distracters from discomfort.

Controversy and change are characteristic of many of the *breathing patterns* employed in the various methods of prepared childbirth. The two basic types of breathing are 1) chest and 2) abdominal, or diaphragmatic. Some childbirth educators feel that abdominal breathing places more pressure on the uterus by having the diaphragm down and the abdomen bulged. However, other educators feel that abdominal breathing prevents pressure on the uterus by relaxing and lifting the abdominal wall off the uterus and that it enhances relaxation because it is the type of breathing used during sleep. Some mothers tend to find abdominal breathing difficult to do as labor progresses, while others find it comfortable throughout labor.

Another area of controversy is related to chest breathing. Among those who teach chest breathing there appears to be a trend toward modification in the use of panting, or rapid superficial breathing.[5,6] Some of the reasons for this are that it is difficult to learn, it may become fatiguing during labor, and it causes hyperventilation in a few mothers during labor. Hence, some childbirth educators have abandoned panting and substituted another breathing rhythm, while other educators have simply solved the problem by teaching a more moderate rate of shallow breathing.

Mothers may be taught to use either abdominal breathing only, chest breathing only, a combination of both, or simply a pattern of breaths with no special attention directed at either abdominal or chest breathing. In general, the rate of breathing increases as labor progresses. Also, during a contraction the rate of breathing may accelerate as the contraction intensifies and decelerate as the contraction subsides.

The mother may breathe only through the mouth or she may inhale through the nose and exhale through the mouth. Any number of combinations of this may be used by any one mother. In addition, breathing may be accompanied by sounds or body movement. One mother may whistle upon exhalation; another may actively and rapidly turn her head to the right as she whispers "ha" and back to the front as she says "hooh."

The nurse will be able to obtain information about the breathing patterns from some mothers simply by asking. Others will not be aware of the breathing pattern they are using and finding helpful. In such cases the nurse must observe the mother carefully. A thorough assessment of breathing patterns helps the nurse anticipate the needs of the mother. If a breathing pattern is not helpful, the nurse will know which patterns are different from the one being used and hence potentially helpful. If the mother will be breathing through her mouth, the nurse can obtain ice chips or a damp cloth to alleviate dry lips and mouth. Some mothers are taught to use a lollipop for this purpose. If the mother uses rapid breathing, the nurse can be alert to reports of tingling in the hands and other initial signs of hyperventilation (carbon dioxide insufficiency). Then the nurse can have a paper bag available for rebreathing carbon dioxide to reverse the process.

Physical activities other than those which fall into the above categories may be used during labor. During a contraction the mother or father may rhythmically massage the abdomen, using some preparation such as talcum powder to keep the skin smooth. The father may rub her lower back between and during contractions. Or, he may employ a maneuver with his hands (learned from a childbirth educator) to raise the abdominal wall during a contraction. The mother may rock her pelvis while standing or lying on her side. The latter appears to be particularly helpful during back labor. Counterpressure is also useful. To achieve this the father may place tennis balls, a rolling pin, his knee or his fist against the lower back.

When the mother is admitted, the nurse also asks her whether or not she has taken *medication* or any other substance for pain relief. The mother may have taken aspirin, codeine, an alcoholic beverage or some other common household item. Or, thinking she was in false labor, she may have taken something previously prescribed for this such as paragoric. If medication was taken, the nurse notes the time, type and amount.

It is always possible that the mother has taken some illegal drug such as marijuana, heroin or a black market drug of unknown composition. The nurse considers this in all cases, not only when the mother "looks like a hippie." Anyone may obtain drugs, and the use of marijuana is widespread. The latter is generally known to those who smoke it as an effective tranquilizer and/or analgesic. The mother who uses illegal drugs may fear legal action against her. Therefore, to increase the likelihood of obtaining an honest answer from a mother who has used an illegal drug, the nurse should always stress that the questions about medication are asked for important reasons. The nurse can explain that it helps the physician determine what other medication can be used safely and what courses of action to take in the event that something unusual happens during labor.

The nurse also inquires about what analgesics and anesthetics the parents may have considered using during labor. The mother may have no knowledge at all about medication, or she and the father may have discussed several possibilities with the obstetrician.

When the nurse assesses each of the foregoing pain relief methods employed by the parents, she determines both their *usage* and their *effectiveness* for the individual mother. Usage refers to which methods the parents used prior to admission, which are being used at the time of admission and what plans, if any, the parents have for using other pain relief methods. What is helpful at the beginning of labor may be useless later.

With regard to effectiveness the nurse wants to know if pain relief methods already used have been helpful either in reducing the perceived intensity of pain or in increasing the mother's tolerance for pain. Naturally, what is helpful for one mother may not be helpful for another.

CURRENT DISCOMFORTS OTHER THAN LABOR. The process of labor may not be the only source of discomfort for the mother. Indeed, there are other diseases or symptoms that may be much more irritating and painful than the concurrent labor. Such discomforts may be associated with the pregnancy itself, a chronic illness, or a recent illness or injury (see Table 16-1, III).

Pregnancy may cause or increase heartburn, hemorrhoids, or varicose veins in the legs or vagina. These and other conditions associated with pregnancy can be extremely uncomfortable for the mother.

The mother may also suffer from a chronic illness such as inflammation of a joint, muscle injury, or allergy. Or, a recent illness or injury may exist. An accident could have resulted in a broken bone, lacerations, corneal abrasion, or a sprained ankle. The mother could have contracted influenza a few days prior to labor.

The nurse assesses sources of discomfort extraneous to labor so that appropriate actions can be taken to provide relief. For example, the mother experiencing heartburn may find it very distressing. But the simple administration of an antacid may enable her to devote her attention and energy to the process of childbirth. Quite likely the mother will have been employing some treatments prior to the onset of labor. The nurse identifies the nature of these and their effectiveness. If the mother has found effective means of handling discomforts, it obviously is expedient for her to use the same methods during labor whenever possible.

CURRENT CONCERNS OTHER THAN LABOR (Table 16-1, IV). The precise time for the onset of labor is rarely predicted accurately. Therefore, it is always possible that significant activities or plans may be interrupted by labor. This may be as minor as leaving a stew partially cooked and forgetting to turn off the flame under the pot. But fear of fire and trying to locate a neighbor to turn off the burner may be an underlying concern of the parents and, therefore, a distraction or a cause for increased anxiety. Or, the onset of labor may interfere with the requirements of the father's occupation. It may have been necessary for him to cancel an important and potentially profitable business appointment.

If the parents have other children, they may be anxious about what will happen to the children during their absence. The parents may have had to leave for the hospital without knowing the exact whereabouts of an older child or without being able to calm the sobbing of a younger child.

The parents may also be concerned about financial arrangements related to hospitalization and the physician's fee, particularly if complications arise such as prematurity or if there is an unexpected multiple birth. More simply, perhaps the parents failed to make recommended financial payments to the hospital during the weeks prior to admission. As a result they may be afraid the hospital will not allow them to stay.

For some reason, realistic or not, the parents may be fearful about the condition of the mother and/or the unborn infant. Because a relative is mentally retarded the parents may be afraid the baby will be born with brain damage. They may fear infant anomalies on the basis of the mother's having had viral infections during pregnancy or having taken certain drugs before she realized she was pregnant. Or, the mother may have a cardiac condition, and both she and her husband may be concerned that she cannot live through labor.

Plans for the care of the baby may be another source of concern. The nurse realizes the newborn can sleep safely in a large box if necessary, but new parents may feel they face an impossible situation because the crib has not arrived. On the more serious side, the mother and/or father may be considering giving up the baby for adoption. The onset of labor may precipitate many feelings about this.

Unexpectedly there may have been a change in some aspect of the parents' plans for childbirth. Their obstetrician may be out of town, or labor may have progressed so rapidly they were unable to reach the hospital of their choice.

It is important for the nurse to recognize these and other areas of potential concern for parents during labor. Obviously the mother or father who is anxious about something other than the process of childbirth will not be able to direct attention toward handling the discomforts, responding to directions, cooperating with examinations and all the other aspects of labor. The nurse often can assist the parents in making plans to handle some sources of concern, or she can help them obtain appropriate assistance.

GOALS AND EXPECTATIONS REGARDING LABOR. Parents who have attended childbirth education classes usually have certain goals and expectations regarding labor. But all patients, whether they realize it or not, have certain ideas about their medical care and their health or illness experiences. A recent study suggests that a therapeutic alliance is established more readily when nurses view patients as partners in planning their care. These investigators suggest that the patient be regarded as a consumer—a consumer of health care. They feel that dictating care is no longer a suitable approach to today's clientele. They state it is the patient's prerogative to accept, modify or refuse care.[7] Clearly, helping the parents to state their personal goals or expectations regarding labor is very pertinent to nursing intervention.

Following are some areas for the nurse to explore with the parents as she plans care with them (Table 16-1, V). In some areas the parents may have no ideas or preferences and will readily accept guidance.

The nurse may encounter extremes in parents' expectations related to pain and pain relief. One mother may expect severe pain and desire that the physician render her practically unconscious throughout labor. Another mother may expect no pain at all and, therefore, no pain relief measures. When discomfort and pain are expected, the parents may believe that the techniques they have been taught to use during labor, such as breathing patterns, will be sufficient assistance for the mother. Their goal may be a completely unmedicated labor. Or, the parents may expect to use the methods they were taught but also to be offered some type of medication if they desire it.

Mention has already been made of some of the possible persons expected to assist during labor. In some cases the father will be expected to remain with the mother from the beginning of labor, during delivery, and through the recovery period following delivery. In other instances the mother will not want the father present. Parents' expectations of the nurse and physician also need to be determined.

Some parents, particularly mothers, want very much to observe the effects of their pushing and the delivery of the baby. Many delivery rooms have mirrors for this purpose. The parents may have brought a camera to take pictures in the labor room and in the delivery room. They may also want someone to take a picture of them with their baby immediately after delivery. Some parents want to tape record the delivery.

An episiotomy is done in most deliveries, but some parents hope for or expect no episiotomy. To achieve this the mother may have done certain exercises daily for weeks prior to labor.

A fully conscious mother almost always wants to touch her newborn as soon as possible. It may be an unexpected but overwhelming urge, or the mother may plan on holding the baby before the cord is cut. She may also expect to be allowed to breast-feed the baby on the delivery table.

In helping the parents express their goals and expectations the nurse is alert to differences between the desires of the mother and father. For example, the father may not want to witness the delivery although the mother wants him in the delivery room. Or, the father may think the mother is unrealistic in her plans for little or no medication. When the nurse observes such differences she helps the parents become aware of them and hopefully formulate compatible goals.

In her assessment of the parents' goals the nurse also notes whether or not these goals have been discussed with the physician. Some goals may be contraindicated for medical reasons. Other goals may require the awareness and cooperation of the physician. In addition hospital policy sometimes places limitations on the parents. For instance, some delivery rooms are so small the hospital must have a policy of excluding the father.

As labor progresses the nurse continues to monitor the patient for any changes in the items listed in Table 16-1. Some aspects of the labor situation may change dramatically, such as the nature of the contractions. There may be a sudden need for modification of pain relief methods. Also, the discomforts and concerns extraneous to labor may be resolved or suddenly may appear when none had existed before.

Prejudices that hamper assessment of pain

SIGNS OF ACUTE PAIN. Precautions must be taken to recognize certain prejudices that may hamper the nurse's assessment of the pain experience. There is a tendency to be prejudiced in favor of recognizing the existence of pain only in those patients who show signs of acute pain, such as perspiration, muscle tension or moaning. The absence of these expressions of pain, as noted previously, does not necessarily mean the patient is not in pain. In fact, the patient may suffer greatly but exhibit only minimal pain expressions.[8]

In childbirth there appear to be two major reasons for minimal pain expressions: 1) the mother may have learned that minimal pain expressions are the expectations of the culture, or 2) activities learned from a method of prepared childbirth may preclude expressions of pain. With regard to the latter, the mother may, for example, practice relaxation; this precludes muscle tension as a sign of acute pain. Use of a breathing pattern and mouthing the words of a song preclude the behavior of moaning. It is often quite difficult, if not impossible, to rely upon signs of acute pain in assessing the laboring mother who is using one of the methods of prepared childbirth. Usually she simply is too busy to show signs of acute pain.

PHYSICAL CAUSE OF PAIN. We also tend to be prejudiced in favor of believing patients only when we know the physical cause of pain.[9] This hampers our understanding of the subjective pain experience. Hence, when the mother states, for instance, that she feels severe pain, her statement must be believed even if it is impossible (from a physical viewpoint) to explain why her labor is so painful. The temptation to judge the mother's discomfort by the results of electronic monitoring of intrauterine pressure must also be avoided.

VALUES OF MOTHER OR FATHER. The mother or father may also harbor prejudices or values that make it difficult for the nurse to assess the pain experience. Either or both of the parents may feel the mother should minimize her responses to pain. The only appropriate response may be felt to be a verbal description of the pain. Some mothers may not even volunteer this much, so they will have to be questioned directly and at regular intervals. Still other mothers may feel the word pain should not be used and that they must not admit to feeling pain. In such cases the other words used may be deceptive. For example, the mother may verbalize feeling "enormous pressure" but refuse to call it painful. Yet the mother may need assistance in coping with this sensation, and measures designed to relieve severe pain may be very appropriate.

Still another type of problem may arise with a father who forcefully tries to impose his own goals upon the mother who does not share his values. In the situation where the father does not want the mother to admit pain or to seek assistance with pain relief measures, the nurse may find that she obtains more accurate information when the father is absent from the room. She may also discover that the mother asks the father to get the nurse, but the father merely stands in the hall and then reports to the mother that the nurse is not available. Of course, the opposite type of situation may exist. The mother may feel perfectly capable of handling the pain and discomforts of labor, but the father may become insistent that she be "put out of this misery."

Components of pain relief

Three components of pain relief will be considered: 1) the gate control theory of the mechanism of pain and pain relief, 2) the uniqueness of pain during childbirth, and 3) aspects of pain relief during labor.

Gate control theory

The mystery and complexity of pain are especially well demonstrated by the fact that no one really knows what neurophysiological mechanism underlies the sensation of pain. Through the ages a number of theories have been advanced, and the most recent of these is referred to as the gate control theory. It was first proposed in 1965 by Melzack and Wall, and has since been expanded.[10,11] Like all theories, it is not absolute truth. Rather, it uses available information to explain the phenomena of pain, suggesting reasons for known facts and offering possibilities where facts are absent.

The gate control theory is constantly subjected to debate, revision and expansion. There are numerous facets to the theory and many ways to categorize them. Hence, the following discussion will focus only on those aspects which seem most pertinent to a basic understanding of the mechanisms of pain and pain relief in childbirth.

As its name implies, the gate control theory proposes that there is a gating mechanism involved in the transmission of pain impulses. A closed gate results in no pain; an open gate, pain; a partially open gate, less pain. This gating mechanism is located in the spinal cord, perhaps in the substantia gelatinosa (a unit of cells which extends the length of the spinal cord). When the gate is closed, the transmission of pain impulses is stopped in the spinal cord—pain does not reach the level of awareness.

The transmission of pain impulses from the spinal cord to cortical awareness can be affected in at least three general ways:

1. *The activity in large and small sensory nerve fibers.* The gate is opened by excitation of small-diameter fibers that carry pain impulses. However, these pain signals can be blocked; i.e., the gate can be closed to prevent or decrease their transmission to the cortex. This can be accomplished by stimulation of large-diameter fibers. Since many cutaneous fibers are large-diameter fibers, stimulation of the skin by rubbing or other means may result in pain relief.

2. *Projections from the brain stem reticular formation.* The reticular activating system regulates or adjusts incoming and outgoing signals, including the amount of sensory input. Somatic inputs from all parts of the body, as well as visual and auditory inputs, are monitored by the reticular system. Although it is not well understood, it appears that the reticular system is influenced by certain sensory input, and on this basis the reticular system then may project inhibitory signals to the spinal cord. That is, the reticular formation may cause the gate to be closed to the transmission of pain impulses. Hence, pain signals would not reach the level of cortical awareness (no pain), or fewer pain signals would reach the brain (less intense pain).

3. *Projections from the cerebral cortex and thalamus.* Signals from the cortex or thalamus can open or close the gate to transmission of pain impulses. This may be done either indirectly by projecting through the reticular formation or directly by projecting to the spinal cord. Cognitive and affective processes are subserved at least in part by neural activity in the cortex and thalamus. Therefore, the individual's own unique

thoughts and feelings can influence the transmission of pain impulses from the spinal cord to the level of cortical awareness. Such thoughts and feelings may include the meaning of the pain, the person's beliefs, anxieties, memories of past painful experiences, and any number of other factors. Thus, input to the spinal cord is evaluated by the individual *before* it is felt as a sensation as well as afterward.

Perhaps the most important contributions made by the gate control theory are its possible explanations for the individuality of the pain experience. One thing has been clear for many years—comparable stimuli or lesions in different people do not produce comparable sensations of pain. In other words, when comparable stimuli are applied to several people, one person may perceive intense pain, another moderate pain and still another no pain at all. The gate control theory suggests mechanisms by which a myriad of factors may determine the existence of pain and influence the nature of a painful experience. In summary, these factors may include not only stimulation of pain fibers but also cutaneous stimulation, other sensory input, thoughts, and feelings.

An appreciation of the gate control theory provides a basis for understanding why each painful event is a unique and largely subjective experience. Fortunately, it also provides a basis for understanding and devising pain relief measures, as will be discussed.

Uniqueness of pain during childbirth

Most of the pain experienced by the general patient population is characterized by one or more of the following anxiety-producing factors. The patient may not know what causes the pain, may not have expected pain to occur, and may not know how to predict the course of the pain, e.g., how long it will last, how severe it will become. Pain may cause the patient to fear some dreaded illness or a long-term change in his lifestyle.

The discomfort and pain of childbirth are unique in that in most cases these common sources of anxiety need not be present. In fact, there are elements inherent in childbirth that are just the opposite of these sources of anxiety. Hence the childbirth experience has a high potential for the achievement of satisfactory pain relief. Following is a brief discussion

of those elements which render childbirth a more manageable pain experience.

ANXIETY-REDUCING KNOWLEDGE. Studies suggest that anxiety is reduced if the person knows when a painful event will occur and how long the discomfort will last.[12] Ordinarily the mother knows the approximate date of confinement and she has some idea of the approximate length of labor. In other words, she knows labor will occur, she knows the expected date within a few weeks, and she knows labor usually lasts a matter of hours, not days.

Even more helpful is the information the mother has once labor has actually begun. With the assistance of a watch she can determine the usual length of her contractions and predict when the next one will occur. In addition she knows that contractions generally become more intense and more frequent as labor progresses. And although her discomfort may increase in intensity, she is not usually in constant discomfort. Between contractions there are periods of relative comfort even during the final phase of labor contractions.

The mother also knows in general the cause of her discomfort. At least she knows it is a normal process that has something to do with the expulsion of her baby and that parts of her body are contracting and stretching to accomplish this. This is quite different from the knowledge possessed by the person who suddenly experiences his first myocardial infarction. Most mothers recognize the onset of labor and do not fear that something harmful or life-threatening is happening.

AN END-PRODUCT. The discomfort of labor is also unique in that there is a tangible end-product—the baby. This outcome, the baby, is something in which there has been deep personal involvement, both emotionally and physiologically. The involvement may have been positive and desirable or unpleasant and unwanted; the birth may be viewed as a good or bad occurrence; the baby may be kept or placed for adoption. Nevertheless, when the baby is born, the discomfort of labor subsides markedly and the event is characterized by physical and psychological closure. Few episodes of pain end so dramatically.

Aspects of pain relief during labor

This discussion of pain relief measures is focused on those other than medication. These pain relief methods may be used either instead of or in addition to analgesics and anesthetics.

The focus is purposefully limited to what the nurse may do for the mother or what she may assist the mother or father to do. Nursing activities related to the use of pharmacologic agents are discussed elsewhere.

METHODS OF PREPARED CHILDBIRTH. A partial list of methods of prepared childbirth appears on page 269; and in the discussion of assessment of the patient in labor some of the examples are taken from these various methods. Methods of prepared childbirth do not necessarily have as their primary objective the management of pain during labor. And certainly they encompass preparation for and assistance with much more than labor. Nevertheless, pain management is inherent in the preparation of the mother and/or father if other objectives are to be met. These objectives may be reduced need for analgesia and anesthesia, an awareness of the birth, or simply a personally satisfying experience for the parents. In any event, each method takes into account that some control of pain is essential. Hence it behooves the nurse to be acquainted with the nature of preparation. Many methods of prepared childbirth require a considerable investment of time and energy on the part of the parents.

The particular method of prepared childbirth used by a mother during labor may have been recommended by her physician, but more often she chooses it herself. Typically the mother and father attend a series of six or more two-hour classes during the last trimester of pregnancy. The series may be free or cost up to $35.00. The classes are usually small, about ten couples, and they are taught by an instructor specially trained in that method. In addition to attending classes and performing other related tasks, the mother and father daily practice certain activities to be used during labor. Some of these activities assist the mother to tolerate pain, or reduce the intensity of pain. Information about the processes of labor is also given in the classes. This tends to reduce anxiety in the mother and father and thereby assist them to cope with pain.

Although the majority of women having babies today have not attended classes in a method of preparation for childbirth, the number of parents seeking childbirth education definitely is increasing. Data is difficult to obtain, but in 1973 the International Childbirth Education Association (ICEA) had 65 member groups. It is estimated that they trained 30,280 couples in the United States that year.[13]

The method of prepared childbirth growing most rapidly is the Psychoprophylactic method (PPM) or Lamaze. In one area of Connecticut, for example, there were two recorded Lamaze deliveries in 1960, 78 in 1965, 590 in 1970, and 1,467 in 1973. In the Los Angeles area in 1963 there was only one Lamaze instructor; in 1973 there were over 75 and they trained about 6,000 couples. In 1974 there were over 100 Lamaze instructors in the Los Angeles area and it was estimated that they would train about 9,000 couples.[14]

Because of the growing popularity of the Lamaze method among laypeople, Table 16-2 summarizes those activities the nurse generally might expect to be used by Lamaze-trained couples during labor for the purpose of handling discomfort or pain. The nurse will encounter variations in these activities since instructors are always making efforts to improve the method and since the individual mother may adapt the method to her own particular needs.

Sometimes the nursing staff tends to spend very little time with Lamaze-trained or otherwise prepared couples. While it is true that some couples may manage quite well on their own, most couples will need some type of assistance. Knowledge of how a mother and father may attempt to cope with pain and discomfort enables the nurse to provide appropriate help. For example, when a breathing pattern has ceased to be effective, the Lamaze-trained mother may need assurance that labor has progressed sufficiently to warrant changing to the next breathing pattern. Or, when the father must leave the labor room the nurse will know how to assume some of his responsibilities such as counting or breathing with the mother.

GOALS AND PRINCIPLES OF PAIN RELIEF. Good pain relief does not necessarily mean the total elimination of painful sensations. In fact, complete abolition of pain is rarely a realistic goal. It is significantly helpful to the patient and often more reasonable to aim at a decrease in the intensity of pain and/or a decrease in the degree to which pain bothers the patient. The latter is closely related to another possible goal of increasing the patient's tolerance for pain.

Two important principles that underlie the accomplishment of these goals are 1) decreasing the pain impulses that reach the cortex of the brain, and 2) managing anxiety. The transmission of pain signals may be interrupted in a number of ways such as decreasing the source

Table 16-2 Summary of Pain Relief Measures

Approximate Progress of Labor	Position	Relaxation	Mother's Activities During Abdominal Massage
Onset to 3 cm., or contractions 5 to 20 min. apart.	Supported comfortably sitting or lying on side.	Inhales deeply at beginning of contraction and relaxes totally upon exhalation. Also takes a deep breath at end of each contraction.	Palms of one or both hands move slowly from pubic area up to umbilicus and out around abdomen down to pubic area.
Dilates from 4 to 7 cm., or contractions 2 to 4 min. apart.	Same as above.	Same as above.	Same as above.
Dilates from 8 to 10 cm., or contractions 1 min. apart.	Same as above.	Same as above.	Omitted.
Delivery.	Same as above except when pushing. For pushing: semi-propped position with back curved, head and shoulders supported by pillows, head forward. If legs not in stirrups, she holds legs under knees with elbows out and brings knees as close to shoulders as possible.	Same as above except omitted when pushing.	Omitted.

Each Contraction in Relation to			Father's Activities Either During or Between Contractions
Eye Focus	Breathing Pattern	Thoughts	
Eyes open and focused on one particular object ("concentration point").	Slow chest breathing, 6 to 9/min., inhale through nose, exhale through mouth.	On inhalation, "In, 1, 2." On exhalation, "Out, 1, 2, 3, 4."	Times frequency of each contraction.
Same as above.	Shallow chest breathing through mouth. Begins slowly, accelerates as contraction intensifies, decelerates as contraction subsides. Breathing is 4/4 rhythm.	Counts each breath in 4/4 rhythm emphasizing count of one, e.g., "1, 2, 3, 4, 1, 2, 3, 4," etc., or silently sings Yankee Doodle, a 4/4 song.	During contractions: At 15-sec. intervals he calls off time that elapses, i.e., "15 sec., 30 sec., 45 sec., 60 sec." until contraction is over. Checks for state of relaxation by moving parts of her body. As need arises may give signals to help increase relaxation, do abdominal massage for her, rub her lower back, breathe in rhythm with her, count aloud in rhythm to her breathing or sing song in rhythm, remind her of eye focus, remind her to deep breathe at end of contraction. If "back labor," may try deep counterpressure to lower back.

Between contractions: Offers encouragement; wipes face with cool, wet cloth; moistens lips and mouth with water, ice chips or lollipop. |
| Same as above. | Shallow chest breathing through mouth. Rhythm of 4, 6, or 8 breaths and then one blow. Begins slowly, accelerates and decelerates with intensity of contraction. If not allowed to push but feels urge to push, blows repeatedly. | Counts each breath according to rhythm selected, e.g., "1, 2, 3, 4, 5, 6, blow." | |
| Same as above except when pushing. Then may focus on mirror, if available, to see results of pushing. | Same as above except when pushing. For pushing: 2 or 3 deep breaths, inhale, hold breath, lean forward, slowly count to 10, release breath. Repeat inhalation and holding to count of 10 until contraction is over or until instructed to stop pushing. | Same as above except when pushing. For pushing: slowly counts to 10 during each breath holding. | Same as above except when pushing. For pushing: stands at mother's back to support her in pushing position. Counts aloud to 10 during each breath holding, tells her to take a deep breath and hold it, then counts to 10 again. |

of noxious stimuli or closing the spinal gate. Likewise there are numerous ways of managing anxiety. The desirable level of anxiety varies with the phase of the pain experience. During labor, or the phase of the presence of pain, it it desirable to have anxiety at as low a level as possible. (In contrast, prior to labor, or during the anticipation phase of pain, a moderate level of anxiety is advantageous since this motivates the patient to plan ways of coping with the impending pain.)

An appreciation of the variety of potentially effective pain relief methods available is enhanced by understanding the relationships between anxiety and pain sensations. It has long been recognized that most types of pain cause some degree of anxiety or fear and that anxiety increases the intensity of pain, or at least renders pain less tolerable and more bothersome. The gate control theory suggests that anxiety opens the gate to pain impulses, thereby actually increasing the intensity of pain. Anxiety may also increase the intensity of pain directly by causing muscle tension. In labor it is obvious that tension in the muscles of the abdomen, perineum, and lower back will increase discomfort.

The interaction between anxiety and pain may become a spiraling process. Pain may cause anxiety, and this anxiety may increase the intensity of pain by causing muscle tension or by opening the gate to pain impulses. Thus, pain increases anxiety, and anxiety increases pain which in turn causes greater anxiety. In this way mild pain and anxiety can eventually become severe pain and panic.

Pain relief measures during labor

Pain relief measures are aimed at interrupting the vicious cycle of pain and anxiety. This may be done by reducing either anxiety or pain impulses. Following is a discussion of specific nursing activities to accomplish this. Some guidelines to the effective utilization of these pain relief measures are:

1. Use a variety of pain relief measures.
2. Use pain relief measures *before* pain becomes severe. (It is easier to prevent severe pain and panic than to alleviate them once they occur.)
3. Include those pain relief measures which the patient believes will be effective.

4. Take into account the patient's ability to be active or passive in the application of the pain relief measure.
5. Regarding the potency of the pain relief measure needed, rely on the patient's behavior as indicative of the severity of pain rather than the known physical stimuli.
6. If a pain relief measure is ineffective the first time it is used during a contraction, encourage the mother to try it at least one or two more times before abandoning it.

Support during labor

From the beginning of labor the mother needs to have someone with her at increasingly frequent intervals and to know that someone is available at all times. Toward the end of labor she needs to have someone with her constantly. The presence, actions and words of this person can be very supportive to the mother. This person may be the nurse, the father or someone else. At times the nurse's greatest contribution is to support the father so that he can in turn support the mother. Specific ways the mother may be supported during labor are discussed on pages 312 to 313.

Support during labor lowers anxiety and increases the mother's ability to handle discomforts. Support, then, is a pain relief measure. It also enhances the effectiveness of other pain relief methods. Hence, it is important that other pain relief measures be implemented within the context of this type of relationship with the mother.

Giving information

As mentioned previously, part of the uniqueness of labor pain is that the mother may possess anxiety-reducing knowledge. If the mother does not obtain this information for herself, the nurse can supply it. For example, the nurse may tell the mother approximately how long it will be before the next contraction and how long that contraction will last. During intense contractions the nurse may "count down" the seconds until the end of the contraction, telling the mother how long it will be until the contraction is over. Or, the nurse may time the contraction so she can reassure the mother by telling her when the contraction has reached its peak and will begin to subside. Information about the progress of labor, e.g., cervical dilatation and descent of the baby, is also important. It serves as a reminder that there is a purpose to labor, that labor does end, and that the end is closer and closer.

Such information not only reduces anxiety but may also motivate the mother to tolerate pain. Especially toward the end of labor when discomfort increases, the knowledge that the ordeal is almost over may enable the mother to tolerate an intensity of pain that she would otherwise find unbearable.

Knowing that she and her baby are not in danger is also, of course, anxiety-reducing. Sometimes the mother finds the forces of labor so unexpectedly powerful that she is fearful of harm. The nurse should periodically reassure the mother that she and her baby are doing well (provided, of course, that this is true). She may say, for example, that the baby's heartbeat is strong and regular. Remembering that discomfort is associated with a normal process and not a life-threatening illness may be helpful to the mother. Briefly and in simple terms the nurse can remind the mother of what is happening, e.g., that each contraction enlarges the opening for the baby.

Understanding what is happening during labor seems to increase the mother's sense of control over the event. Feelings of powerlessness can be anxiety-provoking, so it is important to further feelings of control. This may be done through instructions and explanations that help the mother cooperate with examinations and with the process of labor such as effective pushing. In particular the mother's feelings of control can be strengthened by teaching her about pain relief measures as early as possible. When this has not been done prior to labor the nurse can begin in early labor to explain certain of the following pain relief measures. The mother then knows that pain relief is available, that there are several possibilities, and that to some extent she may choose from among them.

Decreasing sources of noxious stimuli

One source of noxious, or painful, stimuli is abdominal pressure on the contracting uterus. Total skeletal muscle relaxation, discussed in more detail later, relaxes the abdominal muscles and contributes to relieving pressure on the uterus. Pressure may also be prevented by either abdominal breathing or chest breathing. While there is controversy as to which breathing method best relaxes abdominal muscles, the fact seems to be that it depends largely upon the individual mother. Hence, regardless of the breathing method the mother may be using, if she feels it is exerting uncomfortable pressure on her uterus, it seems wise for the nurse to help her learn the other method.

Between contractions the nurse can assist the mother to differentiate between abdominal and chest breathing and learn to use one or the other of the methods. While the mother is lying on her back, she places one hand on her chest, the other on her abdomen. The nurse points out that during an abdominal breath, the abdomen will rise as air is inhaled. During a chest breath, the chest will rise as air is inhaled. The nurse can have the mother practice each breathing method several times. Then the mother can choose the method that seems the most comfortable and/or the easiest. However, there probably is no need for the nurse to assist the mother to differentiate between chest and abdominal breathing as long as the abdominal muscles are not contracted and the mother finds breathing easy and comfortable.

Another obvious method of reducing abdominal pressure is simply by lifting the abdominal wall. The nurse may do this for the mother, or the father may be taught to perform this maneuver. A hand must be kept on the uterus to identify the beginning of the contraction. The instant the uterus begins to contract, the nurse places both hands at waist level with the fingers pointing downward. She slides her hands down and under the mother's back until the fingertips meet at the spinal cord. The nurse then firmly and gently *lifts* until her hands rest between the pelvic bone and rib cage. As the hands are drawn from underneath the back, the hands are turned gradually (without releasing the upward lift) until the fingertips point toward the rib cage. The upward lift must be completed before the contraction reaches its peak. There should be lifting only and *no inward pressure*. When the contraction is over the upward lift is released slowly.[15]

Also possible is a more simple method of abdominal lifting, but it is equally strenuous for the nurse or father. At the beginning of the contraction the fingers are hooked under the ribs and the distended abdomen lifted as the mother inhales. In both methods of abdominal lifting it is important that the mother not arch her back, since this would cause discomfort. Depending upon the amount of pressure exerted by the hand, the latter method may also result in lifting the baby, thus removing the pressure of the uterus on the back.[16]

Decreasing the weight of the uterus and baby on the muscles and bones of the mother's back can decrease considerably the amount of noxious stimuli. This is an especially important and effective pain relief measure when the mother experiences "back labor," i.e., when the occiput of the fetus presses on the mother's sacrum. Regardless of the position of the fetus, a mother in normal labor probably will be more comfortable if she avoids the supine position.

A recent study compared the 30° upright position with the recumbent position during labor. The upright position was recommended for several reasons. Although the intensity of contractions was higher in this position, the contractions did not last any longer, the uterus relaxed more completely between contractions, and the first two stages of labor were shorter.[17] Thus, the duration of discomfort may be shortened by the upright position. This has the added advantage of reducing the danger to mother and infant that usually attends prolonged labor.

Unless there are complications such as a prolapsed cord, the mother should be allowed to choose the position she finds most comfortable. However, if she wants to lie on her back, she probably should have the head of the bed somewhat elevated and her thighs slightly flexed. Besides the 30° upright, or semisitting position, other positions commonly found comfortable during labor are the lateral Sims's and the tailor-sitting. An unusual but increasingly popular position for mothers with back labor is the up-on-all-fours position. It may even succeed in rotating the baby's head to an anterior position. If the baby's head is not in the posterior position, this crawl position may still produce pain relief, especially during transition, when labor is so often felt in the back.

As delivery approaches, most mothers feel the urge to push. However, unnecessary noxious stimuli can be eliminated if the mother understands that it is futile to push early in labor. She also prevents painful stimuli if during delivery she obeys instructions as to when she should and should not push. The urge to push can be almost irresistible. Thus the mother may need some techniques such as blowing or rapid breathing to help her refrain from pushing.

When external electronic monitoring is used the transducer may be a source of discomfort if it is secured in the same position over a period of time. The sensations of discomfort or heaviness may be decreased by moving the transducer as little as ¾ inch.

Distraction

Research studies as well as personal experiences confirm that distraction is an effective method of pain relief. The gate control theory provides some possible explanation. When the cerebral cortex is involved in activity (cortical excitation), the gate may be closed to pain by pain-blocking signals sent to the spinal cord. The cortex may signal a decreased attention to pain impulses. Or, the reticular system in the brain stem may register that there is sufficient incoming stimuli and therefore signal the gate to be closed to further stimuli—painful stimuli in this case.

Regardless of the theoretical mechanism for pain relief through distraction, common sense suggests that pain will be more tolerable if the patient becomes less aware of it—in short, distracted from it. A person may be distracted from pain in an almost limitless variety of ways.

Instructors of methods of prepared childbirth have devised and taught many different means of distraction for use during contractions. It is interesting to note that a large number of these are rhythmic in nature, such as "riding the wave," tapping out the rhythm of a song, rhythmic head movements, and rhythmic breathing. The method of distraction tends to change as labor progresses, seemingly taking into account the increasing intensity of pain and the increasing effort the mother must exert to engage in any activity not related to labor. Thus, as demonstrated by the Lamaze method (see Table 16-2), during transition abdominal massage is eliminated and a relatively more easy breathing pattern is adopted. As a rule, the more intense the pain the more involved the patient must become in the distraction to achieve pain relief. However, the involvement must be compatible with the patient's ability.

Table 16-2 provides examples from the Lamaze method of activities that may serve as distracters. Many of these activities have other purposes as well. The breathing rhythms and purposeful thoughts undoubtedly serve as distracters, but maintenance of rhythmic breathing is also thought to relieve pain by providing adequate oxygenation of the uterus. While relaxation, too, serves other purposes such as anxiety reduction and prevention of abdominal pressure, the mother may find that her concentrated efforts to relax provide a significant distraction. Changing positions and massaging the abdomen require both motor and cognitive effort, and therefore may be distracting. Keeping the eyes open and focused on a particular point is perhaps the purest and simplest distracter. Altogether, the Lamaze-trained mother consciously performs several varied activities with the end result of distraction from pain.

Other breathing patterns for use during contractions are suggested by the Maternity Center Association and are described in Chapter 13, pages 230 to 233.

A brief comparison of the Lamaze method and the Maternity Center Association method reveal some of the ideas common to most methods of prepared childbirth—concentration on relaxation and a rhythmic breathing pattern during contractions.

The nurse needs to be familiar with a variety of distracters that she may suggest to the mother. What is sufficiently distracting for one mother may not be for another. And, a mother may need assistance with distracters even if she has attended classes in a method of prepared childbirth.

Emphasis here will be placed on distracters that are of some proven effectiveness and also relatively easy to teach the mother. Most of the techniques taught in the Maternity Center Association (MCA) method and the Lamaze method meet these criteria. (A review of the information in the page numbers mentioned above and Table 16-2 will assist the reader in the following discussion of these distracters.) Some distracters used in the various methods of prepared childbirth are extremely distracting but difficult to teach quickly once labor is in progress.

Early in labor the mother may be able to distract herself by "walking and talking" through a contraction. As labor progresses, some form of rhythmic breathing pattern is usually helpful. Slow rhythmic breathing is both relaxing and distracting, examples being either the "complete breathing" of the MCA or the "slow chest breathing" of Lamaze. If this is not effective, the nurse may suggest adding some of the distracters of the Lamaze method, e.g., a concentration point, counting during inhalation and exhalation, and/or abdominal massage.

When discomfort intensifies and a more powerful form of distraction is needed, the nurse may teach the mother the "modified complete breathing" of MCA or the accelerating and decelerating "shallow chest breathing" of the Lamaze method. Either of these may result in hyperventilation so the nurse should caution the mother to inform her of any dizziness or tingling. Hyperventilation may be treated by having the mother breathe into a paper bag and suggesting that henceforth she breathe more slowly. Again, more distraction may be added to these breathing patterns by incorporating one or more of the distracters of the Lamaze method—the concentration point, abdominal massage, silent counting or singing in rhythm with breathing. Another effective and relatively easy distracter to employ is finger tapping the rhythm to a 4/4 song, coordinating the rhythm with breathing.

Of all the breathing patterns suggested here, the one most likely to be difficult for the mother to learn during labor is the accelerated and decelerated aspect of the Lamaze "shallow chest breathing." If the mother finds this or any other distracter too difficult or fatiguing, it should be abandoned.

During transition the mother's focus tends to become extremely narrow because of the great increase in the intensity of contractions. Whereas earlier in labor the distracters could be suggested and taught between contractions, there is little time now and it is difficult for the mother to focus on anything but labor. Therefore distracters to be used during transition should be more simple and must be taught prior to the onset of transition. The Lamaze method suggests rhythmic, shallow chest breathing with blowing. Although this breathing pattern includes acceleration and deceleration with the intensity of the contraction, it is an easy breathing pattern to learn and use. The MCA suggests "modified complete breathing" with the further modification of puffing out gently upon exhalation of every third or fourth breath. Simple additions to these breathing rhythms may include coordinated and silent counting and/or use of a concentration point.

When the nurse wishes to assist the laboring mother with pain relief measures in the form of distracters, it is only reasonable to approach the mother between, not during, contractions. The nurse can describe briefly one or two possibilities. This needs to be accompanied by some explanation, such as, "It may seem silly at first, but many mothers find that it makes the contractions less bothersome because it forces them to think of something else." The mother should be asked to decide which one she would like to try first. It usually is most helpful if the nurse first demonstrates the pattern and then has the mother do it. If a song or counting is to be used, it is often much easier for the mother if the nurse counts or sings for her during the first contractions in which the pattern is used.

Certainly not everyone deals with pain in the same way. That is why it is so necessary to involve the mother in a decision about which distracters she would like to use. If the mother does not like any of the distracters discussed in this section, the nurse may creatively invent some others or simply ask the mother for suggestions. Some mothers prefer a form of distraction that is characterized by an inward focus rather than the outward focus of the distracters described here. For example, the mother may stare into space or close her eyes and focus on the forces of her body, concentrating on the contraction being a wavelike force that she envisions herself on top of.

We have not yet begun to uncover and understand fully the various strategies people use to cope with pain. These strategies include much more than distraction, but within the area of distraction there are numerous approaches.[18]

Whatever type of distracters the mother may choose to use during a contraction, the nurse and others must take care not to distract her from using them. Early in labor it may be a helpful distraction to the mother to have someone to talk with during a contraction, but later she may find this irritating because it interferes with other strategies for coping with pain. In any event, the nurse needs to find out from the mother what, if anything, she wants the nurse to do for her during a contraction.

Cutaneous stimulation

Rubbing a painful body part is a universal activity. The gate control theory provides a possible reason for the effectiveness of this and other forms of cutaneous stimulation. As discussed previously, the theory suggests that a gating mechanism in the spinal cord can be partially or completely closed to the transmission of pain impulses to the cortex by stimulation of large-diameter nerve fibers. Because many cutaneous fibers are large-diameter fibers, stimulation of the skin may result in pain relief.

Several types of cutaneous stimulation may be used during labor and may prove to be effective pain relief measures. Rubbing the lower back is common. The Lamaze method describes a type of abdominal massage. The application of heat or cold (with the physician's permission) may be especially comforting to the patient with "back labor."

The above are examples of relatively moderate stimulation of cutaneous fibers. Mild to moderate stimulation is ordinarily more effective than intense stimulation. However, one notable exception is the use of intense pressure over the sacrum during a contraction. The pressure may be applied with the knee or fist, or the mother may lean back (in a semisitting position) on a tennis ball or rolling pin. It has been estimated that pressure so applied during a contraction is equivalent to the pain relief potential of 50 to 100 mg. of meperidine.[19]

Rubbing of any part of the body, even between contractions, possibly may contribute to pain relief. This not only encourages relaxation, but experimentation with cutaneous stimulation shows that it may help close the spinal gate to painful impulses long after its usage and that the painful area need not always be the area of stimulation.[20] An example of the latter is the pain relief felt by the laboring mother when her feet are massaged.

Relaxation

Virtually every method of prepared childbirth heavily emphasizes total skeletal muscle relaxation during labor. Relaxation contributes to pain relief in a variety of ways. Some of these have already been mentioned, such as relaxing the abdominal muscles to decrease the noxious stimuli of pressure on the uterus.

But even when noxious stimuli are not affected directly, skeletal muscle relaxation is itself a pain relief measure. It accomplishes this by interrupting the spiraling process of pain and anxiety. Muscle tension is a response to pain and/or anxiety. Since relaxation is the opposite of muscle tension, it prevents or diminishes tension. The behavioral response of relaxation, therefore, is incompatible with pain-anxiety responses. Some research suggests that a person's evaluation of the intensity of pain is in part a function of her evaluation of her own overt behavioral response to pain.[21] Possibly when the patient observes herself relaxed instead of tense, she evaluates her pain as less intense. Or, relaxation may cause the cortex to send signals to close the spinal gate to the transmission of pain impulses.

Undoubtedly relaxation provides pain relief for other reasons, depending upon the individual patient. For some patients efforts to relax can serve as a distraction from pain. In other patients a state of relaxation may increase suggestibility, causing the patient to accept explicit and implicit suggestions of comfort.[22]

How can the patient achieve total skeletal muscle relaxation? Possibly the most frequently used but most unproductive method is for the nurse to say, "Relax." The verbal cue "relax" may be used effectively with patients who have been trained in relaxation, but to the untrained patient such a command often sounds impossible, if not absurd. The patient's inability to follow such an instruction may engender feelings of powerlessness and failure.

People may be trained in relaxation techniques in many different ways and for many reasons besides childbirth. Relaxation techniques are also used to handle anxiety unrelated to any form of pain, e.g., the tensions of daily living. When the nurse encounters a mother who has been trained in relaxation techniques, she simply finds out how best to assist her. It is particularly helpful to identify those cues which will encourage relaxation if the mother becomes tense. These cues may be verbal, such as "relax," or tactile-kinesthetic, such as touching or moving the tense body part.

If the mother has not been trained in relaxation, the nurse may use some simple techniques that are capable of making a significant difference in the mother's level of relaxation. The nurse first explains to the mother that relaxing during a contraction is very important because it can decrease abdominal pressure on the uterus and also help her feel more calm and generally comfortable. The quickest and easiest ways to promote relaxation are to instruct the mother to take a deep breath or to yawn and to "go limp" or relax as she exhales. The nurse suggests that the mother try one or both of these at the beginning and end of contractions and anytime during contractions that she feels the need to relax. (The patient who chooses to yawn may find it becomes spontaneous and more frequent. Because yawning is highly contagious the nurse may find the same thing happening to her.)

These techniques are effective because they take advantage of conditioned responses. Both a big sigh (deep breath) and a yawn are associated with relaxation.

Relaxation may be furthered by providing support to comfortably positioned and slightly flexed extremities. Also, the nurse may gently move extremities and the head to test for the degree of relaxation. This slight movement enables the mother to feel tense muscles and helps her to relax them.

Assistance with change in expectations and goals

During the relatively brief and rapidly moving events of labor, any unexpected change in the parent's goals or expectations must be handled quickly. Otherwise anxiety may persist or increase, resulting in an increased intensity of pain. Some items listed in Part V of Table 16-1 are examples of areas in which a disturbing change may occur.

Sometimes the mother's personal obstetrician is not available, and a physician unknown to the parents must manage labor and delivery. Or, the mother and father may have expected to be together throughout labor, but perhaps the father cannot be located or is unable to get to the hospital. In some instances the labor suite is too crowded or the delivery room too small to accommodate the father. He may be excluded if there is a lack of personnel to supervise him in the delivery room or if complications of an emergency nature arise. Crowding and lack of staffing may also prevent the parents from enjoying the homelike atmosphere they desire, e.g., a calm environment in which they can eat, visit and walk around.

If external or internal electronic monitoring of the fetus is used, this may be disconcerting to parents for several reasons. The parents may be very fearful if they associate its usage with possible complications. Most hospitals monitor only high-risk situations, but some hospitals routinely monitor all patients. Regardless of the reason for electronic monitoring, the parents may strongly object to the use of such equipment because it renders childbirth less of a natural experience. In addition, external monitoring in particular will make it difficult for the parents to use certain pain relief measures such as abdominal lifting, abdominal massage, and some positioning. Often external monitoring requires that the mother lie quietly on her back. If this is disturbing to the parents, the nurse should, if possible, remove the external monitoring equipment for a few contractions so that the parents can employ some of their pain relief activities.

When a situation occurs that disturbs the parents the nurse encourages them to express their feelings, and she indicates an appreciation of their disappointment. She then explains the reasons for any rules, policies, or circumstances that prevent them from achieving their goals or expectations.

One of the more difficult problems is assisting the parents who are not able to achieve their "ideal" of labor and delivery. This ideal may vary considerably from one couple to another and may consist of any one or combination of goals referred to previously (see Table 16-1 and related discussion). Inability to achieve this ideal labor may cause profound feelings of failure in the mother or father. Also, they may refuse or be very reluctant to accept measures incompatible with their ideal.

Patients who have specific expectations or goals associated with an ideal labor may have arrived at these in a number of ways. But these parents seem most often to be a product of classes that prepare them in a specific method of childbirth. One of the most common criticisms of methods of prepared childbirth is that the mother and father are taught to strive for a particular kind of labor and delivery experience, e.g., no medication, ecstasy over the delivery. The majority of childbirth educators do not currently state such goals. Yet parents, especially mothers, tend to adopt such goals and feel a sense of failure if they are not achieved. The reason for this is not usually related to what the childbirth educator says. Rather the goals are implicit in personal narratives and films to which the mother is exposed.

Written personal labor experiences are found in books and may be available from the childbirth educator's collections about former students. Some methods of childbirth use their own particular film to introduce their method to the parents. Examples are "The Story of Eric," showing the use of the Lamaze method, and "Childbirth for the Joy of It," showing the use of Husband-Coached Childbirth. Viewing these films, it is easy to understand why the mother or father would desire the same "ideal" experience. The films focus not on pain but on the techniques of the particular method of childbirth and on the parents' extreme happiness immediately following delivery. These films are especially persuasive because the parents probably have never seen any other labor.

At the end of the film, with tears of joy in her eyes, the pregnant woman is not likely to want to settle for less than what she has just seen. She may reason, "If those women can give birth that way, I should be able to do it too." Hence, the feeling of failure or not being "good at childbirth" may result if the mother finds that she is unable to go through her own labor as she saw it portrayed in film or in written narratives.

How does the nurse help the mother and father minimize feelings of failure and accept a change in their goals? Throughout childbirth, and particularly when goals must change, the nurse praises the mother and father for their efforts and abilities to handle labor. This promotes feelings of success. For example, the mother may have the goal of an unmedicated labor, but she may find the discomfort intolerable and request medication. If medication is given, the nurse can verbalize that she knows medication was not planned. She can allow the mother to express her feelings and then praise the mother for the success of her efforts up to now and for the length of time medication was not necessary. She may add that the mother's continuing efforts may reduce the amount of medication required.

The mother may, however, choose to handle the above situation in a different manner. She may decide it is in the best interests of herself and her baby for her not to request medication, in spite of how intolerable she finds the pain. Such pain may cause her to become extremely tense and unable to cooperate with examinations or the forces of labor. This may prolong labor and increase the possibility of complications. If medication seems highly desirable, the nurse may find it necessary to use a direct approach with the mother to modify her perceptions of the situation. This may be accomplished by stating how the health team views the situation and pointing out differences in this view and the mother's perceptions. One thing the nurse may point out is that the mother wants to avoid both medication and complications, but the two goals are now incompatible.

This direct approach tends to cause unpleasant psychological tension, called cognitive dissonance. In other words, the mother's goals are at dissonance, or at odds, with one another and with the knowledge received from the nurse. Cognitive dissonance may motivate a person to change. One way to reduce dissonance in this case is for the mother to change her own beliefs to be more consistent with the nurse's opinion.[23]

Another approach to this type of situation is to employ analogy. This may disrupt the mother's denial of what is actually happening, assist her with a clearer understanding of the situation, and/or foster feelings of "normality" about her childbirth experience. Explaining the situation by comparing it with something else allows the mother to distance herself from the actual situation. She is able to understand the problem but avoid the anxiety associated with looking directly at the problem.[24]

Continuing with the former example, the nurse may compare labor to a menstrual cycle. She may say that no two labors are exactly alike, just as no two women have exactly the same menstrual cycle. She may point out that everyone's uterus acts a little differently. The length of a menstrual cycle may be 28 or 32 days, it may or may not be accompanied by cramps, and the flow may vary in length and amount. She may continue by saying that in the same way each labor is individual, a little different from anyone else's. She may add that some women "normally" experience more pain than others. Or she may cite some other symptom or sign that explains the need for a change in the mother's goal.

Aftermath assimilation

After anticipation of pain and the presence of pain, a third and final phase of the pain experience occurs—the aftermath. The pain experience does not end with the cessation of the painful sensations. The patient does not necessarily immediately forget about the pain, especially if it was severe, frightening or in any way disconcerting.

On the maternity unit it is a common observation that mothers talk a great deal about their childbirth experiences. It is a frequent topic of conversation regardless of whether the mother experienced "ecstasy," "failure," or simply relief mixed with satisfaction. Not only may the mother want to talk about the pain, but a variety of feelings resulting from the pain may be present, such as nausea, vomiting, chills, anger or embarrassment. The mother may even have nightmares about the pain.

Clearly, at least some mothers will need assistance during the aftermath phase of the pain experience. The most appropriate nursing action may be to assist the mother with the intellectual and emotional assimilation of her childbirth experience. In a sense the nurse helps the mother relive her labor. The nurse can ask the mother questions that help her discuss her discomforts, emotions, thoughts, overt responses, and the reactions of others during her labor. The nurse needs to be particularly alert and responsive to the mother's needs for support, e.g., praise, confirmation that her perceptions of discomfort are believed by others, or reassurance that her behavior was acceptable. Some patients will need information to help them fill in memory gaps or to correct understandings that are inaccurate and anxiety-provoking.[25]

Assimilation is particularly important to encourage in mothers who may harbor feelings of failure about childbirth. For all mothers assimilation may help maintain or restore a positive self-concept and aid in the ability of the mother to deal with mothering and other impending tasks.

Bibliography

1. Clark, A. L., *et al*: MCH in American Samoa. *Am. J. Nurs.* 74:700-702, April 1974.
2. McCaffery, M.: *Nursing Management of the Patient with Pain.* Philadelphia, J. B. Lippincott, 1972, p. 8.
3. *Ibid.*, pp. 11-24.
4. Copp, L. A.: The spectrum of suffering. *Am. J. Nurs.* 74:491, Mar. 1974.
5. Sasmor, J. L., Castor, C. R., and Hassid, P.: The childbirth team during labor. *Am. J. Nurs.* 73:444-447, Mar. 1973.
6. Ulin, P. R.: Changing techniques in psychoprophylactic preparation for childbirth. *Am. J. Nurs.* 68:2586-2591, Dec. 1968.
7. Burgess, A. C., and Burns, J.: Why patients seek care. *Am. J. Nurs.* 73:314-316, Feb. 1973.
8. McCaffery, M.: Intelligent approach to intractable pain. *Nurs. '73* 3:29, Nov. 1973.
9. *Ibid.*
10. Melzack, R., and Wall, P. D.: Pain mechanisms: a new theory. *Sci.* 150:971-979, 1965.
11. ———: *The Puzzle of Pain.* New York, Basic Books, 1973.
12. Jones, A., Bentler, P. M., and Petry, G.: The reduction of uncertainty concerning future pain. *J. Abnorm. Psych.* 71:87-94, April 1966.
13. Data obtained from ICEA, 1414 NW 85th St., Seattle, WA 98117.
14. Data obtained from The American Society for Psychoprophylaxis in Obstetrics, Inc., 1523 L St., NW, Suite 410, Washington, D.C. 20005.
15. Gamper, M.: *Preparation for the Heir Minded.* Illinois, Margaret Gamper, 1971, p. 48.
16. Bean, C. A.: *Methods of Childbirth.* New York, Dolphin Books, 1974, pp. 103-104.

17. Liu, Y. C.: Effects of an upright position during labor. *Am. J. Nurs.* 74:2202-2205, Dec. 1974.
18. Copp, *op. cit.*, pp. 492-495.
19. Pace, J. B.: Psychophysiology of pain: diagnostic and therapeutic implications. *J. Fam. Practice* 1:4, May 1974.
20. McCaffery, *op. cit.*, 1972, pp. 130-132.
21. Bandler, R. J., Jr., Madaras, G. R., and Bem, D. J.: Self-observation as a source of pain perception.

J. Pers. Soc. Psych. 9:205-209, July 1968.
22. Chertok, L.: *Motherhood and Personality: Psychosomatic Aspects of Childbirth.* Philadelphia, Tavistock Publications and J. B. Lippincott, 1969, pp. 13-16.
23. Miller, J.: Cognitive dissonance in modifying families' perceptions. *Am. J. Nurs.* 74:1468-1470, Aug. 1974.
24. Wacker, M. S.: Analogy: weapon against denial. *Am. J. Nurs.* 74:71-73, Jan. 1974.
25. McCaffery, *op. cit.*, 1972, pp. 193-200.

Suggested Reading

Acupuncture in labor. *Curr. Concepts Pain Analgesia* 1:15, 1975.

BAER, E., DAVITZ, L. J., AND LIEB, R.: Inferences of physical pain and psychological distress. I. *In* Relation to verbal and nonverbal patient communication. *Nurs. Research* 19:388-392, Sept./Oct. 1970.

BEAN, C. A.: *Methods of Childbirth.* New York, Dolphin Books, 1974.

BING, E.: *Six Practical Lessons for Easier Childbirth.* New York, Grosset and Dunlap, 1967.

BOWES, W. A., *et al*: The effects of obstetrical medication on fetus and infant. *Mono. Soc. Res. Child Dev.* 35:1-55, 1970.

BRADLEY, R. A.: *Husband-Coached Childbirth.* New York, Harper and Row, 1974.

BURGESS, A. C., AND BURNS, J.: Why patients seek care. *Am. J. Nurs.* 73:314-316, Feb. 1973.

CHERTOK, L.: *Motherhood and Personality: Psychosomatic Aspects of Childbirth.* Philadelphia, J. B. Lippincott, 1969.

CLARK, A. L., *et al*: MCH in American Samoa. *Am. J. Nurs.* 74:700-702, April 1974.

COPP, L. A.: The spectrum of suffering. *Am. J. Nurs.* 74:491-495, Mar. 1974.

CORAH, N. L., AND BOFFA, J.: Perceived control, self-observation, and response to aversive stimulation. *J. Pers. Soc. Psych.* 16:1-4, Sept. 1970.

DAVENPORT-SLACK, B., AND BOYLAN, C. H.: Psychological correlates of childbirth pain. *Psychosom. Med.* 36:215-223, May-June 1974.

DELYSER, F.: *A Professional's Guide to Prepared Childbirth.* Washington, D.C., American Society for Psycho-Prophylaxis in Obstetrics, Nov. 1973.

DICK-READ, G.: *Childbirth Without Fear.* New York, Harper & Row, 1972.

DIERS, D., *et al*: The effect of nursing interaction on patients in pain. *Nurs. Research* 21:419-428, Sept./Oct. 1972.

GAMPER, M.: *Preparation for the Heir Minded.* Illinois, Margaret Gamper, 1971.

HACKETT, T. P.: Pain and prejudice: why do we doubt that the patient is in pain? *Res. Staff Physician* 18:100-109, May 1972.

HAIRE, D.: The Cultural Warping of Childbirth. Seattle, Wash., International Childbirth Education Association Supplies Center, 1974.

HASSID, P.: PPM derives its effectiveness from the gate control theory. *Am. J. Nurs.* 74:827, May 1974.

HOTT, J.: An investigation of the relationship between psychoprophylaxis in childbirth and changes in self-concept of the participant husband and his concept of his wife. *Image* 5:11-15, 1972.

JACOX, A., AND STEWART, M.: *Psychosocial Contingencies of the Pain Experience.* Iowa, University of Iowa, 1973.

JOHNSON, J. E., AND RICE, V. H.: Sensory and distress components of pain: implications for the study of clinical pain. *Nurs. Res.* 23:203-209, May/June 1974.

KARMEL, M.: *Thank You, Doctor Lamaze.* Philadelphia, J. B. Lippincott, 1959.

KITZINGER, S.: *Experience of Childbirth.* London, Victor Gollancz Ltd., 1972.

KROGER, W. S.: *Childbirth with Hypnosis.* Hollywood, Wilshire Book Company, 1965.

LENNANE, K. J., AND LENNANE, R. J.: Alleged psychogenic disorders in women—a possible manifestation of sexual prejudice. *N. Eng. J. Med.* 288:288-292, Feb. 1973.

LEPPERT, P., AND WILLIAMS, B.: Birth films may miscarry. *Am. J. Nurs.* 68:2181-2183, Oct. 1968.

LIU, Y. C.: Effects of an upright position during labor. *Am. J. Nurs.* 74:2202-2205, Dec. 1974.

Maternity Center Association: *Preparation for Childbearing.* New York, The Association, 1972.

MCCAFFERY, M.: *Nursing Management of the Patient with Pain.* Philadelphia, J. B. Lippincott, 1972.

MELZACK, R.: *The Puzzle of Pain.* New York, Basic Books, 1973.

MILLER, J.: Cognitive dissonance in modifying families' perceptions. *Am. J. Nurs.* 74:1468-1470, Aug. 1974.

NEUFELD, R. W. J., AND DAVIDSON, P. O.: The effects of vicarious and cognitive rehearsal on pain tolerance. *J. Psychosom. Res.* 15:329-335, Sept. 1971.

SASMOR, J. L., CASTOR, C. R., AND HASSID, P.: The childbirth team during labor. *Am. J. Nurs.* 73:444-447, Mar. 1973.

SHEALY, C. N., AND MAURER, D.: Transcutaneous nerve stimulation for control of pain.—A preliminary technical note. *Surg. Neurol.* 2:45-47, 1974.

SIEGELE, D. S.: The gate control theory. *Am. J. Nurs.* 74:498-502, Mar. 1974.

SMITH, B. A., PRIORE, R. M., AND STERN, M. K.: The transition phase of labor. *Am. J. Nurs.* 73:448-450, Mar. 1973.

STERNBACK, R. A.: *Pain: A Psychophysiological Analysis.* New York, Academic Press, 1968.

STRAUSS, A., *et al*: Pain: an organizational-work-interactional perspective. *Nurs. Outlook* 22:560-566, Sept. 1974.

TANZER, D.: Natural childbirth: pain or peak experience. *Psych. Today* 2:17-21, 69, Oct. 1968.

ULIN, P. R.: Changing techniques in psychoprophylactic preparation for childbirth. *Am. J. Nurs.* 68:2586-2591, Dec. 1968.

WACKER, M. S.: Analogy: weapon against denial. *Am. J. Nurs.* 74:71-73, Jan. 1974.

WHITE, J. R.: Effects of a counterirritant on perceived pain and hand movement in patients with arthritis. *Phys. Ther.* 53:956-960, Sept. 1973.

WRIGHT, E.: *The New Childbirth.* New York, Hart Publishing Co., 1966.

analgesia and anesthesia for labor

The discomfort endured by women in childbirth has been related in the historical records since the time of early civilizations. It was not until the middle of the 19th century that medical science introduced anesthesia for delivery.

Recent years have witnessed significant advances in our ability to control the discomfort which can be associated with labor safely and to provide appropriate anesthetic modalities in those situations requiring operative intervention. Since labor and delivery are generally looked upon as physiologic experiences, the choice of anesthesia and analgesia is a controversial area. It involves a great burden of responsibility because two patients, mother and fetus, must be considered, and the duration of the process occupies several hours. The effect of a given agent on maternal physiology, labor itself, placental exchange of oxygen (affected materially by maternal hypotension) and the fetal respiratory system must be carefully considered. Choice of agents, usually elective or semielective, is influenced by maternal attitudes as well as by the physician's bias in favor of one approach over another. A good level of communication among physician, nurse and patient improves the ability to select just the right approach in a given situation, and can make labor and delivery a joyous and satisfactory experience for all involved.

General principles

In spite of the fact that delivery may be several months away when the pregnant woman makes her initial visit to the obstetrician, she is often anxious to know about labor and delivery and anesthesia and analgesia. She may have some rather definite ideas as the result of previous experience, the experience and advice of friends and relatives, or her own research into the matter. Others have no particular opinions but are nonetheless anxious to hear those of the obstetrician. It is well for the physician to advise the patient, at this time, of the several methods which exist, briefly describing each and suggesting reading material, if applicable. Generally, it is well to leave the matter open, especially if the obstetrician has not had an opportunity to get to know the patient. The patient should also be advised that, although she may help to decide upon the type of analgesia or anesthesia for a normal labor and delivery, complications may dictate a change in plans. Having had an initial discussion with the patient, it is well to rediscuss the subject

289

as the time of delivery approaches. The physician and the nurse should help the patient avoid preoccupation with the type of anesthesia and direct her thoughts to the birth of a healthy baby.

Every woman experiences a degree of discomfort during labor, unless there has been an interruption of the nerve supply to the uterus, as would be the case in a paraplegic. This discomfort is the result of several factors, including the stimulation of pressure-sensitive nerve endings in the cervix and ischemia of the uterine muscle during contractions. The level of discomfort of the woman in labor is modified by numerous factors, including previous experiences, prenatal education, emotional stability, parity, fetal size and position, pelvic capacity, and the emotional support of those attending her labor. In addition, there are a variety of analgesic and anesthetic methods which can be used by the obstetrician in conjunction with the anesthesiologist. In every method which will be described, a balance must be struck between the comfort of the patient and possible adverse effects upon the fetus. Any method selected must be clearly outlined to the patient and to the father if he is participating. Departures from the plan, if dictated by the obstetric situation, should also be explained to the patient, if time permits.

Methods

Natural childbirth

This term applies to a rather broad and general philosophy of labor management. Such methods are based upon the principle that, with careful prenatal education, the support of obstetrician, nurses and husband, and the application of controlled breathing and voluntary muscle relaxation, the need for anesthesia and analgesia can be minimized, if not eliminated. The effectiveness of these methods is not based primarily on the physical techniques employed, but rather on the total involvement and acquired knowledge of the patient and her husband, and the interest of the people supporting her.

The methods outlined by the British obstetrician, Grantly Dick-Read, have more recently been replaced in popularity by the Lamaze method or psychoprophylaxis, an approach involving controlled breathing and active participation by the husband. Instructions in the use of such an approach are available in most areas

through private tutors, or an organization known as the Childbirth Education Association. If such instruction is not available, there are a number of books which the obstetrician and his patient may use. Such an approach is not applicable to all patients, and the key to a successful application of the technique is motivation. Those interested only because of intellectual curiosity, or those talked into the idea, generally do poorly. Patients who select this approach should understand that, even though they may fail to get through their entire labor without anesthesia, they have still accomplished something and should not feel guilty. When used successfully, this approach can be a very rewarding experience for all concerned.

Hypnosis

This technique is not used frequently but has some of the same advantages as the natural childbirth approaches, namely, the absence of agents which might depress the fetus. However, the use of hypnosis requires special training for the obstetrician, a patient who is a good subject, and often a considerable amount of prenatal training of the patient.

Narcotics

Narcotics are the most common form of analgesia used in this country. The most common narcotic used is the synthetic compound meperidine hydrochloride (Demerol). Meperidine resembles morphine as an analgesic, although many feel it is less depressant to respiration. The drug may be given intravenously or intramuscularly in doses of 50 to 100 mg. The dose is smaller and the duration of action less when the intravenous route is used. As a general principle, narcotics are withheld until labor is in the active phase. This avoids prolongation of the latent phase. It is also well to avoid a dose of meperidine late in labor. This would produce a high blood level of meperidine in the baby at birth. Although it is often said that an average dose of narcotic will not depress a healthy full-term fetus in an uncomplicated labor, the number of qualifying conditions is such that unnecessary chances are not justified.

Tranquilizers

These drugs, in the form of phenothiazines and other agents (e.g., Phenergan, Largon, Vistaril, Sparine, Valium), have become very popular in recent years. These agents are used in combination with narcotics whose action they potentiate, thus reducing the dose of narcotic to be used. In addition to this action, these drugs are also effective antinauseants and reduce anxiety.

Barbiturates

These are hypnotics and are effective in reducing the tension and fear of the patient in labor. These agents are not analgesics, and they produce excitement rather than sedation if administered alone in the presence of pain. Barbiturates are not well handled by the newborn and should generally be avoided in advanced labor. Thus, these agents are most useful in the patient in early labor whose major problem is apprehension, rather than pain. The more common barbiturates in use are sodium pentobarbital (Nembutal), sodium secobarbital (Seconal), and sodium amobarbital (Amytal). They may be used orally, intramuscularly, or intravenously in doses of 100 to 300 mg.

Scopolamine

This belladonna alkaloid depresses the parasympathetic nervous system and is used in labor because it is also capable of producing amnesia. The latter effect is desired by some patients, although this approach is less popular now than it was several years ago. In the presence of pain, if adequate analgesia is not provided along with scopolamine, excitement, and even hallucinations and delirium, may result. This is a most unpleasant situation, and when it occurs the patient may even sustain injuries as a result of the uncontrolled activity. When the patient is in labor under the influence of this drug, she may respond to the discomfort of contractions by crying out or grimacing but remembers nothing of it when it is over, unless specifically reminded. Every precaution should be taken to protect the patient from injury (this includes side rails on the labor bed) including constant observation.

Regional anesthesia and analgesia

This designation refers to all those techniques which produce anesthesia in the anatomical area supplied by the nerve or nerves blocked. These techniques have the common advantage of reducing discomfort in the mother without significant effect on the fetus. All of these techniques are of course risky if the patient is allergic to one or more of the "caine" drugs, or if the amount used and consequently

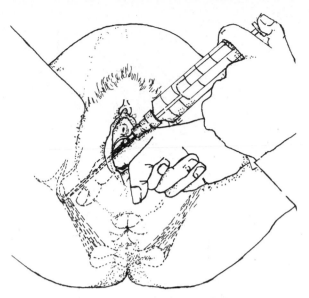

Figure 17-1. Pudendal block done transvaginally with the examiner's finger guiding the needle to the ischial spine and pudendal nerve.

absorbed into the circulation is too great. In questioning a patient regarding reaction to these agents, it is important to ask about previous dental procedures for which they are commonly used.

LOCAL INFILTRATION can be used for performing and repairing episiotomies, as well as for the repair of lacerations. Procaine (Novocaine), lidocaine (Xylocaine) and mepivacaine (Carbocaine) are the commonly used agents, in 0.5 to 1.0 percent solution.

PUDENDAL BLOCK produces more extensive perineal anesthesia, as well as relaxation of the

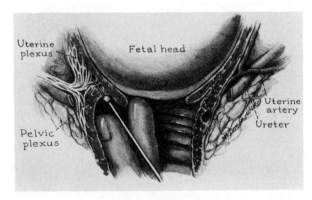

Figure 17-2. Technique of paracervical block. Schematic coronal section (enlarged) of lower portion of cervix and upper portion of vagina showing relation of needle to paracervical region. (Bonica, J. J.: Principles and Practice of Analgesia and Anesthesia, Philadelphia, F. A. Davis, 1967)

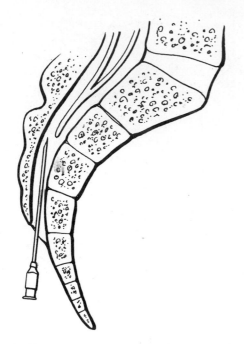

Figure 17-3. Sagittal section of sacral canal, with caudal needle properly placed in the caudal space.

superficial perineal muscles. Although this injection can be made through the perineal skin, it is more comfortable and more successful when the injection is made through the vaginal mucosa directly over the ischial spines (Fig. 17-1). The block is done on both sides just prior to delivery; it does not have any effect on the discomfort of uterine contractions.

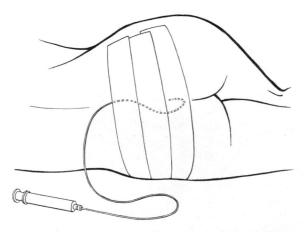

Figure 17-4. Continuous caudal analgesia, catheter method. The patient is in modified Sims's position, with legs properly placed as necessary for "laying" the caudal catheter. The Pitkin's syringe for continuous technique is shown attached to the caudal catheter in place in the caudal canal. Note method of taping the catheter in place.

PARACERVICAL BLOCK is the transvaginal injection of an anesthetic solution on each side of the cervix (Fig. 17-2). This can relieve the pain of uterine contractions for 45 to 60 minutes. The technique is relatively simple to master, is effective in a high percentage of patients, and is especially useful in the multiparous patient whose labor is progressing rapidly. The need for repeated injections when a longer period of analgesia is required makes the technique somewhat cumbersome, although several types of indwelling paracervical catheters are now being used. Transient fetal bradycardia occurs occasionally following the injection and fetal deaths have been reported, probably because of rapid absorption of the anesthesia from the very vascular paracervical area. To avoid this, the total dose and concentration of the anesthetic should be reduced.

CAUDAL ANESTHESIA is a form of analgesia and anesthesia achieved by "blocking" the nerves in the peridural space. The anesthetic agent is introduced into the peridural space via the sacral hiatus. This opening leads to a space within the sacrum known as the caudal canal or the caudal space (Fig. 17-3). The space is really the lowest extent of the bony spinal canal. Through it a rich network of sacral nerves passes downward after the nerves have emerged from the dural sac a few inches above. The dural sac separates the caudal canal below from the spinal cord and its surrounding spinal fluid above.

When the patient is in active phase labor, with the presenting part well down in the pelvis, caudal analgesia may be started. By the addition of anesthetic solution through the indwelling caudal catheter at appropriate intervals, the desired effect can be maintained throughout labor and provide anesthesia for delivery as well.

To insert the catheter, the obstetric patient is placed on her side in a modified Sims's position, with the upper leg well flexed at the hip and knee joints and the lower leg extended (Fig. 17-4). The sacral and coccygeal area is cleansed with an antiseptic solution. The area is surrounded with sterile towels or a sterile drape. The physician wears sterile gloves for the procedure, since it requires aseptic technique. After the pliable needle or fine plastic catheter has been inserted into the caudal space, a test dose of 8 cc. of the local anesthetic solution, such as Metycaine 1.5 percent, Pontocaine 0.15 percent, Xylocaine 1 percent or Nesacaine 3 percent, is injected. When five minutes have elapsed, the following test for spinal anesthesia is made to be assured that the drug has not been injected into the subarachnoid space. If the 8-cc. dose has been accidentally placed in the subarachnoid space, spinal rather than caudal anesthesia will result, and within five minutes the patient will experience difficulty in moving her legs and will also have a sensory block above the pubic symphysis. At this time the physician also will check the anal sphincter for loss of tone and examine the lower extremities for increasing skin temperature. If these two observations prove to be positive (i.e., the anal sphincter is relaxed, and the patient's feet are becoming warmer and dry), they are an indication that the caudal catheter is placed properly in the caudal space. Only after this is certain is the patient given the obstetric dose of 20 to 30 cc. of medication. This will block the afferent sensory nerve supply from the uterus and usually will provide anesthesia to the 10th thoracic dermatome. This level (Fig. 17-5) is at the umbilicus and is required to eliminate the discomfort of uterine contractions. The large volume (20 to 30 ml.) of anesthetic solution in the peridural space is necessary to achieve this level.

At first the patient experiences a sense of fullness along the distribution of the sciatic nerve in one or both legs, which may cause temporary discomfort. About 15 minutes after the injection, relief is obtained from the abdominal discomfort of uterine contractions, and in about 20 minutes the analgesia should be complete. One observes the lower extremities for pronounced vasodilatation and cessation of sweating as one of the first effective signs. The great toe and the ball of the foot are the first parts to develop vasomotor block; thus this area is the first to become pink, warm and dry. The heel will be the last to show these signs. The effect may be unilateral at first, and some minutes may elapse before it affects the other side, or the physician may have the patient lie on the unaffected side to encourage diffusion of the anesthetic agent. The nurse should remember that the physician should be consulted before changing the patient's position to one side or the other during this early stage of analgesia. After anesthesia has been well established, there is usually no contraindication to changing the patient's position so long as the pliable needle or plastic catheter is protected. If the procedure is suc-

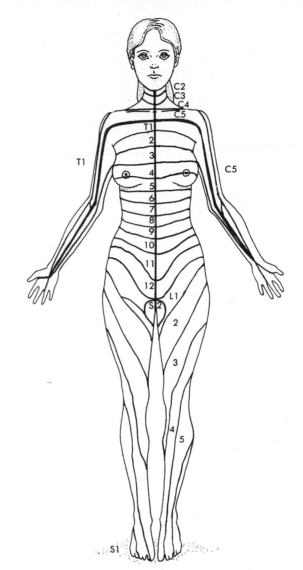

Figure 17-5. Cutaneous dermatomes to illustrate sensory anesthetic levels.

cessful, the patient experiences no pain whatsoever in labor and is not conscious of either uterine contractions or of perineal distention, except for some minor degree of pressure.

Provided that the maternal systolic blood pressure does not fall below 100 mm. Hg, with resulting fetal hypoxia, a continuous caudal has the advantage of exerting the least possible effect on the infant, because it does not cross the placental barrier in significant pharmacologic doses. This factor is an advantage to the premature infant particularly, as well as the fact that caudal analgesia tends to retard rapid and forceful labor and enables the physician to perform an easy, controlled delivery. It also

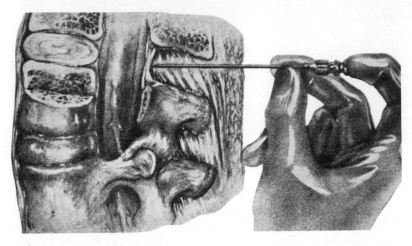

Figure 17-6. Peridural anesthesia. Insertion of needle to ligamentum flavum. (Pitkin, N.: Conduction Anesthesia, ed. 2, Philadelphia, J. B. Lippincott)

lessens the strain of labor for mothers handicapped with heart disease, pulmonary tuberculosis, acute respiratory infections or diabetes.

LUMBAR EPIDURAL is another form of peridural anesthesia in which the space is approached from the lumbar rather than the caudal area. The advantages of this technique as opposed to caudal are technical; the end result for the patient is essentially the same. The anesthetic agents used are the same as those used for caudal, the only difference being that a smaller volume is necessary when injected at the higher lumbar site. Although the anatomy of the lumbar spine is more consistent than that of the caudal area, thus making the injection simpler in some ways, the risk of penetrating the dura and thus obtaining an inadvertent spinal anesthetic is greater.

With the patient on her left side and the legs partially flexed, the lumbar back is cleansed and draped. The skin and ligamentum flavum in one of the lumbar interspaces are infiltrated and a 16 gauge tuohy needle is introduced (Figs. 17-6 and 17-7). The tuohy needle itself is blunted but the stylet is sharp to allow penetration of the skin, subcutaneous tissue and interspinous ligament. The needle is passed through the ligamentum flavum, which offers some resistance. The syringe is aspirated to be sure that the subdural space (containing spinal fluid) has not been inadvertently entered. Proper positioning is tested further by introducing air from a 2-cc. syringe, which should pass without resistance. A plastic catheter is then introduced into the epidural space and the needle withdrawn. Because of the extreme danger of an inadvertent high spinal anesthesia and respiratory paralysis caused by the large amounts of agent to be used, the position of the catheter is checked further. Two test doses of 2 ml. of agent are administered five minutes apart. Either of the test doses would, if the catheter were in the spinal canal, produce a safe low spinal anesthesia. When the catheter is properly located in the peridural space, however, there will be no anesthetic effect. As with caudal anesthesia, skill is re-

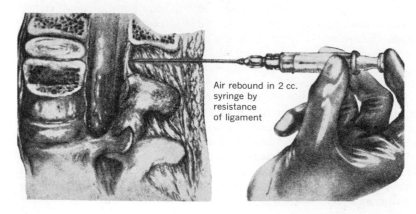

Air rebound in 2 cc. syringe by resistance of ligament

Figure 17-7. Peridural anesthesia, air-rebound technique. When the bevel of the needle rests against the ligamentum flavum, air cannot be injected with ease.

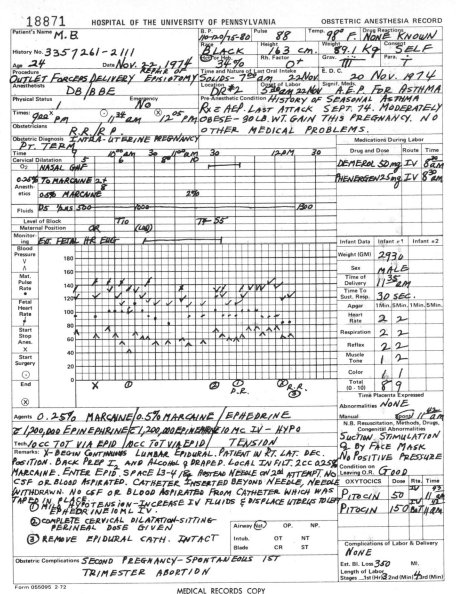

Figure 17-8. Obstetrical anesthesia record during the course of continuous epidural anesthesia. Note the frequency of blood pressure and fetal heart rate recordings.

MEDICAL RECORDS COPY

quired and careful supervision is most important, as long as anesthesia is maintained.

Possible Complications. One of the commonest complications of conduction analgesia for labor is *maternal hypotension*; thus it is important for the nurse or the physician in attendance to keep a constant check on the patient's blood pressure. Blood pressure, pulse and respiration should be recorded at least every minute within the first 15 minutes after each injection of anesthetic agent and at 5-minute intervals thereafter (Fig. 17-8).

Hypotension can be controlled by alertness and prompt action on the part of the attendant. One of the first clues that may alert the nurse that the patient's blood pressure has dropped abruptly is a sudden episode of rather severe nausea, accompanied promptly by the other signs of sudden hypotension. When the mother in labor becomes hypotensive, immediate action should be taken to restore the blood volume to the central circulation. The most expedient measure in this instance is to elevate the patient's legs, either by raising the foot of the bed or merely elevating the legs. The patient may require oxygen at this time. If her blood pressure does not return to normal, she should be turned on her left side (with the foot of the bed elevated) and continue to breathe oxygen. Lying on the left side relieves the uterine pressure exerted on iliac veins and the inferior vena cava, and thus facilitates venous return

analgesia and anesthesia for labor 295

from the lower extremities. Patients receiving caudal anesthesia should have an infusion of 5 percent dextrose in water, started before the block is administered. If hypotension occurs, increasing the rate of this infusion will often correct the situation. If the above measures are not successful, the physician may decide to administer small divided doses of a vasopressor drug.

In addition to the tendency to produce hypotension, other disadvantages of continuous caudal are 1) it increases the frequency of forceps deliveries, 2) it may prolong labor, especially if started too early in labor, and 3) if the anesthesia reaches a high level, uterine atony may result. Caudal anesthesia would be contraindicated in the case of shock or hemorrhage because of its vasodilator tendencies and, for the same reason, it should be used cautiously in toxemia. Any infection of the skin over the sacral area would also be a contraindication to its use. A final disadvantage of the technique is that careful supervision is necessary, placing heavy demands on personnel. If adequate personnel are not available, the technique should not be used.

SPINAL ANESTHESIA is a popular form of obstetric anesthesia in the United States and has the advantage of other forms of regional anesthesia (i.e., good pain relief with little or no effect on the fetus). The term saddle block has been applied to the use of a low-dose hyperbaric (drug heavier than spinal fluid) spinal anesthetic. This technique is used for terminal anesthesia in delivery, generally with a sensory level from T-9 to T-11. This provides a pain-free delivery and does not interfere with uterine contractions. As with most spinal anesthetics, the drug is usually introduced at the L-3—L-4 level. Although the level of anesthesia obtained is to some extent the result of the dose and volume of anesthetic solution used, and to a lesser extent the level of injection, the most important factor is the position of the patient after the injection. To obtain the lower levels in saddle block for vaginal delivery, the injection is made with the patient sitting up, and she remains sitting for 30 to 120 seconds, permitting the hyperbaric solution to fall. Higher dose spinal anesthesia is generally reserved for cesarean sections. Levels of anesthesia from T-6 to T-8 are required. This is achieved by using a larger dose than for saddle block (6 to 8 mg. instead of 4 mg.), and by positioning the patient after the injection. For cesarean section, the injection is usually made with the patient in a lateral rather than a sitting position. Continuous catheter spinal anesthesia has virtually no place in modern obstetric practice.

The major problems with spinal anesthesia are hypotension and headaches. The hypotension is, as it is in peridural anesthesia, the result of sympathetic block and to a great extent is related to the level of anesthesia obtained. Postspinal headache is probably the result of leakage of spinal fluid at the puncture site, with consequent reduction in spinal fluid pressure. This problem occurs more often in the pregnant than the nonpregnant patient, probably because of the natural diuresis which occurs postpartum, and may also involve pressures during uterine contractions. The typical spinal headache, although self-limited (five to ten days), may be incapacitating until it resolves. The treatment includes increase of fluid intake, antihistamines, such as diphenhydramine (Benadryl) and dimenhydrinate (Dramamine), tight abdominal binders, caffeine sodium benzoate, and in resistant cases the injection of dextrose or saline solution into the peridural space.

General anesthesia

This implies the use of an agent, either by inhalation or injection, which will provide analgesia and render varying levels of unconsciousness. As a group, these agents have several problems in common. The first of these problems is that the anesthetic action of the agents is related directly to the blood concentration, and such blood levels are reflected quickly in the fetal circulation. Fetal narcosis and respiratory depression at birth is then a major concern. A second and really serious problem is vomiting and aspiration. The obstetric patient may not have been in a fasting state when labor began, as is the case for elective surgery. When labor begins, intestinal motility and gastric emptying virtually cease. Thus, even though delivery may occur many hours after the last meal, the stomach may still be full and vomiting may occur during induction of anesthesia. This is less likely to occur with agents such as nitrous oxide in analgesic concentration, because in this concentration the cough reflex is maintained. When vomiting does occur, great skill is required on the part of the anesthetist to avoid aspiration. If aspiration occurs, the immediate and most ominous consequence may be respiratory failure and cardiac arrest. Unfortunately, this is one of the leading causes of maternal deaths in the United States. Aspiration pneumonia is a delayed complication of considerable gravity. The remaining problems with the general anesthetics are related to the specific agents and are discussed individually.

NITROUS OXIDE in combination with varying concentrations of oxygen is probably the most common anesthetic agent used for obstetrics in this country. When used in safe concentrations, this gas is not capable of producing total surgical anesthesia but does afford excellent analgesia. Since the level of anesthesia is not profound and consciousness is not lost, especially if the agent is used intermittently with contractions, nitrous oxide poses less risk of vomiting and aspiration. The concentration of nitrous oxide should never exceed 80 percent (with 20 percent oxygen) and preferably should be lower to avoid fetal hypoxia. It is necessary to use either local infiltration or pudendal block for the episiotomy and repair to provide complete anesthesia for that area and obviate the need for prolonged continuous administration of the gas.

TRICHLORETHYLENE (Trilene) is a volatile analgesic agent which is usually self-administered, using an inhalator strapped to the patient's wrist. There is a safety factor with the Trilene mask; the patient will drop the mask as soon as she is sufficiently depressed. Profound surgical anesthesia cannot be obtained in this fashion. If the agent is used in an anesthesia machine with a carbon dioxide absorber, one must be cautious, because an increase in heat may cause the formation of a toxic gas, phosgene. The same precaution applies to patients who have been using Trilene for analgesia and subsequently require surgical anesthesia. Delivery room personnel should not hold the Trilene mask on the patient's face, and its use is contraindicated in patients with heart disease because of a tendency to produce cardiac arrhythmias.

CHLOROFORM is another volatile anesthetic which is now of greater historic than practical interest, having been administered to Queen Victoria in 1853. Since its toxic level is only slightly above that required for anesthesia, its use has been discontinued in American hospitals. The toxicity is cardiac in nature, and arrhythmias are common if epinephrine or oxytocin is used in conjunction with the agent. Advantages include the fact that chloroform is pleasant and rapid and, if necessary, can produce excellent uterine relaxation.

ETHER for many years was the mainstay of obstetric anesthesia. The reasons for the popularity of ether included its safety, because of its slow action, and the fact that distinct stages of anesthesia could be observed. The agent can be administered either by an open drop technique or with a standard semiclosed anesthesia machine. Disadvantages of ether include those of all inhalation agents (i.e., the dangers of vomiting and aspiration); also, ether is irritating to breathe, often causing coughing and a prolonged induction of anesthesia. In addition, ether produces profound uterine relaxation, which is helpful if one is doing a version and extraction or manual removal of a placenta, but is a distinct disadvantage in a normal delivery. Since ether is cleared very slowly from the lungs, the uterine relaxation is prolonged, thereby increasing the postpartum blood loss. Induction with ether takes considerable time, so it is not the agent of choice when deep anesthesia is needed quickly.

CYCLOPROPANE is an anesthetic gas which has the major advantage of being able to produce profound surgical anesthesia very quickly (within a few minutes). It can be administered in relatively low concentrations, thereby maintaining a high oxygen concentration and can, if the level of anesthesia is deep enough, produce uterine relaxation. This gas should never be used unless complete precautions have been taken to avoid an explosion, including conductive shoes or shoe covers. Cyclopropane is usually administered in a closed system machine, and, although very helpful in many obstetric emergencies, it is probably "more anesthesia" than is necessary for a normal vaginal delivery.

HALOTHANE (Fluothane) is a rapid-acting volatile anesthetic agent which produces excellent uterine relaxation very quickly and, for this reason, is probably the agent of choice when such is needed. Fluothane should not be used in patients with liver disease and, like cyclopropane, is probably excessive anesthesia for normal obstetrics.

METHOXYFLURANE (Penthrane) is another halogenated ether which has found use in obstetrics. It does not produce uterine relaxation like halothane and can be used in analgesic concentrations for a normal delivery. As with halothane, a history of liver disease contraindicates its use.

THIOPENTAL SODIUM (Pentothal), the only intravenous agent in use in obstetric anesthesia, is used for vaginal deliveries, as well as cesarean sections. Because pentothal reaches the same concentration in the fetal circulation as in the maternal very rapidly (within five minutes), it is not a popular agent for normal deliveries. Blood levels of barbiturates in the newborn are not usually cleared quickly, and neonatal depression is a problem. Laryngospasm in the mother is also a serious problem which can produce fetal as well as maternal hypoxia, and a skilled anesthetist is essential. Thus, although thiopental is easy to administer, its potential problems are so significant that most obstetricians avoid its use.

Special obstetric anesthesia problems

Breech

Breech presentation poses a particular anesthesia problem. Most obstetricians prefer to have a cooperative patient who can bear down during the second stage, but they also need adequate anesthesia available, if there is difficulty in delivery of the shoulders, or the after-coming head. Caudal, epidural and spinal anesthesia have the problem of impairing the ability of the patient to push. This increases the frequency of breech extractions, with their inherent risk. It is preferable to use local anesthesia or a pudendal block, along with intermittent nitrous oxide analgesia, which permits the patient to bear down, and to have an anesthetist present who is prepared to add a more profound agent such as cyclopropane or halothane, if difficulty occurs with the shoulders or after-coming head.

Cesarean section

Since more complete anesthesia is required before the operation may be started, and since the time required to deliver the baby may be longer than for a normal delivery, there is greater risk of neonatal depression. Several techniques are in common use for cesarean section. Spinal anesthesia has been favored by many because it provides adequate anesthesia without fetal depression. The major problem with spinal anesthesia is the frequent hypotension resulting from the sympathetic block and the uterus compressing the vena cava. Cyclopropane anesthesia with a rapid induction can provide adequate anesthesia but forces the surgeon to proceed rapidly, in an effort to deliver the baby before the gas equilibrates across the placenta. A third technique involves a small dose of thiopental, just sufficient to induce sleep, followed by nitrous oxide and oxygen along with a muscle relaxant such as succinylcholine. This affords adequate oxygenation with minimal fetal depression. In some circumstances, the anesthesia of choice is local infiltration of the abdominal wall. Cesarean section can be accomplished with this approach if the operator is skilled in the use of local anesthesia and avoids undue peritoneal traction. Of course, as with any surgical situation, circumstances will dictate the choice of approach (e.g., one would avoid spinal anesthesia in a patient with bleeding, who would be prone to hypotension. On the other hand, one might select spinal anesthesia in a patient who has recently eaten).

Uterine relaxation

Several obstetrical procedures—internal version, breech extraction, manual removal of the placenta, intrauterine examination, and cervical cerclage operations—require uterine relaxation. Although ether, chloroform, cyclopropane and halothane all can produce such relaxation, halothane does it more quickly and efficiently and is, therefore, the agent of choice.

Suggested Reading

BONICA, J. J.: *Principles and Practice of Obstetric Analgesia and Anesthesia.* Philadelphia, F. A. Davis, 1967.

BUXTON, C. L.: *A Study of Psychophysical Methods for Relief of Childbirth Pain.* Philadelphia, W. B. Saunders, 1962.

DICK-READ, G.: *Childbirth Without Fear.* New York, Harper & Row, 1972.

GOTTSCHALLZ, W.: Anesthesia in obstetrics, *Clin. Ob. and Gyn.* 17, 1974.

MATERNITY CENTER ASSOCIATION: *Psychophysical Preparation for Childbirth: Guidelines for Teaching,* ed. 2. New York Maternity Center Association, 1965.

SHNIDER, S. M., AND MOYA, F.: *The Anesthesiologist, Mother and Newborn.* Baltimore, Williams and Wilkins, 1974.

conduct of normal labor

18

Effective Nursing Care / Onset of Labor / Continuing Care / Examinations in Labor / Conduct of the Stages of Labor / Immediate Care of the Infant / Emergency Delivery by the Nurse / Lacerations, Episiotomy and Repair

Dimensions of effective nursing care

Perhaps at no other time during the maternity cycle is the nurse in such an advantageous position to give nursing care as she is during the time of parturition. It is a unique and humbling experience, this miracle of giving birth, not only for the mother and the father, the main participants, but also for the physician and the nurse who share this experience, and upon whom so much depends. From the parents' point of view, labor looms as a critical period in the process of childbearing; often it is considered by them, and especially by the mother, as the end of a long-drawn-out process rather than the beginning of new life. Hence they attribute enormous significance to events and people who are necessary and helpful to them at this time. They indicate repeatedly that they consider the nurse in particular to be one of those necessary, helpful people. Indeed, she can be if she utilizes the opportunity.

Effective nursing care during labor provides for maximum well-being and comfort for both mother and infant and at the same time allows the father to participate in the process, insofar as he is able, and to derive a sense of satisfac-

tion from that participation. The nursing intervention is purposeful but flexible, based always on the needs of each individual patient, infant and father. To execute such care, the nurse must have knowledge and understanding of the course of normal labor, ability to recognize deviations from the normal, and judgment and ability to cope with stressful and emergency conditions. In addition, she should have a mastery of certain skills, both technical and communicative, which she can apply appropriately to meet the exigencies of the situation. The importance of teamwork between doctor and nurse should not be overlooked, and it is especially important to keep the physician informed through accurate reporting and recording of the progress of the mother in labor.

However, knowledge and technical ability are not sufficient in themselves, for the nurse must also be able to convey warmth and empathy if she is to be really effective. The empathic nurse is able to enter into the feelings of her patient and at the same time to retain her separateness. Thus, objectivity is maintained, which contributes to more effective care. Yet the worth and the individuality of each mother always are recognized. In addition, the nurse ought to be accepting and nonjudgmental regarding the behavior of the mother or the father, realizing that this is a stressful period, and that their usual behavior may be drastically different. She strives to sustain her patient and to reinforce her confidence whenever necessary, thus helping the mother to attain the greatest amount of comfort and satisfaction from the labor experience. By assisting the patient and her husband to mobilize their resources and strengths, she is able to work with them in a positive way and to reinforce their concept of themselves as adequate people.

The mind of the nurse boggles a bit when she is faced with this considerable responsibility; certainly the young student has some trepidation when she is called upon to assume these duties. Yet with competent guidance and instruction she learns to function efficiently in this role. To help the student and/or young graduate prepare for her responsibility, the authors in this chapter have focused on both the patient and the nurse as they move through the successive stages of labor. Although it is the mother who truly delivers her infant, the other important people in this event—the husband, the doctor and ancillary personnel—are not to be forgotten, for they also play important roles.

The nursing process in labor

Implicit in the area of effective nursing care is the ability to initiate the nursing process appropriately through the use of effective clinical judgments. The nursing process embodies such activities as assessment, planning, implementation or intervention and evaluation.[1] Other practitioners have conceptualized the process as including observation, inference, validation, assessment, action and evaluation.[2] As stated previously (see Chapter 12), various terminology has been employed over time to describe nursing practice: nursing diagnosis, clinical judgment, assessment, and the like. All of these constitute in some way the anatomy of nursing care.

Certainly, the ability to initiate the nursing process appropriately through the use of effective clinical judgment is utilized not only in attending the labor patient, but throughout all of nursing. However, the components of the process are specified at this time because the nature of the nursing care during labor and the exigencies under which it is given require a great facility with this process. There is much that is unpredictable in the delivery area. Patients may be admitted with great rapidity; labors may progress in a similar manner. Unforeseen emergencies may occur no matter how well organized and efficient the personnel, and when they do occur, they may be serious. Hence the nurse may be called upon to exercise a great deal of judgment "on her feet" so to speak, without specific direction or the luxury of thinking through the problem. In the midst of crises where human lives are at stake, calm fact finding and judicial deliberations become increasingly difficult. Some of our most crucial problems arise from conflicts between principle and expediency. Hence, we need to have a method so internalized as to be second nature so we can operate without conscious step by step proceedings. Thus, we can arrive quickly at appropriate decisions and conclusions regarding our patients.

The components of the process can help the student understand how nursing practice can be made operational. The various operations have been classified under headings derived from Bloch.[3] One is not to assume that these categories are mutually exclusive or stand alone. Rather, there are constant feedback loops in the process (see Chapter 12). Many authors might consider the data collection part of the nursing diagnosis stage. We present this interpretation as one means of conceptualizing more clearly the nursing process. (See next page.)

As we review the process, it can be seen that components 1 and 2 constitute a reconnoitering stage in which information is gathered and the diagnosis begun. Resources such as the chart, the family, the patient herself, members of the health team and elements in the environment can be utilized. The nurse also may utilize her ability to "role take" to speed up the data collection. (For a detailed definition and explanation of the concept of "role taking" and its application in maternity nursing, see the Turner and Reeder articles in the Suggested Reading.) This term refers to the ability of the nurse to put herself in the place (position) of the patient in order to imaginatively construct the role of the patient, so as to provide herself with appropriate cues for predicting and understanding the meaning of the patient's behavior, and thus, for determining appropriate behavior for herself. The process by which the role of each particular patient is inferred stems from basic knowledge about the patient role in general, prior experience with the individual or others like her, and/or a specific bit of behavior that is being manifested. As the student gains more experience with various individuals involved in the patient role who are confronted with different kinds of health-illness conditions (including maternity patients) she will find her role-taking ability facilitated. As we acquire our data, we become able to decide the existence and extent of a problem. We can say in the most general terms that a problem does exist when there is a health goal to be obtained but the individual (patient) sees no well-defined, well-established means of attaining it. For instance, she may be too ill or weak to help herself. Again, the goal may be so vaguely defined or unclear that the patient cannot determine relevant means of achieving it. Thus, the patient may not understand or know how to accept conditions and instruction regarding achieving the goal of health.

A decision about the existence and extent of the problem initiates the diagnosis. There are many definitions of this term. For our purposes we shall regard a nursing diagnosis as a conclusion based on a systematic and scientific appraisal of an individual's health-illness problem, resulting from critical analysis of her behavior (alone and with others), the nature of the illness and the numerous other factors, environmental, social, psychological, that may affect her condition. This conclusion serves as a guide for our nursing care. It is well to remember also that the statement of the diagnosis may be several words, and more descriptive than etiological. As we find out additional information about our patients we may move from descriptive to more etiological statements. Moreover, there may be several diagnoses relating to a constellation of interrelated problems the patient has; for instance, if the nurse were to write the diagnoses regarding a labor patient the diagnoses might be: "anxiety regarding process of labor"; "elevated temperature"; "inefficient but painful contractions." Finally, one can have the same nursing diagnosis but have different pathological conditions which give rise to it. In the case of a newly delivered infant, for instance, the diagnosis might be "inadequate oxygenation"; the cause for one infant might be a congenital heart defect; for another infant, immature lungs associated with prematurity. Thus, the total interrelationship of all the influencing factors is to be considered as it gives direction to our care plan.

Components of the Nursing Process

Assessment

1. Collection of Data (Subjective, Objective)
   a. Gathering of information on the physical, social and emotional aspects of the health status of the individual and family.
   b. Construction of the data base by: observation, interview, history taking, physical examination, role taking, etc.

2. Definition of the Problem
   a. Making decisions regarding the deficit(s) or potential deficit(s) in the health status of the individual and family.
   b. Making these nursing diagnoses based on clinical judgment and inference.

Intervention

3. Planning the Intervention
   a. Making decision(s) regarding the action(s) believed to be appropriate to effect a solution of the defined problem(s).
   b. Decision(s) include goal setting, priority setting, nursing prescriptions.

4. Implementation of the Intervention
   a. Execution of a nursing regimen by: administering a prescribed medication or treatment, executing a medical regimen, providing comfort measures and physical care, providing health education, providing counseling, providing referral services, coordinating services for the patient.

Evaluation and Reassessment

5. Evaluation of the Intervention— this in turn may lead to further reassessments.
   a. Determining the degree of effectiveness of the action(s) taken in solving the defined problems by: observation, interview of patient status and condition(s), physical examination, reading of current records, etc.
   b. Prediction of future nursing action and patient potential for change.

Components 3 and 4 are concerned with the planning and implementation of knowledgeable intervention in the form of nursing activities which encompass everything from the administration of comfort measures to counseling. These activities are directed toward moving the patient toward increased positive adaptation to the environment. Again, it is important to remember that the implementation also is fluid since it is based upon the diagnosis or diagnoses which may be reassessed at any point in the process. Moreover, as we administer care, the patient's condition will be expected to change, which, upon evaluation, will necessitate possibly new diagnoses and hence modification of care. Therefore, the continuous feedback loops built into the process become apparent.

Component 5 includes both evaluation and prediction facets. A worthwhile evaluation should include an estimation of the results of our past nursing care activities to help us predict the validity of our care for the future. Any statement of the effectiveness and reliability of our actions is best made with qualifications indicating the degree or amount of effectiveness and reliability claimed. *Were all symptoms relieved? What was the extent of the results? On what evidence (observation of self, others, verbal response, cessation of symptoms)? Who was involved (nurse, patient, others)? In what contexts (what else was happening when the action was performed)?* If these points are established, then we can begin to build categories of nursing action that are effective under certain circumstances for certain patients given certain conditions. As we ascertain the extent of our effectiveness we are then in a better position to predict the patient's potential for change toward stability and/or a wellness condition. Thus, we arrive at the nursing prognosis.

The student is encouraged to utilize the Suggested Reading for the articles on the nursing process and clinical judgment for a thorough and varied treatment of the subject. Let us continue with some of the events that the mother will be experiencing.

Prelude to labor

The prodromal signs heralding the onset of labor begin several weeks before true labor commences (see Chapter 15). Lightening may occur any time during the last four weeks of pregnancy; in primigravidas it usually occurs about ten days to two weeks prior to labor. This phenomenon causes a sensation of decreased abdominal distention produced by the descent of the presenting part of the baby into the pelvis. In multigravida this may not occur until the labor has begun. The usually painless Braxton Hicks contractions which have occurred intermittently throughout the latter part of pregnancy may increase so much that

they become annoying. They may cause the mother many restless or sleepless nights that contribute to her gradually increasing tension and fatigue. Since the rise in the anxiety level contributes to heightened awareness, the mother becomes more sensitive to various stimuli: if the baby is generally less active, she may worry; if he moves more than usual, she may worry. She wonders about the 2- to 3-pound weight loss that may occur three to four days before the onset of labor. Ordinarily this may be an occasion of great rejoicing, but now it may give her some concern. Even the increased vaginal mucous discharge may have an ominous significance for her. The spurt of energy that may occur one to two days before labor begins often leads her into activities that are overfatiguing, and she will need anticipatory guidance from the nurse and the physician to help her to set limits on activity.

This is the time to finish packing her suitcase and to simplify her housekeeping duties. She may want to complete meal preparations for the family's use when she is in the hospital; if this is done daily little by little, then it should not become bothersome. Last-minute details for the care of the other children or the functioning of the household can be taken care of at this time. Short walks in the fresh air are a good way to release extra tension without overfatigue. The mother should be encouraged to achieve a happy balance between activity and rest.

During the latter part of pregnancy the mother will have been instructed about what to do when she thinks labor has begun. As term approaches, it is wise for the nurse to explore with the mother her preparations for coming to the hospital. The mother and father should know approximately how long it will take them to reach the hospital and what alternate means of transportation are available if the father is not able to take her. What entrance to the hospital they should use and what admission procedures they must go through also are important. A tour of the ward for the parents can be arranged during the antepartal period so that they can become more familiar with the surroundings.

The onset of labor

Most physicians instruct their patients to notify them if the labor contractions become rhythmic and regular and/or the bag of water breaks. To prepare the patient adequately for what to expect, and to instruct her on an appropriate course of action, it is necessary that the nurse have an understanding of the physiology of labor as well as other factors (p. 170). Since the nurse will be with the patient more constantly than the doctor after the patient is admitted to the hospital, the nurse will be expected also to report on the general character of the labor contractions as well as the other symptoms of labor. First, it must be determined whether the patient is actually in labor. Although this is occasionally a difficult problem to settle, usually a decision can be reached on the basis of the differential points between true and false labor (Table 18-1). It is important that the patient be aware of the difference, too, since it will save herself and the doctor innumerable telephone calls and concern if she does not think every contraction is indicative of true labor.

Admission to the hospital

As previously stated, the mother who has been given adequate antepartal care will have received instruction from the physician or the nurse on what to anticipate when she comes to the hospital to have her baby. If this is the mother's first hospital experience, it will be much easier for her if she has been told about the necessary preliminary procedures, such as any vulvar and perineal preparation, the methods of examination employed to ascertain the progress of labor, and the usual routines exercised for her care in the course of labor. It is important for the mother to understand that she should come to the hospital at the onset of labor; for as labor progresses, these activities are more difficult to carry out and are much more distressing to the patient. If the mother has not had adequate antepartal care to prepare her, then her labor may be rather advanced upon admission and she may not know what to expect. It will then fall to the nurse to reassure this mother and orient her as quickly as possible to the process of labor and the physical environment. In these instances, the nurse will find her ability to make decisive clinical judgments, especially with regard to establishing priorities of care, extremely helpful and necessary.

The preparation for delivery will of necessity vary in different hospitals, since every hospital has its own admission procedure. The nurse should be aware that many details may

Table 18-1 Differential Factors in True and False Labor

True Labor	False Labor
Contractions:	*Contractions:*
Occur at regular intervals	Occur at irregular intervals
Intervals gradually shorten	Intervals remain long
Intensity gradually increases	Intensity remains the same
Located chiefly in back	Located chiefly in abdomen
Intensified by walking	Walking has no effect; often gives relief
Show:	*Show:*
Usually present	None
Cervix:	*Cervix:*
Becomes effaced and dilated (this can be determined by digital examination)	Usually uneffaced and closed

be accomplished in a number of ways. Very few institutions employ precisely the same technique in preparing a mother for delivery. Actually, the differences are in details only, for the principles are the same everywhere—namely, asepsis and antisepsis, together with careful observation of the mother for any deviations from the normal.

Establishment of the nurse-patient relationship

For many a young woman in labor, admission to the maternity unit may mark her first acquaintance with hospitals as a patient. Her immediate reaction may be one of strangeness, loneliness and homesickness, particularly if the father is not permitted to stay with her in the labor room. Regardless of the amount of preparation for this event, whether she is happy or unhappy, whether she wants the baby or not, every mother enters labor with a certain amount of normal tension and anxiety. Moreover, not infrequently mothers are thoroughly afraid of the whole process. This may be attributed in part to the fact that the mother's preparation for childbearing has been limited, or she may have been reared in an environment fraught with mysteries and old wives' tales about childbirth. If she has had previous children, she may have had unfortunate and fear-producing experiences. All these factors make her fear understandable.

In addition, the nurse's contact with the patient during the labor and delivery process is very short term. Thus, the nurse is faced with the problem of providing high quality care in a short space of time. The key to the problem appears to lie in her ability to utilize whatever time she has available, whether it be five minutes or an hour, to provide an atmosphere of receptivity to her patients' needs. Her ability to determine needs lies in her ability in the collection and diagnosis portion of the nursing process. When she implements effective care, her facility with therapeutic communication plus technical understanding and skill are key issues.

There has been a good deal of time and effort spent in nursing research to determine the needs of patients (see Suggested Reading), especially the needs above and beyond those related directly to the physiologic and/or pathologic conditions of the patient. These needs have generally been classified as "emotional" or "psychosocial." Whatever their label, they are especially important for consideration in the maternity patient. Newman's study has indicated that patients when questioned expressed a preponderance of needs that were emotional in origin. These fell into the following general areas: the need to have one's *identity* recognized and maintained in the face of disability, the need to have some *control* over events relating to oneself, and needs deriving from *fear, anxiety* and *loneliness* which become translated into concern for *safety* and *comfort*.[4] Aiken and Aiken point out that, if we as nurses look at patients' behavior as a probable consequence of our own behavior, and if we then view our own behavior as a force to facilitate patients' behavior, we will be in a better position to understand our patients' behavior. Moreover, we will then be better able to devise specific approaches to facilitate change.[5]

ENCOURAGEMENT. Accordingly, one of the first responsibilities of the nurse is to recognize that, in addition to the physical manifestations, there are these psychosocial factors which influence each mother's pregnancy and have a bearing on her individual needs for care (see Chapters 12 and 13). Therefore, every mother deserves encouragement that tends to inspire assurance during her labor. Her discomfort never should be minimized, and an effort should be made to help her to keep in control when her labor is painful. Attention should be directed to the fact that progress is being made, and that her efforts to work cooperatively with her labor are helpful and necessary.

AWARENESS OF PHYSICAL AND BEHAVIORAL SIGNS. In addition, the nurse will want to be constantly alert to the physical and behavioral signs associated with the progress of normal labor. She can be extremely helpful by giving the couple anticipatory guidance in this respect so that they will know what to expect during this experience. At the same time, she will watch vigilantly for any sign that may point to abnormal developments. For instance, an increase in pulse rate, a rise in temperature, excessive bleeding, changes in the character of uterine contractions, passage of meconium with a vertex presentation, or alterations in the fetal heart sounds are changes which may have profound implications for the mother's welfare.

RAPPORT. One of the most highly talked about, yet not well understood, concepts deemed essential to an effective nurse-patient relationship is that of rapport. Rapport may be thought of as a relationship consisting of interrelated thoughts and feelings that include empathy, compassion, sympathy, interest and respect for each individual as a unique human being. One of the crucial components of this type of relationship is empathy; that is, the ability to enter into the life of another person, to accurately perceive her *current* feelings and their meanings.[6] The idea of currency is an important one here. Empathy must involve understanding the current feelings of a patient, not her feelings of sometime in the past. Previous perceptions based on earlier experiences with a patient or patients similar to her can be misleading if they block present understanding of what the patient is currently experiencing.

It is well to examine the difference between empathy and sympathy, another type of human understanding and another component in a rapport relationship. In empathy, the helper "borrows" her patient's feelings in order to fully understand them, but she is always aware of her own separateness and realizes that the feelings of the patient are not her own.

Sympathetic understanding, on the other hand, involves a process in which the helper loses her own separate identity and takes on the patient's feelings and circumstances, experiencing them *as if* they were the helper's *own*. It is a true sharing of feelings without maintaining the separateness that empathic understanding requires. The nurse, for instance, "feels" the mother's discomfort during labor as intensely as she thinks the mother is feeling the pain.

There are several reasons why sympathy does not provide as much help to a patient as does empathy. First, when the nurse absorbs the patient's feelings in terms of how she would feel if she were in a similar position (sympathy), she may not be accurate in her perceptions, for the patient's reaction may be and often is quite different from the nurse's response. For example, the patient may be frightened at the prospect of receiving intravenous oxytocin to augment her labor, but the nurse may not (or vice versa). An empathic attempt to view the patient "as if I were she" will generally yield a much more accurate perception of the true feelings of the patient than does the sympathetic attempt to *absorb* feelings.

Second, the sympathetic taking on of the circumstances of the patient causes involvement of the self to such an extent that the nurse herself may then be in need of help. We have all experienced some situations that reactivated anxieties and old involvements so that we have functioned less effectively than we might have. The old saying that doctors and nurses aren't very "successful" in providing health care for their families is a case in point. In empathy, a nurse's realization that her identity is separate from the patient's enables her to be sufficiently free from the intensity of emotion to help her patient.

Finally, in sympathy, a nurse is preoccupied with her similarities to the patient (or those she imagines that she has), and this interferes with her ability to concentrate on the patient and her point of view. Moreover, sympathy denotes condolence with the patient's viewpoint whereas in empathy, such agreement is not necessarily present. Here the nurse conveys *understanding* of the patient's viewpoint without necessarily agreeing with it.[7]

Perhaps the most important quality necessary for the nurse to begin to empathize with the patient is the ability to identify with the patient. (For an interesting discussion of why student nurses often identify more quickly with certain patients see the Yeaworth article in the Suggested Reading.) Identification has been described as the mechanism which enables a person to take up any attitude toward another's mental life. Certain changes take place in the ego structure when this mechanism is employed resulting in an expansion of ego boundaries to include the attitude once observed in the other and now made a part of one's self. This type of identification is seen in children as they learn their various social roles, for instance. However, in the therapeutic relationship, the altered ego structure is only a temporary experience and remains "ego segregated" but available for reality testing and further thought. Certainly to be able to identify and share with another and then revert to one's own identity requires flexibility of the ego boundaries, and this flexibility can become enhanced with repeated use of the mechanism. After the nurse has attempted to experience the patient's feelings, she must be able to step back, that is, to narrow her ego boundaries back to reality. She then uses her intellectual processes to review what has occurred from three perspectives: 1) what is known about the patient, 2) what is known about herself, 3) what is known from theory. Thus, subjectivity is converted into objectivity and permits valid assessment of needs and problems. In order for effective nursing therapy to be instituted, empathy must operate within a sound conceptual framework, backed by theoretical knowledge and clinical experience. It is a valuable aid in designing and implementing care, but is not to be considered a substitute for careful planning and rational evaluation. Unfortunately, we do not know if and how empathy can be taught or learned. We do know the ability to utilize the identification mechanism has something very vital to do with the empathy process. It is to the identification-empathy-rapport linkage that more research needs to be directed.

In addition to the notion of empathy, the concept of rapport also involves positive communication that contributes to mutual understanding and acceptance. While no "method" or "rules" have yet been determined to establish this positive, therapeutic communication, the student may find the following general behavioral principles useful when attempting to institute an effective relationship. 1) The nurse's verbalization regarding an aspect of the patient's behavior or appearance confronts the patient with the nurse's perception of the immediate situation. This tends to elicit the patient's agreement or disagreement and any subsequent explanation, especially when nondirective probes are used. Here the nurse indicates her attention and concern and the patient has the option of responding. 2) By being alert to the patient's cues regarding her various social roles (mother, wife, possible bread-winner, career woman) and by demonstrating a genuine interest in her roles, the nurse can collect more data upon which an evaluation of her immediate and future needs can be based. This allows the patient to keep her identity and gives her some feeling of control in the situation. 3) Communication can be facilitated when the nurse acknowledges to the mother that she does not understand what she is saying and asks for further clarification. 4) All members of the health team (and family also if appropriate) ought to be informed of any needs of the patient that cannot be handled by the nurse alone; moreover, subsequent actions by personnel (and family) are to be communicated to the patient so that she may recognize that communication lines are open and her needs and problems are recognized and attended to as they arise. This retards feelings of helplessness and loss of control. 5) Therapeutic communication is more likely to be initiated and facilitated if the nurse assumes a relaxed and/or sitting position, *close* to the patient if possible. Standing at the foot of the bed or in the doorway is not conducive to satisfying conversation. In the hustle and bustle of the labor and delivery suite, the nurse often falls into the habit of "popping in and out" with the result that the mother may never have a chance of more than a rhetorical answer to "How are you coming along?" This of course demolishes any attempts at positive communication, and promotes the feelings that many mothers have of the delivery staff as being "too busy to care."

The nurse who establishes rapport with her patient will, then, demonstrate understanding and acceptance of the mother. The mother, in turn, is able to trust the nurse, and an effective nurse-patient relationship is facilitated.

First Impressions. The kind of greeting that the patient receives as she enters the delivery suite is extremely important and sets the tone for future interaction with the health team. Some institutions permit the father to accompany his wife to the area; others prefer to admit the mother first and then let the husband and the wife remain together. When the husband is present, the nurse should be mindful that he is to be considered and welcomed in an appropriate way, as is his wife.

The mother can be made to feel welcome, expected and necessary (remember that it is she who delivers the baby). Thus she and her husband, if he is present, can be called by name and shown personally by the nurse to the labor room that the mother will occupy. Once there, the patient can be helped, if necessary, to undress and to get into bed.

Orientation. The mother and the father will need to know some of what will be expected of them, and what they in turn can expect as participants in this new situation. Hence, the nurse can begin an orientation to the process of labor as well as to the general environment. It is to be remembered that there is no set form or content for this orientation and no set time for the introduction and the continuation of this process; rather the nurse must first explore what the parents do know about the environment and the labor process, so that she can judge what needs to be introduced, reinforced, etc., and when the most appropriate time to do this would be. An easy conversational manner may be employed rather than a rapid-fire explanation of dos and don'ts.

The rationale for any procedures and/or restrictions is always given. The patient should not be overloaded with too much stimuli at one time and should be allowed to absorb any new information and explanation before additional material is presented. The nurse can structure the situation to allow the patient to "feed back" information, so that she knows how much the mother really understands.

Generally, the mother and her husband will need to know what procedures and activities will be performed and the reason for them. In addition, the couple should know the limits of the mother's activity, and what restrictions of food and fluids there will be. What the patient and her husband can expect regarding the progress of labor should be included also (i.e., what will be happening physically, how the mother will be feeling, and how she and her husband can participate in the labor experience. See Table 18-2 and Chapter 15. The father, if present, can be included in any explanations, etc., since he may be participating in the care of his wife. As implied, this orientation will continue throughout the entire course of labor and possibly delivery. The nurse will determine when and how each phase will be instituted, according to the cues given by the mother and father.

Continuing care

After making the mother comfortable in the labor room, the nurse will need to find out some rather specific information regarding the mother's general condition (i.e., the frequency, the duration and the intensity of her contractions, the amount and the character of show, and whether the membranes have ruptured or are intact). At this point it is expedient to learn when the first signs of labor became apparent to the mother and the nature and timing of the uterine contractions from that time. Since the mother's emotional status often has bearing on her physical labor, it is wise to be continuously alert to her behavior—whether she seems *unduly* apprehensive, or whether she is relatively relaxed or calm. Restlessness, excessive conversation, rapid, darting eye movements, arm and body rigidity, and plucking at the bedclothes are all signs of the former. The nurse reports all findings to the physician as soon as possible.

Although the nurse will want to avoid any outward display of rush or hurry, she should proceed with the admission as quickly as possible. It must be remembered that the mother's labor usually will become progressively stronger; hence the more procedures, orientation, etc., that can be accomplished early in labor, while she is able to be more responsive with relative ease, will enhance the patient's comfort and well-being. Also, there generally will be several other people concerned with the care of the mother—the physician, intern, laboratory technician—and they often cannot carry out their activities until the patient is fully admitted. Finally, an expeditious completion of the admission procedures leaves more time for the mother and father to be together before the actual delivery.

PRIOR TO THE PHYSICIAN'S EXAMINATION the nurse will take the mother's temperature, pulse, respiration and blood pressure and listen to the fetal heart tones. A voided urine specimen will be obtained for the admission specimen and will facilitate the physician's vaginal examination. It will be examined for its protein and glucose content. If the patient is allowed to use the bathroom, a receptacle is placed under the toilet seat since the physician will want to have available for examination whatever material may be passed per vagina, as well

as the urine specimen. As soon as possible, a blood specimen is taken to check the hemoglobin or hematocrit concentration. Often the routine serologic testing is done and an additional tube of clotted blood is kept available for use by the blood bank to cross-match a donor if the occasion occurs. If the patient is in labor, the doctor probably will order such procedures as clipping or shaving and cleansing of the vulva.

ENEMA. Unless labor is progressing too rapidly, a cleansing enema may be ordered. The nurse will use the same principles in giving the enema as for any other patient; however, she may find it more difficult to insert the tube because of the pressure of the presenting part of the fetus or of hemorrhoids that the mother may have. Hemorrhoids and/or the strength of the contractions may make the enema discomforting for the patient. It is essential that the nurse let the mother know that she is aware of the possible discomfort, and that she will do all she can to give the enema carefully and comfortably. Giving a step-by-step explanation of the procedure as well as telling the mother specifically what she can do to help to allay the discomfort will go far to alleviate the discomfort. Helpful remarks are: "Let me know when you're having a contraction, and I'll clamp the tubing. Relax your buttocks when you begin to feel the tube being inserted. I'll give this very slowly, so as not to increase cramping. Let me know if it's too uncomfortable, and I can stop the flow for a little while." It is wise for the nurse to ascertain, during the history taking, the state of the mother's bowels. That is, whether or not the mother may be constipated or has been having diarrhea. If the former, then there is a clue that there may be some difficulty in inserting the tubing and/or in retention of the enema. If diarrhea is present, then there may be no need for the enema and infection may be considered.

An admission bath is rarely a routine procedure. Most patients have sufficient warning at the onset of labor to enable them to bathe prior to coming to the hospital. When a bath is deemed desirable, the type used will depend to some extent on the facilities of the hospital. The types usually given are the shower and the sponge bath. The hand spray may be used as an improvised shower when the shower stall is not available.

Table 18-2   Guidelines to Mother's Participation in Labor

What is Happening	Helping Yourself	Breathing Pattern in Contraction	Other Support
Prelude to Labor			
Lightening (2-4 weeks before first baby comes)	Simplify housekeeping		Husband can encourage continued practice of breathing and relaxation techniques
Braxton-Hicks contractions may increase	Have hospital suitcase packed		
Increased vaginal discharge			
Baby less active	Conserve energy		
Excitement about labor may make sleeping difficult	Try different relaxation positions		
Spurt of energy (1-2 days before labor)			
Onset of Labor			
You may notice any one or a combination of:	Check signs; time contractions		Husband can assist with timing of contractions
Regular contractions (felt as backache, pelvic pressure, gas, menstrual cramp, etc.)	Call doctor. He will advise you when to go to the hospital		Husband or other companion offers diversion and relieves possible tension-producing situations in the home
"Show"—vaginal discharge with pink or red tinge	Continue usual activity as long as comfortable		
Leaking of fluid			
You may feel excited and relieved that labor has begun and yet somewhat apprehensive			
Early First Stage			
Cervix effacing, dilatation beginning	When contraction starts, take complete breath and try to relax. Continue slow deep breathing through contraction		No distracting conversation during contractions
Contractions become strong enough so that you feel need to do something	Between contractions rest, read, watch TV, etc.		
Dilatation continuing; contractions becoming somewhat closer and stronger	Relax as much as possible in sitting or lying positions		
Contractions consume your attention	Lie on side, breathe deeply and slowly while rocking pelvis very gently throughout contraction		Firm pressure against lower back or slow deep massage during contractions
Contractions may cause backache			

Late First Stage

Dilatation continuing; contractions becoming closer, markedly stronger, and of longer duration

May worry about ability to see labor through

Assume comfortable position
Switch to modified breathing pattern, if desired
Rest between contractions

Direction in control of relaxation and of breathing rhythm and depth
Face sponged with cool cloth; lips moistened
Use effleurage
(Medication as indicated)

Transition

10-20 strong, long contractions, close together but may be somewhat irregular. These contractions complete dilatation

Rectal pressure may cause desire to bear down

Possible tremors, nausea, heavy perspiration, hiccoughs, sense of panic

Concentrate on breathing control
Use modified breathing
Puff out occasionally if there is urge to push
Don't hold breath! Don't push!

Reassurance about normality of sensations and probable limit of their duration
Remind her this is transition; contractions not endless
Understanding acceptance of possible expressions of irritability
Do not leave her alone at this point!

Second Stage

Contractions change in character, remaining very strong but slightly further apart

Continuing strong contractions pushing baby down against pelvic floor and causing stretching, perhaps burning sensation

May be afraid to push despite desire

Baby's head seen at vaginal opening

As doctor slowly delivers head, there may be strong desire to push

Shoulders are born one at a time. Relief is experienced as birth of baby is completed

Push toward vaginal opening as directed, relaxing pelvic floor and steadily reinforcing work of uterus

Between contractions relax completely

While being moved to delivery room, pant deeply through contractions

When settled on delivery table, push as directed through contractions, remembering to relax pelvic floor and thighs

Rest completely between contractions

Pant to control pushing urge; relax thighs

If requested to push, push very gently

Pillows arranged to support mother in comfortable position for pushing
Direction of pushing effort and encouragement of relaxation between contractions; reassurance that progress is continuing
Keep her informed of downward progress baby is making
(Transfer to delivery room)
(Anesthesia as indicated)
(Episiotomy as indicated)
Direction for controlled pushing and panting

Third Stage

Rhythmical contractions, less intense
Abdomen sensitive
Placenta delivered

Push as directed
Lie back and enjoy baby!

Source: Maternity Center Association: Preparation for Childbearing, ed. 4. New York, 1973, pp. 30-39.

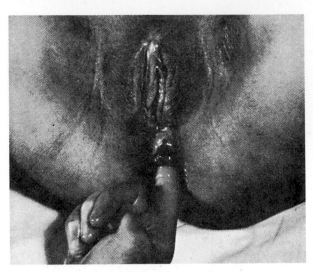
Figure 18-1. Rectal examination, showing flexion of thumb of the gloved hand to prevent contamination of the vulva.

VULVAR AND PERINEAL PREPARATION. The aim in shaving and washing the vulva is to cleanse and disinfect the immediate area about the vagina and to prevent anything contaminated from entering the birth canal. During labor, pathogenic bacteria ascend the birth canal more readily, and every effort should be made to protect the mother from intrapartal infection. In some hospitals a sterile gauze sponge or a folded towel is placed against the introitus to prevent contaminated matter, such as hair or soapy fluid, from entering the vagina during the preparation procedure. In addition, the nurse should be aware that infection from the nasopharynx is possible, and she should avoid unnecessary coughing or talking which might contaminate the vulva from this source.

Some physicians do not require that the mons pubis be shaved because of its distance from the episiotomy area and because of the discomfort that the regrowth of the hair causes; clipping the hair in this area often suffices. Some do not even wish the perineum shaved although episiotomy repair is certainly facilitated in the absence of perineal hair. However, most physicians still require the traditional perineal shave. When this is done, the vulvar hair is lathered prior to shaving to facilitate the procedure and make it more comfortable for the mother. An ordinary safety razor is used, and, beginning at the mons veneris (if the pubic area is included), with the direction of the stroke being from above downward, the area of the vulva and the perineal body is shaved. The nurse can stretch the skin above each downward stroke and permit the razor to move smoothly over the skin without undue pressure. When the entire area anterior to an imaginary line drawn through the base of the perineal body has been shaved, the patient can be turned to her side to enable the nurse to complete the shaving of the anal area. With the upper leg well flexed, the anal area is lathered and shaved, again with a front-to-back stroke. It must always be remembered that anything which has passed over the anal region must not be returned near the vulvar orifice.

The solutions as well as the techniques used in cleansing the genitals will vary in different hospitals, but warm water with soap is probably the most commonly employed.

In washing the genitals, the nurse cleanses thoroughly first the surrounding areas, using sterile sponges or disposable washcloths for each area, and gradually works in toward the vestibule. The strokes must be from above downward and away from the introitus. Special attention should be paid to separating the vulvar folds in order to remove the smegma which may have accumulated in the folds of the labia minora and/or at the base of the clitoris. Finally, the region around the anus is cleansed. It should be emphasized here again that a sponge which has passed over the anal area must not be returned near the vulvar orifice but should be discarded immediately. The patient is instructed not to touch the genitals lest she infect herself.

Examinations in labor

GENERAL. The pulse, respiration and temperature are taken, as previously stated, and are repeated every 4 hours. In cases in which there is fever, or in which labor has lasted more than 24 hours, it is desirable to repeat these observations every two hours. The blood pressure is recorded by either the physician or the nurse and is repeated every hour; in cases of toxemia of pregnancy, this may be done more frequently, according to the physician's instructions. As soon as possible after admission, a complete examination of the heart and the lungs is carried out by the physician to make certain that there are no conditions present which might contraindicate the type of analgesia or anesthesia to be used.

ABDOMINAL. The abdominal examination is similar to that carried out in the antepartal period, comprising estimation of fetal size and position and listening to the fetal heart sounds.

RECTAL AND VAGINAL. Both rectal and vaginal examinations may be performed during labor. They are generally done by the physician, although with special training in some institutions, nurses are given the responsibility for them. It was previously thought that rectal examinations were much safer than vaginal examinations, since they reduced the risk of carrying pathogenic bacteria from the introitus and the lower vagina to the region of the cervix and the lower uterine segment. Studies and general experience show that this supposed advantage of rectal examinations over vaginal examinations has been greatly exaggerated. Nevertheless, rectal examinations do have the advantage of not requiring preliminary disinfection on the part of the physician or the patient.

For either rectal or vaginal examination the patient lies on her back with her knees flexed. The nurse should drape the patient so that she is well protected, but with the perineal region exposed. In making a rectal examination the index finger is used, the hand being covered by a clean but not necessarily sterile rubber glove. As shown in Figure 18-1, the thumb should be fixed into the palm of the hand, because otherwise it may enter the vagina and introduce infection. The finger is anointed liberally with a lubricating jelly and introduced slowly into the rectum. The cervical opening usually can be felt as a depression surrounded by a circular ridge (Fig. 18-2). The degree of dilatation and the amount of effacement are noted. Very often the membranes can be felt bulging into the cervix, particularly during a contraction. The level of the fetal head is now ascertained and correlated with the level of the ischial spines as being a certain number of centimeters above or below the ischial spines. After the completion of the examination the patient's perineum is wiped, and the examiner's hands are washed. The rectal glove is cleansed and sterilized if it is to be reused; otherwise, it is discarded.

The frequency with which rectal examinations are required during labor depends on the individual case; often one or two such examinations are sufficient, while in some instances more are required. The nurse who stays with the mother constantly will find that she becomes increasingly skillful in her ability to follow the progress of labor to a great extent

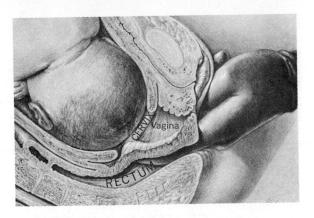

Figure 18-2. Rectal examination, showing how the examining finger palpates the cervix and the infant's head through the rectovaginal septum.

by careful evaluation of subjective and objective symptoms of the mother (i.e., the character of the uterine contractions and the show, the progressive descent of the area on the abdomen where fetal heart sounds are heard, the mother's overall response to her physical labor, etc.).

If the mother is to have a vaginal examination, she may be prepared by cleansing the vulvar and the perineal region in a manner

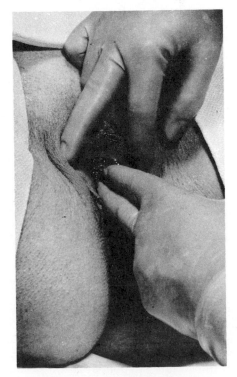

Figure 18-3. Vaginal examination.

similar to that used in preparation for delivery. The physician scrubs his hands as for an operation and dons sterile gloves. Before introducing his fingers into the vagina, he takes care to separate the labia widely in order to minimize possible contamination of his examining fingers if they should come in contact with the inner surfaces of the labia and the margins of the hymen. Then the index and the second fingers of the examining hand are gently introduced into the vagina (Fig. 18-3). Vaginal examination is more reliable than rectal, since the cervix, the fontanels, etc., can be palpated directly with no intervening rectovaginal septum to interfere with the tactile sense. Some authorities feel that the danger of introducing infection into the birth canal is increased with repeated vaginal examinations and thus attempt to limit the number of times the examination is repeated, using it only as necessary.

Conduct of the first stage

The first stage of labor (dilating stage) begins with the first symptoms of true labor and ends with the complete dilatation of the cervix. The physician examines the patient early in labor and sees her from time to time throughout the first stage but may not be in constant attendance at this time. In normal labor his examinations (fetal heart, rectal, and so on) will show that the baby is in good condition and that steady progress is being made. Furthermore, the rate of progress often will give some indication as to when delivery is to be expected. Since the physician is usually unable to be with the mother constantly during this stage, he must rely on the nurse not only to safeguard the welfare of mother and fetus but also to notify him concerning the progress of labor.

Support during labor

As already emphasized, it is important for the nurse to have an empathic supportive attitude toward the mother, so she can interpret the progress of labor and perform certain technical procedures skillfully. It should be pointed out that "supportive care" includes not only aspects of emotional support but also aspects of physical care which in the total context of care contribute to the well-being and the comfort of the mother and hence to her emotional equilibrium. Thus, a sponge bath, oral hygiene, a backrub, an explanation before a procedure,

etc., all enhance her comfort and help the mother to feel that she is a special, worthwhile person. Many of the physical care activities that nurses perform consist, in part at least, of "laying on of hands," which is known to be necessary and helpful to patients in maintaining or reachieving good health. These activities, then, can be valuable entrées in establishing and maintaining rapport and hence an effective relationship. Even the intrusive procedures which are so often painful or distasteful, if done with gentleness and skill, show the patient that her dignity and integrity are respected.

Related to this "laying on of hands" aspect is the effectiveness of the use of touch. Although this has not been explored to any great degree scientifically, its importance was recognized as far back as the mid-19th century. More recently, research indicates that the patient's ability to work effectively with her labor contractions increased when extensive physical contact was introduced and then decreased when physical contact was withdrawn (see Suggested Reading). This contact can take the form of a backrub, allowing the patient to grasp the nurse's hand, stroking the patient's brow, and so on. Indeed, many of the relaxation techniques practiced in the prepared childbirth classes rely on the use of this sense. However, touch need not be used indiscriminately, as excessive and/or inappropriate touching is offensive to many people. The need will vary from patient to patient, and the mother will indicate which type of touch is helpful and who will be the most appropriate person to give it. The nurse must use her professional judgment regarding its use, and her rapport with the patient will help her to make a correct decision. This type of communication can be a way of demonstrating the nurse's concern and empathy, especially when verbal communication is difficult or impossible. It is also an effective means of incorporating the husband into the care and the support of his wife.

The more cheerful, flexible environment of the modern labor room undoubtedly is conducive to putting the patient and her husband more at ease, but this in itself is not enough. Once labor is well established, the mother should not be left alone. The morale of women in labor is sometimes hopelessly shattered, regardless of whether or not they have been prepared for labor during pregnancy, when they are left by themselves over long periods of time. During labor the mother is more sensitive to the behavior of those about her, particularly in relation to her perception of how much concern the personnel about her show for her safety and well-being. As labor progresses, there is a normal narrowing of the phenomenal field, an "inward turning," which results in easy distortion of stimuli and perception. For instance, careless remarks dropped in conversation often are misinterpreted as indicative of negligence or unfeelingness. It is well to remember that comments and laughter overheard in the corridor outside the patient's room may contribute to her uneasiness. Therefore, the nurse must be on guard against unfortunate happenings of this kind.

The nurse will want to be aware that her own anxieties in the situation may be communicated to the patient. The process of labor and the forthcoming delivery will produce normal anxieties which are no more than a healthy anticipation of the events to come (in both patient and nurse). Thus, most patients tolerate their labor much better if they are told the kind of progress that is being made and assured that they are doing a good job working with their contractions. This is part and parcel of the continuing orientation to the labor process that was mentioned earlier.

Another point that is apropos here is the usefulness and the effectiveness of suggestion for the mother in labor. It has been shown that the pregnant woman is extremely passive and vulnerable; this increases her sensitivity and makes her receptive to both positive and negative suggestion from virtually total strangers. The nurse can utilize this suggestibility to great advantage in her supportive care, since the mother responds very readily to suggestions, especially in early labor. The groundwork can be laid at this time for the more complicated instructions that may be necessary later in labor concerning relaxation, breathing techniques and the management of pain.

The mother who has attended antepartal classes that have included exercise and relaxation techniques is usually better prepared for labor, but nevertheless she needs to be coached in utilizing the techniques which will enable her to cooperate with the natural forces of labor. During early labor the patient usually prefers to move about the room and frequently is more at ease sitting in a comfortable chair. She can be permitted and encouraged to do this and whatever else seems to be most relaxing and pleasant to her. If hospital policy permits the father to be in the labor room, his presence can be a valuable asset because of the support that it gives the mother. Several studies have documented the presence of the father during labor as a major source of support for the mother (see Suggested Reading). This not only benefits the mother but also helps the father to feel that he has a more vital role in participating with her in the birth of their child.

PROGRESSION OF ACTIVE PHASE OF LABOR. When the mother begins to mind her labor, she may need help to get into a comfortable position and to relax. During the contractions she can be coached as necessary in the application of the slow deep-breathing technique described in Chapter 13. Regardless of how diligently the mother has practiced the various breathing and relaxing techniques during pregnancy, or the level of her understanding about the physiology of labor, the situation is changed somewhat for her by active labor. Each mother may react in a slightly different way, for each is an individual. Some analgesic medication may be required for the mother's comfort after good labor is established (see p. 290). The nurse may observe in time that as the active phase progresses (i.e., the 7 to 10 cm. dilatation) slow deep breathing becomes difficult for the patient. The mother herself is aware that "her diaphragm won't cooperate." Rapid, shallow breathing (accelerated breathing) with the contractions is usually easier and more effective.

Uterine contractions

The term "pains" has been associated with uterine contractions of childbirth since time immemorial. One finds this term still in common usage, so that even today many young women approach childbirth with fear of pain. It is no easy task to dispel this age-old fear, but throughout the childbirth experience a conscious effort must be made to instill a wholesome point of view in the mother. The nurse will want to avoid the use of the word "pain" whenever possible because of the very connotation of the word, and it is hoped that she will not use it in reference to uterine contractions. It is important to remember, however, that as labor progresses, the contractions often become painful. This is not just a figment of the patient's imagination. Therefore, it is the nurse's responsibility to help the mother to distinguish between the *fear and anticipation* of pain and the *actual* pain she may be experiencing, and to help her to cope effectively.

The contribution that the nurse can make in the management of pain during labor and delivery has already been discussed in Chapter 16. However, we would like to reiterate a few of the major points here in order to reinforce them. We know that studies of pain have demonstrated that the anticipation of pain raises the anxiety level significantly to cause the pain reaction threshold to lower. Thus, the patient reacts sooner to even minimal pain stimuli. The pain is subjectively intensified and even a slight amount of pain seems to be much greater. Furthermore, other sensations are misinterpreted as pain (e.g., pressure, stretching, etc.), which explains why the digital examinations and even the pressure of the nurse's fingers on the abdomen as she times contractions "hurt." Therefore, "everything" is painful, and the heightening of the anticipation of pain in turn increases the response to pain, and soon a vicious cycle is established. The nurse can help to break this cycle or to prevent it from becoming established by intervening at the anticipation-anxiety junction. She does this by reminding the patient when a contraction is over (and the pain is gone), that another contraction is not expected for several minutes: thus, this is the time for the mother to rest and to relax. The anxiety related to the anticipation of pain then is lowered or eliminated (the mother knows now she is free from pain for several minutes and can rest), and the subjective intensification is diminished. It is obvious that the nurse or some other reliable person must be in continuous attendance in order to do this. Moreover, sociocultural factors play an important part in the meaning and interpretation of pain for patients. While pain is basically a physiologic phenomenon, the meaning pain has and the kinds of responses to pain that are deemed appropriate are matters of cultural prescription. Cultural orientations, social conditioning, and sociocultural sanctioning play a large part in molding patterns of response to painful experiences which are modal (i.e., occur most frequently) in a group, and these modal patterns are meaningful in terms of the values and beliefs of a particular group. Therefore, a culture or subculture from which a person comes conditions the formation of her particular reaction patterns to pain, and a knowledge of a group's attitudes toward pain is extremely important to the understanding of the reaction of a particular member of that group. (For a more thorough discussion of the responses and interpretation of pain by various cultural and subcultural groups see Suggested Reading.)

The frequency, the duration and the intensity of the contractions should be watched closely and recorded. The frequency of contractions is timed from the beginning of one contraction until the beginning of the next. The duration of a contraction is timed from the moment the uterus first begins to tighten until it relaxes again (Fig. 18-4). The intensity of a contraction may be mild, moderate or strong at its acme. Since this is a relative factor, it is difficult to interpret unless one is at the mother's bedside. For the sake of description, one might say that during a mild contraction the uterine muscle becomes somewhat tense; during a moderate contraction the uterus becomes moderately firm; during a strong contraction the uterus becomes so firm that it has the feel of woody hardness, and at the height of the contraction the uterus cannot be indented by pressure of the examiner's fingers.

When the mother first becomes aware of the contractions, they may be 15 to 20 minutes

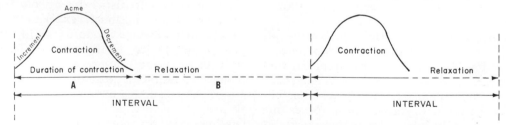

Figure 18-4. The interval and the duration of uterine contractions. The frequency of contractions is the interval timed from the beginning of one contraction to the beginning of the next contraction. The interval consists of two parts: (A) the duration of the contraction and (B) the period of relaxation. The broken line indicates an indeterminate period, since this time (B) is usually of longer duration than the actual contraction of (A).

apart and lasting perhaps 20 to 25 seconds. Since these are of mild intensity, she usually can continue with whatever she is doing, except that she is alert to time the subsequent contractions (to have specific information to give the physician when she calls him). If this is her first pregnancy, he may advise her to wait until the contractions are five to ten minutes apart before coming to the hospital (depending on the other signs of labor). However, if she is a multipara, she will more than likely be told to come to the hospital as soon as a regular pattern of contractions is established (again, depending on other criteria).

As labor progresses, the character of the contractions will change (see Chapter 15). They will become stronger in intensity, last longer (a duration of 45 to 60 seconds) and come closer together (at a frequency of every two to three minutes). One effective method the nurse can employ to time contractions is to keep her fingers lightly on the fundus. The fingers are recommended because they usually are more sensitive than the more calloused palm. However, for some people the whole hand is helpful. It should be emphasized that enough of the fingers should be used to ensure adequate contact with the abdomen; too slight a contact does not enable the nurse to ascertain the contractions accurately.

As the nurse times in this manner, she is able to detect the contraction, as it begins, by the gradual tensing and rising forward of the fundus, and to feel the contraction through its three phases until the uterus relaxes again. The inexperienced nurse can get some idea of how a contraction will feel under her fingertips if she feels her own biceps contract. First, the forearm should be extended and the fingertips of the hand on the opposite side placed on the biceps. Then, the arm is gradually flexed until the muscle becomes very hard, held a few seconds, and gradually extended. This should take about 30 seconds to simulate a uterine contraction. It is not reliable to ask the mother to let you know when a contraction begins, because often she is unaware of it for perhaps five or ten seconds, sometimes even until the contraction reaches its acme. It is important for the nurse to observe the rhythm of the contractions and to be assured that the uterine muscle relaxes completely after each contraction. As the labor approaches the transition, the contractions will be very strong, last for about 60 seconds and occur at two- to three-minute intervals. If any contraction lasts longer than 70 seconds and is not followed by a rest interval with complete relaxation of the uterine muscle, this should be reported to the physician immediately because of its implications for both the mother and her infant (see Chapter 25).

Particularly during the late active phase the need for human contact—someone to hold on to—during the severe contractions will be seen. The mother responds less well to other physical contact, stroking, sponging, etc.; she may even say, "Leave me alone," meaning, of course, "Don't disturb me." However, if it is helpful for her to have someone's hand to hold, she should be allowed to do this if she indicates the need.

Since during the first stage of labor the uterine contractions are involuntary and uncontrolled by the patient, it is futile for her to "bear down" with her abdominal muscles, because this only leads to exhaustion. The mother who has been prepared for "natural childbirth" has been schooled in breathing techniques, such as diaphragmatic breathing or rapid shallow costal breathing, and with coaching from her husband or her nurse is usually able to accomplish conscious relaxation.

With the unprepared mother, a different situation exists. These mothers are often best helped to relax by encouraging and coaching them to keep breathing slowly and evenly during the early contractions, and then to assume a pattern of more rapid and shallow breathing that is most comfortable to them during the late active phase. They will very often need to be reminded not to hold their breath during the contractions. One cannot expect perfection in breathing techniques with these patients; however, this activity gives the inexperienced mother a point of concentration, and her feeling that she is actually participating and "controlling" her labor to some degree is helpful to her. Most mothers in labor, whether they are "prepared" or not, want to cooperate, and the calm, kind, firm guidance of an interested nurse can do much to help the mother utilize her contractions effectively.

Show

This mucoid discharge from the cervix is present after the discharge of the mucous plug. As progressive effacement and dilatation of the cervix occur, the show becomes blood-tinged due to the rupture of superficial capillaries.

The presence of an increased amount of bloody show (blood-stained mucus, not actual bleeding!) suggests that rather rapid progress may be taking place and should be reported immediately, particularly if associated with frequent severe contractions.

A perineal pad is not to be worn during labor because of the nature of the vaginal discharge. The tenacious mucoid discharge frequently comes in contact with the anus and could easily be smeared about the external genitalia and vaginal orifice when the patient moves about the bed or adjusts the pads. A quilted pad placed under the mother's buttocks serves very well to absorb material discharged from the vagina. This pad can be changed frequently and the perineum cleansed as necessary to keep the mother clean and dry.

Evaluation of the fetal heart rate

The behavior of the fetal heartbeat in labor is of great importance. The heart rate can be monitored in a number of ways. The simplest, and still an effective method, is by frequent auscultation using a specialized head stethoscope. The widely used DeLee-Hillis stethoscope or the Leff fetal heart stethoscope are satisfactory for this purpose.

When checking the fetal heart sounds, the nurse listens and counts the rate for one full minute. Checking the rate before, during and after a contraction is important so that any slowing and/or irregularities may be detected.

As previously explained, the fetal heart rate is normally between 120 to 160 beats per minute, except during and immediately after a uterine contraction, when it may fall to as low as 70 to 110. Hon found that in multigravidas the fetal heart rate might fall from 140 to 110-120 beats per minute at the acme of a contraction (see Suggested Reading). In primigravidas the drop is greater, at times reaching 60 to 70 beats per minute (Fig. 18-5). This physiologic bradycardia begins after the onset of a contraction and ends 10 to 15 seconds prior to its end. It is believed to result from compression of the fetal skull by the partially dilated cervix rather than from fetal hypoxia. It appears to occur most commonly between 4 and 8 cm. of cervical dilatation.

It may be difficult to hear the sounds during a contraction, because the uterine wall is tense, and, in addition, it is more difficult for the mother to lie still during this period. But it is particularly important to listen at this time, since these observations inform the listener how the fetus reacts to the contraction. From a clinical standpoint any prolonged slowing should be reported to the obstetrician. Should the slowing be below 100 beats per minute, and should it last more than 30 seconds after the termination of a contraction, then it is no longer considered to be physiologic and is taken as a sign of fetal distress. Occasionally, this prolonged slow rate is accompanied by the passage of meconium, another sign indicative of

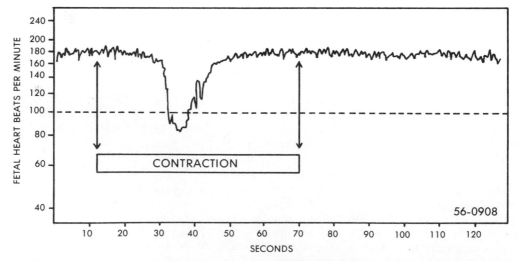

Figure 18-5. Electronic evaluation of fetal heart rates, showing normal slowing of the fetal heart rate during uterine contraction. (Hon, E. H.: Observations on "pathologic" fetal bradycardia, Am. J. Ob.-Gyn. 77:1084, 1959)

fetal distress if it occurs in a vertex presentation. It must be remembered that unless the membranes have ruptured, the meconium will not be apparent. Any unusual observations must be reported to the physician promptly so that measures can be instituted before permanent damage is done to the infant.

Repeated auscultation of the fetal heart sounds constitutes one of the most important responsibilities in the conduct of the first and the second stages of labor (see Chapter 11). During the early period of the first stage of labor the nurse records the fetal heart rate every hour, and once good labor is established, every half hour, or even more often if indicated. During the second stage of labor it is done every 5 minutes and recorded.

The fetal heart tones are checked immediately following the rupture of membranes, regardless of whether they rupture spontaneously or are artificially ruptured by the physician. With the gush of water that ensues, there is a possibility that the cord may be prolapsed, and any indication of fetal distress from pressure on the umbilical cord can thereby be detected.

ELECTRONIC MONITORING. Although monitoring by auscultation has been successful in a majority of cases, it has some shortcomings. It has been demonstrated that, in monitoring the fetascope, listeners tend to be subjective and to normalize the fetal heart rate. Indeed, 20 percent of the observations were found to be inaccurate by 15 beats per minute from the actual heart rate.[8] Moreover, the method does not provide for continuous surveillance.

Electronic monitoring does provide for accurate and continuous appraisal of both intrauterine pressure (IUP) and fetal heart rate (FHR), but its success depends on accurate application of equipment, reliable equipment design, accurate data interpretation and patient acceptance.

There are two categories of patients who are candidates for electronic monitoring. The high-risk mothers (for instance those with eclampsia, diabetes, previous stillbirths) are prime candidates because of the associated fetal morbidity and mortality. The second type of patient is the normal obstetrical patient who develops fetal distress during labor. It is becoming more common to monitor all labor patients, at least externally, in order to ascertain fetal distress early in labor. However, not all hospitals are able to afford or maintain

Glossary

AMPLITUDE of *Contraction*
Pressure exerted by uterus during a contraction; measured from baseline to peak

AMPLITUDE of *Fetal Heart Rate*
Difference in beats per minute between baseline and the minimum or maximum count

FLUCTUATION
Change in fetal heart rate from a baseline rate
Acceleration Transient increase of more than 15 beats per minute
Deceleration Transient decrease of more than 15 beats per minute

TACHYCARDIA
Fetal heart rate of more than 160 beats per minute that persists through at least 2 complete contraction cycles or 5 minutes
Moderate 160 to 179
Severe 180 or more

BRADYCARDIA
Fetal heart rate of fewer than 120 beats per minute that persists through at least 2 complete contraction cycles or 5 minutes
Moderate 90 to 120
Marked 70 to 89
Severe Fewer than 70

REACTIVE BASELINE
Fetal heart rate normally fluctuating more than 5 beats per minute from baseline

RECOVERY TIME
Seconds from end of contraction until fetal heart rate returns to baseline

LAG TIME
Time between peak of uterine contraction and lowest count of fetal heart deceleration

Tips for Buyers

Many brands of monitoring equipment are marketed. When one is considering the purchase of a monitoring system, the following information may be helpful:

The system should be designed to monitor externally and internally.

An ultrasonic transducer should have a wide beam, so that the fetal heart rate signal is not easily lost.

The tachometer should measure each fetal heartbeat instead of taking an average of several beats.

The chart speed should be the standard 3 cm. per minute.

An engineer should evaluate all components of the system.

The manufacturer should be able to supply all needed accessories, such as ultrasonic jelly, catheters, and so forth.

The system should be portable. Some companies sell monitoring carts with drawers to store accessories.

There should be a warranty.

Servicing should be readily available.

The company should permit a trial period before final purchase, and most companies will agree to this.

the various types of devices presently on the market. Thus, judicious buying practices are necessary.[9] (See Glossary, p. 317.)

Continuous monitoring of the IUP and FHR during labor is possible by both internal and external methods. The latter have the advantage of being noninvasive, and can be used in early labor before rupture of the membranes. Moreover, the equipment is relatively simple and can be applied easily.

External Methods. Intrauterine pressure (IUP) is monitored by a pressure transducer called a tokodynamometer. A transducer converts one form of energy to another; this transducer converts sounds and pressure to electrical signals. The tokodynamometer is a flat disk with either a protruding or a flush plunger transducer; it is secured to the mother's abdomen with an elastic belt or a bandagelike belt. As the uterus contracts, the abdominal wall rises and presses against the transducer. The subsequent movement of the plunger is converted into an electrical signal and is recorded on a graph, giving a continuous and permanent record of the frequency and duration of all contractions.

Correct placement of the tokodynamometer is necessary if interpretable data are to be gathered. The transducer is placed over the area where the greatest displacement of the uterus occurs during a contraction (i.e., fundus). Excessive movement and/or materials that interfere with the ability of the transducer to pick up signals or to be positioned correctly lead to poor data. Thus, restless patients or those who are obese are not good candidates for this type of monitoring. Patients who are trying to practice their prepared childbirth techniques sometimes find that the firm straps interfere with their breathing techniques and effleurage and become uncomfortable over time. Thus, explanation for the reason for the procedure, repositioning of the transducer and/or alternate monitoring methods are useful in these patients.

The fetal heart rate (FHR) can be monitored externally by phonocardiography. A crystal contact microphone picks up the fetal heart sounds and emits an audible signal. Again, if either the fetus or mother moves excessively, the signal is poor.

More recently, ultrasonic transducers have been used to monitor FHR. Ultrasound is a high-frequency sound signal and the mechanism, the Doppler shift in the ultrasound energy, can be used to detect movements of remote objects.

A continuous sound signal is sent out from the transmitting crystals and bounces off an object, and a return signal is reflected back to the receiving crystals. In practice, the ultrasonic signal is directed toward the fetal heart. As this organ pumps blood, the movement of the walls of the heart can be detected, since the reflected signal is altered with each heartbeat. This change in frequency is acknowledged by the receiving crystals as a beat and each time a beat is heard an audible signal is heard on the machine. This is often referred to as the Doppler signal.

A cardiotachometer uses the time intervals between the audible signals and, in that way, measures beat to beat FHR. The transducer changes the sound signal to an electrical signal and records it.

In the application of the ultrasonic transducer, the nurse's objective is to locate the area on the abdomen where the best quality of fetal heart tones is heard. This does not mean necessarily the loudest, but rather the sharpest "click-click" sounds, similar to the galloping sound of horses' hooves. To locate the sounds, the nurse will lubricate the face of the transducer with a thin layer of ultrasonic jelly (or will wet the patient's abdomen); then she searches for the area where the sounds are the sharpest. Before the appropriate "click-click" sounds are found, other sounds, such as the umbilical cord or maternal aorta noises, may cause interference, but with practice and perseverance an appropriate signal can be obtained. If possible, it is wise to attach the transducer laterally, rather than medially, on the mother's abdomen since it is displaced less easily in that position.

Internal Methods. It is possible to institute internal monitoring when the cervix is 3 to 4 cm. dilated, the station is −2 or lower and the membranes are ruptured or can be ruptured safely. Although this is an invasive technique, complications are usually rare and of a minor nature, if appropriate technique is observed. Moreover, the data are quantitative —IUP is measured in millimeters of mercury— and are more useful than the qualitative sound data that the external monitoring machines give.

When internal monitoring is done, both the IUP and the FHR are recorded simultaneously. To assess IUP, a soft catheter filled with isotonic sterile saline (so that air will not be introduced into the uterus) is passed through the vagina into the uterus intraamniotically behind the presenting part. It must be situated in the amniotic fluid to measure pressure. The catheter is connected to an external transducer (strain gauge). As the uterine pressure increases with the contractions, fluid pressure in the catheter increases simultaneously and the transducer converts the pressure values into an electrical signal. The change in pressure is recorded on a graph. If the presenting part is too low, insertion of the catheter may be impossible. Also, any bleeding or a low-lying placenta are contraindications for catheter insertion.

When the FHR is monitored internally, a continuous ECG is recorded. A scalp-clip electrode is attached to the presenting part of the fetus—head, buttocks or foot. In a face presentation, the procedure is contraindicated because of possible damage to the infant's eyes. The signal received is actually the fetal ECG and is continuous.

Possible complications include endometritis secondary to a break in sterile technique during catheter insertion. Rarely is there detachment of an undiagnosed low-lying placenta. Sterile fetal scalp abscesses from the electrode have occurred but have responded promptly following either spontaneous or surgical drainage. These can be avoided, however, with the observance of appropriate aseptic technique.

Inserting the catheter and the scalp clip is a relatively uncomplicated procedure. Nevertheless, it is generally the physician's responsibility. Some hospitals are instituting special training programs to educate nurses not only in the interpretation of the electronic data, but also in the insertion of the internal devices (see Suggested Reading). It is apparent that some type of specialized instruction is necessary before the health personnel involved can assume full responsibility for attaching the internal devices. A physician's order is required for the insertion of internal devices.

When internal monitoring is begun, it is performed under sterile conditions with the patient prepped as for delivery. The mother may be placed in one of three positions: lithotomy with her legs in stirrups, lithotomy with her buttocks on a sterile bedpan or on her side with her knees flexed and drawn upward.[10]

INTERPRETATION OF DATA. There are several parameters to be examined when monitoring IUP: amplitude, duration and frequency of contractions as well as a baseline. Baseline, the resting tone of the uterus, is low when the uterus is relaxed and rises with increased tonicity. Bearing-down efforts are recorded as feather-like marks on the curve at the peak of the contraction. Figure 18-6 illustrates these intrauterine pressure recordings.

Several different criteria have been derived by numerous investigators; hence, there is some difficulty in defining and interpreting the FHR. The following discussion derives mainly from the work of Russen et al and O'Gureck et al, which is based on the earlier work of Hon and colleagues.[11]

Initially, the parameters of the FHR and the definitions employed need to be determined (see Glossary, p. 317). Any change in the baseline is termed a *fluctuation* and is either an *acceleration* or a *deceleration*. Other measures to consider are *amplitude, lag time,* and *recovery time.*

When examining an FHR recording, the nurse will check the baseline first for tachycardia, bradycardia or reactivity. A significant FHR baseline value must persist for two complete contraction cycles or for five minutes.

Tachycardia has been associated with asphyxia and is considered to be a compensatory mechanism. Tachycardia is also associated with low Apgar scores when accompanied by decelerations of 50 beats per minute and a frequency over 50 percent. When these conditions occur, oxygen administration is advised, although its actual efficacy is still a matter of debate. If oxytocin is being administered, it is discontinued since it is one of the causes of aberrations in contractions.

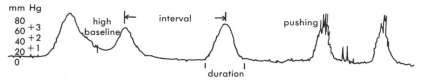

Figure 18-6. Intrauterine pressure recording shows smooth waveforms during three contractions, and featherlike marks when the mother pushes. (Russen, A. W., O'Gureck, J. E., and Roux, J. F.: Electronic monitoring of the fetus, Am. J. Nurs., July 1974)

If the uterus is also hyperactive (i.e., if the intensity of the contractions is more than 50 mm. Hg) in the first stage of labor, or if there are more than five contractions for every ten minutes, the patient is placed in a lateral position to avoid hypotension and improve circulation. The positional change is utilized first, followed by oxygenation by mask. The patient is asked to breathe deeply and slowly. It has been found that tachycardia with deceleration may persist for up to 30 minutes without a *serious* compromise to the fetus. However, it is recommended that after 30 minutes delivery be effected.

Bradycardia is significant depending on its degree. For instance, an FHR fewer than 100 to 120 beats per minute (moderate bradycardia) is *not* associated with significant fetal acidosis. However, congenital heart disease may be reflected by a persistent FHR of 90 to 100 beats per minute. If the FHR tends to drift persistently downward, treatment is instituted to prevent the tones from going below 100. Moderate bradycardia is treated by the administration of oxygen, discontinuing oxytocin and changing the mother to a lateral position. Since this type of bradycardia is felt at this time to pose little threat to the fetus, labor may continue without interference. It must be remembered that various physicians may have different criteria for defining bradycardia and may institute treatment at different stages.

When there is marked bradycardia (FHR 70 to 99), the fetus may become acidotic; the FHR may suddenly drop below 70 beats per minute. In these cases, prompt administration of oxygen, discontinuance of any oxytocin and placement of the mother in a lateral or Trendelenberg (or both) position are treatments of choice. If the marked bradycardia persists, it has been found that 20 minutes is the maximum time from its onset to the delivery of a viable, uncompromised fetus. If decelerations have occurred prior to the onset of bradycardia, insult to the fetus occurs earlier and delivery must be effected as soon as possible.

Oxytocin is a major cause of bradycardia and is always discontinued when there is persistent or marked lowered FHR. Another cause is supine hypotension which is usually precipitated by a regional anesthetic—caudal, epidural, spinal or saddle. However, hypotension can occur in supine, unanesthetized patients. Nursing treatment consists of a lateral position change, preferably to the left side to facilitate emptying of the vena cava into the heart. If an anesthetist is available, treatment may also include ephedrine sulphate, 50 percent dextrose, and elevating the mother's legs at a 90-degree angle to the bed. The Trendelenburg position is *not* used in patients having spinal anesthesia since there is danger that the anesthetic might migrate upward, causing respiratory and cardiac immobility.

Reactivity of the baseline is a final important consideration when one is observing the FHR. A reactive baseline (one which fluctuates more than five beats per minute) without abnormalities in the heart tones is an indication of an apparently healthy fetus. Conversely, a nonreactive or "silent" baseline can indicate serious fetal compromise reflecting an acidotic fetal nervous system unable to make minor parasympathetic and sympathetic responses. Occasionally, for no apparent reason, a healthy fetus will have a silent baseline for 10 to 20 minutes. In these cases, vigorous digital or mechanical stimulation of the fetal scalp is recommended. If the FHR fluctuates in response, the condition is considered transient. If there is no response, the mother's position is usually changed and observations are made to see if she has received any central nervous system depressant (narcotic, magnesium sulphate, etc.). If the baseline remains silent, then all factors are quickly evaluated to make preparations for prompt delivery.

Fluctuations in the baseline of the FHR are the next major consideration. The FHR is considered regular if none of the fluctuations exceeds 15 beats per minute. Accelerated fluctuations may be related to a change in intrauterine pressure and may be of two types: Type 1 or combined acceleration immediately precedes or follows a variable deceleration. It does not seem to be pathologic, although its exact significance is not known. Type 2 or isolated acceleration is not combined with any deceleration pattern and its significance depends on its severity. When there is moderate acceleration, there is an amplitude of fewer than 50 beats per minute. This indicates a responsive nervous system and an anticipated good fetal outcome. Moderate acceleration may appear with stimulation of the fetal scalp and may disappear with medication. Acceleration amplitude of more than 60 beats per minute is considered severe and indicates fetal compromise. These severe isolated accelerations may be due to periodic episodes of fetal hypo-

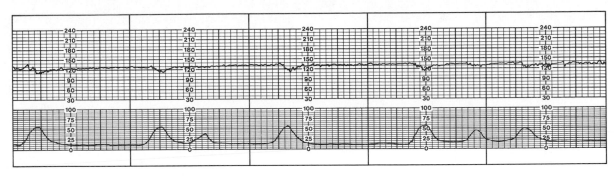

Figure 18-7. Early deceleration. The FHR baseline is the normal range, with normal variability. Uterine activity is normal with oxytocin augmentation. Early deceleration patterns are evident, approximating a mirror image of the uterine pressure curve. The nadir of the early deceleration occurs at the same time as the peak of the uterine contraction. (Parer, J. T., et al: A Clinical Approach to Fetal Monitoring, San Leandro, Calif., Berkeley Bio-Engineering, Inc., 1974)

tension. The nursing management consists of placing the patient in the lateral position and promptly discontinuing any oxytocin. The ultimate aim is suppression of the accelerations.

Another type of fluctuation is that of *deceleration*. This type is also related to change in the intrauterine pressure and several patterns have been described: Early or Type 1, late or Type 2, and variable or Type 3.

An early deceleration (Type 1) shows a waveform that is smooth with a gradual onset and recovery; thus, the waveform appears curvilinear and mirrors the pattern of intrauterine pressure. The pattern also is uniform in appearance from one contraction to the next. Early deceleration begins near the onset of the uterine contraction. The nadir of the deceleration occurs at the peak of the contraction and the fetal heart tones return to the baseline by the end of the contraction. There is no loss of variability in the baseline and no fetal tachycardia; thus the FHR characteristically stays within the normal range during the

deceleration. This type of deceleration is considered benign and of no pathologic significance. It probably represents head compression as the vertex is compressed against the tissues of the birth canal. Early deceleration is mediated by a vagal reflex and the administration of atropine will diminish or eliminate it. It is most frequently seen during the early part of the active phase of labor (Fig. 18-7).

A late deceleration (Type 2) also manifests a smooth, curvilinear, uniform heart rate pattern which mirrors the pattern of intrauterine pressure, but is later in onset than early deceleration. Late deceleration begins as the contraction reaches its peak, and the nadir of late deceleration occurs well after the peak of the contraction—usually about the time the contraction is over. Moreover, the fetal heart rate does not return to baseline until well after the contraction is over. This type of deceleration has been characterized as mild, moderate or severe depending on the magnitude of the deceleration. Usually, the FHR remains in the

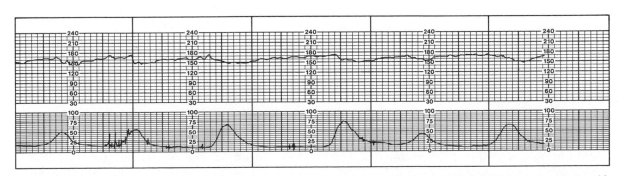

Figure 18-8. Moderate late deceleration. There is a mild fetal tachycardia, ranging between 160 and 170 beats per minute, with decreased variability. Uterine activity is normal. The nadir of late deceleration occurs when the uterine contraction is nearly over. A scalp capillary blood sample had been taken just prior to the first portion of this panel, and mild fetal acidosis was demonstrated, with scalp blood pH 7.21. (Parer, et al: A Clinical Approach to Fetal Monitoring)

conduct of normal labor   321

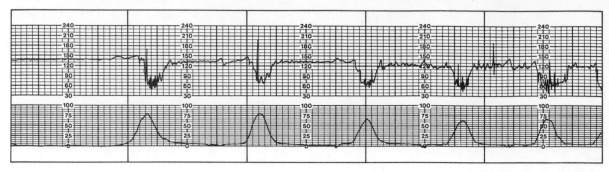

Figure 18-9. Moderate variable deceleration. The FHR baseline is in the normal range, with normal variability. Uterine activity is normal. (Parer, et al: A Clinical Approach to Fetal Monitoring)

normal range unless the deceleration is very severe; it is, however, frequently associated with loss of baseline variability and fetal tachycardia. It is never considered to be normal and is, indeed, an ominous sign of fetal distress. Late deceleration is a hypoxic phenomenon associated with placental insufficiency syndromes and decreased respiratory function of the placenta. The pathophysiologic mechanism is thought to be decreased intervillous blood flow during uterine contractions with a resulting insufficiency in the fetoplacental exchange and intrauterine hypoxia. Each contraction stresses the fetus and continued late deceleration is associated with progressive hypoxia and fetal acidosis. This type of deceleration may be improved by maneuvers which improve uteroplacental blood flow and oxygen transfer across the placenta, such as turning the mother on her side, administering oxygen and correcting maternal hypotension (if present). Reducing uterine activity by discontinuing oxytocin is also indicated. If uncorrected, this type of deceleration is associated with an increased incidence of depressed infants or fetal demise (Fig. 18-8).

Variable deceleration (Type 3) is a nonuniform periodic change in the FHR and bears no consistent time relationship to the uterine contractions. This Type 3 pattern usually occurs during a uterine contraction, but may occur following a contraction or at irregular intervals between contractions. It has a jagged waveform characterized by an abrupt fall in the FHR and then a rapid return to baseline levels rather than the smooth, curvilinear waveform of early and late decelerations. Variable deceleration is often preceded and followed by acceleration and the FHR usually falls to fewer than 100 beats per minute. The mechanism is thought to be due to compression of the um-

bilical cord since this pattern can be reproduced by occlusion of the cord transiently at the time of cesarean section. When severe variable deceleration is present, prolapse of the cord, either overt or occult, should be suspected. Most frequently, however, this pattern is due to impingement of the fetus upon the cord in utero, for instance, the cord lying alongside the fetal shoulder. These patterns usually can be corrected by changing the mother's position, thus relieving the impingement on the cord.

There are three categories of variable deceleration: severe, moderate and mild. In severe variable deceleration, there is a fall in the FHR to fewer than 70 beats per minute for longer than 60 seconds. In moderate variable deceleration, there is a fall in the FHR to either fewer than 70 beats per minute for between 30 to 60 seconds or a fall between 70 to 80 beats per minute for greater than 60 seconds. With mild variable deceleration, there is a fall in the FHR which is less than the above criteria, that is, a fall to any level for less than 30 seconds or a fall to 80 beats per minute or greater for any duration. Mild variable deceleration is usually not a major problem, since it is associated with infants with good Apgar scores. Umbilical cord compression and variable deceleration are associated with respiratory acidosis which can be cleared rapidly through the placenta when this type of deceleration is relieved (Fig. 18-9).

Severe variable deceleration, on the other hand, is very difficult to manage since it is associated with progressive fetal acidosis and low Apgar scores. Moreover, baseline tachycardia and loss of variability are frequently present when the infant is compromised as in fetal cardiac arrest. Fortunately, cardiac activity usually returns spontaneously after a second or two; however, the possibility of fetal demise always exists in these cases (Fig. 18-10).

Since variable deceleration is mediated through a vagal reflex, it may be blunted or abolished by giving atropine. This drug is given if the variable deceleration is so severe as to suggest the possibility of fetal cardiac asystole at the nadir of the deceleration; however, at the present time, there is no definite evidence to support its value clinically.[12]

SPECIAL NURSING CONSIDERATIONS FOR THE MONITORED PATIENT AND FAMILY. Throughout our discussion of electronic monitoring, we have referred to specific measures the nurse can take to help restore normal maternal and fetal functioning as they applied to the various contraction and FHR patterns. There are, however, some basic considerations to be kept in mind regardless of the type of labor the monitored mother may be having. Continuous monitoring should free the nurse to give more and better quality care to her patients. However, it often happens that, with all the apparatus and data that are produced (and must be observed and recorded), there arises a tendency to nurse the machines rather than the mother. Thus, the nurse will want to be aware of this and take special care to relate directly to the patient and her family. Explanations of the monitor and the benefits derived from its use are essential to insure its acceptance by the mother. Ideally, this explanation begins in the prenatal period so that the mother and father can get used to the idea and become familiar with the equipment through tours, films and the like. However, anxiety about the labor and the use of the equipment can be allayed by suitable explanation and assurance at the time of labor. Including the father in any explanations is, of course, also necessary.

Comfort measures and general hygiene, particularly with respect to bladder hygiene, need not be slighted. Backrubs, position changes and repositioning the external monitors (without being asked) all contribute to the mother's comfort and feelings that she is getting personalized care. A 30-degree upright position during labor has been found to be effective in shortening the first and second stages of labor. This position can be employed even if the mother is being monitored.[13] These measures can be employed as a matter of course. Very often, patients are afraid to move lest they disturb the attachments, but the nurse can assure the patient that she may move carefully and can see to it that the mother does, in fact, assume a comfortable and appropriate position. Changes in position can be noted on the graph paper as well as transducer repositioning.

Unless there is fetal distress, observation of the data recordings can be done at about 15-minute intervals and can also be incorporated into other care activities such as checking vital signs, vulvar hygiene and the like. The nurse can place the face of the machine away from her so that both she and the mother will not be tempted to become fixated on the data output.

It almost goes without saying that the nurse will need to be very familiar with the particular equipment in use at her hospital. In-service education, discussion and demonstration by the manufacturer's representative, as well as demonstration by those health personnel who are skilled in its use, are all measures that contribute to successful operation of these finely tuned machines.

It must be remembered also that this equipment can pose a serious safety hazard if not operated properly. Thus, a three-pronged,

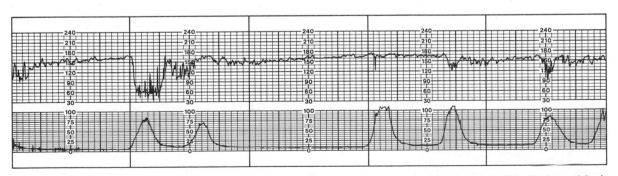

Figure 18-10. Severe variable deceleration. There is a mild fetal tachycardia, with normal baseline variability. Uterine activity is normal. The deceleration is corrected by changing the patient's position. Subsequent deceleration patterns are much less severe. (Parer, et al: A Clinical Approach to Fetal Monitoring)

grounded plug must be used *at all times* and, if more than one piece of equipment is used for the same patient, they should all be plugged into the same power receptacle if possible. Also, operators should avoid touching other metal objects, such as other equipment or plumbing fixtures, at the same time they are handling the monitoring machines. Finally, if a tingling sensation is felt upon touching the patient or the equipment, all devices not necessary to the life of the patient must be unplugged immediately and the situation reported to both the physician and the hospital maintenance personnel.

Other aspects of care

TEMPERATURE, PULSE AND RESPIRATION. The pulse in normal labor is usually in the 70s or the 80s and rarely exceeds 100. Sometimes the pulse rate on admission is slightly increased because of the excitement of coming to the hospital, but this returns to normal shortly thereafter. A persistent pulse rate over 100 suggests exhaustion or dehydration. The temperature and respiration should also be normal. If there is an elevation of temperature over 37.2° C. or 99° F. (orally), or the pulse and respiration become rapid, the physician is to be notified. The temperature is recorded every four hours, or more frequently if indicated. On the other hand, the pulse and respiration are taken every hour.

BLOOD PRESSURE. The blood pressure is recorded every hour during labor. During the first stage of labor there is little change in blood pressure between contractions, but during contractions an average increase of 5 to 10 mm. Hg may be expected. For this reason the blood pressure readings are taken between the contractions. Any unusual recordings of either systolic or diastolic pressure are reported immediately.

FLUID AND FOOD INTAKE. The practice here varies greatly among different physicians and in different institutions. Therefore, the wishes of the physician in charge need to be ascertained before proceeding. In general, it is customary to urge the mother to take water or clear fluids, such as tea with sugar, during the early phase of the first stage of labor, but she is not given solid or liquid foods because digestion is delayed during labor. Evidence that the powers of digestion are impaired at this time is demonstrated by the fact that it is not unusual for nausea and/or vomiting to occur near the end of the first stage of labor. It may be necessary to administer a general anesthetic for the delivery, so that if the patient takes fluid or food shortly before delivery, vomiting and consequent aspiration may occur. On the other hand, in a prolonged labor, it is most important to maintain adequate fluid and caloric intake in order to forestall dehydration and exhaustion, in which case the physician may find it desirable to administer intravenous glucose solutions.

BLADDER. The patient can be asked to void at least every three or four hours. The mother in labor often attributes all of her discomfort to the intensity of uterine contractions and therefore is unaware that it is the pressure of a full bladder which has increased her discomfort. In addition to causing unnecessary discomfort, a full bladder may be a serious

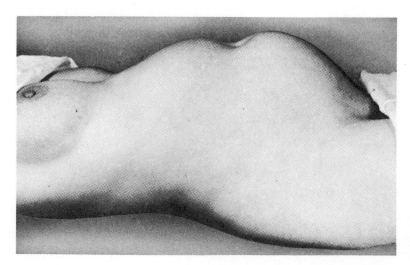

Figure 18-11. Dystocia due to bladder distention. The tremendously distended bladder is plainly seen in the photograph. This patient was sent to the hospital after three days of ineffectual labor at home. The cervix had been dilated, it is believed, for 24 hours, yet no progress had been made. Catheterization of the greatly distended bladder yielded 1,000 ml. of urine. Following this, the infant's head descended at once, and delivery was easy. (Eastman, N. J.: *Williams' Obstetrics*, ed. 11. New York, Appleton-Century Crofts)

impediment to labor (Fig. 18-11) or the cause of urinary retention in the puerperium. If the distended bladder can be palpated above the symphysis pubis, and the patient is unable to void, the physician is to be so informed. Not infrequently he will order catheterization in such cases. Various techniques are used, all designed to maintain strict asepsis.

ANALGESIA. (See Chapter 17.) Before administering the medication prescribed to promote analgesia, the nurse informs the mother that she is going to give her medication which will make her more comfortable and help her in labor. She should encourage the mother to try to rest and assure her that she will not be left alone. It is also wise to tell her that you will remain quietly at the bedside and keep conversation at the very minimum in order for her to get the maximum benefit from the medication. Her bladder can be emptied prior to administering the drugs, and the fetal heart tones and the mother's vital signs can be recorded before and after such medication is given. Once analgesic therapy has been instituted, the mother should not receive fluids or food by mouth and should remain in bed. The environment should be conducive to rest, the room quiet and darkened but with sufficient light to permit accurate observation of the patient. Many institutions require that side rails be applied when the patient is medicated, even though there is someone in attendance. The necessity of this can be explained to both the patient and her husband, so that any undue fears or misinterpretations are avoided. The father, especially, can be alerted to the importance of keeping the rails up if he is attending to any of his wife's needs, since he is not used to their presence and is apt to forget to reapply them if he steps away from the bedside for a time. This can be a difficult experience for the husband. Thus, if he shows the strain at this time, he may welcome the suggestion of having a cup of coffee and a change of scene for a while. If the mother has received scopolamine or other drugs in dosage sufficient to cause her to be heavily sedated, she *never* should be left unattended.

Signs of second stage

There are certain signs and symptoms, both behavioral and physical, which herald the onset of the second stage of labor. These signs and symptoms are to be watched for carefully. They are as follows: 1) The patient begins to bear down of her own accord; this is caused by a reflex when the head begins to press on the perineal floor. 2) Her mood of increasing apprehension, which has been building since the contractions became well established, deepens; she becomes more serious and may appear bewildered by the force of the contractions. 3) There is usually a sudden increase in show that is more blood-tinged. 4) The patient becomes increasingly irritable and unwilling to be touched; she may cry if disturbed. 5) The mother thinks that she needs to defecate. This symptom is due to pressure of the head on the perineal floor and consequently against the rectum. 6) Although she has been "working" successfully with her contractions during most of her labor, the uncertainty that she has been experiencing (since 4 to 8 cm. cervical dilatation) as to her ability to cope with the contractions becomes overwhelming; she is frustrated and feels unable to manage if left alone. 7) The membranes may rupture, with discharge of amniotic fluid. This, of course, may take place any time but occurs most frequently at the beginning of the second stage. 8) The mother may be eager to be "put to sleep"; or if she is given appropriate help, she may narrow her concentration to trying to cope with the contractions and/or pushing according to instructions. It is important to remember that the mother's consciousness is somewhat altered because of the pain, her enforced concentration and possibly medication; therefore, any coaching needs to be short and explicit and may need to be repeated with each contraction. The nurse also must be firm but gentle in setting limits with the mother, so that she can conserve her energy for the second stage. Thrashing about and continued crying only lead to exhaustion, and the mother needs the firm guidance of a skillful person to help her to maintain control. 9) The perineum begins to bulge and the anal orifice to dilate. This is a late sign, but if signs numbered 1, 3, 5, and 7 occur, it should be watched for with every contraction. Only rectal or vaginal examination (or the appearance of the head) can definitely confirm the suspicion. Emesis at this time is not unusual.

In order to spare the mother a hurried trip to the delivery room and permit adequate time to cleanse and drape her properly for the delivery without unnecessary rush, the nurse will want to report promptly any or all of these symptoms which are observed. If these signs are overlooked, a precipitate delivery may occur without benefit of medical attention. In general, primigravidas are usually taken to the delivery room when the cervix is fully dilated, and multiparas when it is 7 or 8 cm. dilated.

Conduct of the second stage

The second stage of labor (expulsion stage) begins with the complete dilatation of the cervix and ends with delivery of the baby. The complete dilatation of the cervix can be confirmed definitely only by rectal or vaginal examination. However, the nurse often is able to make a nursing diagnosis on the basis of her observations of the progress of labor, particularly if she correlates these findings with knowledge of the mother's parity, the speed of any previous labors, the pelvic measurements, and so on, noted in the antepartal record. Although the general rule regarding the optimal time for taking a mother to the delivery room has been stated, it must be remembered that, in addition, the physician will be guided in his decision to give such an order by such factors as the station of the presenting part and the speed with which labor is progressing. If on examination of a primigravida, the physician finds the cervix to be fully dilated but the presenting part of the fetus only descended to the level of the ischial spines (midpelvis), he undoubtedly will want the mother to remain in the labor room to permit the forces of labor to bring about further descent of the fetus before taking the mother to the delivery room. During this period he may want the patient to exert her abdominal forces and "bear down." In most cases bearing-down efforts are reflex and spontaneous in the second stage of labor, but, occasionally, the mother does not employ her expulsive forces to good advantage, particularly if she has had caudal analgesia. The nurse will be asked to coach and encourage the mother in this procedure. The mother's head and shoulders can be raised slightly and supported firmly during the contraction—the father is of great help in this regard and can provide the strength needed for this physical support. The mother's thighs are then flexed on the abdomen, with hands grasped just below the knees when a contraction begins. Instructions should be given to take a deep breath as soon as the contraction begins and, with her breath held, to exert downward pressure

exactly as if she were straining at stool. Pulling on the knees at this time, as well as flexing the chin on the chest, is a helpful adjunct to maintain downward pressure of the diaphragm and to stabilize the chest and the abdominal musculature. In addition, maintaining the legs flexed as for the "push" position deters the mother from pushing her feet against the table or bed. Avoiding such pressure on the feet is important, because it discourages tensing of the gluteal muscles and thus contributes to further relaxation of the pelvic floor. The bearing-down effort should be as long and sustained as possible, since short "grunty" endeavors are of little avail. If at this time the mother is in the delivery room, but her legs as yet have not been put up in stirrups or leg holders, she can be coached in the same manner. In most hospitals the delivery tables have firmly attached hand grips which can be adjusted in position so that the mother can reach them comfortably to pull against, if she wishes. However, in doing so her hands are not free to pull up on her knees with the contraction, so that the nurse or other person in attendance needs to assist her. This can be accomplished by assisting the mother to bring her legs up into position and exerting proper pressure against her knees as she bears down with the contraction. Care should be exercised to grasp the mother's knees from above, since doing so under the knees could exert undesirable pressure on the popliteal veins. At the end of each contraction the mother is assisted to put her legs down and encouraged to rest until the next contraction begins. Usually, these bearing-down efforts are rewarded by increased bulging of the perineum, that is, by further descent of the head. The patient should be informed of such progress, for encouragement is all-important. In certain instances it may be undesirable for the mother to bear down; thus the nurse would not encourage the mother to do so without the physician's request. In these cases, if the mother has an urge to bear down, she can be instructed to pant during each contraction; this will obviate her bearing down since it is impossible to push while panting.

When the mother is ready to be transferred to the delivery room, it is more helpful if the same nurse who has been attending her in labor accompanies her to the delivery room. This transfer will mean a new environment for the patient to cope with under very stressful circumstances. There may be great physical and

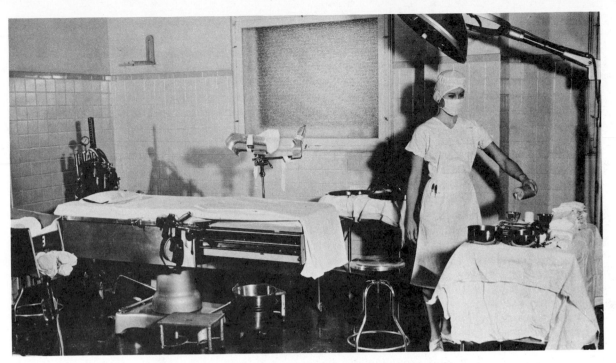

Figure 18-12. The delivery room. Nurse preparing instrument table.

mental exertion called for with little preparation or practice. To the mother in labor who is unfamiliar with such surroundings, the "sterile" atmosphere of the delivery room can be strange, cold and uninviting, with its obstetric furnishings and supplies that become even more foreboding as they reflect the glittering lights of the room. Under such circumstances the sight and the sound of familiar faces and voices, even though partially concealed and muffled by the surgical caps, masks and gowns, do give the patient some sense of continuity and security. Furthermore, by this time the nurse and the patient will have established a communication pattern, each able to pick up the other's more covert cues. Thus, the coaching, guidance and follow-through necessary in the second stage of labor will be expedited if the same person continues with the care.

The nurse will notice that the mother has become increasingly involved in the whole birth process. The seemingly panicky frustration of the late active phase subsides a bit (with appropriate coaching and reassurance), and the patient may experience a sense of relief that the expulsive stage has begun. The desire to push and to bear down is very strong now—uncontrollable, in fact—and the patient generally gets enormous satisfaction with each push. Some patients, however (e.g., those with a highly charged emotional labor), experience acute pain and need all available help and encouragement to continue bearing down. The nurse will note that in most instances there is complete exhaustion after each expulsive effort, and the mother often drops off to sleep, only to be roused by the next contraction. Since consciousness is still altered, it may be difficult for the mother to follow directions readily even though she may want to. Again, repeated, short, explicit directions are required to encourage her to rest or to work, but especially to prepare the mother for the expulsive effort if she is sleeping between contractions and awakens abruptly.

Muscular cramps in the legs are common in the second stage because of pressure exerted by the baby's head on certain nerves in the pelvis. To relieve these cramps, the leg can be straightened and the ankle dorsiflexed by exerting pressure upward against the ball of the foot until the cramp subsides (see Fig. 12-14, p. 211). Meanwhile, the knee is stabilized with the other hand. These cramps cause excruciating pain and must never be ignored.

Good obstetric care during the second stage of labor demands the closest teamwork among physician, nurse and anesthetist. By previous understanding, or more often by established hospital routine, each has his or her own responsibilities in the delivery room, and, if the best interests of the mother and her infant are to be fulfilled, the responsibilities of each must be carried out smoothly and efficiently.

Up to now, the primary focus for the nurse has been on direct patient care. Now she must enlarge her focus to include the obstetrician and other allied professionals; that is, there will be more activities which will require the actual assistance of these persons than was necessary during the first stage of labor. Thus, the nurse must be sensitive not only to the cues sent by the mother but also to those relayed by the other personnel.

Preparation for delivery

PREPARATION OF THE DELIVERY ROOM. There are no two hospitals in which the setup of a delivery room or the procedure for delivery is precisely the same, and this is one phase of the nurse's work which she must learn wholly from actual observation and experience in her own institution. Nevertheless, she can obtain a general idea of the main equipment used from Figure 18-12 on page 327.

The delivery table is designed so that its surface is actually composed of two adjoining sections, each covered with its own mattress. This permits the patient to lie in the supine position until it is desired to put her legs up into stirrups, that is, put her in the lithotomy position. At this time the table is "broken" by a mechanical device. The retractable or lower end of the table drops and is rolled under the main section of the table. Thus ready access is given to the perineal region. Or, if it is desired to deliver the patient in the dorsal recumbent position, the lower portion of the table can remain in place.

The instrument table opposite the foot of the delivery table contains the principal sterile supplies and instruments needed for normal delivery, including, among other articles, towels, sponges, catheter, solutions, basins and the "cord set." The cord set is a group of instruments used for clamping and cutting the umbilical cord, namely, two hemostats, a pair of scissors and a cord tie or clamp. Other instruments often are included, because it may be necessary for the physician to perform an episiotomy or to repair lacerations (p. 349). Other instruments frequently included are two hemostats, two Allis clamps, one mouse-tooth tissue forceps, two sponge sticks, one vaginal retractor, two tenaculae, one needle holder, assorted needles and a pair of obstetric forceps.

A double-bowl solution stand or basin rack generally is used to hold the basins, one for wet sponges and the other to receive the placenta. Emergency instruments, a crib and a resuscitator are part of standard delivery room equipment. Even if the infant does not require resuscitation, the resuscitator affords him a warm, protected environment, and it is a convenient place in which to give him care. To

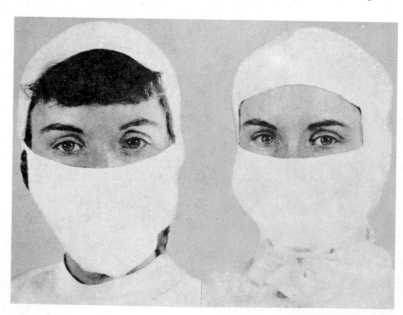

Figure 18-13. (Left) Incorrect method of wearing cap. Bacteria, hairs and other infectious particles can readily fall from exposed hair and contaminate sterile fields. (Right) Correct method of adjusting cap so that all hair is covered.

facilitate the delivery, all equipment should be in readiness at all times.

ASEPSIS AND ANTISEPSIS. Persons who have a communicable disease or persons who have been in contact with a communicable disease should be excluded from maternity service until examined by a physician. The examining physician should certify that the employee is free from infections before he or she is allowed to return to duty. Personnel with evidence of upper respiratory infections or open skin lesions, diarrhea, or any other infectious disease also should be excluded. Furthermore, it is recommended that all persons working in the maternity area should have a preemployment physical examination and such interim examinations as may be required by the hospital.

Of prime importance in the conduct of the second stage are strict asepsis and antisepsis throughout. To this end everyone in the delivery room wears a clean scrubdress, cap and mask, and those actually participating in the delivery are in sterile attire. Masking must include both nose and mouth. Caps are to be so adjusted as to keep *all* hair covered (Fig. 18-13). If the nurse scrubs to assist the doctor, the strictest aseptic technique is observed. The hands are disinfected as carefully as for a major surgical operation. Scrubbing the hands should be started sufficiently early so that full time may be allotted for the scrub, as well as to don gown and gloves.

TRANSFER OF THE MOTHER TO THE DELIVERY ROOM. When the physician deems the birth to be imminent, he will ask that the mother be transferred to the delivery room and prepared for delivery. If the mother is awake, she can be told what is happening and be informed in advance about any procedure. If the husband will not be accompanying his wife to the delivery room, then time is allowed, if possible, for them to bid each other a temporary goodbye. This kind of planning not only is supportive but also enables both to cooperate more fully. Care should be taken to have only one person instruct or coach the mother at any one time. When delivery is imminent, her attention will be limited necessarily, as already illustrated, and the sound of several voices at one time is confusing. If the physician, for example, is coaching, it is well for the nurse not to participate verbally; however, she should remain alert and ready to step into the role whenever it is appropriate.

Prior to the actual transfer to the delivery room, the nurse will find out what type of anesthesia the physician is planning to use. Since the immediate positioning of the patient in the delivery room will depend on the type of anesthesia used, this preplanning will expedite activities during delivery and promote smoother functioning of the team.

Delivery

If spinal anesthesia is to be administered, the patient is turned on her side for the administration. If she is given a saddle block, she may be placed on her side or assisted to a sitting position on the side of the delivery table, with her feet supported on a stool and her body leaning forward against the nurse. Her back should be toward the operator and bowed (the position requires flexion of the neck and the lumbar spine). This principle of cervical and lumbar flexion is used also in the side lying position (see Chapter 17).

Although the positioning and the administration of the anesthesia take only a few minutes, the mother undoubtedly will be extremely uncomfortable due to the severity of the contractions at this time; she can be assured that this discomfort is only temporary, and soon she will be pain-free. The fetal heart tones and the maternal blood pressure are checked frequently—every five minutes or so. In addition, the mother should have her head elevated with two pillows to help prevent the anesthetic level from rising beyond the desired height. So that the anesthetic level may stabilize, the nurse waits for instructions from the anesthetist before putting the mother's legs in stirrups or performing any other manipulations. If the mother is to receive general anesthesia, she lies supine on the table. Local or pudendal anesthesia is administered with the mother in the lithotomy position (see Chapter 17).

As has been previously stated, anesthesia should be administered only by a qualified physician or a nurse anesthetist. This entire subject is discussed in more detail in Chapter 17.

During the time that the anesthesia is being administered, the circulating nurse can uncover the sterile tables, check the resuscitator and attach a sterile suction catheter and oxygen mask, and perform other duties for which she is responsible. Once the anesthesia has been administered, the nurse resumes checking the FHR every five minutes.

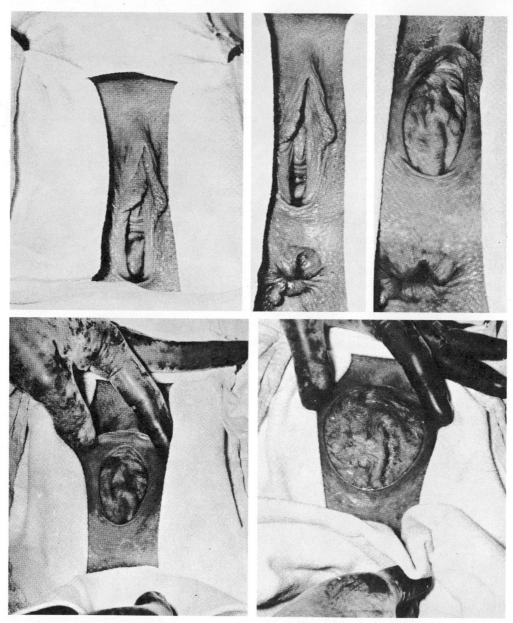

Figure 18-14. (*Upper left*) Proper draping for delivery showing appropriate placement of sterile towels, one of which covers the anus. (*Upper center*) Scalp of the infant detected through a slitlike vulvular opening as the perineal region begins to bulge and the skin over it becomes tense and glistening. Pressure of the descending head causes the anus to become patulous and everted. For purposes of showing changes which take place in the anus, the lower towel has been removed from this and the following photographs. (*Upper right*) Appearance of the infant's head with subsequent contractions. The vulva becomes more dilated and distended by the infant's head so that the opening is gradually converted into an ovoid. (*Lower left*) Control of the progress of the head to preserve the perineum from tearing. (*Lower right*) Further advanced extension of the head. The left hand is used to prevent sudden expulsion of the head as it crowns, while pressure on the infant's chin through the perineum by the right hand expedites extension and delivery. This is Ritgen's maneuver. (The Johns Hopkins Hospital, Baltimore, Md.)

Before elevating the mother's legs into the stirrups, cotton flannel boots which cover the entire leg are put on. In putting the legs of the patient up into stirrups or leg holders, care is taken not to separate the legs too widely or to have one leg higher than the other. Both legs are raised or lowered at the same time, with a nurse supporting each one if the mother is unable to help in the positioning. Failure to observe these principles may result in strain-

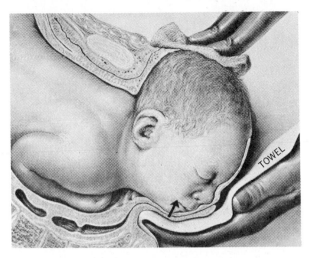

Figure 18-15. Ritgen's maneuver, as it appears in median section. Arrow shows direction of pressure.

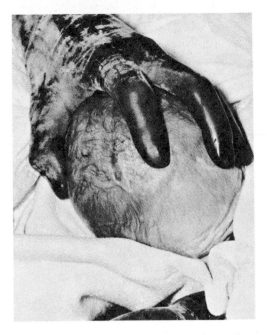

Figure 18-16. Birth of the head. The full hand is used to control the progress with emergence of the forehead and face. (The Johns Hopkins Hospital, Baltimore, Md.)

ing the ligaments of the pelvis, with consequent discomfort in the puerperium. Care should be taken to avoid pressure on the popliteal space, and to angle the stirrups so that the feet are not dependent. More frequently, when a spinal type anesthetic is not used, stirrups are being dispensed with during the delivery itself and the mother is allowed to grasp her knees as she did in the labor room, and she continues to push with the contractions. Stirrups may be employed if there is a repair of an episiotomy or laceration.

If stirrups are used during the delivery, the mother can be given handles to grip and pull on, which aid her in her bearing-down efforts. Wrist straps are attached to these, which are secured about the wrist and allow some limited movement but prevent the mother from reaching up to touch the sterile drapes. The purpose of the handles and the cuffs should be explained to the mother, since many patients often complain about being "strapped down."

With the patient in the lithotomy position, the nurse carries out the procedure for cleansing the vulva and the surrounding area. If the delivery is to be conducted with the mother in the recumbent position, this may be carried out with the knees drawn up slightly and the

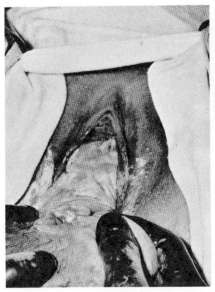
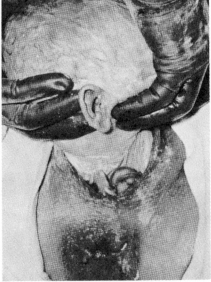

Figure 18-17. Delivery of the shoulders. (Left) The anterior shoulder is brought under the symphysis pubis. (Right) Delivery of the posterior shoulder. (The Johns Hopkins Hospital, Baltimore, Md.)

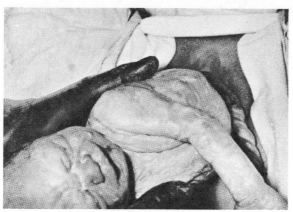

Figure 18-18. Delivery of the infant's body. (The Johns Hopkins Hospital, Baltimore, Md.)

legs separated. Then, the physician, who meanwhile has scrubbed his hands and donned sterile gown and gloves, drapes the patient with towels and sheets appropriate for the purpose (Fig. 18-14).

After the patient has been prepared for delivery, catheterization, if done, is carried out by the physician. Sometimes it is difficult to catheterize a patient in the second stage of labor, since the infant's head may compress the urethra. If the catheter does not pass easily, force never should be employed. Whenever it is possible and appropriate, all procedures, of course, should be explained to the mother as they occur.

As the infant descends the birth canal, pressure against the rectum may cause fecal material to be expelled. The physician will employ sponges (as a rule soaked with saline solution) to remove any fecal material which may escape from the rectum.

Fundal pressure should not be used to accomplish spontaneous delivery or to bring the head deeper into the birth canal. Severe fundal pressure may cause uterine damage or rupture of the uterus.

As soon as the head distends the perineum to a diameter of 6 or 8 cm., the physician often will place a towel over the rectum and exert forward pressure on the chin of the baby's head while the other hand exerts downward pressure on the occiput (Figs. 18-14 and 18-15). This is called Ritgen's maneuver, and allows the physician to control the egress of the head; it also favors extension so that the head is born with the smallest diameter presenting. The head usually is delivered between contractions and as slowly as possible (Fig. 18-16). At this time the mother may complain about a "splitting" sensation due to the extreme vaginal stretching as the head is born. All these measures (control of head by Ritgen's maneuver, extension and slow delivery between contractions) help to prevent lacerations. If a tear seems to be inevitable, an incision which is called an episiotomy may be made in the perineum. This will not only prevent lacerations but also will facilitate the delivery (see p. 349). Immediately after the birth of the infant's head the physician passes his finger along the occiput to the infant's neck in order to feel whether a loop or more of umbilical cord encircles it. If such a coil is felt, it should be

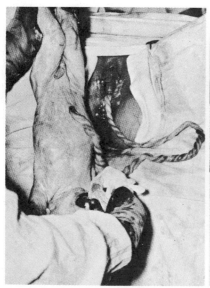

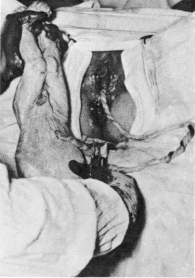

Figure 18-19. (Left) Upon delivery the infant is held in the head-down position to promote drainage of secretions from the respiratory passage. Mucus is gently wiped from the infant's face, then suctioned from the nostrils and the mouth with an ear bulb syringe or other suction device. Note that there is no traction on the cord, which is still attached to the placenta. (Right) The cord is cut between the two Kelly clamps, which have been placed a few inches from the umbilicus. (The Johns Hopkins Hospital, Baltimore, Md.)

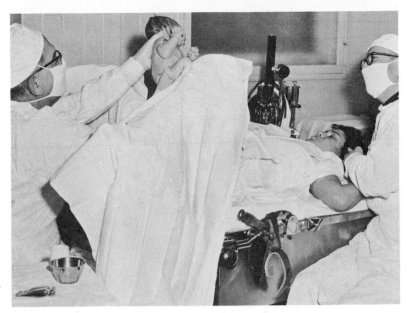

Figure 18-20. Physician lifts infant for parents to see immediately upon delivery.

gently drawn down and, if loose enough, slipped over the infant's head. This is done to prevent interference with the infant's oxygen supply, which could result from pressure of its shoulder on the umbilical cord. If the cord is too tightly coiled to permit this procedure, it must be clamped and cut before the shoulders are delivered; then the infant must be extracted immediately before asphyxiation results. As shown in Figure 18-17, the anterior shoulder usually is brought under the symphysis pubis first and then the posterior shoulder is delivered, after which the remainder of the body follows without particular mechanism (Figs. 18-18 and 18-19). The exact time of the baby's birth should be noted. The infant usually cries immediately, and the lungs become expanded; about this time the pulsations in the umbilical cord begin to diminish. The physician usually will defer clamping the cord until this occurs, or for a minute or so if practicable, because of the marked benefit of the additional blood to the infant. Using sterile instruments, he cuts the cord between the two Kelly clamps, which have been placed a few inches from the umbilicus; then the umbilical clamp or tie is applied. The tie, a sterilized linen tape ligature, is usually applied about an inch from the abdomen, with care to secure it tightly enough to prevent bleeding without its cutting into the cord (Figs. 18-19 and 18-22). A second ligature may be applied for further protection if it is desired, or if it is necessary because of any bleeding. There are several types of umbilical clamps, such as the Kane, the Zeigler and the Hesseltine, which are used extensively in many institutions (Fig. 18-21). With these the possibility of hemorrhage is minimized.

The first 15 minutes after the infant's birth is the most hazardous period of life, when more infants succumb than during any subsequent time. The responsibility for much of the care during this period is delegated to the nurse, so that the physician may devote his

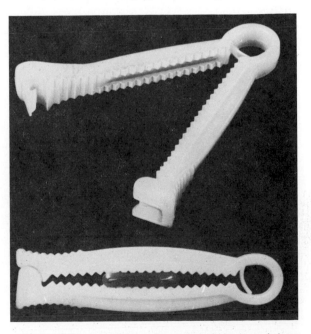

Figure 18-21. Umbilical cord clamp. A double-grip cord clamp in the opened and closed positions. (Hollister, Inc., Chicago, Ill.)

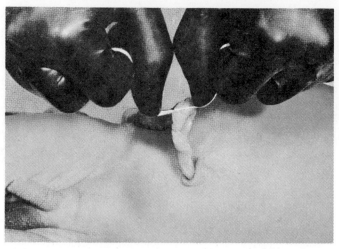

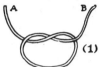 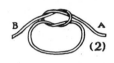

attention to the mother during the third stage of labor (see Chapter 21).

Conduct of the third stage

Delivery of the placenta

The third stage of labor (placental stage) begins after the delivery of the baby and terminates with the birth of the placenta. Immediately after delivery of the infant the height

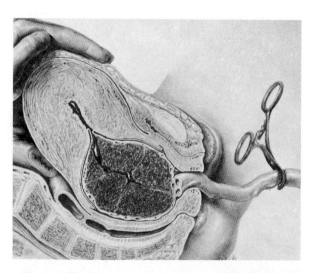

Figure 18-23. Expression of placenta is usually done by the physician, if necessary, but *on his instructions* may be done by an assistant. The *uterus must be hard* if this is attempted. Note that the uterus is not squeezed.

of the uterine fundus and its consistency are ascertained. The physician may do this by palpating the uterus through a sterile towel placed on the lower abdomen, but it is a duty which often is delegated to the nurse, at least while the physician is engaged in clamping and cutting the umbilical cord. The nurse may do so by placing her hand on the abdomen *under* the sterile drape. The uterus should be held very gently with the fingers behind the fundus and the thumb in front. So long as the uterus remains hard, and there is no bleeding, the policy is ordinarily one of watchful waiting until the placenta is separated; no massage is practiced, the hand simply resting on the fundus to make certain that the organ does not balloon out with blood. Since attempts to deliver the placenta prior to its separation from the uterine wall are not only futile but may be dangerous, it is most important that the signs of placental separation be well understood. If the responsibility of "guarding" the fundus is delegated to the nurse, she should watch for signs of placental separation and report such to the physician. The signs which suggest that the placenta has separated are as follows:

1. The uterus rises upward in the abdomen; this is due to the fact that the placenta, having been separated, passes downward into the lower uterine segment and the vagina, where its bulk pushes the uterus upward.

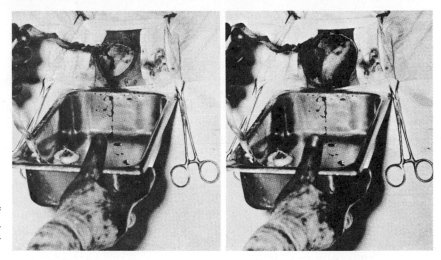

Figure 18-24. Third stage of labor. The delivery of the placenta. (The Johns Hopkins Hospital, Baltimore, Md.)

2. The umbilical cord protrudes 3 or more inches farther out of the vagina, indicating that the placenta also has descended.

3. The uterus changes from a discoid to a globular shape and becomes, as a rule, more firm.

4. A sudden trickle or spurt of blood often occurs.

These signs are apparent sometimes within a minute or so after delivery of the infant and usually within five minutes. When the placenta has certainly separated, the physician first ascertains that the uterus is firmly contracted. He then may ask the patient, if not anesthetized, to "bear down," and the intraabdominal pressure so produced may be adequate to expel the placenta. If this fails, or if it is not practicable because of anesthesia, the physician, again having made certain that the uterus is hard, exerts gentle pressure downward with

his hand on the fundus and, employing the placenta as a piston, simply moves the placenta out of the vagina. This procedure, known as placental *expression*, must be done gently and without squeezing (Figs. 18-23 and 18-24). It never should be attempted unless the uterus is hard; otherwise the organ may be turned inside out. This is one of the gravest complications of obstetrics and is known as "inversion" of the uterus. The physician carries out a careful inspection of the placenta to make sure that it is intact (Fig. 18-25); if a piece is left in the uterus, it may cause subsequent hemorrhage.

Oxytocin and/or ergonovine, or their derivatives, may be administered at the physician's request to increase uterine contractions and thereby to minimize bleeding. These agents are employed widely in the conduct of the normal third stage of labor, but the timing of their administration differs greatly in various

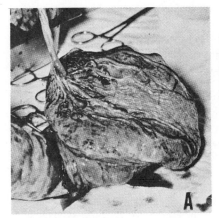
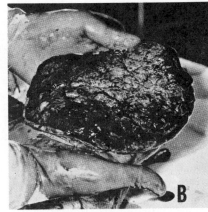

Figure 18-25. Inspecting the placenta: (A) the fetal side, (B) the maternal side. (The Johns Hopkins Hospital, Baltimore, Md.)

conduct of normal labor   335

hospitals. These oxytocics are not necessary in most cases, but their use is considered ideal from the viewpoint of minimizing blood loss and the general safety of the mother.

THE OXYTOCICS. Ergonovine is an alkaloid of ergot. It is a powerful oxytocic; it stimulates uterine contractions and exerts an effect which may persist for several hours. When it is administered intravenously, the uterine response is almost immediate, and within a few minutes after intramuscular or oral administration. This response is sustained in character with no tendency toward relaxation and so is ideal for the prevention and the control of postpartal hemorrhage. This drug will cause an elevation of blood pressure. More recently a semisynthetic derivative of ergonovine, methylergonovine tartrate, has been widely employed because it possesses several advantages over the parent drug. Usually called by its trade name, Methergine, it has the ability to produce stronger and longer contractions and is less likely to cause elevation of the blood pressure. Both drugs when given intravenously may cause transient headache and, to a lesser extent, temporary chest pain, palpitation and dyspnea. These side effects are less likely to occur with intramuscular administration of the drugs.

Oxytocin is another agent which, like ergonovine, causes a marked contraction of the uterus. However, the response of the uterus to oxytocin resembles the response to ergonovine for only the first five to ten minutes; then normal rhythmic contractions of amplified degree return, with intermittent periods of relaxation. The oxytocic fraction separated from posterior pituitary extract is referred to by the name oxytocin; it is widely used because it does not possess the strong vasopressor effects of Pituitrin, which was used more extensively in former years. Oxytocin's most important side effect is its antidiuretic effect which can cause water intoxication if administered intravenously in a large volume of electrolyte-free aqueous dextrose solution. Fortunately the antidiuretic effect disappears within a few minutes after the infusion is discontinued. A synthetic oxytocin injection has been developed and marketed under the brand name of Syntocinon. Its action, dosage and indications are similar to those of oxytocin. Another drug which has been developed is sparteine sulfate (Tocosamine). It is used primarily in dysfunctional types of labor and for induction of labor. When used as recommended, it usually produces a gradual onset of regular uterine contractions similar to that encountered in normal labor. The quality of uterine response cannot always be predicted, however, and cases of uterine rupture following its use have been reported. Increasingly, the use of IM oxytocic preparations during labor is being discarded in favor of the more easily controlled IV route by drip.

On the obstetrician's order the nurse administers the oxytocic intramuscularly, the intravenous medications being administered by a physician. The average doses of the drugs are as follows: oxytocin, 10 units (1 cc.) intramuscularly or intravenously; Syntocinon, 10 units (1 cc.) intramuscularly or intravenously; Tocosamine, 150 mg. (1 cc.) intramuscularly, administered at one and one-half to two hour intervals to maintain satisfactory uterine stimulation until a total of 4 doses (600 mg.) has been given; ergonovine, 0.2 mg. ($\frac{1}{320}$ gr.) or 1 cc. IM or IV; and Methergine, 0.2 mg. ($\frac{1}{320}$ gr.) or 1 cc. IM or IV. Various institutions use the drugs separately or in conjunction as is necessary to produce the desired results. The choice of the oxytocic usually will depend on the anesthetic agent administered. Oxytocin is contraindicated for use with drugs that have a sympathomimetic action.

Conduct of the fourth stage

These first hours after delivery have been described aptly as the "fourth stage of labor."[14] The wearying work of labor per se is completed and the mother and father can look forward to a brief respite before assuming the forthcoming responsibilities of parenthood. This is truly a transition period and many important physical and psychosocial tasks will be begun at this time.

After the delivery has been completed and/or the episiotomy repaired, the drapes and the soiled linen under the mother's buttocks are removed, the lower end of the delivery table is replaced and the mother's legs are lowered from the stirrups *simultaneously* to prevent cramping or twisting of the extremities. A sterile perineal pad is applied and the mother given a clean, warm gown and covered with a blanket to avoid chilling.

Chilling accompanied by uncontrollable shaking often occurs in this early period after delivery. It is uncomfortable and sometimes embarrassing or frightening for the patient but is self-limiting (usually not over 15 minutes) and is not considered an ominous sign. The exact etiology has not been determined, although several explanations have been offered, which include sudden release of intraabdominal pressure after delivery, nervous and exhaustion responses related to the stress of childbirth, disequilibrium in the internal and external body temperature resulting from the waste products of muscular exertion, break in aseptic technique which predisposes to infection, minute circulatory amniotic fluid emboli and previous maternal sensitization to elements of fetal blood. Clean, dry, warm gowns and blankets as well as a warm nondrafty environment help in the prevention and control of this phenomenon. Warm fluids by mouth can be given and are much appreciated for their hydrating and energy-giving effects.

Constant massage of the uterus during this period immediately after delivery is unnecessary and undesirable. However, if the organ shows any tendency to relax, it is to be massaged immediately with firm but gentle circular strokes until it contracts effectively. Relaxation of the uterus is a prime cause of postpartum hemorrhage, and surveillance of the uterus and the amount of bleeding is of extreme importance at this time.

Since the prevention of postpartum hemorrhage is such a crucial factor in the health and well-being of the mother, the nurse will want to be able to identify quickly those patients at risk (most likely) to develop this condition. The following include the most predictive factors associated with postpartum bleeding:

1. Older age and high parity
2. Rapid labor
3. Prolonged first and second stages of labor
4. Operative delivery, i.e., forceps extraction
5. Overdistention of the uterus—polyhydramnios, multiple pregnancy, overly large infant
6. Previous uterine atony and/or associated previous postpartal hemorrhage
7. Other hemorrhagic complications such as abruptio placentae or placenta previa
8. Induced labor
9. Heavy medication during labor and/or general anesthesia
10. Preeclampsia and eclampsia

The nurse will also want to have in readiness an intravenous infusion with an oxytocin for immediate administration in the event that the physician suspects hemorrhage is imminent.

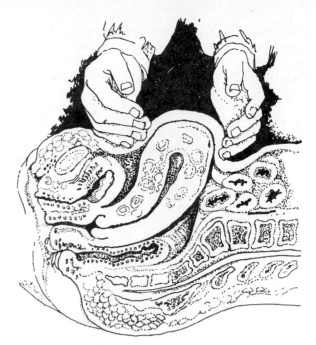

Figure 18-26. Proper method of palpating fundus of uterus during first hour after delivery to guard against relaxation and hemorrhage. The right hand is placed just above the symphysis pubis to act as a guard; meanwhile the other hand is cupped around the fundus of the uterus.

Thus, the first hour following the delivery is a most critical one for the mother, since it is at this time that postpartal hemorrhage is most likely to occur. The fundus is to be checked every five minutes or so and massaged as necessary to insure continued firmness and prevent its ballooning with blood (Fig. 18-26). It is also important for the nurse to be alert not only to the condition of the mother's uterus but also to any abnormal symptoms relating to her general condition. Thus, checking the maternal vital signs are included in the nursing interventions. Blood pressure and pulse are generally checked every 15 minutes until stable and then every half hour for one hour. Thereafter, they are continued every hour for several hours until it is certain that the mother is definitely stabilized. The flow is also checked about every half hour and the amount of pads saturated is recorded.

If the mother is awake, she will usually be eager to have a closer look at her baby and hold it, if this is possible. One should remember that, although she is quite tired, she is usually elated, proud of her accomplishment of giving birth and eager to share this with the baby's father. Whenever possible, all efforts should be made to allow the father, the mother and the infant to share this momentous time together if they so desire.

In some hospitals, the baby is placed in the mother's arms as soon as she is transferred to her bed, and the father is permitted to remain at her bedside while she is in the recovery area. This type of arrangement provides an excellent opportunity to let both the mother and father have a close, thorough look at their baby and to let them begin the necessary process of incorporating it into their family unit. It is important, however, that the nurse keep a watchful eye on the infant during this time before it is transferred to the nursery. Besides making sure the infant's airway is clear and free from mucus, the nurse will want to be sure that the infant is well wrapped in warmed, dry nursery blankets to prevent undue heat loss. Maintenance of body heat is of critical importance to the infant. An uncompromised infant's capacity to produce heat in response to cold stress approaches that of an adult. However, an infant also tends to lose heat rapidly in a suboptimal thermal environment and this is dangerous. Keeping the infant in a warmed incubator or placing it close to the mother's body, allowing it to be held and cuddled while being wrapped securely in blankets, will diminish the heat loss from radiation, conduction and convection, three of the four sources of heat loss for the infant during this period. Thus, the nurse will want to remind the parents to keep the infant well covered, and help them in their efforts so that undue exposure will not occur.

In other institutions, the nursery nurse comes to the recovery area and transfers the infant after the initial visit. In still others, the infant may be transferred immediately after delivery with no initial parental visit. Whatever the practice, the nurse who is attending the family immediately after delivery will be responsible for insuring the safety of the mother and infant and providing the family with the opportunity to be together if they wish to treasure that important occasion.

Immediately after delivery, or perhaps later, the parents, particularly the mother, may relieve tension by giving way to some emotional displays such as laughing, crying, incessant chatter or anger (if all has not gone well or as expected). These emotions often are quite unexpected and shock and embarrass those involved. A calm, accepting, nonjudgmental attitude on the part of the nurse is very effective in allaying any embarrassment and in helping the patient to gain control.

The nurse must remember that the patient is beginning a period that is enormously important; she is, in fact, now a "mother" with all its concomitant responsibilities; glimmerings of this already are reaching the consciousness. This is not the "end" but only the beginning of a whole new role! In addition, she is physically and emotionally exhausted from the great effort she has put forth; thus, there may be a temporary emotional upheaval.

Several comfort measures can be employed to restore calm and to help the mother to relax enough to get some much-needed rest and sleep. A soothing backrub, change of gown and linen, a quiet conversation with the nurse and/or the father in which the patient is allowed to ventilate her feelings, an environment conducive to rest—all are helpful. In addition, a warm beverage can be offered to help to allay undue excitement; since the mother is apt to be extremely hungry and thirsty, this is welcome nourishment as well as a therapeutic soporific.

Many mothers, of course, do not have an emotional outburst per se, although the majority do experience some degree of excitement and elation when the delivery is accomplished. Any of the above nursing activities are suitable also for them. Some patients experience a great need for sleep and drop off as soon as they ascertain that the baby is "all right." If the patient is sleeping continuously or intermittently, she should be allowed to do so, being disturbed only for those nursing observations which are necessary. When she indicates readiness (after the first hour after delivery), her baby can be presented, and she can be allowed to examine and to explore to her heart's content.

The mothers who have not been conscious during the delivery may have rather different reactions than those patients who have participated in the birth process. Often they do not seem to believe that delivery has taken place, or that the baby shown them "is really mine." They will question again and again: "Is it really all over?" "What is it again?" (This refers to the sex of the child.) "Did I have the baby?" The apparent alteration in awareness seems to be related to the anesthesia and the unconsciousness. These patients may need more firm reassurance and contact with their infants to help them realize that they have had a baby. Even though the repeated questioning may become annoying, the nurse will recognize that this is necessary for the mother so that she can begin the important process of disengagement from the symbiotic relationship that she had with her infant during pregnancy. She must now establish the baby as a real entity outside her body rather than inside. All mothers have this task to perform, but it may be harder for the mother who has been delivered under heavy anesthesia, for as far as she is concerned, she was not "there" when it all happened.

Maternal attachment feelings, as we know, do not spring unbound at the time of delivery. Rather, they are developed, often slowly, as is the case in any other developmental process. It is now becoming recognized that the early encounters the mother has with her newborn (which often begin immediately after delivery) pave the way for later maternal responses in the postpartal period and, indeed, throughout life.[15]

Maternal attachment behavior has been defined as the extent to which a mother feels that her infant occupies an essential position in her life. Components of this phenomenon are feelings of warmth or love, a sense of possession, devotion, protectiveness and concern for the infant's well-being, positive anticipation of prolonged contact and a need for and pleasure in continuing transactions. As in other meaningful relationships, there is an acceptance of impositions and obligations intolerable with less important objects and a sense of loss experienced with the infant's actual or imagined absence.[16]

Until recently, research studies have emphasized manifestations of attachment behavior in the child, while processes of maternal and particularly paternal attachment are poorly documented (see Chapter 2). However, there now seems to be a salubrious thrust in that much-needed direction. Rubin has pioneered in this area (see Suggested Reading). More recently, Robson and Moss, for instance, found when studying primiparous mothers that during labor and delivery per se there was a certain dissociation between the mechanics of the birth process and the knowledge that their own infant was being born. The immediate expression of interest in seeing the baby generally reflected concern about its physical appearance and intactness and/or the need to concretize the reality of its existence. Interestingly, the type of anesthesia employed, according to these authors, did not alter what they term a dissociative lack of involvement. However, with the first real contact with the infant, even though it lasted only several minutes, positive feelings of liking, warmth and "feeling good" were expressed by over half the sample. Some hours later in the postpartum period, the mothers attempted to deal with their infants' anonymity by creating some sense that their infants were unique individuals who belonged to them. Thus, they personalized the infant's behavior—"He is waving at me," "She's got my husband's temper," etc. Family resemblance was also imputed as were behaviors that reportedly "inherited."[17]

In a similar vein, Cronenwett and Newmark found that fathers who had attended preparation for childbirth classes and/or were allowed to attend the *delivery* (not just the labor) of their wives rated their overall experiences during childbirth significantly more positively than husbands who had not had these experiences. These fathers also felt that being with their wives during labor (and/or having attended the childbirth preparation classes) affected their marital relationship positively; that is, it strengthened the marital bond. It is less clear how the childbirth classes and being present during delivery affected the bonding of the father to his infant. There was no apparent association in this regard. It may be that the father's reaction is similar to the mother's (i.e., a certain dissociation) in that they are both intent on the mother's labor and not yet able to attend to the infant as a person.[18] While much more research is needed in this very important area of infant-parent bonding, what evidence we have tends to support the practices of preparing the couple for childbirth, allowing fathers to be present during both labor and delivery, and allowing ample opportunities for early and sustained contact between the infant and both parents.

Rising has pointed out that there is a certain openness about the fourth stage of labor that may not occur again during the postpartum period. This openness allows the nurse to make assessments regarding the couple's ability to proceed with integrating the infant smoothly into the family. She and other practitioners have suggested that it may be helpful to utilize a form to systematically record observations of the family unit during the

Table 18-3 Observations of Responses of the Mother During Fourth Stage of Labor

Patient's Name:_____

Please circle appropriate responses:

Verbal Responses
1. Calls baby by name
2. Calls baby affectionate terms
3. Comments on beauty of baby and on realistic defects
4. Voices unhappiness over sex of baby
5. Calls baby "it"
6. Uses unhappy or scolding inflections
7. Asks husband or nurse if baby is all right
8. Talks about baby
9. Answers in monosyllables
10. Complains of difficult labor and delivery
11. Doesn't talk about baby
12. Requests that baby be taken to nursery
13. Seeks considerable support for own discomfort

Nonverbal Responses
1. Looks, reaches out to baby
2. Hugs, touches baby
3. Smiles at baby
4. Kisses baby
5. Undresses baby
6. Doesn't touch baby
7. Doesn't look at baby
8. Pushes baby away
9. Tenses face, arms
10. Sleepy, not drug induced
11. Turns away from baby
12. Turns away from husband, nurse, visitor
13. Positive eye contact, emotional feeling with husband
14. Unresponsive to husband, nurse, visitor
15. Cries unhappily
16. Holds husband's hand
17. Breast feeds baby

First comments made in delivery room by mother about baby:
_____

Visitor with mother during fourth stage:_____
Involvement of husband or visitor:_____
Problems with baby:_____
Subjective opinion of response of mother: Parity:_____

_____   Age:_____
Analgesia within last 4 hrs.:_____   Marital status:_____
Anesthesia:_____   Feeding method:_____
Complications:_____   Service:_____
Significant social history:_____   Race:_____

Behavior of baby:
    Crying: None—periodic—almost continuous
    Affect: Difficult to arouse—dozes—eyes open—very alert

This form helped nurses at Yale focus their observations of mothers and infants the first one or two hours after delivery.
Source: Rising, S.: The fourth stage of labor: family integration. *Am. J. Nurs.* 74:873, May 1974.

fourth stage of labor (Table 18-3).[19] Such an assessment tool is invaluable in providing a focus for observations of behavior and can be further developed as a predictive tool to help determine those couples which may have difficulty in integration.

If the nurse does identify family units as potentially at risk for maladaptive integration, she will want to set aside more time to be with the couple to reinforce any positive responses that they might demonstrate and to give as much encouragement as she can. She will listen attentively as the couple relive their recent experiences (and perhaps their disappointments) and encourage verbalization of these. She can also point out whatever positive realities did occur in the recent event that the parents overlooked or did not view as such. Most importantly, the nurse will want to pass on her observations and interventions to the postpartum personnel so that they may continue with positive interventions. These personnel, in turn, can work closely with community health nurses, or arrange for other follow-up care to encourage subsequent adjustment. This is a time when the nurse needs to use all of her observational skill, time and "laying on of the hands" to foster beginning integration and to begin prescribing future care aimed at consolidating the family unit.

Immediate care of the infant

As soon as the infant is born, measures are taken to promote a clear air passage before the onset of respiration. Often, as the head is delivered, it is necessary to wipe the mucus and fluid from the infant's nose and mouth before it has a chance to gasp and aspirate with this first breath. Babson and Benson recommend that the infant be kept in a face-down position immediately after delivery in order to facilitate the drainage of mucus, blood and amniotic fluid from the oropharynx.[20] A small rubber bulb syringe, or a soft rubber suction catheter attached to a mechanical suction or mouth aspirator, can be used promptly to suction the oropharynx and to remove fluids which may be obstructing the airway. If there seems to be much mucus present, the physician will hold the infant up by the ankles to encourage more mucus to drain from the throat. The mucosal surfaces of the palate and the posterior pharynx should not be wiped with gauze, since its rough texture can lead to abrasions and thus provide a portal of entry for pathogenic organisms. A flexible rubber catheter may be passed by the physician to suction the larynx if the above measures do not clear the mucus well enough.

The baby may not "cry" at once, but it usually gasps or cries after the mucus has been removed, as oxygen by way of the lungs is now needed, since the accustomed supply was cut off when the placental circulation stopped. If crying has to be stimulated, it is to be done with extreme care. As the infant is being held in the head-down position to promote the drainage of mucus from the respiratory passages, gentle rubbing of the infant's back is usually sufficient stimulus to initiate crying. And, in the act of crying, mucus is forced from the nose and the throat, thus enabling the infant to be better able to breathe. Vigorous, external irritants are *unnecessary* and *dangerous* and should not be employed. These include harsh spanking on the soles of the feet and/or buttocks, forcible rubbing of the skin along the spine, alternate hot and cold tubbing of the infant, and dilatation of the anal sphincter. These procedures are obsolete and shocking to the infant.

A sterile receiving blanket is made available to the physician so that he may wrap the infant securely to prevent heat loss. It must be remembered that any room, and particularly the delivery room, is much cooler than the mother's body, and if not properly cared for the infant can become dangerously chilled. Korones and others stress the importance of providing environmental warmth to minimize loss of the infant's body heat.[21] At birth, a major cause of heat loss is the evaporation of amniotic fluid from the infant's skin. Thus, he is to be dried rapidly by the nurse who takes the infant from the physician as soon as the infant's airway is cleared satisfactorily. The baby can be placed in a slight Trendelenberg position (15 degrees) or in a supine position for the immediate appraisal. There are various devices for preventing hypothermia in the infant. They include a warmed incubator, resuscitators that can be warmed and overhead radiant lights. The basic principle behind the use of this equipment is the same—to maintain the infant's body temperature which is related to the amount of oxygen needed by the infant, the control of apnea, and finally an acid-base balance. In addition, all of these various devices provide a convenient place for the nurse

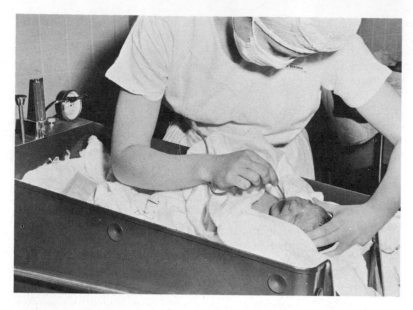

Figure 18-27. Suctioning the newborn in the delivery room.

to proceed with the infant's care. The nurse who is responsible for the infant's care in the delivery room will have cleansed her hands thoroughly with surgical soap or some other similar agent in preparation for the initial assessment of the newborn, preferably while the physician is delivering the infant's head.

Appraisal of the newborn infant

Once the infant has been placed under the radiant lamps (or in the warmed incubator or resuscitator), the responsibility for the infant's care is delegated to the nurse. It cannot be stressed enough that the infant's condition be evaluated accurately immediately after birth and that close observations be continued by the nurse. As she makes her observations, her interpretations of the baby's responses will provide valuable baseline data for subsequent care in the nursery.

One further note of caution is appropriate at this time. Als and Brazelton have made the point that infants whose mothers have been heavily premedicated may respond at delivery with excellent function and optimal Apgar scores. However, these same infants arrive in the neonatal nursery as little as 30 minutes later in a dangerously depressed state of unresponsiveness. Their color, respirations, and muscle tone, as well as their ability to respond to life-threatening mucus in their airways, are so depressed that they need constant nursing care for this transient period of depressed function.[22] This fact has special relevance if the baby is to spend some time with the parents before being transferred to the nursery. The nurse will want to be especially watchful whenever the mother has had a good deal of medication throughout labor or just before delivery.

SUCTIONING. Since it is important to maintain a clear airway for the infant, it may be necessary to suction further mucus from the oropharynx. It is important *not to oversuction* at any time, because this merely deprives the infant of oxygen and irritates the mucous membrane. If further suctioning is necessary, the nurse may use the suction apparatus on the electric infant resuscitator, a bulb syringe, or a soft rubber catheter attached to a DeLee glass trap, which was designed especially for aspirating mucus in the treatment of newborn infants (Fig. 18-27). Care should be taken not to traumatize the tissues of the oropharynx with the tip of the catheter or with forceful suction. When the nasopharynx is obstructed by mucus which must be removed via the nostrils, the nurse may safely pass a small French catheter into the nostril if she avoids using force. The catheter must *not* be inserted far back. If the catheter is directed horizontally, as if passing over the roof of the mouth, instead of directing it upward as for the adult patient, it usually slips into the tiny infant nostril with more ease. If a bulb syringe is used, it should be collapsed before it is inserted in the baby's mouth; otherwise the material in the oropharynx will be forced into the bronchi and lungs when the bulb is collapsed.

THE APGAR SCORING SYSTEM. The Apgar score provides a valuable index for evaluating the newborn infant's condition at birth. Every nurse who is responsible for the care of newborn infants, not merely those in the delivery room, should be familiar with the principles set forth by Apgar for infant evaluation because they provide a simple, accurate and safe means of quickly appraising the infant's condition. The Apgar scoring system is based on the following five signs (ranked in order of importance). In general, they are made at one minute of life and repeated again in five minutes. Each sign is evaluated according to the degree to which it is present and is given a score of 0, 1, or 2 (Table 18-4). The scores of each of the signs then are added to give a total score (10 is maximum).

Heart Rate. This sign is the most important and the last to be absent when the infant's condition is grave. It may be evaluated by palpating the pulsation of the cord or by observing the pulsation where the cord joins the abdomen. Listening to the heartbeat with a stethoscope is surely the most accurate method of ascertaining the beat. The beat may range from 150 to 180 beats per minute during the first few minutes of life; later, within the hour, it usually slows to between 130 and 140 beats per minute. Crying or increased activity will increase the number of beats. If the rate is 100 per minute or under, asphyxia is present, and resuscitation is indicated.

Respiratory Effort. A baby who is responding well cries vigorously and has no difficulty in breathing. "Regular" respiration usually is established in a minute or so. Depressed, irregular respiration or apnea indicates that respiratory difficulty is present, and these signs should be reported immediately so that prompt treatment may be instituted.

Muscle Tone. An infant who has excellent tonus will keep his extremities flexed and resist efforts to extend them. A baby who does not keep his extremities flexed consistently usually has only moderate tonus; one who is flaccid is in extremely poor condition.

Reflex Irritability. Although there are several ways to test this sign, the one most frequently used is a slap on the sole of the infant's foot. This sign can be observed when a vigorous infant is suctioned for mucus by the way in which it resists the catheter. A baby who

Table 18-4 The Apgar Scoring Chart

Sign	0	1	2
Heart rate	Absent	Slow (less than 100)	Over 100
Respiratory effort	Absent	Slow, irregular	Good, crying
Muscle tone	Flaccid	Some flexion of extremities	Active motion
Reflex irritability	No response	Weak cry or grimace	Vigorous cry
Color	Blue, pale	Body pink, extremities blue	Completely pink

Source: Special Committee on Infant Mortality of the Medical Society of the County of New York: Resuscitation of the Newborn. Philadelphia, Smith Kline & French Laboratories, 1963.

is in excellent condition will respond with a vigorous cry. An infant is judged to have a poor response if it cries weakly or merely makes a grimace. If there is a good deal of central nervous system depression, the infant will not respond at all.

Color. Cyanosis is seen in all infants at the moment of birth. As the infant's circulation makes the change from fetal to extrauterine existence and breathing begins, the body of a healthy infant usually will become pink within three minutes (see Chapter 8). Since acrocyanosis usually is present for a short while, even in infants who are in excellent condition, those who have scored 2 for each of the other signs may receive only a score of 1 for this part of the evaluation. This will, of course, influence the total score.

Interpretation. An Apgar score of 7 to 10 indicates that the infant's condition is good. If the infant breathes and cries (or coughs) seconds after delivery, there are usually no special procedures necessary other than those of routine close observation, maintaining a clear airway, and supplying warmth as necessary. A score of 4 to 6 means that the baby is in fair condition. There may be moderate central nervous system depression, some muscle flaccidity and cyanosis; respiration will not establish readily. *These infants must have their air passages cleared and be given oxygen promptly.* Administration of oxygen can best be done by mask, and the flow should not exceed 4 liters. Gentle patting and rubbing with the receiving blanket to dry the infant's body usually acts as an additional stimulus. A score of 0 to 3 denotes an extremely poor condition. Resuscitation is needed immediately (see Chapter 29).

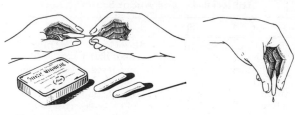

Figure 18-28. *(Left)* Silver nitrate 1 percent solution for the care of the eyes of newborn babies; needle puncture of wax ampule. *(Right)* Showing how to manipulate the ampule in administering the drug. (Eli Lilly and Company)

During the interval following the five-minute Apgar score, the nurse will continue her appraisal of the infant. Auscultation of the chest will ascertain proper position of the heart and normal air exchange. The head and body surfaces are scrutinized for trauma and for obvious congenital anomalies. These can include caput succedaneum, cephalhematoma, or forceps marks. The anterior fontanel is checked for bulging or sunkenness and the head circumference for enlargement or smallness. The skin is also checked for scaling or undue wrinkling indicative of the maturity of the infant. Any jaundice is also noted. The abdomen is palpated for masses and for enlargement of the liver, spleen or kidneys. The genitalia are examined for normal sexuality and the anus for patency. Each of the shoulders is moved while a finger is placed over the clavicle. A crunching sensation (crepitus) indicates a fracture. Before the final clamp is applied to the cord, the physician or nurse will examine it closely to see if it contains the normal number of vessels (two arteries and one vein). The presence of only one artery suggests one or more major congenital malformations. The cut edges of the arteries are seen as two white papular structures, which usually stand out slightly from the surface. The vein is larger, often gaping so that the lumen and thin wall are easily seen. The student is referred to Chapter 5 of the Korones book (see Suggested Reading) for details of the physical assessment and the nurse's responsibilities.

Other aspects of care

CARE OF THE CORD. In many hospitals no dressing is applied after the cord has been clamped or ligated and cut; in others a sterile plain gauze dressing is applied around the cord stump and secured with a binder, which is removed at appropriate times. Regardless of the technique employed, it is imperative that frequent inspection be done to note any signs of bleeding and that strict aseptic precautions be utilized in caring for the cord stump. The method of leaving the cord stump exposed has proved to be very satisfactory. If it is left free, it apparently dries and separates more quickly than when it is kept covered. There is also less irritation of the abdomen and the back, which sometimes results from a moist binder. Some pediatricians think that the abdominal muscles become stronger by not being bound.

CARE OF THE EYES. As soon as the cord is cared for and the infant's respiration is well established, the eyes should receive prophylactic treatment for protection against ophthalmia neonatorum (see Chapter 29). This treatment is so important that at the present time the use of some antibacterial agent is mandatory by statute in all states. Penicillin and silver nitrate are the usual agents employed, although a nonirritating solution of 15 percent sulphacetamide is preferred by some physicians. When silver nitrate is used, it is supplied in wax ampuls containing a 1 percent solution especially prepared for eye instillation (Fig. 18-28).

Instilling drops in the infant's eyes is more easily accomplished if the nurse shades the eyes from the light while putting the drops first in one eye, allowing time for the baby to recover from the shock and the smarting before she puts the drops in the other eye. One of the best methods is to draw down the lower lid gently and carefully instill two drops of the solution in the conjunctival sac, using great care not to drop it on the cornea. After two minutes, when it will have diffused itself over the entire conjunctiva, the lids should again be held apart and the conjunctival sac of each eye flushed gently with normal saline solution or sterile distilled water (Fig. 18-29). Prompt irrigation of the eyes following instillation of silver nitrate drops is said to reduce the incidence of chemical conjunctivitis without affecting prophylactic efficacy. The nurse must take especial precautions against allowing any contamination of the eyes and against dropping any silver solution upon the face. Silver nitrate prophylaxis may cause signs of irritation, such as redness, edema or discharge, but these manifestations are transient and in no way cause permanent damage if the silver nitrate solution used is in correct concentration.

If penicillin is to be used, it can be obtained

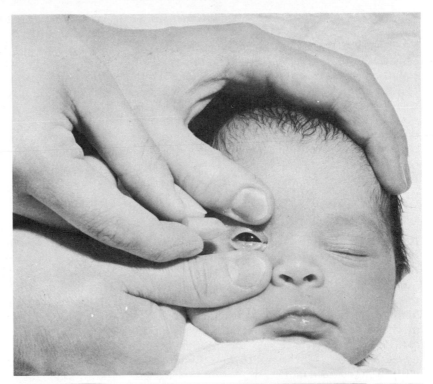

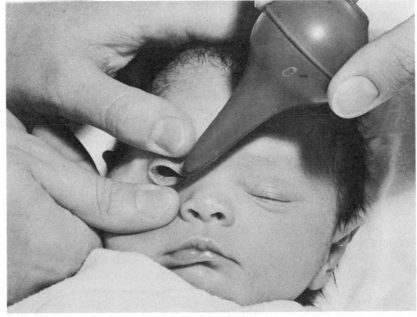

Figure 18-29. Silver nitrate prophylaxis. (*Top*) Instillation of two drops of silver nitrate 1 percent solution from a wax ampule into the conjunctival sac of each eye. (*Bottom*) After the medication has diffused over the entire conjunctiva (two minutes), the conjunctival sac of each eye is gently flushed with sterile distilled water or normal saline solution to remove the excess silver nitrate.

in ophthalmic drops or ointment. The technique for instillation is similar to that for silver nitrate, except that there is no flushing with saline or water. Penicillin is also given intramuscularly for both prophylaxis and treatment of ophthalmia neonatorum. When gonorrheal ophthalmia does develop, it can be cured by penicillin within a few hours, whereas silver nitrate has long since been abandoned for treatment purposes. The incidence of chemical irritation with penicillin ointment or intramuscular injection is much less than with silver nitrate, and the irritation is generally milder. However, some sensitivity reactions have been reported; thus, silver nitrate continues to be used.

HYPOPROTHROMBINEMIA PROPHYLAXIS. Many physicians prescribe that a single dose of phytonadione solution (Aquamephyton) 1.0 mg. (0.5 cc.) be administered intramuscularly during the course of the immediate care of the newborn after delivery. This water-soluble form of vitamin K_1 acts as a preventative measure against neonatal hemorrhagic disease. Amounts of the medication in excess of 1.0 mg. may predispose to the development of hyperbilirubinemia and are to be avoided.

IDENTIFICATION METHODS. Some method of identification of the newborn is applied before the cord is cut or before the baby is removed from the delivery room. Most hospitals use pliable plastic tapes which are applied to the infant's wrist and ankle. These contain the mother's name, physician's name, date, time of birth, and sex of the infant, and often the mother's hospital number. The baby's identification is checked against the mother's each time the baby is brought to her. Linen tapes with similar information are sometimes used. Less frequently used is the string of beads, since only the name can be recorded on it.

In addition, palmprints or footprints may be taken. This method of identification consists of a stainless procedure made on chemically treated, sensitized paper. It is designed to take the palmprints or footprints of the baby and the thumbprint of the mother at the time of delivery and may be repeated at the time of discharge from the hospital. It is a simple, quick and permanent method.

Current practice emphasizes that the newborn should be discharged without removing the identification band. Several states now have laws making it mandatory not to remove the identification bands on hospital premises. The mother should be taught how to remove the band as part of the discharge instructions.

As already discussed in Chapter 1, the registration of the infant's birth is a legal responsibility. It is mandatory that a birth certificate, such as that shown in Figure 1-2, p. 10, be filled out on every birth and submitted promptly to the local registrar.

AFTER THE DELIVERY. After caring for the infant, the nurse will continue to assist the physician with the care of the mother and her infant. If the mother is awake, she may be anxious to have her baby brought near so that she may see it at close range. If she is drowsy,

it may be better to wait until she is more alert. The nurse will be governed by each mother's response at this time. Some mothers want to touch their babies; others are eager to hold their babies at this time, and if this is sanctioned by the physician, there is no reason that it should not be permitted for a brief period. In this instance the nurse will be careful to keep her hand under the infant for support and added protection, should this be necessary, because of the mother's excitement in her first contact with her newborn.

If the infant is well wrapped and warm, it may be kept in a crib at the mother's side until the mother leaves the delivery room. The infant should be kept in a slight Trendelenburg position (at an angle of 15 degrees) to promote drainage of mucus, and on his side to avoid aspiration of this mucus. Care should be taken to avoid placing the infant in an exaggerated Trendelenburg position (almost directly downward), since the relatively large amount of abdominal contents will press against the diaphragm and the partially expanded lungs and may impede the infant's respiratory efforts.

The nurse observes the infant at frequent intervals to make sure that he is breathing properly, that the mouth and the nose are free from mucus, and that there is no bleeding from the cord. Because this period may be a critical one for the infant, many hospitals have facilities, such as a receiving nursery on the labor and delivery division, where the infant is transferred at this time. This not only provides closer supervision and care for the infant but also permits the nurse in the delivery room to devote her undivided attention to the mother.

BAPTISM OF INFANT. If there is any probability that the infant is in imminent danger and may not live, the question of baptism should be considered in cases in which the religion of the family is Roman Catholic; this also applies to some of the other denominations of the Christian church. This is an essential duty and means a great deal to the families concerned, and thoughtfulness in this matter will never be forgotten by them. (It is to be understood that such baptism would be reported to the family.)

The following simple instructions were given by the late Rev. Paul L. Blakely, S.J., Ph.D.

> The Catholic Church teaches that in case of emergency, any one may and should baptize. What is necessary is to make the intention of doing what the Church wishes to do and then to pour the water on the child (the head by

preference) saying at the same time, "I baptize thee in the name of the Father and of the Son and of the Holy Ghost." The water may be warmed if necessary but it must be pure water and care should be taken to make it flow. If there is any doubt whether the child is alive or dead, it should be baptized, but conditionally (i.e., "If thou art alive, I baptize thee . . .").

On page 281 of the Book of Common Prayer of the Protestant Episcopal Church, it is stated: "In cases of extreme sickness, or any imminent peril, if a Minister cannot be procured, then any baptized person present may administer holy Baptism, using the foregoing form" (i.e., the form given above).

Emergency delivery by the nurse

In the course of labor one occasionally encounters the so-called *precipitate delivery*, a rapid spontaneous delivery in which the infant is born without adequate preparations on the part of the physician or the nurse, sometimes even without benefit of their immediate care. This may occur in certain multiparous women, particularly if the soft parts of the pelvis offer little resistance, if the contractions are unusually strong and forceful, or if the mother does not experience painful sensations during labor and thus has inadequate warning that the delivery is approaching. The mother, of course, may suffer lacerations of the tissues as the result of tumultuous labor. The infant is endangered because, in its rapid progress through the birth canal, it may suffer cerebral trauma; or the umbilical cord may be torn in the process of the delivery. In addition, if the mother is unattended, the infant may be in jeopardy from lack of care during the first few minutes of life.

Whether the nurse is caring for a mother in the hospital labor room, making a home visit, or involved in some emergency situation, it is well for her to be prepared for a precipitate delivery. It seldom happens that the nurse is alone with her patient in the hospital when the delivery is imminent; but knowing what to do in such a situation, in the event that the physician is not present, is advantageous for all concerned. In the excitement which may ensue, the nurse's concern for the immediate safety of the mother and the baby usually demands all of her attention.

However, it should be stressed that the nurse's composure and her ability to convey this is one of the cornerstones in a successful delivery. Whenever possible, the nurse is to let the mother know what to anticipate and instruct her as best she can in what she can do to cooperate effectively. Here teamwork with the mother is essential and can be accomplished if the nurse instills confidence by demonstrating her competence in both the physical and the emotional aspects of care. If the father is present, he can be utilized in the care of his wife in whatever capacity seems most appropriate and in accord with his ability. He might help best by taking care of the other children or by calling the physician, or he might be involved directly in some aspect of the delivery. If it seems more desirable that he be away from the immediate vicinity, then the reasons for his leaving should be given. He is not to be dismissed summarily from the situation.

The nurse who is consistently conscientious about applying principles of asepsis and antisepsis will automatically apply them in this instance, to the best of her ability. Usually, there is inadequate time for proper cleansing of the vulva, or scrubbing her own hands and donning sterile gloves, or draping the mother, all of which would be ideal. However, a clean delivery area should be maintained, and, if time and facilities permit, the nurse's hands should be cleansed.

DELIVERY OF THE HEAD. As the head distends the perineum at the acme of a contraction, gentle pressure is exerted against the head to control its progress and thereby to prevent undue stretching of the perineum. This kind of *control* applied to the descending head during each contraction will prevent its sudden expulsion through the vulva, reducing the possibility of consequent complications. *The head must never be held back.* The mother should be encouraged to pant during the contraction to deter bearing-down efforts on her part, particularly as the head, which will be supported by the nurse, is being delivered. Whenever possible, the infant's head should be delivered between contractions.

RUPTURE OF THE MEMBRANES. If the membranes have not ruptured previously, they may remain intact until they appear as a smooth, glistening object at the vulva. If they protrude, they may rupture with the next contraction. But if the membranes have not ruptured before the head is delivered, they must be broken and removed immediately (by nipping them at the nape of the infant's neck) to prevent aspiration of fluid when the infant takes its first breath.

PRECAUTIONS CONCERNING THE CORD. As soon as the head is delivered, the nurse should feel for a loop or loops of cord around the neck and, if any is found, gently slip it over the baby's head, if this can be done easily. But, as stated on page 333, if the cord is coiled too tightly to permit this, it must be doubly clamped and cut (between the clamps) before delivery of the rest of the body. One or more loops of cord around the fetal neck occur in about a quarter of all deliveries.

DELIVERY OF THE INFANT'S BODY. After external rotation of the head, which is usually spontaneous, there is no occasion for haste in the delivery of the body. Gentle downward pressure with the hands on either side of the head may be exerted to direct the anterior shoulder under the symphysis pubis, then reversed upward in order to deliver the posterior shoulder over the perineum. The infant's body now will follow easily and quickly and should be supported as it is born.

IMMEDIATE CARE OF THE INFANT. As soon as the face appears, mucus and fluids should be wiped from the nose and the mouth. Then, after the infant is born, if he does not cry spontaneously, or if there seems to be mucus in the respiratory passages, the infant should be held up by the ankles to encourage the mucus to drain from the nose and mouth. In doing this, care must be exercised to avoid any traction on the umbilical cord and, at the same time, to prevent the infant's head from pressing down against the bed. Drainage of mucus is stimulated when the infant cries but can be encouraged by "milking the trachea" (i.e., with the forefinger, stroking the neck from its base toward the chin). Further stimulation by gentle rubbing of the back may stimulate breathing.

CARE OF THE CORD. There is *no* hurry to cut the cord, so this should be delayed until proper equipment is available. It is a good plan to clamp the cord after pulsations cease (but not imperative at the moment) and to wait for the physician to cut the cord after he arrives. One must always bear in mind that sterile conditions must exist for the cord-cutting procedure; otherwise the infant's safety is jeopardized. Also, the technique for applying the cord tie or umbilical clamp must be assiduously carried out to prevent bleeding from the umbilical stump.

DELIVERY OF THE PLACENTA. When signs of placental separation are apparent, the mother can be asked to bear down with the next contraction to deliver the placenta. Since the danger of hemorrhage is always to be guarded against, the fundus should be massaged after the delivery of the placenta if there is the slightest tendency toward relaxation of the uterine muscles.

When the infant is breathing satisfactorily, he can be placed on his side across his mother's abdomen (with his head kept low to promote postural drainage and his body covered to prevent chilling). This accomplishes several things: the mother is given her baby, she can touch him and is usually enthralled by the close physical contact with him; the warmth of the mother's body prevents the infant from being chilled; and the pressure exerted on the uterus by the weight of the infant helps it to contract.

One must remember to proceed slowly and carefully throughout the delivery. As stated earlier, the nurse's reaction to the situation undoubtedly will be transferred to the mother; If the nurse remains poised and unfaltering, the mother and other people involved are more likely to do so.

Lacerations of the birth canal

During the process of a normal delivery lacerations of the perineum and the vagina may be caused by rapid and sudden expulsion of the head (particularly when it "pops" out), the excessive size of the infant and very friable maternal tissues. In other circumstances they may be caused by difficult forceps deliveries, breech extractions or contraction of the pelvic outlet in which the head is forced posteriorly. Some tears are unavoidable, even in the most skilled hands.

Perineal lacerations usually are classified in three degrees, according to the extent of the tear.

First-degree lacerations are those which involve the fourchet, the perineal skin and the vaginal mucous membrane without involving any of the muscles (Fig. 18-30 A).

Second-degree lacerations are those which involve (in addition to skin and mucous membrane) the muscles of the perineal body but not the rectal sphincter. These tears usually extend upward on one or both sides of the vagina, making a triangular injury (Fig. 18-30 B).

Third-degree lacerations are those which extend completely through the skin, the mucous membrane, the perineal body and the rectal sphincter (Fig. 18-30 C). This type is often referred to as a complete tear. Not infrequently these third-degree lacerations extend a certain distance up the anterior wall of the rectum.

First- and second-degree lacerations are extremely common in primigravidas; their high incidence is one of the reasons that episiotomy is widely employed. Fortunately, third-degree lacerations are far less common. All three types of lacerations are repaired by the physician immediately after the delivery to ensure that the perineal structures are returned approximately to their former condition. The technique employed for the repair of a laceration is virtually the same as that used for episiotomy incisions, although the former is more difficult to do because of the irregular lines of tissue which must be approximated.

Episiotomy and repair

An episiotomy is an incision of the perineum made to facilitate delivery. The incision is made with blunt-pointed straight scissors about the time that the head distends the vulva and is visible to a diameter of several centimeters. The incision may be made in the midline of the perineum—a median episiotomy. Or it may be begun in the midline and directed downward and laterally away from the rectum —a mediolateral episiotomy (Fig. 18-31). In the latter instance the incision may be directed to either the right or to the left side of the mother's pelvis.

As the infant's head distends the vulva, if a laceration seems to be inevitable, the physician undoubtedly will choose to incise the perineum rather than allow that structure to sustain a traumatic tear. This operation serves several purposes:

1. It substitutes a straight, clean-cut surgical incision for the ragged, contused laceration which otherwise is likely to ensue; such an incision is easier to repair and heals better than a tear.
2. The direction of the episiotomy can be controlled, whereas a tear may extend in any direction, sometimes involving the anal sphincter and the rectum.
3. Inordinate stretching and tearing of the perineal musculature is avoided and the incidence of subsequent perineal relaxation with cystocele-rectocele may be reduced. It spares the baby's head the necessity of serving as a "battering ram" against perineal

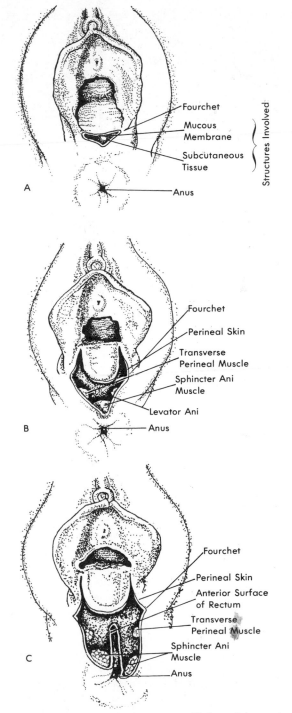

Figure 18-30. (A) First-degree tear. (B) Second-degree tear. (C) Third-degree tear.

obstruction; if prolonged, this "pounding" of the infant's head against the perineum may cause brain injury.
4. The operation shortens the duration of the second stage of labor.

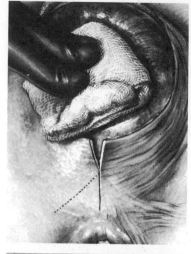
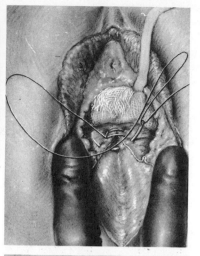
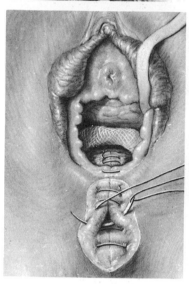
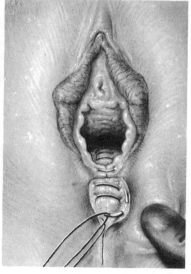

Figure 18-31. Episiotomy. (*Upper left*) Lines of incision for median and mediolateral episiotomy. (*Upper right*) "Tail-sponge" in vagina to occlude bleeding, continuous suture in vaginal mucosa. (*Lower left*) After levator ani muscle has been united by two or more sutures (shown tied and cut), the fascia covering the muscle is sutured. Note the "tail-sponge." (*Lower right*) After suturing to the lowermost angle of the fascia, the round needle is replaced by cutting needle and the running suture continued upward in subcuticular fascia.

In view of these several advantages of episiotomy, many physicians employ it routinely in the delivery of the primigravida.

There are many equally satisfactory methods utilized by different physicians for episiotomy repair. The suture material ordinarily used is a fine chromic catgut, either 00 or 000. The technique employed at the Johns Hopkins' Hospital is shown in Figure 18-31. However many other methods are equally satisfactory.

A round needle and continuous suture is used to close the vaginal mucosa and fourchet, and then laid aside while several interrupted sutures are placed in the levator ani muscle and the fascia. Then the continuous suture is again picked up and used to unite the subcutaneous fascia. Finally, the round needle is replaced by a large, straight cutting needle, and the running suture is continued upward as a subcuticular stitch.

Bibliography

1. Bloch, D.: Some crucial terms in nursing: what do they really mean? *Nurs. Outlook* 22:689-694, Nov. 1974.
2. Carrieri, V. K., and Sitzman, J.: Components of the nursing process. *Nurs. Clin. North Am.* 6:115-124, Mar. 1971.
3. Bloch, *op. cit.*, p. 693.
4. Newman, M. A.: Identifying and meeting patients' needs in short-span nurse-patient relationships. *Nurs. Forum* 5, 1:76-86, 1966.
5. Aiken, L., and Aiken, J.: A systematic approach to the evaluation of interpersonal relationships. *Am. J. Nurs.* 72:863-867, May 1973.
6. Kalisch, B. J.: What is empathy? *Am. J. Nurs.* 73:1548-1552, Sept. 1973.
7. *Ibid.*, pp. 81-83.
8. Wood, E. C.: Studies of the human fetus during normal and abnormal labor. *Int. J. Gyn. Ob.* 8:856-871, 1970.

9. Russen, A. W., *et al*: Electronic monitoring of the fetus. *Am. J. Nurs.* 74:1291-1299, July 1974.
10. *Ibid.*, pp. 1294-1296.
11. *Ibid.*, pp. 1294-1296. Also, O'Gureck, J. F., *et al*: A practical classification of fetal heart rate patterns. *Am. J. Ob-Gyn.* 40:356-361, Sept. 1972.
12. Parer, J. T., *et al*: *A Clinical Approach to Fetal Monitoring*. San Leandro, Berkeley Bio-Engineering, Inc., 1974, pp. 45-52.
13. Liu, Y. C.: Effects of upright position during labor. *Am. J. Nurs.* 12:2202-2205, Dec. 1974.
14. Clausen, J. P., *et al*: *Maternity Nursing Today*. New York, McGraw-Hill Book Company, pp. 526-547.
15. Barnett, C. R., *et al*: The maternal side of interactional deprivation. *Pediatrics* 45:197, 1970.
16. Robson, D. S., and Moss, H. A.: Patterns and determinants of maternal attachment. *Pediatrics* 77:976-985, Dec. 1970.
17. *Ibid.*, pp. 97-98.
18. Cronenwett, L. R., and Newmark, L. L.: Fathers' responses to childbirth. *Nurs. Research* 23:210-217, May/June 1974.
19. Rising, S.: The fourth stage of labor: family integration. *Am. J. Nurs.* 74:870-874, May 1974.
20. Babson, S. G., and Benson, R. C.: *Management of High-Risk Pregnancy and Intensive Care of the Neonate*. St. Louis, Mosby, 1971, p. 149.
21. Korones, S. B.: *High-Risk Newborn Infants: The Basis for Intensive Nursing Care*. St. Louis, Mosby, 1972.
22. Als, H., and Brazelton, T. B.: Comprehensive neonatal assessment. *Birth and the Family J.* 2:3-9, Winter 1974-75.

Suggested Reading

AULD, P. A.: Resuscitation of the newborn infant. *Am. J. Nurs.* 74:68-70, Jan. 1974.

BLAYLOCK, J.: The psychological and cultural influences on the reaction to pain: a review of the literature. *Nurs. Forum* 7:262-274, 1968.

BONICA, J. J.: Obstetric analgesia and anesthesia: recent trends and advances. *N. Y. J. Med.* 70:2079-2084, August 15, 1970.

BRADLEY, R. A.: Fathers' presence in delivery rooms. *Psychosomatics* 111:474-479, Nov./Dec. 1962.

BUXTON, C. L.: *Study of Psychophysical Methods for Relief of Childbirth Pain*. Philadelphia, W. B. Saunders, 1962.

CALDEYRO-BARCIA, R., *et al*: Fetal monitoring in labor. *In* H. M. Wallace, *et al* (ed.): *Maternal and Child Health Practices*, Springfield, Illinois, Thomas, 1973, pp. 332-394.

CHAGNON, L. J., AND HELDENBRAND, C. L.: Nurses undertake direct and indirect fetal monitoring at a community hospital. *JOGN*, Sept./Oct. 1974, pp. 41-46.

CHAMBERS, W.: Nursing diagnosis. *Am. J. Nurs.* 62:102-104, Nov. 1962.

CHRISTIAN, J. R.: Comparison of ocular reactions with the use of silver nitrate and erythromycin ointment in ophthalmia neonatorum prophylaxis. *J. Pediatrics* 57:55-60, July 1960.

CLARK, A. L.: The adaption problems and patterns of an expanding family: the neonatal period. *Nurs. Forum* 5, 1:92-109, 1966.

COHEN, S. N., AND OLSON, W. A.: Drugs that depress the newborn infant. *Ped. Clin. North Am.* 17:835-850, Nov. 1970.

CUMMINS, H., AND MIDLO, C.: *Fingerprints, Palms and Soles*. New York, Dover, 1962.

DE AGUSTINA, J., *et al*: Ward study: The meaning of touch in intrapersonal communication. *In* S. Burd, and M. Marshall: *Some Clinical Approaches to Psychiatric Nursing*. New York, Macmillan, 1963.

DICK-READ, G.: *Childbirth Without Fear*. New York, Harper & Row, 1972.

DURAND, M., AND PRINCE, R.: Nursing diagnosis: process and decision. *Nurs. Forum* 5, 4:50-64.

DWYER, J. M., AND LYNCH, W. A.: Nursing responsibility for decreasing maternal and perinatal mortality and morbidity. *Hosp. Progr.* 48:66-67, Jan. 1967.

GREISS, F. C., JR.: Obstetric anesthesia. *Am. J. Nurs.* 71:67-69, Jan. 1971.

HOFF, F. E.: How any nurse can help. *Am. J. Nurs.* 69:1451-1453, July 1969.

HOMMEL, F.: Nurses in private practice as monitrices. *Am. J. Nurs.* 69:1446-1450, July 1969.

HON, E. H.: Electronic evaluation of fetal heart rates. *Am. J. Ob-Gyn.* 83:333-338, Feb. 1, 1962.

JOLLY, C., *et al*: Research in the delivery of female health care: The recipient's reaction. *Am. J. Ob-Gyn.* 110:291-294, June 1, 1971.

JONES, J. A.: Examining the newborn's eyes, a satisfactory method. *Clin. Pediat.* 7:124, Feb. 1968.

KORONES, S. B.: *High-Risk Newborn Infants: The Basis for Intensive Nursing Care*. St. Louis, Mosby, 1972.

LESSER, M., AND KEANE, V.: *Nurse-Patient Relationships in a Hospital Maternity Service*. St. Louis, Mosby, 1956.

LEVINE, M. E.: Adaption and assessment, a rationale for nursing intervention. *Am. J. Nurs.* 66:2450-2453, Nov. 1966.

LUDEMANN, R. S.: Empathy—a component of therapeutic nursing. *Nurs. Forum* 7:275-288, 1968.

MANNING, R. E.: To do or not to do—a critical review of vaginal examination during labor. *Am. J. Ob-Gyn.* 82:1356-1358, Dec. 1961.

MILLER, J. S.: *Childbirth*. New York, Atheneum, 1963.

MOSS, F. T., AND MEYER, B.: The effects of nursing interaction upon pain relief in patients. *Nurs. Research* 15:303-306, Fall 1966.

MUNDINGER, M. O., AND JOHNSON, G.: Developing a nursing diagnosis. *Nurs. Outlook* 23:94-98, Feb. 1975.

NEWMAN, M. A.: Identifying and meeting patient's needs in short-span nurse-patient relationships. *Nurs. Forum* 5:76-86, 1966.

Psychophysical Preparation for Childbearing: Guidelines for Teaching, ed. 2. New York, Maternity Center Association, 1965.

REEDER, S.: Becoming a mother, nursing implication in a problem of role transition. A.N.A. Regional Clinical Conferences, 204-210. New York, Appleton-Century Crofts, 1968.

REITER, F. K.: The clinical nursing approach. *Nurs. Forum* 5:39-44, 1966.

RICH, O. J.: Hospital routines as rites of passage in developing maternal identity. *Nurs. Clin. North Am.* 4:101-109, Mar. 1969.

RISING, S.: Babies have fathers, too. *Am. J. Nurs.* 71:1980-1981, Oct. 1971.

ROBERTS, C. J.: Developmental and neurological sequelae

of the common complications of pregnancy and birth. *Brit. J. Pre. Soc. Med.* 24:33-38, Feb. 1970.

Rosengren, W. R.: Some psychological aspects of delivery room difficulties. *J. Nerv. Ment. Dis.* 132:515-521, June 1961.

Roy, Sister Callista: A diagnostic classification system for nursing. *Nurs. Outlook* 23:90-93, Feb. 1975.

Saltenis, I. J.: *Physical Touch and Nursing Support in Labor.* Unpublished master's thesis. Yale University, New Haven, Conn., 1962.

Sasmor, J. L., *et al*: The childbirth team during labor. *Am. J. Nurs.* 73:444-447, Mar. 1973.

Smith, B. A., *et al*: The transition phase of labor. *Am. J. Nurs.* 73:448-450, Mar. 1973.

Smoyak, S.: Cultural incongruence: the effect on nurses' perceptions. *Nurs. Forum* 7:234-247, 1968.

Travelbee, J.: What do we mean by rapport? *Am. J. Nurs.* 63:70-72, Feb. 1963.

Tryon, P. A., and Leonard, R. C.: The effect of the patient's participation on the outcome of a nursing procedure. *Nurs. Forum* 3:79-89, 1964.

Turner, R. H.: Role taking: process versus conformity. *In* A. M. Rose (ed): *Human Behavior and Social Processes,* Boston, Houghton Mifflin, 1962, pp. 20-40.

———: Role taking, role standpoint and reference group behavior. *Am. J. Soc.* 61:316-328, Jan. 1956.

Ulin, P. R.: The exhilarating moment of birth. *Am. J. Nurs.* 63:60-67, June 1963.

Van Auken, W. B. B.: Preparing the patient for labor. *Am. J. Ob-Gyn.* 24:318-321, Aug. 1964.

Vellay, P., *et al*: *Childbirth Without Pain,* D. Lloyd, trans. New York, Dutton, 1959.

Williams, B. L., and Richards, S. F.: Fetal monitoring during labor. *Am. J. Nurs.* 70:2384-2388, Nov. 1970.

Yeaworth, R. C.: Identification and maternity nursing. *Nurs. Forum* 7:248-261, 1968.

Yeh, S. Y., *et al*: Obstetrical anesthesia: A study of diazepam during labor. *Am. J. Ob-Gyn.* 43:363-373, Mar. 1974.

Zborowski, M.: Cultural components in responses to pain. *J. Soc. Issues* 8:21-25, 1952.

Conference Material

1. A mother who is contemplating the delivery of her first child is worried for fear that she may not get her own baby if another infant is born at the same time she is delivered. How would you reassure this mother concerning the identification methods for newborn infants?

2. An 18-year-old woman having her first baby is admitted to the hospital in early labor. It is obvious from her behavior that she has had no preparation for this experience and is frightened and apprehensive. What specific measures would you include in your nursing plan for her care?

3. An unwed mother goes into labor, having made no arrangement for the care of her 2-year-old girl and her 12-year-old boy. What resources could you suggest in this situation? What is the responsibility of hospital and community agencies in this case?

4. A couple who have attended Lamaze childbirth education classes find that all patients must be monitored externally during labor at the hospital they have chosen for delivery. What explanation would you give the couple for this practice? What specific measures would you include in your care plan to help the couple practice their relaxation, concentration, etc., and still maintain monitoring?

5. Why is prophylaxis for the eyes of the newborn required by law in all states? How would you go about securing the desired information concerning such legislation in the various states of the United States?

6. You are caring for a mother having her fourth child who is in very active labor. Suddenly, the membranes rupture, and she begins to bear down. As you observe the perineum, you see the infant's head crowning. Since you are alone with this mother at the time, what will you do?

7. A 21-year-old mother at term, who has attended "natural childbirth" classes for a previous pregnancy, comes to the hospital on her physician's instructions because her membranes have ruptured. She is apologetic because her contractions are only 10 to 12 minutes apart, of mild intensity, lasting about 35 seconds and "not really good enough yet to come to the hospital." On examination, her cervix is found to be 2 cm. dilated and 10 percent effaced. Discuss the nursing care you would plan for this mother if she were assigned to your care.

Study Questions for Unit IV

Read through the entire question and place your answer on the line to the right.

1. Give the term of the phrase which best fits each of the following statements:
   A. Enlargement of the external os to 10 cm. in diameter. _____
   B. Maximum shortening of the cervical canal. _____
   C. A type of drug used in obstetrics which blots out memory of whatever occurs under its influence. _____

D. A condition caused by failure of the uterine muscle to stay contracted after delivery. _____

E. A surgical incision of the perineum during second-stage labor. _____

F. Settling of the baby's head into the brim of the pelvis. _____

2. The character and the frequency of uterine contractions and the location of the discomfort experienced by the mother during labor often provide pertinent information regarding the labor.

SITUATION NO. 1: In the case of a multipara who is having discomfort but is not in real labor, which of these symptoms would most probably serve to identify false labor contractions?

A. Discomfort may begin as early as three or four weeks before the onset of true labor.

B. Discomfort occurs three or four days before the onset of true labor.

C. Contractions occur at regular intervals.

D. Contractions occur at irregular intervals.

E. Discomfort is confined to the lower abdomen and the groin.

F. Discomfort is felt in the upper abdomen and the back.

Select the number corresponding to the correct letter or letters.
1. A only
2. A and C
3. A, D and E
4. All of them _____

SITUATION NO. 2: In the case of a primigravida in the beginning of the first stage of labor, which of the following symptoms would most probably describe her labor contractions?

A. Contractions occur at regular intervals.

B. Contractions occur at irregular intervals.

C. Discomfort is confined to the lower abdomen and the groin.

D. Discomfort is located in the lower back and the abdomen.

E. Contractions occur at intervals of from two to three minutes.

F. Contractions occur at intervals of from ten to fifteen minutes.

Select the number corresponding to the correct letters.
1. A and C
2. A, D and F
3. B, C and E
4. All of them _____

SITUATION NO. 3: In the case of a primigravida approaching the end of the first stage of labor, which of the following symptoms would most probably give an accurate description of her labor?

A. Contractions occur at regular intervals.

B. Contractions occur at irregular intervals.

C. Contractions occur at intervals of every one to one and one-half minutes.

D. Contractions occur at intervals of from two to three minutes.

E. Duration of contraction is from 45 to 60 seconds.

F. Duration of contraction is from 50 to 70 seconds.

Select the number corresponding to the correct letters.
1. A, C and E
2. A, D and F
3. B, D and E
4. All of them _____

3. Labor is divided into the first, the second, and the third stages.
   A. When is the first stage of labor considered to be terminated?
      1. When contractions occur at 10- to 15-minute intervals.
      2. When the cervix is completely dilated.
      3. When the baby is delivered.   _____

   B. When is the second stage of labor considered to be terminated?
      1. When the cervix is completely dilated.
      2. When contractions occur at two- to three-minute intervals.
      3. When the baby is delivered.   _____

   C. When is the third stage of labor considered to be terminated?
      1. When the baby is delivered.
      2. When the placenta is delivered.
      3. After the uterus has remained firm for one hour.   _____

4. The nurse is caring for a mother in the accelerated phase of labor who is being monitored internally because of suspected fetal distress. Which of the following observations would you report promptly to the physician?
   A. A silent FHR baseline for 15 minutes.
   B. A consistent reactive FHR baseline fluctuating more than five beats per minute.
   C. Moderate amount of bright blood in the vaginal discharge.
   D. Plugs of blood-streaked mucus in the vaginal discharge.
   E. FHR rate that slows during a contraction but returns to its usual rate of 10 to 15 seconds following contractions.

   Select the number corresponding to the correct letters.
   1. A and C
   2. A, C and E
   3. B, D and E
   4. All of them   _____

5. On admission of the mother to the labor suite, which of the following procedures are usually carried out routinely?
   A. Check mother's temperature, pulse, respirations and blood pressure.
   B. Take the mother to the bathroom and have her void.
   C. Cleanse and shave the vulvar and perineal area.
   D. Listen to the fetal heart sounds.
   E. Prepare the mother for vaginal examination.

   Select the number corresponding to the correct letter or letters.
   1. A only
   2. A and E
   3. A, C and D
   4. All of them   _____

6. Why is an enema frequently given to a mother during the early part of the first stage of labor?
   A. To obtain a stool specimen.
   B. To avoid straining as the mother bears down with contractions.
   C. To cleanse the lower bowel and/or stimulate labor contractions.   _____

7. After the cervix is dilated, and particularly if the membranes have ruptured, what facilities would provide the mother with the greatest degree of comfort and safety to expel an enema?
   A. Use of toilet facilities in bathroom.
   B. Remain in bed and use the bedpan.
   C. Use the bedpan on a chair close to the bed.   _____

8. Often it is the nurse's responsibility to decide when the mother is ready to be moved from the labor room to the delivery room. Which of the following signs would signify to the nurse that the time of delivery is near?

   A. Mother has a desire to defecate.
   B. Increase in frequency, duration and intensity of uterine contractions.
   C. Mother begins to bear down spontaneously with uterine contractions.
   D. Bulging of the perineum.
   E. Increase in amount of blood-stained mucus from the vagina.

   Select the number corresponding to the correct letter or letters.

   1. D only
   2. A, C and E
   3. B, D and E
   4. All of them   _____

9. A physician was busy suctioning mucus from the mouth of the baby immediately after its birth and asked the nurse to let him know as soon as the placenta seemed to be separated. Which of the following would indicate that it was separated?

   A. Gradual descent of the uterus farther into the pelvis.
   B. Protrusion of several more inches of umbilical cord.
   C. Uterus becomes more firm and rounded.
   D. A sudden gush of blood from the vagina.
   E. Large clots of blood slip out of the vagina.

   Select the number corresponding to the correct letters.

   1. A and C
   2. B, C and D
   3. B, C and E
   4. All of them   _____

10. As soon as the physician had clamped and cut the umbilical cord, he handed the infant over to the nurse to care for. Which of the following acts would the nurse perform in the immediate care of the infant?

    A. Place the infant so that he lies in a slight Trendelenburg position in a heated crib or resuscitator.
    B. Wipe the mucus out of the infant's mouth with sterile gauze.
    C. Slap the infant's back and soles of the feet sharply to stimulate crying.
    D. Gently remove all vernix caseosa and blood in drying the infant's body with the receiving blanket.
    E. "Label" infant with required item of identification as soon as he is transferred to the nursery.

    Select the number corresponding to the correct letter or letters.

    1. A only
    2. A and C
    3. B, D and E
    4. All of them   _____

11. After the delivery the infant is cared for by a nurse in the receiving nursery. The nurse who is caring for the mother during the fourth stage of labor would include which of the following in her nursing care plan?

    A. Keep the mother warm and out of drafts.
    B. Express blood clots if they should accumulate in the uterus.

C. Massage the fundus continuously.
   D. Administer ergotrate 0.2 mg. intramuscularly.
   E. Check the mother's vital signs at frequent intervals.

Select the number corresponding to the correct letter or letters.
   1. B only
   2. A and C
   3. A, B and E
   4. All of them _____

12. Possibly the most dangerous stage of labor for the mother is the third stage because of the possibility of postpartal hemorrhage and shock.
   A. Because there is a certain amount of blood loss, hemorrhage is said to take place when the loss exceeds what amount of blood?
      2. 300 cc.
      2. 200 cc.
      3. 500 cc. _____

   B. The most common cause of postpartal hemorrhage is atony of the uterus. What is the first thing to do as a preventive measure if the uterus appears to be atonic?
      1. Take a firm grasp on the uterus.
      2. Massage the uterus firmly.
      3. Administer an oxytocic drug.

13. The physician told the nurse to watch a mother during labor for evidence of a prolapsed cord which he feared might occur.
   A. What type of FHR pattern would be most likely to appear if the cord prolapses?
      1. Combined acceleration waveform.
      2. Isolated acceleration waveform.
      3. Severe variable deceleration waveform.
      4. Late deceleration waveform.
      5. Early deceleration waveform.

   B. If the nurse did suspect the cord to be prolapsed, what position should she put the mother in, with the hope of relieving the pressure on the cord?
      1. Knee-chest position.
      2. Fowler's position.
      3. Sims's position.
      4. A prone position. _____

   C. In addition to changing the mother's position to relieve pressure on the cord, what other measures may the nurse employ if she observes the umbilical cord prolapsed out of the vagina?
      1. Immediately wash the cord with warm antiseptic solution and replace in vagina.
      2. Cover the cord with a wet sponge.
      3. Apply a clamp to the exposed cord and cover with a sterile towel.
      4. Keep the cord warm and moist by continuous applications of sterile saline compresses. _____

   D. What are the chief objectives of the emergency care given when prolapsed cord occurs?
      1. To prevent cold air from prematurely stimulating respiration.
      2. To prevent drying of the cord while it is still pulsating.
      3. To stimulate and restore circulation in the cord by vasodilatation.
      4. To prevent or relieve pressure on the cord. _____

assessment and management of the normal mother-infant dyad

The Physiology of the Puerperium
Nursing Care During the Puerperium
Care of the Newborn Infant

unit V

the physiology of the puerperium

19
Anatomic Changes / Clinical Aspects / Postpartal Examinations

This chapter deals with the study of the anatomic and the physiologic changes that normally occur during the puerperium. Knowledge of the reproductive process concerning pregnancy and labor will serve as a basis for understanding how the generative organs and the various systems of the human body adapt following the delivery.

The term puerperium (from *puer,* a child; and *parere,* to bring forth) refers to the six-week period elapsing between the termination of labor and the return of the reproductive organs to their normal condition. This includes both the *progressive changes* in the breasts for lactation and *involution* of the internal reproductive organs. Although the changes brought about by involution are considered to be normal physiologic processes, they border closely between a condition of health and disease, for under no other circumstances does such marked and rapid involution of tissues occur without a departure from a state of health. For this reason, the quality of the mother's care at this time is important to ensure her immediate as well as her future health.

Anatomic changes
Uterus

INVOLUTION OF THE UTERUS. Immediately following the delivery of the placenta the uterus becomes an almost solid mass of tissue. Its thick anterior and posterior walls lie in close opposition, so that the center cavity is flattened. The uterus remains about the same size for the first two days after delivery but then rapidly decreases in size by a process called involution. This is effected partly by the contraction of the uterus and partly by autolytic processes in which some of the protein material of the uterine wall is broken down into simpler components which then are absorbed.

The Process of Involution. The separation of the placenta and the membranes from the uterine wall takes place in the outer portion of the spongy layer of the decidua, and, therefore, a remnant of this layer remains in the uterus to be cast off in part in a vaginal discharge referred to as the lochia. Within two or three days after labor this remaining portion of decidua becomes differentiated into two layers, leaving the deeper or unaltered layer attached to the muscular wall from which the new endometrial lining is generated. The layer adjoining the uterine cavity becomes necrotic and is cast off in the lochia. The process is very like the healing of any surface; there is oozing of blood from the small vessels on this surface. The bleeding from the larger vessels is controlled by compression of the retracted uterine muscle fibers. The process of regeneration is rapid, except at the site of former placental attachment, which requires six or seven weeks to heal completely. Elsewhere, the free surface of the endometrium is restored in half that time.

The Progress of Involution. The normal process of involution requires five or six weeks, and at the end of that time the uterus regains its normal size, although it never returns exactly to its nulliparous state. One can realize more fully the rapidity of this process by comparing the changes which occur in the weight of this organ. Immediately following the delivery the uterus weighs approximately 2 pounds; at the end of the first week, about 1 pound; at the end of the second week, about 12 ounces; and by the time that involution is complete, it should weigh only about 2 ounces. By observing the height of the fundus, which may be felt through the abdominal wall, the nurse is able to appreciate more fully these remarkable changes. Immediately after the delivery of the placenta the uterus sinks into the pelvis, and the fundus is felt midway between the umbilicus and the symphysis, but it soon rises to the level of the umbilicus (5 or 5½ inches above the pubes); and 12 hours later it probably will be found a little higher. Day-by-day careful measurements will show that it is diminishing in size, so that at the end of 10 days or so it cannot be detected by abdominal palpation. The approximate rate of decrease in the height of the fundus is a little over half an inch or one fingerbreadth a day. Observation of this rate of involution is very important; the physician will want to be informed about any marked delay, especially if accompanied by suppression of the lochia or retention of clots. In measuring the height of the uterus, care should be taken that the observations are made after the bladder is emptied, as a full bladder will raise the height of the fundus.

Apparent indications that involution is not occurring satisfactorily are: the uterus fails to decrease progressively in size, it remains "flabby" and causes the mother much discomfort (see Subinvolution in Chapter 26).

CHANGES IN THE CERVIX. After the delivery the cervix is a soft, flabby structure but, because it is retracting, by the end of the first week it becomes so narrow that it would be difficult to introduce anything the size of a finger. Simultaneously, any lacerations are healing. Once a mother has delivered a child vaginally, the cervix does not assume its pregravid appearance, but the external os remains open in varying degrees, although the internal os is closed. This is one of the characteristics of the uterus of a multiparous woman.

THE LOCHIA. A knowledge of the healing process by which the lining of the uterus becomes regenerated is valuable to the nurse in understanding and interpreting the lochial discharge. At first the discharge consists almost entirely of blood with a small amount of mucus, particles of decidua and cellular debris which escape from the placental site. It should not contain large clots or membrane or be excessive in amount. The discharge lasts about three days and is called *lochia rubra.* As the oozing of blood from the healing surface diminishes, the discharge becomes more serous or watery and gradually changes to a pinkish color, the so-called *lochia serosa.* Toward the tenth day the lochia is thinner, greatly decreased in amount and almost colorless, the so-called *lochia alba.* By the end of the third week the discharge usually disappears, though a brownish mucoid discharge may persist a little longer. Lochia possesses a peculiar animal emanation which is quite characteristic and should never, at any time, have an offensive odor.

The quantity of lochia varies with individuals, but, generally speaking, it is more profuse in multiparas. It is to be expected that when a mother is out of bed for the first time there may be a definite increase in the amount of discharge. Nevertheless, the recurrence of fresh bleeding after the discharge has become dark and diminished in amount, or the persistence of bright blood in the lochia or the suppression of the discharge should be reported to the obstetrician. The daily observation of the amount and the character of the lochia is of the greatest importance as an index of the progress of healing of the endometrial surface.

The pelvis

The vaginal walls, the vulva and all other tissues which have become hypertrophied during pregnancy also undergo a process of involution in their return to normal. The *vagina* requires some time to recover from the distention brought about by the delivery. This capacious passage gradually diminishes in size, although it rarely returns to its nulliparous condition. The *labia majora* and the *labia minora* become flabby as compared with their condition before childbearing. Any abrasions and lacerations of the genital canal caused by the passage of the fetus should heal completely during the puerperium. The *ligaments* that support the uterus, the ovaries and the tubes, which have also undergone great tension and stretching, are now relaxed and will take considerable time to return almost to their normal size and position.

Abdominal wall

The abdominal wall recovers partially from the overstretching but remains soft and flabby for some time. The striae, due to the rupture of the elastic fibers of the cutis, usually remain but become less conspicuous because of their silvery appearance. The process of involution in the abdominal structures requires at least six weeks. Provided that the abdominal walls have retained their muscle tone, they gradually return to their original condition. However, if these muscles are relaxed because they have lost their tone, there may be a marked separation or *diastasis of the recti muscles,* so that the abdominal organs are not properly supported. Rest, diet, prescribed exercises, good body mechanics and good posture may do much to restore the tonicity of these muscles.

The breasts

During pregnancy progressive changes occur in the breasts in preparation for lactation (see Chapter 10). After the delivery the breasts continue much the same for about two days. The breasts secrete a small amount of *colostrum,* which appears as a thin yellowish fluid. It will be remembered that colostrum is formed at the end of pregnancy, and women who carry out special breast care preparation during the last weeks of pregnancy often are able manually to express small amounts of it before the birth of the baby. The nutritive value of colostrum is low in comparison with that of normal breast milk. Colostrum contains more protein (lactalbumin) and inorganic salts but less fat and carbohydrate than human breast milk. During these first days after the delivery breast-feeding is advantageous for both mother and infant. The infant's sucking at the breast helps to stimulate lactation, and, in addition, it stimulates the uterus to contract. These early breast-feeding experiences simultaneously fulfill the infant's need for sucking.

On the third or the fourth day postpartum the breast milk usually "comes in." There is an obvious change in the color of the secretion from the nipples; it becomes bluish white, the usual color of normal breast milk. At this time the breasts suddenly become larger, firmer and more tender as the lacteal secretion is established, causing the mother to experience throbbing pains in the breasts, extending into the axillae. This congestion, which usually subsides in one or two days, is caused in part by the pressure from the increased amount of milk in the lobes and the ducts but even more by the increased circulation of blood and lymph in the mammary gland, producing tension on the very sensitive surrounding tissues. This is sometimes referred to as *primary engorgement.*

Breast milk varies markedly in its quality and quantity, not only in different individuals, but also in the same individual at various times. In general, the amount of breast milk increases as the infant's need for it increases. Nature seems to have coordinated carefully the mother's need for rest and the infant's need for food during the first two days, when only colostrum is secreted. But during this time lactation is definitely stimulated by the infant's sucking, and although the secretion of breast milk would occur naturally, without this stimulation and the complete emptying of the breasts the secretion of breast milk would not continue for more than a few days. If the infant is put to breast consistently, by the end of the first week a healthy mother usually has about 6 to 10 ounces of breast milk a day. By the end of 4 weeks this amount almost doubles, so that she produces about 20 ounces a day. Breast milk is produced on the basis of "supply and demand" (i.e., the amount secreted gradually adjusts in relation to what the baby takes at an average feeding). In time, as the baby grows, the mother may have about 30 ounces of breast milk a day.

The supply of breast milk is dependent on several factors, such as the mother's diet, the amount of exercise and rest she gets, and her level of contentment. An adequate diet for lactation requires increased amounts of protein, calcium, iron and vitamins as well as an ample fluid intake (see p. 390). The mother who is breast-feeding needs a good night's sleep, a rest period in the middle of the day and normal exercise. Worry, emotional tension and too much activity (overexertion and fatigue) have an adverse effect on lactation (see Chapters 12 and 21). In relation to lactation, the actual size of the breast is not as important as the amount of glandular tissue, since the secreting tissues of the mammary gland produce the breast milk and not the fat. It has been verified that certain drugs, if administered to the lactating mother, are excreted in the breast milk, for example, large doses of salicylates, certain cathartics, iodides, bromides, quinine, atropine, and opium.

Clinical aspects

Early ambulation

The normal patient should be encouraged to get out of bed as soon as practical, and certainly within the first 24 hours postpartum. In general, patients feel stronger and psychologically better as a result of early limited activity, and constipation and bladder complications are less frequent. Most important, the incidence of thrombophlebitis and pulmonary embolus has been decreased materially in recent years as a result of early ambulation.

Temperature

Slight rises in temperature may occur without apparent cause following the delivery, but, in general, the mother's temperature should remain within normal limits during the puerperium, that is, below 38° C. (100.4° F.) when taken by mouth. Any mother whose temperature exceeds this limit in any two consecutive 24-hour periods of the puerperium (excluding the first 24 hours postpartum) is considered to be febrile.

It was formerly believed that an elevation of temperature naturally occurred with the establishment of lactation on the third or the fourth day after the delivery, and the so-called *milk-fever* was considered to be a normal accompaniment of this process. At the present time this is considered to be a fallacy. On rare occasions a sharp peak of fever for several hours may be caused by extreme vascular and lymphatic engorgement of the breasts, but this does not last longer than 12 hours at the most.

In judging the significance of a rise in temperature, the pulse rate provides a helpful guide, for in a puerperal patient with a slow pulse, a slightly elevated temperature is not likely to signify a complication. Nevertheless, any rise of temperature in the puerperium should excite the suspicion of endometritis (see Chapter 26).

Pulse

In the early puerperium a pulse rate which is somewhat slower than that at other times is a favorable symptom. The rate usually averages between 60 and 70 but may even become a little slower than this in one or two days after the delivery. This is merely a transient phenomenon, so that by the end of the first week or 10 days the pulse returns to its normal rate. On the other hand, a rapid pulse after labor, unless the mother has cardiac disease, may be an indication of shock or hemorrhage.

Blood

Most of the blood and metabolic alterations characteristic of normal pregnancy disappear within the first two weeks of the puerperium.

After-pains

Normally, after the delivery of the first child, the uterine muscle tends to remain in a state of tonic contraction and retraction. But if the uterus has been subjected to any marked distention, or if tissue or blood clots have been retained in the cavity, then active contractions occur in an effort to expel them, and these contractions may be painful. In multiparas a certain amount of the initial tonicity of the uterine muscle has been lost, and these contractions and retractions cannot be sustained. Consequently, the muscle contracts and relaxes at intervals, and these contractions give rise to the sensation of pain, the so-called "after-pains." These after-pains are more noticeable after a pregnancy in which the uterus has been greatly distended, as with multiple births or hydramnios. They are particularly noticeable in the breast-feeding mother, when the infant is put to breast (because sucking causes release of oxytocin from the posterior pituitary which stimulates the uterus to contract), and they may last for days, although ordinarily they become quite bearable in about 48 hours after delivery. They also occur with increased intensity, following the administration of oxytocic agents such as ergotrate. Often after-pains become so sharp that the administration of a sedative is necessary. Any time that they are severe enough to disturb the mother's rest and peace of mind, the physician should be notified.

Digestion

Although the mother's appetite may be diminished the first few days after labor, the digestive tract functions normally in the puerperium. Her thirst is considerably increased at this time due to the marked diaphoresis associated with the puerperium. Moreover, the fact that the mother has probably gone without fluids for some hours in labor undoubtedly increases her thirst.

Loss of weight

In addition to the 10- or 11-pound loss of weight which results at delivery, there is generally a still further loss of about 5 pounds of body weight early in the puerperium due to the marked diuresis, with its associated loss of body fluid.

Kidneys

The amount of urine excreted by the kidneys in the puerperium is of particular significance. As previously stated, during pregnancy there is an increased tendency of the body to retain water, so that now the tremendous output of urine represents the body's effort to return its water metabolism to normal. Diuresis regularly occurs between the second and the fifth days after delivery, sometimes reaching a daily output of 3,000 ml. After the delivery, in particular, the bladder may distend without any awareness on the part of the mother, especially if she has received any form of analgesia. Therefore, it becomes a major responsibility of the nurse to be alert to signs of a full bladder and thus to prevent distention from occurring.

During the first few days after labor there may be an increase in the amount of nitrogen in the urine. This excretion is due to the breakdown of protein material of the uterine wall during involution. Concerning acetone in the urine—as long as the regimen of "starvation" is not included in the management of labor, the presence of acetone in the urine, related to the incomplete metabolism of body fat, would not occur. Occasionally, during the first weeks of the puerperium the urine contains substantial amounts of sugar, which has no relationship to

diabetes but is due to the presence of lactose, milk sugar, which is absorbed from the mammary glands.

Intestinal elimination

The mother is nearly always constipated during the first few days of the puerperium. This is due to the relaxed condition of the intestinal and the abdominal muscles, in particular, and to the inability of the abdominal wall to aid in the evacuation of the intestinal contents. In addition, if hemorrhoids are present, the mother often is afraid to have a stool because of the discomfort these varicosities cause during elimination.

Skin

It is to be expected that elimination of waste products via the skin is accelerated in the early puerperium, often to such a degree that the mother is drenched with perspiration. These episodes of profuse sweating, which frequently occur in the night, gradually subside and do not require any specific treatment aside from protecting the mother from chilling at such times as they occur.

Menstruation

If the mother does not breast-feed her infant, the menstrual flow probably will return within eight weeks after delivery. Ordinarily, menstruation does not occur so long as the mother is breast-feeding, but this is not a certainty. During lactation the first menstrual period may occur as early as the second month but usually occurs about the fourth month following the delivery. It has been known not to reappear until as late as the eighteenth month. Studies have shown that failure to menstruate during lactation is due to suppression of ovulation, but, since some mothers have been known to become pregnant in the course of breast-feeding an infant, we know that this is not always the case.

Postpartal examinations

The condition of the mother is confirmed before she is discharged from the hospital to make sure that her progress has been satisfactory during the early puerperium. In addition to verifying her vital signs and present weight, observations are made to determine the condition of her breasts, the progress of involution and the healing of the perineal wound. A pelvic examination is deferred, since findings made by palpation of the uterus and inspection of the lochia will give satisfactory evidence as to the progress of involution at this time.

Follow-up examinations

As has been mentioned previously, the reproductive tract should return to its normal condition by the end of the puerperium. In order to investigate the general physical condition of the mother and determine with what normalcy she has completed her maternity experience, she should return to her physician for examination about six weeks postpartum. During the visit the weight and the blood pressure are taken, the urine is examined for albumin, and a blood count may be done. The condition of the abdominal walls is observed, and the breasts are inspected. If the mother is breast-feeding, the condition of the nipples and the degree of lacteal secretion are a significant part of the observation. If the mother is not breast-feeding, the breasts should be observed to see that physiologic readjustments have occurred. A thorough pelvic examination is carried out to investigate the position of the uterus, the healing of perineal wounds, the support of the pelvic floor, and whether involution is complete. In addition, this return examination provides an opportunity for the mother and the obstetrician to discuss any other problems relating to this maternity experience and to discuss methods of family planning (see Chapter 20). If abnormalities are found, they may be treated at this time and arrangements made for further examinations and treatments as necessary. Regardless, most physicians instruct their patients to return in six months for a check-up examination. Many encourage the mothers to return for a check-up again at the end of one year.

Suggested Reading

HELLMAN, L. H., AND PRITCHARD, J. A.: *Williams Obstetrics,* ed. 14. New York, Appleton-Century Crofts, 1970.
GREENHILL, J. P., AND FRIEDMAN, E. A.: *Biological Principles and Modern Practice of Obstetrics.* Philadelphia, W. B. Saunders, 1974.

nursing care during the puerperium

20

Changes and Reactions / Immediate Care / General and Special Physical Care Aspects / The Nursing Couple / Mechanisms in Lactation / Parental Guidance and Instruction

During the last two decades the constantly expanding dimensions of maternity nursing have redirected the emphasis and given new significance to what had become a rather routinized kind of care for the mother, as well as for those who provided the nursing care.

The newly delivered mother is usually a healthy patient who is adjusting physically and emotionally to the experiences of pregnancy and labor. However, in addition, a vastly important developmental phase begins for the mother, her newborn and her family. She must adapt to her infant, as well as to a new family structure.

In the context of total health care, on a continuum,

> Optimal maternal care can be defined as the accomplishment of those measures which are necessary to achieve a state of physical, mental and social well-being, and the maintenance of this state prior to planned conception, during pregnancy, and throughout the postpartal period, not just for the mother and child but for the whole family.[1]

Providing optimal maternal care requires a thoughtful approach to the many facets and factors responsible for high-level wellness of the maternity patient. Her needs for physical care have been greatly modified by the advent of early ambulation following delivery and the subsequent evolution of more simplified maternity nursing procedures. Newly delivered mothers need certain kinds of physical care; for example, in relation to evaluating the progressive changes which occur in the breasts for lactation, as well as the involutional changes of the internal reproductive organs to regain the normal nonpregnant condition. New mothers need nourishment, rest and sleep, and activity tempered with purposeful use of early ambulation.

Increased insight into the psychosocial needs of the newly delivered mother has resulted in greater attention to the emotional aspects of her care. This does not in any sense negate the need for physical care. As has been emphasized previously, the mother, the infant, the father and other children are considered as a family unit. In the hospital the same nurse may not necessarily have the responsibility for caring for the mother and her new baby at the same time (the baby might be cared for by nurses assigned primarily to the nursery). Nevertheless, the infant's care must be considered in relation to the mother's care, and their care in turn must be related to the total family constellation. A very important consideration is the need that the mother and her newly born infant have for each other; and in today's highly organized hospitals, such times do not always coincide with hospital policy or routine.

The simplification of certain aspects of physical care in no way diminishes the need for professional nursing care, for the astute nurse can use physical care activity as a valuable entree in developing a productive nurse-patient relationship. Moreover, she needs to use her observational and communicative skills continuously. The mother's physiologic functioning must be observed accurately, her dependency needs must be met, anticipatory guidance and health teachings must be given according to the mother's readiness to learn, and the developing relationship between the mother and infant should be appropriately observed, guided and nurtured. This may appear to be a gigantic challenge to the nurse. However, the shortened hospital stay for the mother who has had an uncomplicated delivery makes it all the more important to see that she receives the support and kind of teaching she requires concerning the care of her baby and herself, before being discharged to face her new responsibilities. Truly, this is a period when nursing assessment can be utilized most fruitfully.

High-level wellness might well be paraphrased: High-level wellness for the mother and her newly born infant is an integrated method of functioning (interacting) which is oriented toward maximizing the potential of the mother-infant relationship of which this mother-infant dyad is capable. This requires that the mother-infant adaptation be dynamic, but maintains a continuum of balance and purposeful direction within the environment (family) where they are functioning.

Changes and reactions during the puerperium

Immediately after labor, the mother usually experiences a sense of complete fatigue comparable to that which would normally follow any strenuous muscular activity. At the same time, if she has been awake during the delivery of her infant, she may be so exhilarated by the experience and the feeling of relief which accompanies it that she is not aware of being exhausted. She is interested in seeing and holding her baby and visiting with the father. Although this first visit of the family together may be rather brief, it is an experience which is particularly gratifying to the parents. Following this, every effort should be made to help the mother to rest, and with little encouragement she usually passes off into a sound natural sleep. The discomforts and activities which may interfere with sleep, such as soreness of the vulva, hemorrhoids, "afterpains," and frequent postpartal observations, should be expedited and/or mitigated as much as possible.

Many mothers complain of feeling chilled immediately after labor; some appear to have a shaking chill. Such chills may be due in part to nervous reaction and exhaustion. As stated previously, there is some disturbance of equilibrium between internal and external temperature caused by excessive perspiration during the muscular exertion of labor. Some authorities believe that the "chill" may be due partly to the sudden release of intraabdominal pressure which results as the uterus is emptied at delivery. This reaction may be alleviated if the mother is made comfortable in a warm bed and given a warm beverage when possible. If her body does begin to quiver, an extra cotton blanket should be placed over her or tucked close around her body for comfort. Many mothers (and their husbands) are frightened or disturbed by the chill; thus, reassurance by the nurse that this is not an unusual occurrence following delivery is extremely helpful.

Physiologic and psychologic changes

Specific anatomic and physiologic changes already have been discussed in Chapter 19. However, it is well to keep in mind that these alterations occur abruptly and are sizable. They involve profound diminution in circulating blood volume, a weight loss, displacement of internal organs, etc. It is truly marvelous that the new parturient copes so adequately, and that she complains so little.

The normal puerperal course follows a predictable healing and regenerative pattern, one that is not confined to the physical aspects of the patient. A new role must be assumed along with all of its concomitant tasks, new attitudes must be formed, and these adjustments must be undertaken before physical restoration is complete.

As with any regenerative process, energy is involved—energy that is needed to survive and to meet the everyday obligations of the mother's social and individual role. During the time that the mother coped with the increasing demands of labor there was a progressive withdrawal of social energy (i.e., a narrowing of attention and an inward turning). During the postpartal period the reverse process occurs: the mother is slowly able to extend the sphere of physical and psychic energy from herself to others in the immediate environment and then to events and persons outside her immediate environment.

PHASES OF THE RESTORATIVE PERIOD OF THE PUERPERIUM. *Taking-in Phase.* One author[2] has described certain phases that occur during the restorative period of the puerperium. The first of these seems to be a "taking-in" period (this lasts two or three days), in which the mother is passive and dependent. She tries to do what she is told, she gratefully accepts what she is given, and she initiates little or no action; rather she awaits the action of others. She seems to be grateful when decisions are made for her, and even simple decision-making as well as slight physical activity seems to fatigue her. It becomes apparent to the nurse that the needs she expresses are more in relation to herself than in relation to her baby.

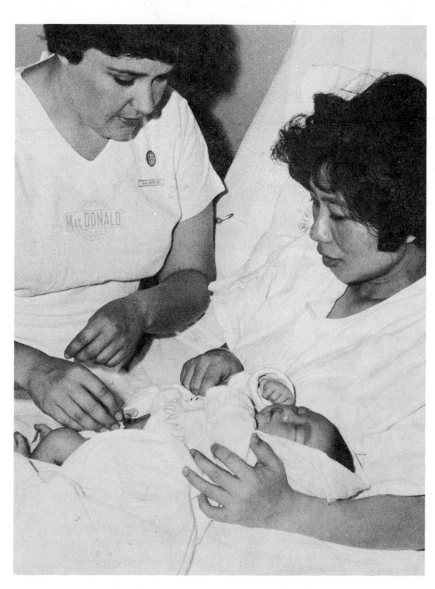

Figure 20-1. Mother observes umbilical cord stump of her newborn. (MacDonald House, The University Hospitals of Cleveland, Cleveland, Ohio)

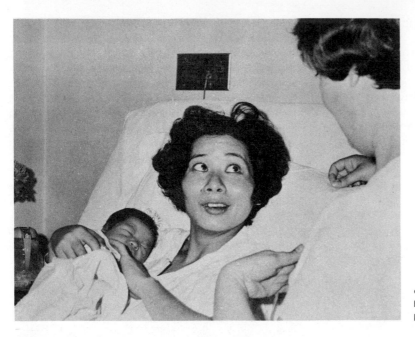

Figure 20-2. Mother learning ways to change her infant's position. (MacDonald House, The University Hospitals of Cleveland, Cleveland, Ohio)

The wise nurse attempts to meet these needs to the mother's satisfaction, thus enabling her to move on to the more complex tasks of mothering her baby (Figs. 20-1 to 20-3).

Sleep and food play an important part during this phase. The mother is far more able to begin the activities required of her if she is allowed to have a well-earned refreshing sleep. If this necessary rest is disrupted, the mother may experience a "sleep-hunger" which may last for several days; this results in irritability, fatigue and general interference with the normal restorative process. Thus, the necessity of appropriate intervention by the nurse to allow the mother to get adequate sleep cannot be stressed enough.

The nurse will note, also, that the mother usually has a good appetite and, in fact, may talk a good deal about food, about either the adequacy or the inadequacy of her meals. In-between nourishment is appreciated and needed (especially by nursing mothers). The concern about food seems to be a part of the mother's general need to be restored. Food, as we know, has tremendous psychologic significance in terms of care-asking and care-giving. The nurse should be especially cognizant of the mother's need for hearty meals and should expedite extra nourishment whenever possible. Moreover, she will want to be aware that a poor appetite often is one of the first symptoms that all is not proceeding normally in the puerperal period.

Psychologic Adjustment. During the "taking-in" phase the mother begins to relive the delivery experience in order to integrate it fully with reality. She is apt to be very talkative at this time, and she may want to know certain specifics and details so that she can form a total picture of what "really happened" during delivery. As she obtains this information, she is able to realize more fully that the pregnancy and the delivery are truly over, and that her baby now is born and is an individual outside of and separate from herself. This is a considerable task and involves rather profound changes in attitudes and feelings. The symbiotic relationship between mother and infant during pregnancy is at an end, and the mother now must identify her child as a separate individual.

Taking-hold Phase. The second phase in the puerperal period has been described as a "taking-hold" phase; that is, the mother strives for independence and autonomy and finally begins to be the initiator. One of her main concerns at this point seems to be her ability to control her bodily functions; her bowels and bladder must perform well, and she takes an active part in seeing that they do. If she is nursing her infant, she is concerned about producing an acceptable quantity and quality of milk. She often will ask the nurses and the doctors anxiously (referring to the milk), "Has it come in yet?" And later she wants to know: "Do you think I have enough?" She cannot have enough explanation and reassurance that she is "performing" well at this time. She wants to walk, to sit, to move as she did before delivery and is very anxious and impatient if she cannot make her body behave as it once did. It is as though she is thinking, "How can I possibly assume all my responsibilities for others if I cannot control my own body?"

Her first mothering tasks are especially important to her, and "failures" (inability to elicit a bubble from her infant, poor sucking response on the part of the baby, her awkwardness in handling her child), no matter how small and expected (by the staff), can send her to the depths of despair. Even the skillful intervention of the nurse seems only to point up her "inadequacy" as a mother. She often will voice her feelings with an "Oh, I'll never be able to bathe her as easily as you do." Or another mother may say: "He always seems to take his milk better when *you* feed him." Conversely, when she succeeds at a task, her delight and relief are wonderful to behold. It is

difficult to imagine (for anyone other than a new mother) how thrilling a hearty bubble from a small infant can be.

Since there is a good deal of anxiety as well as activity in this phase, fatigue and exhaustion may occur if the mother is not helped to set realistic expectations and limits for herself. Since this "taking-hold" phase lasts about ten days, much of it will take place at home.

The nurse can be invaluable in giving the mother, as she appears able and ready to accept it, anticipatory guidance about what to expect and how to manage. During the hospital stay the mother profits greatly from reassurance and explanation regarding the various processes and hour-by-hour events. She finds guidance and reinforcement of appropriate behavior particularly helpful when she attempts to perform her mothering tasks.

When assisting the mother, the nurse must be careful not to impose herself between the mother and her baby (no matter how awkward or maladroit the mother seems). Rather,

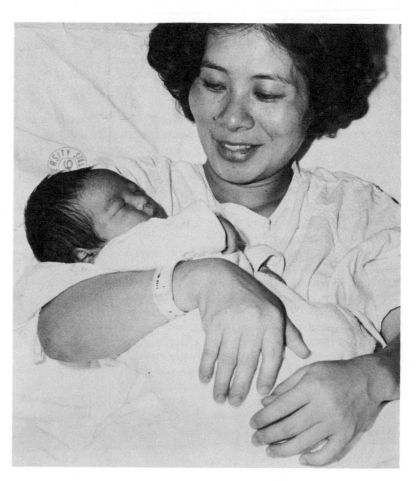

Figure 20-3. Mother enfolds her newborn. (MacDonald House, The University Hospitals of Cleveland, Cleveland, Ohio)

the nurse should allow the mother to perform the actual task (after necessary demonstration or instruction) and then encourage or reinforce whatever behavior was appropriate. In this way she demonstrates that she has confidence in the mother's ability to cope with new tasks. In order to gain skill and confidence in her mothering ability, the mother needs the opportunity to make decisions about the baby's needs as well as guidance regarding his physical care. When she is allowed to find answers to her questions (again with guidance as necessary) and is reassured that her judgment is correct, she is able to feel confident in her ability to perceive needs accurately and to make decisions. Thus, she is better able to meet problems in the future. (See Suggested Reading for a more thorough discussion of changes and behavior during the puerperium.)

POSTPARTAL BLUES. Sometime during the puerperium, for no apparent reason, the mother quite suddenly may experience a "let-down" feeling. She may become irritable and tearful, may even lose her appetite and find it difficult to sleep. These are the usual manifestations of the so-called "postpartal blues"; they usually are very temporary and may occur while the mother is in the hospital or after her discharge. This temporary depression is thought to be related to the hormonal changes that occur during this time and the ego regression that can accompany the increased dependency needs and responsibilities. Discomfort, fatigue and exhaustion certainly contribute to this condition, if they do not actually precipitate it. The mother may release tension by crying and thus become more comfortable. However, since she usually does not know exactly why she is crying, she may feel guilty about this somewhat unaccustomed emotional display.

The nurse can help the mother most effectively if she is able to recognize and to interpret the mother's behavior and, in turn, is kind and understanding. If the mother does want to cry, her privacy should be respected, and she should be assured that this behavior is not only acceptable but therapeutic. Accurate reporting and recording of the mother's emotional state is important at all times. Occasionally a more serious and pathologic psychologic upheaval occurs, and the prodromal signs may become apparent during the hospital stay (see Chapter 26).

SUMMARY. It is well to keep in mind during the early days of the puerperium that although the mother appears to recover with amazing rapidity after the delivery, she is still going through a period of transition. Therefore, she is more vulnerable to stress at this time. Problems that she might otherwise handle with relative ease may stimulate emotionally charged situations as she faces the increased responsibilities for the nurturing and the care of her new baby, family and home. At the same time, the mother's own need for affection and attention may bring about feelings of jealousy and guilt when the major attention more often than not is directed to the infant. Therefore, care should be focused on providing physical rest for the mother as well as an environment that is as free from tension and worry as possible. In addition, the mother should be given as much help as she needs to gain self-confidence in caring for her baby and perceiving his needs. This will mean that the old cliché "routine postpartum care" is not to be taken literally. Nursing care during the puerperium, as during any other period of the childbearing cycle, must be "tailored" to meet the needs of each individual patient.

Immediate care

Intelligent interpretation of the patient's physiologic and behavioral responses is essential to the mother's safety and welfare. Paramount among the physiologic responses is the condition of the uterus. The mother must be observed carefully for bleeding during the first eight hours after labor and particularly during the first hour after delivery.

Considerable information can be gained by palpating the fundus through the abdominal wall to be assured that the uterus remains firm, round and well contracted. At the same time it is also important to inspect the perineal pad for obvious signs of bleeding, as well as to take the pulse and the blood pressure. During the first hour these observations should be made at least every 15 minutes, or more often if indicated. As long as the bleeding is minimal, and the uterus remains firm, well contracted and does not increase in size, it is neither necessary nor desirable to stimulate it. However, if the uterus becomes soft and boggy because of relaxation, the fundus should be massaged immediately until it becomes contracted again. This can be best accomplished if one hand is placed just above the symphysis pubis to act as a guard, as the other hand is

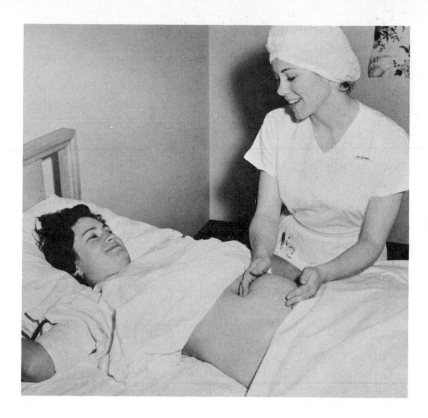

Figure 20-4. Nurse palpating fundus.

cupped around the fundus and rotated gently. It should be remembered that the uterus is a sensitive organ which, under normal circumstances, responds quickly to tactile stimulation. Care must be taken to avoid overmassage, because, in addition to causing the mother considerable pain, this may stimulate premature uterine contractions and thereby cause undue muscle fatigue. Such a condition would further encourage uterine relaxation and hemorrhage. If the uterus is atonic, blood which collects in the cavity should be expressed with firm but gentle force in the direction of the outlet, but only after the fundus has been first massaged (Fig. 20-4). Failure to see that the uterus is contracted before pushing downward against it could result in inversion of the uterus, an exceedingly serious complication.

During the first hour the mother is kept clean, dry and comfortable but allowed to rest as much as possible. At the end of this hour it is usually customary to give the mother a partial bath as necessary and take the temperature, in addition to other vital signs, before transferring her to the postpartal division. The nurse must be constantly alert for any changes in the mother's condition, such as color, character of the pulse, respiration and blood pressure, the status of the fundus and the amount of vaginal bleeding.

General physical care

The daily routine procedures for the postpartal patient vary in different hospitals, but the principles of care are essentially the same. Certain observations should be made and recorded daily. These would include such findings as temperature, pulse and respiration; urinary and intestinal elimination; the physical changes which occur normally in the puerperium. One should note the changes in the breasts, the height and consistency of the fundus, the character, the amount and the color of the lochial discharge and the condition of the episiotomy. Furthermore, it is equally important for the nurse to be alert to the mother's general comfort and well-being—how she rests and sleeps, her activity, her appetite, her emotional status and, particularly, because of its vast influence, how she is adjusting to her role as a new mother.

Temperature, pulse and respiration

The temperature is carefully watched during the first two weeks of the puerperium, as fever is usually the first symptom of an infectious process. And, as has been stated previously, the pulse rate provides a helpful guide in determining the significance of a rise in temperature. These observations are usually made and recorded every four hours for the first few days after delivery, omitting the 2 A.M. observations, which would disturb the mother's sleep. Thereafter, they are made every night and morning, as long as the mother is progressing normally. If the temperature rises above 37.8° C. (100° F.) or the pulse rate above 100, the physician should be notified immediately. Usually, the blood pressure is not checked regularly unless there has been some abnormality. Then observations and recordings are made every two to four hours or more frequently, as indicated.

Nutrition

Very shortly following the delivery, after having gone without food or fluids for some hours, the mother may express a desire for something to eat. Unless she has received a general anesthetic or is nauseated, there is usually no contraindication to giving her some nourishment. She usually enjoys a normal diet.

The two factors which the nurse must bear in mind when considering the mother's diet are: 1) providing for her general nutrition and 2) providing enough nourishing foods to supply the additional calories and nutrients required during lactation. If these nutritional requirements are provided for, the mother's convalescence will be more rapid, her strength will be recovered more quickly, and the quality and quantity of her milk will be better. She will also be more able to resist infections.

Mothers in general, and particularly mothers who are breast-feeding, usually have good appetites and become hungry between meals. For this reason it is advisable to see that they receive intermediate nourishment consisting of a nourishing beverage or a snack three times a day. If the nourishment is in the form of a glass of milk or some milk product, this helps to incorporate the additional milk requirement for the nursing mother.

Rest and sleep

During the puerperium the mother needs an abundance of rest and can be encouraged to relax and sleep whenever possible. This can best be accomplished if she is comfortable and free from worry and other anxiety-producing situations. The need for rest has even more significance for the mother who is breast-feeding, because worry and fatigue inhibit her milk supply. With the exception of the father, visitors can be limited during the first week or so because they can be tiring. A mother who is not getting sufficient rest is usually anxious, and worries over minor things that otherwise might cause her little concern. Furthermore, many emotional problems are often precipitated by sleeplessness and fatigue.

It becomes the nurse's responsibility to adjust the hospital routine whenever possible to provide the mother with uninterrupted periods of rest. Routine procedures can be delayed or rearranged to meet the mother's needs. A bottle-fed infant may be fed occasionally by the nurse if the mother is sleeping and does not want to be awakened. If the mother is unable to nap during the day (and she may not, due to excitement and fatigue), she can be encouraged to rest as quietly as possible for certain continuous periods. The need for rest and sleep may have to be explained and reiterated to her, especially during the "taking-hold" phase, as she is eager to be up and about and may tend to overdo.

Early ambulation

Although early ambulation of the so-called "normal" mother had its inception out of necessity during World War II, experience with this aspect of management of the puerperium has shown that it possesses certain intrinsic advantages to the mother, and as a result it is almost generally accepted today. With this increase in exercise for the newly delivered mother, her circulation is stimulated, and there are fewer complications of thrombophlebitis. Moreover, bladder and bowel functions are improved, with the result that bladder complications leading to catheterization are greatly reduced. Abdominal distention and constipation occur less frequently. The majority of healthy mothers are allowed out of bed in four to eight hours.

If the patient has had a conduction anesthesia which involves entering the dura, she may be kept in a recumbent position for about the first eight hours. It is felt by many physicians that keeping the patient flat in bed for this time helps to prevent the occurrence of a postspinal headache, since headache is precipitated and aggravated when the head is elevated. Postspinal headache is thought to be due to a leakage of the spinal fluid through the puncture hole of the dura, with subsequent decrease in cerebrospinal fluid volume and pressure. Therefore, the use of a small gauge needle for making the puncture, a recumbent position while the puncture hole is sealing, and encouraging the patient to force fluids (to hasten fluid replacement) are all measures which may be helpful in the prevention of this condition.

The first time that any mother is out of bed she can "dangle" for a short time before actually getting up. Then usually she can walk a few steps from the bed and sit in a chair for a brief period. On succeeding times up, she can increase her activity gradually. The newly delivered mother needs someone to assist her in and out of bed and to go with her when she walks to the bathroom. The nurse will want to remain close at hand while the mother is in the bathroom so that she can give immediate assistance if the mother becomes weak or faint.

It is important that the nurse explain the purposes of early ambulation to the mother and help her to learn how she can achieve an effective combination of sitting, walking and lying in bed. All too many mothers feel that once they are out of bed they are "on their own" and expected to take care of themselves entirely. Most of them are afraid of being a nuisance and hesitate to ask for help, whereas others do not realize that help is available. The nurse's attitude is important, for if she acts interested in the mother, demonstrates a desire to help her and makes her feel comfortable, the mother is more likely to ask for help. New mothers, in particular, are sensitive to the attitudes of those responsible for their care. Many of them are experiencing an enforced dependency for the first time in their adult lives and find this difficult. Others become resentful because they feel that they are being forced toward independence too quickly. It is only as the nurse recognizes each patient as an individual that she is able to gain insight in providing for the mother's total nursing needs.

Although it is customary for mothers to be discharged home on the second or third day, it should be remembered that early ambulation and the duration of hospital stay are two entirely different matters. Regardless of the day of discharge, mothers need to be cautioned to proceed slowly at home during the puerperium, resting a large part of the time. If teaching about "getting back to routine gradually" was begun early in the antepartal period, the mother will be better prepared.

Bathing

As previously mentioned, the mother is prone to have marked diaphoresis in the early puerperium, so that she will find the daily bath or shower refreshing and a source of comfort. When the mother showers for the first time, the nurse usually will give the self-care instructions regarding breast care, perineal care and other aspects of physical care. The nurse will be guided by the mother's readiness to learn and she will remember that the mother can absorb only so much information at one time. Subsequently whenever the mother is able to absorb the information, the nurse can explain to the mother about breast care, perineal hygiene, elimination, general activity and hospital routines.

Showers usually are permitted as soon as the patient becomes ambulatory, if such facilities are available. The first time or two that the mother takes a shower, the nurse or the attendant should remain nearby for safety. It is particularly important that a patient who has had a cesarean section be instructed regarding her bathing. Usually, these patients are not allowed to shower even though they are ambulatory, since the incision should be kept dry until it has closed, and/or the sutures have been removed.

Tub baths usually are allowed in two weeks, and some physicians permit tub bathing earlier.

Urinary elimination

The newly delivered mother may not express a desire to void, in part because the bladder capacity is increased as a result of reduced interabdominal pressure. In addition, if the mother has received analgesia or anesthesia during labor, the sensation of a full bladder may be further diminished. The mother should be encouraged to void within the first six to eight hours following the delivery. It is not prudent, however, to adhere to a designated lapse of time to indicate when the mother should empty her bladder, but rather on evidence indicating the degree of bladder distention. It is well to keep in mind that there is an increased urinary output during the early puerperium. Moreover, mothers who have received intravenous fluids, or who are having them, are very likely to develop a full bladder. As the bladder fills with urine, it gradually protrudes above the symphysis pubis and can be observed bulging in front of the uterus. If the bladder is markedly distended, the uterus may be pushed upward and to the side and may be somewhat relaxed. When a hand is cupped over the fundus to massage it and to bring the uterus back to its midline position, the bladder will protrude still further. When the hand is removed, the uterus will return to its displaced position. Further evidence of bladder distention can be gained by palpation and percussion of the lower abdomen, which will reveal a difference in consistency between the uterus and the bladder. The latter will be ballotable and filled with liquid in contrast with the uterus, which will have a firm tone. Such observations are of extreme importance and demand immediate attention. A full bladder is considered to be one of the causes of postpartal hemorrhage, and if the bladder is permitted to become distended, urinary retention will inevitably follow.

Some mothers have difficulty in voiding at first. As a result of the labor itself, the tone of the bladder wall may be temporarily impaired, or the tissues at the base of the bladder and around the urethra may be edematous. When the mother is allowed early bathroom privileges, urinary elimination may present no problem. On the other hand, some efforts may be needed to excite normal urination. First of all, a positive approach, asking the mother, "Will you try..." rather than "Do you feel as if you want to..." is often helpful to get the mother to void. Running water so that the mother can hear it, letting the mother dabble her fingers in water or offering a beverage (preferably warm) are other helps to initiate voiding.

If the mother must be on bedrest, the nurse can assist the mother to void by helping her assume a comfortable position, providing privacy and giving her assurance that she will soon be able to urinate. The nurse will want to offer the mother a bedpan at intervals of two to three hours at first and measure the urine at each voiding during the first day (or days) until it has been established that the mother is emptying her bladder completely. A voiding must measure 100 ml. to be considered satisfactory. At the first voiding, it may be apparent that the bladder has not been entirely emptied. If the bladder is not distended, the mother may be allowed to wait for an hour or so, as the second voiding usually empties the bladder. If, however, the mother continues to void small amounts frequently, one may suspect that she has residual urine, and these voidings are the result of the overflow of a distended bladder. If all attempts fail and the mother cannot void a sufficient quantity, catheterization will be necessary. It is very important to avoid this procedure because of the risk of hospital-induced infection. If, however, the mother is absolutely unable to void, despite astute and persistent nursing intervention, the patient will have to be catheterized.

CATHETERIZATION. Although the procedure for catheterization varies to some degree in different hospitals, the principles involved are essentially the same. Aseptic technique must be maintained throughout to avoid introducing bacteria into the bladder or contaminating the birth canal. If the mother is given routine perineal care prior to beginning the catheterization procedure, the potential danger of infection is further reduced.

Because there is a certain amount of soreness of the external genitalia, the nurse will proceed with extreme gentleness and convey to the mother that she is aware of the additional tenderness. As the labia are separated to expose the vestibule, care should be exercised to prevent pulling on the perineal sutures. The nurse will find that the meatus may be difficult to locate due to the edema and consequent distortion of the tissues; therefore a good light is imperative.

The urinary meatus and surrounding area are cleansed prior to the insertion of the catheter; the nurse proceeds gently, but remembers all the while that a certain degree of friction is necessary for proper cleansing of the area. None of the cleansing solution is permitted to run into the vaginal orifice because of the danger of contaminating the birth canal. Immediately following the cleansing, a dry cotton ball can be placed at the introitus to prevent excretion from the vagina (i.e., blood or lochia) from spreading upward to the urinary meatus, from whence it can be carried into the bladder when the catheter is inserted.

Intestinal elimination

Because the bowel tends to remain relaxed in the early puerperium (as in pregnancy), intestinal elimination may be somewhat of a problem. In view of the sluggishness of the bowels during this time, constipation can be anticipated unless certain measures are instituted to prevent it. Although obstetricians' orders vary, it is common to give a stool softener each night after delivery and/or a laxative or mild cathartic on the evening of the second day following delivery. If a bowel evacuation has not occurred by the morning of the third day, a cleansing enema or a suppository may be prescribed. The latter is very effective and less traumatic for most patients.

If there has been no elimination and especially if the mother has had more extensive perineal repair done, an oil retention enema, followed some hours later by a cleansing enema, sometimes is ordered.

The mother who is breast-feeding will be advised to follow her physician's prescription if laxatives are required to encourage proper elimination after she is discharged from the hospital. Certain laxatives are excreted in breast milk and therefore affect the infant. In addition, the usual measures employed to encourage good bowel habits (i.e., adequate fluid intake, roughage foods in the diet, establishing a habit time, and so on) are to be included in the health teaching.

Special physical care aspects

Throughout the care of the maternity patient, emphasis has been directed to the prevention of infection by application of principles of antiseptic and aseptic techniques. In view of this, the special procedures employed in the care of the mother during the puerperium can be planned so that individual care techniques can be maintained whenever possible. Disposable equipment for such purposes is safe, it utilizes simplified procedures, and it is economical.

Each mother should have her own supplies and equipment kept in a designated place, for her convenience. This is facilitated in hospitals where the physical plan of the postpartal unit provides a bathroom adjoining each room, in which separate shelves are provided for each mother's equipment and supplies. Such practices are important in the overall effort to prevent cross contamination.

Breast care

The care of the breasts during pregnancy has been discussed in Chapter 12. Although some aspects differ after the delivery, depending on whether or not the mother is breast-feeding, the principles of good breast hygiene continue to be of primary importance.

The routine care is directed to maintaining cleanliness and adequate breast support necessary for the normal function of the breasts and the comfort of the mother. Precautions are to be exercised to handle the breasts gently, and above all to avoid rough rubbing, massage or pressure on these organs.

The mother who is bottle-feeding her infant can bathe her breasts daily with mild soap and water; this is done most conveniently at the time of the daily shower or bath. No other special care need be given.

If the mother is breast-feeding, her nipples may be cleansed with clear water if cleansing is thought necessary. It is also recommended that soap not be used on the nipples; even the use of water is unnecessary under most circumstances since the nipple skin itself is cleansed by the natural antiseptic, lysozyme. It is important to instruct the mother not to use any drying agent (such as alcohol, etc.) on her nipples since it tends to remove the secretions of sebum, a physiologic emollient. Under normal circumstances, the best nipple care is provided by the body itself, without outside interference.[3] Additional cleansing before each nursing need not be done but the mother is to be instructed to wash her hands with soap and water, as they will come in contact with the nipples and breast during nursing. In this way precautions can be taken against infection.

The mother can be encouraged to wear a well-fitting supportive nursing brassiere as soon as her milk begins to come (in about the second to fourth day but sometimes earlier). It is wise that she become accustomed to lowering the flaps of the bra occasionally during the day for 15 to 30 minutes to permit air to come in contact with the nipples. The brassiere should not have plastic liners in the cup to occlude air from the nipples. If there is leaking of milk, the mother may use disposable breast pads and change them every time they become damp. This will promote the integrity of the nipples and inhibit infection since milk is a perfect media for many bacteria.

Mothers who are not breast-feeding will also need breast support, and a well-fitting brassiere is appropriate for them also. Usually these mothers will be given some type of lactation-suppressing hormone to help them dry up, and engorgement is not a problem. Occasionally, however, they do suffer this phenomenon and they may experience throbbing pains in the breasts which extend back into the axillae. During this time, analgesic medication may be required for pain relief until the condition subsides in one or two days. Ice bags to the breasts and axillae also are often helpful.

Lactation

The process of lactation is thought to be initiated by the sudden change in the proportion of estrogen and progesterone in the mother's blood level following delivery of the placenta. Thus, placental expulsion is said to stimulate the release of *prolactin*, the lactogenic hormone, from the anterior pituitary. After the infant is put to breast, the stimulation of the nipples by the infant's sucking aids the further release of prolactin. Prolactin, in turn, stimulates milk secretion in the alveoli. The regular, periodic emptying of the milk from the alveoli by the infant's sucking stimulates the continuation of the process of lactation. When the infant is not put to breast, or the sucking stimulus is suddenly interrupted, suppression of lactation is initiated and the breasts become engorged with milk, and very painful.

SUPPRESSION OF LACTATION. The breasts fill with milk initially, unless lactation is suppressed, whether or not the mother nurses her infant. Tenseness and engorgement result as milk fills the breasts. Since the accumulation of milk in the breast inhibits further secretion, engorgement generally subsides in a day or two. However, until the breasts soften the mother may experience considerable discomfort.

In the event that the mother is not going to breast-feed, the physician will prescribe accordingly. Many physicians use estrogenic hormones to suppress the production of the lactogenic hormone. Diethylstilbestrol, an estrogenic hormone, is one of the drugs in use today for this purpose. It usually is given orally during the early postpartal period and is decreased gradually.

Lactation is not always effectively suppressed by the administration of hormones, and there may be a mild transient filling or engorgement either a few days after delivery or later, in one or two weeks. This soon disappears spontaneously. It is important for the nurse to remember that side effects sometimes accompany the administration of hormones. For instance, the androgens have the potential for retarding the onset of menstruation. Uterine bleeding may follow a prolonged course of estrogen therapy. The nurse will observe that after a course of stilbestrol the lochial discharge is heavier and contains a greater proportion of bright red blood.

A combination of hormones such as estrogens and androgens has been widely used to suppress lactation (it suppresses the release of prolactin), prevent engorgement, and reduce the tenderness of the breasts. In addition, these hormones in combination counteract the undesirable side effects of each other. Deladumone-OB is an example of a long-acting estrogen-androgen combination and is given intramuscularly; one injection is all that is necessary. To achieve maximum effectiveness, the antilactogenic hormones must be given immediately after (or just prior to) delivery, since the anterior pituitary begins production of the lactogenic hormone immediately.

If hormones are not used, the breasts usually become engorged two to three days after delivery, and the tenseness and discomfort last from 24 to 48 hours. Since the breasts are not emptied, the accumulated milk suppresses further secretion of milk. As secretion subsides, engorgement wanes, and the breasts become more comfortable.

During the period of engorgement, discomfort may be considerable, and the mother needs to receive as much symptomatic relief as possible. A well-fitting uplift brassiere relieves discomfort from the weight of the breasts and wearing it before the milk "comes in" is helpful. The nurse must remember that the milk is not to be pumped or expressed from the breasts, since this only stimulates the secretion of more milk. In the past it was thought that the application of very tight binders, restriction of fluids and the administration of diuretics all suppressed lactation; these practices are no longer in general use and have been found to be of little value (see Suggested Reading).

Care of the perineum

Perineal care is a procedure employed to cleanse the vulva, the perineum and the anal region as a means of preventing infection, promoting healing of the perineum and making the mother comfortable. In addition, it provides an opportunity for the nurse to inspect the area and the lochial discharge. Regardless of whether or not an episiotomy has been performed, perineal care is to be done as a routine part of morning care, each time that the mother voids, and after each bowel evacuation. The nurse usually attends to this aspect of care until the mother becomes ambulatory; then, after proper instruction, the mother herself may assume this care. However, it should be emphasized that even though the nurse may not be performing the actual procedure, she is to make a point of inspecting the perineum daily, preferably in the morning, to ascertain whether the stitches are healing properly and to check the character and the amount of lochia. If the mother is allowed to shower, these observations should be made first so that the nurse can observe the lochial discharge more accurately.

There has been much discussion concerning the "best way" for the nurse to give perineal care in the time immediately following delivery. The technique for individual care has simplified the procedure to a large measure, but procedures will vary according to hospital routines. Most hospitals maintain that this is a "clean" procedure rather than a sterile one, and that the safety of the mother is ensured if antiseptic precautions are adhered to conscientiously.

Disposable washcloths, cotton balls or gauze sponges may be used for cleansing. When the pubic hair begins to appear, cotton balls tend to catch on the stubble, and particles of cotton remain unless they are picked off. Another variation found is in relation to the cleansing agent, which might be a mild soap or detergent solution.

In preparation for the procedure, the nurse washes her hands thoroughly. After preparing the mother, remove the perineal pad, noting the amount, the odor and the appearance of the lochia, and discard the pad in a paper bag. In both removing the perineal pad and using the sponges or washcloths in the actual cleansing process, always proceed from the front toward the back to avoid contamination of the vestibule from the anal region.

The labia are cleansed first, working from the pubis to the perineum, taking care not to separate the labia with the fingers. The cleansing is done by using a single downward stroke with each sponge, which then is discarded in the paper bag. This cleansing is repeated with as many sponges as necessary. The area then is dried in the same manner.

The cleansing of the anal region can be accomplished most effectively if the mother turns on her side and the buttocks are separated before wiping from the perineum to the anus. If the mother's thighs or buttocks are soiled with profuse lochia, these areas can be bathed with soap and water, for these parts do not have to be cleansed in the same manner as the vulva.

When disposable washcloths are used, the first cloth is soaped and the labia washed down on one side to the perineum and then on the other side. Then the anus is washed last, and the soaped washcloth is discarded. The area is rinsed in the same manner with a second washcloth and dried with a third one. The perineum should be kept clean and dry to promote healing.

The nurse must be mindful of the potential danger of infection if pathogenic organisms ascend the birth canal to the uterus. Care is always exercised to see that none of the cleansing solution seeps into the vagina because of the possibility of contamination. If the washcloths or moist sponges are used, they are not to be dripping wet.

The clean perineal pad is grasped on the outside so that the nurse's fingers do not touch the side which will come in contact with the perineum. Then the pad is applied to the vulva (front to back) and secured to the sanitary belt in front before turning the mother to her side to secure the back tab.

PERINEAL SELF-CARE. The first time the mother is allowed up to the bathroom, the nurse should take her and show her where her equipment is kept and how to do perineal self-care. The principles of personal hygiene which were stressed when the nurse gave the mother perineal care in bed can be reviewed again. Instruct the mother to wash her hands carefully before and after carrying out the procedure. Show her how to assemble the necessary equipment, the paper bag, box of small cleansing tissues and wrapped perineal pad, all of which can be placed on a small stool or table adjacent to the toilet. A box of small cleansing tissues is preferable to a roll of tissue for obvious reasons. Have the mother unfasten the perineal pad she is wearing, and instruct her to grasp it by the tabs and remove it from front to back. This perineal pad is placed in the paper bag, which will be disposed of in a step-on can or other covered waste receptacle. After the mother voids, instruct her to cleanse herself from front to back with tissues, using fresh tissues for each stroke and discarding them in the toilet. The mother can again be instructed how to handle the clean perineal pad so that the inner surface is not contaminated by her fingers, and to put it on from front to back. It should be fastened imme-

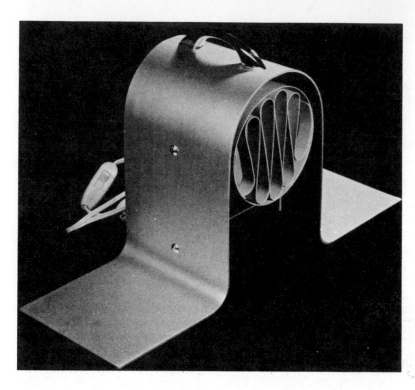

Figure 20-5. Perineal heat lamp. (Dann Manufacturing Company, Cleveland, Ohio)

diately to prevent the pad from moving forward. The toilet is flushed after the mother assumes a standing position to avoid having any of the flushing water spray the perineum.

PERINEAL DISCOMFORT. Following a spontaneous vaginal delivery without laceration, mothers usually do not experience perineal discomfort. It is most likely to be present if an episiotomy has been performed, or if lacerations have been repaired, particularly if the perineum is edematous, and there is tension on the perineal sutures. Almost all primigravidas experience some degree of discomfort from an episiotomy, depending largely on the extent of the wound and the amount of suturing done. For the most part during the first few days, local treatment in the form of dry heat, analgesic sprays or ointments is all that is necessary to alleviate the discomfort. But if the pain is more severe in the first day or so, such treatment may not be sufficient, and analgesic medications may have to be administered by mouth or hypodermic injection. Later on, sitz baths may be ordered if the discomfort persists.

Exposure of the perineum to heat from the perineal lamp not only provides a considerable measure of comfort to the mother but also supplies a safe amount of heat to promote local healing of the perineal wound. The physician may prescribe such treatment for 20- to 25-minute periods, two or three times a day. If a lamp such as the one shown in Figure 20-5 is used, the mother can recline in bed with the lamp between her knees during the treatment, without spreading the thighs too far apart. This lamp is so constructed that the frame can be completely covered with a pillowcase. The excess cover is brought forward over the arch of the frame and tucked securely between it and the shield which is around the bulb. The heat is provided by an ordinary 25-watt light bulb. When the mother has assumed the dorsal recumbent position, the lamp can be easily slipped between her legs and placed about 10 to 12 inches from the perineum. After the perineum is exposed, the bulb is adjusted so that the light shines directly on it. The mother can be completely covered during the treatment, because the arch of the lamp frame acts as a cradle to support the top bedclothes.

Mothers who have discomfort from perineal sutures usually will find it uncomfortable to sit for the first few days. Many of them will be observed sitting in a rigid position, bearing their weight on one side of the buttocks or the other, with obvious discomfort to the back as well as the perineum. Therefore, it is important to teach the mother how to sit comfortably with her body erect. In the sitting position, the perineum is suspended at the lowermost level of the ischial tuberosities, which bear the weight of the body. Thus, in order to achieve a greater measure of comfort, the mother must bring her buttocks together to relieve pressure and tension on the perineum, in the same manner as that described in the exercise for contraction and relaxation of pelvic floor muscles. After assuming a sitting position the mother is instructed to raise her hips very slightly from the chair, only enough to permit her to squeeze her buttocks together and contract the muscles of the pelvic floor, and hold them this way momentarily until after she has let her full weight down again. This exercise will also prove to be helpful to the mother when she is reclining in bed.

The nursing couple

Making the decision

The type of infant feeding is an important decision for the parents to make. Their ultimate choice will be influenced by a variety of factors, physical and psychologic as well as social. Ideally, the subject of the method of infant feeding will be raised during the antepartal period, and the parents will have time and guidance from the doctor and the nurse in making a decision that is most suitable for them.

It is no longer essential that the mother breast-feed her infant to ensure his survival or well-being. The development of modern methods of artificial feeding adequately meet the infant's needs for nutrition and growth. However, breast-feeding has several advantages. Particularly important is the fact that if the mother wants to nurse her infant, this method of feeding can enhance a close relationship between her and her baby.

A variety of factors will influence the couple's decision to breast-feed the infant. The term *couple* is used here deliberately, since the husband's attitudes, feelings and behavior may be as important in terms of decision-making as the mother's. Moreover, they usually have a profound influence on the outcome of the nursing experience. It is wise for the physician and the nurse to explore adequately with the mother (and the father, if necessary) their mutual attitudes, since they are so relevant.

The nurse will note that there seems to be a wide range of commitment to breast-feeding. For instance, some mothers are very eager to nurse their infants; others want to breast-feed but do not feel bad (or "inadequate") if for some reason they cannot. Others try to nurse in spite of the fact that they would prefer to give the baby a bottle; still others flatly refuse to attempt to nurse. Some mothers feel that breast-feeding is too tiring, confining or simply repulsive; many are afraid that it will disfigure their breasts. The mores and pressure of the mother's class and peer group also are important. Bottle-feeding may be the acceptable practice in the community or neighborhood; relatives, friends, and so on, may be either very much for or against breast-feeding. Return to employment for the mother may be a very significant factor.

Certain conditions in both the mother and the infant also can have a bearing on the decision and outcome. The mother's physical condition is particularly important. Diseases and infection (i.e., syphilis, tuberculosis, heart and kidney disease, staphylococcal infections, communicable diseases) generally are contraindications for breast-feeding. Similarly, certain infections and anomalies in the infant may make nursing impossible, or at least temporarily impossible (see Chapter 29). Breast infection or painful, cracked or fissured nipples also may require temporary discontinuance of nursing. Pregnancy usually is considered to be an indication for weaning because of the physiologic strain that it places on the mother.

The attitudes of the physician and nurse influence the couple a good deal; so do the amount and the kind of help that the mother gets in the hospital when she is first attempting to nurse. The willingness on the part of the staff to impart information and to give assistance helps the parents immensely, especially if they have little information about the process or are actually misinformed about it. However, it is unwise to try to persuade a mother to nurse if she has very negative feelings about breast-feeding. This situation often leads to emotional conflicts in the mother and may impede the adjustment between mother and infant.

Mechanisms in lactation

The anatomy of the breasts and the physiology of lactation have been discussed in Chapters 5 and 19, to which the student is referred for a renewal of background understanding of the subject.

SECRETION OF MILK. Two major mechanisms are involved in lactation. The first of these is the secretion of milk. It is believed, as was previously stated, that the hormone luteotrophin (prolactin, LTH, the lactogenic or mammogenic hormone) is responsible for the initiation of lactation. It is thought that the release of this hormone is enhanced by the sucking of the infant. The milk itself is secreted by the alveoli or acini cells. This secretion commences three to four days postpartum and continues for as long as the breasts are sufficiently emptied. Frequency of emptying the breasts also is a very important factor, especially when lactation is becoming established. Thus, both the production of milk and the quantity produced are dependent on *frequent* and *complete* emptying of the breasts. The nurse will recall that if the breasts are not entirely emptied, and the back pressure in the alveoli is not relieved, milk secretion decreases and eventually stops.

When lactation is becoming established, milk secretion can be stimulated by having the infant nurse both breasts at each feeding and by increasing the frequency of the feedings. Care should be taken not to tire the mother unduly. Milk production is slow in some mothers, but it can be stimulated by allowing the infant to nurse both breasts every two to three hours.

MILK-EJECTION REFLEX. This is the second mechanism involved in lactation. This reflex has also been called the expulsion mechanism, the let-down reflex and the draught reflex. It is postulated that the mechanism works in the following way: Impulses from the baby's sucking cause release of oxytocin from the posterior portion of the pituitary. This hormone causes the contractile tissue (myoepithelial cells) around the alveoli to squeeze the milk into the larger ducts and eventually to propel it to the ducts leading to the nipples. Then the milk is removed by the compression and suction action of the baby's nursing. It is important to remember that the let-down reflex can be influenced profoundly by psychic factors and the emotions of the mother. For instance, some mothers find that the let-down reflex is elicited (i.e., their breasts begin to drip milk) by an infant's cry or some other sound, sight, etc., that has become associated with nursing. Often they will say that they can feel their milk "come down" in anticipation of nursing. Fear, worry, pain and tension—all may affect the expulsion mechanism adversely. Thus, it is par-

ticularly important for the nurse to help the mother to avoid these emotional disturbances whenever possible. A relaxed atmosphere for nursing, adequate assistance, effective pain relief, and a supportive attitude on the part of the nurse are essential components of effective nursing care for the mother who is breast-feeding. Sometimes oxytocin is given the mother during early lactation to facilitate the milk flow. It may be administered by injection or by a nasal spray (40 U.S.P. units per ml. of solution). This hormone assists the ejection of milk when the let-down reflex is inhibited (as in times of stress) and also is effective in facilitating the milk flow when the breasts are engorged.

Engorgement

Breast discomfort several days after delivery has been attributed to venous and lymphatic engorgement, which mothers experience in relation to initiation of lactation. More recently it has been proposed that postpartal breast discomfort is attributed to two factors: 1) venous and lymphatic engorgement and 2) filling of the acini with milk. Most studies indicate that breast discomfort occurring during the first three or four postpartal days, the "initial breast engorgement," is due to venous engorgement. The breast discomfort appearing after the third or fourth postpartal day is due to filling of the acini with milk, the so-called "late engorgement." Thus, any treatment during the first few days is directed toward symptomatic relief of engorgement.[4]

The peak incidence of discomfort seems to occur on the fourth or the fifth day postpartum. It is believed that the engorgement is caused by the pressure from the increased amount of milk in the lobes and ducts.

SYMPTOMS. When the milk "comes in," the breasts suddenly become larger, firmer and more tender; consequently, many mothers experience varying degrees of discomfort. Some do not seem to be bothered by this transitory condition (and produce a large quantity of milk), but the majority usually have at least a moderate amount of tenderness and pain. A few experience a great deal of discomfort, with throbbing pains in the breast, extending to the axilla.

The engorgement may distend the breasts so much that the skin appears to be shiny. The tissue surrounding the nipple may also become taut to the extent that it actually retracts the nipple, making it extremely difficult for the baby to grasp the nipple and the areola adequately. It used to be thought that fever was a normal consequence of this condition; however, engorgement is *not* an inflammatory process, and if fever occurs, some other cause should be suspected. Still the breasts may be reddened and feel warm to the touch. They can be very painful, and they become more so when touched or moved.

Although this condition is transitory and usually disappears in 24 to 48 hours, prompt treatment is to be instituted, not only for the mother's comfort but also to prevent the condition from progressing. If engorgement is allowed to become marked, then emptying of the breasts (which is the basis of treatment) becomes very difficult because of the occlusion of the ducts by the surrounding congested tissues and the thick and tenacious character of the retained secretions. Secondary lymphatic and venous stasis may occur because the milk cannot be emptied.

Until this time it has been somewhat difficult to find an objective means for evaluating venous engorgement of the breast. Menczer and Eskin have made a study evaluating venous engorgement of the breast by means of thermography. It is known that the amount of infrared emission from the skin is proportional to its temperature. In this study the infrared emission from the skin of the breast is recorded on a polaroid photographic film. The image is recorded in different shades of gray and black, thus the lighter area of the film corresponds to the skin areas of the breast with increased infrared emission (hot areas).[5]

PREVENTION of engorgement is preferable to treatment and is generally possible with good management. Rooming-in is considered by many to be the best preventive measure. When the mother and infant are together around the clock, engorgement tends to occur less since the baby can nurse in response to the mother's needs as well as his own. If rooming-in is not available, the infant can be taken to the mother as soon as her breasts begin to fill and as often thereafter as is necessary to maintain her comfort. It is important that the mother's requests for her infant be met promptly and with friendliness; she can be reassured that even if the infant may not be hungry immediately, he soon will be.

TREATMENT usually consists of removal of the milk, support of the breast, hot packs and/or ice bags and analgesics for the relief of pain. Removal of the milk may be facilitated by the use of oxytocin before the baby nurses to encourage the let-down reflex. Interestingly enough, this drug sometimes is used to relieve discomfort from engorgement in mothers who are *not* nursing. The way in which the drug relieves pain in breasts that are not being emptied is unclear. In addition, manual expression of the milk and pumping, as well as the use of a nipple shield (to help the baby to grasp the nipple), may be recommended. Some mothers find the use of hot packs 15 to 20 minutes before nursing beneficial in improving the flow of milk. Often ice packs between nursing periods are very useful in alleviating discomfort. A good uplift support for the breasts cannot be stressed enough, particularly during the period of engorgement. Analgesics such as aspirin, propoxyphene (Darvon) or codeine frequently are used for pain relief. These should be given in adequate dosage and with appropriate timing so that the mother can be relatively comfortable during nursing. Since engorgement is transitory, the drugs are needed for a very short time; hence any danger to the infant is minimal.

Initiation of breast-feeding

Depending on the condition of both the mother and the infant, breast-feeding usually is started from 4 to 12 hours after delivery. Since the assessment of relevant data is a part of every nursing care plan, such observations as to the readiness of both mother and baby for breast-feeding are of primary importance. The mother can be encouraged to participate in decision-making which determines breast-feeding practices, insofar as they concern her baby and herself.

Some physicians prefer to give the baby one or two bottle feedings of water before breast-feeding begins. It is felt that this helps the infant to regurgitate any mucus or secretions that have been swallowed during delivery. If mucus is a problem with the baby, postponement of nursing is thought by some to be beneficial until the baby can rid himself of it. Usually, the baby is clear of mucus in 24 hours.

Rather than delaying the initiation of breast-feeding for all babies, it is better to maintain close supervision and guidance of mothers and babies during the early feeding periods.

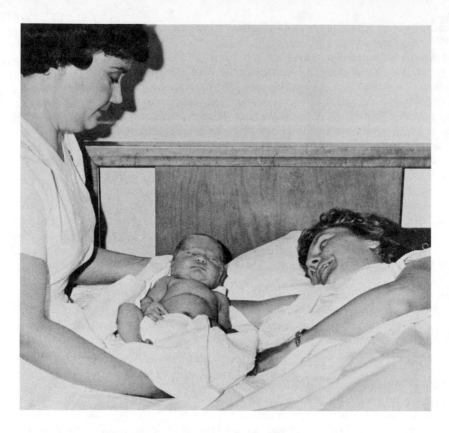

Figure 20-6. Baby handed to mother for feeding. Mother enjoys a look at her baby, a part of the identification processes in maternal claiming. (MacDonald House, The University Hospitals of Cleveland, Cleveland, Ohio)

Following an uncomplicated delivery, some authorities feel that instruction in breast-feeding can begin almost immediately. During the first few hours after birth, the unmedicated infant has a heightened sucking reflex. In view of this, it is felt that every effort is to be made to give the baby the opportunity to suckle, preferably in the delivery room or within an hour or two of delivery. At this early time there is rarely any difficulty in establishing the infant at breast and little need to teach him to suck.[6] Allowing the infant to breast-feed at this early date remains controversial at this time but the general consensus is that as soon as the baby is mucous-free and the mother is rested, breast-feeding can be initiated.

Colostrum will be the chief source of the infant's nourishment until the milk comes in. Putting the infant to breast early is advantageous for both mother and baby, since the sucking stimulates the milk production and helps the uterus to contract; moreover, nursing satisfies the infant's need for sucking. It is important for the nurse to remember that *both* mother and baby must learn how to work as a team in the nursing process. Hence, practice is essential. Even though the mother has breast-fed before, there is a wide range in nursing behavior among infants, and the experience of breast-feeding each infant can be somewhat "new." The mother will need to learn how to handle the infant appropriately, how to interpret cues of hunger and satiety, and how to help the infant to grasp the nipple and to withdraw the milk successfully. The infant, in turn, must learn to associate the nipple with food and to coordinate grasping of the nipple with sucking and swallowing in such a way as to get food successfully. No wonder that mother and baby often take a few days to become adept at this process!

An interested and experienced nurse needs to be immediately available to mothers in their first experiences with their new babies. Maternity nurses in the hospital can play a major role in facilitating the mothers' efforts to breast-feed their babies (Fig. 20-6).

Many of the problems associated with unsuccessful breast-feeding experiences can be prevented or solved through purposeful nursing action. Nurses need to accept the responsibility to help mothers gain knowledge and skill needed to successfully breast-feed their babies.[7]

Preparation of the mother *before* the actual breast-feeding experience plays a large part in giving effective care. This includes instructions about "hand-washing," sterile technique procedures and other rituals associated with the feeding of the infant in the hospital. When the infant is brought to the mother for feeding, the delay from such tasks can be frustrating and stress-producing for both mother and baby.

Whenever it is indicated, the mother should be informed about the feeding reflexes of her infant (see p. 421). During the actual nursing period the nurse can reinforce this information (as necessary) and *show* the mother how to elicit these responses. It is essential that the mother be able to evoke these reflexes herself, since she ultimately must assume total responsibility. Too often the nurse takes over these aspects, and the mother does not get sufficient practice to acquire any skill during these first days in the hospital. It is not easy to "stand-by" and watch the inexperienced mother trying to breast-feed her baby without offering too much interference. But it is necessary to be careful not to disrupt the learning process.

POSITION. Assisting the mother to experiment with various positions which are comfortable during breast-feeding is another important facet of care. The mother is sometimes asked whether she wants to nurse the baby sitting up or lying down. An inexperienced mother does not know this, although she may think she does, and she should be given an opportunity to try various positions, while help is available, and make her own choice.

A method to expedite the nursing process and help the baby learn to suck properly is a technique called alternate massage.

> ...Alternate massage is a procedure of breast-feeding that was developed to prevent common problems of early breast-feeding. The nurse can teach it to any nursing mother. Alternate massage consists simply in alternating massage of the breast with the baby's nursing in order to complete each nursing period. It enables the baby to empty the breast, an achievement that insures the milk supply and at the same time prevents painful breasts and nipples. ...

How to Use Alternate Massage

...Put the baby to breast and observe how he nurses. Usually after the first minute or so the movements of the baby's mouth become long, slow and rhythmic. In this type of nursing the

baby compresses the milk reservoirs with his gums and swallows milk. Such nursing avoids production of sustained negative pressure, which is responsible for injuring the nipple.

After a while you notice that the baby stops nursing, then he goes on as before. As the feeding proceeds, he rests more frequently and the character of the nursing changes from mouth movements that are long, slow and rhythmic to those that are rapid and shallow. Later there are still fewer slow rhythmic mouth movements and more of the sleepy rapid shallow type. It is the shallow kind of nursing that produces sustained negative pressure that hurts the nipple. The baby cannot extract milk from the breast when he nurses in this manner. Indeed he resorts to this kind of nursing only when the milk flows from the breast quite freely.

When the pattern of the baby's nursing changes from long, slow mouth movements to sleeping for the most part or to rapid shallow mouth movements, start alternating breast massage with the baby's nursing. Do not remove the baby from the breast; simply slip your hand to the back and middle portion of the breast near the armpit and gently massage the breast several times. While the breast is being moved the baby usually stops nursing, then responds by nursing with long, slow strokes. He may take only two or three strokes, however, because he can quickly pick up the milk that the massage has caused to move from the alveoli to the milk reservoirs. Then repeat the massage and permit the baby to nurse again. Often you will find the breast softening beneath your fingers. When one area softens, move your fingers to a new position and continue alternating breast massage with the baby's nursing until the entire breast has been softened.

It is important not to use breast massage until the character of the baby's nursing has changed from long, slow mouth movements to sleeping for the most part or to rapid shallow nursing. If massage is used before this time, the milk flows too fast for the baby to manage....[8]

To nurse satisfactorily, the infant needs to be held properly by the mother; although some mothers seem to know how to support a baby at the breast, many are awkward, and definite instructions are helpful. Both the mother and the baby must be comfortable and in such a position that the baby can grasp the nipple *and the areola* without any undue effort. If only the nipple is grasped, the baby will not be able to draw out the milk; moreover, the mother's

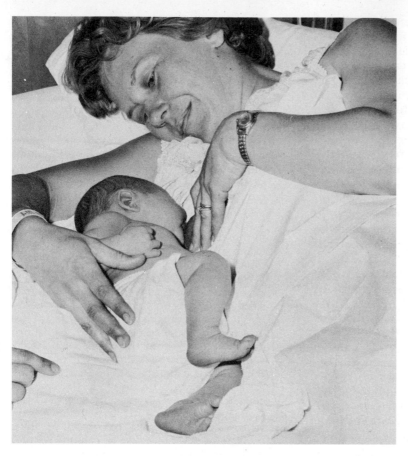

Figure 20-7. Both mother and infant should be comfortable during the nursing period. (MacDonald House, The University Hospitals of Cleveland, Cleveland, Ohio)

nipples are likely to be damaged. If the mother is lying down (Fig. 20-7), she should be on her side with her arm raised and her head comfortably supported. The baby lies on his side, flat on the bed or so supported that he can grasp the breast easily. If the mother prefers to sit up to nurse, she can use a comfortable chair and a stool to support her feet, as necessary. It is often helpful to place a pillow under the arm that is supporting the infant (to reduce the tension on the muscles, Fig. 20-8); or to place a pillow under the baby to raise him to a sufficient height so that he may reach the breast easily. If the stitches of the episiotomy are bothersome, a rubber ring or a pillow under the mother's buttocks may be helpful. The nurse may have to work with the mother a bit to be sure that she is comfortable. Often mothers in their eagerness to get the baby on the breast become very tense and assume quite uncomfortable positions (although they assure the nurse that they are "comfortable"). Patience and gentle reminding on the part of the nurse encourages these mothers to relax more readily.

ORIENTATION OF INFANT. After being placed beside the mother, the baby needs to be allowed a little time to become accustomed to the new environment and to hunt for the nipple. The baby should not be forced to nurse immediately, especially if he is hesitant or shows disinclination. If the rooting reflex is well developed (and as he smells the milk), the baby will turn toward the nipple or any object that brushes the cheek. Thus, if the mother or the nurse touches his cheek gently with the nipple, he will turn toward it, open his mouth and grasp it. Sucking usually follows closely thereafter. If the infant seems to have some difficulty in finding and grasping the nipple, although he seems to be eager, the mother or nurse can gently cup a hand around the baby's head and guide him to the nipple. Care should be taken, however, not to touch his cheek or to force his head, since he will only turn away and resist the pressure. In addition, he may cry, and a crying baby tends not to grasp a nipple successfully even though he may be hungry.

SUCKING BEHAVIOR OF INFANT. Babies will exhibit a wide variety of sucking behavior. Some, after finding the nipple, suck vigorously without stopping until they are satisfied. Others may suck vigorously for a time, appear to sleep or to rest and then resume sucking. Still others mouth the nipple before actually sucking but eventually nurse well. Others seem rather disinterested in the whole thing and dawdle throughout the nursing period. When the milk comes in, however, a change usually is noted, and even these infants begin to nurse more in earnest.

The important point here is that individual differences do exist in infants, apparently from birth; hence care must be taken to allow for these differences. To try to force the infant into a style or speed that is not his will only result in screaming, resistance and refusal; the nursing period should be adapted to the infant and not the infant to the nursing period. Mothers, especially, are appreciative of learning about this; often they think there is "*a* way to nurse" and do not realize the differences in eating behavior that infants have. Giving mothers anticipatory guidance and instruction in this aspect of nursing a baby is a very important component in nursing care.

If the infant is to suck effectively, he must place the nipple well back in his mouth, close his lips tightly around the areola, and squeeze the nipple against his palate with his tongue. He then can compress the lactiferous sinuses behind the areola and draw the milk into his mouth by sucking. He empties the breast through a combination of compression and suction. As he nurses, he moves his jaws up and down to compress and empty the sinuses; his tongue, as it draws the nipple back against the palate, suctions the milk from the nipple. Swallowing occurs when enough milk has been obtained to induce the reflex. This activity is carried on rhythmically, interspaced with periods of rest, until the infant is satisfied.

When the nurse assists the mother, she needs to be sure that the baby has the nipple on top of his tongue and that enough of the areola is in his mouth to prevent damage to the nipple. If he has a good grasp, his jaws will move up and down regularly, and sucking and swallowing movements can be seen in his cheeks and throat. If his grasp is poor, sucking and swallowing may be infrequent and/or absent, although his jaws may continue to move. If the nurse notes that the breast tissue

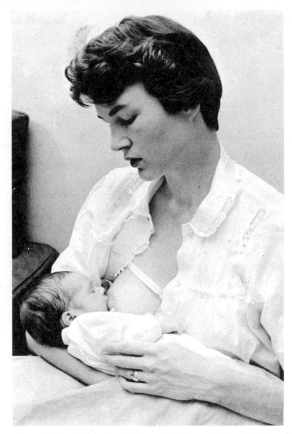

Figure 20-8. Babies nurse better if the mother is relaxed and both mother and baby are comfortable.

seems to press against the infant's nose and thus obstructs his breathing, she can instruct the mother to take her forefinger and gently compress the tissue so that it no longer impinges on the infant's nose. Care should be taken not to pull the nipple away from the infant in this maneuver.

Usually, getting the nipple in his mouth and tasting the milk seem to increase the baby's interest and ability to nurse. If the infant does not seem too interested or adept, moistening the nipple by expressing a few drops of colostrum or milk often encourages sucking.

Occasionally, a breast shield (Fig. 20-9) may be used to start the infant nursing if for some reason he cannot grasp the nipple. Continued use of this appliance is unwise, since the breasts cannot be emptied because the lacteal sinuses are not compressed during the nursing. The shield can be useful during the first few minutes of nursing to draw the nipples out if they are flattened by engorgement or inversion. Usually, however, even inverted nipples become

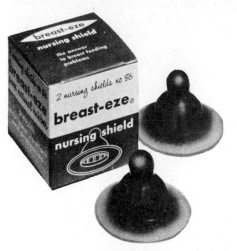

Figure 20-9. Nursing shield. (The Pyramid Rubber Company, Ravenna, Ohio)

prominent if the alveolar area is compressed gently by the fingers before nursing; they generally evert more when the infant sucks. The shield may be used also for a short period if the mother's nipples become sore; some nipple pain is experienced by most women during the first days of nursing, but generally it subsides as milk secretion begins, and the baby becomes satisfied. Mothers often state that the pain disappears when the let-down reflex occurs. The care of sore nipples is discussed below.

GIVING SUPPORT AND SUPERVISION. If the infant has taken the nipple without difficulty and has been sucking well for several minutes, the nurse can feel fairly assured that no further assistance is necessary *at this time.* If she leaves the mother and infant, however, she will place the bell cord within reach and instruct the mother to ring if she feels that she needs further help. Moreover, she needs to make a point of looking in occasionally to observe the progress of the two. Letting the mother have reasonable periods of managing the nursing process by herself will instill confidence in her, but she never should be left without adequate instruction and reassurance. Often, the presence of the nurse is all that is necessary to give the mother the necessary encouragement.

The nurse will want to remind the mother that the first week is a time of learning for the nursing mother and child. Unfortunately, the shortened hospital stay only diminishes the time that professional assistance can be given. Therefore, a referral to a public health agency may be indicated, and this possibility can be explored with the mother before she leaves the hospital. If the infant does not seem to respond satisfactorily to the nursing situation during the time that he is in the hospital, he should not be forced. As previously stated, a crying, upset baby will not take a nipple well; rather, he needs to be cuddled and soothed until he becomes quiet. If the baby still refuses or cannot nurse after about 10 or 15 minutes of effort on the part of the nurse and mother, it is better to stop and to try again when the baby seems to be more ready. If the infant does not appear to be hungry, it is permissible to omit a feeding. Often, after a few days, an infant who has been disinterested and resistant to the breast suddenly takes hold and begins to nurse with vigor. Since the mother can become very discouraged when her baby is nursing poorly, it is important that the nurse support the mother in her attempts to continue nursing. Patience, reassurance and adequate guidance are key factors in helping the mother over this initial adjustment.

Care of the nipples

Too much emphasis cannot be placed on the care of the nipples to facilitate breast-feeding. Cleanliness is a cardinal principle. Thus, keeping the nipples clean and dry is basic to keeping them in good condition.

Sore nipples are a frequent complaint during the mother's early breast-feeding experience, and so she can be instructed to report any discomfort in order that corrective measures may be instituted at once.

Sore nipples can be treated after each nursing period with the application of a bland cream or ointment, such as lanolin or a commercially prepared compound (e.g., Massé Nipple Cream or Vitamin A and D Ointment). Many hospitals advocate the use of a thermalite (therapeutic) lamp for tender or cracked nipples; the affected breast is exposed for 20 to 30 minutes twice a day. The mother can be advised that even the exposure of the breast to fresh air for similar periods is beneficial.

When a sore nipple is examined, it may be found to be fissured (cracked) or to have a small erosion or blister. Interestingly, more frequent feedings day and night have been recommended in these cases to prevent overstrenuous sucking and to keep the breasts from becoming too full and thus making the nipple difficult to grasp easily.[9] Letting the nipples dry after nursing by exposing them to air and the judicious use of a nipple cream have also been recommended for helping control this condition. Manual expression of the milk to relieve engorgement can also be instituted if the sore nipples are due to this problem. Cracked and raw nipples afford an easy portal of entry for pathogenic bacteria to gain access to the breast and to cause infection. If mastitis or abcess occurs, the physician usually suggests termination of breast-feeding. This is not always the case, however, since with the aid of antibiotics some women are permitted to continue.

Length of nursing time

The infant will begin nursing, from one to five minutes, from one or both breasts. Gradually, the time is increased according to the tolerance of the mother's nipples. When lactation is well established, the nursing period is approximately 20 minutes, although there may be a wide variation, depending on the infant's sucking pattern. When the breasts are full and the milk flow is easily ejected, the breast usually is emptied in the first five minutes or so of nursing. The baby may continue to suck, or he may fall asleep. If the infant continues to suck for an inordinately long time (30 to 45 minutes), this may be an indication that there is not enough milk present, and that he is still hungry, or it may be an indication that he sucks intermittently and therefore takes longer to get the milk. Again, he may wish merely to suck, even though he is not hungry. If secretion of milk is not the problem, it is wiser to let him proceed at his own pace than to attempt to hurry him, so long as nipple irritation does not occur. Sometimes the let-down reflex is so active that the milk literally streams, and the baby not only does not have to suck very hard but may have difficulty in swallowing fast enough to keep up with the stream. Placing the baby in a more upright position is sometimes helpful in preventing choking in these cases. He may have to nurse a bit, stop, and then continue as he learns to cope with the increased stream.

BUBBLING. The mother can be instructed in the technique of bubbling her infant. This may be done when she changes breasts, or midway and at the end of the feeding period. If the infant has had difficulty in beginning to nurse, it is usually better to bubble him at the end of the feeding. Breast-fed babies tend not to swallow as much air as bottle-fed infants; hence the need for bubbling usually does not present much of a problem.

SCHEDULE. A self-regulatory or self-demand schedule is the usual accepted practice today, especially for breast-fed babies; that is, the baby is fed when he indicates hunger by crying and body posture. The infant cries when he is hungry because actual contractions in his stomach cause him pain. If he is fed when he cries and is experiencing pain, he learns to associate food with the relief of pain. Thus food (and the mother who supplies it) become pleasant factors in his life. If, on the other hand, he is made to wait until "time" for feeding, he may not nurse well because he is exhausted from crying or has lost his feeling of hunger. Similarly, if a baby is "sleepy" and not allowed to wake up sufficiently by himself, he also will not nurse well and will soon resent efforts made to wake him up. Slapping the soles of his feet, spanking his bottom and the like generally are not effective. These infants may want to nurse only every six to eight hours for the first few days; later they enjoy more frequent nursing periods.

Most average-sized babies regulate themselves on an *approximate* four-hour schedule. Smaller infants may prefer three hours. However, the nurse and the mother must remember that a wide variation will exist; the interval at times may be from two to six hours and sometimes as long as eight hours. Usually, however, there will be six to eight feeding in 24 hours. Each infant also will vary his own schedule. For instance, after a few days the mother may notice that the infant wants to eat every two hours or so. She usually can meet the demand, since frequent nursing stimulates the milk production. Care is to be taken that her nipples do not become sore because of strenuous sucking, or that she does not become fatigued. The nurse will want to be particularly careful in observing mother and baby during this time. If the mother does evidence the above signs, then the nurse may suggest that a bottle be given for one feeding so that the mother may rest.

COMPLEMENTAL FEEDINGS. This subject has long been controversial. Some physicians (and mothers) feel that giving the infant any artificial feedings diminishes the success of breast-feeding and is extremely detrimental to establishing and maintaining lactation (see Sug-

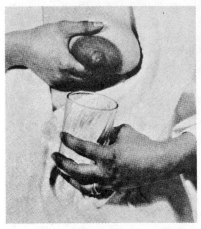
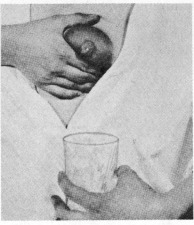
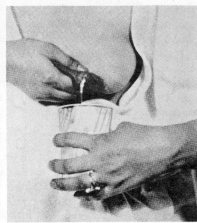

Figure 20-10. (*Left*) First position in the expression of breast milk from a large, pendant breast, showing the thumb and fingers properly placed and pressing backward. (*Center*) Second position, showing the thumb and finger pressed deeply into the breast, at the same time compressing the breast well behind the nipple. This deeper pressure is necessary in a round, virginal-shaped breast. (*Right*) Second position, showing compression of the breast between the thumb and fingers, well behind the nipple, and the milk coming in a stream. Care is exercised to avoid pinching or bruising the breast tissue.

gested Reading). Others feel that there are legitimate indications for an occasional artificial feeding. A variety of feedings may be used (i.e., plain water, glucose water, dilute formula, full-strength formula). If the mother is to use complemental feedings when she gets home, the nurse will want to be sure that she understands their preparation, the kind and the amount of feedings, and the indications for their use.

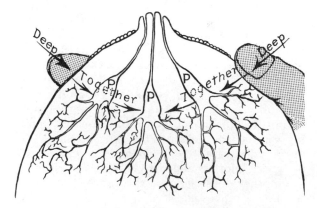

Figure 20-11. Illustrating the movements needed to force milk out of the little pockets (P) in which it collects. Place a finger and a thumb on opposite sides of the nipple at "Deep." Press deeply into the breast in the direction of the black arrows. Then compress the breast together in direction of the arrows toward center point "P." This will force the milk out of the ducts in streams. "Deep" and "together" express in two words the motions required. (After U. C. Moore, Nutrition of Mother and Child)

Expression of milk

There are some instances in which the mother is desirous of breast-feeding, but for certain reasons the infant cannot be "put to breast." There are also situations in which the breast-fed infant is not able to empty the breast completely. At such times it becomes necessary to utilize artificial means to empty the breasts of milk; otherwise, if this condition is allowed to persist for several days, lacteal secretion is inhibited, and the future milk supply may be jeopardized.

The hands of the person expressing the milk are washed thoroughly with warm water and soap and dried on a clean towel. Since the daily care of the breast is designed to maintain cleanliness, the same cleansing ritual required before putting the baby to breast would be utilized here.

MANUAL EXPRESSION. This can be done by nurse, but it is preferable to teach the mother how to carry out this procedure while she is in the hospital. In this way she can have guided practice under the supervision of the hospital nurse, so that when she has to do it after she returns home, her confidence and ability will be increased.

A sterile glass or wide-mouthed container is to be in readiness before beginning, and if the milk is to be fed to the infant, a sterile bottle and cap also will be needed. It may be desirable first to massage the breast for a few seconds to stimulate the flow of milk, and in such instances it is helpful to lubricate the hands with a drop of mineral oil. Breast massage should be done with a gliding movement of the hands. The pressure exerted should be firm, even, and, above all, gentle. First, place one hand on top of the other above the breast, then as they are drawn apart turn the fingers downward and encircle the breast. As the hands sweep forward toward the areola, they should cup the breast, drawing it forward and upward, and glide off without ever touching the areola or the nipple. If the breast is pendulous, care should be taken to allow it to fall gently.

One hand is used to support the breast and to express the milk; the other, to hold the container which will receive the milk. Although some authorities advocate that the right hand be used to milk the left breast, the decision as to which hand is used should depend on how the mother can accomplish this with the greatest of ease. The forefinger is placed below and the thumb above the outer edge of the areola. The forefinger is to be kept straight so that pressure can be exerted between the middle of this finger and the ball of the thumb. As they are alternately compressed and released, with the area of the collecting sinuses between them, milk is forced out in a stream (Figs. 20-10 to 20-12). It is of paramount importance here to avoid pinching and possibly bruising the breast tissue. The fingers should not slide forward on the areola or the nipple during the milking process. However, they must be moved in clockwise fashion around the areola, each time compressing and releasing the fingers on that area, so that all the collecting sinuses may be emptied.

Many authorities advocate this method of emptying the breasts rather than using the breast pump, because the action more nearly simulates the action of the infant's jaws as he nurses. Furthermore, since no mechanical equipment is required, it is a method which can be readily used when necessary after discharge from the hospital.

ELECTRIC-PUMP EXPRESSION. Several types of electric breast pumps employing the principle of intermittent negative pressure are sometimes used in hospitals (Fig. 20-13). These are used much less now than formerly because of their potential danger of traumatizing the breast tissue. Nevertheless some physicians still employ them to empty the breasts of milk, and thus the nurse will need to be cognizant of

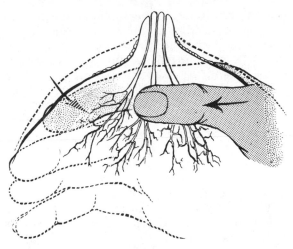

Figure 20-12. Diagram showing the method of expressing the milk from the breast, as the mother would view it from above, by compressing the milk pockets between the thumb and forefinger. The three unused fingers are used to support the breast. This represents the second or "together" motion. (After U. C. Moore, Nutrition of Mother and Child)

their potential danger as well as familiar with the particular pump that she is using. Electric breast pumping must always be done under professional supervision; the mother is never to be left alone to pump her own breasts in this manner.

Low suction is purported to express the milk without discomfort or injury. For whatever purpose the electric breast pump is used, the suction should be increased gradually to

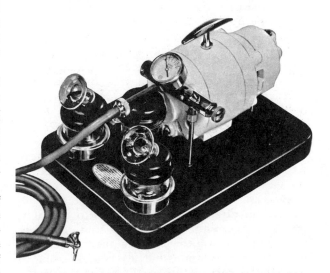

Figure 20-13. Electric breast-pump. Suction system provides vacuum up to 15" of mercury. Control allows patient to regulate degree of suction to her requirements and comfort. (Gomco Surgical Manufacturing Corp., Buffalo, N.Y.)

nursing care during the puerperium   389

prevent irritation to the nipple and needless pain which, in turn, might cause anxiety in the mother and retard the flow of milk. Suction should be intermittent to simulate the sucking of the infant. It takes approximately 5 to 12 minutes to empty a breast completely, depending on the stage of lactation, but pumping should be stopped as soon as milk ceases to flow. A breast should never be pumped longer than 10 minutes at any one time. However, if the mother experiences back or chest pain, an indication that the breast is dry, the pumping should be stopped immediately.

The breast milk obtained is measured and the amount recorded. When only one breast is pumped at a time, the record should indicate whether it was the right or the left, so that the next time the other breast can be pumped. If the milk is to be fed to the infant, it can be poured into a sterile nursing bottle, labeled with the infant's name, the time and the date and refrigerated immediately. To ensure further safety in the hospital, milk that is saved for an infant in this way is sterilized before it is fed.

The electric breast-pump machine may be used for more than one mother and thus should be washed with soap or detergent each time that it is used. In addition, certain removable parts, such as the breast-pump bottle and cap, the breast funnel and the rubber connection tubing, must be washed thoroughly, wrapped and autoclaved immediately after use.

HAND-PUMP EXPRESSION. At times a hand breast-pump may be used. Suction is obtained by alternately collapsing and releasing the rubber bulb. The principles of use and action are the same as those for the electric pump. Since this appliance is used also for more than one mother, it should be washed thoroughly in soap or detergent, rinsed and autoclaved.

Hygiene of the mother

REST AND ADEQUATE NUTRITION. Perhaps these two are the most important considerations for the lactating mother. The detrimental effects of fatigue and worry already have been discussed. In the hospital the nurse is able to act as a buffer between the mother and some of these problems. In addition, the mother is relieved of household responsibilities and is able to have meals served to her. When she leaves the hospital, she no longer has this somewhat protected environment. Thus, it is important that the nurse make sure that the parents under-

stand the importance of rest and adequate nutrition, and that the parents have made adequate plans to provide for them. If it is at all possible, the mother should have help at home. Her main energies then can be directed to the care of the infant and giving attention to her husband and other children. Housekeeping chores will have to be simplified and the mother's activity restricted so that she will get sufficient rest. Since her sleep will be broken at night, naps during the day become particularly *essential*—they should not be considered a luxury. Without adequate rest, the milk supply soon will be reduced to a dribble. If heretofore the woman has been very active, she may need special help to realize the importance of naps and rest periods. It is helpful, also, if visitors (including relatives) are restricted; they can become fatiguing to the mother, and they may be a source of potential infection to the newborn.

DIET. The daily diet of the lactating mother should be similar to that taken during pregnancy, with the addition of about 700 calories and amounts of the various nutrients (protein, calcium, iron, vitamin A, thiamine, riboflavin, niacin, vitamin B_6, vitamin B_{12}, and ascorbic acid) as recommended by the Food and Nutrition Board of the National Research Council. These increased requirements of the diet during lactation can be supplied with the addition of a pint of milk, one serving of vegetable and one of citrus fruit, an egg and one large serving of meat. Foods which the mother knows from experience disagree with her should be avoided; but the old belief that certain foods eaten by the mother will cause colic in her infant is now discredited. However, as previously stated, certain drugs may be excreted in the mother's milk in sufficient quantity to affect the breast-fed infant.

Caloric allowances must be adjusted for the variation in energy requirements which result from differences in the body size of women. Another important consideration in determining additional energy requirements for lactation is that they be proportional to the quantity of breast milk produced, and compatible with maintenance of the mother's weight. Since the quantity of breast milk produced varies from woman to woman, the caloric intake needs to be adjusted in relation to the mother's actual milk production. The basic diet can be supplemented by approximately 120 calories for each 100 ml. of breast milk that is produced. Let us assume that a mother has an average yield of breast milk of 850 ml. per day. In this instance an additional allowance of up to 1,000 calories might be utilized.

The National Research Council recommends an additional 20 Gm. of protein per day in the mother's diet. This allowance should be estimated according to the quantity of breast milk secreted and the protein content of this milk.

The vitamin and mineral intake should be adjusted also to supply the needed amounts for lactation. The average riboflavin content, for example, is approximately 40 mg. per 100 ml. of human milk. The World Health Organization Expert Committee on Nutrition in Pregnancy and Lactation assumes the average daily human milk secretion to be 850 ml., with an upper limit of 1,200 ml.

Vitamins B_6 and B_{12} have been added to the list of recommended daily dietary allowances in the 1968 revision. The increased need of vitamin B_6 for lactation is indicated by the amount of vitamin B_{12} in human milk (approximately 0.1 mg./liter). During lactation 2.5 mg. of vitamin B_6 is required in the mother's diet.

The value of a high protein diet to the mother cannot be stressed enough. The mechanism by which food is converted into milk protein is not very efficient; therefore, approximately 2 Gm. of food protein is needed to produce 1 Gm. of milk protein. The greater part of this protein intake (98 Gm. daily) should be in the form of animal protein, since this type supplies all the essential amino acids.

A high fluid intake also is necessary for milk production. Between 2,500 and 3,000 ml. is recommended for the mother engaged in usual activity under pleasant environmental conditions. More may be required in hot weather or with physical exertion. This fluid intake should include a good deal of water as well as other beverages. Many mothers find that taking a beverage prior to nursing facilitates the let-down reflex.

If the mother's diet was adequate in pregnancy, then additions rather than changes are all that will be necessary. It is important that the nurse ascertain that the mother is aware of these additions. If she is not, then guidance must be given. Often nursing mothers do not realize that their nutritional needs increase even over the needs of pregnancy, and they try to go back to their prepregnant diet. Increasing the milk intake to at least 1½ quarts daily will meet the additional protein, thiamin, riboflavin, calcium, phosphorus and niacin needs. Supplementing the citrus fruit recommendations in pregnancy with generous servings of other fruits and vegetables will meet the vitamin C requirements. An adequate vitamin D intake can be obtained by supplementing the vitamin-D-rich foods recommended during pregnancy. To further ensure optimum vitamin and mineral intake, many physicians will prescribe that the vitamin supplement capsules taken during pregnancy be continued.

The mother's weight is one of the best criteria in determining adequate caloric intake. It should remain stationary; wide fluctuations will necessitate adjustment of her diet, usually in carbohydrate and fat intake (this statement is based on the assumption that she has an adequate protein intake). The mother may take all foods in moderation as long as they agree with her. The old notion that certain foods (chocolate, the "strong" vegetables such as cabbage, onions, garlic) were excreted through the milk and would upset the baby is no longer universally held.

Debatable Items. Some physicians feel that certain foods, such as berries and chocolate, may produce an allergic reaction in the baby. If the mother has any question regarding these matters, she should consult her physician. Alcohol may be taken in moderation; many mothers find that a glass of wine or beer before nursing relaxes them considerably and facilitates the let-down reflex. Smoking is to be avoided for the reasons stated previously.

DRUGS. Many drugs are excreted in the milk, and it is particularly important for the mother to consult her physician before she attempts any self-medication, *even though she has taken the drug before.* Small doses of aspirin, milk of magnesia, mineral oil and some of the bulk-producing laxatives usually may be taken without passing harmful effects to the infant; however, it is well to advise the mother to inform her doctor if she feels she must continue to use any of them.

Weaning

Occasionally, it becomes necessary to wean the baby suddenly. In these cases the physician may follow the regimen for "drying up the breasts" as described on page 376. Most often, weaning is done gradually. There does not appear to be any "best" time for this procedure. Sometimes, with the introduction of solid foods, the infant tends to take the breast

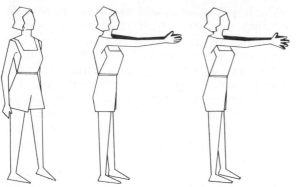

Figure 20-14. Breast exercise. After breast-feeding has been discontinued the breasts seem to be soft and flabby. These simple exercises may help to restore firmness of tissues because they involve the pectoral muscles which lend secondary support to the breasts. Stand with feet apart, toes turned in slightly, abdomen in and up, buttocks tucked under, and head held high. Hold fingertips together, with arms at shoulder level. Press fingers together sharply and firmly. Relax and repeat ten times.

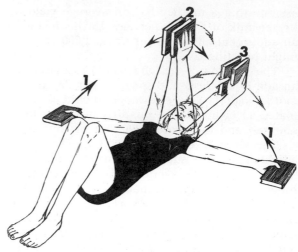

Figure 20-15. Breast exercise. Lie flat on back with knees and thighs flexed to place spine firmly on the floor. Abdomen is kept flat. Breathe naturally and do exercises slowly. (1) Holding a small book in each hand, stretch arms out level with shoulders. (2) Raise arms forward from body to bring books together, keeping arms straight. Lower arms to outstretched position. (3) Raise arms forward as in 2; then carry them, held straight together, to floor behind head. Return arms to outstretched position. Repeat. Stop all exercises before feeling tired.

less, and the milk supply consequently will diminish. However, many infants appear to relish solids and still continue to nurse well. It is essential to good health that the baby have solid foods by the age of six months or so. By this time the iron reserve has been depleted, and foods rich in protein and iron are particularly important. Provided that the baby receives a varied diet that includes meat, eggs, fruits and vegetables, there is no indication for weaning other than the natural inclinations of the mother and the baby. The process can be done gradually, with a cup and/or bottle offered in place of the breast. As the stimulation decreases, so does the milk supply, and lactation gradually ceases. Usually no engorgement ensues; if any should occur, the mother should be instructed to consult her physician.

Breast exercises

Mothers are sometimes concerned about the temporary increase in the size of the breasts during lactation. When breast-feeding has been discontinued, the breasts soon approximate their previous size and firmness, particularly if needed support has been maintained. There are exercises which, if done regularly, may be helpful. The breast itself is made up of glandular tissue and fat, and since there is an absence of elastic tissue, exercises cannot directly hasten the return of the breasts to their former state. However, exercises that involve the pectoral muscles may be helpful, because these muscles lend secondary support to the breasts (Figs.

20-14 and 20-15). These exercises may be started when the mother is no longer breast-feeding, should be limited at first and increased only as the mother can tolerate them without fatigue.

Parental guidance and instruction

A considerable amount of health supervision throughout the mother's pregnancy is devoted to anticipatory guidance, not only to provide for her immediate care, but also to help her plan and prepare for the time when she takes her new infant home from the hospital. A good foundation to facilitate this transition has been laid in this way, but it may lose some of its effectiveness unless certain aspects are reinforced in the immediate puerperium.

Each mother's understanding and ability will vary, depending largely on her background and previous experiences. Undoubtedly, the primipara who has not been accustomed to infants will have much to learn about the care and handling of her new baby. On the other hand, the multipara may feel uncertain about the response of an older child to the new baby and thus require guidance in understanding and dealing with sibling rivalry. Many mothers need to know more about their own care;

others need to know how to facilitate certain adjustments within the home or the family group. If the mother knows what she can expect and what to do, she usually can handle simple problems which might otherwise cause fear or apprehension.

Proper care for the mother during the puerperium emphasizes the need for rest, nourishing food and protection from worry. Parents, as a rule, seem to be under the impression that once the delivery is over, normality is restored and they can resume their usual activities immediately. However, it is agreed that it may be weeks before the generative organs have returned to normal size and position, and the emotional and endocrine adjustments may be even more delayed.

Since the nurse is in close and continuous contact with the mother, she can assume the responsibility of giving this anticipatory guidance and/or reinforcing it, or delegating that part which might be done more suitably by others. One of the most important points to be emphasized is that the mother should proceed *as slowly as possible* in the postpartal period at home. The general feeling of well-being and the excitement of having the baby, together with the emotions aroused in the "taking-hold" phase, all too often provide so great a stimulus that the mother has a tendency to overdo. If there are other children in the household, especially toddlers, the demands on the mother may be considerable.

If it is at all possible, the major responsibilities of housekeeping should be taken over by a "helper," so that the mother can be more relaxed and devote herself primarily to caring for her new infant and spending more time with the immediate family. At this time family relationships can be strengthened if the mother is not overwhelmed with apprehension and fatigue. The subject of household assistance needs to be explored thoroughly with the mother (and if necessary, the father). The parents may need help in realizing what possibilities and alternatives they have in this matter. Some parents, for instance, manage very nicely when the father takes some vacation-time and assumes management of the household. However, it must be remembered that not all fathers are able (or willing) to shoulder this considerable task. Other couples can rely on parents, in-laws or relatives for a time. Still others must hire outside help; in these cases the expense and consequent budget-

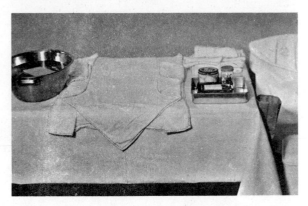

Figure 20-16. Setup used for baby bath demonstration in the mothers' classroom. Note paper bag for discarded cotton balls, pillowcase for a laundry hamper and step-on can for diaper pail. (MacDonald House, The University Hospitals of Cleveland, Cleveland, Ohio)

ing may have to be discussed. If outside help is employed, then the mother may have some question as to whether a housekeeper or a "nurse" (to take care of the baby) would be more desirable. This, of course, will depend on many factors. Most mothers find that when they are relieved of the heavy housekeeping chores, the "care" of the baby is relatively easy and provides an opportunity to get thoroughly acquainted with the new addition to the household.

The nurse should not "recommend" one type of helper over another. Rather, she can explore the subject with the mother, point out the alternatives that the parents have, and let them make the final decision. This approach would also be appropriate for any other aspect of guidance.

By the time that the mother leaves the hospital she should have at least a basic understanding of her own condition and status, and she ought to know what physical and emotional changes to expect. In addition, she should be familiar with the daily care of her baby and know what to expect of him, together with any other important details related to his care. Parents also need to know how and where to contact the physician if before the next scheduled visit there should arise any medical problem pertaining to either the mother or the infant.

Since the present-day maternity stay is rather short, some type of follow-up service often is desirable and necessary. Therefore, parents need to be offered information about the services of the public health nursing agency

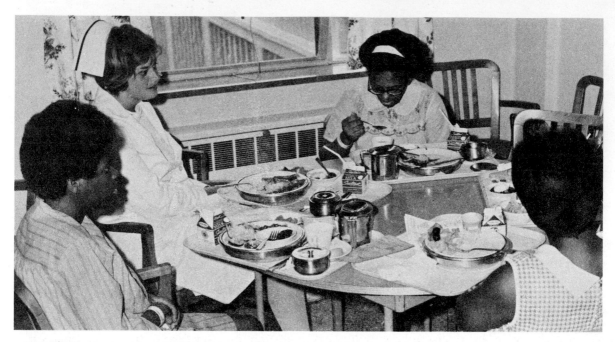

Figure 20-17. Luncheon "round table" for small group of mothers to learn about their own care and their baby's through guided group discussions. (MacDonald House, The University Hospitals of Cleveland, Cleveland, Ohio)

in their community, and how they may use these services. In cases of obvious need a referral to an agency should be instituted before the patient leaves the hospital.

Fathers who have participated in parents' classes are usually much more conscious of this period and prepared for it. Often they plan their time at home so that they can assume some of the responsibilities. It is not so much physical help that is needed as it is the satisfactions gained by the mutual "sharing" engendered by the partnership. If the mother takes special care to express her appreciation of her mate's awareness and consideration, then this initial readjustment period becomes less tedious and truly gratifying to both.

Individual teaching

Regardless of the fact that a mother may attend all the group classes offered in the maternity hospital, each mother should be given individual help to learn how to handle and care for her infant while she is in the hospital, particularly if this is her first baby. Many new mothers are timid at first because they do not know what to expect of their infants, or they are afraid of what they will do to them because of their own feelings of inadequacy. A mother who has had no previous experience with infants will need some guided practice in chang-

ing diapers, dressing her baby and handling the infant in general. (Fig. 20-18). Rooming-in units provide an environment in which the mother can have such an experience over an extended period of time. However, even in situations where the infants are kept in a central nursery, the nurse will want to plan to spend some time with the mother, in addition to the regular feeding periods, to help her learn to care for her baby. If hospital staffing permits the time, it may be desirable for some mothers to bathe their own infants at the bedside, under the nurse's guidance, before leaving the hospital. There is no reason that such practices should violate the "clean nursery technique" if they have been properly planned. A rooming-in experience is undoubtedly beneficial for mother, father and baby. But when this is not possible because of hospital facilities or policies, a daily extended visiting period can be extremely helpful. In this way the parents and the baby can become better acquainted in the security of the maternity division, where experienced personnel are near at hand to answer the parents' questions and to offer advice.

Postpartal exercises

Certain exercises are advantageous to the mother during the postpartal period to strengthen the abdominal muscles and to promote involution and a general sense of well-being (Fig. 20-19).

Discharge instructions

Before the mother is discharged from the hospital, the physician will give her instructions about her care and the rate at which it is prudent for her to resume normal activities in the following weeks at home. She is told to avoid any heavy work and to get as much rest as possible during the next three weeks. Her schedule can be planned to include morning and afternoon rest periods and adequate sleep at night. Stair climbing should be limited until the second week at home. If the mother is advised to take exercises to strengthen abdominal and perineal muscles, the physician will specify when they may be started and the frequency with which they are to be done. The hair may be washed at any time, and tub baths or showers are permissible. The mother usually is advised not to have intercourse or to take a vaginal douche until after the "six-week check-up" to prevent infection and trauma to the newly healing organs and structures. Instructions concerning eating habits and regulation of the bowels are discussed.

If the medical care of the infant is being supervised by a pediatrician, he may give the home-going mother instructions concerning her baby; otherwise this is taken care of by the obstetrician. The mother needs to be given specific information about feeding, skin care, clothing, sleep, bowel habits, behavior and the early growth and development of her infant.

Many hospitals provide printed instructions for home-going maternity patients. When these are used, it is the responsibility of the nurse to make sure that the mother understands them before she leaves the hospital.

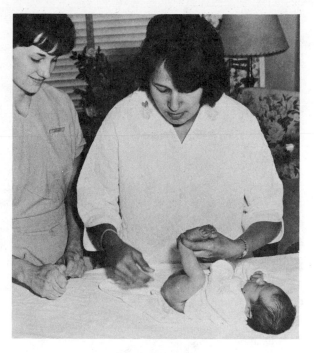

Figure 20-18.   Individual care.

The maternity programs of most public health agencies include home visits by the nurse. When a referral has not been made by the hospital nurse, the mother can be informed that such services are available in the community and told how to secure them if she should need help with the care of the baby.

The importance of follow-up care for both mother and baby is stressed. The mother is instructed that it is essential for her to keep the appointment for her "six-week check-up." The infant can be checked in four weeks and regularly thereafter by a private physician or in one of the well-baby clinics sponsored by the department of health.

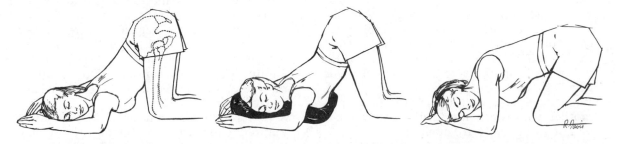

Figure 20-19.   Knee-chest position may be advised by the physician if the uterus has not returned to its almost normal position. *(Left)* CORRECT—Chest resting on bed, thighs perpendicular to surface. *(Center)* INCORRECT—Chest on pillow, thighs slant away from body. *(Right)* INCORRECT—Resting on elbows, thighs slant inward toward body.

Bibliography

1. Peckham, B.: Optimal maternal care. *Am. J. Ob-Gyn.* 33:862-868, June 1969.
2. Rubin, R.: Pueperal change. *Nurs. Outlook* 9:753-755, Dec. 1961.
3. Countryman, B.: Breast care in the early puerperium. *JOGN* 2:36-40, Sept./Oct. 1973.
4. Menczer, J., and Eskin, F.: Evaluation of postpartum breast engorgement by thermography. *Am. J. Ob-Gyn.* 33:260-263, Feb. 1969.
5. *Ibid.*
6. Countryman, B., *op. cit.*, p. 37.
7. Iffrig, Sister M. C.: Nursing care and success in breast feeding. *Nurs. Clin. North Am.* 3:353, June 1968.
8. *Ibid.*
9. Countryman, B., *op. cit.*, p. 38.

Suggested Reading

ADELS, M. J., AND ROGERS, S. F.: Use of a new nonnarcotic analgesic for postpartum pain. *Am. J. Ob-Gyn.* 84:952-955, Oct. 1, 1962.

AYD, F. J.: The teenager and contraception. *Ped. Clin. North Am.* 16:355-361, May 1969.

BRADBURY, B.: Preventing the diaphragm baby syndrome: a matter of teaching and time. *JOGN* 4:24-32, March-April 1975.

CAHILL, I.: *Child-Rearing Practices in the Culture of Poverty.* NLN Convention Papers, 1967.

DAW, E., *et al*: Lactation inhibition. *Nurs. Mirror* 136:18-19, June 29, 1973.

EPPINK, H.: An experiment to determine a basis for nursing decisions in regard to time of initiation of breastfeeding. *Nurs. Res.* 18:292-299, July 1969.

EVANS, R. T., *et al*: Exploration of factors involved in maternal physiological adaptation to breastfeeding. *Nurs. Res.* 18:28-33, Jan.-Feb. 1969.

MILLINGTON, M., *et al*: For high risk infants and their parents: postnatal discussion groups and well-baby clinics operate in storefront. *JOGN* 4:42-46, Jan./Feb. 1975.

NEWTON, N., AND NEWTON, M.: Psychologic aspects of lactation. *New Eng. J. Med.* 277:1179-1188, Nov. 30, 1967.

REEDER, S.: Becoming a mother—nursing implications in a problem of role transition. ANA Regional Clinical Conferences, 1967, pp. 204-210.

RICH, O. J.: Hospital routines as rites of passage in developing maternal identity. *Nurs. Clin. North Am.* 4:101-109, March 1969.

RUBIN, R.: Basic maternal behavior. *Nurs. Outlook* 9:683-686, Nov. 1961.

——: Puerperal change. *Nurs. Outlook* 9:753-755, Dec. 1961.

——: Maternal touch. *Nurs. Outlook* 11:828-831, Nov. 1963.

——: The family-child relationship. *Nurs. Outlook* 12:36-39, Sept. 1964.

——: Food and feeding—a matrix of relationships. *Nurs. Forum* 6:195-205, Spring 1967.

WEIR, R., AND FELDMAN, W.: A study of infant feeding practices. *Birth and the Family J.* 2:64-65, Spring 1975.

YUNEK, M. J.: Postpartum care is more than a routine. *Nurs. Outlook* 17:50-52, Jan. 1969.

ZACHA, M. C.: Nursing goals in working with families under multiple stress. *Nurse Clin. North Am.* 4:69-75, March 1969.

THE WOMANLY ART OF BREASTFEEDING. Franklin Park, Illinois, LaLeche International, 1973.

Conference Material

1. The patient's husband is severely injured the day after her infant is born. What provision can be made by the hospital to keep the patient informed about conditions at home and the care of her three other children?

2. What instructions should be given to the primipara and her husband concerning her care following delivery and discharge from the hospital? How can the public health nurse participate most effectively in this family's care?

3. What approach would you use to help a mother who was undecided about whether or not to breast-feed her infant?

4. Why is the postpartal examination important? What is the nurse's role in relation to the examination?

5. A mother tells the nurse that she wants to breast-feed her baby for six to eight months because she knows that she cannot become pregnant so long as she is nursing. How can the nurse reply?

6. What are the pros and the cons of early discharge of the maternity patient?

7. How can the nurse help a nursing mother so that she can make her limited food budget provide well-balanced meals for the family? The family consists of the mother, the father (employed as a factory worker) and two small children.

8. A young mother is concerned that her two-year-old child will be jealous of the new baby. How can this problem be handled?

care of the newborn infant

21

Physiology of the Newborn / Characteristics of the Newborn / The Environment of the Newborn / Nursing Care of the Newborn / Infant Feeding / The Mother and Her Newborn

From the standpoint of maternity care, the infant will be considered through the neonatal period (the first four weeks of life).

During pregnancy, the unborn infant has been protected and nourished by his mother, but at birth he suddenly becomes an "independent" individual and undergoes the most profound physiologic changes that are encountered at any period of life. Some of these alterations are immediate, and all permanent and, therefore, significant.

Since these first days and weeks are so critical, the nurse is called on to give expert nursing care when assuming care of the newborn. The nurse must use the utmost care in handling the baby, keeping him warm and protecting him from exposure and injury. She must also make accurate observations and record and report them. Communication and teaching skills are utilized, since she must ensure the infant's future well-being by helping the parents to develop an understanding of their baby's needs and to acquire skill in his care. In this way their concept of themselves as adequate parents is reinforced. The nurse also must be aware that some parents need assistance in developing healthy attitudes regarding childrearing practices, so that the infant can make a satisfactory emotional and social adjustment. A close parent-infant relationship must be fostered (and provision made for this in the hospital environment), and communication must be maintained between the nurse and the parents. Thus, the care of the newborn infant presents an interesting challenge to those in maternity nursing.

Physiology of the newborn

The infant must pass through approximately six overlapping stages before he becomes entirely adapted to extrauterine life. During these stages he is in a *transition* period which he must negotiate successfully if he is to survive and to develop normally. The first step or stage begins with labor, when the fetus receives the stimulation from the uterine contractions and the changes in pressure as the membranes rupture. As he passes through the second step, he encounters a variety of foreign stimuli—light, sound, heat, cold, gravitation, and the like. In the third stage, he must begin breathing. Stages four and five require profound changes and reorganization in the functioning of the organ systems and metabolic processes. Here he must initiate respiration, change from fetal to neo-

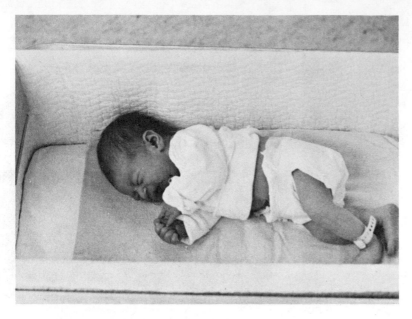

Figure 21-1. A healthy newborn infant four hours after birth. (Woman's Hospital Division, Hospital of the University of Pennsylvania, Philadelphia)

natal circulation, alter hepatic and renal function, and pass meconium. Stage six demands further reorganization of the metabolic processes to achieve a viable, steady state. This includes changes in blood oxygen saturation, reduction of enzymes, diminution in postnatal acidosis, and recovery of the neurologic tissues from the trauma of labor and delivery. Since these changes take time, it is no wonder that the infant's natal day is so crucial to his life and future well-being.

Respiratory changes

During the fourth month of pregnancy, the infant apparently attempts respiratorylike movements. Some authorities feel that amniotic fluid is aspirated during this activity; others feel that the lungs actually manufacture amniotic fluid. At any rate, amniotic fluid seems to pass in and out of the lungs. Yet during gestation the lungs perform no other function.

INITIATION OF RESPIRATION. With birth, however, profound changes occur. Now the lungs must exchange the oxygen and the carbon dioxide in the blood, work previously performed by the placenta. Exactly what initiates respiration is as yet unclear. It is believed to be a combination of physical, sensory, and chemical factors, but precisely how each of these influences the other and to what degree is not known exactly. There is some evidence to indicate that the sudden change from intrauterine to extrauterine life produces enough physical stimulation to prompt respiration. It may be that the passive motion of the joints and the squeezing of the infant's thorax during delivery, as well as his spontaneous movements after birth, also contribute to minute ventilation and influence the other physical and sensory factors. It is worth noting in this regard that mothers of the various mammalian species, as they vigorously lick and cleanse their offspring after delivery, do, in fact, seem to apply a deliberate mechanical sensory stimulation to their young.

The chemical changes that occur in the blood as a result of the transitory asphyxia that occurs during delivery seem to be of paramount importance. These include a lowered oxygen level, an increased carbon dioxide level, and a lowered pH. If the asphyxia is prolonged, depression of the respiratory center ensues rather than stimulation, and resuscitation is usually necessary (see Chapter 29). A vigorous infant often breathes seconds after birth and certainly within one minute of delivery.

A great effort is required to expand the lungs and to fill the collapsed alveoli. Surface tension in the respiratory tract, as well as resistance in the lung tissue itself, the thorax, the diaphragm, and the respiratory muscles must be overcome. Moreover, any obstruction (i.e., mucus, and so on) in the air passages has to be cleared. The first active inspiration comes from a powerful contraction of the diaphragm, which creates a high negative intrathoracic pressure, causing a marked retraction of the ribs because of the pliability of the baby's thorax. This first inspiration distends the alveolar spaces which heretofore have been filled with fluid. Any remaining fluid that is left is reabsorbed rapidly if the pulmonary capillary blood flow is adequate, since it is hypotonic and passes easily into the capillaries. After several minutes of breathing, lung expansion should be complete.

RESPIRATION IN FIRST AND SECOND PERIODS OF REACTIVITY. A healthy infant begins life with intense activity. This phase has been designated by some authorities as the first period of reactivity. In this phase the infant exhibits outbursts of diffuse, purposeless movements which alternate with periods of relative immobility. At this time respiration is rapid (reaching as high as 80 breaths per minute), and there may be *transient* flaring of the alae nasi; retraction of the chest and grunting are not uncommon. Tachycardia also is present, at times reaching 180 beats per minute in the first minutes of life and thereafter falling to an average of 120 to 140 beats per minute.

After this initial response, the baby becomes relatively quiet and does not respond intensely to either internal or external stimuli. He relaxes and may fall asleep. His first sleep occurs on an average of two hours after birth and may last anywhere from a few minutes to two to four hours.

When he awakes, he is again hyperresponsive to stimuli, and he begins his second period of reactivity. His color may change rapidly (from pink to moderately cyanotic), and his heart rate responds to stimulation, becoming rapid. Oral mucus may be a major problem in respiration during this period. Choking, gagging, and regurgitation alert the nurse to the presence of mucus, and appropriate intervention must be taken (see Chapter 29). Since the length of the second period of reactivity is variable, the nurse must be particularly alert for the first 12 to 18 hours of the infant's life.

CHARACTER OF NORMAL RESPIRATION. As the infant adapts successfully to extrauterine life, his respiration usually ranges from 35 to 50 breaths per minute. They are easily altered by internal and external stimuli. Normally, his respiration is quiet and shallow. This can be observed most accurately by watching the movement of the abdomen, since his respiratory activity is carried out largely by the diaphragm and the abdominal muscles. Periods of dyspnea and cyanosis may occur suddenly in an infant who is breathing normally (even after the transition period and after several days). This *may* indicate some anomaly or other pathologic condition and should be reported promptly. Therefore, the nurse should notify the physician if the respiration drops below 35 or increases beyond 50 when the infant is at rest, or if dyspnea or cyanosis occur.

Circulatory changes

The anatomic changes that occur with birth have been discussed previously in Chapter 8. The nurse will recall that a rapid change takes place, with oxygenated blood being distributed in a manner similar to that of circulation in an adult.

TOTAL BLOOD VOLUME. The amount of time between birth and the clamping of the umbilical cord is an important factor in determining the amount of the infant's total blood volume. For instance, the baby receives an additional 50 to 100 ml. of blood if the cord is clamped and cut after pulsations have ceased. This is due to the fact that as the uterus contracts, it pumps blood from the placenta into the baby's circulation. The increased blood volume is quickly readjusted through the elimination of excess fluid.

THE PERIPHERAL CIRCULATION of the newborn is somewhat sluggish. It is felt that this accounts for the residual cyanosis of the infant's hands, feet, and circumoral area. The nurse will note that these areas often remain mildly cyanotic for one or two hours after delivery. The general circulatory lability probably accounts for the mottled appearance of the baby's skin when it is exposed to air and for the "chilliness" of the infant's hands and feet.

THE PULSE RATE, like the rate of respiration, also is labile and generally follows a pattern similar to that of the respiration. When the respiration is rapid, the pulse tends to be rapid; similarly, when the respiration slows down, so does the pulse. Since the pulse is affected by both internal and external stimuli, the nurse can be more accurate if she counts the *apical* pulse rate while the baby is quiet. The normal rate is usually 120 to 150 beats per minute, but it may rise to 180 with crying and other intense activity. When the infant is asleep, the rate may range from 70 to 90 beats per minute.

THE BLOOD PRESSURE is characteristically low, being around 80/46 at birth and rising to 100/50 by the tenth day. Since the extremities of the newborn are so small, accurate auscultation is difficult. If any accuracy is to be obtained, proper equipment is essential. A cuff 1 inch wide should be used and should cover two-thirds of the upper arm or thigh.

ERYTHROCYTE COUNT AND HEMOGLOBIN CONCENTRATION. The newborn infant has a much higher erythrocyte and hemoglobin level than an adult. The erythrocyte level ranges between 5,000,000 and 7,000,000 per microliter, and the hemoglobin level is usually 15 to 20 Gm. per 100 ml. of blood. These higher rates are needed by the baby in utero for adequate oxygenation. After birth the need no longer exists, since the lungs are functioning, and a gradual decrease takes place, particularly during the second and the third weeks of life. There is usually a slight *increase* in these concentrations on the first and the second postnatal days; this is due in part to the extra amount of blood received through delayed clamping of the cord and to the subsequent readjustment of the blood volume. The gradual decrease in the erythrocyte count and the hemoglobin concentration results in a *physiologic* neonatal anemia, which disappears spontaneously. Clinical symptoms usually do not appear (except in cases of nutritional problems and/or infection), and no therapy is needed. The lowest counts are reached when the infant is three months old, when the hemoglobin level ranges between 11 and 12 Gm. per 100 ml. of blood, and the erythrocyte count between 4,000,000 and 4,300,000 per microliter; after that there is a gradual increase.

Physiologic Jaundice. Another effect of the destruction of the red blood cells is the so-called physiologic jaundice which usually is seen on the second or the third day of life. It is thought that an increase in serum bilirubin results from the breakdown of the red blood cells, and this, together with a temporary inability to remove the bilirubin, results in the jaundice. The condition usually begins to subside on the sixth or the seventh day, and it should disappear by the second week of life. A bilirubin concentration of 13 mg. per 100 ml. of blood is beyond the physiologic limit and a total serum bilirubin above 18 to 20 mg. per 100 ml. is termed hyperbilirubinemia (see Chapter 29). Since the physiologic jaundice is not usually manifest until the infant is two or three days old, the nurse must be alert for any signs of jaundice before that time, especially in the first 24 hours of the baby's life. This latter type of jaundice may be pathologic and should be reported immediately so that treatment can be instituted.

BLOOD COAGULATION. Immediately after birth the intestinal tract of the infant does not harbor the bacteria necessary to help to synthesize the very important substance, vitamin K. Other substances important in blood coagulation are manufactured in the liver and are under the influence of vitamin K; these substances are temporarily diminished. Thus the infant suffers from a transitory deficiency in blood coagulation. This condition occurs between the second and the fifth postnatal days and returns to normal spontaneously in several more days. Some physicians feel that this deficiency can be minimized or prevented by the administration of a small dose of vitamin K_1 at the time of birth (see Chapters 18 and 29).

WHITE BLOOD CELLS. The normal newborn has a wide range in the total number of white blood cells. A leukocytosis (15,000 to 45,000 cells per microliter) is present at birth, with polymorphonuclear cells accounting for a large percentage of the total count. During the first few days after delivery there is a considerable decrease in the total count, as well as a shift in the type of predominating cell. The polymorphonuclear neutrophils decrease, and the lymphocytes increase, so that by the end of the first week the lymphocytes predominate.

Temperature regulation and metabolic changes

THE TEMPERATURE-REGULATING MECHANISM of the newborn infant is not fully developed at birth; thus his heat production is somewhat low, and he responds readily to environmental heat and cold stimuli. At birth his body temperature is assumed to be the same or higher than that of his mother; however, at birth it may drop 1 or 2 degrees despite the application of external heat and blankets. With chilling, the drop is even more precipitous and dangerous for the baby. If the infant is given adequate covering and protection, the temperature soon begins to rise, and it returns to normal in about eight hours. The nurse should keep in mind how easily the infant responds to environmental cold and heat and avoid subjecting the baby to wide variations in temperature.

BASAL METABOLISM. Since the surface area of the newborn is large in comparison with his weight, his basal metabolism per Kg. of body weight is higher than that of an adult.

Thus his *caloric requirements* are high during infancy. About 50 to 55 calories per pound of body weight per day suffice in the beginning. However, because of the increase in activity during the neonatal period and the energy requirements needed for the baby's rapid growth at this time, an increase in the caloric requirements may be needed after several days. Caloric needs will vary a good deal, even for infants of the same age and weight. Activity seems to be a determining factor. An infant who moves about a good deal, cries, and so on, will need more calories than his more phlegmatic counterpart. The infant's caloric needs usually are based on weight-gain, well-being and satiety. A caloric intake of about 110 to 120 calories per Kg. of body weight per day (50 to 55 calories per pound per day) is usual after the first few days.

The infant's *fluid requirement* also is greater per Kg. of body weight than that of an adult. This is due to his increased muscular activity, caloric intake, and basal metabolism.

TRANSITORY FEVER OF THE NEWBORN. This condition sometimes occurs between the second and the fourth day of life. It is caused by a low fluid intake and the usual fluid loss that occurs in the immediate postnatal period. The temperature may rise as high as 38.9 to 40° C. (102 to 104° F.), the skin is dry, the fontanels may be depressed, the urinary output may be decreased, and a weight loss may occur. This condition is found most often in infants who do not take their feedings well (or who do not suck well) or in those who take only small, infrequent feedings. Both the fever and the subsequent side effects can be remedied by increasing oral feedings (i.e., giving the baby water between milk feedings or administering parenteral fluids).

Neurologic changes

The nervous system of the newborn is immature; that is, it is neither anatomically nor physiologically fully developed. Although all neurons are present, many remain immature for several months, and some, for years. Thus, the infant is uncoordinated in his movements, is labile in his temperature regulation, and has poor control over his musculature: he "startles" easily, is subject to tremors of the extremities, and so on. However, during the neonatal period, development is rapid, and as the various nerve pathways controlling the muscles are used, the nerve fibers connect with one another.

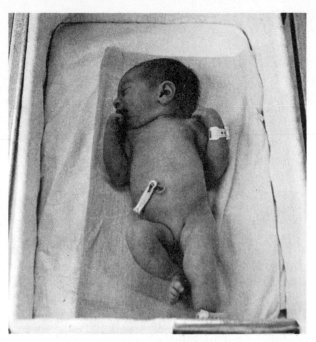

Figure 21-2. Moro reflex.

Gradually, more complex patterns of behavior emerge, and the higher cerebral levels begin to function.

REFLEXES are important indices of the baby's normal development, for their presence or absence at certain times reflects the extent of normality in the functioning of the central nervous system.

The *Moro* or *startle reflex* indicates an awareness of equilibrium in the newborn (Fig. 21-2). This reflex should be elicited when the baby is lying quiet. A sudden stimulus, such as a change in position, a jarring of the crib, a jerking of the blanket or clothes, or even a loud noise (which jars his position) causes the baby to draw up his legs, to bring his arms forward in an embracing motion, and usually to cry. The movements should be symmetrical. If they are not, injury to the part that lags should be suspected. The Moro reflex should be present at birth; normally it disappears by three months of age. If it cannot be elicited at birth, edema of and/or injury to the brain may be present. As the edema subsides, the reflex returns, and it should be demonstrable on the day following delivery. If frank brain damage has occurred, the reflex will be absent for several days; if the damage is not too severe, the reflex will return in three or four days. Occasionally, the reflex is present at birth

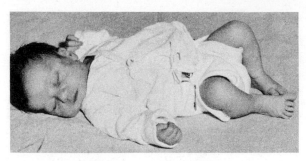

Figure 21-3. Tonic neck reflex.

but disappears over the first days. Increasing cerebral edema or slow intracranial hemorrhage then are suspected.

When the *tonic neck reflex* is elicited, the infant assumes a "fencing" position; that is, he lies on his back with his head rotated to one side. The arm and the leg on the side to which he is facing are partially or completely extended, and the opposite arm and leg are flexed (Fig. 21-3). This reflex also disappears in a few months, since it is another manifestation of the immaturity of the newborn's nervous system.

Several reflexes are involved in feeding. The *rooting reflex* causes the baby to open his mouth and turn his head toward anything that touches his cheek. This is helpful when he is searching for food. Brushing his cheek with the mother's breast, for example, enables him to find the nipple for nursing. The *sucking reflex* (Fig. 21-4) stimulates sucking movements whenever anything brushes the infant's lips. Normally, this reflex is present at birth and accompanies the *swallowing reflex,* absence of

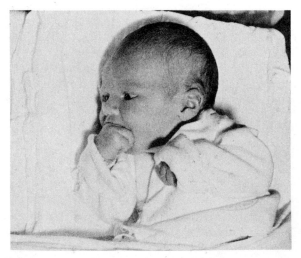

Figure 21-4. Sucking reflex.

which indicates immaturity, narcosis, brain injury, or retardation. Moreover, if it is not stimulated, it ceases to exist. The *gag reflex* operates when the infant takes more into his mouth than he can swallow. He can cough or hiccup a little if fluid does go "down the wrong way."

Since the infant is not well coordinated, he may have difficulty in bringing several of these reflexes into play at the proper moment, and he will need help from his mother or nurse. For instance, he may succeed in finding the nipple when he attempts to nurse, but if he gets the nipple under his tongue, successful sucking and swallowing are inhibited. It is important that the mother understand these feeding reflexes, so that she can help her infant. Often the inexperienced mother, in her anxiety to assist the infant to nurse, attempts to turn his head toward the breast by pushing on his cheek. The rooting reflex therefore is elicited, and the infant promptly turns his head in the opposite direction. This causes no end of consternation for both mother and baby.

The *grasp reflex* is present at birth in both the hands and the feet (Fig. 21-5). The infant will grasp any object placed in his hands, cling briefly, and then let go. Even at birth he may be able to hold onto an adult's forefinger so securely that he can be lifted to a standing position. Although the baby cannot actually grasp with his feet, stroking the soles causes the toes to turn downward as though trying to grasp. The grasping movements are a reflex action at birth, but with practice and experience they soon become voluntary and purposeful.

The *stepping* or *dancing reflex* is another action that is present at birth but soon disappears. This reflex causes the infant to make little stepping or prancing movements when he is held upright with his feet touching a surface. After this reflex diminishes, the infant will not attempt stepping motions until he is ready to stand and to walk. However, he does exercise the leg muscles a great deal and seems to derive much enjoyment from waving and kicking his legs about.

The next group of reflexes might be termed protective, since they are necessary and at times essential to the preservation of the newborn's safety. The *blinking reflex* occurs when the infant is subjected to a bright light. The *cough and the sneeze reflexes* clear his respiratory passages. The *yawn reflex* draws in additional oxygen. These, together with the infant's ability to cry when uncomfortable, to withdraw from painful stimuli, to resist restraint, and so on, are all defensive measures. As the baby grows and develops, these together with the other reflexes mentioned either diminish or become more highly developed according to the need. Thus, the infant's behavior patterns become more complex and highly developed.

Gastrointestinal changes

It is well for the nurse to remember that the newborn, to be able to swallow, must have his food placed well back on his tongue, since he does not have the ability to transfer food from his lips to his pharynx. This means that the nipple should be placed well inside the infant's mouth. Sucking is facilitated by strong sucking muscles and ridges or corrugations in the anterior portion of the mouth. In addition, the *sucking pads* (deposits of fatty tissue in each cheek) prevent the collapse of the cheeks during nursing and further make sucking effective. This fatty tissue remains (even when fat is lost from the rest of the body) until sucking is no longer essential to the baby's getting food. The salivary glands are immature at birth and manufacture little saliva until the infant is about three months old.

STOMACH, INTESTINES, DIGESTION. The capacity of the newborn's stomach is rather difficult to measure, since the feedings may empty easily into the duodenum even before the feeding is completed. The capacity has been estimated to be approximately 50 to 60 cc. The cardiac sphincter is not as well developed as the pyloric sphincter, and hence the baby should be "bubbled" several times during the feeding so that any swallowed air can be eructed.

The newborn's intestinal tract is proportionately longer than that of an adult. Although it contains a large number of secretory glands and a large surface for absorption, its elastic tissue and musculature are poor and not fully developed. Furthermore, nervous control is variable and inadequate. Nevertheless, the infant digests and absorbs a tremendous amount of food in proportion to his body weight.

Most of the digestive enzymes seem to be present and adequate, with the exception of pancreatic amylase and lipase. These last are somewhat deficient for several months but eventually reach a normal amount. The infant can digest simple foods more easily, but has a difficult time with the more complex starches.

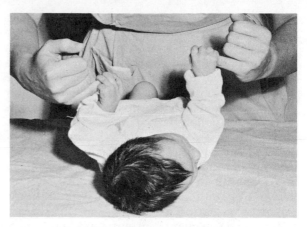

Figure 21-5. Grasp reflex.

Protein and carbohydrates are easily absorbed, but fat absorption is poor.

Regurgitation; Vomiting. The nurse and the mother will note that often the baby regurgitates (spits up) soon after a feeding. Sometimes regurgitation happens as long as 60 minutes after a feeding. This occurs because of the imperfect control of the cardiac sphincter and the immaturity of the nervous control. Activity also seems to be implicated, since the more active infant tends to spit up more often and for longer periods than the more quiet infant. The condition can be minimized by bubbling the infant well during and after feedings and by avoiding overfeeding. Handling the infant gently (and as little as possible) after feedings and placing him on his right side with his head and trunk elevated slightly are also helpful measures.

Occasionally, actual vomiting occurs during the first several days after birth. It is felt that this may be due to the secretions and material that were swallowed by the infant during delivery. Another cause is the swallowing of air by the infant during a feeding. This condition should subside within two or three days (with proper feeding, bubbling, and positioning) and requires no special treatment. If the condition persists, however, or if the vomiting is of a projectile nature, the physician should be notified immediately (see Chapter 29).

STOOLS. The baby's stools change daily during the first week of life, and their changes and amount should be recorded accurately.

Kidney function and urinary excretion

The kidneys of the newborn function quite efficiently at birth. During fetal life, even though the placenta takes care of waste excretion, they become functional, and urine can be found in the bladder of the fetus as early as the fourth month of gestation. Excretion begins during the ninth week of gestation. Since the baby has urine in his bladder at birth, he may void at delivery; but sometimes urination is delayed for as long as 12 to 24 hours. Voidings during the first days after birth may be scanty and somewhat infrequent (unless edema is present) until feeding increases the fluid intake and consequent output. The number and the amount of voidings gradually increase until the infant is urinating as many as 30 times a day after the immediate postnatal period (see p. 420). With the development of bladder control, the frequency again decreases. The urine of the newborn (after the first voiding) has a high specific gravity and may appear to be quite cloudy due to the mucus and urate content, as well as its high concentration. As the infant takes an increasing amount of fluid, the specific gravity gradually drops, and the cloudiness disappears, leaving the urine the usual straw color and almost odorless. Uric acid excretion is high in the newborn period, and this substance, when excreted on the diaper, may appear as reddish or "brick-dust" stains. Since the material looks like blood, it is sometimes thought that the infant is suffering from hematuria (see p. 420).

Changes in hepatic function

During fetal life, the liver performs an important role in blood formation, and it is thought that it continues this function to some degree after birth. Later in the neonatal period the liver produces substances that are essential in the coagulation of the blood (see p. 400). If the mother's iron intake has been adequate during pregnancy, enough iron will be stored in the infant's liver to carry him over the first months of life when his diet (primarily milk) is iron-deficient. About the fifth month, however, the baby's iron reserve is depleted, and unless foods containing iron are given, a deficiency will ensue.

Characteristics of the newborn

Immediately after birth, or within the next few hours, the physician will give the infant a complete physical examination. This usually includes: head (fontanels, overriding of skull bones), eyes, mouth (palate, gums, tongue), heart, lungs, abdomen, extremities, genitalia, and anus. The measurements of the infant are noted, such as the circumference of the head and the shoulders, and the weight and the length. The average full-term boy baby weighs from 7 to 7½ pounds (about 3,300 Gm.) at birth; girl babies weigh a little less. The average length of a full-term infant at birth is about 20 inches (51 cm.).

The physician will scrutinize the infant carefully for any deformity (e.g., cleft palate, clubfoot), injury (e.g., cephalhematoma, fracture of the clavicle) or abnormality (e.g., tonguetie, phimosis). If a malformation or an injury is found, the physician will advise concerning the infant's care and will assume the responsibility for telling the parents about their baby.

General appearance

The nurse should be familiar with the characteristics of the normal newborn in order to be able to distinguish them from the abnormal. For example, certain symptoms which might be cause for concern in an older child (e.g., rapid rate and rhythm of respiration), when observed in a newborn infant, may merely represent normal neonatal physiology. Also, it is well for the nurse to look at the baby from the mother's viewpoint. The healthy newborn infant has many characteristics which momentarily may look unusual to her. The nurse should be ready to talk with the mother about her baby and to answer her questions. A daily inspection sponge bath affords the nurse an excellent opportunity to observe the infant's anatomy and behavior, and thus to become familiar with the infant.

POSITION AND MOVEMENTS. The newborn infant usually lies with his arms and legs flexed, or tending to imitate the position that he has been accustomed to in utero. When the infant is awake, he sucks, yawns, sneezes, blinks, and stretches. His movements for the most part are purposeless. For the first day or two he sleeps most of the time, but even while he is relaxed and quiet, he occasionally may exhibit some coarse, jerky movements. During the first few weeks of life he may lie with his head turned to one side and the arm and leg on that side extended, while the other arm and leg are drawn up (tonic neck reflex). If he is awakened suddenly or startled by jarring or a loud noise, he will thrust his arms out in an "embracing motion" (Moro reflex).

HEAD. The infant's head is large, comprising about one-quarter of his size, and with cephalic presentations may initially appear to be asymmetrical because of the molding of the skull bones during labor (Fig. 21-6). The suture lines between the skull bones and the anterior and the posterior fontanels can be palpated easily (see Fig. 14-1, p. 244). When the nurse's hand is passed over the fontanels, the areas should feel soft but neither bulged nor depressed. The anterior fontanel, the diamond-shaped and larger of the two (normally 2 to 3 cm. wide and 3 to 4 cm. long), may feel smaller for the first several days when there is marked overriding of the skull bones. The posterior fontanel is triangular in shape and is located between the occipital and the parietal bones. It is smaller than the anterior fontanel and may be almost closed at birth. Occasionally, the scalp is covered with a thick growth of hair which sheds for the most part before the permanent hair appears.

The face is small and round, and the lower jaw appears to recede.

EYES AND VISUAL PERCEPTION. The eyes are closed much of the time but will open spontaneously if the infant's head is lifted (a valuable point to remember when one wants to inspect the eyes). The infant from birth can see and discriminate patterns as the basis for form perception. This capacity is rather limited by imperfect oculomotor coordination and inability to accommodate for varying distances. Moreover, the eye, the usual pathways, and the visual part of the brain are poorly developed at birth. Nevertheless, although the baby's vision is much less acute than an adult's, a good deal of visual experience is possible for him. Babies love faces and soon learn to recognize mothers' faces. Visual patterning seems to be particularly stimulating or interesting to the infant, more so than color or brightness alone. For instance, he will show a preference for a face or a solid object rather than a blob of light or a bright color. Thus, even the newborn sees a patterned and organized world which he explores discriminatingly (albeit with his limited means). When and how his visual contact with environment makes a lasting impression on his behavior remain topics for future research. Most mothers do not realize that their infants can see as well as they do, and they appreciate being informed of this fact. In addition, some mothers become exceedingly anxious when they observe strabismus or nystagmus in their in-

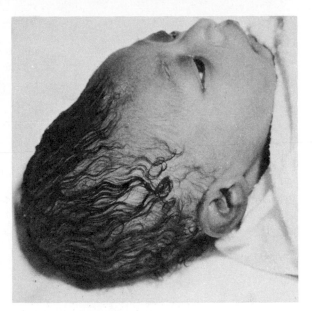

Figure 21-6. Molding of the head.

fants, but they should be reassured that this lack of coordination is normal during the first few months of life.

All babies' eyes are blue or a slatey gray color at birth. By the time the infant is three months old, they have achieved their permanent color, although complete pigmentation of the iris does not occur until the infant is about one year old. Since the lacrimal glands may not be functioning at birth, the baby does not usually shed tears when he cries. Tears may not appear for several weeks and sometimes for several months. There may be some edema of the lids and/or purulent discharge caused by the silver nitrate (see p. 415). The changes in the vascular tension of the eyes during delivery sometimes cause small areas of subconjunctival hemorrhage. These areas disappear spontaneously in one or two weeks and are not significant.

EARS AND HEARING. The ear and the nerve tracts for hearing are anatomically mature at birth, and the newborn can hear after his first cry. Hearing apparently becomes acute within several days as the eustachian tubes become aerated, and the mucus in the middle ear disappears.

LIPS, MOUTH, CHEEKS. The lips are sensitive to touch, and any stimulation of this nature usually elicits the sucking reflex. Moreover, the rooting reflex is well developed, so that when the cheek is stroked on one side the infant will turn his head in that direction. In conjuction

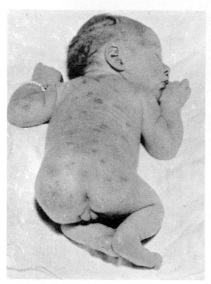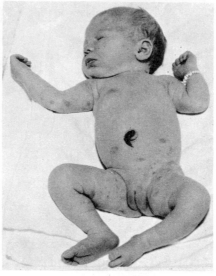

Figure 21-7. Erythema toxicum. This "newborn rash" develops more frequently on the back, the shoulders and the buttocks. (MacDonald House, The University Hospitals of Cleveland, Cleveland, Ohio)

with sucking, a labial tubercle may be present on the center of the upper lip, as well as the sucking pads (fat) in the cheeks. At this time the tongue does not extend far beyond the margin of the gums because the frenum is normally short. A mother's concern that her baby is tonguetied is usually unwarranted.

It is well known that during the first two months of life the newborn infant has a great need to suck and will usually suck on anything that comes in contact with his lips. Newborn infants can suck while sleeping and nonnutritive sucking can have a quieting effect on excited babies. One study, in which infants sucking on pacifiers were tested during ordinary restful sleep, revealed that sucking renders the sleeping infant unresponsive to external stimuli.

Body; Skin. The infant's neck is short. His chest is round and slightly smaller in circumference than his head. The breasts may be engorged initially and may even secrete "witch's milk." This condition, like menstruation, a vaginal tag or enlarged labia in girl babies, is due in utero to stimulation by maternal hormones and will disappear spontaneously. In boy babies the scrotum appears to be relatively large, and the prepuce is long and adherent to the glans penis (this separates in several months). The abdomen is round and protruding due to the relative size of the abdominal organs and weak muscular structures. The respiratory movements are largely diaphragmatic, and breathing is rapid, shallow, and irregular.

The infant's skin appears to be thin and delicate and is often dry and peeling. The baby's color may be pink, reddish, or pale, becoming very ruddy when he cries. Initially, the hands and the feet are quite blue, due to the sluggish peripheral vascular circulation, but this cyanosis of the extremities soon disappears, often within a few hours. Vernix caseosa, a white cheesy material which has been a protection to the skin while the fetus is floating in amniotic fluid in the uterus, may be apparent, particularly in the creases of the body. Also, on the body there may be large areas of fine downy hair called lanugo. Milia may be present on the nose and the forehead, and small flat hemangiomas may be apparent on the nape of the neck, the eyelids or over the bridge of the nose. These so-called stork bites, clusters of small capillaries, usually disappear spontaneously during infancy.

In nonwhite infants, dark bluish areas are usually apparent on the buttocks or the lower back. These "mongolian spots" have no relationship to mongolism and will disappear spontaneously during late infancy. A pilonidal "dimple" resulting from an irregular fold of skin sometimes is seen in the midline over the sacrococcygeal area.

Miscellaneous conditions

At times, the following conditions are seen in the normal newborn infant. Although they are not serious, they do represent some deviation from what is "usual." Moreover, they often cause concern in the parents; thus the nurse should be familiar with them to be able to

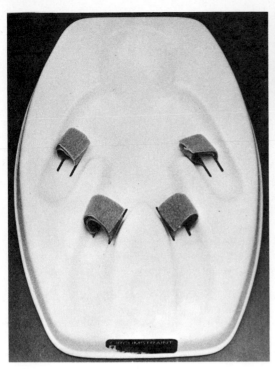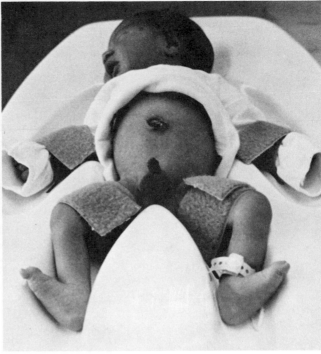

Figure 21-8. Preparation of the infant, restrained for circumcision. (*Left*) Board as used in many hospitals for circumcision. (*Right*) The infant, restrained on the board with towels, ready for circumcision.

answer any questions that the parents may have and give appropriate reassurance.

ICTERUS NEONATORUM. This is an exceedingly common condition during the first week of life and, as the name implies, is characterized by jaundice. Physiologic jaundice is dependent on the normal neonatal rise in the serum bilirubin level (see p. 400). It makes its appearance, as a rule, on the second or the third day of life and disappears without treatment about the sixth or the seventh day. Almost one baby in three shows icterus, which is often due to physiologic jaundice. Most authorities attribute it to inadequate liver function and the destruction of red cells which takes place during the first week of life. The mother may be assured that the condition is due to a normal process and will clear up within a few days.

ERYTHEMA TOXICUM. Sometimes referred to as the newborn rash, erythema toxicum is a blotchy erythematous rash which may appear in the first few days of life (Fig. 21-7). The erythematous areas, which develop more frequently on the back, the shoulders and the buttocks, have a small blanched wheal in the center. The cause of this skin disturbance is obscure, and no treatment is necessary. The rash is transient and likely to change appreciably within a few hours, and it may disappear entirely within a day or so.

MILIA are pinpoint-sized, pearly white spots which occur commonly on the nose and the forehead of the newborn infant. When touched gently with the tip of the finger, these spots feel like tiny, firm seeds. They are due to retention of sebaceous material within the sebaceous glands, and if they are left alone, will usually disappear spontaneously during the neonatal period. Mothers often mistake milia for "whiteheads" and may attempt to squeeze them if the nurse or the physician has not warned them against such practice.

PHIMOSIS. In many male infants the orifice in the foreskin of the penis is so small that the foreskin cannot be pushed back over the glans. This condition is known as phimosis. Although it is rarely of sufficient degree to obstruct the outflow of urine or to cause any immediate symptoms, it is undesirable because it prevents proper cleanliness. Phimosis may be corrected either by stretching the orifice of the foreskin with a hemostat, or by circumcision. Both procedures are carried out by the physician, but sometimes the nurse is asked to stretch the

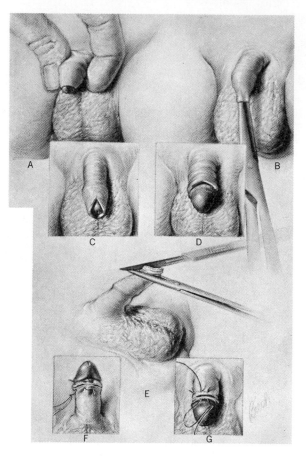

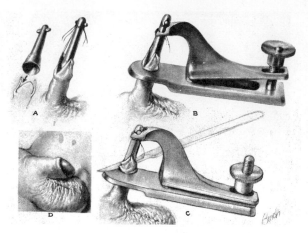

Figure 21-10. Technique of circumcision with Yellen clamp. After cleansing area and stripping back prepuce as shown in Figure 21-9, the cone of the Yellen clamp is placed over the glans and the prepuce put on a stretch with sutures (A). The prepuce is now drawn through the beveled hole of platform (B). Screwing down clamp crushes prepuce, producing hemostasis. Three to five minutes of such pressure is necessary to prevent subsequent bleeding. The excess of the prepuce is then cut away (C) and the clamp removed (D). (Yellen, H. S.: Am. J. Ob.-Gyn. 30:146)

Figure 21-9. Technique of circumcision, using hemostat, scalpel, and sutures. After cleansing penis and surrounding area, the prepuce is stripped back with the help of a partial dorsal slit (A to D). The prepuce is now clamped and excessive prepuce cut off (E). The suture material used in plain 00 or 000 catgut in a very small needle (F and G).

foreskin gently every day after having first received detailed instructions from the physician. Preparation of an infant for circumcision, two common methods of performing the operation, and postcircumcision inspection are depicted in Figures 21-8 to 21-11.

BREAST ENGORGEMENT. Engorgement of the breasts is common during the neonatal period in both male and female infants (Fig. 21-12). It is due to the same causes that bring about mammary engorgement in the mother—that is, endocrine influence. In the case of the infant, the breasts have been acted on throughout pregnancy by the estrogenic hormone which passes to them through the placenta from the mother. This is the same hormone which prepares the mother's breasts for lactation. When

it is withdrawn after birth, changes in the infant's breasts take place similar to those in the mother.

Mammary engorgement in the newborn subsides without treatment, but sometimes it persists for two or three weeks.

MENSTRUATION occasionally occurs in newborn girls and is due to estrogenic hormone, as just described. It usually amounts only to slight spotting and need cause no special concern.

The environment of the newborn

Prevention of infection

The prevention of infection is of paramount importance in caring for the newborn. Everyone who is in contact with infants—including parents and personnel—must assume this responsibility. Staff should take special care to instruct parents so that their activities conform to the prevention of infection. The basis of "good" technique in handling the infant is thorough handwashing with an antiseptic detergent or soap. Some institutions require scrubbing with a brush; others feel that detergent, water, and friction are sufficient. Whichever the procedure, meticulous handwashing is essential, whether the infant is cared for in the central or regular nursery or in a rooming-in

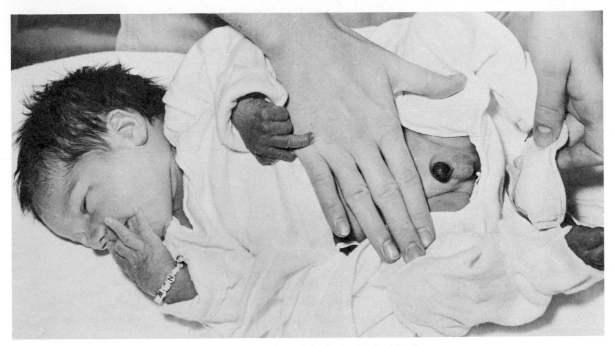

Figure 21-11. Postcircumcision inspection for bleeding.

situation. Parents and staff should be especially careful to wash their hands before a feeding and after a diaper change. The parents will need instruction about the importance (and technique) of proper handwashing, and reinforcement should be given as necessary during the hospital stay.

As with personnel in the delivery room (see Chapter 18), all nursery staff should have a pre-employment physical examination and a yearly physical examination thereafter to minimize the possibility of spreading infection from the staff among the newborn. In addition, any staff member who contracts *any* infection (i.e., respiratory, gastrointestinal, skin lesions, and the like) should remain away from the nursery and contact with the newborn until the infection is gone *completely*.

If the mother manifests signs of infection and has been in contact with her infant, the infant will be isolated from the other babies (usually in the isolation or observation nursery) and will be removed from the mother's presence until her disorder is treated and cleared. Since the mother may be concerned about being separated from her baby and miss him, the importance of the precautions should be explained thoroughly. If the mother is concerned about continuing breast-feeding (and her condition permits), her breasts can be pumped to ensure stimulation and a continued supply of milk. Her milk is discarded, however, as an added precaution, until her infection subsides. The mother who has not had contact with her infant before she evidences signs of infection, will also be separated from her infant, and the foregoing explanation and management of feeding is applicable to her as well.

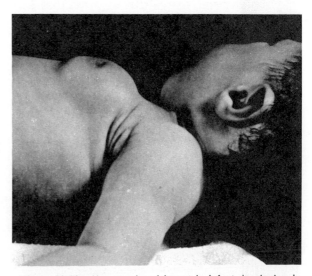

Figure 21-12. Hypertrophy of breast in infant developing in the neonatal period.

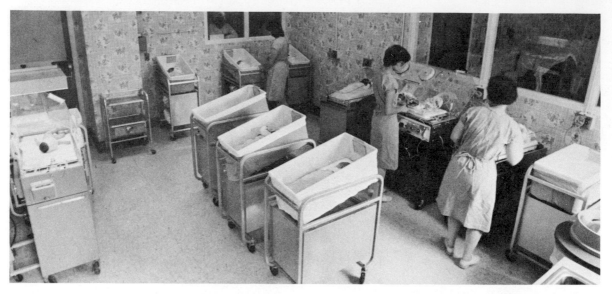

Figure 21-13. Term newborn nursery. (Woman's Hospital Division, Hospital of the University of Pennsylvania, Philadelphia)

Babies who are delivered outside a hospital are not admitted to the regular newborn nursery. They usually are cared for in the observation nursery or with the mother in a rooming-in situation.

To further reduce the hazards of infection from outside sources, the number of visitors may be restricted in the maternity area, and no visitors are allowed in the nursery proper. Children also are excluded from the maternity unit, since various infections and particularly communicable diseases are so prevalent among them. To further ensure cleanliness, members of the staff wear special gowns when they care for infants. These gowns should be short-sleeved so that a thorough scrub or wash may be given the hands, the forearms, and the elbows, and the gowns should be changed for each "shift" and more frequently if soiled. Masks are no longer worn, since they must be changed every 20 to 30 minutes to be effective, and, in fact, they can become a reservoir of bacteria when not applied and changed properly. Occasionally, the mother will be instructed to wear a mask in tending the baby if she has had a recent cold, or if she develops a cold when she goes home. The nurse should make certain that she understands the principles underlying the application and the wearing of the mask and especially that she be aware of how her hands can be contaminated in adjusting and tying it. Even at home a clean mask should be worn each time the need arises, and the mother should be instructed to wash her hands each time after she adjusts it.

Types of care for the newborn

THE CENTRAL NURSERY SYSTEM. The central or general newborn nursery on the postpartal division is designed for the care of a variable number of healthy newborn infants (Fig. 21-13). In this system the infants are brought to their mothers at certain specified times during the day—generally for feeding and/or visiting. The staff assumes the responsibility for all the care of the babies. Some authorities feel that the separation of mother and child (and father) in this manner results in an unnatural fragmentation of the family at a momentous time for building family unity. Also with the emergence of the many drug-resistant organisms that abound in the hospital environment, the danger of epidemics (whenever a large aggregate of persons collect) is enhanced. Certainly, in a central nursery system the contact among the mother, the infant, and the father is not as extensive as it would be in a rooming-in plan. However, the hospital's physical plant may make a central nursery arrangement the only type feasible. Moreover, some mothers prefer the type of care that is given under a central nursery system for a variety of reasons. At any rate, some type of central nursery usually is found in most hospitals. Control of the physical facilities and stringent personnel policies accomplish a good deal of protection of the newborn so managed. For instance, cribs should be placed at least 2 feet apart with 3-feet-wide aisles between the cribs. Limiting the number of infants in a nursery from 8 to 12 is also helpful. Requiring all personnel to put on clean gowns before entering the nursery, limiting the number of individuals who may enter the nursery, and requiring strict adherence to nursery aseptic technique on the part of nursery personnel all aid in protecting the infants. Washing the hands and arms to the elbows and scrubbing the fingernails thoroughly before entering the nursery, as well as washing the hands carefully before and after handling each baby, afford additional protection.

The central nursery is a so-called clean nursery. But it must be understood that there is a difference in nursery technique between what is considered to be nursery clean and what is considered to be baby clean (i.e., what is clean for an individual baby). There should be no common equipment, such as a common bath table, used in providing care for the babies. There should be provisions in the nursery so that individual technique can be followed. Each infant should have his own crib and general supplies, so that he can be given such care as his daily inspection bath or be diapered or dressed in his own bed. Most cribs are constructed with a built-in cabinet for the infant's own supplies (clean diapers, shirts, and linens) and a drawer to hold the containers for cotton balls, safety pins, thermometer, and so on. When such cribs are not available, improvised units for the infant's crib should be obtained so that individual-care techniques can be carried out.

If there is any evidence of a questionable infection at the time of delivery, if the infant is born on the way to the hospital, or if the infant is suspected of having an infection of the eyes, the skin, the mouth, or the gastrointestinal tract, the infant should not be admitted to the central nursery but should be kept in isolette isolation.

OBSERVATION NURSERY. Maternity hospitals should have an observation nursery where infants suspected of developing an infectious condition may be kept until the presence or absence of infection is determined. When a definite diagnosis of infection is made, the infant must be transferred immediately to an isolation nursery away from the maternity division.

Aside from the fact that infants in the sus-

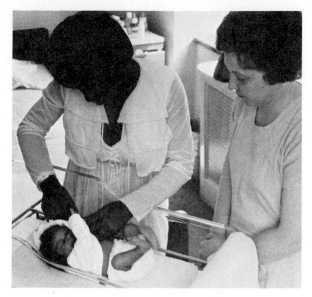

Figure 21-14. Rooming-in. (Woman's Hospital Division, Hospital of the University of Pennsylvania, Philadelphia)

pect or observation nursery must be segregated from others, and naturally require closer supervision and care because of suspected infection, their nursing care otherwise should be like that given a healthy newborn infant.

ROOMING-IN. This term has been applied to the plan of having the new infant share his mother's hospital unit so that they may be cared for together. This type of arrangement has come to mean much more than caring for the mother and the infant in the same unit of space. Rather, it implies an attitude in maternal and infant care that supports parental education and is based on recognition and understanding of the needs of each mother, infant and family. Rooming-in often is discussed as if it were a modern innovation. Historically, however, all mothers back to Paleolithic times "roomed-in" until the central nursery was instituted during the first two decades of the 20th century. Nevertheless, rooming-in as it is practiced today does represent a departure from the concept of the traditional central nursery (Fig. 21-14).

Attitudes in maternal and infant care have changed, in part because of increased insight into the needs of the mother, her baby, and the family as a unit. Rooming-in plays an important part in the family-centered approach to maternity care, for it not only provides an environment which fosters a wholesome, natu-

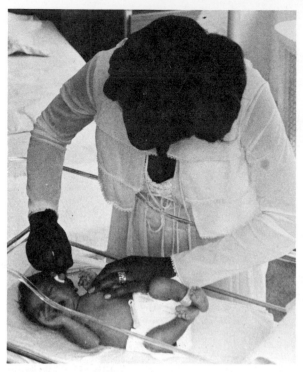

Figure 21-15. Rooming-in arrangement. Mother has opportunity to learn about her new baby. (Woman's Hospital Division, Hospital of the University of Pennsylvania, Philadelphia)

The newborn infant must be protected from sources of infection regardless of where he is cared for. The same basic principles for asepsis employed in the nursery must be followed in infant care in the rooming-in unit. Some years ago Dr. Edith Jackson said that it was possible to provide "the essential psychological satisfactions" which the mother and baby derive from a rooming-in experience "without losing the hard-won safeguards to physical health."[1] This has been demonstrated, for epidemic infections, such as diarrhea and skin infections, which sometimes occur in large hospital nurseries have not been observed in rooming-in programs.

Individual mothers must be taken into consideration as to whether or not they should have rooming-in. Some mothers will want to have their babies with them most of the time so that they can get to know them and learn to care for them under the guidance of the nurses and the physicians. Others, particularly multiparous mothers, may not want rooming-in because they feel that this is an opportunity for rest and freedom from responsibility. Many mothers feel that they would enjoy rooming-in but hesitate because they do not feel sufficiently able to assume the care or the responsibility for the baby at this time. These mothers need help, of course, to understand that the nurse is there to help them, and that they do not have to take over any more of the infant's care than they feel able or want to do. It is interesting to note that research has indicated that these negative feelings and qualifications are not as significant or widespread as one might think.[2]

ral mother-child relationship from the very beginning, but it also affords unlimited opportunities for the parents to learn about the care of their baby (Fig. 21-15).

To have a rooming-in program function successfully requires administrative planning and sound preparation of the entire hospital staff and the parents who use it. Generally, it demands a different architectural arrangement. Adequate space must be allowed for the mother's unit to accommodate the regular equipment needed for her, as well as that needed for the infant's care. Different physical plans for rooming-in arrangements have been developed, some units to accommodate one mother, others for as many as four of them. Each rooming-in unit should have an adjoining nursery and its own workroom. Where it has not been feasible to make major changes in the physical plan of a maternity hospital to provide for continuous rooming-in, some hospitals have adopted a modified rooming-in program, providing extended time for the mother and her baby to be together during the day but otherwise utilizing the central nursery.

Nurses with understanding and interest often can anticipate the mother's needs and desires and can be of invaluable help to her. Much of the practical care of the new baby must be learned by the new mother during her brief hospital stay to supplement the theoretical knowledge she has gained during the antepartal period. At this time the mother usually needs close supervision and guidance from the nurse so that she may develop confidence in her own ability to handle and care for her baby (Fig. 21-16). The father, also, may share in some of these experiences and learn much about his baby and his baby's care (Fig. 21-17). With this kind of preparation, parents of first babies in particular do not feel so helpless when they return home. These shared experi-

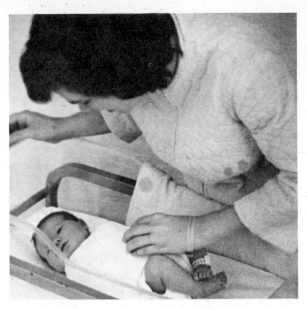

Figure 21-16. Maternal touch in an initial contact of mother with her newborn. (Woman's Hospital Division, Hospital of the University of Pennsylvania, Philadelphia)

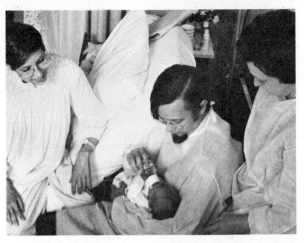

Figure 21-17. Rooming-in unit. Mother is assisting father to feed their baby as nurse observes. (Woman's Hospital Division, Hospital of the University of Pennsylvania, Philadelphia)

ences undoubtedly contribute to an excellent foundation for stable and secure family relationships.

Nursing care of the newborn

Initial care

In the delivery room the initial care has been given to the infant's eyes and the cord, and appropriate identification has been added. The baby should be observed to see that he is kept warm (a most important detail), that respiration is normal, that color is good, and that there is no bleeding from the cord (see Chapter 18).

It is customary in many maternity hospitals today to provide a "receiving" nursery on the labor and delivery division so that closer supervision and care for the infant may be assured immediately following the delivery.

Observations

As previously stated, the infant's natal day is the most hazardous during the postnatal period. Therefore, it is important that the nurse take particular care with her observations during the first 24 hours of the baby's life. The receiving or transition nursery in the labor or the nursery sections affords an excellent physical environment (similar to that of

recovery room care for adults) for the extensive observations that are necessary. In particular, high-risk babies (infants who have been exposed to or have experienced a prolonged labor, difficult labor, fetal distress, maternal complications during pregnancy and/or labor, respiratory distress, and so on) need intensive observation and often special equipment for their care, such as incubators, suction equipment, and the like.

BEHAVIOR AND PHYSIOLOGIC RESPONSES. Because these responses are indicative of normal reactions in the newborn, they should be observed and recorded, as well as any abnormal signs. For instance, the frequency and the type of cry are important, since the infant aerates his lungs in this way. Moreover, the type of cry may be indicative of cerebral damage (see Chapter 29). In a vigorous, normal infant, the cry should be lusty and should occur especially when the baby is handled or moved. If this does not happen, and the infant seems "sleepy" or depressed, it may be necessary to stimulate him to cry every hour or more frequently, depending on the degree of depression. This response may be aroused by changing his position or rubbing his back, head, or feet. Occasionally, with a drowsy infant it becomes necessary to slap or rub the soles of the feet *gently* to elicit the necessary cry. The time of the baby's first stool and voiding should be noted, to indicate proper excretory function. It is sometimes necessary for the nurse to check with the delivery room records to see whether the infant voided or defecated at delivery. Finally, the newborn's general activity, muscle tone and reflexes (especially the Moro and the sucking reflexes) should be observed. A healthy infant will be active, evidence good muscle tone, and respond with behavior appropriate to the various reflexes (see pp. 401 to 403).

RESPIRATION AND COLOR. These should be given close attention, for they are good indices of whether or not the newborn is experiencing respiratory insufficiency. Dyspnea, rapid respiration exceeding 50 breaths per minute, and persistent cyanosis should be reported to the physician. Since mucus in the nasopharynx often causes respiratory distress, the nurse should be particularly watchful for its presence. Gagging, vomiting, breath holding, retraction of the head, choking, and cyanosis are all signs of the presence of mucus, which is particularly prone to develop in the second period of reactivity following the first sleep. Postural drainage and the technique for aspirating mucus are explained in Chapter 29.

CONDITION OF THE CORD. This should be noted; any oozing or hemorrhage should be reported immediately, and the cord should be reclamped or retied as indicated. Oozing more often occurs between the second and the sixth hours of life and frequently is associated with crying or the passage of meconium.

THE BABY'S SKIN should be observed also for pallor and jaundice as well as cyanosis. Pressing the skin with a finger often enables clearer visualization of jaundice. The blanching that occurs with the maneuver provides a contrast that shows up the icteric color more clearly. The significance of pallor and jaundice in the first 24 hours is explained in Chapter 29.

THE INFANT'S TEMPERATURE should be checked frequently (every hour), and particularly if external heat is being applied. Even though the infant's temperature may have been quite low at first, he responds readily to external changes in temperature. Therefore, care must be taken that he does not become overheated. If the baby is placed in an isolette, the temperature of the isolette should be checked at frequent intervals.

Continuing care

CLEANSING. The daily cleansing of the infant affords the nurse an excellent opportunity for making the observations that are necessary during the immediate postnatal period. The materials used for the bath, its frequency, and so on, may vary from institution to institution. Several decades ago the daily soap and water and oil baths were replaced with merely wiping off excess vernix with dry or slightly moist cotton balls. The diaper area was cleansed as necessary. However, in view of the increase in staphylococcal infections in newborn nurseries, in many centers an initial sponge bath with a liquid detergent containing 3 percent hexachlorophene is used, with special attention to the cord and genital areas. For the remainder of the baby's stay, he is cleansed with plain warm water on cotton balls. Alcohol is sometimes placed on the cord. Just prior to discharge, the sponge bath with hexachlorophene may be repeated. Daily hexachlorophene baths are no longer recommended because of suggestive evidence of CNS damage following prolonged exposure. Thus some cleansing of the infant occurs daily, and the nurse should utilize the opportunity to inspect the baby thoroughly.

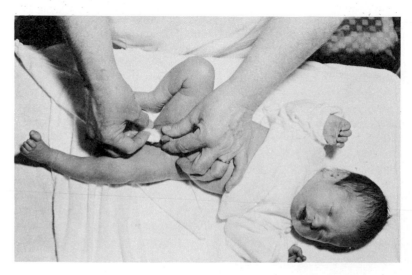

Figure 21-18. Retracting foreskin for cleansing penis (uncircumcised). (MacDonald House, The University Hospitals of Cleveland, Cleveland, Ohio)

ASSESSING THE MOTHER'S UNDERSTANDING. In the verbal exchanges with the mother during the daily care of the baby, it is important that the nurse assess the mother's understanding and her skill in caring for her infant. Any basic principles or procedures related to infant care that the mother finds necessary and useful should be part of the nurse's teaching plan for the mother during her hospital stay. A referral to a community health agency may be necessary to ensure appropriate follow-up, particularly if the mother is inexperienced. The following principles of care can be conveyed easily to the mother (and the father when he is present).

EYES. In the daily care of the baby, no special treatment other than necessary cleansing with sterile water is given the baby's eyes unless there is a discharge. Any redness, swelling, or discharge should be reported and recorded on the chart. There may be some reaction from the medication used for prophylaxis against ophthalmia neonatorum, but the physician will prescribe treatment if necessary.

CORD. Babies do not receive a tub bath until the cord has separated, and the umbilicus has healed. A cord dressing is considered to be unnecessary in most hospitals, since exposure to the air enhances drying of the cord; nevertheless, it is still used in some institutions. If a cord dressing is used, it is removed when it becomes soiled, or when the baby is taken to the nursery for its initial bath. If the cord is

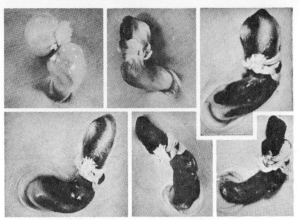

Figure 21-19. The umbilical cord drying.

left exposed to the air, some physicians prefer that the base be wiped with alcohol daily to encourage drying further and to discourage the possibility of infection.

No attempt should be made to dislodge the cord before it separates completely. If there is a red inflamed area around the stump or any discharge with an odor, this condition should be recorded and brought to the physician's attention immediately. The cord usually becomes detached from the body between the fifth and the eighth days after birth, but its detachment may be delayed until the twelfth or the fourteenth day without causing any concern (Figs. 21-19 and 21-20). When the cord drops off, the umbilicus is depressed somewhat and usually free from any evidence of inflam-

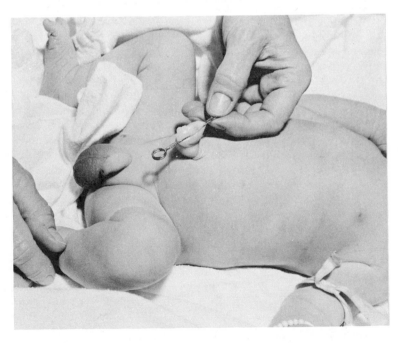

Figure 21-20. Inspection of cord stump.

mation. No further treatment is necessary, except to keep the part clean and dry. When inflammation is present, the physician will give specific orders for care.

ADHERENT FORESKIN. In a male infant, adhesions between the prepuce and the glans penis are very common. The foreskin may be extended beyond the glans. Reduction to a very small opening is called phimosis (see p. 407). A curdy secretion, *smegma*, may form in considerable amount and collect under the prepuce behind the glans. Also, small amounts of urine may be retained. Any of these conditions favor irritation and, if found, should be reported to the obstetrician. He may perform the delicate operations of separating the adhesions, stretching the prepuce, or circumcising the baby.

The manipulation following dilatation and retraction is difficult at first, and should be done gently. The foreskin must be replaced immediately; if not, edema may result, rendering the replacing difficult.

CARE FOLLOWING CIRCUMCISION. When the newborn infant is circumcised, the main principles of postoperative care are to keep the wound clean and to observe it closely for bleeding (see Fig. 21-11, p. 409). For the first 24 hours the area is covered with a sterile gauze dressing to which a liberal amount of sterile petrolatum has been added.

Mothers are naturally anxious about their babies at this time, so, as soon as it is feasible after the circumcision has been done, the nurse should take the baby to his mother for a brief visit. She can be reassured that the procedure has not been very painful for her child. The infant will cry during the operation, but this is due as much to the necessary restraints as to the discomfort. Occasionally, a local anesthetic will be used, but generally the procedure is performed without it. Thus, the infant may be fed immediately after the circumcision, and both mother and baby seem to enjoy the comfort that the feeding and cuddling bring. It is unwise, however, to keep the baby away too long from the careful observation of the nurse.

The infant's diaper should be applied so that only one layer of the material covers the penis. This lessens the danger of masking any bleeding that might occur. In changing the infant's diaper the nurse should hold his ankles with one hand so that he cannot kick against the operative area. Unless the physician orders otherwise, the circumcision dressing can be removed postoperatively when the infant voids for the first time. Cleansing must be done gently but can be accomplished as necessary with cotton balls moistened with warm tap water. A fresh sterile petrolatum dressing usually is applied to the penis each time the diaper is changed for the first day. The penis must be observed closely for bleeding, and during the first 12 hours should be inspected every hour. It is advisable to place the infant's crib where he can be watched conveniently. Moreover, to keep all the nursing personnel alerted, some signal, such as a red tag, can be attached to the identification card on the crib. If bleeding occurs, usually it can be controlled with gentle pressure. If bleeding persists, the physician should be notified immediately.

Since the length of the maternity stay has been considerably shortened, circumcision may be done on the second or the third postnatal day or even before the baby leaves the delivery room. To overcome the transitory coagulation deficiency, some physicians administer vitamin K_1 at birth. Sometimes the operation is performed on the day preceding discharge; therefore the nurse should ascertain the physician's wishes for aftercare and make certain that the mother knows how to care for her newly circumcised infant. Generally, the care will be the same as that described.

CARE OF FEMALE BABIES. Similar adhesions sometimes are found about the clitoris in female infants and, when observed, should be reported to the obstetrician. The smegma which may accumulate between the folds of the labia should be gently and carefully cleansed with moistened cotton balls, using the front-to-back direction and a clean cotton ball for each stroke. Occasionally, a slight bloody discharge may come from the vagina (see p. 408). This usually is due to a hormonal reaction and rarely reappears; cleanliness is the only treatment necessary. Very infrequently, the discharge may be caused by injury; if the discharge persists, it should be reported to the physician.

WEIGHT. The baby should be weighed on the birth date and every day or every other day thereafter. If the infant remains in the hospital longer than five days, he should be weighed at intervals prescribed by the medical staff. His weight should be recorded accurately.

During the first few days after birth the infant may lose 5 to 10 percent of his birth weight. This is due partly to the minimal intake of nutrients and fluid and partly to the loss of excess fluid. About the time the meconium begins to disappear from his stools, the weight begins to increase, and in normal cases does so regularly until about the tenth day of life, when it may equal the birth weight. Then the baby should begin to gain from 4 to 6 ounces per week during the first five months. After this time the gain is from 2 to 4 ounces weekly. At six months of age, the baby should be double his birth weight, and he should triple it when he is a year old. This is one way to note the baby's condition and progress; when the baby is not gaining, that fact should be reported to the physician. Besides gaining regularly in weight and strength, the baby should be happy and good-natured when awake and inclined to sleep a good part of the time between feedings.

PULSE AND TEMPERATURE. The clinical record of a normal baby should show a variation in pulse of 120 to 150. Only experience can teach a nurse to count an infant's pulse rate accurately (see p. 399). Touching his wrist will generally startle him and noticeably accelerate the heartbeat. The pulse can always be felt at the temporal artery to best advantage, particularly during sleep. The rectal temperature may normally vary a whole degree (see p. 400). A premature baby, who may have a temperature below that of a normal baby, will stabilize his temperature within 24 to 72 hours somewhere between 96 and 98° F., depending on his weight—the smaller the baby, the lower the temperature will be.

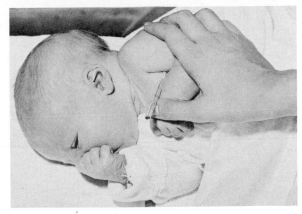
Figure 21-21.   Taking axillary temperature.

CRYING.   After the baby is born and has cried lustily, he becomes quiet and usually sleeps. After the eyes, the cord, and the skin have received the necessary care, he is dressed and placed in a warm crib and usually does not cry unless he is wet, hungry, ill, or is moved. A nurse soon will learn to distinguish an infant's condition and needs from the character of his cry, which may be described as follows. A loud, insistent cry with drawing up and kicking of the legs usually denotes colicky pain; a fretful cry, if due to indigestion, will be accompanied by green stools and passing of gas; a whining cry is noticeable when the baby is ill, premature, or very frail; a fretful, hungry cry, with fingers in the mouth and flexed, tense

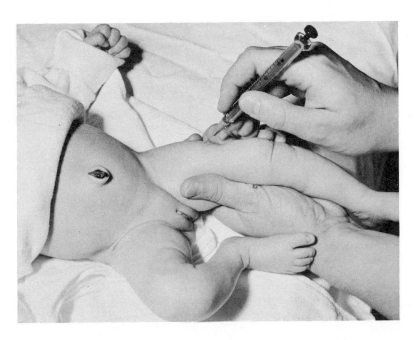
Figure 21-22.   IM injection for infant.

extremities, is easily recognized; and there is a peculiar, shrill, sharp-sounding cry which suggests injury. A nurse should make every effort to recognize any deviation from the usual manner in which a baby announces his normal requirements. Moreover, she should convey this information to the mother, since it is essential that the mother learn to interpret her infant's cues. The newborn has only his posture and his voice at this time to inform others of his needs.

Hypertonic Babies. Occasionally, the nurse will find that an infant seems to be fussy from birth. He appears very active, startles easily, cries readily and more frequently (and apparently for no reason), is alert and awake much of the time, and in general does not fit the usual pattern of activity, feeding, and sleeping described. Some physicians term these babies *hypertonic*, that is, they do not seem to be able to relax as well as other infants. The parents, particularly, may find their adjustment to their new baby difficult and anxiety provoking until they are informed (or learn by trial and error) that this is "normal behavior" for this child. Too often they assume they must be doing something "wrong," since despite their efforts, their baby remains fussy, tense, and crying. The nurse can be very helpful to the parents in giving them anticipatory guidance about their baby's behavior and helpful ways in which he can be soothed. She should inform the physician of her observations so that he may advise the parents appropriately. These infants usually respond favorably to being held securely. Thus, wrapping them snugly with a receiving blanket, cuddling them securely, changing their position slowly and surely rather than quickly all help to allay undue tenseness. Of course, rocking the baby and walking with him are particularly successful measures, but no parent can or should do this over protracted periods of time.

Any new activity or procedures should be introduced to this kind of infant slowly. For instance, when he is given a tub bath for the first time, he should be placed in a small amount of water very slowly and each lower extremity immersed gradually. This will help him to be less frightened and startled. The parents should not consider an occasional evening out a luxury; rather it should be considered a necessary item in the care of their baby. These infants do place greater demands on their parents than do infants of a more placid nature, and a short time away from the baby does wonders in restoring the perspective and good humor of the parents.

CARE OF THE SKIN. The skin is thin, delicate, extremely tender, and very easily irritated. Since the skin is a protective covering, breaks in its surface may initiate troublesome infection; hence skin disturbances constitute an actual threat to the baby's well-being.

The new baby does not perspire, usually, until after the first month, and he does not react to cold by having "goose flesh." In warm weather, or if the baby is dressed too warmly, he may develop prickly heat, a closely grouped pinhead-sized rash of papules and vesicles, on the face, the neck, and wherever skin surfaces touch. Fewer clothes and some control over the room temperature will help to relieve the discomfort.

Bathing. In the majority of hospitals today, elaborate procedures for bathing the infant have been discarded. It is recommended, as previously stated, that the skin be cleansed every other day with sterile cotton or a soft washcloth, and warm water. Blood is removed from the skin after the delivery, but no attempt is made to remove the vernix caseosa thoroughly unless it is stained with blood or meconium. The vernix caseosa serves to protect the skin and disappears spontaneously in about 24 hours. If it remains in the creases and folds of the skin longer than two days, it is apt to cause irritation. In this case gentle wiping usually removes it sufficiently. An inspection bath should be given, at which time the infant can be "spot cleansed" as needed with the moistened cotton balls. The use of strong soap, oil, and baby powder is discouraged by many pediatricians because of the sensitivity of the newborn's skin. The nurse should pay particular attention to cleansing (and drying) the scalp and all creases at the neck, behind the ears, under the arms, the palms of the hands and between the fingers and the toes, under the knees, the soles of the feet, and in the groin, the buttocks, and the genitals.

Basic Principles. Each nurse will develop her own manner of bathing the newborn according to her manual dexterity, the size and the activity of the infant, and the facilities available. Several basic principles should be observed.

First, all equipment, clothing, and supplies should be assembled so that the infant never is left alone or exposed unduly. Safety pins should be closed and placed out of the reach of the baby. Receptacles for soiled clothing, cotton balls, and so on should be available.

Second, care should be taken so that the environment is free from drafts and warm enough (i.e., 75 to 80° F.). The nurse should not have to interrupt the bath to close a door or a window. The water for the bath should be about 98 to 100° F. Water that feels warm to the elbow is approximately that temperature.

Third, in giving the bath the nurse should proceed from the "cleanest" areas to those that are "most soiled." Thus, the eyes are bathed first, then the face, ears, scalp, neck, upper extremities, trunk, lower extremities, and finally the buttocks and the genitals. Each of these in turn is washed, *rinsed well*, and dried. To prevent undue exposure, a portion of the infant can be undressed at one time, bathed, and then redressed.

Finally, *the infant never should be left alone*, even on a large work area; one hand should be kept on him at all times.

Demonstration and Practice. Each mother should have an opportunity to observe a demonstration of a sponge bath and, if at all possible, to give a bath to her infant. The various principles enumerated above can be conveyed to the mother readily. In addition, the nurse should explore with the mother what facilities are available in the home so that the necessities can be met and undue expense and difficulty avoided. For instance, a large drainboard which can be washed and padded adequately (and is a comfortable height for handling the infant) can be utilized for the bath area. A large pan or basin does very well for the bathtub in the early weeks; it should be kept only for the baby's use. Thus, the extra expense of special equipment can be minimized.

On returning home, a daily sponge bath using a soft washcloth and mild soap is recommended until the cord has fallen off and the area is healed. After this, a tub bath can be given. The mother is also advised to wash the baby's hair when she gives the baby a sponge bath. The same soap the baby is washed with, or any brand of baby shampoo can be used. She should be told not to put any kind of baby oil in the hair, as this may predispose to "cradle cap."

The cord tie should be left in place until the cord drops off; the clamp is removed in 24 hours, provided that the umbilical stump has dried sufficiently. The nurse should observe whether the skin is clear, pink, cyanotic,

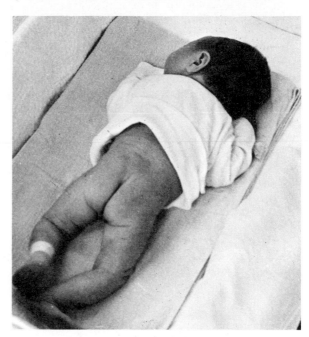

Figure 21-23. Exposing buttocks to air.

blotchy, or jaundiced and if there is dryness present.

Buttocks. Sometimes, despite good nursing care, the infant's buttocks become reddened and sore. A diaper rash may occur which is caused by the reaction of bacteria with the urea in the urine. This in turn causes an ammonia dermatitis. The most important prophylaxis lies in keeping the diaper area clean and dry. Sometimes, petroleum jelly, baby oil, or a bland protective ointment, such as vitamin A and D ointment, is prescribed by the physician. Pastes may not be advised, because they are much more adhesive than ointments and thus create cleansing problems.

A simple treatment which is often effective is merely to expose the infant's reddened buttocks to air (Fig. 21-23) and light several times a day, using care to keep the infant covered otherwise. Warm daylight may be all that is necessary, although the use of a *lamp* treatment is more effective, and at the same time provides a measure of warmth. An ordinary gooseneck lamp with a screened bulb (no stronger than 40 watts) can be placed on the table so that it is a foot or more away from the infant's exposed buttocks. The light may be used for 30 minutes at a time. Because the skin is already irritated, the nurse should exercise care not to burn it further by using too strong a bulb or placing the light too close.

If the condition occurs at home, the treatment described above also is appropriate, and the mother can be so instructed. Boiling the diapers is another effective measure, since this destroys the bacteria. However, many of the detergents and conditioners used today have antibacterial agents in them; these may be effective in washing the diapers. Care should be taken to rinse the diapers thoroughly, since the residue of the detergent in itself can be irritating. In this respect, the modern diaper services have very effective facilities; many sterilize diapers and entire layettes as part of the service.

SLEEPING. The baby will need rest and sleep with as little handling as possible. If he is well and comfortable, he usually sleeps much of the time and wakes and cries when he is hungry or uncomfortable. He may sleep as much as 20 hours out of 24 (although this varies considerably from infant to infant). It is not the sound sleep of the adult; rather he moves a good deal, stretches, and at intervals awakens momentarily. Since he responds so readily to external stimuli (and this may make him restless), his clothing and coverings are important. They should be light in weight, warm but not too warm, and free from wrinkles and "bunches." His position should be changed frequently when he is awake. He can be placed on either side or on his abdomen, especially when he is ready for sleep. If he is positioned on his back, someone should be present, for if the baby regurgitates, he is more likely to aspirate in this position. As he gets older and learns to roll over, he will assume the position that he likes most for sleep.

INTESTINAL ELIMINATION. During fetal life the content of the intestines is made up of brownish-green tarlike material called meconium. It is composed of epithelial and epidermal cells and lanugo hair that probably were swallowed with the amniotic fluid. The dark greenish-brown color of the meconium is due to the bile pigment. During fetal life and for the first few hours after birth, the intestinal contents are sterile. Apparently, there is no peristalsis until after birth, because normally there is no discoloration of the amniotic fluid.

Stools. For the first five or six days, the stools gradually change from meconium to transitional stools (after which they become the regular milk stools). During this time the color of the stools changes from tarry black to a greenish black, to greenish brown, to brown-

ish yellow, and thence to greenish yellow. The transitional stools are composed of both meconium and milk stools; hence their variation in color. After the transitional stools the color gradually changes to a soft yellow of a smooth pasty consistency with a characteristic foul odor if the infant is formula-fed. Stools of breast-fed infants tend to be golden yellow and of mushy consistency. Most newborns pass the first stool within 12 hours of birth—nearly all have a stool in 24 hours. If an infant has not passed a stool by this time, intestinal obstruction must be considered as a possible reason for the delay, and the baby must be observed closely. The number of daily stools on about the fifth day of life is usually four to six. As the infant grows, this number decreases to one or two each day. The type of stool may be influenced by the mother's diet. However, there may be slight variations from the normal, which may have little significance if the baby appears to be comfortable and sleeps and nurses well. If the baby's stools have a watery consistency, are of a green color, contain much mucus, and flatus is being passed, the condition may be evidence of some digestive or intestinal irritation and should be reported to the physician. The number, color, and consistency of stools should be recorded daily on the baby's record.

URINARY ELIMINATION. Urinary activity of the fetus is evidenced by the presence of urine in the amniotic fluid. The baby usually voids during delivery or immediately after birth, but the function may be suppressed for several hours. However, if the baby does not void within 24 hours, the condition should be reported to the physician, as retention of the urine may be due to an imperforate meatus. After the first two or three days the baby voids from 10 to 15 times a day. When the urine is concentrated, red or rusty stains on the wet diaper may be due to uric-acid crystals in the urine.

Infant feeding

The newborn's ability to handle food

One of the major physiologic adaptations which the infant must make in the transition from intrauterine to extrauterine life concerns the source of his nourishment and the ability to take food into his body, to digest it, and to assimilate it. During prenatal life the nutritive substances for growth and handling of waste products are provided for by means of the placental circulation (see Chapter 8). Thus, prior to birth the gastrointestinal tract has not been required to utilize muscle, chemical, or absorptive activity in handling food. The digestion and the absorption of food is, like the respiration of air, a function that the infant has had no opportunity of practicing during its fetal career. Following delivery not only must the gastrointestinal tract begin abruptly to process a rather large amount of food, but the infant must begin to suck and swallow to take the food into his stomach. The infant's capacity to take the food in and digest it is adequate when the food is appropriate (i.e., breast milk or milk formula) and when it is appropriately given.

CERTAIN IMPORTANT CONSIDERATIONS in relation to the development of the infant's digestive apparatus and infant feeding will be recalled here, because they have a direct bearing on feeding practices.

Sucking and Swallowing Reflexes. The infant's ability to take in food through his own efforts demands the ability to suck and to swallow. At birth the sucking and swallowing reflexes are already present, and normally they are quite strong. It is known that the swallowing reflex, as well as peristaltic movements in the stomach, become active during the last two months of fetal development, because bits of vernix caseosa and lanugo are found with other debris in the meconium stool. The nurse who has witnessed the birth of babies can easily recall how the infant is able to swallow mucus, and how sometimes, even while the initial care is being given in the delivery room, the infant will begin to suck on anything that gets near his mouth.

Stomach and Intestines. At the time of birth the infant's stomach is small, its capacity is approximately 50 to 60 cc., but it is capable of considerable dilatation. During feeding the infant's stomach is able to stretch to at least three or four times its approximate capacity. It is not merely distended by the amount of food taken in (i.e., milk), but also by the amount of air the infant swallows as he sucks the milk or cries. In the act of crying, the infant tends to gulp in air.

The gastric musculature is somewhat deficient at birth. In contrast, the glandular structures in the mucosa are present, although shallow in contrast with those of the adult. The relatively greater length of the intestinal tract and the weakness of the abdominal muscula-

ture to serve as a supporting structure explain in part the reason that considerable distention of the stomach is possible.

Although gastric digestion is not considered to be a factor of primary importance to the nutrition of the newborn infant, many of the findings reported by Clement Smith in his textbook could be useful in the consideration of infant feeding schedules. For example, the stomach empties more slowly in the newborn period than any other time in life. However, the distended stomach is able to adjust its content by promptly emptying some or all of its content into the duodenum. A number of the studies on gastric motility have demonstrated wide individual differences in emptying time. The major portion of the feeding usually leaves the stomach in less than three or four hours, although the greater portion of this occurred one and one-half to two hours after the meal. In some instances, the emptying time of the infants' stomachs took more than eight hours. It was found also that the introduction of a second feeding before the stomach was empty caused portions of the first feeding to remain somewhat longer in the stomach than if the stomach was emptied from the last feeding before the next was offered. Another important finding is that human milk leaves the stomach somewhat more rapidly than cow's milk, although a formula made of cow's milk which has been boiled leaves the stomach more rapidly than that which is fed without this additional preparation.

INFANT NUTRITION. In the last several decades progress in scientific developments has made artificial feeding (formulas) very much like human breast milk in chemical composition. Although it is generally considered that the best food for the baby is that designed by nature—human breast milk—the individual differences in mothers and babies must be considered in the practical situation. It is the mother who makes the decision of how she wants to feed her baby, and the nurse should support her in this decision.

Some advantages of feeding breast milk are: it is exactly the correct chemical composition for babies, is constantly available (and no preparation is necessary), is at an even temperature, is free from bacteria, and causes a lower incidence of allergy, and contains beneficial antibodies and other substances that protect the infant against infection.

In artificial feeding, the differences in ca-

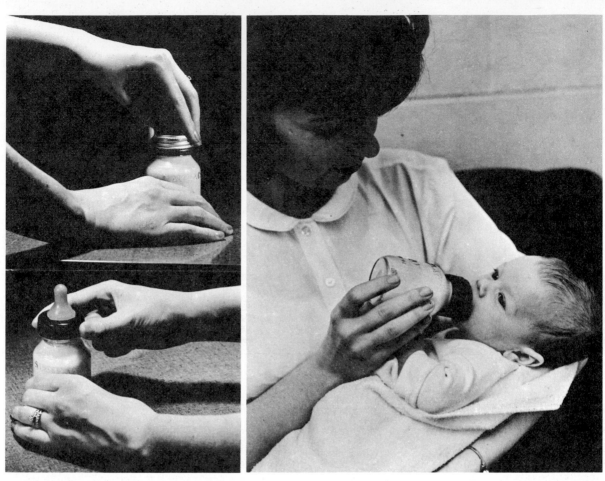

Figure 21-24. The ready-to-use commercially prepackaged sterilized formula provides a safe, simple three-step feeding for the convenience of the mother at home. At feeding time, *(left, top)* remove lid, *(left, bottom)* apply sterilized nipple, and *(right)* feed the baby. Ross Laboratories, Columbus, Ohio)

loric allowances required for various infants will depend on: 1) the individual nutritional needs and 2) the infant's rate of growth. All of the infant's nutritional needs, except that for growth, can be met by providing 33 calories per pound per day. When the component necessary for growth is added, approximately 42 calories per pound per day will be required. One might anticipate that by the time some infants are 10 to 14 days old, they may consume 55 calories per pound per day, but this should not be followed rigidly.

SELF-REGULATORY FEEDINGS. A permissive feeding regimen for newborns means that babies should be offered as much formula or feeding as they seem to want and should not be forced to take the amount prescribed unless forcing has been specifically ordered by the responsible physician.

The variation in baby readiness and the desirability of individualizing the time of start-ing feedings needs to be stressed. The time of initiating feedings will depend on evidence of the infant's hunger and the readiness of the baby. Once the first feeding has been offered, the routine or prescribed schedule for offering feedings should be followed.

The permissive feeding regimen for breast-fed newborns may require even more flexibility. A mother who is breast-feeding may desire to begin breast-feeding her baby before the time specified by hospital routine for the first water feeding, as sometimes happens when the nursery requires that the first feeding be water and given by the nurse prior to other feedings. Unless there is a maternal complication or contraindication, every baby should visit his mother at each feeding time, starting with the first feeding of "breast" or "bottle," but excluding the 2 A.M. feeding period for the first visit unless the mother wants to see her baby at this time.

COMPOSITION OF HUMAN MILK. Breast milk, as it leaves the mother's breast, is a sterile fluid. It should have an alkaline or possibly a neutral reaction, but never an acid reaction. Colostrum cells should be absent after the twelfth day, and the fat globules should be small, numerous and of uniform size.

Milk is a natural emulsion and consists of about 10 percent of solids and 90 percent of water. The solid substances are fat, sugar, proteins, and salts. The fat of milk is the cream, the sugar is the kind known as *lactose*, or *milk-sugar*, and the protein makes up the bulk of the curd.

Artificial feeding

Although breast-feeding is again gaining favor, formula feeding has become the predominant mode of nurture for infants born in American hospitals today.

The most significant change to come into the hospital newborn nursery in more than 50 years (i.e., since the advent of the central nursery system) is the use of disposables and unit packaging. This includes ready-to-feed formulas in disposable containers (Fig. 21-24).

Prepared milk mixtures in throw-away containers with sterile nipple units attached represent the newest development in infant feeding in the hospital. The prepared milk mixtures are said to have features which improve on evaporated milk or whole milk formulas.

In artificial feeding it is necessary to modify the milk to approximate as nearly as possible the chemical and the physical characteristics of human milk. When human milk and cow's milk are compared, the difference in fat and protein content needs to be considered. Cow's milk is diluted, and therefore carbohydrate is added to the newborn infant's formula. It is generally accepted that even normal fat in milk (3.5 percent) is poorly tolerated. Thus, cow's milk is diluted essentially to lessen the fat component of the formula. In addition, when whole milk is diluted, the casein curd is more flocculent in the infant stomach and thus aids in the digestion of milk. In diluting the formula, the carbohydrate of milk is also diluted inadvertently and should be restored to the original amount (4.5 percent) or more to furnish additional calories for optimal nutrition and weight gain. The added carbohydrate may be in the form of granulated sugar, corn syrup, or a commercially prepared carbohydrate modifier. Added carbohydrate permits normal metabolism of fats, allows protein to be used to build new tissues instead of serving to provide calories, and encourages normal water balance.

The physician will prescribe the formula for the infant and give specific directions concerning its use. Various milk formulas are used today: diluted pasteurized milk with added carbohydrate, diluted evaporated milk with or without carbohydrates added, fresh skim milk, powdered skim milk, or one of the brands of prepared milk preparations (see Table 21-1).

Table 21-1 Comparative Data on Relative Components in Human Milk, Cow's Milk and Evaporated Cow's Milk in Normal Dilution

| Type of Milk | Normal Dilution | | Approximate Percentage Composition in Normal Dilution (Gm. per 100 ml.) | | | |
	Ratio	Cal./Oz.	Protein	Fat	CHO	Minerals
Human Milk, average	undiluted	20	1.2	3.8	7.0	0.21
Cow's Milk, market average	undiluted	20	3.3	3.7	4.8	0.72
Cow's Milk, evaporated (many brands)	1:1	22	3.8	4.0	5.4	0.8
Commercial Premodified Milks:						
Infant Formula, Baker	1:1	20	2.2	3.3	7.0	0.6
Bremil with Iron, Borden	1:1	20	1.5	3.5	7.0	0.5
Modilac, Gerber	1:1	20	2.2	2.7	7.8	0.4
Enfamil, Mead	1:1	20	1.5	3.7	7.0	0.3
Similac with Iron, Ross	1:1	20	1.8	3.4	6.6	0.4
SMA S-26, Wyeth	1:1	20	1.5	3.6	7.2	0.25

Source: Adapted from Vaughn, V. C., III, M.D., and McKay, R. J., M.D. (eds.): *Nelson Textbook of Pediatrics*, ed. 10, Philadelphia, W. B. Saunders Co., 1975, p. 174.

Of these milk formulas, the most widely used formula is diluted evaporated milk with added carbohydrate. It should be noted that evaporated milk has several advantages: It is safe because it is sterilized in an unopened can, it is convenient to store, the cost is relatively low, and the formula is simple to prepare. An evaporated milk formula for the newborn infant is usually made up of one part evaporated milk diluted with two parts of water and carbohydrate in sufficient amount to meet the required calories.

ESSENTIAL NUTRITIONAL REQUIREMENTS are a basic consideration in the computation of a formula for the newborn infant. Certain "rules of thumb" concerning nutrients and formula computation are as follows:

1. *Proteins.* One-and-one-half ounces of cow's milk per pound of body weight equals 1.5 Gm. of protein per pound, which equals one-tenth of body weight.
2. *Carbohydrates.* One-tenth ounce per pound of body weight equals 1 ounce per 10 ounces of milk prescribed, which also equals 1 percent of the body weight. One-third of the carbohydrate should be derived from the milk of the mixture, and the remainder added in the form of starch or sugar. Later in the first year, the carbohydrate is given in the form of a starch cereal, and the carbohydrate in the milk formula may be reduced at that time.
3. *Fats.* Anywhere from 3 to 5 percent is included, no specific amount being stipulated. If the fats are restricted, a larger amount of protein or sugar, or both, is required for energy sources. The suitable quantity of fat is supplied in amounts of milk which furnish the required amounts of protein. An excess of fat is not to be desired.
4. *Minerals.* An adequate mineral-salt intake is supplied to any infant when 1½ ounces of milk per pound of body weight are given. Enough iron is stored in the liver of the normal infant (from the hemoglobin breakdown after birth) to suffice until about the fourth or fifth month. This deficiency is usually made up by the addition of the solid food supplements (egg yolk, fortified cereals, vegetables, and fruit) which are usually added before this time, except in the completely milk-fed infant who refuses or is not offered these iron-containing foods in the first year.
5. *Water.* The requirement for water varies from 10 to 15 percent of the body weight, or may be expressed as 1½ to 2½ ounces per pound of body weight. This is supplied in the milk itself, in the diluent of the milk mixture, and supplemented to instinctive demands by offerings of water and fruit juices between feedings.
6. *Calories.* The average requirement for growth in the first year is 50 calories per pound of expected weight, two-thirds of this caloric need being supplied by the milk and one-third by the added carbohydrate.

FORMULA COMPUTATION. A simple problem with which to apply the basic rules of formula computation would be the food needs of an infant weighing 10 pounds at two months of age, having weighed 6 pounds at birth. This infant would probably take 3 ounces more than his age in months (2) which would be (2 months plus 3 equals 5) 5 ounces per feeding. In 24 hours he probably would be satisfied with five feedings; hence, he would need 25 ounces in a total 24-hour period.

Example—Whole Milk Mixture

1½ oz. whole milk per lb. of body weight (10 lb.)	Milk, 15 (fluid) oz. = 300 cal.
1 oz. CHO [carbohydrate] per 10 oz. milk used	Cane sugar, 1½ oz. = 180 cal.
Diluent to make up total 24-hour amount	Water, 10 (fluid) oz.
5 feedings of 5 oz. each	25 (fluid) oz. = 480 cal.

Calorically, this should effect normal growth since it provides 48 calories per pound. Should it not provide normal weight increase of about 5 to 7 ounces per week, or should the infant fail to be satisfied by evidencing signs of hunger, the milk proportion could be increased, or the total amount be enlarged, or additional CHO added, or all of these procedures could be changed to fit the particular infant's specific needs.

In calculating a formula with evaporated milk and a corn syrup for the same hypothetical infant, the construction would be as follows:

1 oz. evaporated milk per lb. body weight	Evap. milk, 10 (fluid) oz. = 440 cal.
1/10 oz. CHO per lb. body weight	Corn syrup, 1 (fluid) oz. = 120 cal.
Diluent to make up total 24-hour amount	Water, 14 (fluid) oz.
5 feedings of 5 oz. each	25 (fluid) oz. = 560 cal.

With this mixture the calories are increased to 56 per pound, which might easily be tolerated by the infant, especially if he were active and hungry and needed more food.

DIRECTIONS FOR MAKING FORMULA. The hands should be washed before assembling the equipment. All equipment used for the preparation of the formula should be kept separate (Fig. 21-25). If bottled milk is used, the outside of the bottle should be washed with soap and cool water as soon as received, and the bottle should be placed in the refrigerator. If canned milk is used, the top of the can should be washed with soap and water, using friction, and thoroughly rinsed. Hot water should be poured over the top just before it is opened. All equipment should be washed thoroughly in warm soapy water and rinsed well so that no milk film remains to hold bacteria.

BOTTLES AND NIPPLES. The 8-ounce bottle is a good size to use and should be graduated in ounces and half ounces so that it will be possible at all times to know exactly how much food the baby has taken. A sufficient number of bottles and nipples should be sterilized to supply the feedings for the 24-hour period. It is always safer to have one or two extra bottles and nipples in reserve in case of breakage.

The shape of the bottle should be such that every part of the inner surface can be reached with a brush to facilitate cleaning.

The holes in the nipple are usually small, but they may be made the required size by heating a fine sewing needle with its eye fixed in a cork (used as a handle). The point is held in the flame until red hot, then accurately plunged into one of the three holes and withdrawn quickly. The procedure needs practice before holes of proper size can be made. Some nipples have crucial incisions instead of punctured holes to prevent them from clogging.

The test of proper hole size is made by holding the bottle, filled with milk and with the nipple attached, upside down. The milk should escape drop by drop, and if it runs in a stream, the hole is too large. The objection to the large hole is that the baby nurses too rapidly, which causes indigestion, colic, and other disorders. If the stream is very rapid, the baby may have difficulty in swallowing.

ASEPTIC METHOD. In this method, the bottles, nipples, nipple caps, and equipment used in making the formula are sterilzed before the formula is prepared. The mother will need a glass or enamel pitcher in which to mix the formula, a measuring cup, measuring spoons, tablespoon (to mix the formula), funnel (depending on the size of the bottle mouth), can opener (if canned milk is used) and some kind of tongs that can be sterilzed. The tongs will be used as a forceps to handle the equipment. These items, together with the bottles, caps, and nipples are placed in a large pan or sterilizer half full of water and boiled vigorously for ten minutes. The equipment and the bottles, nipples, and so on, may be done separately if the sterilizer cannot accommodate such a large load. Care should be taken to place the forceps in such a way that the handles can be reached

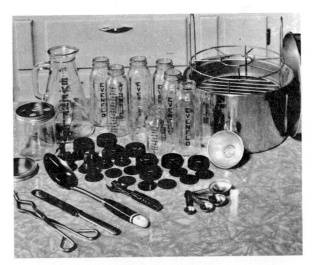

Figure 21-25. Formula equipment. Sterilizer with bottle rack and tight-fitting lid; six 8-ounce nursers (for formula) and two 4-ounce nursers (for water and orange juice) complete with nipples, caps, and sealing disks; quart-sized formula pitcher with clearly marked graduations; nipple jar with perforated (for sterilizing) and solid lids; long-handled tongs; table knife; long-handled mixing spoon; can opener; set of measuring spoons and a funnel-strainer. (Pyramid Rubber Company, Ravenna, Ohio)

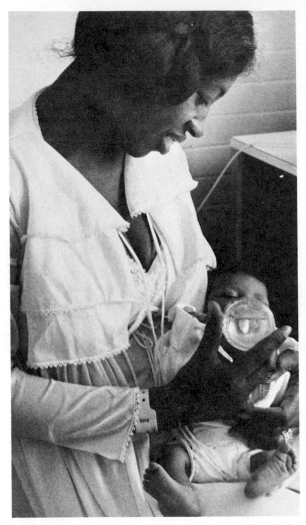

Figure 21-26. Mother feeds formula to her newborn baby. Note correct angle for holding baby's bottle. (Woman's Hospital Division, Hospital of the University of Pennsylvania, Philadelphia)

boil rapidly in the bottom of the sterilizer for 25 minutes. In this method, formula, bottles, nipples, and protectors are all sterilized in one operation. Before the formula is refrigerated, the screw collar should be made secure. The majority of hospitals use the autoclaving method, but in the home the procedure immediately above is used. In each method, the formula must remain sterile and the nipple untouched and sterile until it reaches the baby's mouth.

There are various kinds of bottles and nipples on the market, many of which are sold as units (bottle, nipple, and nipple protector).

HUNGER. If the baby is not getting enough food, he will wake before his regular nursing time and be obviously hungry. He will cry and fret, refuse water with apparent disgust, and when a feeding is offered, seize the nipple ravenously and nurse with great vigor. Often for the very young infant, increasing the amount of feeding is all that is necessary. For an older infant, increasing the concentration of the formula and/or its amount may be necessary. Solids sometimes are introduced at this time to help allay the hunger. Occasionally, a baby appears to be hungry between feedings when in reality he is only thirsty. He may be given a small amount of tepid boiled water to satisfy his thirst.

BUBBLING. After five minutes or so, or in the middle and at the end of each feeding, the infant should be held in an upright position and his back *gently* patted or stroked (Fig. 21-27). Pounding the baby on the back vigorously is neither effective for bubbling him nor conducive to his well-being. The change in position (from semireclining to upright) is the important factor in eliciting a bubble. Often holding the infant upright and pressing him against the breast is all that is necessary. Because the new infant's gastrointestinal tract is labile, milk may be eructated with gas bubbles. Care should be taken to ensure adequate bubbling before the infant is placed back into the crib, thus preventing milk regurgitation.

REGURGITATION. Regurgitation, which is merely an overflow and often occurs after nursing, should not be confused with vomiting, which may occur at any time and is accompanied by other symptoms. This regurgitation is the means of relieving the distended stomach and usually indicates that the baby either has taken too much food or has taken it too rapidly.

easily after sterilization. If the mother must reach into the water for them, she contaminates the water, and hence, the materials being sterilized. After sterilization the formula is made according to directions. A specific amount of the formula is put into each bottle. The bottles are then nippled, capped and refrigerated.

TERMINAL STERILIZATION. In this method, the formula is prepared under a clean but not aseptic technique. The equipment, bottles, nipples, and nipple caps are washed thoroughly but are not sterilized. The formula is prepared and poured into the bottles, and the nipples and the caps are applied loosely. They then are placed in the sterilizer, covered with a tight-fitting lid and sterilized by having the water

Assisting the mother feeding her infant

The feeding of the baby is one of the first tasks which must be achieved in the mothering role. The young inexperienced mother undoubtedly will need guidance, assistance, and emotional support in feeding her new baby whether she feeds him by breast or by bottle. The help given by the nurse in the first feeding experiences not only helps the mother to deal with her anxiety in handling the new baby and in coping with the manipulative problems related to feeding him, but it lends her the emotional support that she so desperately needs in surmounting her own stress in the situation. The mother who has never handled a small infant before, being confronted with a sleepy or a squirmy infant, can feel all the more inadequate as she realizes that the responsibility to nourish this "bundle of joy" is hers.

THE ENVIRONMENTAL CLIMATE surrounding the feeding of the baby should be peaceful and unhurried (see Figs. 20-7 and 20-8, pp. 384 and 385). The mother should be rested and ready. She should not have been rushed through a previous task, such as the morning bath or other daily care routine procedures, to meet a deadline imposed by the baby's feeding schedule. The nurse who brings the baby to his mother should avoid hurrying him to his mother's bedside, pushing the crib into the room, and leaving at once with the remark, "I'll be back to give you your baby as soon as I get the other babies out." Meanwhile, the mother looks at her hungry fretful baby in his crib, and often she is afraid to pick him up lest she be reprimanded for failing to wait for the return of the harassed nurse.

EXPANDING CONTACTS WITH THE BABY. When babies are kept on a routine feeding schedule in the conventional maternity hospital, the mother's contacts with her baby are sometimes limited to the feeding period. It is unfortunate when the mother feels she must begin to feed her baby the moment she takes him into her arms. Feeding often takes up most of the time mothers and infants are together in the hospital, leaving little opportunity for their getting acquainted otherwise. Smith has described a plan whereby the demand feeding regimen to meet the needs of the individual baby was successfully achieved in a maternity hospital.[3] To provide some flexibility in the routine schedule, babies easily could be brought to their mothers at least 15 minutes before the feeding

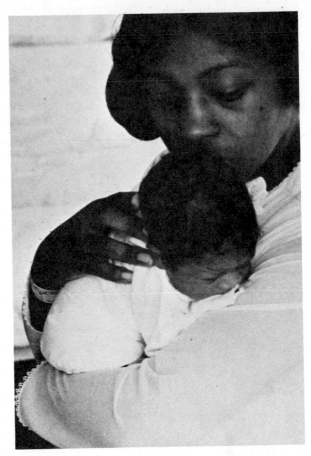

Figure 21-27. Bubbling the baby. (Woman's Hospital Division, Hospital of the University of Pennsylvania, Philadelphia)

time and left with them for a similar period of time afterward, if the mothers so desired, without disrupting hospital routine. This plan would relieve some of the mother's stress at the beginning of the feeding period by allowing her more freedom to hold the baby leisurely, look at him or fondle him as she chooses. For mothers who are breast-feeding, this contact would have a positive effect on the let-down factor.

GETTING INSIGHT INTO THE MOTHER'S GOALS AND PROBLEMS. One must always bear in mind that each mother has her own goals in each new maternity experience. The astute nurse will utilize opportunities to assist the mother in achieving the mother's goals in accordance with the mother's individual capacity. Some time spent in purposeful conversation with the mother in addition to the time when her baby is with her may help the nurse to gain further

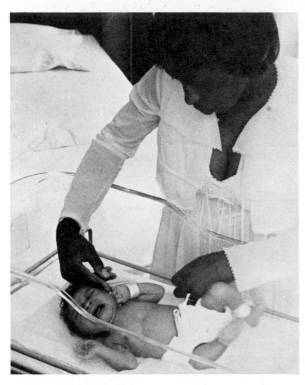

Figure 21-28. Mother uses her fingers to stroke her baby's cheek. (Woman's Hospital Division, Hospital of the University of Pennsylvania, Philadelphia)

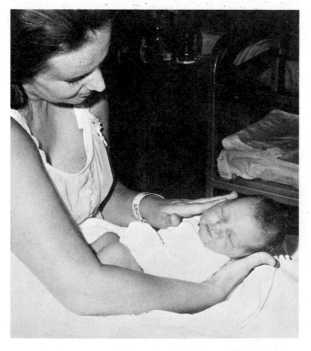

Figure 21-29. Mother uses her fingers to stroke cheek of her sleeping baby. (MacDonald House, The University Hospitals of Cleveland, Cleveland, Ohio)

insight into the mother's concerns. Even when hospital staffing is limited, the nurse who organizes her activities thoughtfully usually can find the "extra" time to accomplish what she considers to be the most important components of patient care.

One of the most obvious ways for the nurse to support the mother in the feeding experience is to stay with the mother until both mother and baby are settled, and then, in leaving the bedside to let the mother know that she is immediately available. The nurse who takes time to listen to what the mother is saying and to observe the interaction between the mother and baby often can identify problems that the mother is experiencing.

For example, the nurse left Mrs. Bee comfortably feeding her 2-day-old son. When she returned to the room ten minutes later, Mrs. Bee looked up and said, "He only sucked for 2 minutes and now he's asleep. Look at him. Is his skin a little yellow? I can't make him take any more." Most mothers will verbalize their concerns, though they may not ask directly for help. In this instance the nurse responded with concern, "You wonder if he's had enough to eat?" The mother responded as she looked down at the baby, "Yes," and then went on to talk about her awkwardness in handling the baby and the bottle at the same time. She said, "I wonder whether perhaps I have tired the baby."

The nurse meets the mother's concern half way by her inquiry. At the same time, she must use judgment not to create concerns that do not exist. Responding to the mother's remarks in a way that leaves the conversation open and encourages the mother to express her concerns is not only helpful to the mother, but also likely to give the nurse important clues about what the mother at the moment feels are "problems." The words that the nurse uses to speak with the patient are important, but even more important is the feeling communicated in this interaction between two people.

The mother and her newborn

With the birth of her baby the mother must assume a new role, along with all its concomitant tasks and responsibilities. Moreover, these adjustments must be undertaken before physical and psychologic restoration from pregnancy and labor is complete. Since the adaptation to motherhood usually evolves as a slow, often

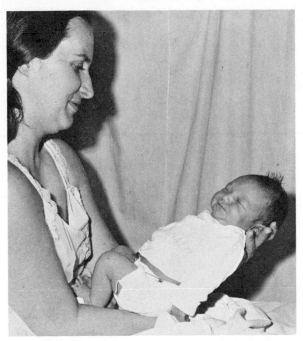

Figure 21-30. Mother holds sleeping baby on her forearm to look at him. (MacDonald House, The University Hospitals of Cleveland, Cleveland, Ohio)

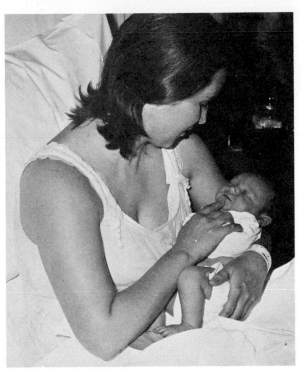

Figure 21-31. Mother cradles baby in her arm. (MacDonald House, The University Hospitals of Cleveland, Cleveland, Ohio)

unconscious modification of the individual's attitudes and activities, the professionals who provide for the mother's and the infant's care in the hospital are not always cognizant of what mother and baby experience in the early days of homecoming.

The literature on the development of maternal behavior (see Suggested Reading) tends to support the fact that primigravidas are generally more awkward and anxious and have more early concerns about their abilities to care for their newborn than do multiparas. One cannot assume that because the newly delivered mother seemingly makes a "good adjustment" during the first days after birth in the hospital that the adaptation will be smooth and uncomplicated after she returns home. This early period of adjustment—particularly during the first week of the infant's life—is a crucial one. Thoughtful nursing intervention at this time can make a significant contribution to the welfare of the family. Therefore it becomes important to ask what the nurse in the hospital might do to prepare the mother more adequately for coping with problems that she may encounter on going home with her new baby.

Carpenter interviewed mothers of first-born infants to determine the kinds of help they needed for themselves and their babies in the first months at home following delivery.[4] She reported that mothers in the lower socio-economic groups not only have more difficuties than their more affluent neighbors, but are also less likely to have assistance from relatives or friends, or the services of a private physician. In relation to their own health, concerns most frequently mentioned were about the condition of the perineum and breasts, fatigue and depression. The mothers expressed needs in relation to feeding and other care-taking activities for their babies. In addition, they felt they needed better understanding of the baby's behavior, especially the normal ranges of infant behavior.

Presently, more seems to be known about maternal attitudes and practices in general than about the specifics of maternal behavior —at least that assumption can be made from what appears in the literature. How do mothers interact with their babies? What clues can be observed of mother and baby in a reciprocal relationship that inform us about the nature of the indentification process? (See Figs. 21-28 to 21-31.) To provide appropriate nursing care it becomes important to know, for example, how mothers behave when they feed their babies.

Some mothers care for their babies as if they are very fragile things. These mothers are task-oriented and approach routine care of their babies completely separate from social interaction. Their interaction, for example, does not evoke the baby's smiles or vocal responses.

Maternal touch has reciprocal value for both mother and infant. The mother uses her fingers, hands and arms to explore and fondle her baby as she begins to establish a relationship with the baby. As she caresses the baby she is going through identification processes with him which assist her in "claiming" him as her baby. This is significant for the infant in his growth and learning. For the maternity nurse these understandings should make the difference in the quality of her care. Mothers should not only be given the opportunity to look at and learn to care for their babies in an unhurried fashion while they are in the hospital, but they should have planned opportunities for social experiences with their babies. In many maternity hospitals mothers must wait until the nurse, or her assistant, hands the baby to his mother to be fed, and then relinquish him to the nursery personnel when he has hardly finished feeding because this is the "routine."

Mother's concerns about their babies

Every new mother experiences concerns to some degree about caring for her newborn infant. The mother who has had other babies may feel quite confident in performing the mothering tasks for the baby, but at the same time she may wonder how on returning home she ever will be able to manage her time and energy to give all the children and her husband what they need and what she would like to give them. On the other hand, the mother with her first baby may have many early concerns about fulfilling the infant care activities, such as feeding and bathing the baby, if she has had little or no experience.

FEEDING THE BABY. This is a major concern during the first weeks. The mother's questions usually are related to the amount and the frequency of feeding. The first days after delivery the mothers ask how to prepare formula, but by the end of the week they are more interested in getting answers to questions about how to feed the baby, how often to feed, and the amount of feeding. Mothers who are breast-feeding want to know about the adequacy of their milk supply. "Is he getting enough?" is a frequent question.

BATHING THE BABY is another task that mothers must learn to carry out, one that often causes concern. At first the task itself seems most important, thus, how to bathe the baby (i.e., the procedure, seems most urgent). But after new mothers have had some experience in handling their infants, they are more interested, as homegoing approaches, in learning how they are going to hold a squirming, soapy baby during his bath, and how to bathe him in a tub.

THE BABY'S CRYING is of greater concern to mothers after the first week of life. When the baby spends most of his time in the hospital nursery, the mother may not get a chance to hear him cry, and she may wonder whether he can. One mother was ready to go home from the hospital (on her fifth postpartal day) and had never heard her baby cry. As the nurse wheeled his crib into the room that morning, the baby was crying lustily from hunger. The mother's face lighted up with great satisfaction as she said, "Now I *know* he can cry!" Mothers want to know why the baby is crying. With appropriate anticipatory guidance in the hospital, they can be helped to learn about the infant's communication through crying and how to interpret various kinds of crying.

OTHER CONCERNS. According to Adams, "concerns are areas of special interest or worry to mothers as indicated by questions pertaining to particular areas of care." Other questions they ask are related to care of the navel and/or circumcision, sleeping, taking the baby outdoors for the first time, hiccups, weight gain, rashes. Fathers, too, have concerns about tasks they must learn, particularly how to hold and to handle the new baby.

THE RELATION OF TEACHING TO AREAS OF CONCERN. An understanding of how new parents view their problems with infant care activities must underlie any preparation for teaching mothers and helping them to learn about their babies and their care. The small group demonstrations of the infant bath and formula preparation are rather basic, but they need to include time for mothers' questions to be answered. There is a real need to have small group discussion conferences for new mothers, where they can initiate the conversation in the presence of a professional nurse who can act as a discussion leader or resource person.

Clinical study: a nurse and a new mother

A clinical study in maternity nursing was carried out for the purpose of studying the nurse-patient interaction and nursing intervention with a young primigravida during the early puerperium. There was conscious evaluation of the nurse-patient interaction by the nurse during the relationship. Also, there was an attempt to apply psychosocial concepts to this situation by reflecting on the psychodynamics of behavior. Because Olive Rich's writings have particular significance for maternity nurses, she has graciously consented to share them with the authors for use in this textbook (see Suggested Reading).

The clinical experience

The patient selected, a 24-year old primigravida, had no major complications during pregnancy, labor, or delivery. The nurse had daily contacts with the patient for seven days, beginning with the day of delivery and extending through the day of discharge. The nature of the contacts varied. At times the contact was solely for verbal and nonverbal interaction; at other times other facets of nursing care were included (e.g., assisting the mother with breast-feeding and teaching her how to carry out manual expression of breast milk). After the mother's discharge, the nurse had three significant contacts with the patient in her home and three significant contacts by telephone. In the course of this experience, there was only one direct interaction of the nurse with the patient alone. The patient had the same roommate throughout her hospital stay, and at home her mother and mother-in-law were both present— the latter intermittently—during the first two contacts with the nurse.

This clinical nursing study is directed to an examination of the possible dynamics involved when a patient who has made a good adjustment in the hospital suddenly encounters major problems on arriving home with her new baby. During the early postpartal days the patient's behavior was assessed by several staff members in the hospital setting as confident, mature, "doing just fine," and physically able and calm. In contrast, after the first 52 hours at home the young mother found herself fatigued and depressed. As she summarized it: "I just wasn't prepared for all this."

So that the student can understand and evaluate the nursing intervention, a fairly detailed description of the patient in the hospital and on the nurse's first visit to the home will be presented. As a further basis of understanding, concepts of the psychodynamics of pregnancy and childbearing as presented by selected authors will be discussed. Application will be made to this unique patient situation in the areas in which data are available. Finally, there will be some evaluation of the means of nursing intervention that were utilized and some reflective questioning about what other measures might have been of further help in preparing this mother for being at home with her baby.

The first seven days

The nurse's first contact with Mrs. X was on the afternoon of her day of delivery. Although Mrs. X had been in labor for more than 24 hours and had not slept for about 36 hours, she was sitting up in bed, making preparations to have her baby for a visit. She had seen her baby briefly on two previous occasions but had not held him. The nurse brought the baby from the nursery, placed him in his mother's arms, and waited for her comments. At first she looked and looked, not touching the baby's face but holding him quite securely.

PATIENT: "I don't know why, I expected him to be a towhead. I was when I was born. (*After a pause*) I don't see any forceps marks. They've trimmed his fingernails. Are his eyes blue?"

NURSE: "Most babies' eyes tend to be more blue than brown at first. What color would you say your eyes are? Your husband's eyes?"

PATIENT: "Mine are hazel. His are brown."

NURSE: "It is possible that you could each have the characteristic of blue eyes to pass on to a child."

PATIENT: "He looks like his daddy."

NURSE: "What part of him? Can you tell?"

PATIENT: "No, not really. His nose maybe."

NURSE: "You can unwrap him if you'd like."

PATIENT: "He has big feet. Look at his long toes."

Mrs. X continued for about the next 30 minutes to hold the baby quite comfortably and to comment about him in a similar vein. Little pauses threaded her observations as she went on: "He was a very active baby when I was carrying him. What's he doing? Is he hiccupping? What can he really see? He has a nice pink color. Does he have a bridge in his nose? I was born without one. Has he been given water yet? His ears are so big! At least they seem to be, in relation to his head."

The questions and comments were stated rather matter-of-factly with a certain objectivity and a seeming lack of involvement, as though she were commenting on any baby in the nursery. Mrs. X did not speak to the baby, kiss him, or show much change in voice or face during the first prolonged encounter with her baby. The nurse remained with the mother the entire time and offered once to take the baby back to the nursery, assuming that she might be tired, but she wanted to keep him longer.

These observations of the mother's first holding of the baby are presented in considerable detail because they introduce Mrs. X's continued relationship with her baby as the nurse saw it in the hospital. Mrs. X, of course, gained skill in handling the baby but continued to relate to him in a matter-of-fact manner. No spontaneous expression of delight in her child was observed.

Mrs. X made an apparently rapid physical recovery from childbirth. Even on the day of delivery she was able to sit on her episiotomy and did not complain of perineal pain. The gastrointestinal and urinary systems readily assumed normal functioning. The mother made no complaint of afterpains, even when nursing the baby. She had only minimal engorgement of the breast tissue and only occasional nipple tenderness during her seven days in the hospital. Mrs. X's perception of her postpartal status was similar to this. On the day after delivery she was sitting on the side of her bed, with her legs hanging down. The nurse attempted to intervene.

NURSE: "Some mothers like to sit that way for feeding their babies. But they don't think about the fact that they've no backrest and no support for their arms, and that their feet hang down without support. They don't understand why they're tired until after it happens. Wouldn't you like to lie down in your bed or sit in the arm chair for feeding the baby?"

PATIENT: "No, I'm just fine. I feel good. I felt just fine all during pregnancy. You know, I worked until the seventh month."

On another occasion:

NURSE: "I see you have skim milk."

PATIENT: "That was my only problem during pregnancy—weight gain. I must have gained 30 to 35 pounds."

Other persons commented about Mrs. X's well-being. Her mother said, "I'm proud of how well she's done." The obstetrician spent a minimal amount of time with her during his hospital rounds. She had few questions and had "no problems." The pediatrician commented, "That's the kind of mother it takes to be successful with breast-feeding—one who's calm and doesn't get all flustered." Her roommate, who had a 16-month-old child whom she had breast-fed for several months, commented, "She's *so* mature." Whenever other nurses were asked about Mrs. X, they would report, "Oh, she's doing real well. She's just fine."

Mrs. X appeared to adjust with minimal difficulty to her first mothering task, that of feeding the baby. The baby nursed the first time the breast was offered and at fairly frequent intervals during the prelactation period. Mrs. X didn't appear to be upset about some of the baby's sleepy times during this period. She would hold the baby, but not overstimulate him or urge him to nurse. There were no problems concerning the configuration of the breast or nipple for breast-feeding. About the third postpartal day Mrs. X had some engorgement, and by the next day she had milk enough to effect a gain in the baby's weight. He continued to gain, and she was kept informed about his daily gain in weight until they were discharged from the hospital.

Although the nurse observed that Mrs. X did not express much spontaneous delight in her baby, the following interaction should be noted:

PATIENT: "Will the baby be coming to me at 2 o'clock this morning?"

NURSE: "You don't have milk yet, do you? There's no reason to disturb your rest until you have milk for the baby. Do you want to tell the nursery nurse, or should I?"

PATIENT: "I think I would like to have him —just to hold him."

NURSE: "Are you sure you don't need the rest? The purpose for bringing him at 2 A.M. is for his feeding and your comfort in relieving the milk, once it comes in. You may have him, if this is what you wish."

PATIENT: "I would like to have him."

Mrs. X said that she could use the signal system to call for anyone or to ask for anything during her hospital stay, but that it wasn't necessary; she had whatever she needed. From observation and discussion it seemed that Mrs. X was offered the "usual" guidance given to a new mother by the nurses. She had some assistance the first few days during the feeding periods, and she was included in a demonstration class for mothers on bathing the baby. She was presented with the possibility of her baby's being in her room for two to three hours in the afternoon for an "extended visit." (During this time the mother has the opportunity to observe her baby, to diaper and dress him, and to feed him if she desires.) Mrs. X took advantage of the extended visit during the last two afternoons she was in the hospital.

There were several instances of cues which verbally portrayed some of Mrs. X's need for instruction and guidance. The following exchange occurred in the first meeting:

NURSE: "I would like to help you with getting acquainted with your baby and with being a new mother."

PATIENT: "Sure. I don't know very much."

Several days later:

PATIENT: "I don't know just what I'm supposed to eat when I'm breast-feeding."

Then, several days later:

PATIENT: "They're going to bring him in to be with me from 1 to 4 P.M. tomorrow afternoon. I can diaper him and dress him. I need this kind of opportunity."

And still later:

NURSE: "Some doctors have printed instructions about their views of baby care."

PATIENT: "I hope mine does. There's so much I need to know."

On the second day of the extended visit experience the nurse came into the room and found the babies of both mothers asleep.

PATIENT: "I've had a busy time changing diapers and shirts."

NURSE: "What went on?"

PATIENT: "Well, he was messy before the feeding, so I changed him. Then I nursed him for five to six minutes, and he needed changing again. I had his clean diaper partly on him, and he voided all over his shirt and diaper. So I changed his shirt for the first time. There are three dirty diapers and a dirty shirt in the paper sack. They should have brought me a shopping bag!"

This was stated with a bit of humor accompanied by a moderate degree of frustration in the voice. (The nurse did not attribute any particular significance to these comments at this time.)

The patient expressed some concern and frustration about the length of her labor.

PATIENT: "Just how do you tell how long labor is? I had my first contraction at 3 A.M. on Sunday, and the baby wasn't born until 5 A.M. on Monday."

NURSE: "It's hard to judge when labor begins. Some of the early contractions are helping to thin and soften the cervix—and are useful. We call that prelabor. They don't accomplish anything very dramatic, though."

PATIENT: "I had a lot of back pain. I finally called the doctor, and he said to come into the hospital. But they slowed down when I got here. It would have been easier to stay at home longer. I had hardly dilated at all when I got here. If I'd been home, I could have been up and around. I was lucky, though. I was able to be up to the bathroom. There's no place to walk. I guess they don't like you walking up and down the corridors up there. The doctor had to give me something to stimulate labor, but then it wasn't too long—about three or four hours."

NURSE: "I don't know how one prepares a first-time mother for labor. Was it anything like you expected?"

PATIENT: "You can read a lot, and people can tell you. But you don't really know what to expect until you experience it yourself. I'm glad it's over, though, because I didn't know what it would be like."

NURSE: "I think mothers have two kinds of feelings about labor. They're eager to have it begin—"

PATIENT: "They're anxious to have the baby here."

NURSE: "They're tired of carrying that heavy uterus around. It's awkward."

PATIENT: "That never bothered me. I always felt fine."

NURSE: "Was that your main impression, that labor was long, and there was a lot of back pain?"

PATIENT: "Yes. I had no pains in the front, only pain in the back. I don't remember too clearly, because they gave me some medication to sleep. Dr. O said it would be a long time."

On another occasion (following the attendance of both patients in the room at the baby bath demonstration on Mrs. X's fourth postpartal day):

PATIENT: "They used the baby of another one of Dr. O's patients, one who delivered just 50 minutes after I did. There was a sort of race to see who'd get to the delivery room first."

NURSE: "You made it."

PATIENT: "Yes, but she'd come in only a few hours before."

NURSE: "And you'd been at work for at least 20 hours."

PATIENT: "Yes, and then some. I hope it won't be so long the next time. It shouldn't, should it?"

NURSE: (*To patient's roommate*) "Is it, Mrs. A? Was it as long this time?"

PATIENT'S ROOMMATE: "No, but I have rather short labors. My first was only eight-and-one-half hours, and this one was five hours."

NURSE: "That's right. You're the one who has babies quite easily."

PATIENT: "You're lucky!"

Further discussion about labor continued (not all included here).

NURSE: "At least you're ready to have one more."

PATIENT: "Yes."

PATIENT'S ROOMMATE: "When I had my first baby, I said on the delivery table, 'Well, I'm ready to have another.'"

PATIENT: "I don't think I'd have said that."

NURSE: "But by the fourth day you are ready."

PATIENT: "Maybe even two days ago I'd have said it."

In summary, the nurse's evaluation of the patient at the time of homegoing was as follows:

1. She experienced a minimal amount of (physical) discomfort, less than what the nurse had observed in the immediate puerperium of a primipara in a long time.
2. She was concerned about her baby's welfare, although she related to him with some degree of objectivity and distance. She proceeded with the mothering skills of feeding, dressing, and handling him with considerable naturalness and lack of apparent frustration. She didn't request much assistance from the nursing or medical staff in relation to her care or the baby's.
3. She seemed to have realistic plans for managing when she went home. Her mother-in-law lived with them and could assist with cooking, cleaning, and answering the telephone. Her mother would come at intervals to assist with the laundry and heavier duties. Her husband would be there evenings and nights, and she would take care of herself and the baby.

The more dominant themes would lead one to assume that she would manage at home in a similar manner with maturity, calmness, and matter-of-factness. The nurse herself would always have assumed so, had she not been privileged to see Mrs. X at home on the ninth postpartal day.

After first 52 hours at home

The nurse called the X residence about 6:15 P.M. on the day after the mother's discharge from the hospital. This time was selected to fit into the family's usual 5:15 P.M. dinner hour, as described by Mrs. X during her hospital stay. The purpose of the nurse's call was to determine whether this would be a suitable time to visit the family at home. Mrs. X's mother-in-law answered the telephone but soon called her son, because Mrs. X was feeding the baby.

PATIENT'S HUSBAND: "Hello."

NURSE: "Good evening. How's the new father?"

HUSBAND: "Pretty good."

NURSE: "I had mentioned to your wife that I might stop today, but that I would call first to see how things were going."

HUSBAND: "She's running a little behind schedule. We're going to have our dinner as soon as she's finished feeding the baby."

NURSE: "Perhaps I should wait and come tomorrow—or another time."

HUSBAND: "The baby was kind of fussy around 2."

NURSE: "2 P.M.?"

HUSBAND: "No, 2 A.M. this morning. I guess she was up most of the night with him."

NURSE: "Has she had any rest today?"

HUSBAND: "Not too much. Her mother said she would come over for a while this evening."

The conversation continued a short while. The nurse indicated that she would call again the next day to ascertain an appropriate visiting time. The nurse telephoned about 1:30 P.M. the following day.

PATIENT: "How are you?"

NURSE: "How are *you* is the question."

PATIENT: "I guess I'll survive."

NURSE: "You guess you'll survive?"

PATIENT: "I've just finished feeding him. He

seemed hungry. He nursed for about 20 minutes. I'm getting him settled now."

NURSE: "How did it go last night?"

PATIENT: "He slept real well from about 11 P.M. to 2:15 A.M."

NURSE: "That was over three hours."

PATIENT: "Then he had a fussy period after I fed him. He didn't go back to sleep until about 4:30. I gave him some water. He took about 2 ounces. Then I had to wake him about a quarter to 8."

NURSE: "That was pretty good. He slept more than three hours *that* time."

PATIENT: "My husband was up with me, too."

There was further telephone discussion about feeding, and the nurse made arrangements to come for a visit within the next few hours.

Mrs. X was seated in an armchair. The front of her dress was open, but the brassière was in place. The baby was dressed in a kimono and wrapped in a receiving blanket. Mrs. X looked pale and tired. She didn't look up right away. The nurse sat down on a hassock near the mother's chair.

NURSE: "How are things going by now?"

PATIENT: "I just wasn't prepared for all this. I felt so good in the hospital."

PATIENT'S MOTHER: (*Rubbing lotion on creases of infant's arms and legs*) "I told Mary when she was pregnant that she ought to go to some classes, and she said, 'What do I want to go to classes for?'"

NURSE: "I don't really know *how* parents can be prepared for these early days. Classes help some, but perhaps one needs to experience them. I don't know if you can really get prepared!"

PATIENT'S MOTHER: "I think he's growing. I think I can see him growing."

NURSE: "You think you can see him change each day?"

PATIENT'S MOTHER: "Yes, I think I'm enjoying the baby more than Mary. She's so tired—and she has the responsibility."

Mrs. X excused herself. While she was gone, her mother commented:

PATIENT'S MOTHER: "She hasn't had much sleep. She's very tired. Everything's so new to her. I came over Monday night a while so she could get some rest. Now I helped with the laundry and bathed the baby just before his feeding."

Mrs. X returned with her mother-in-law and introduced her to the nurse. She sat down in the living room now, where the four adults were seated, and where the baby was asleep in his bassinet.

NURSE: (*To patient*) "I see you have something here to drink."

PATIENT'S MOTHER: "She's not eating very well. Says she's not hungry. I made her a steak sandwich for lunch. She only ate half of it—and some salad and some milk."

NURSE: "When you're so tired, it's hard to be interested in food."

PATIENT: "I just have to force myself. I'm not hungry."

NURSE: "What about fluids? Are you drinking plenty?"

PATIENT: "I'm drinking quite a bit. Milk, fruit juices, water."

NURSE: "How has today gone in comparison with yesterday?"

PATIENT: "Everything's so new. Things all seem to come at once. I don't know where to start. I've never been around babies much. Some people have younger brothers and sisters; others have baby sat. I never did much of that, at least not with such a small baby. Not even with my niece and nephew. My sister-in-law was so protective that even my mother couldn't get close to the baby."

NURSE: "There are a lot of young women who haven't had the benefit of caring for small babies."

PATIENT: "Everything's so new. I just want to do the right thing." (With this statement her eyes became watery and red, and the tears nearly spilled over.)

MOTHER-IN-LAW: "Mary's doing a fine job."

NURSE: "You had some question last night about how long the baby was nursing, and how to keep him awake. How has this been today?"

The discussion continued with details for feeding and other events surrounding the baby.

PATIENT: "Last night my husband said, 'You're never going to breast-feed another baby!'"

NURSE: "Why do you think he said that?"

PATIENT: "He compares our baby with my brother's child, who takes 8 ounces from the bottle and sleeps all night. He forgets that he's a 2-month-old baby!"

The discussion focused for a while on bathing the baby.

PATIENT: "I haven't done that yet. I'll need to take hold. There's so much I don't know about. It's different seeing it done than doing it."

NURSE: "Perhaps right now, if you're tired, it's just as well to let someone else bathe him. *You're* the only one who can feed him. Others can do some of the other things."

PATIENT: "I'm used to work. It's not that. I worked in an office for six years. I began to work even when I was in high school, when I was 15. You grow up fast under those circumstances."

NURSE: "You probably needed to have things pretty carefully scheduled, to work full time and to manage a house and take care of your husband."

PATIENT: "You can say that again."

NURSE: "Now you have a squirming, crying bundle that doesn't fit into any schedule. Remember, Dr. M said he's not even sophisticated enough to know he shouldn't have his fussy periods at night."

PATIENT: "If you only knew when it would *end*, you know—not even on the day, but which *week*."

NURSE: "If there were only some limits which you could count on, you mean, knowing that sleeping through the night would happen by such and such a time."

PATIENT: "It's not knowing that's hard."

Further conversation revealed that Mrs. X had expressed some of her feelings by crying, and that her husband had found her weeping when she'd gotten up to be with the baby during a fussy time at night. The nurse gave some guidance about scheduling, feeding, placement of the baby's crib, and she answered questions of Mrs. X and her mother. It was near the dinner hour, and the nurse made plans to visit again in a few days.

Just by chance Mrs. X's mother met the nurse in a distant part of the hospital. The following remarks are excerpts from the mother's comments: "My daughter was so sure of herself during pregnancy. I wanted her to go to prenatal classes to learn about babies, but she didn't want to.... She feels so inadequate. I wasn't prepared for her depression. She seems to feel so inadequate about the bath."

The expressed concerns of Mrs. X's mother added weight to the previous question of what was happening to cause such a marked change in Mrs. X's behavior and performance in her new role. What facets of nursing care in the hospital could have been utilized to prepare Mrs. X more adequately for coping with problems on her return home?

At the beginning of the third day, 52 hours after she returned home, Mrs. X seemed to experience the low point of her "depression." The following day the baby began to sleep longer between feedings. Mrs. X began to get more rest, her appetite improved, she felt stronger, and she bathed her baby. There were still frustrations and problems to be handled, but they seemed to be more manageable. For instance, on Monday of her second week at home, the nurse telephoned at 3:30 in the afternoon to see whether she might stop for a visit. Mrs. X said that everything was topsy-turvy, and that she was still trying to get herself dressed. However, she had bathed the baby, and she was preparing dinner. The following week the nurse made her third visit to the home. It was her first contact with the patient alone. Although the nurse was aware that the "right moment" had probably passed for helping Mrs. X with the distress she expressed by nearly crying, she did introduce the subject. The following interaction occurred with some expression of feeling, but there was no weeping or overt manifestation of anxiety as the "first 52 hours" were discussed.

NURSE: "You've been home a little more than a week now. Is it what you expected? Anything like what you envisioned it would be?"

PATIENT: "I had *no* idea what to expect. I was never with small babies. I just didn't know how much time and work a baby would take. It's a 24-hour responsibility."

NURSE: "Those first days must have been pretty difficult. You must have felt a bit helpless at not knowing what to do when the baby cried."

PATIENT: "Yes, they were. Sunday wasn't so bad. I'd just come home, and people were around. My mother was here. But then Monday mother had to work, and my husband went to work, I was alone with the baby except for my mother-in-law. I knew how to change a diaper, but that was about all. I wanted to do the right thing for the baby."

NURSE: "I'm sure a mother wants to respond to her baby's needs, but deciding what is the right thing is hard. It is a lot of responsibility, to be a mother, a parent."

PATIENT: "I think we're getting acquainted. I can tell his cry when he's hungry; I can tell when he has gas by the way he draws up his legs."

NURSE: "You are more certain about making decisions as to what to do for him? You can decide when he needs milk—or water?"

PATIENT: "Yes. This week is so much better than last."

NURSE: "Did other things bother you those first days—beside not knowing what to do with the baby? The house?"

PATIENT: "Well, yes. I do have certain ways of doing things, and when other people help, they can't know how you do them. I've always been very healthy."

NURSE: "So you're not accustomed to having people help you?"

PATIENT: "No, I've always been quite independent. I've worked since I was 15. I worked until my seventh month of pregnancy. I felt so well in the hospital."

NURSE: "Yes, we kept talking about that, and kept looking for some problems, but—"

PATIENT: "There weren't any. Not even my stitches hurt after the second day."

NURSE: "When you came home, you hit a low point."

PATIENT: "I wasn't prepared for being so depressed. I guess it's called the 'baby blues.'"

NURSE: "Some people have this experience in the hospital. Did it happen to you there?"

PATIENT: "Not really—maybe only once. One evening my husband didn't come to see me because he wasn't feeling well, but he didn't tell me until later. That upset me, because I wish he'd tell me. Maybe I could do something to help him."

NURSE: "You probably haven't felt so helpless in a long time as you did those first several days."

PATIENT: "No, I haven't. If we have another baby, I'd know more what to expect...."

It may be helpful to have further information about Mrs. X and the significant people in her environment. Mrs. X is the younger of two children born to parents of different religious faiths. Although her father is in the family picture, Mrs. X did not once refer to him. Mrs. X's mother, on the other hand, has played an active role. She visited her daughter in the hospital and assisted her daughter with household tasks on the days in which she was not working. The mother commented that her daughter has always been a "good girl," and that she never had to worry about her when she was out on a date. If she were going to be late, she'd always call. Some of the interactions previously shared might provide some clues about her opinion of her daughter's adequacy as a mother.

There is little information about Mrs. X's brother except that he has been to college, is married, is the father of two children, and lives with his family in a nearby suburb. On the other hand, Mrs. X mentioned twice that she had gone to work when she was 15 (there are gaps in information here as to the reason for working and the nature of her work). On graduation from high school Mrs. X went to work as a bookkeeper and continued to work in that position through the seventh month of her pregnancy.

Mr. and Mrs. X have been married for several years. Mr. X, who is nine years older than his wife, has been employed as a craftsman with the same company for the past 13 years. Mrs. X spoke with delight in her voice and her face when she told that her husband was thinking of painting a banner with the words "Welcome home, Mary and Johnny." On the day of discharge from the hospital, when the nurse first saw them together, they seemed to relate with warmth but with a certain self-consciousness and reserve. He was attentive in helping her into the car.

The nurse observed the new parents together briefly on two occasions in their home. On the day Mrs. X was so depressed, she eagerly listened for sounds of the car as the time for her husband's homecoming drew near. When he did come into the living room, she immediately offered to get his slippers. On another occasion he slipped his arm around her waist as she was in the kitchen warming a bottle of water for the baby. The X's are not in financial distress; they have two cars, hospitalization insurance, more than adequate equipment for the baby, and are buying a new suburban home.

They are eager to move into their new home. The advent of the baby has crowded them, since Mr. X's mother also lives with them in their two-bedroom house. This necessitates placement of the baby's equipment in their bedroom and the baby in the living room. Mrs. X's mother is an elderly woman who has a serious chronic illness. Mrs. X expressed her desire to contribute toward making a home for her mother-in-law and making her life as pleasant as possible. She commented several times on how well she and her mother-in-law got along. When the nurse was in the home, Mrs. X's mother-in-law was friendly and courteous, but she kept busy with her household tasks instead of joining in the conversation.

Comments and conclusions

The concept that pregnancy is a period of disequilibrium and maturational crisis needs to be reiterated to professionals working with women during the childbearing cycle. This may need special emphasis in relation to the woman who has an uncomplicated pregnancy and childbirth experience, since it is usually the woman with problems and complications who occupies the major portion of the nurse's attention. Pregnancy involves profound physiologic and psychologic changes. An intensive longitudinal study of 15 women during pregnancy and the first year after delivery was conducted by Bibring *et al* in Boston. The theoretical framework on which the study is based is as follows:

> Pregnancy is a crisis that affects all expectant mothers, no matter what their state of psychic health. Crises, as we see it, are turning points in the life of the individual, leading to acute disequilibria which under favorable conditions result in specific maturational steps toward new functions. We find them as developmental phenomena at points of no return between one phase and the next when decisive changes deprive former central needs and modes of living of their significance, forcing the acceptance of highly charged new goals and functions. Pregnancy as a major turning point in the life of a woman represents one of these normal crises, especially for the primigravida who faces the impact of this event for the first time. We believe that all women show what looks like remarkable, far-reaching psychological changes when they are pregnant. The outcome of this crisis, then, has profound effects on the early mother-child relationships.[5]

The final results of the study have not been published, but they may contribute significantly to understanding the nature of the crisis and the maturation expected.

Bibring states that the crisis does not end with the birth of the baby but continues into the puerperium and perhaps beyond:

> The findings that crisis continues, more or less so, beyond parturition offer strong support in favor of the proposition that the frequent problems in the early mother-child relationship are partly due to an as yet incomplete reorganization of the mother's psychic equilibrium at the time of delivery.[5]

Deutsch agrees that the crisis period extends beyond the delivery of the baby.[6]

Pregnancy and childbirth could be discussed much more extensively as a general crisis, but it may be more helpful to investigate some of the possible components of the crisis and to reflect on those which may be applicable to Mrs. X's situation. The first several post-hospital days illustrate an obvious crisis period for Mrs. X.

Components of the crisis situation

A very complex component of the crisis and disequilibrium has to do with the relationship of psychosexual development and maternal feelings.

Deutsch[6] writes extensively about motherhood, pregnancy, confinement and lactation in relation to Freud's concepts of psychosexual development. For example, breast-feeding the baby may arouse the erogenous area of the nipple and create sexual sensations. The nursing mother may be confused by the aroused sexual feelings and the feelings of love and responsiveness as she nurses her baby.

There is limited data from which to assess Mrs. X's situation in regard to the psychosexual component. Mrs. X appeared to be rather matter-of-fact about the process of breast-feeding. She would prepare the nipple for feeding in the presence of her roommate and the nurse, and she allowed the nurse to touch her breast to assist the baby in obtaining proper grasp of the areola. She practiced the technique of manual expression of breast milk at the same time her roommate was practicing, although a certain degree of privacy was planned during this teaching-learning experience.

Mrs. X did not ask questions of the nurse or the obstetrician concerning the appropriate time for renewing sexual intercourse in relation to the process of vaginal and perineal healing. The nurse introduced the subject, and Mrs. X seemed to appreciate the guidance offered, since the obstetrician had not included this in his homegoing instructions.

On three different occasions the subject of subsequent pregnancies and child spacing was indirectly introduced by giving information in relation to breast-feeding and ovulation. Mrs. X did not pursue the topic with further discussion or questions. She seemed to remain somewhat guarded and reserved in all of the relationships, and thus one would expect that she would maintain this reserve in the area of psychosexual material.

Closely aligned with the psychosexual component of the crisis is Caplan's description of the change in equilibrium between the ego and the id. He likens the usual relationship of id and ego to an iceberg, the portion above the surface being the ego and the portion below the surface being the id. During pregnancy the iceberg turns upside down and allows id material to come to the surface rather easily. Fantasies and wishes are consciously expressed with a relatively minimal production of anxiety.

Caplan describes the pregnant woman as a kind of battery that needs to be charged. If those significant to her are not able to meet her needs for being nurtured, she may have more difficulty in extending herself to her child during those early months when the child has many needs but gives little to the mother in response to the fulfillment of those needs.

There is very little data about Mrs. X's period of pregnancy except that she felt fine and continued to work until the third trimester of pregnancy. One would, however, question the degree to which she was allowed to be dependent and to receive care during the early puerperium in the hospital. She did "take in" rest and food, but on the day after delivery she was already taking her own bath in the shower. She had no obvious or particular reasons to request or demand nursing or medical care. One could question whether she might have been better fortified to cope with the baby at home if there had been more attention to the "battery-charging" process.

There are clues that Mrs. X is a "giving" person who does not ask much for herself. She was accustomed to giving herself to a job and to her family. She invested herself in her mother-in-law to provide "pleasant moments" for a woman with a serious illness. She invested herself in her husband in proper feeding ("He's not been served a TV dinner since we were married!") and in caring ("Would you like your slippers?"). She might well have had some conflicting feelings about the reversal in role with these significant people. It might have been easier for her to receive care from hospital personnel, because helping is an expected part of their function; but to receive care from those to whom she usually extended herself was quite a different situation.

Another component of the crisis of childbearing is the inescapable revival of feelings about the woman's relationship with her own mother. This relationship is always influenced by guilt feelings. The degree to which further independence from her mother is sought is somewhat in direct proportion to the extent of her guilt feelings. She is caught between two poles: that of needing her mother or a mother substitute in providing care and guidance in the new role of motherhood, and that of asserting that she is now the mother.

> The fate of the identification with the mother is another factor that determines the course of pregnancy. In every instance the capacity for motherhood is related to this identification. The ego of the pregnant woman must find a harmonious compromise between her deeply unconscious identification with the child, which is directed toward the future, and her identification with her own mother, which is directed toward the past. Wherever one of these identifications is rejected, difficulties arise. In the first case the fetus becomes a hostile parasite, in the second the pregnant woman's capacity for motherhood is weakened by her unwillingness to accept her identification with her own mother.[6]

Many questions could be raised about Mrs. X's mother's advice that she attend some classes during pregnancy and her daughter's expressed lack of need and interest in attending prenatal classes. The question of why Mrs. X refused to attend classes has many facets. It is interesting to note the mother's response on the "52nd hour," the day of frustration and depression: "I told her when she was pregnant she ought to go to some classes." Perhaps Mrs. X did not need to depend on her mother too much during pregnancy or in the hospital period. She did indeed need her mother in the early days at home. She needed her to do the laundry, to bathe the baby, and to give guidance in understanding the needs of her child. How could Mrs. X work through becoming a "coequal" with her own mother in terms of motherhood when she felt so helpless and inadequate in meeting her baby's needs?

Mrs. X's responses in "I just wasn't prepared for this.... I just want to do the *right* thing," may communicate something of ego inadequacy in relation to motherhood. She once commented ironically, "They call babies a bundle of joy!"

She was afraid to do certain things for the baby. The day after she had bathed the baby for the first time:

PATIENT: "It wasn't so bad once I did it.

I just was afraid to be by myself to bathe him. I was afraid I wouldn't know what to do—like I couldn't get under one of his arms. So my sister-in-law says, 'Just skip it this time.'"

NURSE: "You were afraid you might hurt him."

PATIENT: "I had so much more confidence after I'd done it."

Something of the extent of her fear may be understood by the fact that it was *seven days* after she had given the first bath that she ventured to give the bath when she was alone. Similarly, she waited to give vitamins to the baby until her husband was at home with her. This is quite in contrast with her observation of the nurse's handling of the baby when he was regurgitating some mucus on his first day of life. When the nurse asked her if she'd know what to do, she said: "Just turn him on his side to get the mucus out—so it doesn't get in his throat."

Perhaps it is somewhat artificial to attempt to describe components of a crisis experience. Certainly in the actuality of a situation these components overlap and merge. However, for the purpose of attaining a closer understanding of the patient in order to help her to achieve her goals, there is value in investigating all aspects of the situation. For practical purposes it might be said that Mrs. X's crisis is a fairly predictable one. Therefore, the nurse's anticipatory guidance will be of immense benefit to the new mother during a necessarily critical period of her life.

Bibliography

1. Jackson, E. B.: Should mother and baby room together? *Am. J. Nurs.* 46:17, 1946.
2. Ringholz, S., and Morris, M.: A test of some assumptions about rooming-in. *Nurs. Research* 10:196-199, Fall 1961.
3. Smith, C. S.: Demand feeding in the newborn nursery. *Nurs. Outlook* 6:514-515, Sept. 1958.
4. Carpenter, H. M.: *The Need for Assistance of Mothers With First Babies During the Three-Month Period Following the Baby's Birth.* New York, Columbia University, 1965.
5. Bibring, Grete, *et al*: A study of the psychological processes in pregnancy and of the earliest mother-child relationships. *Psychoanal. Stud. Child* 14:25-26, 1959.
6. Deutsch, Helene: *Psychology of Women.* New York, Grune & Stratton, 1945.

Suggested Reading

General

AMERICAN ACADEMY OF PEDIATRICS: *Hospital Care of Newborn Infants*, ed. 5. Evanston, Illinois, The Academy, 1971.

AMERICAN ACADEMY OF PEDIATRICS: *Recommendations for Day Care Centers for Infants and Children.* Evanston, Illinois, The Academy, 1973.

BABSON, S. G.: Feeding the low birth weight infant. *Pediatrics* 79:494, 1971.

BLAKE, F., WRIGHT, F. H., AND WAECHTER, E. H.: *Nursing Care of Children*, ed. 8. Philadelphia, J. B. Lippincott, 1970.

BRACKBILL, Y., AND THOMPSON, G. G.: *Behavior in Infancy and Early Childhood.* New York, The Free Press, 1967.

ESTOK, P. J.: What do nurses know about breast feeding problems? *J. Ob-Gyn. Neonat. Nurs.* 2:36-39, 1973.

FENNER, A., AND LIST, M.: Observations of body temperature regulation in young premature and full-term newborns while being connected to a Servo control temperature unit. *Biol. Neonate* 18:330, 1971.

HALL, R. T., AND OLIVER, T. K.: Visual estimate of body temperature in neonates. *JAMA* 218:1700, 1971.

HALSTEAD, L.: The use of crisis intervention in obstetric nursing. *Nurs. Clin. North Am.* 9:69-76, 1974.

HAYNES, U.: A developmental approach to case-finding. Children's Bureau Publication #449, Washington: U.S. Government Printing Office, 1967.

HERDOVA, A.: Nursery evaluation of the newborn. *Am. J. Nurs.* 67:1669-1671, Aug. 1967.

HEY, E.: *The Care of Babies in Incubators. In* D. Gairdner and D. Hull (eds.): *Recent Advances in Poediatrics*, ed. 4. London, J. & A. Churchill, 1971.

KEITEL, H. G.: Preventing neonatal diaper rash. *Am. J. Nurs.* 65:124-126, May 1965.

KNAFL, K.: Conflicting perspectives on breast feeding. *Am. J. Nurs.* 74:1848-1851, 1974.

OLIVER, T. K., JR.: Temperature Regulation and Heat Production in the Newborn. *Pediatr. Clin. North Am.* 12:765, 1965.

PARMALEE, A. H., JR., *et al*: Infant sleep patterns from birth to 16 weeks of age. *Pediatrics* 65:576-582, Oct. 1964.

PRYOR, K.: *Nursing Your Baby.* New York: Harper & Row, 1963.

RICH, O. J.: Hospital routines as rites of passage. *Nurs. Clin. North Am.* 4:101-109, Mar. 1969.

———: Personal communication to authors, 1965.

———: *Clinical Study of a Primipara's Initial Adaptation to Mothering.* USPHS Grant STIMH 7988-03, unpublished, 1965.

RIKER, A. P.: *Breastfeeding.* Public Affairs Pamphlet No. 353S, New York, Public Affairs Pamphlets, 1964.

RINGHOLZ, S., AND MORRIS, M.: A test of some assumptions about rooming-in. *Nurs. Research* 10:196-199, Fall 1961.

ROSSI, A. S.: Transition to parenthood. *J. Marriage and Fam.* 30:26-39, Feb. 1968.

RUBIN, R.: Basic maternal behavior. *Nurs. Outlook* 9:683-686, Nov. 1961.

———: Puerperal change. *Nurs. Outlook* 9:753-755, Dec. 1961.

———: Maternal touch. *Nurs. Outlook* 11:828-831, Nov. 1963.

———: The family-child relationship and nursing care. *Nurs. Outlook* 12:36-39, Sept. 1964.

STEMBERA, Z. K.: Umbilical blood flow in healthy newborn infants during the first minutes after birth, *Am. J. Ob-Gyn.* 91:568-574, Feb. 15, 1965.

STERN, E., *et al*: Sleep cycle characteristics in infants. *Pediatrics* 43:65, Jan. 1969.

VAUGHN, V. C., McKAY, R. J., AND NELSON, W. E.: *Nelson Textbook of Pediatrics.* Philadelphia, W. B. Saunders, 1975.

WOLFF, P. H., AND SIMMONS, M. A.: Nonnutritive sucking and response thresholds in young infants. *Child Develop.* 38:631-638, 1967.

The Mother and Her Newborn Infant

ADAMS, M.: Early concerns of primigravida mothers regarding infant care activities. *Nurs. Research* 12:72-77, Spring 1963.

ANTHONY, E. J., AND BENEDEK, T.: *Parenthood: Its Psychology and Psychopathology.* Boston: Little, Brown, 1970.

BARNES, G. R., JR., *et al*: Management of breast feeding. *JAMA* 151:192-199, Jan. 17, 1953.

BENSON, L. G.: *Fatherhood: A Sociological Perspective.* New York: Random House, 1968.

BIBRING, G. L., *et al*: A study of the psychological processes in pregnancy and of the earliest mother-child relationship. *Psychoanal. Stud. Child* 16:9-72, 1961.

BOWERS, R.: *Touch—A Pilot Study in Clinical Teaching.* Maternal Child Nursing Conference, University of Pittsburgh School of Nursing, pp. 31-33, June 1966.

BOWLBY, J.: *Maternal Care and Mental Health.* Geneva, World Health Organization, 1952.

BRODY, S.: *Patterns of Mothering.* New York, Internat. Univ. Press, 1956.

CAPLAN, G.: *An Approach to Community Mental Health.* New York, Grune & Stratton, 1961.

CLARK, A.: The beginning family. *Am. J. Nurs.* 66:802, April 1966.

———: The adaptation problems and patterns of the expanding family, the neonatal period. *Nurs. Forum* 5:92-109, 1966.

DISBROW, M. A.: *Factors Involved in Successful Breast Feeding.* USPHS Grant GN7901, unpublished, 1962.

EVANS, R. T.: *Needs Identified Among Breastfeeding Mothers.* ANA Clinical Sessions, 1968, pp. 162-171.

EVANS, R. T., *et al*: Exploration of factors involved in maternal physiological adaptation to breastfeeding. *Nurs. Research* 18:28-32, Jan./Feb. 1969.

IFFRIG, SISTER M. C.: Nursing care and success in breast-feeding. *Nurs. Clin. North Am.* 3:345-354, June 1968.

KEANE, V. R.: Nursing care of the family after delivery. *Bull. Am. Coll. Nurs. Midwifery* 9:56-63, Fall 1964.

KLAUS, M. H., AND KENNELL, J.: Mothers separated from their newborn infants. *Pediatr. Clin. North Am.* 17:1017, 1970.

McELIN, T. W., *et al*: The microbiological environment of a rooming-in maternity. *Am. J. Ob-Gyn.* 83:907-917, April 1964.

MOORE, L., AND WHITE, G. D.: Comparisons of teaching methods in maternal and infant care. *Nurs. Outlook* 13:74-76, May 1965.

NEWTON, M., AND NEWTON, N.: The normal course and management of lactation. *Clin. Ob. and Gyn.* 5:44-63, Mar. 1962.

———: Psychologic aspects of lactation. *New Eng. J. Med.,* Nov. 30, 1967.

PARENT-CHILD RELATIONSHIPS: *The Role of the Nurse.* New Brunswick, N. J.: Rutgers University, May/June 1968.

RICHARDSON, S. A. (ED.): *Childbearing: Its Social and Psychological Aspects.* Baltimore: Williams & Wilkins, 1967.

VONRUDEN, J.: *Relation Between Acceptance by the Nurse of the Feeding Method and Alleviation of Guilt Feelings in the Mother.* ANA Regional Clinical Conferences, 1966.

Study Questions for Unit V

Read through the entire question and place your answer on the line to the right.

1. Soon after the mother was normally delivered, she complained of feeling chilly. The nurse observed that she was having a chill. In addition to reporting this to the physician, which of the following measures would the nurse carry out?

   A. Provide external warmth to the mother with blankets.
   B. Give a heart stimulant.
   C. Prepare to give oxygen.
   D. Give a hot drink.
   E. Place the mother in shock position.

   Select the number corresponding to the correct letter or letters.
   1. A only
   2. A and C
   3. A and D
   4. B and E

   _____

2. If a mother making satisfactory progress has a pulse rate of 90 immediately before delivery, what average rate or rates would be considered to be favorable soon after delivery?

   A. 60
   B. 70
   C. 80
   D. 90
   E. 100

   Select the number corresponding to the correct letter or letters.
   1. C only
   2. A, B and C
   3. C, D and E
   4. All of them   _____

3. The appearance of the lochial discharge normally changes during the process of involution. In the space provided after the descriptive phrase in Column 2, place the letter of the period of time in Column 1 that corresponds to it.

Column 1		Column 2	
A. First day		1. Clotted blood with strings of membrane	_____
B. From one to two days		2. Brownish color; thin, scanty	_____
C. From four to seven days		3. Blood mixed with small amounts of mucus	_____
D. From eight to fourteen days		4. Pinkish color; moderate amount	_____
E. Third week		5. Yellow, creamish color	_____
F. Seventh week		6. Dark-brown with occasional bright-red	_____
G. Not at all		7. Characteristic stale odor	_____
		8. Characteristic foul odor	_____

4. A good understanding of the physiologic changes taking place in the mother during the puerperium is a basis for good nursing. Which of the following processes are believed to accomplish involution of the uterus?

   A. The contraction of stretched muscle fibers
   B. The elimination of endometrium along with blood and serous discharge
   C. The casting off of a portion of the spongy layer of the decidua
   D. The generation of new endometrial lining from the layer of decidua attached to the muscular wall
   E. The formation of new endometrium

   Select the number corresponding to the correct letters.
   1. A, B and D
   2. A, C and D
   3. C and E
   4. All of them   _____

5. The nurse should be able to evaluate the observations she makes of her patient's condition. Which of the following changes in the height of the fundus would you consider to be indicative of normal progress of involution?

   A. Twelve hours after delivery—1 cm. above umbilicus
   B. Second day after delivery—6 inches above pubis
   C. Fourth day after delivery—3 inches above pubis
   D. Eighth day after delivery—2 inches above pubis
   E. Tenth day after delivery—1 inch above pubis

   Select the number corresponding to the correct letter or letters.
   1. A only
   2. A and C
   3. B, D and E
   4. All of them   _____

6. Which of the following seem to be the advantages gained from early ambulation after delivery?
   A. Improves bowel and bladder function
   B. Mothers seem to regain their strength more readily
   C. Minimizes the chances of hemorrhage
   D. Hastens involution of the uterus
   E. Eliminates incidence of thrombophlebitis

   Select the number corresponding to the correct letters.
   1. A and B
   2. A, C and D
   3. B, C and E
   4. All of them
   _____

7. Although the precedures for perineal care vary from hospital to hospital, in what respects do they all agree?
   A. Requiring the nurse to carry out surgical aseptic technique
   B. Endeavoring to protect the patient against infection from external sources
   C. Using forceps to handle sponges in cleansing vulva
   D. Requiring that each sponge be used for one stroke only
   E. Requiring that perineal pads be sterile when applied

   Select the number corresponding to the correct letters.
   1. A and E
   2. A, B and C
   3. B, D and E
   4. All of them
   _____

8. To keep the nipples in good condition for breast-feeding, which of the following should be included in their daily care?
   A. Keep the nipples clean and dry.
   B. Wash with warm water once a day.
   C. Wash with mild antiseptic solution prior to each feeding period.
   D. Cover the nipples and areola with clean plastic breast squares to prevent contamination.
   E. If nipple is sore, discontinue breast-feeding until tenderness subsides.

   Select the number corresponding to the correct letters.
   1. A and B
   2. A, C and D
   3. B, D and E
   4. All of them
   _____

9. The neonatal period constitutes one of the most important periods of life because of the profound physiologic changes which occur. Which of the following statements concerning these alterations are correct?
   A. Certain of these physiologic changes are immediate; some are delayed.
   B. All of these physiologic changes are immediate.
   C. All of these physiologic changes are permanent.
   D. Certain of these physiologic changes are temporary.

   Select the number corresponding to the correct letters.
   1. A and C
   2. A and D
   3. B and C
   4. B and D
   _____

10. Which of the following reasons best explain why the maternity hospital should adopt the rooming-in plan for the mother and her newborn?
    A. All mothers need the experience gained thereby.
    B. Selected mothers and babies may profit where the plan could be adopted.
    C. All mothers want this type of service.
    D. Most infants cry too much in a central nursery.
    E. All infants need this added attention.

    Select the number corresponding to the correct letter or letters.
    1. A only
    2. B only
    3. A, C and D
    4. B, C and E   _____

11. What type of initial bath usually is given the newborn infant?
    A. Tub bath
    B. Spray bath
    C. Oil bath
    D. Sponge bath with a 3 percent hexachlorophene solution and warm water
    E. Cleansing of the genitals with warm water and sterilized cotton   _____

12. What is the reason for selecting this method of skin care in the above question?
    A. The infant's skin must be washed thoroughly to prevent irritation.
    B. It stimulates circulation.
    C. Special oils provide nourishment to the tissues.
    D. It prevents infection.
    E. It lessens the amount of staphylococcus colonization of the infant's skin and nasopharynx.

                                                              _____

13. What is the usual procedure for the daily care of the genitals of the male infant who is not in need of circumcision?
    A. Wash externally with soap and water; otherwise let alone.
    B. Retract and cleanse under the foreskin with cotton ball moistened with warm water. Replace foreskin over glans after cleansing.
    C. Retract and cleanse under the foreskin with alcohol.
    D. After cleansing, apply sterile petrolatum under the foreskin.
    E. Stretch the prepuce and lubricate with mineral oil.   _____

14. What is the principle underlying the concept of demand feedings for the newborn infant?
    A. Maintaining a regular four-hour schedule to establish eating habits
    B. Feeding the infant every two to three hours to stimulate digestion
    C. Fitting individual feedings to individual needs
    D. Permissive feeding schedule causes less conflict with the mother's household activities
    E. More frequent feedings assure an adequate nutritional intake   _____

15. The young mother asks how she will know when her baby is hungry. Which of the following responses would be most appropriate for the nurse to reply?
    A. "All crying indicates hunger."
    B. "Feed the baby whenever he is awake."
    C. "He will cry, fret, and suck on anything in contact with his lips."
    D. "Offer him water first; if he refuses the water, feed him."   _____

16. The appearance of a healthy newborn infant's stools normally will change during the neo-natal period. Which of the following types of stools, in sequence of appearance, would the nurse observe in the healthy infant?

   A. Dark, tarlike
   B. Clay-colored, soft
   C. Mottled greenish-brown, soft
   D. Smooth, yellow
   E. Green, curdy

   Select the number corresponding to the correct letters.
   1. A and D
   2. A, C and D
   3. B, C and E
   4. All of them _____

17. How does the composition of mother's milk compare with cow's milk?

   A. Human milk contains more protein.
   B. Human milk contains less protein.
   C. Human milk contains more carbohydrate.
   D. Human milk contains larger fat globules.
   E. Human milk contains less iron.

   Select the number corresponding to the correct letters.
   1. A and C
   2. A, C and E
   3. B, C and D
   4. B, D and E _____

operative procedures in obstetrics

Operative Obstetrics

unit **VI**

operative obstetrics

A number of special procedures which the physician may use to assist the mother in labor and delivery come under the heading of operative obstetrics. These include episiotomy and repair of lacerations, the application of forceps or vacuum extractor, destructive operations on the fetus, version, cesarean section, and induction of labor.

Episiotomy and repair of lacerations

Except for clamping and cutting the umbilical cord, episiotomy is the most common operative procedure performed in obstetrics. In view of the fact that this incision of the perineum, made to facilitate delivery, is employed almost routinely in primigravidas, the procedure has been discussed in the section on the conduct of normal labor (see Chapter 18).

Lacerations of the perineum and the vagina which occur in the process of delivery (see Fig. 18-30, p. 349) have also been discussed previously, because some tears are unavoidable, even in the most skilled hands. The suturing of spontaneous perineal lacerations is similar to that employed for the repair of an episiotomy incision but may be more difficult because such tears often are irregular in shape with ragged, bruised edges.

Forceps

Some of the common types of obstetric forceps are illustrated in Figures 22-1 to 22-4. The instrument consists of two steel parts which cross each other like a pair of scissors and lock at the intersection. The lock may be of a sliding type, as in the first three types shown,

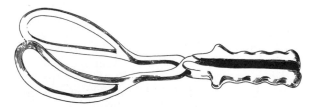

Figure 22-1.   Simpson forceps.

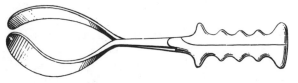

Figure 22-2.   Tucker McLane forceps.

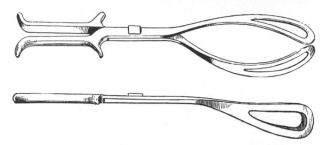

Figure 22-3. Kielland forceps. (Top) Front view. (Bottom) Side view.

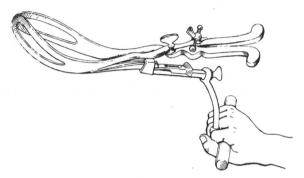

Figure 22-4. Tarnier axis-traction forceps.

or a screw type, as in the Tarnier instrument. Each part consists of a handle, a lock, a shank, and a blade; the blade is the curved portion designed for application to the sides of the baby's head. The blades of most forceps (the Tucker McLane is an exception) have a large opening or window (fenestrum) to give a better grip on the baby's head, and usually they have two curves: a cephalic curve, which conforms to the shape of the baby's head, and a pelvic curve, to follow the curve of the birth canal. Axis-traction forceps, such as the Tarnier, have a mechanism attached below which permits the pulling to be done more directly in the axis of the birth canal. An axis-traction handle is also available for use on standard forceps.

The two blades of the forceps are designated as right and left. The left blade is the one which is introduced into the vagina on the patient's left side; the right blade goes in on the right side. If the nurse is assisting the obstetrician, she should articulate and disarticulate the forceps and make sure that she knows which blade is which.

It may become necessary to deliver the baby by forceps for reasons related to the mother's welfare (maternal indications), or because of conditions associated with the baby's condition (fetal indications). Among the more common maternal indications are: Malposition of the fetal head, toxemia of pregnancy, threatened rupture of the uterus, and inability of the mother to push after full dilatation of the cervix, because of conduction anesthesia, exhaustion, or heart disease. The chief fetal indication for forceps delivery is fetal distress, as suggested by a slow, irregular fetal heart. Many obstetricians, however, deem it desirable to deliver almost all primigravidas with forceps electively, in the belief that the operation spares the mother many minutes of exhausting bearing-down efforts and relieves pressure on the baby's head. This is usually referred to as "elective forceps."

Forceps operations are never attempted unless the cervix is completely dilated. Forceps delivery is contraindicated unless the vertex is engaged (i.e., the greatest biparietal diameter of the fetal head is at, or has already traversed, the pelvic inlet). Usually, but not always, when engagement has occurred, the vertex is at or below the ischial spines. In the vast majority of cases today, the forceps delivery is carried out at a time when the baby's head is on the perineal floor (visible or almost so) and internal rotation may have already occurred, so that the baby's head lies in a direct anteroposterior position. This is called *low forceps*, or "outlet forceps." When the head is higher in the pelvis but engaged, its greatest diameter having passed the inlet, the operation is called *midforceps*. If the head has not yet engaged, the procedure is known as *high forceps*. High-forceps delivery is an exceedingly difficult and dangerous operation for both mother and baby and is rarely done. The obstetrician will inform the nurse of the type of instrument he wishes to use. Autoclaving is the usual type of sterilization employed, and several pairs of the generally approved forceps, each encased in suitable wrappings, are autoclaved and kept in the delivery room for immediate use. The other instruments needed for a forceps delivery are the same as those required for a spontaneous delivery, plus those necessary for repair work (see Chapter 18).

Anesthesia is recommended, but in low-forceps deliveries it may be light, and in many institutions this type of operation is performed successfully under pudendal block anesthesia. The patient is placed in the lithotomy position and prepared and draped in the usual fashion. After checking the exact position of the baby's head by vaginal examination, the physician will introduce two or more fingers of his right hand into the left side of the vagina; these fingers will guide the left blade into place and at the same time protect the maternal soft parts (vagina, cervix) from injury. Taking the left blade of the forceps in his left hand, he introduces it into the left side of the vagina, gently insinuating it between the baby's head and the fingers of his right hand (Fig. 22-5). The same procedure is carried out on the right side, and then the blades are articulated. Traction is not continuous but intermittent (Fig. 22-6); and between traction, the obstetrician will partially disarticulate the blades in order to release pressure on the baby's head. Episiotomy is almost routine nowadays in these cases.

Vacuum extractor

Occasionally, an instrument known as the vacuum extractor is used in place of the forceps. The vacuum extractor consists of a metal cup that is applied to the fetal head and tightly affixed there by creating a vacuum in the cup through withdrawal of the air by a pump (Fig. 22-7). Cups are supplied in various sizes. The largest cup which can be applied with ease is selected for use. Vacuum is created slowly, and the suction creates an artificial caput within the cup, providing a firm attachment to the fetal scalp. Traction can then be exerted by means of a short chain attached to the cup, with a handle at its far end.

Version

Version consists of turning the baby in the uterus from an undesirable to a desirable position. There are two types of version: external, and internal.

EXTERNAL VERSION. This is an operation designed to change a breech presentation into a vertex presentation by external manipulation of the fetus through the abdominal and the uterine walls. It is attempted in the hope of averting the difficulties of a subsequent breech delivery. Obstetricians find the procedure most successful when done about a month before full term; it often fails, however, either because it proves to be impossible to turn the fetus around, or because the fetus returns to its original position within a few hours. Some obstetricians disapprove of it altogether.

INTERNAL VERSION. Sometimes called internal podalic version, this is an operation designed to change whatever presentation may

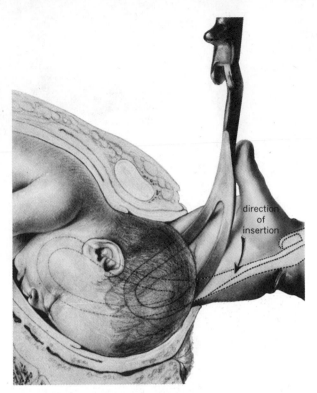

Figure 22-5. Insertion of forceps blade.

exist into a breech presentation (see Fig. 22-8). With cervical dilatation complete, the whole hand of the operator is introduced high into the uterus, one or both feet are grasped and pulled downward in the direction of the birth canal. With his external hand the obstetrician may expedite the turning by pushing the head upward. The version usually is followed by breech extraction (p. 500). Internal version

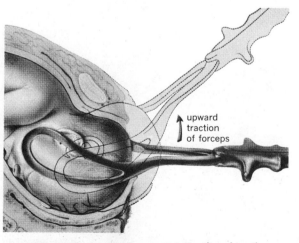

Figure 22-6. Applied forceps and direction of traction.

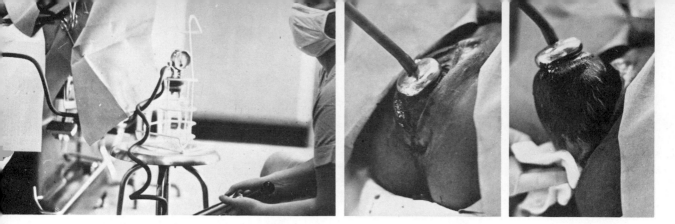

Figure 22-7. Application of the vacuum extractor and delivery of the fetal head.

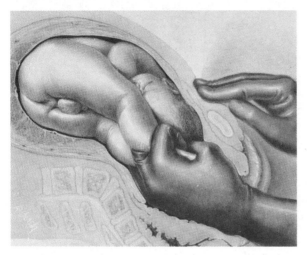

Figure 22-8. Internal podalic version. Elbow length gloves are usually worn for this operation.

finds its greatest usefulness in cases of multiple pregnancy in which the birth of the second twin is delayed, or when the second twin is in a transverse lie. It is now almost never used in other circumstances.

Cesarean section

Cesarean section is the removal of the infant from the uterus through an incision made in the abdominal wall and the uterus. The main indications for cesarean section fall into five groups: 1) disproportion between size of the fetus and that of the bony birth canal, that is, contracted pelvis (p. 502), tumor blocking birth canal, and so on; 2) certain cases in which the patient has had a previous cesarean section, the operation being done because of

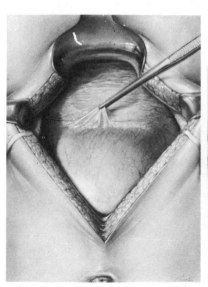

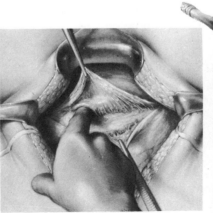

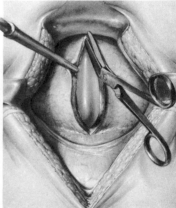

(Caption appears on facing page)

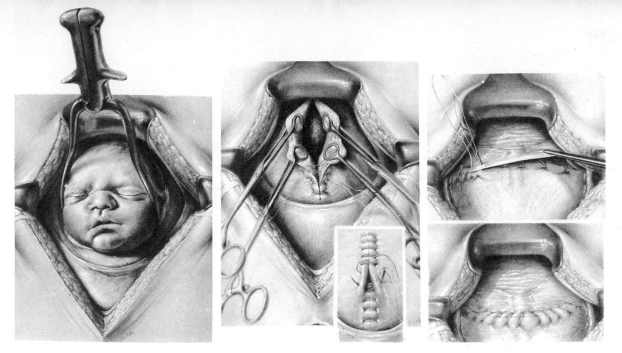

Figure 22-10. Low cervical cesarean section. (*Left*) Extraction of baby with forceps. Oxytocin (1 cc.) intramuscularly is usually given as soon as the head is delivered. (*Center*) After delivery of baby and placenta, edges of the lower segment incision are grasped with ring forceps and sutured. (*Right*) After upper peritoneal flap is pulled down over the uterine wound and sutured, the lower flap is pulled upward and sutured with running suture.

fear that the uterus will rupture in labor; 3) certain cases of very severe toxemia of pregnancy, but rarely in eclampsia; 4) certain cases of placenta previa and premature separation of the normally implanted placenta; 5) fetal distress, actual or impending. When a cesarean section is done prior to the onset of labor, as the result of a prearranged plan, it is called *elective* cesarean section (as with elective low forceps, the obstetrician is not forced to perform the operation immediately, but elects to do it as the best procedure for mother and baby).

Main types of cesarean section

Although there are four types of cesarean section, the lower segment section is usually the operation of choice. In this operation, the uterus is entered through an incision in the lower segment. Other types of cesarean section include the classical cesarean section, in which the incision is made directly into the wall of the body of the uterus; the extraperitoneal cesarean section, in which the operation is arranged anatomically, such that the incision is made into the uterus without entering the peritoneal cavity; and cesarean-hysterectomy, which involves a cesarean section of any variety followed by removal of the uterus.

THE LOW SEGMENT CESAREAN SECTION. This procedure is usually the operation of choice for a number of important reasons. Since the incision is made in the lower segment of the uterus, which is its thinnest portion, the opera-

Figure 22-9. Low cervical cesarean section. (*Left*) High Trendelenburg position, bladder empty, with catheter in place. The peritoneum over lower portion of uterus is picked up with tissue forceps to determine how far up it is loosely attached to uterus. A transverse incision of the peritoneum, slightly concave downward, is to be made about 1 inch below the point where the peritoneum is firmly attached to the uterus.

(*Center*) The lower edge of the incised peritoneum is picked up by the tissue forceps and gently stripped off the underlying uterine segment by finger dissection.

(*Right*) The upper flap of loose peritoneum has been stripped from the underlying muscle by finger dissection and is held back by a retractor. A small incision with a scalpel is made at the upper end of the lower uterine segment and carried downward with bandage scissors.

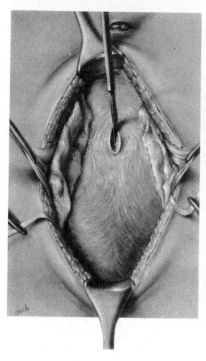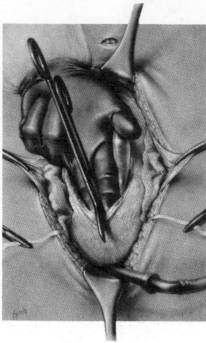

Figure 22-11. Classic cesarean section. (*Left*) Uterus packed off with warm, moist gauze pads. Start of incision with knife. (*Right*) Continuation of incision with bandage scissors.

tion is associated with minimal blood loss, and the incision is easy to repair. The lower segment is also the area of least uterine activity, and thus the possibility of rupture of the scar in a subsequent pregnancy is lessened. Since the incision can be properly peritonealized, the operation is associated with a lower incidence of postoperative infection. The initial incision (the abdominal cavity having been opened) is made transversely across the uterine peritoneum, where it is attached loosely just above the bladder. The lower peritoneal flap and the bladder are now dissected from the uterus, and the uterine muscle is incised either vertically or transversely. The membranes are ruptured, and the baby is delivered. After the placenta has been extracted and the uterine incision sutured, the lower flap is imbricated over the uterine incision (Figs. 22-9 and 22-10, p. 453). This two-flap arrangement seals off the uterine incision and is believed to prevent the egress of infectious lochia into the peritoneal cavity.

CLASSICAL CESAREAN SECTION. A vertical incision is made directly into the wall of the body of the uterus; the baby and the placenta are extracted, and the incision is closed by three layers of absorbable sutures (Figs. 22-11 and 22-12). Thus, this approach requires trav-

ersing the full thickness of the uterine corpus. It is still recommended in certain circumstances. It is particularly useful when the bladder and lower segment are involved in extension adhesions resulting from a previous cesarean section, and occasionally is selected when the fetus is in a transverse lie or when there is an anterior placenta previa.

EXTRAPERITONEAL CESAREAN SECTION. By appropriate dissection of the tissues around the bladder, access to the lower uterine segment is secured without entering the peritoneal cavity. The baby is delivered through an incision in the lower uterine segment. Since the entire operation is done outside the peritoneal cavity, neither spill of infected amniotic fluid nor subsequent seepage of pus from the uterus can reach the peritoneal surfaces. This approach was used extensively in the preantibiotic era, but is rarely employed today.

CESAREAN SECTION—HYSTERECTOMY. (Synonym: Porro's operation). This operation comprises cesarean section followed by removal of the uterus. It may be necessary in certain cases of *premature separation of the placenta*, in patients with multiple *fibroid tumors of the uterus*, and in some circumstances is done electively for sterilization purposes.

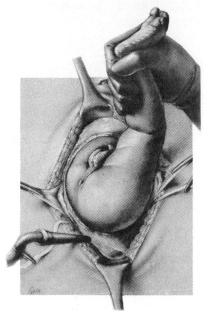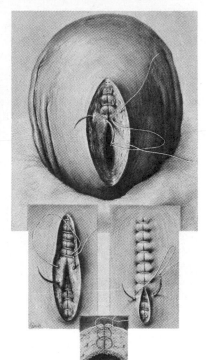

Figure 22-12. Classic cesarean section. (*Left*) Delivery of infant. (*Right*) Method of suturing uterus.

Preparation

Preparations for cesarean sections are similar to those for any other abdominal operation, except that in these cases it includes preparations for the care of the infant. An elective cesarean section allows ample time for a physical examination, routine laboratory studies, typing and crossmatching blood, and other customary procedures. However, if there is an emergency, or if labor has started, then such preparations must be made with expediency. In any event, the usual hospital procedure should be followed.

Nursing care

When the patient is admitted for an elective cesarean section, nursing care which is routine for any waiting mother (e.g., checking fetal heart tones and being alert to prodromal signs of labor) is employed. A short time before the operation the abdomen is shaved, beginning at the level of the xiphoid cartilage and extending out to the far sides and down to the pubic area. A retention catheter is inserted to ensure that the bladder remains empty during the operation and attached to a constant drainage system. One should make certain that the catheter is draining properly before the procedure. The preoperative medication usually ordered is atropine. The use of narcotic drugs prior to delivery is avoided because of their depressant effect on the infant, but these medications should be readily available. Oxytocic drugs (e.g., oxytocin and ergonovine) should be ready in the operating room so that they can be administered promptly on the verbal order of the obstetrician when the infant is born.

In addition to the preparation of the operating room for the surgical procedure, preparation for the care of the infant must be accomplished. There must be a warm crib and equipment for the resuscitation of the infant. An infant resuscitator, equipped with heat, suction, oxygen (open mask and positive-pressure), and an adjustable frame to permit the proper positioning of the infant is most useful. A competent person should be present at cesarean section to give the infant initial care and to resuscitate, if necessary. This person may be a professional nurse, but in many hospitals today it is customary to have a pediatrician present so that he may take over the care of the infant as soon as it is born and thus free the obstetrician to devote all of his attention to the mother.

Usually postoperative care is the same as that following any abdominal surgery. It is well to remember that the patient who has had a cesarean section has had both an abdominal operation and a delivery. The patient must be watched for hemorrhage, as after any delivery. The perineal pad must be inspected frequently. If the abdominal dressings are bulky, it may be difficult to palpate the fundus to see if the uterus is well contracted, but if the dressings are not massive, and do not extend above the level of the umbilicus, the nurse may feel the consistency of the fundus. Oxytocics may be ordered to keep the uterus contracted and to control bleeding. The vital signs should be checked regularly until they have stabilized, and if there is any indication of shock or hemorrhage, it should be reported promptly. Although there may be no visible signs of external hemorrhage, one would suspect internal hemorrhage if the pulse rate becomes accelerated, the respiration increases in rate, or the blood pressure falls, bearing in mind, of course, that the drop in blood pressure could be due to the effects of some types of anesthetic drugs.

If the retention catheter is to remain in place until the following morning, it should remain attached to "constant drainage" and should be watched to see that it drains freely. Intravenous fluids are usually administered during the first 24 hours, although small amounts of fluids may be given by mouth after nausea has subsided. A record of the mother's intake and elimination is kept for the first several days or until the need is no longer indicated.

Sedative drugs should be used to keep the mother comfortable and encourage her to rest. Her position in bed during the early postoperative hours may be dictated by the type of anesthesia that she received. She should be encouraged to turn from side to side every hour. Deep breathing and coughing should also be encouraged to promote good ventilation. Today most mothers delivered by cesarean section are allowed early ambulation. It is felt that this contributes considerably to maintaining good bladder and intestinal function.

The father should be permitted to visit as soon as it is feasible. The mother will be anxious to see her infant, too, and it should be brought to her as soon as she is able to see it. The nurse should remain with the mother while she has her infant with her.

The general care of the mother will be similar to that given any postoperative or postpartal patient. Daily breast care and perineal care are carried out per routine. The mother may have the afterpains, engorgement of the breasts, and the emotional reactions which often accompany a normal delivery.

Destructive operations

Destructive operations (designed for the most part to reduce the size of the baby's head and thus to expedite delivery) are rarely done in modern obstetrics. Even in large maternity hospitals many years may pass without a single destructive operation. This salutary state of affairs is attributable in part to the widespread extension of prenatal care, in part to better management of women in labor, and in part to the availability of cesarean section, which makes it safe to effect abdominal delivery even in neglected cases. In the event that a destructive operation is necessary, the obstetrician will choose the necessary instruments.

Induction of labor

Induction of labor means the artificial bringing on of labor after the period of viability. Induction of labor is indicated when continuation of pregnancy would affect maternal health, or when there are conditions in the mother which would affect fetal well-being. Complications of pregnancy which may require induction include toxemia, diabetes, hemolytic disease, and postmaternity (see Complications of Pregnancy). In some centers, labor is induced electively at term for convenience.

MEDICINAL INDUCTION. Since it was believed that the intestinal peristalsis produced by a cathartic is somehow transferred to the uterus, with the consequent initiation of uterine contractions, castor oil has long been employed to induce labor. It was often followed by the administration of a hot soapsuds enema. While this is a harmless approach, it usually fails.

An efficient and safe method for the induction of labor is the administration of oxytocin by intravenous drip. The properties of this oxytocic agent and its use in the third stage of labor have already been discussed on page 336. Since oxytocin has dangerous potentialities when administered to a pregnant woman, the dosage used is always extremely small. Administration by intravenous drip assures a uniform, although infinitesimal, concentration of the agent in the bloodstream. The amount of oxytocin being administered can be readily controlled and is governed by the response of the uterus. Oxytocin has also been administered intramuscularly, but this approach is no longer recommended. Since the response of a given patient is not predictable, there is no way to select an appropriate intramuscular dose.

For the intravenous administration of oxytocin, the physician will usually ask for a flask containing 500 ml. of 5 percent glucose to which he will add the quantity of oxytocin indicated. The intravenous equipment is set up as usual so that the number of drops flowing per minute can be closely observed in the observation tube. This is extremely important, and the physician will specify the precise number of drops per minute which he wishes employed. Initially, the drip should be run very slowly—4 to 5 drops per minute. The rate of administration should be increased gradually thereafter, always being governed by the response of the patient (Fig. 22-13). To avoid a sudden infusion of oxytocin during placement of the intravenous, a piggyback system is usually recommended. After an infusion of 5 percent D+W is running, the solution containing the pitocin is introduced for a second intravenous setup by placing the needle into the rubber adaptor of the infusion already in place. The amount of pitocin delivered can then be regulated—increased, decreased, or discontinued—without interfering with the continuity of the IV delivery system.

The administration of oxytocin to a gravida carries certain hazards, and it is obligatory for her safety and that of the baby that a physician or a nurse be in constant bedside attendance to make certain that the number of drops flowing per minute does not change and to watch for certain untoward effects. The observer must check the rate of flow of the oxytocin solution at frequent intervals to make certain that it remains constant. The duration and the intensity of each uterine contraction must be watched closely and recorded. Any contraction lasting over 90 seconds indicates that the quantity of solution is too great, and the rate of flow should either be decreased or tentatively discontinued altogether. Furthermore, the fetal heart rate should be counted and recorded. It will be recalled that the fetal heart tones should return to their normal rate and rhythm within 15 seconds or so after the termination of a contraction, and any persistence of fetal bradycardia is another indication for discon-

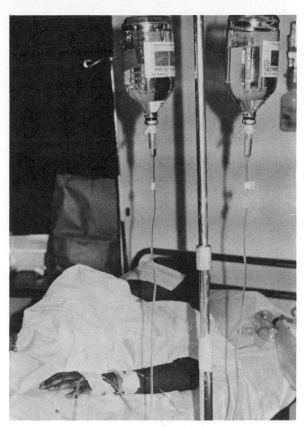

Figure 22-13. Administration of pit drip with piggyback technique.

tinuation of the oxytocin drip. In the event that the nurse should be left alone with the patient while the intravenous-drip oxytocin technique is being employed, and she observes any abnormalities in the uterine contractions or the fetal heart tones, she should turn off the solution *immediately* and report her findings to the physician. The major advantage of the oxytocin drip is that it may be discontinued immediately in the event that untoward effects should be observed—an obvious safety factor.

ARTIFICIAL RUPTURE OF THE MEMBRANES. Amniotomy, or artificial rupture of the membranes, is a common method of enhancing labor. Amniotomy has also been used to induce labor. When the patient is near term and the cervix is favorable, it is almost always followed by labor within a few hours. The membranes serve as a barrier against bacterial invasion. For this reason, once this barrier has been eliminated by amniotomy, delivery should be accomplished expeditiously. Many obstetricians now feel that the primary use of amniotomy for labor induction is tantamount to burning one's bridges, and that the procedure should be delayed until after the initiation of good contractions with intravenous pitocin.

Amniotomy is accomplished after placing the patient in the lithotomy position and carrying out antiseptic preparation of the vulva. The first two fingers of one hand are inserted into the cervix until the membranes are encountered. A long hook, similar to one blade of a disarticulated vulsellum tenaculum, or an Allis clamp, is inserted into the vagina, and the membranes are simply hooked and torn by the tip of the sharp instrument. As much fluid as possible is allowed to drain. The quality of the fluid should be noted. Normally, it is watery-clear. Fetal heart tones should be checked immediately after amniotomy; extra care should be exercised, as there is an increased possibility of cord prolapse.

So far as the nurse is concerned, these obstetric operations do not differ greatly from any other surgical procedures. The direction of these operations is entirely the responsibility of the physician, and the nurse's share consists of these three responsibilities: 1) having everything in readiness beforehand, 2) giving reassuring advice to the patient and her family, and 3) making sure that no opportunity is lost in rendering all possible assistance to the physician.

Suggested Reading

FIELDS, H., SMITH, K., AND GREEN, J.: *Induction of Labor.* New York, Macmillan, 1965.

HELLMAN, L. M., AND PRITCHARD, J. A.: *Williams Obstetrics,* ed. 14. New York, Appleton-Century Crofts, 1971.

Conference Material

1. A mother, Para 2, is admitted to the hospital at 42 weeks' gestation for induction of labor. Her membranes have been artificially ruptured and intravenous oxytocin has been started. Discuss the nursing care of this mother from this time until she is in active labor.

2. What specific nursing care would you give to a mother who sustained a third-degree perineal laceration as the result of a precipitous labor?

3. A 38-year-old gravida 5 had an uneventful pregnancy until the last trimester, when she developed preeclampsia. Now, at term, she is admitted to the hospital because of suspected abruptio placenta and, after consultation, is to have an emergency cesarean section. Discuss the nursing care of this mother from time of admission until she is taken to the operating room for surgery.

4. A primigravida, who has three-year-old adopted twins, is delivered by low cervical cesarean section because of pelvic injuries received in an auto accident six years earlier. Discuss the nursing care of this mother following cesarean section.

Study Questions for Unit VI

Read through the entire question and place your answer on the line to the right.

1. Which of the following structures are involved when an episiotomy is performed?
   A. The vaginal mucosa
   B. The levator ani muscle
   C. The glans clitoris
   D. The cardinal ligament
   E. The fourchet

   Select the number corresponding to the correct letter or letters.
   1. A only
   2. A and B
   3. A, B and E
   4. All of them

2. Obstetric forceps are frequently used to facilitate delivery. In which of the following conditions would it be indicated to deliver the infant by forceps?
   A. The cervix fails to dilate completely.
   B. The mother has heart disease.
   C. The mother has a contracted pelvis.
   D. Prolapse of the umbilical cord.
   E. Passage of meconium-stained amniotic fluid in vertex presentation.

   Select the number corresponding to the correct letters.
   1. A and B
   2. B, D and E
   3. C and E
   4. All of them _____

3. Which of the following principles should be observed in the use of intravenous oxytocin to stimulate labor?
   A. The condition of the fetus must be satisfactory.
   B. It should be used only in cases of secondary uterine inertia.
   C. It should not be given to a multipara who has had four or more full-term pregnancies.
   D. It should be used in cases of borderline pelvis.
   E. A responsible person should be in constant attendance while the mother is receiving intravenous oxytocin.

   Select the number corresponding to the correct letters.
   1. A and B
   2. A, C and E
   3. B, D and E
   4. All of them _____

4. What specific treatment should be included in the care given a mother who has had a repair of a third-degree laceration of the perineum?
   A. Give daily routine perineal care.
   B. Serve a soft diet until the fifth postpartal day.
   C. Omit enemas until the fifth postpartal day.
   D. Limit activities in regard to early ambulation.
   E. Encourage the mother not to sit erect until wound has healed.

   Select the number corresponding to the correct letter or letters.
   1. A only
   2. A, D and E
   3. B, C and D
   4. All of them _____

5. After a cesarean section, which of the following symptoms might indicate that the patient is having excessive bleeding?
   A. Accelerated pulse and respiration and drop in blood pressure
   B. Pain and tenderness in operative area
   C. Abdominal distention
   D. Sanguineous drainage from the abdominal wound and the vagina
   E. Apprehension and restlessness

   Select the number corresponding to the correct letters.
   1. A and B
   2. A, C and D
   3. A, D and E
   4. All of them _____

6. In caring for a mother who has been delivered by cesarean section, which of the following are usually employed to keep the uterus contracted and control bleeding?
   A. Oxytocic drugs
   B. Gentle massage of the fundus if it becomes relaxed
   C. Icebag to the operative area
   D. Pressure dressings and tight abdominal binder
   E. Keep the patient flat in bed for the first six hours postoperatively

   Select the number corresponding to the correct letter or letters.
   1. A only
   2. A, C and D
   3. B, C and E
   4. All of them   _____

assessment and management of disorders associated with childbearing

unit **VII**

Complications of Pregnancy
Coincidental Diseases and Pregnancy
Complications of Labor
Complications of the Puerperium
Fetal Diagnosis and Treatment
Care of Low Birth Weight and Preterm Infants—
Intensive Care
Disorders of the Newborn

complications of pregnancy

23

Toxemias of Pregnancy / Hemorrhagic
Complications / Hyperemesis Gravidarum

Regardless of the fact that from a biologic point of view childbearing is considered to be a normal process, the borderline between health and illness is less distinctly marked during this time because of the numerous physiologic changes that occur in the mother's body during the course of pregnancy. The importance of early and continued health supervision during pregnancy is paramount for the total well-being of the mother and her infant, for such preventive care makes possible the early detection of warning signals of potential pathologic conditions, so that serious problems can be averted or controlled by prompt treatment (see Chapter 12).

Certain "common complaints" are experienced by most expectant mothers to some degree; these are the so-called minor discomforts of pregnancy, which in themselves are not serious but nevertheless detract from the mother's feeling of comfort and well-being. Since these discomforts are usually related to normal physiologic changes occurring within the mother's body and are not in themselves pathologic, they have been included in the chapter on antepartal care (see Chapter 12). However, minor discomforts, if neglected, may lead to a major complication.

The maternal disorders associated with pregnancy may be considered from the standpoint of the complications of the pregnancy itself and from the standpoint of the complications that are related to the coincidental diseases which occur during pregnancy. There are only a few major complications of pregnancy, but they present a serious health problem (e.g., the toxemias of pregnancy). The coincidental diseases which may occur during pregnancy are those which might occur at any other time as well. The pregnant woman is subject to any disorder or disease which might affect a nonpregnant person. However, when these illnesses arise coincident to pregnancy, the disorder is likely to complicate the pregnancy, the disorder itself may be aggravated by the pregnancy, or both effects may result. (See Chapter 24.)

Certain complications of pregnancy may seriously jeopardize the health of both the mother and her unborn infant. The complications which affect the mother primarily and the maternal aspects of those having dual implications will be discussed in this chapter. Although dramatic progress has been made in reducing maternal as well as perinatal morbidity and mortality, some problems remain un-

Table 23-1 Infant Deaths Caused by Neonatal Disorders Arising from Certain Diseases of the Mother During Pregnancy, United States, 1970

Cause of Death*	Number of Deaths
Toxemias of pregnancy	198
Maternal diabetes	267
Maternal rubella	17
Toxoplasmosis	4
Other or unspecified diseases of mother during pregnancy	174
Total	660

* Classified according to the Eighth Revision of International Lists, 1965.

Source: Department of Health, Education and Welfare: Vital Statistics of the United States, 1970, Vol. II, Part A, Table 1-23, Washington, D.C., U.S. Government Printing Office, 1974.

solved. Despite expanding social programs, a great many underprivileged women receive inadequate or no prenatal care. In contrast to those women with optimal care, these have an increased rate of complications, morbidity, and mortality, both maternal and perinatal.

A review of statistics compiled by the U.S. Department of Health, Education and Welfare in 1974 indicates that there was, in 1970, an overall maternal mortality rate of 21.5 per 100,000 live births: 14.4 for the white population and 55.9 for nonwhites. In all 15.4 percent were due to toxemia, 13.8 percent to sepsis (of which 75 percent were abortion-related) and 10.4 percent to hemorrhage. Although these figures represent a relative decrease in these classical causes of maternal mortality as compared with earlier years, toxemia, sepsis and hemorrhage still head the list by a substantial margin. Maternal complications also have a significant influence on perinatal morbidity and mortality. The major causes of infant death, as related to maternal disease, are listed in Table 23-1.

Toxemias of pregnancy

The toxemias of pregnancy are disorders encountered during gestation, or early in the puerperium, which are characterized by one or more of the following signs: hypertension, edema, albuminuria, and in severe cases, convulsions and coma. Despite decades of intensive research, the cause of toxemia is still unknown. The name itself would give rise to the

supposition that these conditions are due to circulating toxins in the blood, derived presumably from the products of conception; but this is probably not correct. Whether toxemia represents an exaggeration of the various physical changes which normally accompany pregnancy, or whether it depends on some entirely new deviation from the normal course of pregnancy, is still one of the most important unsolved problems in the whole field of human reproduction.

The toxemias of pregnancy are a very common complication of gestation, being seen in 6 or 7 percent of all gravidae. They rank among the three major complications (hemorrhage, puerperal infections and the toxemias of pregnancy) responsible for the vast majority of maternal deaths and account for some 1,000 maternal deaths in the United States each year. As a cause of fetal death they are even more important. It can be estimated conservatively that at least 30,000 stillbirths and neonatal deaths each year in the United States are the result of toxemias of pregnancy. The great majority of these deaths are related to prematurity.

The huge toll of maternal and infant lives taken by the toxemias of pregnancy is in large measure preventable. Proper antepartal supervision, particularly the early detection of signs and symptoms of oncoming toxemia and appropriate treatment, will arrest many cases and so ameliorate others that the outcome for baby and mother is usually satisfactory. The nurse is often the first to encounter the early signs and symptoms, not only in the hospital outpatient department, but also on home visits, and it is of utmost importance that she be constantly on the lookout for them so that treatment may be instituted at the earliest possible moment.

Classification

The toxemias of pregnancy have heretofore been classified in many forms. In 1952 The American Committee on Maternal Welfare revised its classification as follows:

1. Acute toxemia of pregnancy
   A. Preeclampsia
      1. Mild
      2. Severe
   B. Eclampsia

2. Chronic hypertensive (vascular disease with pregnancy)
   A. Chronic hypertensive vascular disease without superimposed acute toxemia
      1. Those cases in which hypertension was definitely known to exist before the onset of pregnancy
      2. Cases of early hypertension before the 24th week
   B. Chronic hypertensive vascular disease with superimposed toxemia
3. Unclassified toxemias

ACUTE TOXEMIA OF PREGNANCY is divided into two stages: *preeclampsia* (the nonconvulsive stage) and *eclampsia* (the convulsive stage). The condition is classified as *preeclampsia* when, after the twenty-fourth week of pregnancy, a gravida who previously has been normal in the following respects develops sudden elevation of blood pressure, albuminuria or edema (one or more of the symptoms). Certain criteria have been established to divide preeclampsia into two groups: "preeclampsia mild" and "preeclampsia severe," depending on the symptoms. In *preeclampsia mild*, the systolic blood pressure is found to be 140 mm. Hg or more, or is elevated 30 mm. or more above the usual level; the diastolic pressure will be 90 mm. Hg or more, or is elevated 15 mm. or more above the usual level. Abnormal blood pressures must be observed on two occasions or more at least six hours apart, because a single reading may be misleading. The albumin in the urine is small in amount but must be of sufficient degree on two or more successive days. Persistent edema involving the hands and the face is present. The condition is classified as *preeclampsia severe* if any one of the following signs or symptoms is present: 1) a systolic blood pressure of 160 mm. Hg or more, or a diastolic pressure of 110 mm. or more; 2) marked albuminuria; 3) oliguria; 4) cerebral or visual disturbances; 5) pulmonary edema or cyanosis. Once the preeclamptic patient has a convulsion, she passes into the stage called *eclampsia*.

CHRONIC HYPERTENSIVE VASCULAR DISEASE, sometimes called essential hypertension, is a disease which is not peculiar to pregnancy. When pregnancy aggravates the already existing hypertension so that the gravida with this chronic process develops an acute elevation of blood pressure and a significant degree of albuminuria, the condition is called *chronic hypertensive vascular disease with superimposed acute toxemia*. This disease is seen in all stages of gestation but is prone to occur between the twenty-fourth and thirtieth weeks. Furthermore, the symptoms may increase in severity to the stage of eclampsia.

Preeclampsia

As has been stated in the previous classification of the toxemias of pregnancy, preeclampsia is characterized by a sudden elevation in blood pressure, albuminuria and edema in a gravida who previously has been normal in these respects. It is the forerunner or prodromal stage of eclampsia; in other words, unless the preeclamptic process is checked by treatment or by delivery, it is more or less likely that eclampsia (convulsions and coma) will ensue. Characteristically, preeclampsia is a disease of the last two or three months of pregnancy and is particularly prone to occur in young primigravidae. The underlying disease processes of preeclampsia and eclampsia are probably identical, the chief difference being that the latter goes on to convulsions and coma, whereas the former does not.

SIGNS AND SYMPTOMS. The earliest warning signal of preeclampsia is sudden development of hypertension. Accordingly, the importance of frequent and regular blood pressure estimations during pregnancy cannot be emphasized too strongly. The absolute blood pressure reading is probably of less significance than the relationship it bears to previous determinations and to the age of the patient. For example, a rise from 110/70 to 135/85 in a young woman is a more urgent danger signal than a rise from 135/85 to 150/90 in a patient of 35.

The next most constant sign of preeclampsia is sudden, excessive weight gain. If cases of preeclampsia are studied from the viewpoint of fluid intake and output, it is at once apparent that these sudden gains in weight are due entirely to an accumulation of water in the tissues. Such weight gains, in other words, represent latent edema and almost always precede the visible face and finger edema which is so characteristic of the advanced stages of the disease. From what has been said, it is apparent that scales are essential equipment for good antepartal care. Weight gain of 1 pound a week or so may be regarded as being normal. Sudden gains of more than 2 pounds

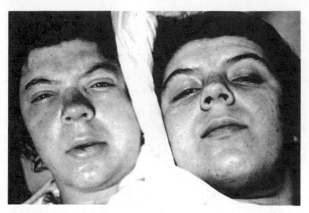

Figure 23-1. (Left) Facies in preeclampsia. Note edema of eyelids and facial skin and general coarsing of features. (Right) Same patient ten days after delivery.

a week should be viewed with suspicion; gains of more than 3 pounds, with alarm. Weight increases of the latter magnitude call for more frequent blood pressure determinations, and if these latter are also abnormal, hospitalization with intensive treatment is indicated. In investigating suspected edema, it is well to ask the patient if her wedding ring is becoming tight, since finger and facial edema is a more valuable sign of preeclampsia than is swelling of the ankles. In the facies of a patient with outspoken preeclampsia, the eyelids are swollen, and, associated with the edema, marked coarseness of the features develops (Fig. 23-1).

The sudden appearance of *albumin in the urine*, with or without other findings, always should be regarded as a sign of preeclampsia. A complete urinalysis, including a microscopic examination, will help to exclude infection as a cause of proteinuria. Usually it develops later than the hypertension and the gain in weight and for this very reason must be regarded as being a serious omen when superimposed on these other two findings.

But the very essence of preeclampsia is the lightninglike fulminance with which it strikes. Although the above physical signs of preeclampsia usually give the physician ample time to institute preventive treatment, it sometimes happens that these derangements develop between visits to the office or the clinic, even though they be only a week apart. For this reason it is imperative that all expectant mothers be informed, both verbally and by some form of printed slip or booklet, in regard to certain danger signals which they themselves may recognize. Insofar as the toxemias of pregnancy

are concerned, the following symptoms demand immediate report to the physician: 1) severe, continuous headache; 2) swelling of the face or the fingers; 3) dimness or blurring of vision; 4) persistent vomiting; 5) decrease in the amount of urine excreted; and 6) epigastric pain (a late symptom).

It should be emphasized that the three early and important signs of preeclampsia, namely, hypertension, weight gain and albuminuria, are changes of which the patient is usually unaware. All three may be present in substantial degree, and yet she may feel quite well. Only by regular and careful antepartal examination can these warning signs be detected. By the time the preeclamptic patient has developed symptoms and signs which she herself can detect (such as headache, blurred vision, puffiness of the eyelids and the fingers), she is usually in an advanced stage of the disease, and much valuable time has been lost. Headache is rarely observed in the milder cases but is encountered with increasing frequency as the most severe grades are met. In general, patients who actually develop eclampsia often have a severe headache as a forerunner of the first convulsion. The visual disturbances range from a slight blurring of vision to various degrees of temporary blindness. Although convulsions are less likely to occur in cases of mild preeclampsia, the possibility cannot be entirely eliminated. Patients with severe preeclampsia should always be considered as being on the verge of having a convulsion.

TREATMENT. Prophylaxis is most important in the prevention and the control of preeclampsia. Since in its early stages preeclampsia rarely gives rise to signs or symptoms which the patient herself will notice, the early detection of this disease demands meticulous antepartal supervision. Rapid weight gain or an upward trend in blood pressure, although still in the "normal" range, are danger signals. Every pregnant woman should be examined by her obstetrician every week during the last month of pregnancy and every two weeks during the two previous months. The most promising prophylaxis of the disease lies in reduction of sodium intake and curtailing weight gain in all pregnant women. Finger edema is a frequent forerunner of preeclampsia, which may precede the hypertension by several weeks and is a valuable warning sign.

Ambulatory Patient. When the patient's symptoms are mild (i.e., there is minor elevation of blood pressure with minimal or no signs of edema and proteinuria), treatment may be instituted at home in the hope that symptoms will abate. During this period the patient should be examined by the physician at least twice a week, and she should be given a strict regimen to follow, as well as careful instructions in regard to symptoms to report promptly. The patient's activities should be restricted, and she should understand that bed rest during the greater part of the day is most desirable. Sedative drugs, such as phenobarbital, may be prescribed to encourage rest and relaxation, the dosage being dependent on the severity of the condition. Of major importance is a salt-poor diet. Therefore, the patient should be instructed so that she understands which foods have appreciable sodium content and therefore must be excluded from her diet, in addition to the fact that no salt may be added to her food in the kitchen or at the table. The diet should be well balanced but restricted in caloric content if the patient's weight gain indicates the need. It should contain ample protein, particularly lean meat, eggs and a quart of milk daily. Fluid intake should be maintained at 2,500 ml. daily; in hot weather, at 3,000 ml. Carbonated beverages should be avoided because of their sodium content.

The restriction of sodium in the diet of the preeclamptic patient is directed at reducing the edema. Even in normal nonpregnant persons an increased intake of sodium chloride causes water retention. Pregnant women, particularly gravidae suffering from preeclampsia, show a marked tendency to retain sodium, and there is reason to believe that this tendency of the tissues to retain sodium is closely correlated with their tendency to hold water. To superimpose still more sodium in the diet on this already existing sodium and water retention is obviously unwise. Since the accumulation of sodium and water precedes the development of hypertension and proteinuria in preeclampsia, the control of such retention is sufficiently important that diuretic therapy is indicated on an ambulatory basis if dietary measures fail. Such diuretic regimens are described later.

Although some have suggested that routine therapy with thiazide diuretics would prevent toxemia in a group of high-risk patients, it has now been clearly established that this is not true and that diuretic therapy in pregnancy is not indicated unless there is symptomatic edema, or one is treating chronic hypertension.

Hospital Patient. In the event that the patient's condition does not respond promptly to ambulatory treatment, she should be hospitalized without delay. A systematic method of study should be instituted upon admission to the hospital. A general physical examination and history should be obtained promptly, followed by constant vigilance for the development of such symptoms as headache, visual disturbances and edema of the fingers and the eyelids. Body weight should be obtained on admission and every other morning thereafter. Blood pressure readings should be taken every four hours except between midnight and morning, unless the midnight blood pressure has risen. Daily fluid intake and output records should be kept, and urine specimens sent to the laboratory daily for analysis for albumin and casts. Retinal examination is always included as part of the admission physical examination and is done every two to three days thereafter, depending on the findings. Blood chemical determinations are also included. Once the patient is admitted to the hospital, complete bed rest is essential.

Drugs and Diet. Even in milder cases, minimal doses of sedative drugs are helpful. Phenobarbital, 32 mg. (½ grain), may be given four times a day, or twice this dosage in cases of moderate severity. The dietary regimen previously described should be adhered to, or it may be indicated to restrict the sodium chloride to less than 3 Gm. daily. In such cases it may become necessary to substitute one of the commercial sodium-free milk powders in place of regular milk, since a quart of milk itself contains about 1.25 Gm. of sodium chloride.

In the case of symptomatic edema diuretic therapy may be indicated. The most commonly used diuretics today are the thiazides, such as chlorothiazide (Diuril), 0.5 to 1.0 Gm. daily, or hydrochlorothiazide (Esidrix), 50 mg. daily. These drugs increase the excretion of both sodium and water without producing acidosis, but at the same time, when given in adequate doses, cause a marked loss of potassium. If not recognized, potassium depletion may become symptomatic, causing fatigue and muscular weakness. This problem can be avoided by administering supplemental potassium, or with dietary measures such as an increased intake of citrus fruit and juices. Some physicians avoid the problem by administering the drugs intermittently (three days out of five, or five out of seven). Occasionally, a patient may become refractory to the thiazides, in which case there are even more potent drugs available, such as ethacrynic acid (Edecrin) or furosemide (Lasix). It is important to be sure that the problem is only one of refractoriness to the diuretic and not a true worsening of the toxemia, which would certainly require more drastic measures than a change in diuretics.

When severe preeclampsia develops, immediate and intensive therapy is imperative. Sedation is of major importance to forestall convulsions. The dosage of drugs employed should be regulated so that they produce drowsiness and sleep, from which the patient can be easily awakened, and also suppress the hyperactive reflexes of the patient. The drug most often used as a sedative and an anticonvulsant under these circumstances is magnesium sulfate. In addition to being an excellent anticonvulsant, magnesium causes vasodilatation and, therefore, is also effective in lowering blood pressure. For rapid action, an IV dose of 20 to 30 ml. of a 10 percent solution (2 to 3 Gm.) is used. Very often the drug is given intramuscularly in doses of 10 to 20 ml. of a 50 percent solution (5 to 10 mg.). The dose is divided, half given into each buttock, and often 1 to 2 ml. of 1 percent procaine is added to the injection to minimize discomfort. A repeat dose of magnesium sulfate should not be given unless the reflexes and respiratory rate have been checked, since it depresses both. The antidote is calcium, and an ampul of calcium gluconate should always be readily available when magnesium is being administered.

The barbiturates can also be used, the dose being larger (60 to 120 mg. every four to six hours) than for mild cases and the route of administration parenteral. If the patient is in labor, it is well to avoid barbiturates because of their depressant effect on the fetus. Although many use morphine in the management of severe preeclampsia, it would seem best reserved for the patient who has the added stimulus of pain (i.e., labor). Minimizing this stimulus will certainly reduce the likelihood of a seizure.

Another drug which is an effective anticonvulsant is diazepam (Valium) in 5- to 10-mg. doses intramuscularly or, if the situation warrants, intravenously.

Delivery. Despite all efforts, the condition may persist to a marked degree, and in that event induction of labor may become necessary for the welfare of mother and infant (see Chapter 22). In occasional instances when preeclampsia is severe and fulminating and conditions for induction of labor are not favorable, cesarean section may be the procedure of choice.

POSTPARTUM. The signs and symptoms of preeclampsia usually abate rapidly after delivery, but the danger of convulsions does not pass until 48 hours have elapsed postpartum. Therefore, continuation of sedation throughout this interval is indicated. In the majority of cases the elevated blood pressure as well as the other derangements have returned to normal within ten days or two weeks. In about 30 percent of cases, however, the hypertension shows a tendency either to persist indefinitely or to recur in subsequent pregnancies. For this reason the prolonged follow-up of these patients is highly important.

NURSING CARE. The nurse's responsibility in the detection and care of cases of preeclampsia is manifold. Since this complication of pregnancy is common and may occur antepartally, intrapartally or postpartally, it is important for the nurse to observe all maternity patients closely for the first indication of early symptoms, as well as to be quick to recognize and report any evidence pointing to an aggravation of the process. The early symptoms and the manifestations related to more severe preeclampsia, such as persistent headache, blurred vision, spots or flashes of light before the eyes, epigastric pain, vomiting, torpor or muscular twitchings, are all vastly important. Data collected in relation to these symptoms in addition to an accurate record of weight gain, fluid intake and elimination, diet and attitudes and behavior, when it is accurately recorded, can assist the physician in evaluating the symptoms and planning the course of therapy.

In setting the therapeutic atmosphere, the nurse should see that the environment is as comfortable and pleasant as possible. The patient should be in a single room, free from the stimuli of noise, strong lights and the presence of unnecessary equipment which might frighten her. To the best of her ability, the nurse must protect the patient from needless traffic into the room; otherwise, the coming and going of personnel to the bedside may be so constant that it could interfere with the efficacy of the treatment being carried out. Every effort should be exerted to relieve the patient's anxiety, which sometimes is brought about by apprehension regarding her illness or may be due to concern for the welfare of her family at home.

Regardless of the severity of the toxemia, certain responsibilities are carried out by the nurse. Medications ordered must be administered promptly, the prescribed diet should be supervised, a careful record of intake and elimination kept, blood pressure readings and basal weights taken, specimens collected and labeled accurately, and observations of slight symptoms or change in condition should be reported immediately, both verbally and on the patient's record. Since rest is a major consideration in the care of this patient, the nurse should plan a schedule of activities so that the patient is disturbed as little as possible. Medications, treatments and nursing procedures should be administered at the same time as far as the physician's orders will permit, but always with the thought in mind that only as much as will not overtire the patient should be planned for any one time. When any treatment is ordered, the procedure is best carried out after sedation has been administered. Before heavy sedation is initiated, any removable dentures or eyeglasses should be removed and stored in a secure place. If the patient is not in labor, the nurse must be alert to watch for signs of labor, particularly after sedation has been given. Any time an intravenous fluid is administered, if the physician has not specified the rate at which the fluid is to flow, it should be given slowly.

The nurse should see that the equipment necessary for the safe and efficient care of the patient is immediately available and in good working order. A padded mouth gag should always be ready for use at the bedside to prevent the patient from biting her tongue in the event that a convulsion develops. Trays for catheterization equipment and for the administration of special medications constitute part of the necessary equipment. Since water retention plays such a large role in the disease, and urinary output is likely to be diminished, an indwelling bladder catheter may be ordered to ensure accuracy in obtaining output from the kidneys. Since the urinary output must be watched carefully, it is imperative to see that the retention catheter is draining properly at all times. In severe cases suction apparatus should be readily available for aspirating mucus, as well as equipment for the administration of oxygen, should symptoms such as cyanosis or depressed respiration indicate the need.

Eclampsia

CLINICAL PICTURE. As indicated, the development of eclampsia is almost always preceded by the signs and symptoms of preeclampsia. A preeclamptic patient, who may have been conversing with you a moment before, is seen to roll her eyes to one side and stare fixedly into space. Immediately, twitching of the facial muscles ensues. This is the *stage of invasion* of the convulsion and lasts only a few seconds.

The whole body then becomes rigid in a generalized muscular contraction; the face is distorted, the eyes protrude, the arms are flexed, the hands are clenched and the legs are inverted. Since all the muscles of the body are now in a state of tonic contraction, this phase may be regarded as the *stage of contraction*; it lasts 15 or 20 seconds.

Suddenly the jaws begin to open and close violently, and forthwith the eyelids also. The other facial muscles and then all the muscles of the body alternately contract and relax in rapid succession. So forceful are the muscular movements that the patient may throw herself out of bed, and almost invariably, unless protected, the tongue is bitten by the violent jaw action. Foam, often blood-tinged, exudes from the mouth; the face is congested and purple, and the eyes are bloodshot. Few pictures which the nurse is called upon to witness are so horrible. This phase in which the muscles alternately contract and relax is called the *stage of convulsion*; it may last a minute or so. Gradually the muscular movements become milder and farther apart, and finally the patient lies motionless.

Throughout the seizure the diaphragm has been fixed with respiration halted. Still no breathing occurs. For a few seconds the woman appears to be dying from respiratory arrest, but just when this outcome seems almost inevitable, she takes a long, deep, stertorous inhalation, and breathing is resumed. Then coma ensues. The patient will remember nothing whatsoever of the convulsion or, in all probability, events immediately before and afterward.

The coma may last from a few minutes to several hours, and the patient may then become conscious; or the coma may be succeeded by another convulsion. The convulsions may recur during coma, or they may recur only after an interval of consciousness, or they may never recur at all. In the average case, from five to ten convulsions occur at longer or shorter intervals, but as many as 20 are not uncommon. Convulsions may start before the onset of labor (antepartum), during labor (intrapartum) or anytime within the first 48 hours after delivery (postpartum). About a fifth of the cases develop postpartally.

Upon physical examination, the findings of eclampsia are similar to those in preeclampsia, but exaggerated. Thus, the systolic blood pressure usually ranges around 180 mm. Hg and sometimes exceeds 200 mm. Hg. Albuminuria is frequently extreme, from 10 to 20 Gm. per liter. Edema may be marked but sometimes is absent. Oliguria, or suppression of urinary excretion, is common and may amount to complete anuria. Fever is present in about half the cases.

In favorable cases the convulsions cease, the coma lessens, and urinary output increases. However, it sometimes requires one or two days for clear consciousness to be regained. During this period eclamptic patients are often in an obstreperous, resistant mood and may be exceedingly difficult to manage. A few develop actual psychoses. In unfavorable cases the coma deepens, urinary excretion diminishes, the pulse becomes more rapid, the temperature rises, and edema of the lungs develops. The last is a serious symptom and usually is interpreted as a sign of cardiovascular failure. Edema of the lungs is readily recognizable by the noisy, gurgling respiration and by the large quantity of frothy mucus which exudes from the mouth and the nose. Toward the end, convulsions cease altogether, and the final picture is one of vascular collapse, with falling blood pressure and overwhelming edema of the lungs.

Like preeclampsia, eclampsia is a disease of young primigravidae, the majority of cases occurring in first pregnancies. It is more likely to occur as full term approaches and is rarely seen prior to the last three months. Eclampsia is particularly prone to develop in twin gestations, the likelihood being about four times that in single pregnancies.

PROGNOSIS. Eclampsia is one of the gravest complications of pregnancy; the maternal mortality in different localities and in different hospitals ranges from 5 to 15 percent of such cases. The outlook for the baby is particularly grave, the fetal mortality being about 20 percent. Although it is difficult in a given case to forecast the outcome, the following are unfavorable signs: oliguria; prolonged coma; a sustained pulse rate over 120; temperature over 103° F.; more than ten convulsions; 10 or more Gm. of albumin per liter in the urine; systolic blood pressure of more than 200; edema of lungs. If none of these signs is present, the outlook for recovery is good; if two or more are present, the prognosis is definitely serious.

Even though the patient survives, she may not escape unscathed from the attack but sometimes continues to have high blood pressure indefinitely. This statement applies to both preeclampsia and eclampsia. Indeed, about 10 percent of all preeclamptic and 5 percent of all eclamptic patients are left with chronic, permanent hypertension. It is of even more importance to note that a still larger percentage of these women (about 50 percent of preeclamptics and 30 percent of eclamptics) again develop hypertensive toxemia in any subsequent pregnancies. This is known as "recurrent" or "repeat" toxemia. These facts make it plain that careful, prolonged follow-up of those mothers who have suffered from preeclampsia or eclampsia is imperative. Moreover, the prognosis for future pregnancies must be guarded, although, as the figures indicate, such patients stand at least an even chance of going through subsequent pregnancies satisfactorily.

PRINCIPLES OF TREATMENT. Since the cause of eclampsia is not known, there can be no "specific" therapy, and treatment must necessarily be empirical. By "empirical" treatment is meant the utilization of those therapeutic measures which have yielded the best results in other cases. It is thus based on experience. Since the experience of different doctors and different hospitals varies considerably, the type of therapy employed from clinic to clinic differs somewhat in respect to the drugs used and in other details. However, the general principles followed are almost identical everywhere. For the nurse to memorize some particular regimen of therapy, as given in this textbook or as used in this or that hospital, will serve little purpose in her later career and conduces to an undesirable rigidity of attitude. However, she should grasp thoroughly the general principles involved. These are enumerated as follows:

1. Prevention. Let it be emphasized again that eclampsia is largely (but not entirely) a preventable disease. Vigilant antepartal care and the early detection and treatment of

preeclampsia will do more to reduce deaths from eclampsia than the most intensive treatment after convulsions have once started.

2. Termination of Pregnancy. Although the precise cause of preeclampsia and eclampsia is not known, it is quite clear that since they do not occur except in pregnancy, the one sure "cure" is to render the patient nonpregnant. In almost all instances of eclampsia, efforts to effect delivery should be undertaken as soon as the patient is stabilized. This involves control of seizures as well as hyperreflexia, by adequate doses of anticonvulsants and the initiation of diuresis. It is often helpful to monitor central venous pressure in addition to urinary output in an attempt to optimize fluid balance. Efforts to accomplish delivery before the patient is stabilized may result in increased maternal morbidity and mortality. The method of delivery should be by the most expeditious route. Prolonged attempts at induction in the face of an unripe cervix are not indicated; however, the possibility of vaginal delivery should not be discounted even at early gestational age since for unexplained reasons the cervix often quickly becomes favorable for induction. Occasionally the obstetrician is faced with the dilemma of an eclamptic with an immature fetus. Although it is tempting to try to prolong the pregnancy in the interest of bringing about greater fetal maturity, such attempts are generally unsuccessful, with impaired placental function and failure of the fetus to prosper.

3. Sedation. The purpose of administering sedative drugs is to depress the activity of the brain cells and thereby stop convulsions. The drugs most commonly employed are described below.

MAGNESIUM SULFATE. This drug is an excellent central nervous system depressant, and therefore anticonvulsant, and also a smooth muscle relaxant which causes dilatation of peripheral blood vessels and thereby reduces blood pressure. For these reasons it is probably the most common drug used in eclamptic patients. The routes of administration, doses and precautions have already been discussed. Since the situation with the eclamptic patient is so urgent, the drug is most often given intravenously, at least initially.

BARBITURATES. Rapid-acting drugs, such as intravenous sodium amobarbital (Amytal) (0.3 to 0.6 Gm.), are often used to control the seizure, while subcutaneous doses of sodium phenobarbital (Luminal) (0.1 to 0.3 Gm.) may be used subsequently.

DIAZEPAM (VALIUM). Intravenous diazepam has now become one of the standard approaches to seizure control. Although there is no evidence to date of ill effects in the fetus and newborn, use is rather recent and therefore safety is still being evaluated.

MORPHINE. Large doses of morphine sulfate have been used in the past but morphine is a relatively ineffective anticonvulsant. Its efficacy is related to its analgesic effect in reducing painful stimuli rather than a direct anticonvulsant effect.

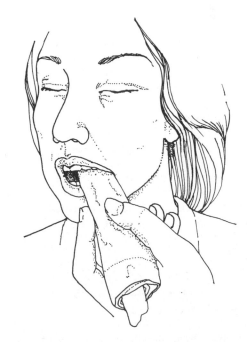

Figure 23-2. Improvised mouth gag inserted between jaws of eclamptic patient to prevent tongue injury. (Putnam, Tracy J.: Convulsive Seizures, Philadelphia, J. B. Lippincott)

complications of pregnancy   471

4. Protection of Patient from Self-injury. The eclamptic patient must never be left alone for a second. When in the throes of a convulsion, she may crash her head against a bedpost or throw herself onto the floor; or she may bite her tongue violently. To prevent the latter injury, some device should be kept within easy reach which can be inserted between the jaws at the very onset of a convulsion. A piece of heavy rubber tubing, a rolled towel or a padded clothespin is often employed (Fig. 23-2). The nurse must take care in inserting it not to injure the patient (lips, gums, teeth) and not to allow her own finger to be bitten.

Eclamptic patients must never be given fluids by mouth unless thoroughly conscious. Failure to adhere to this rule may result in aspiration of the fluid and consequent pneumonia.

5. Protection of Patient from Extraneous Stimuli. A loud noise, a bright light, a jarring of the bed, a draft—indeed, the slightest irritation—may be enough to precipitate a convulsion.

6. Promotion of Diuresis. When an eclamptic patient begins to excrete substantial quantities of urine, the outlook is encouraging. Accordingly, efforts are generally made to stimulate renal activity. This is most often done by the intravenous administration of hypertonic glucose solution, usually about a 20 percent solution in amounts ranging from 200 to 500 ml.

Often now mannitol (25 to 50 Gm.) by intravenous "push" dose is used to promote diuresis. Efforts to induce a diuresis are safer if the patient's central venous pressure is being monitored. Should the CVP be high (above 12 cm. H_2O), the use of osmotic diuretics such as 20 percent glucose of mannitol, or indeed large volumes of fluid, is risky and could well result in cardiac overload and pulmonary edema.

NURSE'S RESPONSIBILITIES IN ECLAMPSIA. The nurse's responsibilities in the management of a case of eclampsia are serious. Some of them have already been mentioned in the discussion of treatment. Although eclampsia usually is regarded as the climax to a mounting pre-eclamptic toxemia which has been present, the nurse must remember that it is occasionally observed as a fulminating case in an apparently normal woman who may develop severe

symptoms in the span of 24 hours. In the event that eclampsia occurs, the best quality of nursing care is necessary. The attack may come on at any time, even when the patient is sleeping. During the seizure it is necessary to protect the patient from self-injury. Never leave the patient for an instant unless someone is actually at the bedside to relieve you. Gentle restraint should be used to guide the patient's movements whenever necessary to prevent her from throwing herself against the head of the bed or out of it. Canvas sides, as well as pads at the head and the foot of the bed, are helpful. The padded mouth gag should be inserted between the upper and lower teeth at the onset of a convulsion to prevent the tongue from being bitten. Regardless of the fact that the nurse is exceedingly "busy" with the patient when a seizure occurs, she should make careful and complete observations of the duration and the character of each convulsion, the depth and duration of coma, the quality and the rate of pulse and respiration and the degree of cyanosis. A careful record should be kept so that this information can be used by the physician in treating the patient. During the coma which follows, care must be taken to see that the patient does not aspirate. It is understood, of course, that one never gives an eclamptic patient fluids by mouth unless it is certain she is fully conscious. The position of the patient in bed should be such that it promotes drainage of secretions and the maintenance of a clear airway. It may be necessary to raise the foot of the bed of the comatose patient a few inches to promote drainage of secretions from the respiratory passage. When this measure must be resorted to, it is particularly important to watch for signs of pulmonary edema, which would be aggravated by this position. The head of the bed may need to be elevated to relieve dyspnea. Even though the patient should be disturbed as little as possible, her position should be changed at hourly intervals.

The patient should be protected from extraneous stimuli. Light in the room should be eliminated except for a small lamp, so shaded that none of the light falls on the patient. Although the room should be darkened, the light should be sufficient to permit observations of changes in condition, such as cyanosis or twitchings. A flashlight, directed well away from the patient's face, may be used during catheterization and rectal installations and during the physician's examinations. Sudden noises, such as the slamming of a door or the clatter of a tray as it is placed on a table, and jarring of the bed must be avoided, because they are often sufficient stimuli to send the patient into convulsions. Only absolutely necessary conversation should be carried on in the room, and this should be in the lowest tones possible.

The fetal heart tones should be checked as often as time will permit. Also, the nurse must watch for signs of labor. In eclampsia this may proceed with few external signs, and occasionally such a patient gives birth beneath the sheets before anyone knows that the process is under way. Be suspicious when the patient grunts or groans or moves about at regular intervals, every five minutes or so. If this occurs, feel the consistency of the uterus, watch for "show" and bulging and report your observations to the physician. Convulsions which occur during labor may speed up this process, and more rapid preparation for delivery should be made. During the delivery, the same atmosphere of quiet should be maintained, and glaring lights should be kept away from the patient's face.

Throughout the care of the eclamptic patient a careful account of fluid intake and output should be recorded, along with all the other observations and pertinent data. And, since further complications of pregnancy may occur in eclampsia, the patient should be observed for signs and symptoms of cerebral hemorrhage, abruptio placentae, pulmonary edema and cardiac failure.

Preeclampsia and eclampsia have been discussed in some detail because the nurse's role in the management of these conditions is extremely important.

Chronic hypertensive vascular disease

As the name implies, this is a process in which high blood pressure is present before pregnancy. Difficulty is encountered in establishing such a diagnosis, because many women are not seen between pregnancies and blood pressures are, therefore, not recorded. Also, there is normally a decrease in blood pressure during the second trimester which could mask a preexisting hypertension, if the patient does not report for care until the fourth or fifth month of gestation. The diagnosis is justified if hypertension is detected prior to the twenty-fourth week of gestation. Most often patients with chronic hypertension are multiparae and commonly over the age of 30.

At least 75 percent of such patients are able to successfully complete their pregnancies, with no significant change in the status of their hypertension. Fifteen percent develop superimposed preeclampsia, an occurrence which carries an ominous fetal prognosis (20 percent mortality), and even an increase in maternal mortality (1 to 2 percent).

The treatment, then, for the majority of those patients with benign chronic essential hypertension is no different than for the nonpregnant patient. It includes salt restriction, diuretics, restricted activities, sedation and antihypertensives. The pregnancy is allowed to run its normal course under such circumstances. In the case of superimposed preeclampsia, after 24 to 48 hours of intensive medical therapy, pregnancy termination is generally indicated. Even though the fetus may be preterm, its chances for survival under these circumstances are generally better outside the uterus. In a small number of patients the hypertension will be so severe, with evidence of kidney involvement, severe retinal changes, or cardiac involvement, that therapeutic abortion might be considered if the patient comes to medical attention in the first trimester. It is also well to consider the advisability of postpartum tubal ligation in this group of patients who are generally older, with established families, and for whom additional pregnancies may represent a serious health hazard. This, of course, can only be a recommendation, the final decision resting with the patient and her husband.

Hemorrhagic complications

The causes of bleeding in pregnancy are usually considered in relation to the stage of gestation in which they are most likely to cause complications. Frequent causes of bleeding during the first half of pregnancy are abortion, ectopic pregnancy and hydatidiform mole. Although hydatidiform mole is a less common cause (it occurs once in about 2,000 pregnancies), it is nevertheless important, because uterine bleeding is its outstanding symptom. The two most common causes of hemorrhage in the latter half of pregnancy are placenta previa and abruptio placentae.

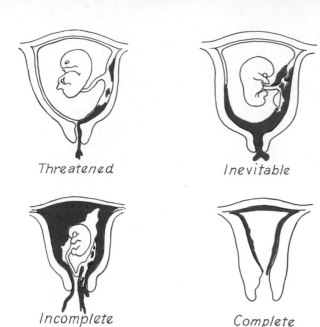

Threatened

Inevitable

Incomplete

Complete

Figure 23-3. Stages of abortion. (Cooke, Willard R.: Essentials of Gynecology, Philadelphia, J. B. Lippincott)

Abortion

DEFINITIONS. Abortion is the termination of pregnancy at any time before the fetus has attained a stage of viability, that is, before it is capable of extrauterine existence.

It is customary to use the weight of the fetus as an important criterion in abortion. Infants weighing 1,000 Gm. (2 pounds, 3 ounces) or less at birth possess little chance for survival, whereas those above this weight have a substantial chance of living. Thus, many authorities regard a pregnancy which terminates when the fetus weighs 1,000 Gm. (about 28 weeks of gestation) or less as an abortion. On the other hand, a small percentage of infants weighing 1,000 Gm. or less do survive. Modern advances in the management and care of preterm infants have made it possible for smaller and smaller infants to survive, so fetuses weighing only 800 to 900 Gm. (1 pound, 13 ounces to 2 pounds) may live. For this reason many authorities now maintain that fetal weight of 1,000 Gm. or less but more than 400 Gm. is classified as immature, and that fetal weight of 400 Gm. (about 20 weeks of gestation) or less constitutes an abortion. It is obvious, therefore, that how the termination of pregnancy is classified in different hospitals will depend wholly on the interpretation to which they subscribe. In summary, the following definitions are generally used. The termina-

tion of pregnancy at any time when the fetus weighs 400 Gm. or less is defined as an *abortion*. Infants weighing between 401 and 1,000 Gm. are called *immature*.

A preterm infant is one born after the stage of viability has been reached but before it has the same chance for survival as a full-term infant. By general consensus, an infant which weighs 2,500 Gm. or less at birth is termed *preterm*; one which weighs 2,501 Gm. (5½ pounds) or more is regarded as *full term*.

It is well to remember that preterm labor does not refer to abortion. *Preterm labor* is the termination of pregnancy after the fetus is viable but before it has attained full term. Although the cause of many preterm labors cannot be explained, the condition can be brought on by maternal diseases, such as chronic hypertensive vascular disease, abruptio placentae, placenta previa, untreated syphilis or a mechanical defect in the cervix.

As a measure to bring about greater uniformity in the interpretation of the terms *abortion*, *miscarriage* and *viability*, the World Health Organization, in 1950, introduced certain new definitions which, in effect, would substitute the term *early fetal death* for abortion and would tabulate all live births and fetal deaths in four groups, according to length of gestation.

TERMINOLOGY OF ABORTION. The term abortion includes many varieties of termination of pregnancy prior to viability but may be subdivided into two main groups, namely, spontaneous and induced. *Spontaneous abortion* is one in which through natural causes the process starts of its own accord. *Induced abortion* is one which is artificially induced whether for therapeutic or other reasons. Induced abortion has been considered on pp. 456 to 458. The laity often use miscarriage to designate spontaneous abortion, and the nurse will do well in discussing the matter with patients or relatives to use that term.

In medical parlance, the word miscarriage is rarely employed.

Threatened Abortion. An abortion is regarded as threatened if a patient in early pregnancy has vaginal bleeding or spotting; this may or may not be associated with mild cramps. The cervix is closed. The process has presumably started but may abate (Fig. 23-3).

Inevitable Abortion. Inevitable abortion is so called because the process has gone so far that termination of the pregnancy cannot be prevented. Bleeding is copious, and the pains are more severe. The membranes may or may not have ruptured, and the cervical canal is dilating.

Incomplete Abortion. An incomplete abortion is one in which part of the products of conception has been passed, but part (usually the placenta) is retained in the uterus. Bleeding usually persists until the retained products of conception have been passed.

Complete Abortion. Complete abortion is the expulsion of the entire products of conception.

Missed Abortion. In a missed abortion the fetus dies in the uterus, but, instead of being expelled, it is retained indefinitely. The term is generally restricted to cases in which two months or more elapse between fetal death and expulsion. During this period the fetus undergoes marked degenerative changes. Of these, maceration, or general softening, is the most common. Occasionally it dries up into a leatherlike structure (mummification) and very rarely it becomes converted into stony material (lithopedion formation). Symptoms, except for amenorrhea, are usually lacking, but occasionally such patients complain of malaise, headache and anorexia. Hypofibrinogenemia, a hemorrhagic complication, may result (see p. 482).

Habitual Abortion. By this term is meant a condition in which spontaneous abortion occurs in successive pregnancies (three or more). This is a most distressing condition, some women having six or eight spontaneous abortions.

CRIMINAL ABORTION. Criminal, or perhaps better stated, extra-hospital (or extra-clinic) abortion is the termination of pregnancy outside of appropriate medical facilities, generally by nonphysician abortionists, regardless of the validity of the indication. The frequency of such abortions is not precisely known but has dropped precipitously in the United States following the Supreme Court decision of 1973. In years past, estimates ranged from 200,000 to 1,200,000 per year in the United States. In most urban areas, abortions were responsible for the majority of maternal deaths, with estimates of 800 to 5,000 abortion deaths per year. Attempts at producing abortion are generally made by the ingestion of drugs such as quinine or castor oil, which usually do nothing, or if taken in sufficient quantities to produce an abortion place the woman in serious jeopardy. Another common approach involves the placement of a foreign body, such as a urethral catheter, into the uterus with or without the instillation of toxic substances. Severe infection, often with shock and kidney failure, is a common consequence of such crude efforts at pregnancy termination. Patients so affected surely are some of the most critically ill the nurse may ever have to care for and, unfortunately, they sometimes succumb in spite of the best efforts of all concerned.

CLINICAL PICTURE. About 75 percent of all spontaneous abortions occur during the second and the third months of pregnancy, that is, before the twelfth week. The condition is very common; it is estimated that about one pregnancy in every ten terminates in spontaneous abortion. Almost invariably the first symptom is bleeding due to the separation of the fertilized ovum from its uterine attachment. The bleeding is often slight at the beginning and may persist for days before uterine cramps occur; or, the bleeding may be followed at once by cramps. Occasionally the bleeding is torrential in nature, leaving the patient in shock. The uterine contractions bring about softening and dilatation of the cervix and expel the products of conception either completely or incompletely.

CAUSES. What causes all these spontaneous abortions—so tragic and shattering to so many women? If the evidence is reviewed with some perspective and with full fairness to all concerned, it is the inevitable conclusion that most of these abortions, far from being tragedies, are blessings in disguise, for they are Nature's beneficent way of extinguishing embryos which are imperfect. Indeed, careful microscopic study of the material passed in these cases shows that the commonest cause of spontaneous abortion is an inherent defect in the products of conception. This defect may express itself in an abnormal embryo, in an abnormal *trophoblast* (p. 108) or in both abnormalities. In early abortions, 80 percent are associated with some defect of the embryo or trophoblast which is either incompatible with life or would result in a grossly deformed child. The incidence of abnormalities passed after the second month is somewhat lower but not less than 50 percent. Whether the germ plasm of the spermatozoon or the ovum is at fault in these cases, it is usually difficult, if not impossible, to say. Abortions of this sort are obviously not preventable and, although often bitterly

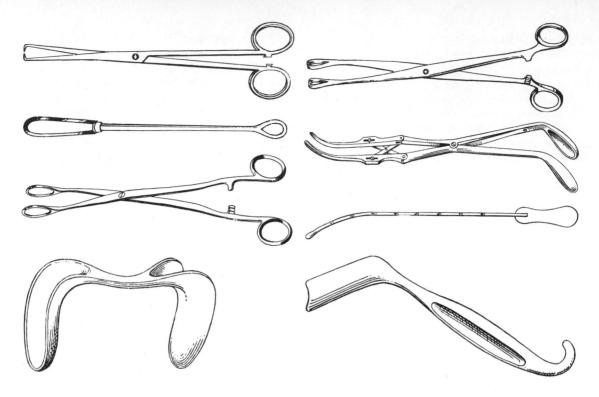

Figure 23-4. (*Left, top to bottom*) Bullet forceps used in grasping the lips of the cervix. Sims's sharp curette, a scraper or spoonlike instrument for removing matter from the walls of the uterus. Sponge holder. Sims's speculum for inserting into the vaginal canal so as to expose the cervix to view. (*Right, top to bottom*) Placental forceps with heart-shaped jaws. Modified Goodell-Ellinger dilator used for enlarging the canal of the cervix. Uterine sound. Schroeder vaginal retractor for drawing back the vulvar or vaginal walls during an operation.

disappointing to the parents, serve a useful purpose.

Spontaneous abortions may be due to causes other than defects in the products of conception. Severe acute infections, such as pneumonia, pyelitis and typhoid fever, often lead to abortion. Heart failure is another etiologic factor. Occasionally, abnormalities of the generative tract, such as a congenitally short cervix or uterine malformations, produce the accident. Retroposition of the uterus rarely causes abortion, as was formerly believed. Many women tend to explain miscarriage on the grounds of injury of one type or another, or excessive activity. Different women exhibit the greatest variation in this respect. In some the pregnancy may go blithely on despite falls from second-story windows and automobile accidents so severe as to fracture the pelvis. In others a trivial fall, anxiety or overfatigue may appear to be related to abortion, but there is obviously no way to determine a cause-and-effect relationship.

TREATMENT. The severity of the symptoms manifested in threatened abortion will determine the treatment prescribed. If the patient is having only a slight vaginal bleeding or even spotting, without pain, she should be advised to stay in bed, eat a light well-balanced diet, and avoid straining at bowel evacuation and the use of cathartics. If she appears to be apprehensive, a mild sedative may be given. Some physicians do not restrict activity, based on the concept that the uterus is well insulated from outside influences. Uniformly the patient should be advised to save all perineal pads, as well as all tissue and clots passed, for inspection. In cases where bed rest has been prescribed, if the bleeding disappears within 48 hours, the woman may get out of bed but should limit her activities for the next several days. Coitus should be avoided for two weeks following the last evidence of bleeding. In cases in which pain accompanies the vaginal bleeding, the prognosis for saving the pregnancy is poor. Usually bleeding is observed first, and a few hours, sometimes days later, uterine contractions ensue. This is often treated by absolute bed rest and narcotic drugs (paregoric, morphine, etc.). When the pain and the bleeding increase, the patient should be hospitalized, if this has not already been done. If the abortion is incomplete, ordinarily efforts are made to aid the uterus in emptying its contents. Oxytocin may be administered, but if this is ineffectual, surgical removal of the retained products of conception should be done promptly. Active bleeding may make this urgently necessary. Many times the tissue lies loose in the cervical canal and can simply be lifted out with ovum forceps; otherwise, curettage of the uterine cavity must be done. The instruments commonly used in completing an incomplete abortion are shown in Figs. 23-4 and 23-5. The suction curet may also be used. If evidence of infection is present (fever, foul discharge, or suspicious history of criminal abortion), evacuation of the uterus should be delayed only long enough to obtain appropriate studies (especially smears and cultures) and to initiate antibiotic therapy. Such prompt and aggressive management of the patient with an infected abortion will effectively reduce the incidence of more serious complications such as septic shock, thrombophlebitis, and renal failure, and will reduce morbidity and hospital stay as well.

NURSE'S RESPONSIBILITIES IN ABORTION CASES. Bleeding in the first half of pregnancy, no matter how slight, always must be considered as threatened abortion. The patient must be put to bed and the physician notified. An episode of this nature is indeed distressing to the expectant mother, many times alarming. The nurse should bear in mind that although the emotional support she gives her patient is important, she must never try to reassure her that "everything will be all right," because in fact the patient may lose this pregnancy. Perineal pads and all tissue and blood clots passed by the patient should be saved. The physician will wish to examine these to determine the amount of bleeding and, when tissue has been passed, to examine the products of conception to ascertain, among other facts, whether or not the abortion is complete. If bleeding is so copious as to be alarming, elevate the foot of the bed (shock position) while awaiting the physician's arrival. If surgical completion of the abortion is to be carried out, the same aseptic regimen is carried out as for delivery.

All cases of abortion carried out in nonmedical hands must be regarded as potentially infected, and strict antiseptic precautions must be carried out to prevent spread of infection to others. In caring for a woman who has had such an abortion recently, or one whose history is suspicious, the nurse may find it difficult to handle her own feelings so that she does not reflect a judgmental attitude. It is helpful to remember that it is not within the province of the nurse to pass moral judgments as she gives nursing care. In such situations the nurse should direct her concern to the gravity of the patient's illness. Occasionally circumstances make it possible for the nurse to be of definite educational help both to her patients and to the public.

Incompetent cervical os

A mechanical defect in the cervix, incompetent cervical os, has gained recognition as a cause of late habitual abortion or preterm labor. When repeated termination of pregnancy in the second trimester is due to an anatomic factor such as this, surgical treatment may make fetal salvage possible. One of the various

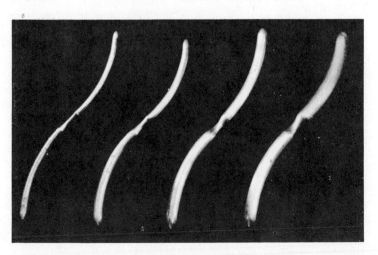

Figure 23-5. Hegar dilators of graduated diameters from 5 to 12 mm. Larger sizes are also used.

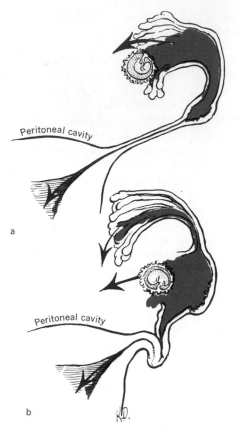

Figure 23-6. (a) Tubal abortion, showing passage of the products of conception, together with much blood, out the fimbriated end of the tube. (b) Rupture of tubal pregnancy into peritoneal cavity. There is an outpouring of blood into the abdomen from vessels at the site of the rupture.

treatments used to prevent relaxation and dilatation of the cervix when it is incompetent to carry on a "good" pregnancy is the modified Shirodkar technique. In this, the vaginal mucous membrane is elevated and a narrow strip of some material such as Mersilene is carried around the internal os of the cervix and tied. Then the vaginal mucosa is restored to its original position and sutured. This is the most popular of several so-called "cerclage" procedures used in the management of the incompetent cervix. The procedure may be done between pregnancies, if the diagnosis is clearly established, or during pregnancy. When done during pregnancy, it is usually elected to wait until the early part of the second trimester (14 to 16 weeks) to avoid the possibility of having to remove the suture if a spontaneous first trimester abortion occurs.

Postoperatively, the main concerns are rupture of the membranes and uterine contrac-

tions. If the membranes rupture, the suture must be removed and the uterus emptied because of the risk of infection. If contractions ensue, an effort to control the contractions is in order, and the most effective means for such control is intravenous alcohol. Attempts to control contractions should not be persistent if they are not effective promptly, since there is a risk of uterine rupture. Decisions regarding the type of delivery a patient is to have are generally based upon the position of the suture when the patient reaches term or labor begins. If the suture is in good position, with the cervical closure maintained, cesarean section may be elected to preserve the suture for future pregnancies. If the suture has loosened or rolled down on the cervix, it is not adequate for subsequent pregnancies. In that case, it is removed when labor begins and vaginal delivery is permitted.

Ectopic pregnancy

An ectopic pregnancy is any gestation located outside the uterine cavity. The majority of ectopic pregnancies are tubal gestations. Other types, which make up about 5 percent of all ectopic pregnancies, are interstitial (in the interstitial portion of the tube), cornual (in a rudimentary horn of a uterus), cervical, abdominal and ovarian gestations.

About once in every 300 pregnancies the fertilized ovum, instead of traversing the length of the fallopian tube to reach the uterine cavity, becomes implanted within the wall of the fallopian tube. This condition is known as "ectopic pregnancy" (literally, a pregnancy which is out of place) or as "tubal pregnancy" or "extrauterine pregnancy." Since the wall of the tube is not sufficiently elastic to allow the fertilized ovum to grow and develop there, rupture of the tubal wall is the inevitable result. Rupture most frequently occurs into the tubal lumen with the passage of the products of conception, together with much blood, out the fimbriated end of the tube and into the peritoneal cavity—so-called tubal abortion. Or, rupture may occur through the peritoneal surface of the tube directly into the peritoneal cavity; and, again, there is an outpouring of blood into the abdomen from vessels at the site of rupture (Fig. 23-6). In either case, rupture usually occurs within the first 12 weeks.

Occasionally an ectopic pregnancy may develop in that portion of the tube which passes through the uterine wall, a type known as "interstitial pregnancy." In very, very rare instances, the products of conception, after rupturing through the tubal wall, may become implanted on the peritoneum and develop to full term in the peritoneal cavity. This extraordinary occurrence is known as "abdominal pregnancy." Surprisingly enough, quite a few living infants have been delivered in such cases by means of abdominal incision.

Ectopic pregnancy may be due to any condition which narrows the tube or brings about some constriction within it. Under such circumstances the tubal lumen is large enough to allow spermatozoa to ascend the tube but not big enough to permit the downward passage of the fertilized ovum. Among the conditions which may produce such a narrowing of the fallopian tube are previous inflammatory processes involving the tubal mucosa and producing partial agglutination of opposing surfaces, such as gonorrheal salpingitis; previous inflammatory processes of the external peritoneal surfaces of the tube, causing kinking, such as peurperal and postabortal infections; and developmental defects resulting in a general narrowing of the tubes.

In cases of ectopic gestation the woman exhibits the usual early symptoms of pregnancy and, as a rule, regards herself as being normally pregnant. After missing one or two periods, however, she suddenly experiences pain which is knifelike in nature and often of extreme severity in one of the lower quadrants. This is usually associated wih slight vaginal bleeding, commonly referred to as "spotting." Depending on the amount of blood which has escaped into the peritoneal cavity, she may or may not undergo a fainting attack and show symptoms of shock.

Ectopic pregnancy is a grave complication of pregnancy and is an important cause of maternal death. Moreover, if a woman has had one ectopic pregnancy and subsequently becomes pregnant, she is more likely to have another such accident.

In the vast majority of cases the tube has already ruptured, and the fetus is dead when the patient is first seen by the physician. It is the rupture which produces the acute clinical picture. The treatment is removal of the tube, supplemented by blood transfusion. Occasionally the ovary must be removed with the tube. Under certain circumstances in which subsequent fertility must be maintained, the tube may be preserved by merely removing the

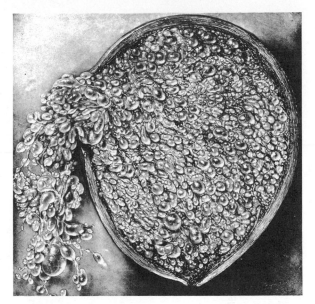

Figure 23-7. Hydatidiform mole. (Eastman, N. J.: William's Obstetrics, New York, Appleton)

pregnancy. This latter approach, called salpingotomy, is applicable if the contralateral tube is badly diseased or has been previously removed and it is the patient's wish to preserve fertility.

During the transportation of such a patient to the hospital or in the interval when the patient is awaiting operation, the nurse can be of immeasurable assistance in combating the shock that is frequently present. An intravenous infusion should be maintained so that blood or plasma expanders can be administered as needed. This along with elevation of the foot of the bed and maintenance of body heat by means of hot-water bottles and blankets may help to save the patient's life.

Hydatidiform mole

Hydatidiform mole is a benign neoplasm of the chorion in which the chorionic villi degenerate and become transparent vesicles containing clear, viscid fluid. The vesicles have a grapelike appearance and are arranged in clusters involving all or part of the decidual lining of the uterus (Fig. 23-7). Although there is usually no embryo present, occasionally there may be a fetus and only part of the placenta involved. Hydatidiform mole is rather an uncommon condition, occurring about once in every 2,000 pregnancies. The pregnancy appears to be normal at first. Then bleeding, a usual symptom varying from spotting to that of a profuse degree, occurs, so that one might suspect threat-

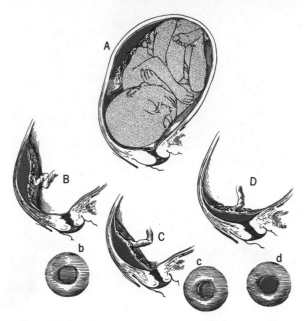

Figure 23-8. The three types of placenta previa, showing position of the placenta in relation to the internal os (B, C, and D) contrasted with normal placental insertion (A). (Below, b, c, and d) On vaginal examination the placenta can be felt during effacement and dilatation of the cervix in low implantation, partial and complete placenta previa.

ened abortion. If the patient does not abort, the uterus enlarges rapidly, and profuse hemorrhage may occur, at which time these vesicles may be evident in the vaginal discharge. Vomiting in rather severe form may appear early. Severe preeclampsia, a complication which does not usually occur until the later months of pregnancy, may appear early in the second trimester. The treatment consists in emptying the uterus. The approach used for evacuation of uterine contents varies, depending on the size of the uterus at the time molar pregnancy is diagnosed. If the uterus is less than the size of a ten-week gestation, dilatation of the cervix, followed by curettage, either by curet or suction, is the usual procedure. This must be carried out with great care, to avoid injury to the uterine wall, which is weakened and spongy due to the growth of the mole. If uterine size is larger, labor is stimulated with a continuous oxytocin infusion. After a portion of the uterine contents have been expelled, curettage is carried out to evacuate uterine contents completely. The tissue obtained must be carefully evaluated by the pathologist, as although mole is a benign process, choriocarcinoma, an extremely malignant tumor, sometimes compli-

cates the picture. For this reason also, follow-up care is very important in cases of molar pregnancy.

Placenta previa

Although abortion is the most frequent cause of bleeding early in pregnancy, the most common cause during the later months is placenta previa. In this condition the placenta is attached to the lower uterine segment (instead of high up in the uterus as usual) and either wholly or in part covers the region of the cervix. There are three types, differentiated according to the degree to which the condition is present (Fig. 23-8):

1. *Total placenta previa,* in which the placenta completely covers the internal os;
2. *Partial placenta previa,* in which the placenta partially covers the internal os;
3. *Low implantation of placenta,* in which the placenta encroaches upon the region of internal os, so that it can be palpated by the physician on digital exploration about the cervix, but does not extend beyond the margin of the internal os.

Painless vaginal bleeding during the second half of pregnancy is the main symptom of placenta previa. The bleeding usually occurs after the seventh month. It may begin as mere "spotting" and increase, or it may start with profuse hemorrhages. The patient may awaken in the middle of the night to find herself in a pool of blood. The bleeding is caused by separation of the placenta as the result of changes which take place in the lower uterine segment during the later months. This separation opens up the underlying blood sinuses of the uterus from which the bleeding occurs.

Fortunately, placenta previa is not a very common condition, occurring about once in every 200 deliveries. It occurs much more frequently in multiparae than in primigravidae. Placenta previa always must be regarded as a grave complication of pregnancy. Until recent years it showed a maternal mortality of approximately 10 percent. Modern methods of management, plus the more liberal use of blood transfusion, have reduced this figure considerably. The outlook for the baby is always dubious, not only because the placental separation interferes with the infant's oxygen supply, but also because many of these babies are very premature when delivery must necessarily take place.

TREATMENT. The presence of a placenta previa causes two main problems for the mother: bleeding and obstruction of the birth canal. For the baby, the most significant concern is prematurity. These problems provide the guides to treatment.

1. *Conservative* management is in order when the fetus is premature (by weight or dates) and the bleeding is not excessive. The natural history of placenta previa is such that uncontrolled bleeding is not likely to occur with the first episode. There may be, in fact, several episodes of bleeding, starting early in the third trimester, before there is sufficient bleeding to force the obstetrician to intervene and terminate the pregnancy. Thus, under such circumstances, bed rest and observation will often result in cessation of the bleeding and provide valuable days for the maturation of the fetus. Often, a technique for placental localization may be employed. Such techniques include isotope scans, amniography, abdominal x-rays, and ultrasound. It is also important that the obstetrician rule out other causes of bleeding under these circumstances. A speculum examination of the vagina is generally carried out to rule out other sources of bleeding such as cervicitis, cervical polyps, vaginal lacerations, etc. The examiner will *not*, however, insert a finger through the cervix under these circumstances, since such a maneuver might well precipitate bleeding and therefore the delivery of a premature infant.

2. An *active* approach is indicated if the fetus is at term by size and dates, if labor has begun, or if bleeding is sufficient to threaten the mother. Then, the patient is taken to the operating room where a "double setup" examination is performed. This means that everything is prepared for an immediate cesarean section, should the examination confirm the diagnosis. This precaution is necessary, since digital examination of the cervix might precipitate increased bleeding. In all instances of total and partial placenta previa, and in most instances of low implantation of the placenta, cesarean section is the approach of choice for delivery. In an occasional case of low implantation, especially if the baby is small, the obstetrician may elect to rupture the membranes in the hope that the presenting part may enter

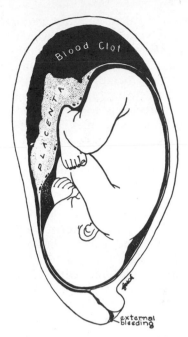

Figure 23-9. Abruptio placentae with large blood clot between placenta and uterine wall.

the pelvis and control the bleeding by compressing the area of placenta which has separated. If this does occur, vaginal delivery may sometimes be accomplished.

Bleeding, shock and infection are the main dangers. Before the arrival of the physician, the nurse should keep a solicitous eye on the amount of bleeding and the pulse rate and watch for signs of oncoming shock (pallor, increased pulse rate, cold extremities, and so on). Should the bleeding be profuse, elevation of the foot of the bed and application of external heat may forestall shock. In determining the amount of bleeding, the patient should be instructed to report feeling the escape of fluid from the vulva. The nurse, in turn, should inspect the pad or bed frequently for hemorrhage.

Abruptio placentae

Abruptio placenta (meaning that the placenta is torn from its bed) is a complication of the last half of pregnancy, in which a normally located placenta undergoes separation from its uterine attachment. The condition is frequently called "premature separation of the normally implanted placenta"; other synonymous terms such as *accidental hemorrhage* (meaning that it takes place unexpectedly) and *ablatio placentae* (ablatio means a carrying away) are sometimes used. Bleeding may be apparent, in

complications of pregnancy   481

which case it is called *external hemorrhage*; or bleeding may be concealed, in which case it is called *concealed hemorrhage*. In other words, if a separation occurs at the margin, the blood is apt to lift the membranes and trickle down to the cervical os and thus escape externally. If the placenta begins to separate centrally, a huge amount of blood may be stored behind the placenta before any of it becomes evident (Fig. 23-9). Although the precise cause of the condition is not known, it is frequently encountered in association with cases of toxemia of pregnancy.

Premature separation of the normally implanted placenta is characterized not only by bleeding beneath the placenta but also by pain. The pain is produced by the accumulation of blood behind the placenta, with subsequent distention of the uterus. The uterus also enlarges in size as the result of the accumulated blood and becomes distinctly tender and exceedingly firm. Because of the almost woody hardness of the uterine wall, fetal parts may be difficult to determine. Shock is often out of proportion to blood loss, as manifested by a rapid pulse, dyspnea, yawning, restlessness, pallor, syncope, and cold, clammy perspiration.

TREATMENT is dependent upon the condition of the fetus and the mother at the time the diagnosis is made. If the fetus is alive, prompt delivery is in order and should be by cesarean section, unless vaginal delivery can be accomplished promptly. If the fetus has already succumbed, this is usually an indication of an extensive placental separation. The complications of abruptio placenta to be described subsequently are all time-related and occur with greater frequency with more extensive separation. Therefore, although a vaginal delivery is desirable with a dead baby, one should not persist for too long.

FURTHER COMPLICATIONS. Hemorrhagic shock is a common complication and demands vigorous treatment with blood replacement and control of the bleeding by emptying the uterus in the most expeditious manner. Occasionally, with a severe abruption, a coagulation defect, *hypofibrinogenemia*, develops. This complication is also seen with other entities such as amniotic fluid embolus, prolonged retention of a dead fetus, and septic abortion. It is brought about by the entry into the circulation of thromboplastin from the uterus and placenta, which causes small fibrin clots in the capillaries and consumes fibrinogen, leaving the patient with nonclotting blood. Treatment involves the use of heparin (to prevent fibrin clots), blood and fibrinogen replacement, and termination of the pregnancy. Also, in severe abruptions, when coagulation is impaired, there is extensive bleeding into the uterine muscle, producing the so-called Convelaire uterus. Such a uterus occasionally does not contract well after delivery, causing further bleeding and even necessitating hysterectomy. Finally, *renal failure* may result, either on the basis of acute tubular necrosis or bilateral cortical necrosis. In the latter case, the outlook is grave.

Mistaken diagnosis of hemorrhage

A false alarm concerning hemorrhage is sometimes due to a normal "show" at the beginning of labor. It simply means that dilatation of the cervix has begun, causing slight bleeding. No treatment is required. However, the nurse should reassure the patient and watch to determine whether or not the bleeding which is present is more than the normal show.

"Supine hypotensive syndrome"

Many pregnant women, if placed in the supine position in the last trimester, suffer a fall in blood pressure. In some of these women the drop is so great as to simulate shock due to blood loss. The chief cause of supine hypotensive syndrome is failure of venous return of blood from the legs and the pelvis as a result of the compression exerted by the enlarged uterus on the inferior vena cava. The condition can be corrected promptly by having the patient lie on her side rather than on her back.

Hyperemesis gravidarum

A mild degree of nausea and vomiting, morning sickness, is the most common complaint of women in the first trimester of pregnancy. This manifestation is considered in the realm of a minor discomfort rather than a complication, and it usually responds to measures discussed in Chapter 12. It is uncommon today for this mild form of nausea and vomiting to progress to such a serious extent that it produces systemic effects (i.e., marked loss of weight and acetonuria), but when it becomes thus exaggerated, the condition is *hyperemesis gravidarum*, sometimes called pernicious vomiting. Because even the gravest case of hyperemesis starts originally as a simple form of nausea, all cases of nausea and vomiting should be treated with proper understanding and judgment, and none should be regarded casually. When simple remedies do not prove to be effective, and symptoms of hyperemesis appear to be imminent, the patient should be hospitalized for more intensive treatment. Appropriate measures should be taken to rule out other disease such as cholecystitis, hepatitis, peptic ulcer and gastroenteritis. At the present time less than 1 pregnant woman in 300 has to be admitted to the hospital because of this complication of pregnancy, and indeed, the grave cases of hyperemesis gravidarum are becoming rare. The recovery of those who are admitted to the hospital is usually rapid.

CAUSE. It is currently recognized that during pregnancy there are certain organic processes which are basic to all cases of vomiting, regardless of whether the symptoms are mild or severe. The endocrine and metabolic changes of normal gestation, fragments of chorionic villi entering the maternal circulation and the diminished motility of the stomach might well give rise to clinical symptoms.

It has long been thought that hyperemesis gravidarum is in large measure a *neurosis*. The term "neurosis," it will be recalled, is employed very loosely to designate a large array of conditions in which symptoms occur without demonstrable pathologic explanation, the symptoms being due, it is thought, to a disturbance of the patient's psyche. As many examples show (quite apart from pregnancy), nausea is often psychic in origin. For instance, a repellent sight, an obnoxious odor or the mere recollection of such a sight or odor may give rise to nausea and even vomiting. Our general use of the adjective "nauseating" to depict a repulsive object is further acknowledgment that an upset mind may produce an upset stomach.

CLINICAL PICTURE. The clinical picture of the patient suffering from pernicious vomiting varies in relation to the severity and the duration of the condition. In any event, the condition begins with a typical picture of morning sickness. The patient experiences a feeling of nausea on arising in the morning; she may even be unable to retain her breakfast, but she recovers in a few hours and has no further episodes until the next morning. With the majority of these patients this pattern persists for a few weeks and then suddenly ceases.

A small number of patients who have "morning sickness" develop persistent vomiting which lasts for four to eight weeks or longer. These patients vomit several times a day and may be unable to retain any liquid or solid foods, with the result that marked symptoms of dehydration and starvation occur. *Dehydration* is pronounced, as evidenced by a diminished output of urine and a dryness of the skin.

Starvation, which is regularly present, manifests itself in a number of ways. Weight loss may vary from 5 pounds to as much as 20 or 30 pounds. This is tantamount to saying that the digestion and the absorption of carbohydrates and other nutrients have been so inadequate that the body has been forced to burn its reserve stores of fat in order to maintain body heat and energy. When fat is burned without carbohydrates being present, the process of combustion does not go on to completion. Consequently, certain incompletely burned products of fat metabolism make their appearance in the blood and in the urine. The presence of acetone and diacetic acid in the urine in hyperemesis is common. In severe cases considerable changes associated with starvation and dehydration become evident in the blood chemistry. There is a definite increase in the nonprotein nitrogen, uric acid and urea, a moderate decrease in the chlorides and little alteration in the carbon dioxide combining power. Then, too, vitamin starvation is regularly present, and in extreme cases, when marked vitamin B deficiency exists, polyneuritis occasionally develops, and disturbances of the peripheral nerves result.

The severe type of vomiting may occur in either acute or chronic form. With prompt, persistent and intelligent therapy, the prognosis of hyperemesis is excellent.

TREATMENT AND NURSING CARE. The principles underlying the treatment of hyperemesis gravidarum are as follows: 1) combat the dehydration by liberal administration of parenteral fluids; 2) combat the starvation by administration of glucose intravenously and thiamine chloride subcutaneously and, if necessary, by feeding a high-caloric, high-vitamin fluid diet through a nasal tube; 3) combat the neurosis by psychotherapy, sedatives and supportive measures.

Although it may be necessary on occasion to treat cases of hyperemesis in the home, hospitalization is urgently desirable, because isolation from relatives, change of atmosphere and better facilities for intravenous medication confer unusual benefits in this condition. During the first 24 hours in the hospital it is customary to withhold all food and fluids by mouth in order to give the gastrointestinal tract as complete a rest as possible. Glucose solution, usually in 10 percent concentration, is administered intravenously and, in addition, normal saline solution intravenously. The total fluid intake should approximate or exceed 3,000 ml. in the 24 hours. The nurse must keep a careful record of the exact quantity of fluids given, the amount of urine excreted and the quantity of the vomitus. Sedation is accomplished either by hypodermically administered barbiturates or by the rectal instillation of some barbiturate drug such as sodium amobarbital, 3 grains (0.2 Gm.) every 6 hours. Thiamine hydrochloride, 50 mg. daily hypodermically, supplies the most urgent vitamin needs during the first 24 hours. All visitors are excluded during this period, including husband and relatives.

After such a regimen for 24 hours, dry toast, crackers or cereal are given by mouth in small quantities every two or three hours. Fluids are given on alternate hours in small amounts (not over 100 ml. at a time); hot tea and ginger ale usually are tolerated better than plain water. If no vomiting occurs, the amounts and the variety of the food are increased gradually until the patient is on a regular soft, high-vitamin diet. The intravenous administration of fluids may have to be continued for several days, depending on the oral intake.

The success of the treatment will depend in large measure on the tact, the understanding and the attitude of the nurse. Although optimism must be the keynote of the nurse's approach to the patient, this must be coupled with a plainly avowed determination to conquer the complication. The patient must be led gradually to understand that, in the treatment of vomiting, the nurse knows no such word as "failure." Not a few of these patients are in psychologic conflict because of family, financial or social difficulties, and many are averse to the whole idea of pregnancy. If one can only get to the root of these difficulties in a tactful, empathic way, and help the patient to become reconciled to becoming a mother, a great deal will have been accomplished.

The nurse must exercise great care in preparing and serving trays for patients suffering from hyperemesis. The portions should be extremely small and attractively arranged. Cold liquids such as ginger ale or lemonade must be ice-cold; and hot foods, such as soups, cocoa and tea, must be steaming hot, since lukewarm liquids may be nauseating. It is best not to discuss food with the patient, even when serving the tray, but simply to assume that she will enjoy it and talk about other matters. At all times keep the emesis basin out of view, since the sight of it may start vomiting. Likewise, the smell of food may be nauseating; accordingly, the patient's room should be kept well aired and should be as far from the food preparation area as possible.

If vomiting continues despite these measures, as it rarely does, the physician may institute nasal feeding. A small rubber tube (Levin tube) is inserted by the physician through a nostril and on down into the stomach. The tube is strapped to the patient's cheek, connected with an overhanging bottle and left in place. By this means, large amounts of vitamin-rich liquid foods may be administered. The secret of success with nasal feeding lies in very slow but constant introduction of food into the stomach. The apparatus should be so arranged that the number of drops per minute passing through the tube can be counted. This should not exceed 50 per minute. Even this slow rate, it may be noted, yields about 200 ml. per hour.

Even the most severe cases of hyperemesis will usually respond favorably to the treatment described if patience and persistence are exercised; but, in extremely rare instances, the patient may continue to vomit despite all efforts, and such grave signs may develop that the physician is forced to the conclusion that further continuation of pregnancy will be at the cost of the woman's life. The following signs are grave omens and, especially when several are present, may call for therapeutic abortion if it has been decided that the mother is to be removed from danger: 1) jaundice; 2) delirium; 3) steadily rising pulse rate to levels of 130 or above; 4) fever of 101° F. (38.4° C.) or above which persists despite liberal fluid intake; and 5) hemorrhages in the retina, as observed by the physician during ophthalmoscopic examination.

Suggested Reading

MONIF, G. R., ED.: *Infectious Diseases in Obstetrics and Gynecology.* New York, Harper & Row, 1974.

ROVINSKY, J. J., AND GUTTMACHER, A. F.: *Medical, Surgi-cal, and Gynecological Complications of Pregnancy,* ed. 2. Baltimore, Williams & Wilkins, 1965.

SHEEHAN, H. L., AND LYNCH, J. B.: *Pathology of Toxemia of Pregnancy.* Baltimore, Williams & Wilkins, 1973.

coincidental diseases and pregnancy

24

Hematologic Disorders / Heart Disease / Diabetes Mellitus / Disturbances in Thyroid Function / Renal Disease / Ptyalism / Infectious Diseases

It has been said wisely that the pregnant woman can have any disease which her non-pregnant counterpart can have except for infertility. One must be aware that many disease states are modified by the physiologic changes of pregnancy. Pregnancy may alter the classical clinical picture of a disease state and, indeed, some of the normal physiologic changes of pregnancy mimic disease. Therapeutic approaches must be altered in some cases, especially with regard to possible effects on the fetus. For most coincidental diseases, the effects of pregnancy on the disease and of the disease on pregnancy are negligible and do not influence the management of either. Some diseases, however, have profound fetal effects, as discussed in Chapter 27; others have a predominantly maternal effect; and some, such as diabetes, affect both. The more common diseases in the latter two categories will be discussed in this chapter.

Hematologic disorders

Iron deficiency anemia

Iron deficiency anemia is the most common hematologic disorder in pregnancy. Because of the expanded blood volume there is an element of hemodilution with a resultant fall in hemoglobin concentration unless the need is met by augmented hematopoesis. There is, in addition, the fetal requirement for iron to contend with. Since many women have depleted iron stores as the result of regular menstrual blood loss, these added demands often result in total depletion of storage iron and the development of overt anemia. The socioeconomically deprived patient with poor general nutrition is more susceptible to this condition.

In most patients with mild to moderate anemia, the signs and symptoms are few and often indistinguishable from the normal symptoms of pregnancy. Such patients are detected by frequent antepartum hemoglobin or hematocrit determinations. Severely anemic patients are symptomatic and in the most severe cases can even develop heart failure as a result of the anemia.

Treatment for mild to moderate cases consists of an iron-rich diet and an oral iron compound such as ferrous sulfate or gluconate. Similar recommendations hold for the nonanemic gravida as prophylaxis. Injectable iron therapy is rarely required since absorption is generally not a limiting factor. More often a failure to respond to oral iron therapy is the result of failure to take the medication (iron tends to produce gastrointestinal symptoms) or a concurrent folic acid deficiency. In severe cases transfusion may be required, especially if labor and delivery are imminent.

Folic acid deficiency

Folic acid deficiency can produce severe anemia in pregnancy. In its full-blown form there is also a reduction in white cells and platelets. Treatment consists of oral folic acid and diet. Prevention is achieved by the inclusion of folic acid in prenatal vitamin-mineral supplements.

Hemoglobinopathies

Hemoglobinopathies present special problems in pregnancy. Sickle cell trait, although not considered a disease, does predispose to urinary tract infection. The genetic implications should be explained to the patient after evaluating the husband's hemoglobin pattern. Sickle cell-C disease is generally innocuous in the nonpregnant woman, producing, at worst, a mild anemia. During pregnancy, however, life-threatening hemolytic crises can occur. Sickle cell anemia (S-S disease) is generally manifest before childbearing and in contrast to sickle cell-C disease, crises occur in the nonpregnant state as well. One must consider not only the impact of pregnancy in precipitating crises, but also the genetic outlook and the fact that patients with S-S disease have a limited life expectancy. Childbearing might well be limited or, in fact, avoided completely after appropriate counseling of these patients. Treatment in the case of sickle trait consists of looking for and treating urinary tract infection, while in the case of S-C and S-S disease more drastic measures may be necessary. Folic acid supplements are indicated because of the rapid turnover of red cells. In the case of patients with previous crises or the occurrence of crises during pregnancy, multiple transfusions are sometimes used to suppress the patient's marrow from forming the abnormal cells and permit her to exist on transfused cells during the period of risk (pregnancy and the puerperium).

Heart disease

Although rheumatic heart disease has for some time been the most common type of heart disease in pregnancy, recognition of the role of streptococcal infection and its appropriate therapy has reduced the frequency of rheumatic fever and its cardiac consequences. Besides reducing the incidence of heart disease in pregnancy generally, this has brought about a relative decrease in the frequency of congenital heart disease as a pregnancy complication. Still another dimension has been added by cardiac surgeons, as there are now appearing surgically treated patients, even some with valve replacements. For most types of heart disease, the major threat imposed by pregnancy is that the increasing blood volume will precipitate congestive heart failure. With appropriate therapy and restriction of activities, however, most patients can tolerate that stress and carry a pregnancy to a successful conclusion. The exception might be that individual falling into functional class IV (symptomatic at rest) in the first trimester, especially if she does not have a surgically correctable lesion. It is now the very rare cardiac patient who should be considered for therapeutic abortion on medical grounds.

Appropriate therapy demands close cooperation between the obstetrician and cardiologist, and the nurse may play a major role by coordinating information for the patient as well as providing day-to-day patient supervision. Treatment is governed to a considerable extent by the functional capacity of the patient, and rest is one of the most important ingredients, with total bed rest being necessary in some advanced cases. Digitalis, diuretics and salt restriction may all be required, depending upon the severity. In the case of valvular lesions, penicillin prophylaxis may be required, and antibiotic coverage is often expanded at delivery, when the possibility of endocarditis is even greater. As for all patients with heart disease, any respiratory infection can be devastating and consequently patients should avoid any predisposing situation and report even a sore throat or cold to the nurse and/or physician.

Since the onset of heart failure may be insidious, it behooves the nurse to be alert to the signs and symptoms. These might include inability to carry on normal activities, increased dyspnea on exertion and paroxysmal nocturnal dyspnea, tachycardia, palpitations and cough, especially if productive of blood or rusty sputum. Very special problems are presented by the patients with valve prostheses, since they require anticoagulant therapy. Sodium warfarin (Coumadin) and related drugs are contraindicated because they cross the placenta; this requires changing such patients to heparin therapy for the duration of pregnancy.

Diabetes mellitus

Diabetes mellitus illustrates well the interplay between the altered physiology of pregnancy and the pathophysiology of disease. In contrast to the majority of disease states which do not alter or are not affected by pregnancy, there is a significant change in the course of diabetes when pregnancy supervenes, and diabetes has a profound effect on the course of pregnancy as well as on the product of the gestation. In addition to participating in the regular medical and prenatal care of the diabetic gravida, the nurse can serve a very important counseling role, and therefore should be thoroughly familiar with this combination of events. Care is a team effort and must involve cooperation among obstetrician, internist, pediatrician, nurse and nutritionist.

In recent years, the number of pregnant diabetics has apparently increased. This is because with modern management, diabetics are now able to conceive and maintain pregnancies, and also because there is presently an increased recognition of the milder forms of gestational diabetes.

Although there is some debate as to whether the oral or intravenous glucose tolerance test should be used as the diagnostic standard in pregnancy, most authorities prefer the three-hour oral test. Although this test is more sensitive than the intravenous one and therefore likely to overdiagnose in mild cases, such patients will generally receive nothing more than diet therapy, certainly not a harmful approach.

Known prepregnancy diabetics do not require diagnostic glucose tolerance tests nor should they be subjected to them. On the other hand, there are large numbers of patients in whom gestational diabetes might be suspected because of the following: previous large babies, family history of diabetes, glucosuria, obesity, and unexplained pregnancy wastage. In these patients the appropriate screening test is a two-hour postprandial blood sugar. Fasting blood sugars are not adequate since the fasting sugar is normally reduced in pregnancy in the first trimester. When a normal value is obtained initially, the patient should be screened for diabetes again in the second and third trimesters. Abnormal values indicate the need for a full glucose tolerance test. A special diagnostic problem occurs when a patient is not suspected of being diabetic until after delivery, as might be the case if she delivered an unusually large baby or an unexplained stillborn. Since the diabetogenic effects of pregnancy disappear quickly following delivery, a normal glucose tolerance test 48 to 72 hours postpartum is not necessarily reassuring. The so-called steroid enforced glucose tolerance test in which cortisone is administered prior to the testing may bring out the abnormality.

A number of confusing terms have been applied and definitions are in order. Prediabetes and latent diabetes are terms which pertain to that period of time prior to the establishment of the diagnosis. Gestational diabetes designates those patients in whom the diagnosis is first made during pregnancy, and often becomes undetectable following delivery. The most universally used classification of diabetes is that by White, which is as follows:

CLASS A—glucose tolerance test diabetes
CLASS B—onset: over age 20
     duration: 0-9 years
     vascular disease: 0
CLASS C—onset: age 10-19
     duration: 10-19 years
     vascular disease: 0
CLASS D—onset: under age 10
     duration: 20+ years
     vascular disease: calcification
      in legs, retinitis
CLASS E—patients with calcified pelvic vessels
CLASS F—patients with nephritis

Although this classification has some pitfalls in that duration of disease and vascular disease are not always absolutely parallel, in general perinatal wastage is a function of the class. The wastage is invariably greater in Classes D, E, and F, those patients with vascular disease, and less in Classes A, B, and C. It should also be noted that mothers with significant vascular involvement have small rather than large-for-date babies.

Careful medical management of the pregnant diabetic is the key to successful outcome. The initial evaluation should include examination of the optic fundi for detection of vascular disease, and also a urine collection to detect asymptomatic bacilluria, a precursor to overt pyelonephritis, to which the diabetic is especially prone. Diet is of paramount importance, and the nurse must be prepared to assist the patient in this area. The caloric requirement for the normal-weight patient is approximately 2,200 calories with 1 to 1.5 Gm. of protein per Kg. of body weight. In the case of many gestational diabetics who are overweight, total calories must be reduced to control blood sugar. It is difficult to go below 1,500 calories and still maintain adequate protein intake and a palatable formulation. Standard diabetic diets tend to lack the protein needed in pregnancy. Occasionally one needs to increase carbohydrate and total calories because of the patient's activities, or in some cases of juvenile diabetes, the large amount of glucose lost in the urine. Food costs and ethnic dietary habits must also be considered.

Although diet alone may control many gestational diabetics, if the two-hour postprandial sugar exceeds 150 to 160 mg. percent, despite the diet, insulin therapy is indicated. Although occasionally used, the oral hypoglycemics are not cleared for use in pregnancy. Progressive insulin resistance is characteristic of pregnancy and it is not unusual for insulin requirements to increase as much as four-fold. This commonly necessitates the use of evening as well as morning doses of insulin to achieve good control.

Obstetrical management involves evaluation of fetal well-being and decisions regarding the timing and method of delivery. Since the major target of diabetes pathology is in the small blood vessels, it is not surprising that the placenta may also be involved and therefore placental insufficiency and even fetal death may result. This result is very much less common in gestational than prepregnancy diabetics and is the basis for the common practice of delivering diabetic patients three to four weeks prior to the expected date of confinement. This is not, however, necessary if one can identify the fetus at risk by a technique such as serial 24-hour urinary estriol determinations (see Chapter 27). In those patients with no evidence of fetal compromise and who are otherwise stable (good diabetic control, absence of toxemia and significant hydramnios), pregnancy may be allowed to go to term, with careful surveillance. The method of delivery is a matter of obstetric judgment at the time. Early deliveries are more often by cesarean section because the cervix is not prepared for induction, and even at term there is an increased need for section because of the mechanical problems created by the fetal macrosoma. During vaginal deliveries fetal size may cause problems in the form of shoulder dystocia.

The problems of the diabetic offspring are discussed in detail in Chapter 27. However, it is important to realize that even under the best of circumstances the perinatal mortality is two to three times that in the nondiabetic, and pregnancy is a very major undertaking for the diabetic and her family.

Disturbances in thyroid function

Hyperthyroidism is probably the second most significant endocrinopathy in pregnancy, second only to diabetes mellitus. Although the totally uncontrolled hyperthyroid woman is likely to be anovulatory and thus unable to conceive, many with milder disease do conceive, and some patients with hyperthyroidism present for the first time during pregnancy. If the condition is uncontrolled during pregnancy, spontaneous abortion and premature labor are common. Diagnosis may be somewhat of a problem in milder cases since some thyroid enlargement and confusing hyperdynamic symptoms occur in normal pregnancy. Laboratory studies may also be confusing since there is increased protein binding of thyroid hormone in pregnancy resulting in higher values for studies such as the protein bound iodine and total T_4, with lower T_3 uptake. Multiple studies and newer methods, however, can overcome the confusion.

Once popular surgical treatment (subtotal thyroidectomy) has been replaced by medical approaches except in special cases (reaction to the antithyroid drugs, unusually large dosage requirements, etc.). The problem with medical therapy is that the antithyroid drugs do cross the placenta and if doses are excessive the fetal thyroid can be suppressed, leading to fetal goiter or even cretinism. This is best avoided by maintaining the level of control at high normal levels, although some have suggested that therapy with methimazole (Tapazole) or propylthiouracil be combined with thyroid extract to avoid that problem. Patients with exophthalmic goiter produce a substance called LATS (long acting thyroid stimulator), which is a gamma-g globulin. This does cross the placenta and if present can cause hyperthyroidism in the newborn.

Hypothyroidism and parathyroid disorders are reported in pregnancy but are rare. Adrenal, pituitary, and ovarian disorders generally result in infertility.

Renal disease

Almost all forms of acute and chronic renal disease have been reported in association with pregnancy. Not infrequently, specific diagnosis is difficult during pregnancy since proteinuria and hypertension may mimic preeclampsia, and also because definitive studies such as renal biopsy and intravenous urography are contraindicated. Chronic renal disease, especially if accompanied by hypertension, may be associated with fetal growth retardation and increased perinatal mortality.

The most common renal problem in pregnancy is urinary tract infection. Anatomic changes as well as hormonal effects cause narrowing of the lower ureter with dilatation of the upper ureter and renal pelvis. These changes result in delayed emptying and an increased risk of infection. The risk increases as pregnancy progresses and continues into the puerperium. Symptoms include chills, fever, frequency, dysuria and pain in the area of the kidney. Severity may vary from extremely mild to extremely toxic, with nausea, vomiting and abdominal distension. Uterine irritability is an important complication of pyelonephritis. The correlation is sufficiently common that it is wise to look for urinary tract infection in any patient with premature labor.

In order to treat the patient adequately, a carefully collected midstream clean catch urine specimen must be obtained. The adequacy of this specimen depends upon the care taken by the nurse in instructing the patient. An examination of the urinary sediment as well as a culture and antibiotic sensitivity studies should be carried out. In addition to the selection of an appropriate antibiotic, it is imperative that a good fluid intake be maintained, parenterally if necessary. Antimicrobial therapy should be continued for 7 to 10 days even if the response is good, and the urine should be recultured following the cessation of therapy. Recurrences are common, causing some authorities to recommend long-term suppressive antimicrobial therapy.

Asymptomatic bacturia in pregnancy is significant because of its high association with subsequent pyelonephritis and consequently should be treated. Association with other obstetrical problems such as prematurity has been suggested, but it is likely that these are simply coincidental findings in a group of high-risk patients.

Ptyalism

Although this is one of the rarer complications of pregnancy, it is one which is most annoying to the patient and very stubborn in resisting treatment. It is due entirely to altered innervation or changes in nerve control and is characterized by an enormously increased secretion of the salivary glands. Women at times have been known to discharge as much as 2 quarts of saliva daily from this cause. This complication, if it occurs at all, usually appears in the early months of pregnancy and lasts a considerable time, but, fortunately, it is inclined to cease spontaneously. It is seen in highly nervous women of low vitality and is likely to cause great mental depression and to interfere with nutrition.

The treatment consists in building up the general health and the administration of such medication as may be prescribed by the physician. The use of astringent mouthwashes often contributes to the patient's comfort. Any treatment may seem to be inadequate, and the condition is most disagreeable.

Infectious diseases

Although most infectious diseases have no established specific ill effects on mother or baby, there are those with profound effects. Diseases with particular fetal effects are discussed in Chapter 27.

The common cold

Susceptibility to acute upper respiratory infections is apparently greater during pregnancy. Therefore, the pregnant woman should make every effort to avoid contacts with these infections. When she does acquire a cold, prompt medical attention is usually desirable, because the common cold often precedes more serious conditions affecting the upper respiratory tract.

Prescribed medication should be used in preference to the various antihistamine drugs obtainable without a prescription. Rest in bed helps the individual and aids in checking the spread of the disease.

Influenza

Although the pregnant woman is not more likely to contract influenza, she is more prone to the development of complicating pneumonia, especially if she is in the third trimester with elevated diaphragm and pulmonary compromise. The development of pneumonia represents a serious threat to the gravida. In the face of an epidemic involving a specific strain of influenza virus, immunization with a killed or attenuated virus vaccine is indicated. Nonspecific polyvalent vaccines are probably ineffectual.

Measles

Ill effects are not commonly noted in pregnancy, but pregnant women who contract measles are said to be more likely to have premature labors. No other definite effects are reported, although eruptions have been noted on infants at birth.

Typhoid fever

Typhoid fever, which is now relatively rare in the United States, may cause serious complications in pregnancy, resulting in abortion, prematurity and infant mortality. Immunization is not contraindicated during pregnancy, and antityphoid vaccine should be administered when necessary.

Smallpox

Smallpox is fortunately a rare disease at this time. Cases of abortion and prematurity increase with the severity of the attack, especially with the hemorrhagic type. As in measles, smallpox may be transmitted through the placenta, for eruptions may be present in live births.

Tuberculosis

The average case of tuberculosis in itself has only a slight effect on the course of pregnancy, since it rarely predisposes to abortion, premature labor or even stillbirth. (Fortunately, the disease is seldom acquired congenitally, although a small number of authentic cases have been reported in which, in addition to a tuberculous condition of the placenta, tubercle bacilli were found in the cord blood, together with tuberculous lesions in the baby.) Medical opinions differ, but the consensus is that pregnancy does not exert an adverse effect on tuberculosis. Some authorities think that this disease becomes aggravated by pregnancy, and that only a patient in an arrested case should consider becoming pregnant. Pregnancy is undertaken with some risk, for although a tuberculous lesion may remain latent for an indefinite time, provided that the natural resistance is not overtaxed, it must be noted that pregnancy is one of the factors often responsible for overtaxing the resistance sufficiently to convert a latent, inactive lesion into an active one. Maintenance of the proper hygiene, nutrition and excellent surroundings so that health is conserved in every possible way will do much to prevent activity in a latent focus. Other authorities deny that the tuberculosis is necessarily aggravated by pregnancy, basing this belief on statistics of a large series of tuberculous patients who have progressed satisfactorily in pregnancy.

The symptoms of tuberculosis in pregnancy do not differ materially from those which accompany the disease in other conditions. During the early months of gestation the characteristic anemia and general malnutrition of tuberculosis are usually pronounced, but in the latter months there is often considerable improvement. Too often, however, this is followed by a rapid decline after delivery.

Treatment with the modern antituberculosis drugs, streptomycin, isoniazid (INH), and PAS, has completely altered management in general, as well as during pregnancy. New advanced cases are rare and a majority of patients are managed as outpatients. Treatment of active cases generally consists of streptomycin, 1.0 Gm. daily for three to four weeks, then 1.0 Gm. twice weekly. Isoniazid, 300 mg., and PAS (para-aminosalicylic acid), 12.0 Gm. daily, are given in divided doses. No deleterious effects on the mother or the infant have been reported. Labor and delivery are conducted in a normal fashion, avoiding inhalation anesthesia, and mother and baby are separated if disease is active. Breast-feeding is unwise even in inactive disease. Some authorities recommend INH therapy in the third trimester and puerperium for the inactive patient who has had active disease within two years of pregnancy.

Tuberculosis detection should be the concern of all physicians, and since the obstetrician sees a number of young women who might otherwise have no medical supervision, he has a responsible role. If the patient has had a recent chest x-ray (within six months), a repeat is not necessary unless there are symptoms which suggest a pulmonic process. Many obstetricians prefer screening patients with a tuberculin skin test. This eliminates the need for an x-ray in nonreactions. Appropriate procedures for shielding the fetus should be used whenever a pregnant woman is x-rayed.

Poliomyelitis

This disease generally does not complicate pregnancy or delivery, except in the very unusual cases in which respiratory paralysis develops; in these rare cases cesarean section has given satisfactory results. Fortunately, the fetus rarely contracts the disease. Of about 80 cases reported during pregnancy, less than one fifth occurred in the first trimester. A milder form of infection of poliomyelitis is attributed to a different virus, the Coxsackie virus, which produces less paralysis but is often unrecognized.

Syphilis

The major hazard of syphilis in pregnancy was, in the past, the occurrence of intrauterine infection and late abortion or stillbirth. Congenital syphilis has now been reduced nearly to the point of elimination. The antenatal blood test for syphilis is required by law and, except for the instances in which prenatal care is nonexistent, maternal syphilis should be detected and adequately treated, thereby protecting the fetus.

Syphilis can occur in any stage during pregnancy. The primary and secondary stages are usually apparent because of their lesions. In latent syphilis, the diagnosis is based upon a positive serology; the most difficult problem occurs when the serology is repeatedly positive and the patient denies a history. Biologic false positives do occur in a number of circumstances, but, fortunately, new, more specific tests are now available which can be used in the questionable case.

Treatment is indicated in the following circumstances:

1. When a diagnosis of early syphilis is made, regardless of stage.
2. When late symptomatic syphilis is discovered.
3. When latent syphilis is diagnosed by repeated positive serologic tests and the patient's history corroborates the diagnosis, and when there has been either inadequate or no treatment.
4. When the diagnosis is made by repeated positive tests, even though the history does not confirm, and when either the more specific tests are not available or there is not time for adequate therapy. Retreatment in subsequent pregnancies is necessary if there is any doubt about the adequacy of previous therapy.

The treatment consists of a course of penicillin in the total dose of 6 million units (12 million for neurosyphilis), or a suitable substitute if penicillin allergy exists. Both mother and baby should be carefully followed by serologic tests postpartum. It is important to know that even the unaffected baby will have a positive test because the mother's test is positive; however, the titer in the baby will be lower than that of the mother and will become negative within three months.

Gonorrhea

This disease should be studied by the nurse with the other infectious diseases; but, because of the consequences of gonorrheal infection to the mother at the time of labor and during the puerperium, as well as the risk of permanent injury to the baby's eyes at the time of birth, this disease is of special concern to the maternity nurse.

The disease is caused by *Neisseria gonorrhoeae*, an organism which may attack any mucous membrane but most commonly affects the mucosa of the lower genital tract. The endocervical glands and urethra are common foci, but for complete detection, the anus and oropharynx should be cultured. Gonorrhea is spread by sexual contact and in the majority of women remains asymptomatic except for a nonspecific vaginal discharge. This is particularly the case in pregnancy, in which the normal route of spread through the endometrial cavity to the tubes is occluded by the pregnancy. The rate of asymptomatic carriers in pregnancy is reported to be as high as 5 to 10 percent in many clinics. Although gonorrhea causes few problems for the patient during pregnancy, it can produce serious puerperal infection if present in the cervix at the time of delivery. Routine gonorrhea cultures are recommended during pregnancy. Gram-stained smears are suggestive but not conclusive in women. The treatment of asymptomatic gonorrhea involves a single injection of 4.8 million units of procaine penicillin preceded by 1.0 Gm. of probenecid to produce the high level of penicillin needed to eradicate the increasingly resistant gonococcus. Cure should be proven by reculture and one should be alert to the possibility of reinfection. Sexual partners should be evaluated and treated appropriately.

The organism can infect the infant's eyes at birth, and if prophylactic treatment of the eyes is not adequate, blindness may result.

Suggested Reading

ROVINSKY, J. J., AND GUTTMACHER, A. F.: *Medical, Surgical, and Gynecological Complications of Pregnancy,* ed. 2. Baltimore, Williams & Wilkins, 1965.

STANDER, R. W. (ED.): Blood dyscrasias in pregnancy. *Clin. Ob. and Gyn.* 17, 1974.

WIESNER, P. J., AND TYLER, C. W.: Venereal disease in obstetrics and gynecology. *Clin. Ob. and Gyn.* 18, 1975.

complications of labor

Dystocia Due to Abnormalities of Labor Mechanics / Hemorrhagic Complications / Prolapse of Umbilical Cord / Amniotic Fluid Embolism / Multiple Pregnancy

Complicated labor requires sensitive and astute nursing care, for it represents a period of great stress for the laboring woman, her partner, nurses and physicians. The principles of nursing care during normal labor (see Chapter 18) also apply when the labor is complicated, with certain modifications depending upon the nature of the problems. The nurse's ability to use clinical judgment is crucial, as the nursing diagnoses and care deriving from these may be of life-saving significance for both the mother and the infant. Assessment skills including observation, interviewing and physical examination provide important data as to the nature and extent of the problem. Reporting, recording and professional intercommunication promote accurate decision making and implementation of appropriate treatment. Physical and emotional supportive measures assist the mother and father to understand and cope with the unusual events in the labor experience, which is often prolonged and painful.

Dystocia due to abnormalities of labor mechanics

Dystocia, or difficult labor, can result from abnormalities in the machinery of labor. When there is cessation or delay of progress in the labor process due to such abnormalities, it is termed *mechanical dystocia* and may be caused by one of these three major conditions:

1. Uterine dysfunction, subnormal or abnormal uterine forces that are not adequate to overcome the natural resistance which the maternal soft parts and bony pelvis present to the passage of the baby through the birth canal.
2. Faulty fetal presentation or developmental anomalies of the type which prevent entrance to or passage of the baby through the birth canal.
3. Variations in the size or shape of the bony pelvis which create an obstacle to the entrance or descent of the baby.

Frequently two or more of these conditions occur together, for faulty fetal presentation or a contracted maternal pelvis are often associated with uterine dysfunction. Or, a contracted pelvis may cause an abnormal fetal presentation. To further understand the nature of these problems, the process of labor can be thought of as divided into three components, each of which must be normal for progress to be made and birth to occur. The *forces*, including uterine contractions with the addition of maternal "bearing down" during the second stage, must be of adequate strength and muscle activity must be coordinated. These forces propel an irregular object, the infant or *passenger*, through the birth canal or *passage*. The passenger must be of appropriate size and shape, and able to undergo the necessary maneuvers to pass through the different dimensions of the birth canal. The passage must also be of normal size and configuration, not presenting any undue obstacles to the descent, rotations and expulsion of the baby.

Thus, when nature tries to propel an infant through the birth canal and fails to do so, there can be one of three causes for the failure: the forces are inadequate (uterine inertia); or the position of the infant is at fault; or there is disproportion between the size of the infant and that of the birth canal.

Uterine dysfunction

DEFINITION. In normal labor a latent phase of several hours' duration occurs first, in which effacement and a small amount of dilatation take place. An active phase follows this, in which progressive, accelerated dilatation occurs. This is followed by a phase of deceleration or slowing just before full dilatation (see Chapter 15). A significant prolongation of any of these phases is termed uterine dysfunction.

The term *uterine inertia* has been used to describe a dysfunctional labor. Inertia was classified as either primary or secondary. Primary inertia occurred at the onset of labor (i.e., the contractions were of poor quality and ineffectual) and was due to unknown causes. Secondary inertia occurred later in labor and was felt to be related to maternal exhaustion. However, increasing knowledge regarding uterine action and the phases of labor indicates that it would be more appropriate to discuss the topic in terms of dysfunction as it relates to the phases of dilatation. The two terms inertia and dysfunction are used interchangeably to some extent. If inertia is used, primary inertia should refer to prolongation of the latent phase and secondary inertia should indicate a prolongation or abnormality of the active phase.[1]

CAUSES. When there is failure to progress despite the presence of uterine contractions, one of the first factors to consider is whether or not the patient is actually in labor. Braxton-Hicks contractions in late pregnancy are not infrequently experienced by the woman as relatively strong and regular, and may be easily mistaken for true labor. Progressive cervical changes must be present to signify true labor, as effective contractions gradually accomplish effacement and dilatation. Appearance of bloody show assists in the diagnosis of labor, particularly when it accompanies cervical changes. Without these other signs to confirm labor, uncomfortable uterine contractions signify false labor. For the diagnosis of dystocia, cervical changes must have occurred and progressed, only to have continued progression in effacement and dilatation slowed or halted at some point.

The chief causes of uterine dysfunction are injudicious use of analgesia (i.e., excessive or too early administration of the drugs), minor degrees of pelvic contraction, and fetal malposition of even a small degree such as a slight extension of the head as seen in some occiput posterior positions. Similarly, postmaturity and large size of the infant have been found to be significantly related to dysfunctional labor. These conditions may occur singly or in combination in cases of dysfunction. Other factors that are associated with this condition include overdistension of the uterus, grand multiparity, excessive cervical rigidity and maternal age. The latter group of factors has been shown to play an etiological role although not such an important one as was once believed. The cause is often unknown. Considering the possible role of cortical steroids in the initiation of labor, and their relation to stress states, the effects of emotional factors in dystocia cannot be overlooked when no other cause is apparent. More research at the cellular level will have to be done to obtain increased definitive knowledge concerning the etiologic factors in this condition.

COMPLICATIONS. The complications of uterine dysfunction are unfortunate for both mother and infant. Fetal injury and death are the most serious outcomes of this disorder. For the mother, exhaustion and dehydration may occur if labor is allowed to become too prolonged. Elevation of the maternal temperature and pulse are the clinical signs that herald the onset of secondary complications. Acetonuria is another sign of exhaustion and dehydration. These symptoms are to be reported immediately. Generally, in patients having dysfunctional labor, supportive intravenous therapy and electrolyte replacement are instituted before this syndrome occurs. Intrauterine infection is another common maternal complication in these types of labor; broad-spectrum antibiotics are the usual choice of treatment. It is particularly important not to allow intrauterine infection to occur, since it contributes heavily to the increased perinatal mortality. In addition, dysfunctional labor appears to have some long-term consequences. Research has indicated that difficult labors and deliveries have a deleterious effect on future childbearing.[2] Apparently, the more difficult the labor and delivery, the less inclination there is to have future children. In addition, the fear and anxiety that are engendered by a complicated childbirth become a special concern of the health team if these patients do have subsequent children.

Types of uterine dysfunction

There are two types of uterine dysfunction, *hypertonic* and *hypotonic*. In order for the pregnant uterus to perform effectively in labor, the fundus and upper segment contract while the lower segment (isthmus and cervix) relaxes from its active tone maintained between contractions. Incoordinate uterine action, in which both segments contract at the same time, causes hypertonic dysfunction. Hypotonic dysfunction occurs when the two segments are synchronized but the tone or tension of the muscles is inadequate, with weak and ineffective contractions.

HYPERTONIC UTERINE DYSFUNCTION. The muscles of the uterus maintain a greater than normal state of constant tension in this type of dysfunction, but the contractions themselves are of poor quality with distortion of the normal distribution of forces. Although these contractions are inefficient from the standpoint of accomplishing dilatation, they are extremely painful. It is particularly important to help these mothers to distinguish between the anticipation of pain and the actual pain (see Chapter 18), for as labor wears on, and no progress is made, the mother's strength and ability to cope with the contractions diminish, and hence the pain seems to be intensified. The anxiety and fear which are generated can easily lead to panic, which is detrimental to resumption of a successful labor course.

It is of paramount importance for the nurse to be able to accurately evaluate the intensity of labor contractions. At the height of an excellent uterine contraction it is impossible to indent the uterine wall with one's fingertips, and during a fairly good contraction it may be possible to cause some slight indentation; but if the uterine wall can be indented easily at the height of a contraction, it is a poor one. In evaluating the intensity of a labor contraction, reliance should be placed on this tactile examination and not on the amount of "complaining" done by the patient about her pain.

Treatment for this type of dysfunctional labor generally consists of rest and fluids. When medication is indicated to produce the needed rest and relaxation, an injection of 16 mg. of morphine may be prescribed, because it usually stops the abnormal contractions. In addition, a 0.1- to 0.2-Gm. dose of a short-acting barbiturate may be administered. Intravenous fluids are utilized to maintain hydration and electrolyte balance, and in most instances normal labor resumes when the patient awakens.

Oxytocin is generally ineffective in treating this type of dysfunction. With the uterus in a constant state of increased muscle tone, oxytocin presents the danger of causing an even greater resting tension, which might interfere with fetal oxygenation. Additionally, it does not correct the incoordinated action of the two segments, which is underlying this problem. However, if labor does not ensue after sedation, oxytocin may be tried in about one half the usual dosage. It must be immediately discontinued if signs of fetal distress occur, or if normal labor does not supervene. Cesarean section is usually employed if either of these situations develops.

Complications. Fetal distress tends to appear quite early in labor when there is hypertonic dysfunction. Fetal heart rate must be carefully monitored, and other signs of distress, such as meconium-stained amniotic fluid, noted. Occasionally in cases of hypertonic dysfunction, membranes will have been ruptured 24 hours or more without effective labor. In this situation, bacteria are likely to ascend into the uterus and give rise to infection. This is *intrapartal infection* and is a serious complication. It is signaled by a rise in temperature, often in association with a chill. Because of this danger, it is customary to take temperatures every two hours in patients whose labors have lasted more than 24 hours or who have ruptured membranes. Even an elevation of half a degree should be reported at once to the physician. Intrapartal infection is much more likely to occur if the membranes have been ruptured for a long time. As previously stated, treatment is usually in the form of antibiotics. Oxytocin also may be used in these cases in spite of its adverse effects (it tends to increase the hypertonicity of the muscle). Cesarean section is resorted to if fetal distress occurs.

HYPOTONIC UTERINE DYSFUNCTION. After the onset of true labor, contractions in hypotonic dysfunction decrease in strength and the tone of the uterine muscles is less than usual. Minimum uterine tension during the resting stage is about 8 to 12 mm. Hg in the normally functioning uterus, while normal labor contractions reach an intrauterine pressure of 50 to 60 mm. Hg at acme. These values are reduced in hypotonic dysfunction, and contractions are not strong enough to effect dilatation. Contractions may become farther apart and irregular.

Dysfunction often is nature's protection against pelvic contraction and abnormal fetal position, and signifies the need for careful assessment for these factors. Thorough vaginal examination to determine position of the presenting part, dimensions of the pelvis, and state of the cervix will usually be done by the obstetrician. The cervix will be at least 3 cm. dilated if the diagnosis of hypotonic dysfunction in the active phase of labor is correct. X-ray pelvimetry is often done for accurate measurement of the pelvis and to confirm abnormal fetal position or abnormalities of development. A typical curve in the fetal cervical spine called "goosenecking" is pathognomonic of hypotonic dysfunction, indicating the characteristically poor uterine forces.[3] This condition usually occurs in the accelerated or active phase, or even during the second stage of labor; the contractions become infrequent and of poor quality, and the uterus is easily indentable at the acme of a contraction.

Treatment. Early and accurate diagnosis of hypotonic dysfunction is a major factor in reducing fetal death and injury. If a marked degree of disproportion exists (see p. 502), or if there is an uncorrectable malposition, then cesarean section will be employed to effect delivery. If these conditions are not present, stimulation of labor is generally the treatment of choice rather than "watchful waiting" for more effective labor to resume spontaneously. The main reason for this is the increased perinatal loss and injury which accompany unduly prolonged first or second stages of labor.

If membranes are intact, initial treatment includes artificial rupture. This procedure alone may stimulate effective labor contractions. Should strong, regular contractions with progressive effacement and dilatation or fetal descent fail to occur, or if membranes are already ruptured, oxytocin augmentation is usually employed. Ten units of oxytocin are mixed with 1,000 ml. of 5 percent glucose in water for controlled intravenous drip. Initially the infusion is begun at a flow of 5 drops per minute (about 3 to 5 mU. oxytocin), as this amount will not initiate tetanic contractions in true hypotonic dysfunction unless there is hypersensitivity to the drug. Contractions and fetal heart rate are carefully evaluated, and if no problems develop, the infusion can be gradually increased up to 15 to 20 drops per minute (yielding about 20 mU. oxytocin). Flows above this rate are rarely necessary, for if effective contractions are not initiated by this dosage of oxytocin, greater amounts are also unlikely to do so, and present serious dangers to both the baby and the mother.

A constant infusion pump is often used to administer oxytocin, as this method enhances the precision of dosage. The *Harvard pump* or *Ivac peristaltic pump* are two types in common use. The oxytocin solution in a separate bottle flows into a syringe mounted on the pump, which delivers an exact amount of solution depending on the drip rate set. This solution can be piggybacked into a plain glucose infusion, if the two-bottle setup is used. Although the pump method allows more precise regulation of the oxytocin flow than simply adjusting clamps attached to the intravenous tubing, both approaches require constant and careful monitoring. Clamps can slip and the pump can malfunction. The dangers of an excessive dosage of oxytocin include uterine tetany with resultant fetal hypoxia, or rupture of the uterus with fetal anoxia and maternal hemorrhage and shock.

Oxytocin stimulation is contraindicated in cases of fetal-pelvic disproportion, overdistension of the uterus, and great parity (para 5 and over). Signs of fetal distress must be carefully watched for, and the infusion immediately slowed or stopped if these occur. Use of external or internal monitors is often mandatory when oxytocin stimulation of labor is employed (see Chapter 18). With internal monitoring, the strength of contractions as well as continual rate of the fetal heart may be constantly evaluated. Occasionally intramuscular or buccal oxytocin is used, but these methods do not allow accurate control of blood levels, either to accomplish effective contractions or to avoid dangers of excessive dosage. Sparteine sulfate (Tocosamine) sometimes is used as an alternative to oxytocin to stimulate labor. It is given in repeated doses until satisfactory uterine action is achieved; however, there are limits to the total dosage that can be used (see p. 336).

Complications. Untreated hypotonic uterine dysfunction exposes the mother to the dangers of exhaustion, dehydration, and intrapartum infection. Signs of fetal distress often do not appear until intrapartum infection has developed. While treatment of intrauterine infections with antibiotics offers protection to the mother, this is of little value to the fetus. Nursing observations include assessment of the mother for signs of infection, as previously discussed.

NURSING CARE. In addition to observing and reporting the maternal and fetal conditions as noted above, nursing care includes explanations and support for the parents. Labors of this type are extremely discouraging for the mother and the father. The diagnostic procedures as well as the therapy will take a certain amount of time, and carrying out these measures will require patience and waiting on the part of everyone concerned. It is essential that the couple know and understand this fact. The physician and the nurse need to spend sufficient time with the parents to explain what is happening in depth and in terms that are appropriate for them. It is very possible that repeated reinforcement of the explanations, progress, etc., will be needed. Feedback from the parents should be encouraged, so that their level of understanding and acceptance can be ascertained. The normal tension and anxiety found in any labor certainly will be intensified, and it is important that it not be compounded by fantasy or misunderstanding. Since dysfunctional labor is so variable, it is often impossible (and unwise) to give the parents any definite reassurances as to when effective labor will commence. Yet some kind of boundaries must be placed on when this ineffective phase will end, and progress will begin, so that the mother will have some goal to look forward to and to work for. Therefore, it is important to reassure the patient, reminding her that her case is not absolutely unique (patients think after many hours that theirs is the longest labor in obstetric history), that certain specific measures are known and can be taken to help

effective labor to begin, and that she will be receiving competent medical and nursing care throughout her labor.

An explanation of the plan for treatment will enable the parents to anticipate more realistically what is in store and therefore reassures them that certain definite measures are available and are being employed.

In addition, all the comfort measures which promote relaxation should be utilized. Sponge baths, various positioning, soothing backrubs, clean, dry linen, quiet conversation, reading or other diversionary activities as well as a quiet restful environment are all appropriate. However, isolating the patient in a dark room on the premise that she needs sleep or rest only contributes to her fear unless she is actually sleeping, and then frequent observations are needed to see when she awakens. Human contact is one of the most important items of "treatment" in cases of complicated labor and should never be neglected. The presence of the same person, nurse and/or physician, is very helpful for the reasons already mentioned in Chapter 18. Coaching the mother in breathing patterns and relaxation techniques also will conserve her strength.

The physician may want the patient to have fluids by mouth, or he may order intravenous infusions to maintain hydration and electrolyte balance. A total of 2,000 ml. or more of intravenous fluid may be given in 24 hours.

If oxytocin stimulation of labor is used, the patient must have someone in attendance at all times during the infusion. Every uterine contraction is to be timed and fetal heart tones are to be taken after each contraction or every five minutes. Maternal blood pressure and pulse are checked every half hour. As the physician specifies the dosage, the nurse (or other attendant) ascertains that the infusion is running at the prescribed drops per minute and reports any maternal or fetal aberrations immediately. Many institutions have an "Oxytocin Record" or a "Pitocin Sheet" on which there is space for recording times, amount and frequency of the oxytocin given, fetal heart tones, maternal blood pressure and pulse, frequency, intensity and length of contractions, and other relevant comments. This type of sheet gives an easily accessible record of the patient's progress during the infusion.

Recording and reporting the physiologic signs and symptoms cannot be stressed enough during these infusions. However, supportive care is also to be maintained. Adequate explanation and reassurance can be given, and since the nurse will be with the mother continuously this time can be utilized to good advantage to establish a relationship of rapport. While the infusion will stimulate contractions (and therefore, discomfort), the mother and her partner often look upon this treatment optimistically for it marks the end of a desultory, ineffective period in labor and brings with it promise of termination of a difficult time. This positive attitude can especially be reinforced if the nurse provides explanation and assurance.

Abnormal fetal positions

PERSISTENT OCCIPUT POSTERIOR POSITIONS. The fetal head usually enters the pelvic inlet transversely and therefore must traverse an arc of 90° in the process of internal rotation to the direct occiput anterior position. (See Figs. 5-5 and 5-7, p. 68).

In about a quarter of all labors, however, the head enters the pelvis with the occiput directed diagonally posterior, that is, in either the R.O.P. or the L.O.P. position. Under these circumstances the head must rotate through an arc of 135° in the process of internal rotation.

With good contractions, adequate flexion and a baby of average size, the great majority of these cases of occiput posterior position undergo spontaneous rotation through the 135° arc just as soon as the head reaches the pelvic floor. This is a normal mechanism of labor. It must be remembered, however, that labor is usually prolonged, and the mother has a great deal of discomfort in her back as the baby's head impinges against the sacrum in the course of rotating. Nursing intervention is aimed at relieving the back pain as much as possible. Sacral pressure, backrubs and frequent change of position from side to side can be helpful, and they should be employed to the degree that seems to be well-tolerated by the patient. In a minority of cases, however, perhaps 5 or 10 percent, these favorable circumstances do not exist, and rotation may be incomplete or may not take place at all. If rotation is incomplete, the head becomes arrested in the transverse position, a condition known as *transverse arrest*. If anterior rotation does not take place at all, the occiput usually rotates to the direct occiput posterior position, a condition known as *persistent occiput posterior*. Both transverse arrest and persistent occiput posterior position represent deviations from the normal mechanisms of labor.

Some controversy persists in the management of persistent occiput posterior. When labor progresses, although first and second stages tend to be prolonged in primigravidas, management the same as for occiput anterior positions results in no increased risk to the fetus although there may be increased incidence of midline episiotomy extensions and postpartum infection in the mother. Premature operative intervention, particularly if the station is high, seems contraindicated. Forceps rotation on the perineum is appropriate to reduce lacerations if this can be easily accomplished.

Sometimes the mechanical problem associated with abnormal uterine action is an abnormal position of the presenting head. Hence, these conditions of posterior or transverse arrest of the occiput appear to have, in some cases, an adverse effect on uterine behavior. Here the malposition is the cause rather than the effect of uterine inefficiency. This conclusion can be verified by the following findings. 1) When the fetal head is rotated or rotates spontaneously, uterine action improves. 2) Oxytocin therapy for dysfunction associated with an occipitoposterior position does not cause the infant's head to rotate.

It should be remembered that the uterus of the multigravid patient usually reacts to mechanical obstruction by becoming more active and ultimately rupturing itself. On the other hand, when the primigravid uterus encounters resistance it nearly always responds by inertia or incoordinate behavior. It is imperative then, that the obstetrician rule out mechanical obstruction before deciding that labor is prolonged due to idiopathic faulty uterine action. Since disproportion may be slight and therefore easily overlooked, only the most careful observation and study can disclose the important association between faulty uterine action and smallness of the pelvis or large size of the baby. The nurse can make an important contribution in this diagnosis by her continuous and critical observations of the character and frequency of the contractions, the amount of the mother's discomfort, her vital signs and general condition, and the fetal heart rate.

BREECH PRESENTATIONS. The breech is the presenting part in 3 to 4 percent of deliveries (see Chapter 14), and is more common when the baby is premature or there is multiple gestation. The reasons for breech presentations are not always apparent, although associated factors include great parity, twinning, hydramnios, hydrocephalus, and placenta previa. Recent studies indicate no positive correlation between breech presentation and contracted pelvis.[3]

There is no significantly increased danger for the life of the mother in breech presentations, although there is increased incidence of lacerations of the birth canal, episiotomy extensions, cesarean sections, and postpartum infections. Labor is not prolonged, contrary to previous belief.[4] For the infant, however, there is considerably increased risk of both death and injury in comparison to vertex presentations. Uncorrected perinatal loss is about 12 percent in the United States, and when corrected for congenital anomalies and maternal disease, fetal loss is still three times higher in single breech than in vertex. Traumatic morbidity is 12 times higher, including fractures, dislocations, and peripheral nerve injuries.[5] Although pulmonary morbidity (pneumonitis, atelectasis, or respiratory distress syndrome) occurs with similar frequency in both breech and vertex, brain damage from asphyxia resulting in neurological abnormalities at one year is increased in breech infants.[6]

The major cause of perinatal death results from trauma sustained in delivery. Tentorial tears and subsequent intracranial hemorrhage are twice as common in breech presentations as they are in cephalic presentations. The symptoms and nursing care associated with these conditions are discussed in Chapter 29. Lesions of the spinal cord and extrusion of the medulla into the foramen magnum also account for a goodly portion of deaths. In footling presentations, prolapse of the umbilical cord (see p. 508) is common. Even in the most skilled hands, and considering only full-term infants, about 1 breech infant in 15 succumbs as the result of delivery.

Unrecognized fetopelvic disproportion is the primary cause of the increase in perinatal mortality and morbidity in breech deliveries. Recommendations for medical management to reduce these complications include accurate x-ray pelvimetry, at least mean normal pelvic measurements and fetal size to permit trial labor, constant monitoring of fetal heart rate for signs of asphyxia, and cesarean section for

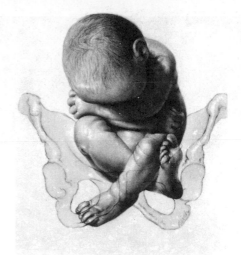

Figure 25-1. Footling breech.

estimated fetal size of above 8.5 pounds, minimal fetopelvic disproportion, failure to progress in labor, and signs of fetal distress.[7,8]

Classification. Breech presentations are classified as follows:

1. *Complete*, when the feet and the legs are flexed on the thighs, and the thighs are flexed on the abdomen, so that the buttocks and the feet present (see Fig. 14-2   p. 245).
2. *Footling*, when one or both feet present through the cervix (Fig. 25-1).
3. *Frank*, when the legs are extended and lie against the abdomen and the chest, with the feet meeting the shoulders, and the buttocks present (Fig. 25-2).

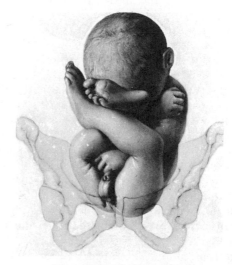

Figure 25-2. Frank breech.

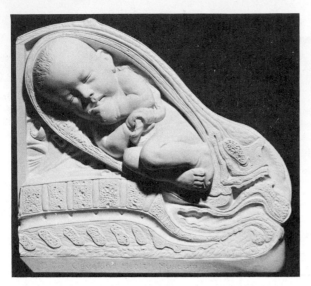

Figure 25-3. Breech presentation. (Dickinson-Belskie model. Cleveland Health Museum, Cleveland)

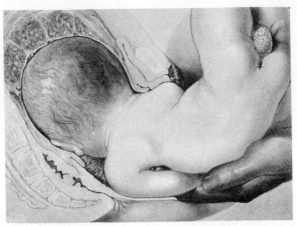

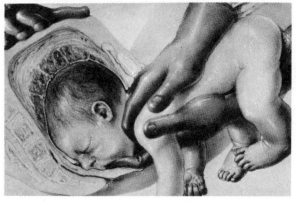

Figure 25-4. (Top) Extraction of posterior shoulder in breech delivery. (Bottom) Extraction of head in breech delivery (Mauriceau maneuver).

Delivery. With strong contractions, particularly in multiparae, breech cases may be delivered spontaneously, or at least with very little aid by the attendant. The breech is pushed through the vulva as the result of the mother's bearing-down efforts and rises upward in front of the symphysis pubis. With the emergence of the trunk, the legs descend, the attendant simply receiving them and steadying the breech. With further bearing-down efforts, the shoulders are expelled; then, as the attendant holds up the body, the head is extruded with the face directed back at the perineum (Fig. 25-4).

However, in the majority of breech cases, especially in primigravidae, it is necessary for the physician to give more aid than is indicated above, and, as a rule, this amounts to extraction of the shoulders and the head after the umbilicus has appeared (Fig. 25-4). It is to be remembered that there is a fundamental difference in a vertex and breech presentation. In the former, the head, which is the largest portion of the infant, is born first, and is followed by successively smaller portions. In a breech presentation, however, the process is reversed, with successively *larger* portions of the infant being born; thus, the buttocks, shoulders and the head represent, in effect, three "births" each preceded by its own internal rotation.

The frank breech usually is a better dilating wedge than a complete breech because the buttocks impinge more closely on the margins of the dilating cervix. However, the complete breech is more satisfactory for immediate delivery if medical assistance becomes necessary, since a foot can be brought down readily for traction. Converting the other types of breech presentations to a complete breech is not done routinely, however, unless there is some abnormality of the mother or infant that makes immediate delivery likely.

Extraction may be employed, and the application of Piper forceps to the aftercoming head is considered a conservative and reliable approach to breech delivery. Similarly, cesarean section is a safer approach and yields better results for the baby than a difficult extraction. It is recommended that cesarean section be employed in cases of breech presentation with concomitant uterine dysfunction, pelvic contractions, large infant and in primigravidae over 35 years of age.

Occasionally, cases of precipitate breech delivery may fall to the care of the nurse. These cases are uncommon and, when they do occur, seldom give rise to difficulty, because the very fact that they are precipitate presupposes a small infant, excellent expulsive forces and a capacious birth canal. As the breech emerges, it is received and is steadied with a sterile towel and sterile hands, and the mother is urged to bear down strongly. This usually will effect delivery of the shoulders in cases of this sort, but if it does not, the arm which is the more posterior is drawn out of the vagina by passing the first and the middle fingers over the infant's shoulder, down the arm to the elbow, and then drawing the forearm and the hand across the face and the chest and out. The other arm is delivered in the same way; and then, to favor the birth of the head, the body of the baby is raised upward in a vertical position. If there is any great delay, the nurse may place two fingers into the baby's mouth, with the trunk resting on the palm of the same hand and the legs straddling her forearm. Then, with the other hand, upward and outward traction is made on the shoulders, while firm downward pressure is made by an assistant on the lower abdominal wall. As with any other emergency delivery by the nurse, the nurse's composure and teamwork with the patient are important cornerstones to a successful outcome (see Chapter 18).

In breech presentation the infant often passes meconium from the rectum during the course of labor, and after the membranes are ruptured, and the liquor amnii has escaped, the nurse may find the black, tar-colored material coming from the patient's vagina. She needs to ascertain that the presentation is, in fact, a breech, for if such a phenomenon occurred in a vertex presentation, it would be an indication of probable fetal distress.

Explanation and appropriate reassurance are important for mothers who have breech presentations, as they are for any patient having an abnormal presentation or complicated labor of any type. Many patients are steeped in old wives' folklore of the fearfulness of a breech birth and become exceedingly anxious and terrified as soon as they find out (or overhear) that theirs is this type of presentation; the same is often true of their partners, and the anxiety and fear that are communicated between them can impede the patient's working effectively with her labor. With modern obstetric techniques and knowledge, labor need not be prolonged or exceptionally painful.

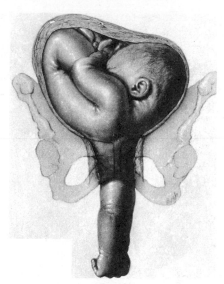

Figure 25-5. Shoulder presentation with prolapse of arm.

SHOULDER, FACE, AND BROW PRESENTATIONS. In shoulder presentations the infant lies crosswise in the uterus instead of longitudinally (see Fig. 14-2 p. 245). This complication occurs about once in every 200 cases and is seen most often in multiparae. Not infrequently an arm prolapses into the vagina, making the problem of delivery even more difficult (Fig. 25-5).

Shoulder presentation is a serious complication, with a slightly increased maternal mortality rate and an extremely high perinatal mortality with vaginal delivery—about 30 percent for term infants. External version in late pregnancy or early labor is occasionally successful, especially in multiparae, in converting the shoulder to a longitudinal lie. Internal podalic version and extraction is a very hazardous procedure (see Chapter 22), the second most common cause of rupture of the uterus, and associated with high perinatal mortality. Its use is justified only in carefully selected cases. Virtually all transverse presentations should be delivered by cesarean section, which reduces perinatal mortality to about 4 percent.

Face presentations are also seen about once in every 200 cases. They usually terminate spontaneously, the face coming through the vulva with the chin anterior. As edema of the scalp is common in vertex presentations (caput succedaneum), so in face presentations the presenting part, the face, becomes greatly swollen and purplish. This disappears within a few days. Brow presentations are even more rare and are much more difficult to deliver because the largest diameter of the fetal head, the occipitomental, presents. They frequently convert themselves into face or occipital presentations. Because the majority of brow presentations occur with premature infants and because of the transient nature of the remainder, spontaneous or forceps deliveries are usually possible. In the case of persistent brow presentation at term, cesarean section becomes the delivery of choice.

Disproportion

CONTRACTED PELVIS. Disproportion between the size of the infant and that of the birth canal (commonly spoken of as cephalopelvic disproportion) is caused most frequently by contracted pelvis. The pelvis may be contracted at the inlet, the midpelvis or the outlet. In the case of inlet contraction, the anteroposterior diameter of the inlet is shortened to 10 cm. or less, or the greatest transverse diameter is 12 cm. or less. The sacrum is broader and less concave from side to side, thinner from behind forward and shorter from above downward. Inlet contraction is most often due to rickets, a fact indicating how much good may be accomplished by the prevention of rickets in infants and children through an adequate intake of vitamin D. Contracted pelvis due to rickets is much more common among black peoples than among whites. In midpelvic contraction, the distance between the ischial spines is diminished; it is often found in conjunction with outlet contraction. In outlet contraction, the angle formed by the pubic rami is narrow, and the ischial tuberosities are close together; it thus resembles a male pelvis insofar as the outlet is concerned. This type of pelvic contraction occurs with equal frequency in white and black peoples, but its cause is not known. It is not only likely to hinder the egress of the infant at the outlet but also may be responsible for deep lacerations, since the narrow pubic rami tend to push the infant's head posteriorly in the direction of the rectum.

One purpose of antepartal care is to detect pelvic contraction during pregnancy, so that—long before labor begins—some intelligent decision can be reached about how best to deliver the infant. Of course, in a case of extreme pelvic contraction, cesarean section is obligatory. But all gradations of contracted pelvis are encountered, and, depending on the size of the infant and other factors, many patients with moderate degrees of the condition can be delivered vaginally without difficulty.

In doubtful cases, the physician may give the patient a "trial labor," that is, four to six hours of labor to ascertain whether or not with adequate contractions the head will pass through the pelvis. For these patients labor may be even more anxiety-provoking than usual (depending in part on the extent and the depth of supportive antepartal counseling), and if cesarean section is the ultimate outcome, there may be a great deal of disappointment and perhaps even a feeling of failure. The warm empathic attitude of the nurse is particularly needed with these patients. Frequent reports on the progress of labor should not be overlooked when the progress is favorable; if it is not, then explanation and anticipatory guidance regarding cesarean section may be given. The health team does the patient a disservice in avoiding the subject if progress is not made in labor.

OVERSIZE BABY. Excessive size of the infant is not commonly a cause of serious dystocia unless the fetus weighs over 4,500 Gm. (10 pounds). About 1 infant in 100 will fall in this class. The trauma associated with the passage of such huge infants through the birth canal causes a decided increase in fetal mortality; this has been estimated as 13 percent (almost 1 in 7), in contrast with the usual death rate of 4 percent for normal-size infants. Uterine dysfunction is frequent in labors with excessive-size infants, because the head becomes not only larger but harder and less malleable with increasing weight. Even though these infants are born alive, they often do poorly in the first few days because of cerebral hemorrhage, and must be watched closely for signs of that condition (see Chapter 29).

Excessive size of the fetus is usually due to maternal diabetes, large size of one or both parents, or multiparity. Postmaturity due to prolonged gestation is not thought to be an important cause of excessive-size infants. Tremendously large infants, weighing over 13 pounds, are extremely rare, and almost all are born dead. Most oversized babies are boys. Although studies have shown a relationship between maternal diet and growth and survival of the fetus, it is doubtful that strict regulation of diet during pregnancy can significantly reduce excessive growth of the infant. However, large women who are heavy tend to have excessive weight gain during pregnancy and also larger babies, and in this way weight gain is associated with large babies.

SHOULDER DYSTOCIA. One serious complication of an oversize infant is shoulder dystocia. After the head has passed through the pelvic canal, the infant's unusually large shoulders may arrest at either the pelvic brim or the outlet. The incidence of shoulder dystocia is 1.7 percent in infants over 4,000 Gm., with mortality of about 16 percent. The time between delivery of the head and delivery of the body must be short to reduce infant deaths, but too vigorous traction on the head or neck can cause serious damage. At times deliberate fracture of the clavicle may be necessary and life-saving to the baby.

HYDROCEPHALUS. Hydrocephalus, or an excessive accumulation of cerebrospinal fluid in the ventricles of the brain with consequent enlargement of the cranium, is encountered in 1 fetus in 2,000, approximately, and accounts for some 12 percent of all malformations at birth. Associated defects are common, spina bifida being present in about one third of the cases. Varying degrees of cranial enlargement are produced, and not infrequently the circumference of the head exceeds 50 cm., sometimes reaching 80 cm. The amount of fluid present is usually between 500 and 1,500 ml., but as much as 5 liters has been reported. Since the distended cranium is too large to fit into the pelvic inlet, breech presentations are exceedingly common, being observed in about one third of such cases. Whatever the presentation, gross disproportion between the size of the head and that of the pelvis is the rule, and serious dystocia is the usual consequence. This is a tragic and serious complication of labor, and the obstetrician will find it necessary, as a rule, to puncture the cranial vault and aspirate as much of the cerebrospinal fluid as may be necessary to permit delivery. This procedure in itself does not injure the child. Nevertheless, fetal mortality is very high, 70 percent (this percentage includes very mild forms of the disease).

Births of this type are a terrible tragedy for all concerned; the mother must undergo a difficult labor at great risk to herself, the father will suffer with her, the fetus may expire, and the physician and the nurse must cope with a grave crisis with a poor prognosis. It is often difficult to describe the emotional climate at this time; perhaps it is impossible if one has not experienced a similar loss or disappointment. A state of emotional shock prevails, in which disbelief, noncomprehension and, sometimes, denial prevail. This is a situation in which the nurse will be called on to exercise nursing skill to the utmost, not only during labor but after the delivery, and particularly if there is an obvious abnormality, or if a fetal demise occurs. The components of care that are useful in helping the parents in such a crisis are discussed fully in Chapter 29.

Hemorrhagic complications

Hemorrhage is probably a more important cause of maternal death in the United States than the 14 percent that statistics indicate, because national vital statistics are based only upon the *immediate* cause of death. In this way, a woman who hemorrhaged after labor, had her resistance to infection lowered, contracted postpartum infection, and died would be classified as a death due to infection; although hemorrhage was the real underlying cause. The major causes of hemorrhage associated with childbearing are placenta previa and abruptio (see Chapter 23) and uterine atony.

Postpartum hemorrhage

Hemorrhage during the postpartum period is the most common cause of serious blood loss associated with pregnancy, and causes about one fourth of all maternal deaths from hemorrhagic complications. The debilitation and lowered resistance which often accompany it are related to postpartum infections, another leading cause of maternal death. To a large extent, death from postpartum hemorrhage is preventable if the condition is diagnosed early and treated aggressively.

DEFINITION AND INCIDENCE. Postpartum hemorrhage is commonly defined as loss of more than 500 cc. of blood during the first 24 hours after giving birth. However, ordinary blood loss following vaginal delivery frequently is slightly more than 500 cc. by accurate measurement. Most obstetricians estimate the amount of bleeding at delivery, and studies show that estimated blood loss is usually only about one half of actual loss. Therefore, an *estimated* blood loss over 500 cc. serves to alert the nurse and physician that the patient has bled excessively and is in danger of postpartum hemorrhage.

Bleeding of this degree occurs once in every 20 or 30 cases despite the most skilled care. Hemorrhages of 1,000 cc. and over are encountered once in about every 75 cases, whereas blood losses of even 1,500 and 2,000 cc. are encountered less frequently. Postpartum hemorrhage is a fairly common complication of labor. Moreover, it is one with which the nurse must be intimately familiar, as nurses are expected to assume an important role in the prevention and treatment of the condition.

THE THREE CAUSES. In order of frequency, the three immediate causes of postpartum hemorrhage are:

1. Uterine atony.
2. Lacerations of the perineum, the vagina and the cervix.
3. Retained placental fragments.

Clotting defects as well as obstetrical accidents such as inversion of the uterus can also be classified as causes, but they are much less common and are of a more indirect nature.

Uterine atony is by far the most common cause. The uterus contains huge blood vessels within the interstices of its muscle fibers, and those at the placental site are open and gaping. It is essential that the muscle fibers contract down tightly on these arteries and veins, if bleeding is to be controlled. They must *stay* contracted down, for only a few seconds' relaxation will give rise to sudden, profuse hemorrhage. They must stay *tightly* contracted down, because continuous, slight relaxation gives rise to continuous oozing of blood, one of the most treacherous forms of postpartum hemorrhage.

In a study of 56 maternal deaths from pregnancy-related hemorrhage over a nine-year period in California, 19 were due to uterine atony. The majority of these women died within four hours of delivery, possibly before the seriousness of their bleeding was recognized. Generally, these patients were older multiparas with spontaneous term deliveries; most of their deaths were avoidable had the hemorrhage been diagnosed earlier and adequate blood and fibrinogen replacement instituted in time. Most of their babies survived.[8]

Lacerations of the perineum, the vagina and the cervix are naturally more common after operative delivery. Tears of the cervix are particularly likely to cause serious hemorrhage. Bright red arterial bleeding in the presence of a hard, firmly contracted uterus (no uterine atony) suggests hemorrhage from a cervical laceration. The physician will establish the diagnosis by actual inspection of the cervix (re-

tractors are necessary) and, after locating the source of bleeding, will repair the laceration.

Perineal and vaginal tears also contribute to postpartal blood loss. In addition, perineal tears may do great damage in destroying the integrity of the perineum and in weakening the supports of the uterus, the bladder and the rectum. Unless these lacerations are repaired properly, the resultant weakness, as the years go by, may cause prolapse of the uterus (called by the laity "falling of the womb"), cystocele (a pouching downward of the bladder) or rectocele (a pouching forward of the rectum). These conditions, which originate from perineal lacerations at childbirth, give rise to many discomforts and often necessitate operative treatment.

Lacerations of the birth canal sometimes occur during the process of normal delivery, and may be unavoidable even in the most skilled hands (see Chapter 18).

Retained Placental Fragments. Small, partially separated fragments of placenta may cause postpartum hemorrhage by interfering with proper uterine contraction. Careful inspection of the placenta to determine whether a piece is missing should be routinely carried out at delivery. If a portion is missing, exploration of the uterus is indicated to remove the placental fragment. In the case of continued postpartum bleeding, retention of placental fragments is generally ruled out by manual exploration. However, this is rarely a cause of immediate postpartum hemorrhage, and is more commonly implicated in late hemorrhage in which profuse bleeding occurs suddenly a week or more after delivery.

PREDISPOSING FACTORS. There are certain factors which predispose to postpartum hemorrhage, so that to a certain extent it may be anticipated in advance. Among these, one of the most important is the size of the infant. With a 9-pound infant, the chances of postpartum hemorrhage are five times as great as they are with a 5-pound infant. Excessive bleeding is twice as common in twin pregnancy. Hydramnios (excessive amount of amniotic fluid) is another predisposing factor. It has been shown, however, that with the careful use of oxytocin in the placental stage and special care to achieve effective contraction in this stage, that the incidence of hemorrhage due to overdistention can be reduced considerably. Operative delivery with deep general anesthesia, prolonged labor with maternal exhaustion, and mismanagement of the third stage of labor greatly increase the likelihood of this complication. Other conditions in which postpartum hemorrhage is extremely frequent are high parity and premature separation of the placenta and placenta previa. Finally, internal podalic version is followed by a very high incidence of hemorrhage. Thus, it is recommended that blood transfusions be ready for *immediate* use if this procedure must be attempted.

CLINICAL PICTURE. Excessive bleeding may occur prior to the birth of the placenta, but it is seen more commonly thereafter. Although it is occasionally torrential in character, the most common type is a continuous trickle—minute by minute. These small constant trickles are not alarming in appearance; consequently, no one may become concerned and no action may be taken.

Such hemorrhages are particularly treacherous for this reason. The condition of the patient determines the amount of blood loss which can be tolerated, with exhaustion from prolonged labor or antecedent anemia or chronic disease reducing the ability of the body to compensate. When hemorrhage has been profuse enough, the pulse becomes rapid and thready, the skin pallid and clammy; chills and disturbed vision occur. As shock deepens air hunger develops with restlessness and sweating; then unconsciousness and death may follow. The pulse and blood pressure may not change significantly until large amounts of blood have been lost; then the vascular mechanism fails and shock ensues. Vascular collapse may lead to death when intravenous infusion cannot be maintained for blood replacement. Cardiac arrest may also occur at this point.

Beecham, a Philadelphia physician, in his survey of 52 deaths from postpartum hemorrhage which occurred in that city, found the average interval between delivery and death in this series was 5 hours and 20 minutes. Only 6 patients, 11.5 percent, died within 2 hours of delivery, and none in less than 1½ hours. In other words, there would have been ample time for intensive treatment in any of these cases, had the attendant been alert to how much blood was being lost.

TREATMENT. The first and most important thing to do is to grasp the uterus and massage it. This must be continued until the uterus assumes a woody hardness; if the slightest relaxation occurs, the massage must be reinstituted. In many cases the uterus stays contracted most of the time but occasionally relaxes; it is therefore obligatory to keep a hand on the fundus constantly for a full hour after bleeding has subsided. When the uterus is well contracted, care should be taken *to avoid overmassage,* because such practice contributes to muscle fatigue, which in turn further encourages uterine relaxation and excessive bleeding. Even then the danger is not over, since relaxation sometimes occurs two or more hours after delivery; in these cases the uterus may balloon with blood, with very little escaping externally. Accordingly, the consistency, size and height of the uterus should be checked frequently until several hours have elapsed. Ordinarily, the height of the fundus after delivery will be about at the level of the umbilicus. If the uterus becomes distended with blood, or if the bladder becomes full and presses upward against the uterus, causing it to rise in the abdomen, then the fundus can be palpated several centimeters above the umbilicus. The nurse must make absolutely certain that she is actually massaging the uterus and not a roll of abdominal fat or a distended bladder (see pp. 337, 371). When properly contracted, the uterus should feel like a small-to-medium-sized hard grapefruit. Frequently, a big, boggy, relaxed uterus is difficult to outline through the abdominal wall, and it may be necessary to push the hand well posteriorly toward the region of the sacral promontory to reach it. The very fact that the uterus is hard to identify usually means that it is relaxed.

Allaying Anxiety. The frequent massage and deep palpation are often painful to the mother; at best they are disturbing, since they come at a time when she wants nothing more than to rest and sleep after her great effort. If she is awake and alert, then the continued attention and scrutiny may increase her anxiety. It must be remembered that apprehension is a natural concomitant of hemorrhage and shock. Quick and efficient nursing observations and appropriate explanation and reassurance help allay the mother's and her partner's concerns.

This aspect of nursing care may be difficult to implement. If the mother or the father expresses concern and questions the activity by asking "What's wrong?" then the nurse can say simply, "The uterus has a tendency to relax, and must be massaged so that it will contract down as it should." Usually, such a statement will suffice. This will indicate the reason for the continued activity without associating hemorrhage and its fearsome consequences with the actions of the attendants. If the mother drifts off to sleep between the nurse's observations, then the nurse can gently rouse her by speaking her name before commencing massage, so that the mother is not awakened abruptly to the painful sensation of someone squeezing her abdomen.

Other Aspects of Care. Vital signs will be required every 5 to 15 minutes, and any variation, however slight, is to be reported immediately. One way that the nurse can keep a more accurate account of the blood loss is to keep a perineal pad count. In doing this one counts the number of pads saturated, how fully they are saturated, and the time it took for the saturation to occur. Thus, the nurse's notes might read: "Two pads ¾ saturated in 20 minutes." This type of report is more helpful to the physician than a more general, vague statement like, "Saturating perineal pads quickly."

If the bleeding occurs prior to delivery of the placenta, the physician may find it necessary to extract the placenta manually. (A change of gloves as well as gown may be called for to ensure strict asepsis, since the uterine cavity is to be invaded.) Oxytocics will invariably be requested, ergonovine or oxytocin or both intramuscularly. One or the other of these may be given intravenously. Blood transfusion will undoubtedly be instituted. The blood group of *all* maternity patients should be known before labor and crossmatched blood should be available for those in whom hemorrhage is anticipated or appears imminent. Seeing that the bloodtyping is carried out, ordering and calling for the cross match and the blood to be sent to the unit are usually responsibilities of the nurse. Time is of the essence for these patients; therefore the nurse must preplan and establish priorities with rapidity.

If oxytocin therapy fails to stop the bleeding, the physician probably will carry out bimanual compression of the uterus. This provides the most efficient means of compressing the site of bleeding. Packing the uterus with gauze, a procedure once considered valuable to promote hemostasis in such cases, is seldom utilized today. It is considered by many authorities (e.g., Eastman, Hellman, Cosgrove, Leff and Berkeley) to be inadequate and conducive to infection. If shock threatens, the Trendelenburg position should be employed, external heat applied, and preparations for blood transfusion made.

In the handling of a case of postpartum hemorrhage, the nurse often assumes the important tasks of massaging the uterus, giving oxytocics, helping with the transfusion and caring for the infant. The nurse must be prepared to act quickly and efficiently if the lives of these bleeding mothers are to be saved.

If postpartal hemorrhage should occur after the physician has left, the nurse should grasp the uterus at once, press out as much blood as possible and begin gentle, but vigorous, massage, sending word, of course, to the physician. If massage fails to stop the bleeding, the physician usually will not object if the nurse gives the patient an intramuscular injection of ergonovine or oxytocin. If possible, this arrangement should be understood beforehand.

LATE POSTPARTUM HEMORRHAGE. Occasionally, postpartum hemorrhage may occur later than the first day following delivery. These late postpartum hemorrhages may take place any time between the second and the twenty-eighth day, are usually sudden in onset and may be so massive as to produce shock. Late postpartum hemorrhage is fortunately uncommon, occurring perhaps once in 1,000 cases. While this condition is relatively uncommon, it is most dangerous because the mother will usually be home, often alone, and without professional attendance. Thus, if the hemorrhage is massive, she may be in immediate danger; even if the bleeding is not great, there is still considerable difficulty getting medical assistance, and all of this can produce a great deal of anxiety and fatigue. Arrangements must be made for the care of the infant even if the mother is to be seen only for a short while in the emergency room. Partners must be contacted, transportation arranged, and often myriads of other details worked through before the mother can receive medical attention. This is why it is so important that the mother know where she can readily contact her physician should she need him in an emergency. Moreover, it becomes clearer why the mother should have help in the person of someone who is readily available and responsible for the first weeks of the puerperium.

Factors which most often cause these late hemorrhages are retention of placental fragments, recurrent bleeding from lacerations or episiotomy and subinvolution of the placental site. The latter condition is especially interesting because as yet the pathogenesis is unknown. The regeneration of the placental site takes longer than the rest of the uterus. It is accomplished in about six weeks as compared with about 21 days for the rest of the endometrium. The regeneration of the placental site begins from the remains of the epithelial glands; if these are not viable, then regeneration must occur from the spread of the surrounding epithelial tissue in the rest of the uterus. Until the site is firmly epithelialized, sloughing of clots may cause bleeding. Certain factors have been found to be associated with clot sloughing and hemorrhage, among them low grade fever, a history of abortion or uterine bleeding during pregnancy, hormonal influences, and the absence of breast-feeding. Often, however, none of these factors are found to be present, and the reason for the subinvolution remains a mystery. The physician will probably want to examine the patient. He may then carry out instrumental dilatation of the cervix at which time he will remove any placental fragments that are present with a curet or ovum forceps or repair any lacerations or incisions.

Use of ultrasonic scanning of the uterus to detect the presence of retained products of conception, thus avoiding unnecessary curettage, has been suggested.[9]

If the mother must return to the hospital, this will no doubt upset to some degree the beginning relationship with the newborn. If the mother is nursing her infant and it is within a two-week period after delivery, the physician often can arrange to have the mother room-in with her infant for the short one- or two-day hospital stay. If the mother is bottle-feeding, then relatives, husband or "mother's helpers" can help in the interim until the mother's return. The nurse will want to remember that much of the mother's apparent anxiety and/or desire to return home as quickly as possible arises from these often abrupt and temporary arrangements that she has had to make. Understanding and counseling the mother to help her get adequate rest upon her return home is one of the helpful measures that the nurse can offer.

Rupture of uterus

Rupture of the uterus is fortunately a rare complication, but when it does occur, it constitutes one of the gravest accidents in obstetrics, since almost all of the infants and about a third of the mothers are lost. In this condition the uterus simply bursts, because the strain placed upon its musculature is more than it can withstand. It may occur in pregnancy but is far more frequent in labor. In modern obstetrics the most common cause is rupture of the scar of a previous cesarean section. Accordingly, when one is observing labor in a patient who has had a previous cesarean section, the possibility of this accident always should be borne in mind. Other contributing factors include prolonged and/or obstructed labor, certain faulty presentations, multiparity, traumatic delivery, such as version and extraction, and the injudicious use of oxytocin in labor. The incidence of uterine rupture is increasing, reported as one per 1,216 deliveries in 1963 and one per 927 in 1971. The more frequent use of oxytocin in grand multiparous patients and the greater number of cesarean sections in obstetrical complications are the major factors contributing to this increase. Rupture of the cesarean scar in a subsequent labor is always a danger; thus the dictum "once a cesarean, always a cesarean" continues to be valid.[10]

When rupture occurs, the patient complains of a severe, sudden, lancinating pain during a strong labor contraction. The rupture may be complete or incomplete; pain and abdominal tenderness are usually present in both cases. If there is complete rupture, regular contractions cease, since the torn muscle can no longer contract. There is an outpouring of blood into the abdominal cavity and sometimes into the vagina. The uterus may be palpated abdominally as a hard mass lying alongside the fetus. The patient soon exhibits signs of shock.

If the rupture is incomplete, the contractions may continue, and the signs of shock may be delayed, since the blood loss is slower. As soon as the diagnosis of rupture of the uterus is made, rapid preparations for an abdominal operation should ensue, since hysterectomy is the usual treatment. In addition, antibiotics are administered to combat infection, and blood transfusions are given to replace blood loss and to alleviate shock. Since this accident gravely compromises the lives of both the infant and the mother, prevention, early diagnosis, prompt treatment, blood transfusions and antibiotics are essential components in improving the prognosis. The nursing care will be essentially that for any complicated delivery and postpartum hemorrhage. Whenever possible it is advisable to have the nurse who has been attending the mother during labor remain with her until the anesthetic for the cesarean section is given. This will provide some measure of continuity of care and help in reassurance and comfort of the parents.

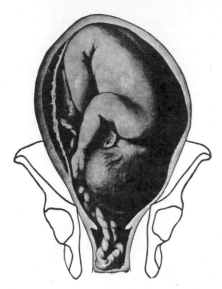

Figure 25-6. Prolapse of the umbilical cord (Bumm). As the head comes down, the compression of the cord between the fetal skull and the pelvic brim will shut off its circulation completely.

Inversion of uterus

Inversion of the uterus is a rare and highly fatal accident of labor in which, after the birth of the infant, the uterus turns inside out. Shock is profound, and hemorrhage may occur, in many cases causing the death of the mother. This rare complication is mentioned here only to stress the two common causes: 1) pulling on the umbilical cord and 2) trying to express the placenta when the uterus is relaxed. In the former case, the traction on the attached placenta simply pulls the uterus inside out, while in the latter the hand pushes the relaxed muscular sac inside out. The umbilical cord *never* should be pulled on, and the uterus *never* should be pushed upon unless it is firmly contracted.

Disorders of placental attachment

Other important causes of bleeding associated with pregnancy and labor are placenta previa and abruptio placentae. These have been previously discussed as complications of pregnancy in Chapter 23. However, at times the first signs of these problems occur during labor, and the nurse in the delivery suite must be familiar with their diagnosis and management. The cardinal sign of *placenta previa* is painless, bright red vaginal bleeding. If partial separation occurs after the onset of labor, contractions may confuse the situation; identification depends upon accurately assessing the extent of vaginal bleeding. Overt hemorrhage

with huge blood loss is not difficult to diagnose, but it requires fine judgment to decide when bloody vaginal discharge ceases to be heavy "show" and becomes potential hemorrhage. It is wise to report any vaginal bleeding which the nurse believes is excessive to the physician, and to refrain from digital examination of these patients.

Abruptio placentae can be a true obstetrical emergency if the area of separation is extensive. The signs that alert the delivery room nurse to this complication include a hypertonic uterus which does not relax well between contractions, an area of extreme sensitivity when the uterus is palpated, sudden sharp and persistent uterine pain, and symptoms and signs of shock which seem greater than the observable blood loss would indicate. An extremely hard, boardlike uterus which cannot be indented and which does not relax indicates a severe degree of placental separation and bleeding.

Marginal sinus rupture was formerly treated as a separate clinical entity, but now is felt to be a mild type of abruptio placentae in which slight separation occurs at the edge of the placenta. The marginal sinus is located under the edge of the placenta, and is one of the large maternal sinuses bathing the placental villi. If the placenta separates at a point along its margin, this maternal sinus is disrupted and bleeding occurs. There is usually no increased pain or uterine tension, and the amount of vaginal bleeding may vary considerably. If the area of separation is small, as it usually is in marginal sinus rupture, there is no danger of hypoxia to the fetus and generally no changes in fetal heart rate. When there is excessive vaginal bleeding during labor, and placenta previa and abruptio have been ruled out, the most probable cause is a small marginal separation of the placenta.[11]

Prolapse of umbilical cord

In the course of labor, the cord prolapses in front of the presenting part about once in every 400 cases. It is a grave complication for the fetus, since the cord is then compressed between the presenting part and the bony pelvis, and the fetal circulation is shut off (Fig. 25-6). Any factor which prevents proper adaptation of the presenting part to the maternal pelvis predisposes to prolapse of the cord. The accident occurs more commonly in shoulder and footling breech presentations, and less often with frank breeches and multiple pregnancy. In cephalic presentations, it rarely occurs unless there is pelvic contraction or excessive development of the fetus. There is an increased incidence with prematurity, probably because the small fetus is poorly fitted to the pelvic inlet. Prolapse frequently occurs following rupture of the membranes when the head, the breech or the shoulder is not sufficiently down in the pelvis to prevent the cord from being washed past it in the sudden gush of amniotic fluid. After the membranes rupture, the cord comes down, and it may be either a concealed or an apparent prolapse. In the latter instance, the diagnosis is made when the cord is seen; but when the cord is not visible, the correct diagnosis is made when the patient is examined and the cord is felt, or examination of the fetal heart reveals distress due to pressure on the cord. This is why it *must* be a routine practice to listen to the fetal heart sounds immediately after the membranes rupture and again in about 10 minutes. When fetal heart rate is monitored internally, a characteristic slowing of the fetal heart with onset early during the contraction and persistence of bradycardia beyond the end of contraction are suggestive of cord compression.

The immediate treatment of cord prolapse is to minimize the pressure of the presenting part upon the cord and the resultant impaired umbilical circulation. The head of the bed or table should be lowered, or the patient placed in a knee-chest position to raise the level of the hips above the shoulders and allow the presenting part to gravitate away from the pelvis. Additionally, the presenting part may be pushed upward by pressure from a sterile gloved hand in the vagina. The physician and other staff must be notified at once so emergency procedures can be instituted. No attempt should be made to reposition the cord, and with a live baby near term the goal of therapy is to effect delivery as soon as possible. If dilatation is incomplete, immediate cesarean section yields the best results for fetal salvage. In occasional carefully selected cases, prolapsed cord in vertex presentations with nearly complete dilatation can be delivered with minimal trauma to mother and infant using vacuum extraction.[12] Perinatal mortality with cord prolapse, which is usually about 26 percent, can be reduced to 5 to 10 percent when delivery is accomplished within one-half hour after diagnosis. More frequent vaginal examinations, checking fetal heart after rupture of membranes, and active rapid treatment combine to reduce mortality.

This particular complication is not painful for the mother; however, it can be very frightening, for many patients realize it can result in their infant's death. Also whether they realize the grave implications or not, the various antic positions and quickened responses of the attendants give them an indication that all is not well. Therefore, again, the calmness, warmth and efficiency of the nurse can do much to reassure the patient that all possible measures are being taken to bring the situation under control. It goes without saying that these patients never should be left unattended, and their partners, if they are present, should be treated with consideration. It is difficult, when any crises occur, to deal with the relatives of the patient with appropriate thoughtfulness, since most of the energy is directed toward meeting the pressing (and often lifesaving) demands of the situation. However, it must be remembered that the patient and her family are considered as a unit, and a few moments usually can be found to provide essential information.

Amniotic fluid embolism

At any time after the membranes have ruptured there is a possibility that amniotic fluid may enter the gaping venous sinuses of the placental site as well as the veins in the cervix, be drawn into the general circulation and in this way reach the pulmonary capillaries. Since the amniotic fluid invariable contains small particles of matter, such as vernix caseosa, lanugo and sometimes meconium, multiple tiny emboli may reach the lungs in this manner and cause occlusion of the pulmonary capillaries. This complication, amniotic fluid embolism, is almost invariable fatal and, as a rule, causes the death of the mother within one or two hours. Fortunately, this tragic condition is rare, occurring only once in many thousand labors.

The clinical characteristics of the condition are sudden dyspnea, cyanosis, pulmonary edema, profound shock and uterine relaxation with postpartum hemorrhage. A highly important feature of amniotic fluid embolism is a diminution in the fibrinogen content of the blood, or hypofibrinogenemia. The mechanism is similar to, if not identical with, that which

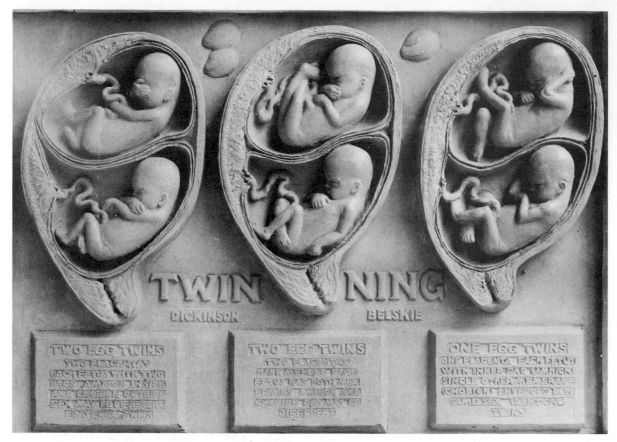

Figure 25-7. One-egg and two-egg twins. (Dickinson-Belskie models, Cleveland Health Museum, Cleveland)

occurs in abruptio placentae and missed abortion, as described on pages 475 and 480.

The treatment consists of oxygen therapy, blood transfusion and the intravenous administration of fibrinogen, but, as indicated, this is usually futile.

Multiple pregnancy

When two or more embryos develop in the uterus at the same time, the condition is known as multiple pregnancy. Twins occur approximately once in every 93 white births and 73 nonwhite births. Triplets occur approximately once in 9,400 births; and quadruplets, once in 620,000.

Types of twins

Twins may be identical (monozygotic) or fraternal (dizygotic). Identical twins *are* identical because they come from a single egg; hence they are called "single-ovum twins." Fer-tilization takes place in the usual way, by a single spermatozoon, but then, very early in the ovum's development, it divides into two identical parts instead of continuing as a single individual. Such twins are always of the same sex and show close physical and mental resemblances. Nonidentical or fraternal twins result from the fertilization of two ova by two spermatozoa and are therefore *double-ovum twins* (Fig. 25-7). Such twins, according to chance, may be of the same sex or of opposite sexes; and the likelihood of their resembling each other is no greater than that of any brother and sister.

Basically, two types of placentae exist in twins, those with monochorial (one chorion) and those with dichorial (two chorions) membranes. Also, the placentae may be fused, separate or a single disk and there may be one or two amnions. Each fetus usually has its own umbilical cord, however. The possible combinations thus include:

1. Monozygotic (identical)
   a. Diamniotic monochorionic (two amnions, one chorion). Common.
   b. Diamniotic dichorionic (two amnions, two chorions). 30 percent.
   c. Monoamniotic monochorionic (one amnion, one chorion). Very rare.
2. Dizygotic (fraternal or nonidentical)
   a. Diamniotic dichorionic (two amnions, two chorions).

Examination of the fetal membranes is used to assist in diagnosing the zygosity of twins, but is not always accurate. Only monozygotic twins can have a single chorion, so this establishes identical twinning. Two chorions are always present in dizygotic twins, but are also the placentation of about 30 percent of monozygotic twins. If the sexes are different, the twins are obviously fraternal; but if twins are the same sex and dichorionic, the diagnosis is uncertain.[13] The usual twin placentations are shown in Figure 25-8. In the United States, 33 percent of twins are identical.

Causes of twinning

Of the two types of twins, only the cause of dizygotic twinning is partially understood. The frequency of monozygotic twins is about the same throughout the world. Dizygotic twins, the result of multiple ovulation, vary with maternal age, racial group, genotype of the mother, and possibly some environmental factors. Dizygotic twinning increases with maternal age up to a maximum at 37 years, then falls sharply. The Nigerian Yoruba tribe has an unusually high dizygotic twinning rate, and women were found to have significantly increased preovulatory FSH secretion related to the number of sets of twins they produced. Certain families have recurrent dizygotic twinning, which is thought to be related to higher gonadotropin secretion rates. Only a history of twins in the mother is significant, however, for the mates of male twins do not have an increased rate of twinning. In Finland the peak of twin conceptions is in July, when it is felt that continuous exposure to light leads to hypothalamic stimulation with resultant polyovulation.[14]

Thus there seems to be a relationship between gonadotropin secretion and dizygotic twinning as a result of multiple ovulation. This is compatible with the increasing phenomenon of quintuplet or sextuplet pregnancy following use of infertility drugs such as *clomiphene*, an

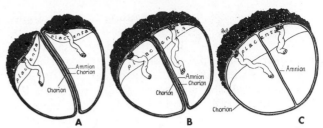

Figure 25-8. Single- and double-ovum twin differences. A and B, double-ovum twins; there are two chorions; in B the two placentas have fused. C, single-ovum twins; there is only one chorion and one placenta.

agent which releases pituitary gonadotropins. Multiple pregnancy after treatment with these agents is as high as 44 percent. Predominantly dizygotic twins are conceived, but numerous triplets and higher multiple births do occasionally occur. Polyovulation is related to the dosage of clomiphene. The higher the number of fetuses, the greater the probability of premature labor and its complications of fetal loss, an additional tragedy for the couple who have suffered through many years of infertility.

Diagnosis

In the majority of instances (but not all) it is possible for the physician to make a diagnosis of twins by abdominal examination during the last few months; in doubtful cases, a roentgenogram may be necessary to settle the question. Twins are suspected whenever uterine size is greater than ordinarily expected for any point in pregnancy. In addition, the palpation of three or four large parts in the uterus, the appearance of two fetal heart tones, of differing frequency, and the history of twins "running in the family" all serve to alert the obstetrician and nurse to the possibility of a multiple pregnancy.

Twins are likely to be born about two weeks before the calculated date of delivery. Even though pregnancy goes to full term, twins are usually smaller than single infants by nearly 1 pound; however, the outlook for such infants, provided that the pregnancy continues into the last month, is almost as good as that for single infants.

Aspects of multiple pregnancy

The patient with a multiple pregnancy faces greater discomforts and greater hazards than does a woman with a single pregnancy. The latter weeks of a twin pregnancy are likely to be associated with heaviness of the lower abdomen, back pains and swelling of the feet and the ankles. Abdominal distention makes sleeping difficult, and therefore the physician may prescribe a hypnotic. A well-fitting maternity girdle will make daytime more comfortable. Because of the excessive abdominal size, the patient may find that frequent small feedings are more suitable than the usual three larger meals a day. The nurse can be very helpful in giving the mother anticipatory guidance regarding these matters during the antepartal period.

Moreover, there are serious complications which these patients are particularly prone to develop: premature labor, toxemia and postpartum hemorrhage. Coitus probably will be restricted during the last three months of pregnancy to mitigate the possibility of early labor. Also, travel will be curtailed, since labor may begin at any time without warning, and delivery in strange surroundings may be hazardous. The mother will be encouraged to take frequent afternoon rests and to avoid activities involving physical strain.

The antepartal course of these patients should be followed with special care for signs of toxemia. Thus, the mother's antepartal visits usually will be more frequent to ensure meticulous supervision. A low-salt diet and diuretics will be ordered when indicated. In addition, iron may be prescribed, since anemia is usual in multiple pregnancy.

Postpartum hemorrhage is twice as common in twin pregnancy, although mechanical difficulties in labor are less frequent than might be expected. Uterine dysfunction, however, is encountered rather often. A spontaneous delivery is particularly desired in instances of twins, since this type of delivery results in less blood loss and maternal morbidity and a greater likelihood of healthy, undamaged infants.

Delivery

When the first baby is born, the physician usually has to rupture the membranes of the second twin. Then with combined vaginal and abdominal manipulation, he turns the infant to either a breech or a vertex presentation. *Judicious* abdominal pressure is used to propel the presenting part through the birth canal and effect either a spontaneous delivery or forceps or breech extraction. Occasionally, a version and extraction (see p. 451) may be necessitated if the vaginal and abdominal maneuvers are unsuccessful.

As soon as the second twin is delivered, the physician will order an oxytocic to be given, and the nurse assists the obstetrician in observing the fundus carefully for distention due to an accumulation of blood. An intravenous infusion of glucose usually will be administered prophylactically. To guard against uterine atony and blood loss, after the placentae are expressed, oxytocin will be added to the infusion to ensure a firmly contracted uterus.

Nursing care

As with any delivery, the nurse will have the responsibility of supportive care for the patient as well as assisting the physician in whatever activities are indicated. Since these infants are apt to be small, oxygen and/or resuscitative measures may be necessary. The care will be similar to that for the premature baby (see Chapter 28). Any supplies and/or equipment that may be needed (resuscitator, oxygen apparatus, etc.) should be procured early in the delivery and kept in readiness (but out of the patient's sight, if possible). Maternal vital signs as well as the fetal heart tones should be checked frequently.

Especially in the case of undiagnosed twins (i.e., the presence of twins is not discovered or suspected until labor and delivery), there is frequently a decided psychologic and economic (albeit somewhat delayed) shock to the parents. Emotionally, one additional child may be desired and acceptable; two may impose a burden, particularly if this pregnancy was to be "the last." The parents may wonder if they can manage the care of two newborn infants simultaneously. Problems may be compounded in feeding, especially if the mother is desirous of nursing her infant. In addition, two of everything must be provided, instead of one, and this additional cost may put a strain on the budget. In terms of long-range planning, the present housing may be inadequate, especially if the children are of different sexes and eventually will require separate rooms. The cost entailed in additional construction and/or new housing is considerable. None of these problems is insurmountable and can be worked through satisfactorily in time. Some parents need an understanding and empathic person to help them over the initial adjustment period. In some cases they may need the help of a social worker or a public health nurse to help them plan for the unexpected new baby. Many parents seem to adjust nicely through being able to ventilate their surprise (and, in some cases, chagrin). Certainly the professional nurse is able and qualified to give this type of support.

Bibliography

1. Hellman, L. M., and Pritchard, J. A.: *Williams Obstetrics*, ed. 14. New York, Appleton-Century Crofts, 1971, p. 838.
2. Jeffcoate, T. N., *et al*: Inefficient uterine action. *Surg. Gyn. Ob.* 95:257, Sept. 4, 1952.
3. Hellman and Pritchard, *op. cit.*, pp. 843, 859, 624-625.
4. Phillips, R. D., and Freeman, M.: The management of the persistent occiput posterior position. *Am. J. Ob-Gyn.* 43:171-177, Feb. 1974.
5. Rovinsky, J. J., Miller, J. A., and Kaplan, S.: Management of breech presentation at term. *Am. J. Ob-Gyn.* 115:497-513, Feb. 15, 1973.
6. Benson, W. L., Boyce, D. C., and Vaughn, D. L.: Breech delivery in the primigravida. *Am. J. Ob-Gyn.* 40:417-428, Sept. 1972.
7. Rovinsky, Miller, and Kaplan, *op. cit.*; Benson, Boyce, and Vaughn, *op. cit.*
8. Hammond, H.: Death from obstetrical hemorrhage. *Calif. Med.* 117:16-20, Aug. 1972.
9. Malvern, J., Campbell, S., and May, P.: Ultrasonic scanning of the puerperal uterus following secondary postpartum haemorrhage. *J. Ob-Gyn. Brit. Comm.* 80:320-324, Apr. 1973.
10. Klein, T., and O'Leary, J. A.: Rupture of the gravid uterus. *J. Reproductive Med.* 6:43-47, May 1971.
11. Hellman and Pritchard, *op. cit.*
12. Altaras, M., *et al*: The use of vacuum extraction in cases of cord prolapse during labor. *Am. J. Ob-Gyn.* 118:824-830, Mar. 15, 1974.
13. Benirschke, K., and Chung, K. K.: Multiple pregnancy. Part I. *New Eng. J. Med.* 288:1276-1284, June 14, 1973.

Suggested Reading

BOCK, J. E., AND WIESE, J.: Prolapse of the umbilical cord. *Acta Obstet. Gynec. Scand.* 51:303-308, 1972.

FRIEDMAN, E. A.: Labor: *Clinical Evaluation and Management.* New York: Appleton-Century Crofts, 1967.

JEFFCOATE, T. N. A.: The causes of abnormal uterine action in labour. *Aust. N.Z.J. Obstet. Gynaec.* 5:222-227, Nov. 1965.

JEFFREY, R. L., BOWES, W. A., AND DELANEY, J. J.: Role of bed rest in twin gestation. *Ob-Gyn.* 43:822-826, June 1974.

McFEE, J. G., *et al*: Multiple gestations of high fetal number. *Am. J. Ob-Gyn.* 44:99-106, July 1974.

complications of the puerperium

Puerperal infection

When inflammatory processes develop in the birth canal postpartally, as the result of bacterial invasion of these highly vulnerable areas, the condition is known as puerperal infection. It is really a postpartal wound infection of the birth canal, usually of the endometrium. As is true of other wound infections, the condition often remains localized but may extend along various pathways to produce diverse clinical pictures. Febrile reactions of more or less severity are the rule, and the outcome varies according to the portal of entry, the type, the number and the virulence of the invading organisms, the reaction of the tissues and the general resistance of the patient.

Puerperal infection is one of the most common causes of death in childbearing. Frequently used (but less satisfactory) synonyms are puerperal fever, puerperal sepsis, puerperal septicemia and childbed fever.

Causative factors

The vast majority of puerperal infections are caused by the streptococcus, but most of the well-known pathogenic bacteria—such as the staphylococcus, the colon bacillus and the Welch bacillus—may be responsible for the disease. The anaerobic streptococcus, of all the various strains of streptococci, has been found to be the most common causative agent of puerperal infection. This organism is often found in the vaginas of normal pregnant women and offers no symptomatology. Since these microbes are nonpathogenic, normal inhabitants of the birth canal, the determining factor in their becoming pathogenic appears to be trauma and devitalization of the maternal tissues. This finding bodes for greater gentleness and restraint during the labor and delivery process. It is to be remembered that hemorrhage at the time of labor or thereafter also takes its toll of maternal strength and tissue resource. Therefore, *hemorrhage and trauma* during labor and delivery are to be considered the two main predisposing causes of puerperal infection.

The late Dr. John Osborne Polak, of Brooklyn, N. Y., used to teach that there are "eleven direct causes" of puerperal infection—the ten fingers and the nasopharynx. He meant by this that the attendants themselves are most likely to carry infection to the parturient uterus. The physician may inadvertently do so in two ways.

515

In the first place, gloved and sterile though the hands may be during the vaginal examinations or the operative manipulations, bacteria already in the vagina may be introduced upward into the uterus. In the second place, the hands and the instruments used may become contaminated by virulent streptococci as the result of droplet infection, dispersed by the obstetrician or some of the attendants, and in this manner may be responsible for introducing bacteria into the birth canal. Even in modern obstetrics, the latter is a very common mode of infection, and unless the utmost vigilance is used in masking all attendants in the delivery room (both nose and mouth) and in excluding therefrom all persons suffering or recovering from an upper respiratory infection, it is a constant source of danger.

Although a less common means of transfer today than a few decades ago, careless physicians and nurses have been known to carry bacteria to the parturient from countless extraneous contacts—from other cases of puerperal infection, from suppurative postoperative wounds. from cases of sloughing carcinoma, from patients with scarlet fever, from infants with impetigo neonatorum, and from umbilical infections of the newborn. The physician may have the infection on his own person, such as an infected hangnail or felon.

Coitus late in pregnancy is more common than ordinarily believed and may introduce extraneous organisms to the birth canal or carry upward bacteria already present on the vulva or in the lower vagina.

During the second stage of labor, the chances of fecal matter being transferred to the vagina are great, another constant source of danger.

Following completion of the third stage of labor, the site of previous placental attachment is a raw, elevated area, deep red in color and about 4 cm. in diameter. Its surface is nodular, due to the presence of numerous gaping veins, many of which are occluded by clots. These form excellent culture media for bacteria. Furthermore, at this time, the condition of the entire endometrium is peculiarly favorable to bacterial invasion, since it is less than 2 mm. thick, is infiltrated with blood and presents numerous small wounds. Since the cervix rarely escapes some degree of laceration in labor, it is another ready site for bacterial invasion. Vulvar, vaginal and perineal wounds offer still other possible portals of entry.

In addition to traumatic labor and postpartal hemorrhage, other causes in this respect are prolonged labor, prolonged rupture of the membranes, retention of placental tissue and preexisting conditions, such as anemia, which lower the mother's general resistance to disease.

Prevention of infection

The prevention of infection throughout the maternity cycle has been emphasized in foregoing sections as an important factor in the maintenance of health and the prevention of disease. During pregnancy, blood studies are done routinely and iron prescribed as necessary, not only for the immediate value but also because anemia predisposes to puerperal infection. A great deal of emphasis is placed on health teaching at this time, particularly in regard to general hygiene. The patient is advised to avoid all possible sources of infection. Some physicians advise against tub baths in the last weeks of pregnancy, because it was thought erroneously that the bath water might introduce surface bacteria from the body into the vagina, particularly in multiparas. It is well for the nurse to recognize that this idea is still prevalent in many circles, although it is now believed to have no validity. The greatest hazard of tub baths in these last weeks of pregnancy arises because climbing in and out of the tub is awkward and sudden changes in balance might result in a fall and, thus, the likelihood of physical trauma. Coitus and vaginal douches are usually avoided during the last six weeks of pregnancy. Contacts with upper respiratory infections should always be avoided.

During labor, care should be exercised to limit bacteria from extraneous sources. In the hospital, cleanliness and good housekeeping are imperative, but, nevertheless, individual care technique reduces the chance of contamination from other patients. Each patient should have all of "her own" equipment, which includes her own bedpan. This bedpan should be cleansed after each use and sterilized once a day. Scrupulous hand washing on the part of all personnel after contacts with each patient will do much to prevent the transfer of infection from one patient to another. The strictest rules should be enforced for surgical cleanliness during labor and delivery. No one with an infection of the skin or the respiratory tract should work in the maternity department. The nasopharynx of attendants is the most common source of contamination of the birth canal. Masks usually should be worn any time that the external genitalia are exposed for examination or treatments, in the labor room as well as in the delivery room. To be effective, masks must cover the nose and the mouth and be clean and dry; thus they must be changed frequently and should not hang around the neck when not in use.

During the puerperium the same careful precautions should be carried out. For many days following the delivery, the surface of the birth canal is a vulnerable area for pathogenic bacteria. The birth canal is well protected against the invasion of extraneous bacteria by the closed vulva, unless this barrier is invaded. Patients, therefore, are to be taught the principles of perineal hygiene and how to give themselves self-care. The nurse should remember never to use the fingers to separate the labia in giving perineal care, because this permits the cleansing solution to enter the vagina.

Types of puerperal infection

Generally speaking, puerperal infection can be divided into two main types: 1) *local lesion processes* and 2) *extensions of the original lesion process*. When a lesion of the vulva, the perineum, the vagina, the cervix or the endometrium becomes infected, the infection may remain localized in these wounds. However, the original inflammatory process may extend along the veins (the most common way) and cause thrombophlebitis and pyemia, or through the lymph vessels to cause peritonitis and pelvic cellulitis.

LESIONS OF THE PERINEUM, THE VULVA AND THE VAGINA. These lesions are highly vulnerable areas for bacterial invasion in the early puerperium and so may become infected. The most common of these is a localized infection of a repaired perineal laceration or episiotomy wound. The usual symptoms are elevation of temperature, pain and sensation of heat in the affected area and burning on urination. The area involved becomes red and edematous, and there is profuse seropurulent discharge. If a wound of the vulva becomes infected, the entire vulva may become edematous and ulcerated. Infections involving the perineum, the vulva and the vagina cause the patient considerable discomfort and alarm. These local inflammatory processes seldom cause severe physical reactions, provided that good drainage is established, and the patient's temperature remains below 38.4° C. (101° F.). To promote good drainage, all stitches may be removed so that the surface is laid open. Because the drainage itself is a source of irritation and contamination, the wound must be kept clean and the perineal pads changed frequently. Care must be exercised in cleansing the wound to see that none of the solution runs into the vagina. It is understood, of course, that vaginal douches would never be given at this time. Treatments by such means as sitz baths or the perineal heat lamp are generally used for the relief of pain. Antibiotics are prescribed to combat the infection. If drainage is impaired, the patient not only will have more pain but also may have a chill, followed by a sudden elevation of temperature.

ENDOMETRITIS. This is a localized infection of the lining membrane of the uterus. Bacteria invade the lesion, usually the placental site, and may spread to involve the entire endometrium. When endometritis develops, it is usually manifest about 48 to 72 hours after delivery. In the milder forms the patient may have no complaints or symptoms other than a rise in temperature to about 38.4° C. (101° F.) which persists for several days and then subsides. On the other hand, the more virulent infections are often ushered in by chills and high fever, with a comparable rise in pulse rate. In the majority of severe cases the patient experiences a chilly sensation, or actual chills, at the onset and often complains of malaise, loss of appetite, headache, backache and general discomfort. It is not unusual for the patient to have severe and prolonged after-pains. The uterus is usually large and is extremely tender when palpated abdominally. The lochial discharge may be decreased in amount and distinguished from normal lochia by its dark brown appearance and foul odor. In some cases, particularly those caused by the hemolytic streptococcus, the lochia may be odorless. If the infection remains localized in the endometrium, it is usually over in about a week or 10 days. But when extension of the infection occurs to cause peritonitis, pelvic thrombophlebitis or cellulitis, the disease may persist for many weeks, often with dramatic temperature curves and repeated chills.

Treatment depends on the severity of the condition. Mild cases with temperature under 100° F. and no chills are best handled by simple measures. Fowler's position facilitates lochial drainage. Ergonovine four times daily for two days promotes uterine tone, and forced fluids provide additional support. The lochia is cultured and the patient is treated with the appropriate antibiotic. Isolation is desirable to protect other patients and to afford the mother greater rest. In this group it is unnecessary to discontinue breast-feeding.

In severe cases, breast-feeding is discontinued not only because it exhausts the mother but also because it is usually futile in the presence of high fever.

PELVIC CELLULITIS, OR PARAMETRITIS. This is an infection which extends along the lymphatics to reach the loose connective tissue surrounding the uterus. It may follow an infected cervical laceration, endometritis or pelvic thrombophlebitis. The patient will have a persistent fever and marked pain and tenderness over the affected area. The problem is usually unilateral but may involve both sides of the abdomen. As the process develops, the swelling becomes very hard and finally either undergoes resolution or results in the formation of a pelvic abscess. If the latter occurs, as the abscess comes to a point, the skin above becomes red, edematous and tender. Recovery is usually prompt after the abscess is opened.

THROMBOPHLEBITIS. This is an infection of the vascular endothelium with clot formation attached to the vessel wall. It may be of two types: pelvic thrombophlebitis, an inflammatory process involving the ovarian and the uterine veins, or femoral thrombophlebitis, in which the femoral, the popliteal or the saphenous vein is involved. The latter type of thrombophlebitis has been spoken of as phlegmasia alba dolens (painful white inflammation) and also very frequently as "milk leg"—a term once given to the condition by physicians in the belief that it was due to the collection of milk in the affected leg. Early ambulation may be a factor in preventing this complication.

Femoral Thrombophlebitis. This condition presents a special group of signs and symptoms. It is a disease of the puerperium characterized by pain, fever and swelling in the affected leg. These symptoms are due to the formation of a clot in the veins of the leg itself, which interferes with the return circulation of the blood. When this condition develops, it usually appears about 10 days after labor, although it may manifest itself as late as the 20th day. As in all acute febrile diseases occurring after labor, the secretion of milk may cease when phlegmasia alba dolens develops.

The disease is ushered in with malaise, chilliness and fever, which are soon followed by stiffness and pain in the affected part. If it is in the leg, the pain may begin in the groin or the hip and extend downward, or it may commence in the calf of the leg and extend upward. In about 24 hours the leg begins to swell, and although the pain then lessens slightly, it is always present and may be severe enough to prevent sleep. The skin over the swollen area is shiny white in color.

The acute symptoms last from a few days to a week, after which the pain gradually subsides, and the patient slowly improves.

The course of the disease covers a period of four to six weeks. The affected leg is slow to return to its normal size and may remain permanently enlarged and troublesome.

The prognosis is usually favorable. However, in some of the very severe cases, abscesses may form and the disease may become critical and produce fatality. Since the clot tends to be attached to the vessel wall somewhat loosely, there is a tendency for the clot to dislodge and produce a pulmonary embolism which also is fatal in the majority of cases.

The treatment of femoral thrombophlebitis consists in rest, elevation of the affected leg, and analgesias as indicated for pain. Anticoagulants, such as heparin and dicumarol, may be prescribed to prevent further formation of thrombi. Antimicrobial drugs may be used in cases where more generalized infection is known or suspected. A "cradle" is used to keep the pressure of the bedclothes off the affected part. Some physicians prefer to use a light in the cradle believing that the heat promotes comfort. Others use icebags along the course of the affected vessels. Surgical treatment may be indicated in some severe and/or nonresponding cases and consists of incision of the affected vessel, removal of the clot, and repair of the vessel. Ligation of the major vessels is sometimes resorted to as a preventive measure for pulmonary embolism. Under no circumstances should anyone rub or massage the affected part. The leg should be handled with the utmost care when one is changing dressings, applying a bandage, making the bed or giving a bath. As the acute stage subsides, nourishing food and the most carefully regulated hygienic conditions are needed to build up the patient's strength. As recovery is usually tedious, skillful nursing care is required to preserve the tissues of the body.

Pelvic Thrombophlebitis. This is a severe complication in the puerperium. The onset usually occurs about the second week following delivery with severe repeated chills and dramatic swings in temperature. The infection is usually caused by anaerobic streptococci, and although it is difficult to obtain a positive blood culture, bacteria are present in the bloodstream during chills. Antimicrobial therapy is used, and is effective in treating most strains of this organism; as long as the chills and the fever persist, blood transfusions may be given. Heparin and dicumarol may be prescribed to prevent the formation of more thrombi. A further problem is likely to arise with metastatic pulmonary complications, such as lung abscesses or pneumonia.

These patients are often depressed, discouraged and feel physically unwell. Their nursing may have been interrupted and all of the great emotional and physiologic changes discussed in Chapter 20 are compounded by the illness. Astute nursing care at this time is particularly essential. Accurate observing, recording and reporting, and paying particular attention to details of the physical care aspects are extremely important in helping to resolve the disorder and to prevent further complications. Supportive care to help the mother (and family) work through the depression and discouragement is another crucial aspect of care. The principles outlined in the discussion of grief are appropriate here.

PERITONITIS. Peritonitis is an infection, either generalized or local, of the peritoneum. Here, as a rule, the infection reaches the peritoneum from the endometrium by traveling via the lymphatic vessels; but peritonitis may result also from the extension of thrombophlebitis or parametritis. The clinical course of pelvic peritonitis resembles that of surgical peritonitis. The patient has a high fever, rapid pulse and, in general, has the appearance of being profoundly ill. She is usually restless and sleepless and has constant and severe abdominal pain. Hiccups, nausea and vomiting, which is sometimes fecal and projectile, may be present. Antimicrobial therapy is given to combat the infection, analgesic drugs for discomfort and mild sedative drugs to relieve the restlessness and apprehension. If there is intestinal involvement, oral feedings are withheld until normal intestinal function is restored; meanwhile, fluids are administered intravenously. Blood transfusions and oxygen therapy may be indicated for sup-

portive treatment. The record of intake and output must be kept, and, in order to be of value to the physician, the elimination of fluids from the skin by sweating should be estimated.

Signs and symptoms

It is highly important that the nurse recognize and report early signs and symptoms of puerperal infection so that proper treatment may be instituted without delay. When puerperal infection develops, one of the first symptoms usually seen is a rise in temperature. Although temperature elevations in the puerperium may be caused by upper respiratory infections, urinary tract infections and the like, the majority are due to puerperal infection. Puerperal morbidity is the term used to include all puerperal fevers. The Joint Committee on Maternal Welfare in this country has defined puerperal morbidity as a "temperature of 100.4° F. (38° C.), the temperature elevation to occur on any two of the first ten days postpartum, exclusive of the first 24 hours, and to be taken orally by a standard technique at least four times daily." The symptoms may vary, depending on the location and the extent of the infectious process, the type and the virulence of the invading organisms and the general resistance of the patient. The affected area is usually painful, reddened and edematous and the source of profuse discharge. The patient may complain of malaise, headache and general discomfort. As mentioned above, the temperature is elevated, and in the more severe infections, chills and fever may occur. In its typical form each of the clinical types of puerperal infection presents a very characteristic set of signs and symptoms, although occasionally one form of the disease is combined with another. The distinctions between these different types of infections are of importance, because the clinical course, the treatment and the prognosis depend on the particular form of infection. For this reason these aspects of the various puerperl infections have been discussed in the preceding pages.

Treatment

The use of antimicrobial therapy has brought about radical changes in the treatment and the prognosis of puerperal infection. These drugs are effective in combating most of these infections, but, nevertheless, the management and the care of patients with puerperal infections are highly important and demand the utmost in skill. Penicillin is effective against the hemolytic streptococcus, the Welch bacillus and the staphylococcus. Since penicillin is not effective against the colon bacillus and certain strains of staphylococci, a broad-spectrum antibiotic may be prescribed for infections caused by these organisms. Many types of antimicrobials are available, some specifically for the gram positive or negative organisms and the penicillin resistant organisms; therefore, the physician has a wide range of products in his armamentarium upon which to draw. The selection and dosage of these drugs will depend upon the severity of the disease and the type of offending organism. Sensitivity series will often be done to help determine the above. Uterine cultures are taken to gain information about the organism; and in severe cases blood cultures may be taken, but if they are to be of real diagnostic value they must be taken at the time of the chill. The infected lesions are treated the same as those of any surgical wound. Drainage must be established, and since this discharge is of a highly infectious nature, care must be taken to see that it is not spread, and that all contaminated pads and dressings are wrapped and burned.

The curative treatment, of course, will be directed by the physician, but good nursing care is essential. The patient should be kept as comfortable and quiet as possible, for sleep and rest are important. Conserving the patient's strength in every way, along with giving her nourishing food and appropriate amounts of fluids, will help to increase her powers of resistance. To promote drainage the head of the bed should be kept elevated, a measure which also contributes to the patient's comfort.

Care must be exercised to prevent the spread of the infection from one patient to another. Isolation of infected patients from others is desirable in order to protect the healthy maternity patients. Ideally, the patient with puerperal infection should be away from the maternity divisions. If it is impossible to arrange for such complete segregation, the nurse must consider every patient with puerperal infection as "in isolation" and follow scrupulous technique accordingly. Regardless of the situation, the nurse who is caring for a patient with puerperal infection (or any infection, for that matter) should not attend other maternity patients. The hands of all attendants need special attention and should be scrubbed thoroughly

after caring for a mother who has an infection. In certain cases strict isolation technique, with special gowns, masks and rubber gloves, is essential. Clean isolation gowns, masks and gloves should be available for all persons who attend the isolated patient and after being used should be left in the room and disposed of in special hampers or containers. Under no circumstances should this apparel be worn outside the patient's room. Since it is assumed that the nurses who care for these patients are fully acquainted with principles of good isolation technique, this aspect of care will not be pursued further here.

Pulmonary embolism

Pulmonary embolism is usually due to the detachment of a small part of a thrombus, which is washed along in the blood current until it becomes lodged in the right side of the heart. In many cases the thrombus originates in a uterine or a pelvic vein, although its origin may be in some other vessel. When the embolus occludes the pulmonary artery, it obstructs the passage of blood into the lungs, either wholly or in part, and the patient may die of asphyxia within a few minutes. If the clot is small, the initial episode may not be fatal, although repeated attacks may prove so. The condition may follow infection, thrombosis, severe hemorrhage or shock, and it may occur any time during the puerperium, especially after sudden exertion.

SYMPTOMS. The symptoms of pulmonary embolism are sudden intense pain over the heart; severe dyspnea; unusual apprehension; syncope; feeble, irregular or imperceptible pulse; pallor in some cases, cyanosis in others; and eventually air hunger. Death may occur at any time from within a few minutes to a few hours, according to the amount or degree of obstruction to the pulmonary circulation. If the patient survives for a few hours, it is likely that she may recover.

TREATMENT. The treatment consists, first of all, in preventing the accident by careful attention to all details of surgical asepsis and to the proper management of labor and delivery. Following delivery, early ambulation may be an additional prophylactic measure, since circulatory stasis is undoubtedly a causative factor. In some instances it is almost impossible to prevent a fatal attack, because the patient may be recovering without elevation of temperature and without complications and yet, on the seventh or tenth day, she suddenly cries out, passes into a coma and succumbs.

When embolism occurs, rapid emergency measures to combat anoxia and shock must be carried out promptly. Oxygen is administered without delay, and anticoagulants are given. Morphine may be helpful to relieve the patient's apprehension and usually is given. It is essential that the patient be kept absolutely quiet and on her back, for the slightest movement may cause fatal results. If the patient survives the attack, absolute rest is mandatory, in the hope that meanwhile the clot may be absorbed. Dicumarol and heparin therapy will be continued to prevent recurrent emboli. During this time the patient must be kept warm, quiet, comfortable and as free from worry as possible. She may be given a light, nourishing diet during early convalescence.

Subinvolution of the uterus

Subinvolution is the term used to describe the condition which exists when normal involution of the puerperal uterus is retarded. The causes contributing to this condition may be 1) lack of tone in the uterine musculature, 2) imperfect exfoliation of the decidua, 3) retained placental tissue and membranes, 4) endometritis and 5) presence of uterine fibroids. Subinvolution is characterized by a large and flabby uterus; lochial discharge prolonged beyond the usual period, sometimes with profuse bleeding; backache and dragging sensation in the pelvis; and disturbance of general health until corrected. Since this abnormality is the result of local conditions, an important phase of the treatment rests in correcting the causative factor. Oxytocic medication, such as methylergonovine (Methergine) or ergonovine, may be administered to maintain uterine tone and prevent the accumulation of clots in the uterine cavity. Curettage is employed to remove any retained placental tissue or secudines. Endometritis will require antimicrobial therapy. If the uterus is displaced, it may delay normal involution and is usually corrected by a suitably fitting pessary.

Early ambulation is believed to have decreased the incidence of subinvolution. And, since it is recognized that breast-feeding stimulates uterine contractions, the fact that the mother is *not* breast-feeding plus the fact that she is usually taking a lactogenic suppressing drug, may be influencing factors when subinvolution occurs.

Hemorrhage

These complications are discussed in Chapter 25.

Vulvar hematomas

Blood may escape into the connective tissue beneath the skin covering the external genitalia or beneath the vaginal mucosa to form vulvar and vaginal hematomas, respectively. The condition occurs about once in every 500 to 1,000 deliveries. Vulvar hematomas manifest themselves by severe perineal pain and the sudden appearance of a tense, fluctuant and sensitive tumor of varying size covered by discolored skin. When the mass develops in the vagina, it may temporarily escape detection, but pain and the patient's inability to void should alert the nurse to this complication. Since these symptoms may also be indicative of other types of complications, the nurse will want to make a careful examination of the perineum so that she may make an accurate report to the physician. As we have already seen, the new parturient has great difficulty in localizing any pain that she may have. Therefore the nurse usually will have to explore with the mother as to the nature and location of her discomfort, gradually moving from more general statements to those which are specific and more accurate. When the doctor has been informed of the situation, he will undoubtedly perform a vaginal examination which confirms the diagnosis. Small hematomas are usually treated supportively and allowed to resolve of their own accord. However, if the pain is severe or the tumor enlarges, incision and evacuation of the blood, with ligation of bleeding points and packing, will be required.

Disorders of the breast

Certain aspects of many of the following subjects have been presented in Chapters 19 and 20. Here the discussion is centered on complications.

Engorgement of the breasts

Any time after the third postpartal day, after lacteal secretion has been established, engorgement of the breasts may occur. The onset is usually rapid, and, as the breasts become distended, dilated veins may be visible under the skin, and on palpation the breasts feel hard and nodular. This condition, commonly called "caked breasts" by the laity, is likely to occur in mothers who are breast-feeding as well as in those who are not. At one time it was believed that this was brought about because the lobules of the breast gland became overdistended with milk, but engorgement is really an exaggeration of the normal venous and lymph stasis of the breasts which occurs in relation to lactation (see Chapter 19). The breasts become tense and swollen for a day or so, with the result that the mother experiences throbbing breast pains which may extend into the axilla. The breasts are sometimes so immensely distended and painful that some analgesic medication, such as codeine, may be required. The condition may be relieved by supporting the breasts properly with a firm uplift breast binder or brassiere, worn day and night, and by applying icecaps at intervals over the affected areas. When the breasts are well supported, they are not only more comfortable but also, if they are pendulous, the support aids in preventing congestion caused by the interference with the circulation. Immediate treatment of engorged breasts is important, because if the condition is allowed to persist, it may threaten the nursing mother's future milk supply. With prompt attention the engorgement usually subsides after 24 to 48 hours. If the mother is breast-feeding, the regular emptying of the breasts by suckling and adequate breast care then will be all that is necessary.

The mother who is desirous of breast-feeding may have additional problems when she is trying to nurse her infant. Because of the fullness of the breasts and the simultaneous flattening of the nipple, the infant may be unable to get a proper grasp on the areola and nipple. Sometimes the use of the breast pump (at very low pressure) for only a few minutes prior to the feeding will bring the nipple out sufficiently to permit the infant to grasp it. It must be remembered that too vigorous use of the breast pump or frequent and prolonged nursing periods are irritating to the breast, as well as highly discomforting to the mother. When the engorgement is pronounced, it may be helpful to apply hot compresses to the breasts for about 15 minutes before the nursing period.

"Drying up" the breasts

When the mother is not breast-feeding, for one reason or another, measures are usually taken to inhibit lacteal secretion. This is discussed in Chapter 20.

Abnormalities in mammary secretion

It is obvious to the nurse who has had experience taking care of new mothers and their infants that there are marked individual variations in the amount of milk secreted by the breasts in almost every case. In most instances it depends on the degree of development of the glandular portions of the breast rather than on the individual's general health or the physical appearance of these organs. A mother with large, well-formed breasts may be eager to breast-feed her infant but produces such a meager quantity of breast milk that she is unable to do so. On the other hand, another mother with small, flat breasts may have a remarkably good milk supply and be able to suckle her infant successfully. Obese women with exceedingly large breasts, the bulk of which is fatty tissue, usually do not have a good supply of breast milk for their infants.

When there is an absolute lack of mammary secretion, the condition is called *agalactia*. This condition rarely occurs and is seldom seen. As a rule, there is at least a small amount of mammary secretion, but it is so scant that, despite all efforts to stimulate lactation, the quantity would be inadequate to supply the nourishment required for the infant. Since in the later instance it is a case of hyposecretion rather than an absolute lack of it, perhaps in time it will be more properly called hypogalactia. One point should be made clear here. When one speaks of abnormalities in mammary secretions, this does not refer to temporary episodes which may momentarily affect lactation but in no way affect the mother's ability to continue with breast-feeding. For example, many new mothers, especially primiparas, who have been breast-feeding their infants quite successfully in the hospital find that when they are discharged home there is a sudden diminution in their milk supply. More than likely this is due to the anxiety and fatigue involved with the experience, because once they are settled and rested at home, the milk supply usually resumes normally. This happens so frequently, in fact, that the nurse will want to apprise the mother of this possibility and include planning for adequate household organization and rest for the mother as part of her regular postpartum counseling.

Occasionally the other extreme in lactation is observed (i.e., the mammary secretion is excessive, so-called *polygalactia*). When this secretion is so copious that it constantly leaks from the nipples, it is called *galactorrhea*. The latter condition is not common, but when it does occur, it may be hazardous to the mother's health if it continues over a prolonged period. The condition is best treated by measures which are similar to those used to "dry up" the breasts. In addition, the failure to empty the breasts completely at each feeding may help to check the excessive secretion.

Abnormalities of the nipples

Variations in what is considered to be normal in the nipple, which is cylindrical in shape and projects well beyond the center of the areolar surface, are not unusual and present no difficulty until the mother wants to breast-feed her infant. The *flat nipple* (i.e., a slightly rounded projection above the breast surface) or the *depressed nipple* (i.e., one which is slightly depressed below the breast surface) are difficult for the infant to grasp with the mouth. The *inverted nipple* is the most pronounced variation, because this nipple is actually inverted, and in this state it is impossible for the infant to grasp it. When these abnormalities exist, the mother should begin corrective measures during pregnancy, such as described elsewhere (p. 200). Afterward, the use of an electric breast pump or a rubber nipple shield at the beginning of each nursing period may be of value to help draw the nipple out. This may require considerable patience and persistence on the part of the mother, but with encouragement and help from the nurse, she may be successful. However, a real danger may arise if persistent efforts at breast-feeding are attempted and are unsuccessful, because the breasts become engorged and/or the nipples become sore, with resultant fissures or erosions on the surface. These raw, cracked sur-

face areas make breast-feeding a very painful experience for the mother and, moreover, provide a portal of entry for pathogenic bacteria which may give rise to mastitis.

Mastitis

Mastitis, or inflammation of the breast, may vary from a "simple" inflammation of the tissues around the nipple to a suppurative process which results in abscess formation in the glandular tissue. Mastitis is always the result of an infection, usually caused by *Staphylococcus aureus* or hemolytic streptococcus organisms. The disease in most instances is preceded by fissures or erosions of the nipple or the areola, which provide a portal of entry to the subcutaneous lymphatics, although under conducive conditions organisms present in the lactiferous ducts can invade the tissues and cause mastitis.

SYMPTOMS. Puerperal mastitis may occur any time during lactation but usually occurs about the third or fourth week of the puerperium. There is usually marked engorgement of the breast preceding mastitis, although engorgement per se does not cause the infection. When the infection occurs, the patient complains of acute pain and tenderness in the breast and often experiences general malaise, a chilly sensation or, in fact, may have a chill followed by a marked rise of temperature (to 105°) and an increased pulse rate. On inspection the breast appears hard and reddened. The obstetrician should be notified at once and treatment instituted promptly in the hope that resolution may take place before the infection becomes localized as an abscess.

TREATMENT. Puerperal mastitis is preventable, for the most part, by prophylactic measures. An important measure is initiated when the expectant mother learns about breast hygiene and begins to take special care of her breasts during the latter months of pregnancy (see Chapter 12). After delivery, appropriate breast care will further help to prevent the development of lesions, but if they do occur, proper treatment must be given promptly. Any time the mother complains of sore, tender nipples, they should be inspected immediately. At this time there may be no break in the surface, but if the condition is neglected, the nipple may become raw and cracked. The alert nurse often can detect even a very small crack in the surface of the nipple if she inspects it carefully. Once a break in the skin occurs, the chances of infection mount, because pathogenic organisms are frequently brought to the breast by the hands or may reach the breast from the patient's nightgown or bedclothes.

With early treatment by antibiotics, the inflammatory process may be brought under control before suppuration occurs. A broad spectrum antibiotic is effective in treating acute puerperal mastitis if the therapy is started promptly, and often symptoms subside within 24 to 48 hours. The breasts should be well supported with a firm breast binder or well fitted brassiere. While the breasts are so painful, small side pillows used for support may give the mother some measure of comfort. Icecaps may be applied over the affected part, but if in time it becomes apparent that suppuration is inevitable, heat applications may be ordered to hasten the localization of the abscess. Most obstetricians advise that breast-feeding be discontinued immediately in cases of mastitis.

If the treatment outlined above is unsuccessful, measures will have to be taken to remove the pus when abscess formation occurs. The obstetrician may prefer in some cases to aspirate the pus rather than resort to incision and drainage. When incision and drainage are done, the incision is made radially, extending from near the areolar margin toward the periphery of the gland, in order to avoid injury to the lactiferous ducts. After the pus is evacuated, a gauze drain is inserted. Following the operation the care of the patient is essentially the same as that for a surgical patient. Complete recovery is usually prompt.

Epidemic puerperal breast abscess

During the last decade a type of puerperal breast abscess has been seen, both in this country and abroad, which is unlike the type described above. In this new manifestation the offending organism is also *Staphylococcus aureus*, but is an antibiotic-resistant strain which has been identified by bacteriophage typing as 52/42B/80/81 and called the "epidemic" strain. Another difference is related to the portal of entry of these microorganisms. In these cases there is no history of nipple lesions, and the infection is introduced through apparently normal lactiferous ducts in the breast, not through the connective tissue. An infant who has been exposed to the epidemic strain

of the staphylococcus, and has the organisms present in the nose and throat, can introduce the infection to the mother's breast in the process of nursing. Once these organisms are introduced into the mother's breast, milk provides a superb culture medium for them. Efforts to prevent puerperal mastitis cannot be limited to the care of the mother's breasts but must extend to the hospital nursery, where the infant may acquire the virulent organism. In the nursery such equipment as soap-solution containers, cribs, mattresses, blankets, and linens, as well as floors, can harbor the organisms. Some methods to help control the spread of infection at its source include rigid nursery aseptic technique on the part of all personnel, measures to prevent the spread of organisms from infant to infant, such as proper spacing of cribs, and the exclusion of carriers from the maternity divisions as soon as they are identified. It should be remembered that in maternity hospitals the nasopharynx of newborn infants tends to become readily infected with *Staphylococcus aureus,* and, moreover, the infection may persist for some weeks after the infant leaves the hospital. Where intensive studies have been carried out and puerperal mastitis or breast abscess appeared after discharge from the hospital, the cultures of the mothers' nares on admission to the hospital did not show evidence of the epidemic strain of the organism. In these cases the infants were the source of infection, because the offending organism was cultured from the nose, the throat and the skin of the infants.

SYMPTOMS. The symptoms of epidemic puerperal breast abscess develop slowly and subtly and usually appear about the third or the fourth week after delivery. The condition is characterized by high fever; the breast becomes very tender, swollen and indurated and suppurates rapidly. The surface of the breast may not be consistently reddened because the abscess is often deep. In some cases the infection may involve more than one portion of the breast, or both breasts.

TREATMENT AND CARE. The underlying principles for the care of this form of breast abscess are essentially the same as those described for puerperal mastitis. Breast-feeding should be discontinued immediately, for obvious reasons. The offending organism here is often antibiotic-resistant as the staphylococcus develops antibiotic resistance easily. When suppuration occurs in the breast, incision and drainage are usually done as soon as localization of the abscess becomes evident, in order to limit the extent of tissue destruction. When this has been done, special measures must be employed for the control of infection. To protect the surrounding area of the breast, it should be washed with a soap containing hexachlorophene, because such cleansing reduces the occurrence of staphylococci to some degree. This soap is also advocated for hand washing and baths. When warm moist applications to the wound are prescribed, vigilance and care must be exercised so that the underlying skin does not become macerated. Aside from the unnecessary discomfort that this would cause the mother, such maceration would provide another portal of entry for microorganisms. When such infections occur, in either the mother or the infant, the nurse should emphasize health teaching in her care of the mother, not only concerning hygienic measures for the prevention of skin infections but also the urgency for prompt treatment of any member of the family if carbuncles, boils, burns or other skin lesions develop.

The *epidemiologic aspects* of antibiotic-resistant infections of infants and their mothers are far-reaching and a major problem, because when these infections occur, nearly all the hospitals in the community may be affected for varying periods of time. A few years ago this was considered a "hospital" infection, but now it may be found throughout a general community. Once the organism is introduced into a family, this organism can be the cause of disease in the family over a long period of time. For example, the infant may acquire the infection in the maternity nursery, four weeks later the mother may develop a breast abscess, and five months later the father may develop a boil—all caused by this epidemic strain of staphylococcus. Flaws in nursery "clean technique" in hospital nurseries have long been cited as the cause of spreading skin infections in the newborn, but when these epidemic infections have occurred in hospital nurseries, and the staff has scrutinized their technique and improved it whenever possible, the results have not been as gratifying as one would hope for, because the epidemics have disappeared and appeared again after a period of time. In fact, large numbers of infections have occurred despite meticulous nursery technique. It must be remembered that these infections are not confined to the maternity service but may be spread by carriers to or from other clinical services in the hospital as well as to other members of the family and the community. The infection is thought to be airborne and is easily spread by droplet contamination from the nasopharynx of carriers of these microorganisms. Scrupulous technique in giving patient care in the hospital is undoubtedly an important factor in prevention and control, in both the nurseries and postpartal divisions, but this alone will not solve the problem. The housekeeping functions which are routine in every institution are of vast importance, from the standpoint of both procedure and personnel, and should be investigated and improved as much as possible. The nurse will find it advantageous to pursue the current literature regarding antibiotic-resistant staphylococcal infections, because there is a wealth of information in the professional journals.

Bladder complications

The two most common bladder complications in the puerperium are retention of urine and residual urine. In the former, the patient is unable to void at all; in the latter, she is able to void certain amounts of urine but is unable to empty the bladder. If these conditions are allowed to persist, then infection of the bladder (cystitis) and/or the kidneys (pyelitis) may develop.

The nurse will remember that the overhydration of the mother that was necessary for the growth and development of the fetus during pregnancy diminishes rapidly after delivery. The two main avenues for the diminution of the circulating blood volume are the skin and the kidneys. Consequently, the newly delivered mother perspires copiously and excretes large quantities of urine within 24 to 48 hours of delivery. As much as *500 cc. to 1,000 cc.* may be voided at *each* urination; that is, as we know, two to three times what is usual in the non-parturient. The nurse will want to be particularly careful of bladder hygiene at this time because of the increase in urinary production and the danger of overdistention. Thus, one should not wait for any designated time to elapse to indicate when the bladder should be emptied; rather one nurse should observe for evidence indicating the degree of bladder distention, because the bladder may fill in a shorter span of time than has been specified. This fact should be reported to the physician if the patient is unable to void since a catheterization order will be needed.

Retention of urine, or the inability to void, is more frequently seen after operative delivery. It often lasts five or six days but may persist longer. The main cause is probably due to edema of the trigone muscle, which may be so pronounced that it obstructs the urethra. Very temporary urinary retention may be due to the effects of analgesia and anesthesia received in labor. As already stressed, the nurse should make every effort to have the patient void within six hours after delivery (see Chapter 20). If the patient has not done so within eight hours, the physician usually will order catheterization. In some hospitals this is routine if voiding has not occurred within eight hours postpartum.

Because of the trauma of labor and/or operative delivery the bladder usually is not as sensitive to distention as it was prior to pregnancy and delivery. Overdistention and incomplete emptying may occur; thus, the problem of residual urine frequently results. Repeated catheterization may be necessary for several days although in these persistent cases, the physician may request that an indwelling catheter be inserted which will provide constant drainage.

When the mother continues to void small amounts of urine at frequent intervals, the nurse may suspect that these voidings are merely an overflow of a distended bladder, and that there is residual urine there. The physician will order catheterization for residual urine, and, to be completely accurate, this must be done within five minutes after the patient voids. If 60 cc. or more of urine still remains in the bladder after the patient has voided, it is usually considered that the voiding has been incomplete. It is not uncommon for the catheterization to yield 800 cc. or more of residual urine. Large amounts of urine (from 60 to 1,500 cc., as shown by catheterization) may remain in the bladder, even though the patient may feel she has completely emptied the bladder when she voided. The condition is due primarily to lack of tone in the bladder wall and is more likely to occur when the mother's bladder has been allowed to become overdis-

tended during labor. A distended bladder requires prompt attention because of the resultant trauma; moreover, it may be a predisposing cause of postpartal hemorrhage.

In many cases of residual urine the patient is without symptoms other than frequent, scanty urination, but in others there may also be suprapubic or perineal discomfort. The treatment of this condition is usually confined to catheterization after each voiding until the residual urine becomes less than 30 cc.; in severe cases constant drainage by means of an indwelling catheter may be employed.

The normal bladder is very resistant to infection, but when stagnant urine remains in a traumatized bladder, and infectious organisms are present, there is danger of cystitis. When cystitis occurs, the patient often has a low-grade fever, frequent and painful urination and marked tenderness and discomfort over the area of the bladder. The physician will order a catheterized specimen of urine for microscopic examination, and if pus cells are present in association with residual urine, the diagnosis of cystitis is confirmed. Since it is important in the presence of bladder infection to avoid accumulations of stagnant urine in the bladder, an indwelling bladder catheter may be inserted. In addition, antimicrobia agents are prescribed, and fluids should be forced.

If the infection spreads and involves the ureters and kidneys, the patient has a high fever and chills and a good deal of pain over the affected kidney(s). Diagnosis and treatment are essentially the same as for cystitis.

It will be the nurse's responsibility to obtain the urine specimens which are used for the microscopic examinations and occasionally cultures. The technique of catheterization already has been discussed in Chapter 20.

However, some physicians do not wish their patients catheterized, especially if the mother is having no particular difficulties in voiding. They feel that this procedure only enhances the possibility of promoting more infection. Therefore a "clean catch" specimen may be requested. Different terminology exists for this procedure in various parts of the country; but the procedure is essentially the same. It consists of the collection of a "clean" urine specimen that is uncontaminated by lochia. One method for this type of collection is as follows:

The patient is requested not to void for at least two hours and to drink as much fluid as she can in the meantime. Then she is taken to the bathroom (or placed in a sitting position on a bedpan if she cannot ambulate) and the vulva and introitus are cleansed. A large sterile cotton ball is placed over the introitus. The mother is then requested to void a little urine forcefully into the toilet or bedpan; but *not to empty her bladder*. Next, a sterile urine specimen or sterile basin is placed under the stream and a specimen of urine is caught. It is sent to the laboratory for examination. Surprisingly, this method yields very good results with respect to uncontaminated specimens, if done carefully with the continued supervision of the nurse. It avoids the possibility of introducing bacteria into the bladder at the time of catheterization.

Suggested Reading

GREENHILL, J. P., AND FRIEDMAN, E. A.: *Biological Principles and Modern Practice of Obstetrics.* Philadelphia, W. B. Saunders, 1974.

SANTAMARINA, B. A. G. (ED.): Symposium on sepsis in obstetrics. *Clin. Ob. and Gyn.*, 13, 1970.

SWEET, R. L., AND LEDGER, W. J.: Puerperal infectious morbidity. *Am. J. Ob-Gyn.* 117:1093, 1973.

fetal diagnosis and treatment

Richard H. Schwarz, M.D.

Determination of Fetal Age / Evaluation of Fetal Well-Being / The Role of the Nurse in Genetic Counseling / Specific Fetal Problems / Fetal Treatment

27

As recently as 20 years ago, evaluation of the fetus and its environment was virtually limited to the animal laboratory or to the vivid imaginations of a few obstetricians. There were some exceptions, such as the transabdominal aspiration of amniotic fluid which was practiced before the turn of the century, but at that time the procedure was used only therapeutically, in cases of severe polyhydramnios. Amniography, an x-ray technique with radiopaque dye placed in the amniotic fluid, was introduced in 1930, but fell into disrepute because the dye used was irritating and caused premature labor. Thus, until recently, obstetricians relied almost entirely upon physical observations, such as palpation and measurement of the uterus to assess fetal growth, and auscultation of the fetal heart tones to evaluate fetal distress. X-rays were used to determine fetal position and the presence of major bony abnormalities. Little can be determined about fetal well-being from such techniques.

In the past decade, the amniotic cavity has been invaded with increasing frequency, and a battery of fetal diagnostics has been developed. But the practice of intrauterine medicine has advanced beyond diagnostics, now covering treatment and genetic assessment as well. Not only is the body of scientific information expanding geometrically, but systems for health care delivery are also changing rapidly. As the birthrate has been reduced by improved contraception, legalized abortion, and a desire among families for fewer children, there has been a heightened interest in the quality of new life. For economic reasons, many obstetric units lack the sophisticated equipment and personnel to deliver appropriate care to any but the uncomplicated full-term pregnancy. As a result, the concept of regionalization, which is rapidly being developed throughout the United States, has evolved. Regional facilities, located so as to be accessible to all obstetricians and their patients, would have available sophisticated equipment and laboratories and neonatal facilities and personnel, including obstetric anesthesiologists, nurse specialists, and adequate medical and surgical consultants. Although in recent years the concept of transfer of the sick newborn to a regional center has been accepted, consideration is now being given to the transport of the high-risk gravida and her fetus.

Implicit in such a system is the ability to identify the high-risk patient sufficiently well in advance to permit transfer to a regional center.

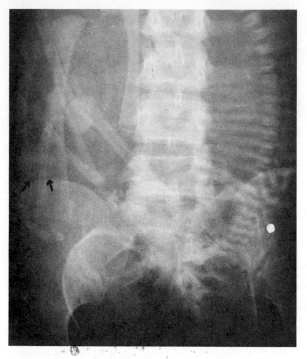

Figure 27-1. Abdominal x-ray showing a fetus with calcification of both the distal femoral and proximal tibial epiphyses (arrows).

determination of fetal age and the evaluation of fetal well-being, including prenatal diagnosis of congenital disease. Fetal treatment is more limited, but developing rapidly.

Determination of fetal age

Although it is customary to determine the period of gestation and estimated date of confinement from the first day of the last menstrual period by Naegle's rule, this method is fraught with error for various reasons, including failure to remember exact dates, irregular cycles, bleeding in the first trimester, and late registration for prenatal care. In the case of the uncomplicated patient, not knowing the exact length of gestation may not represent a serious problem. However, in the high-risk patient for whom timing of the delivery is critical, the information is vital. Thus, the degree to which the determination is pursued depends upon the clinical situation.

Means for determining fetal age

PHYSICAL MEASUREMENTS. Estimation of uterine size by pelvic examination in the first trimester is very helpful, whereas determination of uterine size in the second trimester is less valid. Measuring the fundal height above the pelvic symphysis at each visit can give useful information about growth or lack of growth, but not about the exact period of gestation. Estimation of fetal weight is notoriously inaccurate, with the greatest error at the high and low weights. Other physical determinants include first auscultation of the fetal heart and serial examinations of the cervix to determine effacement and dilatation. As with all physical evaluations, there is considerable individual variation, and consequently such evaluations are not totally reliable unless they are all in agreement.

X-RAY STUDIES. Radiographic studies can be helpful in determining maturity. If both the distal femoral and proximal tibial epiphyses are calcified, one can be assured of a mature fetus (Fig. 27-1). However, if they are not calcified, one cannot assume immaturity, since there is considerable variation based on sex, race, and fetal weight, along with technical problems related to the position of the fetal knee relative to the maternal skeleton.

ULTRASOUND. Ultrasound is a useful recently developed modality. By means of the B mode scan, it is possible to measure accurately the

Factors which contribute to such a designation include age, social status, nutritional status, past obstetric performance, maternal disease, genetic factors, and the like. Scoring systems and even computer programs have been developed for the identification of at-risk patients. Additional risk factors may develop intrapartum, such as hemorrhage, infection, and disproportion. It is not surprising that perinatal outcome is poorest when a patient designated high-risk antepartum develops an intrapartum complication. The second poorest results come from prenatally normal patients who develop an unexpected intrapartum problem. Antepartum high-risk patients who develop no intrapartum problems do better, presumably because they receive more meticulous attention.

To achieve the best results, we must focus attention on the fetus as a patient throughout the period of gestation, not just transiently during labor and the delivery process. This effort may be indirect, by concentrating upon the health of the mother, or it may involve direct intervention, as in the case of the antenatal diagnosis of congenital disorders. Fetal medicine at this time is largely a diagnostic field with the major areas of concern being the biparietal diameter of the fetal skull, and given a fetus which is appropriate in size for the period of gestation, the fetal weight can also be estimated. In assessing fetal growth retardation, serial measurements taken between 20 and 30 gestational weeks provide the best information concerning fetal growth rate. Although this noninvasive method has gained considerable popularity because of its assumed safety for the fetus, it is probably wise to withhold final judgement until long-term follow-up becomes available. This technique is also extremely useful for other purposes, including placental localization, confirmation of fetal death, and early diagnosis of pregnancy.

ENDOCRINE STUDIES. Of all the assays available, estriol (or total estrogens) and human placental lactogen (HPL)—also known as human chorionic somatomammotropin (HCS)—are the most popular. Both have normal curves which rise progressively during pregnancy; however the range of normal is wide, and, consequently, these techniques are less valid in determining fetal age than fetal well-being. It is possible for a given value to be in the normal range for both 35 and 40 weeks, and, as a result, the age differentiation cannot be made. Both serum and 24-hour urine samples are assayed.

AMNIOTIC FLUID STUDIES. Transabdominal amniocentesis has become a standard technique in modern obstetric practice (Fig. 27-2). But it must not be regarded as a totally innocuous procedure and should be undertaken only on the basis of well-founded indications. Potential complications include fetal bleeding, placental disruption, Rh sensitization, and fetal puncture. The frequency of these complications is poorly recorded and is greatly influenced by such factors as the experience of the operator and the use of ultrasound to localize the placenta, but is probably in the 1 percent range. Given a sample of amniotic fluid, the following determinations are useful in evaluating fetal age:

Gross Appearance. The presence of large amounts of vernix caseosa generally indicates maturity, and meconium is often present in the significantly postdate pregnancy. Neither is sufficiently consistent, however, for precise age estimation, and meconium may be present as a sign of fetal distress in less than mature pregnancy.

Cytology. The cells in amniotic fluid come from both the fetus and the membranes. The

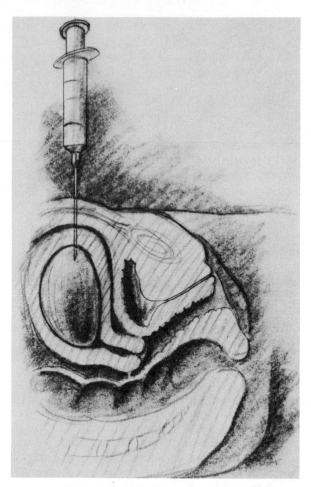

Figure 27-2. Amniocentesis. (Povey, W. G.: *A Guide to Family Planning.* Department of Obstetrics and Gynecology, University of Pennsylvania, 1971)

bulk of fetal cells are desquamated squamous cells from the skin; cells from the respiratory, urinary, and gastrointestinal tract are also present. If amniotic fluid is mixed with a vital stain for fat (Nile blue sulfate) and a smear is made, a varying number of the squamous cells will take up the stain and appear orange on the smear. These cells normally first appear at 34 to 35 weeks of gestation and increase in number as term is approached. Fifteen to twenty percent generally indicate a mature fetus, while at term 50 percent fat-containing cells and free-fat droplets are the rule.

Creatinine. The concentration of creatinine in amniotic fluid gradually increases with maturity of the fetal kidneys, increasing their ability to excrete creatinine and also of the increasing muscle mass of the fetus which causes an increase in creatin to creatinine

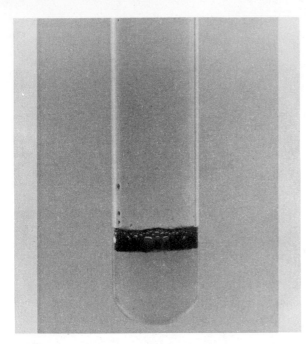

Figure 27-3. Shake test. Note bubbles at the surface maintained by surfactant in the amniotic fluid.

metabolism. Values of 2 mg. per 100 ml. are indicative of fetal maturity.

Bilirubin. Although the determination of bilirubin in amniotic fluid by spectrophotometry has its greatest application in evaluating the fetus in Rh sensitization, it can also be applied in evaluating the age of the fetus in nonsensitized patients. Because of the maturation of the fetal liver and the placenta, the concentration of bilirubin in amniotic fluid is progressively decreased toward term, with the ΔOD_{450} falling to 0.010 by 36 weeks, and disappearing at 37 to 38 weeks. This evaluation is not sufficiently valid to be used as the sole standard, but does complement the other assays.

Osmolality. Although amniotic fluid in early pregnancy is isotonic with maternal plasma, as pregnancy progresses the fluid becomes more hypotonic, presumably because of the increasing contribution of fetal urine. Values of 250 mOsm per liter per kg. or less are generally associated with maturity, but variation is considerable.

Phospholipids. As the fetal lung matures, there is an abrupt increase in the synthesis of surfactant. This material, of which a major constituent is the phospholipid lecithin, eliminates the stickiness of the alveolar membranes per-

mitting the air spaces to remain open once expanded. The presence of sufficient quantities of surfactant eliminates the risk of the respiratory distress syndrome, the greatest hazard to the premature. Not only can surfactant be measured in pulmonary fluids, but its presence can be detected by measuring the lecithin concentration in amniotic fluid as well. Several techniques have been developed, but the most popular is the lecithin sphingomyelin (L/S) ratio.

This method employs thin layer chromatography to separate the two phospholipids. Because the concentration of sphingomyelin is relatively constant, the increase in surfactant at maturity will be reflected as an increase in the L/S ratio. Values of greater than 2:1 indicate pulmonary maturity and are consistently associated with the absence of significant respiratory distress. This level is reached at approximately 35 weeks in normal pregnancy, but may occur even earlier in abnormal pregnancy. The "Shake test" is an alternate rapid method for evaluating the presence of surfactant. Serial dilutions of amniotic fluid are shaken with ethyl alcohol. If sufficient surfactant is present, bubbles will be maintained at the surface at dilutions of 2:1 or greater (Fig. 27-3). Regardless of the technique used, phospholipid measurement is the most valid of current estimates of maturity since it assesses the lung rather than a less vital system, such as the skin. Even though it may not be possible to give an exact week of gestation, one can determine the risk to the fetus were delivery to occur at that time, and this is obviously the more critical question.

Evaluation of fetal well-being

In a variety of circumstances it is necessary, or at least desirable, to evaluate the health of the intrauterine patient. Observations may be needed over a period of time, as in the case of such maternal diseases as diabetes and hypertension, or the need may be for intensive short-term observations during labor. Still another approach is the single early pregnancy study in the case of prenatal diagnosis of congenital disorders. Although currently, fetal evaluation is selectively used only in those pregnancies determined to be at risk, it is likely that in the future there will be screening evaluation of all fetuses, as well as routine fetal monitoring in labor for all patients.

Antepartal fetal evaluation

Having identified that a given fetus may be in jeopardy for any given reason, the obstetrician is faced with a dilemma. In most cases there is little specific to be done to improve the fetal status except to control maternal disease. Most often the obstetrician is faced with a choice between affecting a premature delivery and facing the hazards of prematurity, or permitting prolonged intrauterine life with a potential for fetal death. Fortunately, the studies are generally reassuring, and the pregnancy can be allowed to continue. When intervention is indicated because the studies indicate severe jeopardy, more often than not the result is a sick neonate. Studies in this category are limited to the third trimester, since an abnormal value prior to that time would be of no clinical value, the decision to intervene being obviated by nonviability. An exception to the latter rule occurs in Rh sensitization, in which intrauterine transfusion is feasible as early as 24 weeks.

Endocrine assays

ESTROGENS. Levels of all three of the basic estrogens—estradiol, estrone, and estriol—rise progressively in the mother's blood and urine during the course of normal pregnancy. Prior to accurate chemical assays, biologic tests for these compounds led to considerable confusion because of their relative potency, estradiol being extremely potent, estrone intermediate, and estriol biologically weak. However, with chemical assay the level of estriol shows the greatest rise during pregnancy.

In recent years, the origin of estriol in pregnancy has been well worked out. The precursors are formed in the fetal adrenals, modified to some extent by the fetal liver, and converted to estriol by the placenta. Also, in order to have normal amounts of estriol in the urine, maternal renal function must be normal. Thus, urinary estriol determinations in late pregnancy are not just an index of placental function, but really of the fetoplacental unit, and also may be modified by maternal kidney function. The pattern of normal estriol excretion is illustrated in Figure 27-4. It should be remembered that the values will vary from laboratory to laboratory. Urinary estriol studies are valuable in assessing fetal well-being in a number of conditions, including diabetes, hypertension, and postdate pregnancy. They are not of

value in problems of Rh immunization. Blood estriol determinations are now becoming more readily available and have two distinct advantages: 1) the nuisance of the 24-hour urine collection is eliminated, and 2) the levels are not influenced by maternal renal function. However, one must be aware of the diurnal variation (high in the morning, lower in the afternoon) in blood estriol levels, and specimens should be obtained at the same time each day. The pattern for blood estriol levels during pregnancy is essentially the same as that of urinary values; however, the quantities are in micrograms rather than milligrams. Amniotic fluid estriol values have proven to be of some use in the management of Rh sensitized pregnancies.

PROGESTERONE. This steroid hormone is also produced in progressively increasing amounts during a normal pregnancy, at first by the corpus luteum, but later predominantly by the syncytial trophoblasts of the placenta. Although blood assays are available, the most practical assay is for urinary pregnanediol, the major metabolite of progesterone. Levels of pregnanediol rise progressively throughout pregnancy and fall off with delivery. However, pregnanediol assays are not generally useful in the management of problem pregnancies, since progesterone does not require fetal precursors. Therefore, production can continue and be normal even after an intrauterine fetal death has occurred.

HUMAN CHORIONIC GONADOTROPIN (HCG). This hormone, produced by the trophoblast, normally peaks in early pregnancy and falls off to relatively low levels in the second and third trimesters. It is the basis for most pregnancy

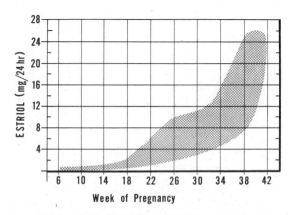

Figure 27-4. Pattern of urinary estriol excretion in normal pregnancy.

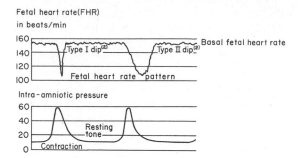

Figure 27-5. Patterns of fetal bradycardia (Type I and Type II dips).

tests, as well as for the follow-up of hydatid moles and choriocarcinoma, but is of limited value in problem pregnancies. An exception occurs in the case of severely affected erythroblastotic infants. Because of placental hypertrophy, HCG values may be quite high; however by the time these values are reached, the fetus is usually beyond salvage.

HUMAN PLACENTAL LACTOGEN (HPL). HPL, or human chorionic somatomammotropin (HCS) is produced specifically by the placenta. It has many characteristics of human growth hormone but can be measured by immunoassay. Both serum and urine assays are available and values rise progressively in normal pregnancy in much the same pattern as that of estriol. Levels are abnormally high in diabetic pregnancies whereas they are low in other instances of fetal compromise. HCS has not provided a replacement for estriol but is complementary, and an assay is now readily available at modest cost.

MATERNAL BLOOD STUDIES. A number of enzymes increase in concentration in maternal serum during pregnancy. The most useful of these is the heat stable fraction of alkaline phosphatase (HSAP), a placental product. In most pathologic situations values are low, with the exception of preeclampsia, in which case abnormally high values are found. Cystine aminopeptidase, an oxytocinase, also rises progressively and may have reassuring value if normal. Diamine oxidase rises early but has a flat late pregnancy curve which reduces its value in fetal assessment.

PHYSIOLOGIC STUDIES. It is not possible to measure directly in the human fetus those placental functions which are most critical, namely the transfer of oxygen, carbon dioxide, and essential nutrients. Numerous indirect approaches have been tried without much success until the recent introduction of stress tests; the most popular being the oxytocin challenge test (OCT). The basic principle of this test is that, with each uterine contraction, pressure in excess of 30 mm. Hg is exerted upon the uteroplacental circulation. Therefore, if that circulation is inadequate for any reason, a hypoxic stress for the fetus will result. Thus, by producing uterine contractions while monitoring the fetal heart rate continuously, one can detect such distress by the occurrence of late decelerations or Type II dips (Fig. 27-5). Although there is need to accumulate more experience with the OCT, current thought is that a negative test indicates the fetus will do well for the subsequent week, barring acute problems. Problems with the OCT include logistics, the lack of standardization (external monitoring cannot quantitate contraction pressures), and inability to detect acute changes when the test is performed on a weekly basis. Nonetheless, it represents a simple approach, adaptable to any hospital situation, and requires no complicated laboratory backup. Other forms of stress tests being evaluated include maternal exercise and administration of less than ambient oxygen mixtures. Still other workers are evaluating nonstressed antepartum monitoring as a means of fetal evaluation. All are promising, but much work needs to be done.

AMNIOTIC FLUID STUDIES. With one major exception, amniotic fluid studies are more helpful in age determination and genetic evaluation than in assessing well-being. The major exception is in the Rh-immunized pregnancy in which measurement of the bilirubin concentration by spectrophotometry is the best guide to the degree of fetal anemia (see section on hemolytic disease). Another indication is in suspected chorioamnionitis. The presence of polymorphonuclear leukocytes in a gram-stained smear of amniotic fluid is diagnostic.

AMNIOSCOPY. The insertion of a lighted speculum into the cervix in late pregnancy can provide useful information by detecting the presence of meconium in the amniotic fluid. The examination can be repeated at regular intervals, but its disadvantages are that fluid samples cannot be obtained for analysis, and also that inadvertent rupture of the membranes may occur precipitating labor and delivery.

Detection of congenital defects
Antenatal diagnosis of congenital disorders is a special category of evaluation of well-being.

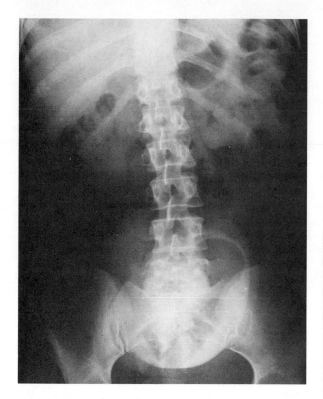

Figure 27-6. Amniogram outlining 16-week fetus with normal skull.

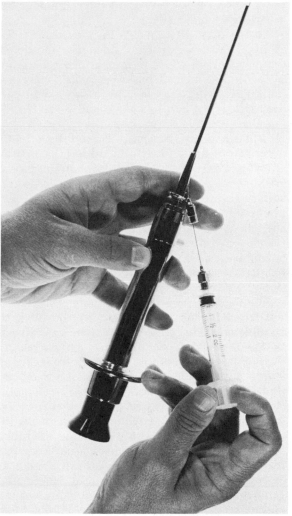

Figure 27-7. Amnioscope. Experimental endoscope for transabdominal amnioscopy with needle for aspiration.

Couples at risk may be identified by the previous birth of an affected child, by population screening studies, such as for Tay-Sachs disease, or by some other cause for concern, such as advanced maternal age. Prenatal diagnostic studies are applicable in several broad areas: the chromosomal diseases, sex-linked disorders, inborn errors of metabolism, and a few miscellaneous multifactoral problems. Additional indicators are being added at a steady rate.

Although amniotic fluid analysis is the main tool in prenatal diagnosis, other methods are in use. Ultrasound scanning and amniography (instillation of radiopaque dye into the amniotic fluid) are helpful in ruling out anencephaly and meningomyelocele (Fig. 27-6). Transabdominal amnioscopy which is now an experimental procedure (Fig. 27-7) will very likely permit careful fetal visualization, aspiration of fetal blood, and fetal biopsy in the near future.

The cells in amniotic fluid constitute the major source of information, and they are largely desquamated squamous cells from the fetal skin. There are also cells from the amnion and the fetal urinary, gastrointestinal, and respiratory tracts. Since many of the desqua-

mated cells are nonviable, it takes time to grow them in tissue culture to the point of chromosome or biochemical analysis. The average time is three weeks for karyotype and four weeks for chemical studies, which can pose problems with regard to the gestational age if abortion is indicated. This is further compounded by the fact that amniotic fluid volume generally does not permit safe amniocentesis before 15 to 16 weeks.

CHROMOSOMAL DISORDERS. These constitute the majority of indications for amniocentesis. In most centers 50 percent of the procedures are done for the age-associated risk of Down's syndrome. An additional 25 percent are done because of a previous affected child (recurrence risk of 2 percent), and the remainder for a variety of indications.

SEX-LINKED DISORDERS. In the absence of ability to make a specific diagnosis, the determination of fetal sex may provide some guidance. In X-linked diseases such as Duchene's muscular dystrophy, one can assume a 50 percent risk if the fetus is male and none if it is female.

BIOCHEMICAL DISORDERS. These inborn metabolic errors are almost uniformly inherited as autosomal recessives. Ever increasing numbers are amenable to antenatal diagnosis. Most result in severe mental and physical retardation in the affected child while the carrier parents are phenotypically normal. Fortunately, from the diagnostic standpoint the heterozygote can be differentiated from the affected as well as from the normal by the degree of critical enzyme activity (normal 100 percent, heterozygote 50 percent affected absent). Couples at risk are most often identified by the birth of an affected child, although in some cases, such as Tay-Sachs disease, they may be uncovered by population screening studies. By utilizing amniocentesis and prenatal diagnosis they can reproduce selectively only normal or heterozygous children, provided that they are willing to terminate the 25 percent of pregnancies in which affected fetuses are detected. Because more cells are required for the assay than for karyotyping, the time from amniocentesis to diagnosis is longer, averaging four weeks.

Of all the other diseases which are detectable in the miscellaneous category, the open neural tube defects (anencephaly and meningomyelocele) are most important because of their frequency and a 3 to 5 percent recurrence rate. Techniques for evaluation include ultrasound, amniography, and measurement of alpha fetoprotein. Ultrasound and amniography can definitely rule out anencephaly as early as the fifteenth or sixteenth week of gestation, while meningomyelocele is a more difficult problem. Levels of alpha fetoprotein have been found to be elevated in the serum and amniotic fluid with open neural tube defects. Serum assays may prove useful for screening, while amniotic fluid determination is helpful in definitive prenatal diagnosis. Experience with this technique has been encouraging in that false negative results have generally been linked to small skin-covered meningoceles, a group of lesions with a good surgical outlook. Thus, the combination of ultrasound, amniography, and alpha fetoprotein assay can provide reasonable reassurance to these very anxious couples.

The prenatal diagnosis of a number of other important diseases is imminent. With the perfection of amnioscopy and techniques for obtaining fetal blood samples, the diagnosis of the hemoglobinopathies (sickle cell disease and thalassemia) will be possible. Amnioscopy will also secure the diagnosis in a number of visible defects such as facial clefts, extremity defects, and the like. Fetal skin biopsy will speed the time to karyotype and biochemical diagnosis. The role of the nurse in this area deserves special consideration.

The role of the nurse in genetic counseling

With increasing use of prenatal diagnosis of genetic disorders, some needs are emerging, and with this a new nursing role is developing.

In dealing with these families, a consistent approach has been developed and the functions of the role can be identified.

The nurse may facilitate communication between patient and the other members of the professional team. The nurse is able to coordinate care, providing joint counseling sessions with the geneticist and the obstetrician when indicated. This level of communication encourages a consistent approach to the counseling and avoids variations in interpretation that could otherwise occur.

The nurse may also facilitate communication within the team, including the laboratory. The major tool for team communication is a regular conference. Each patient is presented and every member of the team can contribute to the planning of care. Each individual has a unique contribution to make. As the team conference is held only at intervals, obviously not all of the information is available for decision making at any given time. By facilitating communication within the team, the coordinating nurse may help to keep the team members aware of progress and problems.

The most important aspect of the nurse's role is patient counseling. The majority of the prenatal counseling can be done adequately by the nurse counselor. If the family situation is complicated or if the diagnosis is unclear, the counseling should be done by a physician. Virtually all patients who seek genetic counseling are referred from other physicians. Often there is little time for prolonged contact because of the gestational age at the time of the initial visit. When calls are received, the goal is to assess the reason for the request for consultation. How was the patient referred—by her physician, by a friend, or because of publicly available knowledge? Why does she want prenatal diagnosis and what is her concept of what can be accomplished? Families come with a widely divergent amount of knowledge.

Specific examples serve to highlight the decision-making process. A 35-year-old primigravida was referred for amniocentesis by her obstetrician, having been told that she presented an increased risk of having a "mongol" (Down's syndrome or trisomy 21). She did not have specific figures, nor did she know anything about the procedure, but she was very apprehensive about having a defective child. She was counseled about the risk of mongolism at her age, 1:300 at most, the risk of the procedure—perhaps a 1 percent risk of a spontaneous abortion, and the length of time to the diagnosis, three to four weeks. She was advised to discuss this with her husband again and to call in several days. She called back the next day to make the appointment and expressed anger that her physician's advice had been questioned. It was explained that her decision to seek counseling was supported, but it was felt that she and her husband should make decisions only after having all of the available facts. This was a serious undertaking and not to be approached without understanding the risks. She did admit that she had thought about it more and had come to the conclusion that they could cope with a spontaneous or therapeutic abortion of a defective fetus much better than they could cope with a mongoloid child.

Other patients are extremely well informed. They possess a great deal of information and ask sophisticated questions such as, "What is the culture failure rate?" Their dilemma may be to chance a mongoloid child or risk a spontaneous abortion.

Others are advised to call for information while still in the process of adapting to the pregnancy. They may still feel ambivalent about continuing or terminating the pregnancy. In some cases the reassurance that prenatal diagnosis can bring may influence the older couple to continue to term. There seems to be general knowledge that an older woman has a greater chance of having an abnormal child. In addition, the older woman has greater concern for her own health and ability to undergo both pregnancy and delivery. In discussing prenatal diagnosis, the risk can be discussed in specific terms and diagnosis of defects specifically related to age can be offered.

For example, a patient called on the advice of her obstetrician because she was told that she was pregnant. Her youngest child was 15 and she had thought she was menopausal at age 43. On discovering she was 14 weeks pregnant she and her husband were shocked. They had vague knowledge that it was unwise to have children after 40. A therapeutic abortion at this stage was not acceptable, but both felt they were not capable of caring for a retarded child in their middle years and that this would impose an unfair burden on their other children. They would elect to abort a defective fetus. The fact that this patient, at age 43, had approximately a 2 percent risk of having a mongoloid child was new to her. Actually, this was a lower age-related risk than she had expected. The amniocentesis was uneventful. By the time the results were available, the family had resigned themselves to another child and were looking forward to the rejuvenation this seemed to promise. The karyotype was normal, and the pregnancy continued without anxiety over a defect related to age.

Because most patients are referred, they are usually prepared for prenatal diagnosis. Some, however, have no prior knowledge. This situation is often complicated by late presentation for prenatal care. When a woman arrives for the first visit at 16 weeks gestation, there is very little time to assimilate information before making a decision. It has been general experience that many such patients refuse amniocentesis rather than cope with this new idea. In discussing this postpartum, they have stated that they tried very hard to put information provided by the genetic counselor out of mind. One must be sensitive to the fact that providing genetic information can increase anxiety. When a family makes a decision not to undergo prenatal diagnosis, they should be supported in this decision. In that case, the positive aspects of the statistics are emphasized. For a 40-year-old woman, a 1 percent chance of having a child with Down's syndrome also means a 99 percent chance of having a child without Down's syndrome.

In offering prenatal counseling, a family pedigree is prepared in order to identify familial conditions that might be amenable to prenatal diagnosis, or which should be explored further with the family. A family referred for antenatal diagnosis because they have one child with Down's syndrome will serve to emphasize the importance of a complete evaluation. The patient was 28 years old, a gravida 3, para 2, and in the fifteenth week of gestation. There was a family history of Down's syndrome, but the child had not been karyotyped. A chromosomal analysis was suggested for the child in order to rule out a familial translocation. Family history revealed that the husband's father, one uncle, and his oldest brother had been hospitalized with Huntington's chorea, a lethal debilitating hereditary disease which appears in later life. The husband had never been counseled regarding this. This family was advised that the husband had a 50 percent chance of developing this disease; therefore, his child had a 25 percent chance of developing this disease. In contrast, the couple's risk of having a second child with Down's syndrome was only 1 percent. Following counseling and after further discussion with their own physician, the couple concluded that the more significant risk was Huntington's chorea and elected to abort this pregnancy and to proceed with sterilization.

After assessing the reason for referral and determining the amount of information already possessed, the nurse counselor informs the patient about antenatal diagnosis. The risk of having an affected child is discussed first. If the patient is an older woman with a 1 percent risk of having a child with Down's syndrome, the prognosis for an affected child is explained. This 1 percent risk is put into perspective in relation to the risk at age 20 (1:1000) and the 3 percent risk within the general population of birth defects which are not diagnosable prenatally at the present time. Couples with a family history of specific genetic disease, for example, Tay-Sachs disease or muscular dystrophy, have often been previously counseled and usually know the facts well.

It is felt that there is about a 1 percent risk that amniocentesis will cause a spontaneous abortion. Most parents express concern over the possibility of injury from needle puncture of the fetus. It is explained that there is a relatively large amount of fluid compared to fetal size, and the fetus will float freely and actually move away if the needle should come close. Damage to a fetus as the result of needle puncture during amniocentesis for prenatal diagnosis is extremely unlikely. However, since amniocentesis is a blind procedure, there is no absolute guarantee that the baby will not be pricked.

Once the balancing of risks has been explained, the nurse can evaluate the available information with the couple. The specific condition that is of concern is explored first. If the parents are carriers of Tay-Sachs disease, enzyme assays are done on the fetal cells and an affected child can be detected. In addition, a chromosome analysis is done. It is now also possible to assay the fluid for alpha fetoprotein to determine the presence of an open neural tube defect.

Although more than 60 conditions can be diagnosed prenatally, all of these determinations are not done in a given pregnancy. These assays are time consuming and costly, and it is not possible to obtain a sufficient number of cells through tissue culture in a reasonable time to perform extensive screening procedures.

In most cases, when normal results are available the family will know that the child does not have an open neural tube defect and that the child has normal chromosomes. In addition, they will know the sex of the child. There are mixed feelings about revealing the sex of the child. Concern has been expressed that the couple may then use this information for sex selection, and proceed to abort the child of an unwanted sex. However, since this information is available, it is usually given to those couples who wish to know. With all of this information, the couple still does not have assurance that this child is normal. The majority of birth defects are not reflected in the chromosomes.

A certain amount of anxiety is caused by contemplating the procedure itself, and so it should be described in some detail. Ultrasound examination is done several hours before the amniocentesis. The only preparation necessary is a full bladder. If an anterior placenta is described, the radiologist selects the area which is clearest and marks the patient's abdomen to identify the safest site for puncture. With an anterior placenta, the risk of placental injury is increased.

Amniocentesis itself takes about five minutes. The patient is instructed to void first. The abdomen is prepped with iodine and draped. Approximately 2 cc. of local anesthetic is infiltrated, and a needle is inserted through the uterine wall into the amniotic cavity. Amniotic fluid will often spill spontaneously when the amniotic sac is tapped. One to 2 ml. of the fluid is discarded as a precaution against obtaining maternal cells. If blood is obtained at first, the fluid is allowed to clear before collecting the specimen. Twenty to 25 ml. of amniotic fluid are withdrawn and the needle is removed. The puncture site is covered with a Band-Aid. Although most patients are somewhat apprehensive, few complain of pain. The main discomfort is caused by the local anesthesia. The sensation, otherwise, is pressure deep in the pelvis. As always, keeping the patient informed during the course of the procedure is helpful in relieving anxiety.

After completion of the procedure, the patient is instructed to remain in the office for from 20 to 30 minutes. She may experience mild uterine cramping for several hours. If she had any vaginal spotting or leakage of amniotic fluid, she is instructed to go to bed and call the obstetrician immediately. If the procedure has been accomplished without problems, there is no restriction of usual activity.

The tests that are done are very reliable, but as with any laboratory procedure, there is a margin of error. If the fluid is contaminated by maternal cells it is possible that the mother's cells will be cultured, not the fetus'; there is no way to differentiate between maternal and fetal cells. Occasionally the amniotic culture fails to grow. There may have been very few cells in the original specimen. In that event it may be necessary to repeat the amniocentesis several weeks after the first tap.

Another main concern occurs when information that is unexpected is obtained. For example, the test may be done to rule out mongolism (trisomy 21) but reveal a trisomy 18, or a chromosomal abnormality that is not understood. This seldom happens, but when it does, the implications must be carefully and completely reviewed with the family.

In all, genetic counseling provides a great deal of information for the couple to deal with. After imparting this, with time for questions, it is important to explore both partners' reaction to this information. This may not be done in the first session, but after they have had an opportunity to talk about this and perhaps to contact their obstetrician again. The nurse is interested in how the family is handling the balancing of risks. One would expect a 40-year-old primagravida to be seriously concerned about the risk of the procedure. In contrast, a young mother with one mongoloid child is usually prepared to accept any risk to avoid another affected child. If, however, the patient accepts the test only on the advice of her physician, her feelings should be explored further and she should realize that in the last analysis the decision is hers. The attitude of the couple regarding therapeutic abortion at 20 weeks gestation is important. If abortion is unacceptable to them, they should seriously consider the risk of fetal diagnosis to a potentially healthy baby, as well as the disadvantage of prior knowledge that the pregnancy will result in the birth of an abnormal child. Although therapeutic abortion is not generally discussed in detail, it is essential to know what the family would do with the information derived from amniocentesis. If the family does have specific questions about terminating a pregnancy at 20 weeks gestation, these should be answered.

The patient's apprehension peaks with the tap and falls off with successful completion. Anxiety again increases in about three weeks, as the time for obtaining the results draws near. The amount of support needed during this period varies with the emotional stability of the family and the kind of support they can provide for themselves. In general, those families with a high risk of an affected fetus are most in need of ongoing professional contact.

Follow-up is also important. The accuracy of prenatal diagnosis is not confirmed until the baby is born. After delivery, the nurse may wish to discuss reactions to amniocentesis once again. Several patients state they would never undergo amniocentesis again because of the anxiety caused by the length of time until the diagnosis was made. Most feel that prenatal diagnosis had made the pregnancy much easier and had relieved worries about having an affected child.

Intrapartum evaluation of fetal well-being

Although the concept of the labor and delivery unit as an intensive care area for mother and fetus has been slow in evolving, and hospitals have for some curious reason been more willing to invest in monitoring equipment to be used in coronary care units on octagenarians with minimal life expectancy, now most hospitals have acquired some fetal monitoring equipment. The future will undoubtedly bring routine fetal monitoring for most patients in

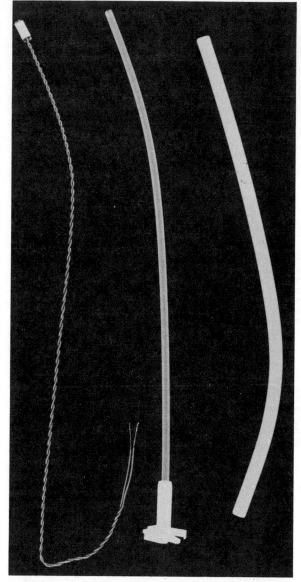

Figure 27-8. Scalp electrode and introducer for fetal heart monitoring.

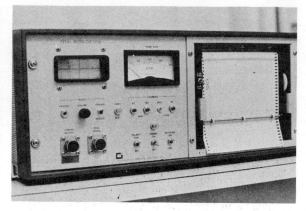

Figure 27-9. Fetal monitor showing chart recorder for both fetal heart rate and contractions.

labor, regardless of risk status, along with improved equipment to provide simple, non-invasive approaches which can be readily utilized by nurses. Intrapartum monitoring can be considered in two categories—physical (mostly heart rate) and biochemical.

Physical monitoring

Various approaches have been developed for monitoring of the fetal heart rate, none of which has yet achieved the ideal. Early efforts have been directed to the use of the fetal electrocardiogram. To provide a usable signal for the cardiotachometer (the instrument for recording of heart rate), it was necessary to obtain direct fetal contact, generally by the transcervical application of electrodes to the fetal scalp. Efforts to record the ECG externally over the maternal abdomen were frustrated by the overpowering maternal ECG signal. Recently this approach has been made clinically applicable by a computer technique which electronically subtracts the maternal signal, leaving the fetal pattern to trigger the rate meter.

Another approach which has been used is phonocardiography amplification of the actual sounds as recorded by a microphone. This has the advantage of being noninvasive, the microphone simply being applied to the mother's abdomen, but has the disadvantage of amplifying all sounds and thereby not providing a clear signal for the tachometer.

Perhaps the most common noninvasive approach in clinical use is the Doppler ultrasound instrument. In simple terms, a low energy ultrasound beam is transmitted toward the fetus. This beam is reflected back when it strikes an interface between substances of differing density (in this case, the heart or major vessels and their contents, blood). The angle of reflection is a function of the difference in densities, and since in this case the density varies with pulsation, a signal can be achieved which can activate the tachometer. A number of transducer designs have been developed in an effort to provide a better focus on the fetal heart with less chance of losing the signal with maternal or fetal movement or uterine contractions (Fig. 27-8).

Recording methods are similar, regardless

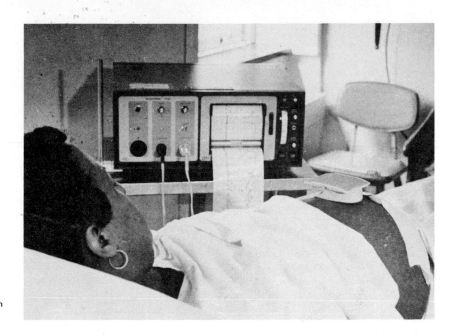

Figure 27-10. Fetal monitor with external transducer attached.

of the method employed in obtaining the signal. Continuous paper strip recorders are the most practical and have the advantage of allowing reinspection of the tracing, and a permanent record (Fig. 27-9). The oscilloscope, even with a "memory" for a given time period, provides a quick visual tracing and is useful for teaching and screening, but does not provide a permanent record.

There is usually a simultaneous recording of uterine contractions, either by an external tocodynamometer (Fig. 27-10) or by an internal transcervically placed strain gauge transducer. This recording is critical because of the importance of the relationship between periodic heart rate changes and contractions in interpreting their significance.

The location of monitors on the labor floor is also the subject of considerable discussion. So called central station monitoring with multiple chart recorders or oscilloscopes at the nurses' station connected to the various labor rooms has been popularized. This is a useful adjunct but is in no way a substitute for bedside monitors and even more important, bedside nursing. Without proper direct supervision and evaluation by trained personnel, fetal monitoring is useless. The obstetric nurse cannot be replaced by a machine. Other optional modifications now available on monitoring equipment include high- and low-rate alarms and even automated interpretation of abnormal patterns.

ABNORMAL PATTERNS. The most significant patterns are the periodic ones and they include:

Early Decelerations, or Type I Dips (Fig. 27-11). This pattern has a wave which is the mirror image of the contractions and is caused by increased fetal intracranial pressure. This is a physiologic response on the part of the fetus to maintain cerebral blood flow, is commonly seen in late labor as the fetal head descends into the pelvis and is not associated with any increased fetal morbidity or mortality.

Late Decelerations or Type II Dips (Fig. 27-12). In this pattern the deceleration begins as the contraction nears its peak and the rate does not return to baseline until after the contraction has ended. There is commonly a baseline tachycardia when this pattern is seen. The tachycardia is caused by fetal hypoxia and is brought about by the initial release of catecholamines, while the deceleration in rate is a vagal response. The relationship to contractions is based upon the fact that contractile pressures normally reach from 40 to 50 mm. Hg in the first stage of labor and higher in the second stage. If the uteroplacental circulation is deficient, the addition of such pressures will sufficiently compromise the already inadequate placental circulation to cause hypoxia and the response as described. Unless this situation is the result of a transient and correctable situation, such as maternal hypoxia secondary to anesthesia, a persistent late deceleration pattern is an indication for prompt delivery by

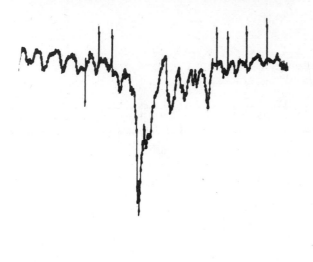

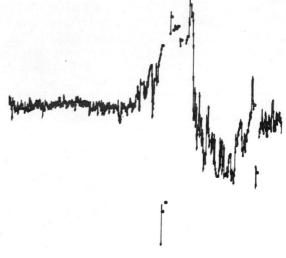

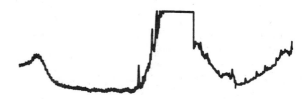

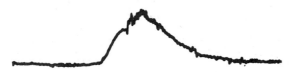

Figure 27-11. Early deceleration (Type I dip). Wave form is reciprocal of the contraction pattern.

the most expeditious means. In the oxytocin challenge test, this pattern constitutes a positive test and provides evidence of uteroplacental insufficiency.

Variable Decelerations (Fig. 27-13). This pattern is one in which there is no consistent relationship between the decelerations in fetal heart rate and uterine contractions. It is thought to be associated with umbilical cord compression and commonly can be eliminated by changing the patient's position (turning to one side or another). Variable decelerations can be classified according to their depth and duration as mild, moderate, or severe (see

Table 27-1). If persistent, the status of the newborn can be directly related to this classification. When moderate or severe variable decelerations persist, labor should not be allowed to continue without biochemical monitoring in addition.

Another consideration in the interpretation of fetal heart rate patterns is the normal pattern in relation to uterine contractions (beat-to-beat variation). This pattern is normal as a healthy fetus will display some change in heart rate from beat to beat. Loss of this variation is an ominous pattern indicating fetal jeopardy. Caution must be exercised in making an interpretation of beat-to-beat changes depending upon the method of recording. Direct fetal scalp tracings are best for making such interpretations. Most systems employing Doppler transducers incorporate a system which rejects signals indicating variation outside certain limits. This provides a nicer tracing but obviates any evaluation of beat-to-beat change.

The question of which patients should be selected to monitor and by which techniques is often raised. It is clear that patients indentified as high risk should have intrapartum fetal monitoring, but the fact that the second highest perinatal morbidity occurs in the group of low-risk patients who develop intrapartum complications makes a strong case for routine monitoring of all patients in labor. At this time, noninvasive techniques have reached a level of sophistication which clearly makes them adequate for routine monitoring of low-risk patients. In the high-risk patient, or in any patient with a suggestion of an abnormal wave pattern, the invasive (scalp electrode) approach is indicated unless precluded by the condition of the cervix or fetal position. The more recently developed helix type electrodes are easy to apply and are associated with a relatively low complication rate in the neonate. The commonly seen complications are scalp hematomas and abscesses. Data with regard to monitoring and maternal morbidity do not seem to indicate a significant increase.

BIOCHEMICAL MONITORING. The availability of fetal blood for analysis would obviously afford invaluable information in assessing the status of the fetus at any time during gestation. Unfortunately, by currently applicable techniques this is only practical during labor, when the cervix is dilated, the membranes ruptured, and the presenting part (preferably the vertex) is well engaged in the pelvis. Given those conditions, however, using a special speculum a small incision can be made in the fetal scalp and a sample collected in a long heparinized capillary tube (Fig. 27-14). Although scalp blood samples have been assayed for a variety of contents for both clinical and research purposes, measurement of pH is at this time the only assay which has well-defined clinical value. The Po_2 and Pco_2 change more slowly and there-

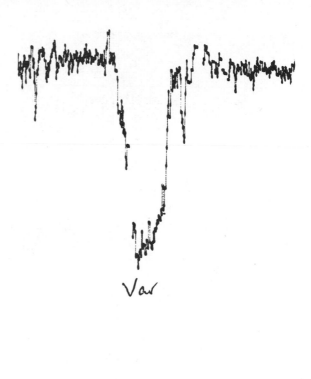

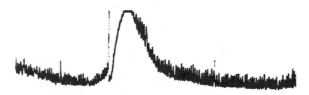

Figure 27-13. Variable decelerations. These have no consistent relationship to contractions.

fore do not acutely reflect fetal status. Acidosis occurs in the hypoxic fetus as a result of anaerobic metabolism with accumulation of lactate and pyruvate. Fetal scalp pH levels above 7.25 are normal while values below 7.20 indicate acidosis and may serve as justification for intervention. Values between 7.20 and 7.25 are

Table 27-1 Principles of Grading Variable and Late Decelerations

Criteria of grading	Mild	Moderate	Severe
Variable deceleration			
Level to which FHR drops and duration of deceleration	<30 sec. duration irrespective of level >80 b.p.m. irrespective of duration 70-80 b.p.m. <60 sec.	<70 b.p.m. >30<60 sec. 70-80 b.p.m. >60 sec.	<70 b.p.m. >60 sec.
Late deceleration			
Amplitude of drop in FHR	<15 b.p.m.	15-45 b.p.m.	>45 b.p.m.

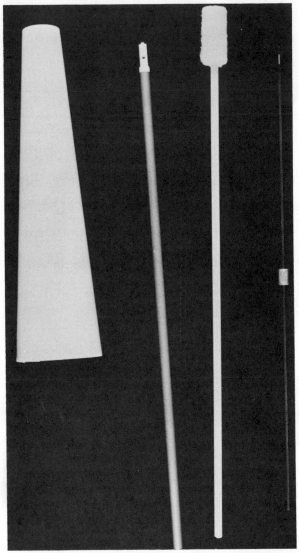

Figure 27-14. Scalp sampling equipment includes plastic speculum, scalpel, sponge, and heparinized capillary tube.

scalp hematomas and abscesses. Occasional reports of persistent bleeding from the scalp would have been noted, but this complication is avoidable with appropriate case selection.

Specific fetal problems

A number of complications of pregnancy have a particular impact on the fetus. Among these are conditions which can be grouped together as causes of acute fetal distress, generally manifest during labor. A second category of chronic fetal problems may be manifest antepartum as well as intrapartum.

Acute fetal distress

The fetus commonly signals its distress in one of three ways. The most important signal is fetal heart rate alteration and the abnormal patterns which have already been described. The presence of meconium in the amniotic fluid with a cephalic presentation indicates at least transient distress. The appearance of meconium is not significant with a breech presentation, and even with a cephalic presentation does not indicate continuing jeopardy unless there are other signs of distress such as heart rate changes or an acidotic scalp pH. There is an additional concern when there is meconium in that, especially with thick meconium, respiratory efforts on the part of the fetus may result in aspiration of the material and significant neonatal respiratory morbidity. The third signal, albeit less reliable, is alteration in fetal movement. Increased movement is sometimes seen with acute distress and obviously absence of movement is ominous.

The common causes of fetal distress can be grouped as follows:

FETAL	prematurity
	congenital malformations
MATERNAL	preeclampsia-eclampsia
	diabetes
	chorioamnionitis
	hypotension
	prolonged or abnormal labor
PLACENTA	placenta previa
	abruptio placenta
CORD	prolapse
	compression
	short cord
	true knot

considered borderline and should be repeated. One important source of potential error is maternal acidosis; if there is any suspicion of that problem, a concomitant maternal sample should be evaluated. The most frequent indication for determination of scalp blood pH is persistent, moderate, or severe variable decelerations. In such patients, an acidotic scalp pH is an indication for immediate cesarean section if vaginal delivery is not imminent, while normal values may permit continued labor and repeated scalp sampling. Scalp pH evaluation may also be helpful in the case of questionable or intermittent late decelerations. Complications include

Management of acute fetal distress has essentially been covered in relation to the management of the various heart rate abnormalities and of course generally involves prompt delivery by the most expeditious means, unless the cause is transient and correctable (e.g., supine or anesthesia-related hypotension). It is important to recognize that heart rate monitoring can also identify those patterns and situations in which intervention is not necessary and thereby avoid unnecessary cesarean section. In most institutions, although the acquisition of monitoring units results in an initial increase in the cesarean section rate, experience with the techniques ultimately reduces the rate. Supportive measures which may be taken while preparation for delivery is made include administration of oxygen and glucose to the mother, the latter being the sole metabolite for the fetal brain.

Chronic fetal problems

Although some of the causes of chronic fetal problems were also listed as causes of acute fetal distress, it is more appropriate that they be discussed in relation to their long-standing influence on pregnancy and the fetus. There are other maternal and/or fetal conditions whose effects are exclusively chronic. A number of these pregnancy complications also have significant maternal effects, which are discussed in other chapters.

HEMOLYTIC DISEASE. This is one of the complications of pregnancy in which there may be devastating fetal effects with virtually no maternal risk. Although the fetal pathology of severe hemolytic disease had been described before the turn of the century, the exact nature of the problem was not known until after the discovery of the Rh factor in 1940. The disease is most unusual in that within 30 years the cause, treatment, and methods for prevention have been worked out. Most of the attention has been focused on the Rh factor as a cause, but the ABO blood groups may also cause a form of hemolytic disease, as do other lesser-blood groups.

The incidence of hemolytic disease is related to the occurrence of blood groups. In the white population, 15 percent are Rh negative, while in blacks this figure is only 5 percent; therefore, the frequency of Rh hemolytic disease is much less in blacks. Approximately 13 percent of American marriages have the "setup" for Rh problems (Rh negative wife, Rh positive husband), and 22 percent have the combinations for ABO disease. Ninety-eight percent of all fetal hemolytic disease is related to either Rh or ABO incompatibilities. Fetal involvement with hemolytic disease occurs from 1 in 100 to 1 in 150 deliveries. These figures will be reduced in the future with the preventive measures now available.

The pathogenesis of Rh hemolytic disease is based upon the fact that, even though the maternal and fetal circulations are normally completely separated, breaks in this barrier permit the entry of fetal red cells into the maternal circulation during the second and third trimesters and at delivery in up to 50 percent of pregnancies. Such breaks also occur with abortions beyond six to eight weeks of pregnancy. If these cells are Rh positive (containing the Rh+ or D antigen), the mother may react to this mismatched "mini-transfusion" by forming protective antibodies. Since the formation of antibodies takes time, and since the unsensitized woman probably does not react until after she delivers, there is rarely a problem in the first pregnancy unless the patient has received a mismatched transfusion in the past. Antibodies formed as the result of the first exposure persist for life. When the woman becomes pregnant again, and the fetus is Rh positive, she will respond with rapid antibody formation as soon as she is exposed to Rh positive cells. Thus, once antibodies have been formed, all subsequent pregnancies with Rh positive infants will be a problem.

There are two types of Rh antibodies. The larger (gamma M, or 19S) type does not cross the placenta as readily as the smaller (gamma g or 7S). In the case of ABO disease where the mother who lacks the antigen has the antibody (e.g., type O has neither A nor B antigen, but has both anti-A and anti-B antibodies; type A has A antigen and anti-B antibody, and so on), these naturally occurring antibodies are the large 19S variety. Also, since these antibodies require a break in the placental barrier to get into the fetal circulation, and since this is most likely to occur at the time of delivery of the placenta, ABO disease is almost always more mild than Rh, and rarely is the child stillborn or severely affected at birth. In addition, because the AB antigens are present in all body cells, this tends to absorb excess antibody and reduce the effect on the red cells. However, in Rh disease, there are both 19S and 7S antibodies (the result of sensitization). The 7S anti-

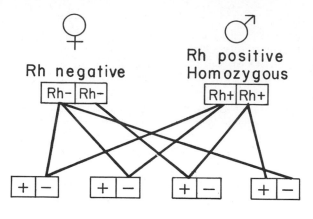

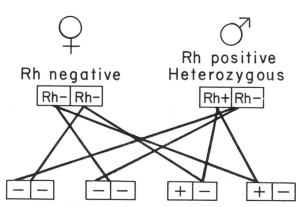

Figure 27-15. Inheritance patterns for the Rh factor.

The inheritance of Rh blood type follows the simple dominant recessive rules, with Rh+ being a dominant. Each individual receives two genes (one from each parent) to determine Rh blood type. It is necessary to receive two Rh negative genes to be negative, whereas one can be Rh positive with one Rh positive and one Rh negative gene (heterozygous), or two Rh positive genes (homozygous). Thus, if the husband is heterozygous, there is a 50-50 chance of having an Rh negative child, and therefore, an unaffected one (Fig. 27-15). If the father is homozygous, all offspring will be Rh positive and subject to hemolytic disease.

In the ABO system, an individual may have genes for A, B, AB, or no antigens. Thus, the contribution to the offspring may be either A or B or none. For example: type O individuals receive neither A nor B genes from the parents; a type A individual may receive an A gene from each (AA), or an A from one and none from the other (AO). The same is true for the type B individual (BB or BO). The AB individual receives an A from one parent and a B from the other.

All pregnant patients should have a blood group determination, at least with the first pregnancy. If adequate records are available, this need not be repeated with subsequent pregnancies. Should the patient be Rh negative or type O (the most common maternal type for ABO disease), the husband's blood should also be typed. If he is Rh positive, a genotype may be done to determine whether he is homozygous or heterozygous. Also, the Rh negative woman's blood should be examined for the presence of antibodies to the Rh factor (D). This is accomplished by the indirect Coombs test and is reported in dilutions (e.g., positive 1:2, 1:4, 1:8, and so on). If the initial screening or titer is negative (i.e., shows no antibodies), this should be repeated at approximately 30 and 36 weeks of pregnancy. If both of those titers are negative, it is safe to assume that there will be no significant problem and to permit the pregnancy to run its normal course. If the titer is positive, it becomes necessary to decide how seriously the fetus is affected (i.e., how anemic it is). Since it is not possible to approach the fetus directly and do a hemoglobin or hematocrit, less direct means must be used. In the past, the physician merely repeated the antibody titer, watching for a rise and, combining this with the patient's past history arrived at a plan of management.

bodies cross readily into the fetal circulation by a facilitated transport mechanism, and are responsible for the destruction of the fetal red blood cells. This produces anemia, and if it is severe enough, heart failure results in an edematous, hydropic infant, and possibly a stillbirth. While the fetus is in utero, the mother is able to remove the breakdown products of the red cells (bilirubin) and handle them in her own liver; therefore, the baby is not born jaundiced. However, once separated from the mother, the baby must handle the continuing breakdown of red cells, and its liver, especially in prematures, lacks the necessary enzymes to do this efficiently. The affected newborn rapidly develops jaundice and, if untreated, brain damage may result from the deposition of the bile pigments in vital areas of the brain (kernicterus). This is the severest form of pathology, but it must be kept in mind that it is not only possible but likely that an Rh negative woman may have one, two, or even more pregnancies without significant difficulty.

It has now been well established that the severity of the hemolytic anemia in the fetus can best be determined by the quantity of bilirubin in the amniotic fluid, that is, the higher the bilirubin level, the lower the fetal hemoglobin. Thus, amniocentesis with analysis of the bilirubin in the fluid is the best basis for making therapeutic decisions in the sensitized patient. Because the quantity of bilirubin is small in the mildly or unsensitized patient, standard techniques for measuring bilirubin cannot be used, and therefore a spectrophotometric approach is used. Bilirubin produces an optical density peak at 450μ and it is the height of this peak or the ΔOD_{450} which is used to evaluate fetal involvement (Fig. 27-16). Amniocentesis is used to evaluate the fetus in all patients with significant sensitization. In most laboratories there can be determined a significant antibody titer below which fetal morbidity is unlikely. Although this varies from institution to institution, titers above 1:8 to 1:16 are generally considered significant. Amniocentesis is usually instituted at from 24 to 25 weeks since intrauterine transfusion is impractical before that, although in instances with previous early stillbirths, the procedure may be instituted as early as 20 weeks. The frequency of repeated amniocenteses is determined by the level of the ΔOD_{450}, weekly taps being indicated if values are high. The common method for evaluating the ΔOD_{450} is the Liley chart illustrated in Figure 27-16. Values in the lower zone for the particular gestation indicate a mildly or even unaffected fetus, while those in the middle zone indicate an affected fetus, but one not in immediate danger of death. Values in the upper zone suggest the fetus will not survive 10 to 14 days without intervention. Management decisions are not based on single values but rather the trend. If the ΔOD_{450} remains in the lower zone, no interference is indicated, and the pregnancy can be allowed to proceed to term. If the values remain in the middle zone, the fetus is best delivered as soon as there is evidence of maturity, especially of the lung, by using the L/S ratio. Upper zone values dictate immediate intervention by delivery if beyond 33 to 34 weeks or by intrauterine transfusion if before that gestational age. This dramatic procedure was first described in 1963 by Liley and involves the instillation (Fig. 27-16) under fluoroscopic control of Rh negative red cells into the peritoneal cavity of the fetus in utero. The fetus is able to absorb these intact cells. If the proce-

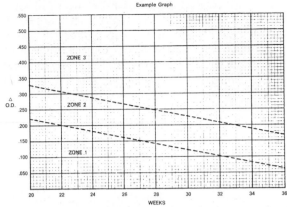

Figure 27-16. Liley graph for relating ΔOD_{450} to weeks of gestation in determining severity of hemolytic disease.

dure is repeated successfully every 10 to 14 days until the point of maturity (approximately 34 to 35 weeks), a stillbirth may be avoided. Only 40 to 50 percent of treated fetuses can be salvaged because the procedure is rather gross, especially in the smaller fetus, and often the fetus is very sick when the procedure is initiated. Of course, these results are far better than no survivors, which could be anticipated without the procedure.

The pediatric management of the newborn involves the use of exchange transfusion to correct anemia and to reduce the bilirubin concentration, this obviating the brain damage of kernicterus. Exchange transfusion is often supplemented by administering albumin to provide more binding sites for bilirubin, and the use of light or phototherapy which controls the rate of increase of bilirubin by converting it to other apparently innocuous pigments. The management of the newborn may be enhanced by the administration of drugs. such as phenobarbital, to the mother prenatally. This drug in relatively small doses can induce in the fetus the synthesis of enzymes necessary to conjugate bilirubin and thereby make the newborn better able to deal with the jaundice.

The ability to prevent Rh sensitization is now an established fact, with human anti-D globulin (Rhogam) having been commercially available since 1969. This material can bring about the clearance from the maternal circulation of Rh positive fetal cells and thereby prevent sensitization. It should be given to all unsensitized Rh negative patients who have delivered Rh positive babies, or untypeable pregnancies such as stillborns, ectopic pregnancies, or spontaneous or therapeutic abortions. Anti-D globulin is of no value in already sensitized patients. It is recommended that it be given within three days of delivery. Failures to prevent sensitization are almost invariably related to the inadequacy of the dose to clear all the fetal red cells. It is important especially in term pregnancy, to establish the adequacy of the dose, either by demonstrating that the fetal cells have been cleared or by the detection of the presence of antibody 48 hours after the administration of anti-D globulin. The latter, which is established by a positive indirect Coombs test, indicates that excess globulin has been given and therefore the cells present have been cleared. If the indirect Coombs is negative at 48 hours, an additional dose of anti-D globulin should be given to assure protection. It seems clear that in the future the only patients who become sensitized will be those who either fail to receive anti-D globulin or who receive an inadequate dose.

DIABETES MELLITUS. This entity is considered in greater detail in Chapter 24. It is important, however, to recognize the fetal effects of the disease. Because glucose crosses the placenta readily and insulin does not, high blood sugars in the mother cause high levels in the fetus which result in hypertrophy of the insulin-producing islets in the fetal pancreas. The combination of glucose and insulin is responsible for the increased size of fetuses in diabetic pregnancies. The magnitude of the size increase is inversely related to the adequacy of diabetic control. This macrosomia makes the likelihood of mechanical problems and fetal injury at delivery greater. In addition, the increased fetal insulin production continues following delivery, resulting in hypoglycemia after the loss of maternal glucose supplies. Diabetic newborns are also more prone to hypocalcemia and jaundice.

Another significant fetal effect of diabetes is the increase in congenital malformations. There is a threefold increase in all anomalies with six times the number of lethal defects. The diabetic offspring is also more prone to eventually develop diabetes, particularly if there are multiple occurrences of diabetes in the family. The precise genetic mechanisms in diabetes are not clear at this time.

Finally, since diabetes has profound vascular effects, it is not surprising that it also affects the vasculature of the placenta, and in certain cases results in placental insufficiency and fetal death. This is the basis for the common practice of early delivery in diabetics, an approach which is not routinely indicated if fetal well-being can be evaluated by appropriate studies such as urinary estriol determinations. This latter approach permits the selection of the fetus in jeopardy for early delivery and avoids the risks of prematurity for the majority of infants not at risk.

Thus, it is apparent that the hazards of being born to a diabetic mother are great. Despite the best of care, the perinatal mortality ranges between 10 and 15 percent, a level at least three times that for the nondiabetic.

PROLONGED PREGNANCY. The average duration of pregnancy is 280 days from the first day of the last menstrual period, or 267 days from the time of conception if the menstrual cycle is of average length. Only 5 percent of women deliver on the actual due date, although most will deliver within 10 to 14 days in either direction from the date. Since the placenta has a normal life span equal to the duration of pregnancy, one may justifiably be concerned that if the due date is exceeded by more than two weeks, the aging placenta may no longer be able to support the fetus adequately. Fortunately, in most instances the placenta is capable of such support. In fact, in a great number of patients who are postdates, the date represents a miscalculation or faulty memory. In addition to those postmature pregnancies in which there is placental insufficiency, there is another group of late pregnancies in which the placenta functions well and the fetus becomes oversized, creating potential mechanical problems in labor and delivery.

If the circumstances, including the status of the cervix, the size and position of the baby, and the size of the maternal pelvis are all favorable, induction of labor should be carried out when a pregnancy exceeds the due date by two weeks. If there is any question about the dates, some of the methods for determining fetal maturity suggested in the section on fetal diagnosis should be applied (pp. 530 to 532). If, on the other hand, conditions are not favorable for the induction of labor, one must utilize means for ascertaining the well-being of the fetus. Twenty-four hour urinary estriol determinations are helpful in this regard. If the values are in the normal range, interference is not necessary, and one may await more favorable conditions for induction. If the value is low and this is confirmed by a repeat determination, delivery by cesarean section is indicated. The oxytocin challenge test is also helpful as a backup study. Evaluation of amniotic fluid is also useful in these cases. The fluid around the fetus affected by postmaturity is scant in volume and heavily stained with meconium. Thus, amniocentesis can provide additional confirmatory information.

The affected postmature (sometimes called dysmature) newborn has a typical appearance. It is long for its weight, appearing to have lost weight. The finger- and toenails are long and stained with meconium, as are the cord and membranes. These infants are especially prone to distress during labor and to respiratory problems in the neonatal period.

On the surface, it would seem simple to determine the due date and when a pregnancy has gone beyond that point, but there are a number of pitfalls. Many patients do not record or cannot recall when they had their last period. Others have long cycles, with ovulation and conception occurring later than the fourteenth day. This is especially true in patients discontinuing oral contraceptive therapy, in whom the first ovulation may not occur until four to six weeks after the last withdrawal flow. One must assess these factors carefully before overtreating a patient for supposed postmaturity.

PREECLAMPSIA-ECLAMPSIA. (See Chapter 23 for maternal aspects). Although the signs of preeclampsia (hypertension, edema, and proteinuria) and eclampsia (convulsions in addition to the above) are primarily maternal, fetal interests cannot be ignored. In fact, once full-blown preeclampsia is manifest, a progressive placental insufficiency develops rather rapidly. If the pregnancy is not terminated, the fetus may fail to grow and even die in utero. On occasion, a patient with severe preeclampsia may seem to be so well controlled that one is tempted to allow the fetus to remain in utero and mature. This decision is fraught with the risk of failure of the fetus to prosper, and possibly a stillbirth; and in most cases it is unwise. Should such a course be elected, one must use some index of fetal well-being, such as urinary estriol, to follow the pregnancy. The perinatal wastage in preeclampsia is largely dependent upon the stage of pregnancy at which the process develops and, therefore, on the degree of maturity of the infant delivered. If toxemia does not develop until after the thirty-sixth week of gestation, the perinatal loss should be quite low. Perinatal loss is high when convulsions (eclampsia) occur. The older studies give the rate as 50 percent, while more recent reviews place it at 20 percent.

CHRONIC HYPERTENSION. Approximately 75 percent of women with benign essential hypertension go through pregnancy with no problems, either maternal or fetal. Unfortunately, some 15 percent develop preeclampsia. When this happens, the fetal prognosis is very poor, especially if it occurs at a time when the fetus is significantly premature (at the end of the second trimester, for example). The perinatal mortality rate in this group is approximately 20 percent. In the case of the hypertensive mother without superimposed preeclampsia, the fetal risk is not great, but it is greater than that for women with normal blood pressure. Because of this, it is recommended that all hypertensive patients be followed with estriol determinations in the third trimester, in order to identify that occasional benign hypertensive patient whose fetus is in jeopardy, and for whom preterm delivery is indicated. There is, in addition, an increased frequency of abruptio placentae in these hypertensive patients, with the added perinatal wastage of that problem.

INFECTIONS AFFECTING THE FETUS. There are a number of infectious diseases which are significant if they occur during pregnancy. Some are important because of their direct effects upon the fetus; others have an indirect effect. The indirect effect is usually abortion or premature labor in the presence of, or as a result of, a high fever in the mother. The most well-documented infection with a fetal effect is *German measles* (*rubella*).

The overall risk of congenital malformation in the newborn of the woman who gets rubella in the first trimester is 20 percent. This risk is greatest in the first four weeks (60 percent), gradually falling off up to twelve weeks, then decreasing even more dramatically. The common defects involve the heart, the eyes, and hearing, although there are a number of others. The question of therapeutic abortion is one which is somewhat controversial, but most feel it is justified if a documented case of rubella occurs in the first eight weeks, and probably up to twelve weeks of pregnancy. When a woman is exposed to rubella in the first trimester, it is important to determine whether the woman has had the disease and is, therefore, immune. This can be done by an examination of the patient's blood for the presence of antibodies to the virus. If the antibody level or titer is high enough, this means the patient is immune and need not worry. If the titer is below the critical level, the patient is not immune and must be carefully watched for the development of the infection. Most authorities do not recommend the use of gamma globulin for the patient exposed to rubella, because the gamma globulin may only modify or mask the infection without preventing the effects on the fetus. Fetal infection with the rubella virus may also occur beyond the first trimester. Such infections do not result in congenital malformations, but often, in fetal viremia with hemorrhagic manifestations. The future is now much brighter with the recent development of the rubella vaccine. Large-scale immunization has been started in children and should in time eliminate the problem. For the time, the use of vaccine in adults should be limited to those women who are not immune (as evidenced by antibody studies) and are at particular risk because of occupation, such as school teachers or pediatric nurses. Since the teratogenic properties of the attenuated virus in the vaccine are unknown, pregnancy must be avoided for three months after its administration.

Other important intrauterine infections are *toxoplasmosis* and *cytomegalovirus*. Both of these infections can produce intrauterine growth retardation and result in the delivery of severely damaged children. Infection with these agents should be suspected when growth lags, although there is no effective therapy which can be applied after fetal infection has occurred. It is important to recognize that toxoplasmosis can be spread by infected pets, particularly cats, and the pregnant patient should be very careful in handling them. The newborn with rubella and cytomegalovirus is highly infectious and special care should be taken if nonimmune pregnant nurses are working in newborn nurseries.

Syphilis, although somewhat less common now, can infect the fetus, bringing about severe pathology, while the herpes simplex virus, if residing in the vagina, can infect the fetus during the birth process. The latter can be avoided by cesarean section prior to rupture of the membranes. Premature labor and spontaneous abortion can be precipitated by a number of maternal infections such as *measles*, *influenza, pyelonephritis, pneumonia, typhoid,* and *cholera.*

Intrauterine infection as the result of premature rupture of the membranes is probably the most common infectious threat to the fetus. It is well recognized that the frequency of such infection parallels the length of the time from rupture of the membranes to the onset of labor. Infection of the fetus occurs by way of the amniotic fluid to the fetal tracheobronchial tree. as well as from the membranes and placenta through the cord vessels, producing fetal sepsis. The organisms most commonly involved are anaerobic streptococci and gram-negative bacilli. Since it is difficult to achieve therapeutic levels of antibiotics in the amniotic fluid once the patient becomes febrile, the treatment is delivery either by induction or cesarean section. More important, however, is the prevention of infection. This is accomplished by delivery (most often by induction, but by section if necessary) of any patient with premature rupture of the membranes whose fetus is larger than 1500 to 1800 grams. This weight range is selected because in most clinics the survival data for babies of that size are such that the risk of delivery and prematurity appears to be less than the risk of intrauterine infection. Recent data have suggested however, that with premature rupture of the membranes, the fetal lung may mature within 24 to 48 hours and therefore a delay may be indicated. This effect, along with the effect of glucocorticoids administered to the mother, in maturing the fetal lung has yet to be clearly established.

FETAL GROWTH RETARDATION. This is one term applied to the clinical syndrome in which the fetus fails to prosper in utero. The terms dysmaturity, placental insufficiency, small-for-date babies, uteroplacental insufficiency, and stunted fetus have also been applied. The syndrome may occur with maternal diseases such as diabetes with severe vascular involvement, chronic renal disease, and chronic hypertension with renal involvement. Intrauterine infection with rubella, toxoplasmosis, and cytomegalovirus are causes. The most severe retardation is produced by multiple congenital malformations. In some cases the syndrome may be idiopathic and recurrent. In general, the earlier in gestation that retardation is apparent, the poorer the outlook. At birth these babies appear to have lost subcutaneous fat, their skin is often wrinkled, and the finger- and toenails are long. The amniotic fluid, cord, and nails are heavily stained with meconium. The stillbirth rate is high and the frequency of respiratory problems in the newborn is increased. The most significant management problem from the obstetrical viewpoint is the antepartal differentiation of the growth retarded fetus from a premature of appropriate size. After delivery, this differentiation is less difficult and can be based on weight (particularly weight gain patterns), certain developmental criteria, such as ear cartilage development and plantar skin creases and behavior patterns. The question of erroneous menstrual dates often arises and this necessitates the use of the method described under fetal diagnosis. Once the diagnosis is suspected, some search for an etiology is indicated. Heroic approaches to the fetus are certainly not indicated if a diagnosis of congenital rubella or cytomegalovirus infection has been established. If, on the other hand, there appears to be no ominous diagnosis, the fetus must be evaluated and followed with an index of well-being, such as urinary estriol, and delivery timed appropriately. In the presence of uteroplacental insufficiency, fetal tolerance to labor may be reduced and the need for cesarean section increased. After birth, newborns with late pregnancy growth retardation and without infection or malformation tend to thrive and rapidly catch up in size to their peers. Those newborns with early pregnancy retardation have reduced cell numbers as well as cell size and tend to remain small.

DISPROPORTIONATE TWIN DEVELOPMENT. Twins with disparity in size may be accounted for by the fact that there can be a connection between the two circulations. This is especially true in single-ovum twins. When this happens in early pregnancy and one heart pumps more strongly than the other, there may be monopolization of a larger area of the placenta by one twin and thus a disparity in size. Such twins are not only greatly different in size at birth, but the smaller one is often anemic and may require transfusion. The larger twin may be hypervolemic and require a phlebotomy to prevent heart failure and jaundice. This type of placental anastomosis, when it occurs in double-ovum twins, accounts for those rare situations known as "chimerism," in which an individual may have two populations of cells, as evidenced by blood groups or sex chromatin. The other important clinical significance of disparity in twin sizes is that difficulties may be encountered in delivery if the smaller of the twins is delivered first through a cervix that is not completely dilated.

Fetal treatment

The art of fetal treatment is at this time, far less well developed than fetal diagnosis. The most common approach to the fetus by the obstetrician is to select an appropriate time for delivery, convert the fetus to a newborn, and thereby turn over the active treatment to the neonatologist. Perhaps the most important approach to the fetus is to provide appropriate support throughout the pregnancy. This includes adequate diet prenatally, as well as glucose and oxygen during labor, especially if there is fetal distress.

Treatment in the case of a positive prenatal diagnosis of congenital disease is generally limited to therapeutic abortion. However, in some instances of metabolic errors, maternal dietary modification may be effective in protecting the fetus with an enzyme defect.

Many drugs administered to the mother cross the placenta into the fetal circulation. Transplacental passage is generally a function of the molecular size of the drug; substances with molecular weights less than 500 crossing readily by simple diffusion. Although most often there is concern regarding the deleterious effects of drugs on the fetus, in some instances one can achieve a desirable therapeutic effect. In the case of the sensitized Rh negative patient, it is possible with certain drugs to induce the fetal liver to produce the enzymes required for bilirubin conjugation. This allows the newborn to cope better with the jaundice and reduces the need for exchange transfusion. The most effective drug is phenobarbital in small doses (15 mgm. QID) for one or two weeks prior to delivery.

Another example of fetal drug therapy is the recently described use of glucocorticoid therapy to induce the production of surfactant in the fetal lung and thereby reduce the risk of respiratory distress syndrome in premature babies. The evidence suggests that if a steroid (Betamethazone was used in the original study) is given to the mother and delivery can be held off for at least 48 hours, the effect will occur. To date no deleterious effects have been demonstrated, but more experience is necessary to confirm the original work.

Intrauterine fetal transfusion in Rh disease is the most publicized form of fetal treatment. Hopefully, the use of Rhogam will ultimately eliminate the need for this rather crude procedure.

The future undoubtedly holds many advances in this area—from the prenatal correction of congenital defects to the even more unbelievable unscrambling of genetic mishaps. There may well be treatments of maladies which are presently unknown in this rapidly developing area of fetal medicine.

Bibliography

1. Barnes, A. C.: *Intrauterine Development.* Philadelphia, Lea & Febiger, 1968.
2. Thompson, J. S., and Thompson, M. W.: *Genetics in Medicine,* ed. 2. Philadelphia, W. B. Saunders, 1973.
3. Abdul-Karim, R. W. (ed.): Human fetal medicine. *Clin. Ob. and Gyn.* 17, 1974.
4. Thompson, H. E. (ed.): Diagnostic ultrasound. *Clin. Ob. and Gyn.* 17, 1974.
5. Osofsky, H. J.: High risk pregnancy with emphasis upon maternal and fetal well-being. *Clin. Ob. and Gyn.* 16, 1973.
6. Simpson, J. L., and Christakos, A. C.: Genetics for the obstetrician and gynecologist. *Clin. Ob. and Gyn.* 15, 1972.
7. Stern, L.: Perinatal biology. *Clin. Ob. and Gyn.* 14, 1971.

the high-risk infant: low birth weight and premature

28

Classification / Etiology / Identification / Assessment of Gestational Age / Characteristics and Physiology / Care of Infants and Parents / Growth and Development

The birth of an infant "before its time" has long posed a problem to the helping professions. Nearly one half of neonatal deaths occur in infants who weigh less than 2,500 Gm. (5½ pounds) and who, for the most part, are born a month or more before term. The general category "prematurity" ranks as the eighth cause of death in the United States, and is considered by many authorities as the single largest problem in contemporary obstetrics and pediatrics as well as public health.

Over the past 10 to 15 years, a sizable body of knowledge and scientific base has developed in the field of perinatology. Recently more precise classifications of the types of small and/or immature infants have permitted a shift from standardized management according to birth weight to an individualized approach based upon the extent of growth and development and the specific problems of the particular baby. As more of these sick and at risk newborns survive, the questions of normality and intactness at a later age gain significance. There are few firm answers at present, and no practical way to shorten the long interval between early treatment and evaluation of outcome in survivors. However, favorable reports of long-term outcome are beginning to appear, and

give support to continued development of perinatal specialties.

Sophisticated technology and complex equipment are increasingly key elements in the care of high-risk infants as special centers for perinatology develop. While these contribute greatly to infant survival, the problems of low birth weight and prematurity will not be solved until the larger social concerns are remedied, for the association between poor socioeconomic status and high perinatal risk still is the predominant influence in eventual outcome as well as incidence and recurrence.

Classification of infants by birth weight and gestational age

In the past, all newborns weighing 2,500 Gm. or less were termed *premature*, and those weighing more were designated *full term*. This approach assumed that intrauterine growth rates were essentially the same for all fetuses, and that birth weight thus corresponded to gestational age. A considerable amount of data have now accumulated to demonstrate the inaccuracy of this assumption, and the two dimensions of *birth weight* and *gestational age* are now considered separately. Standards for

Table 28-1 Premature Infant Classified by Weight and Gestational Age

	5 lb. 8 oz. (2,500 gm.) or less			Over 5 lb. 8 oz. (2,500 gm.)	
	Less than 3 lb. 5 oz. Group I	3 lb. 5 oz. to 5 lb. 8 oz. Less than 37 Weeks Group II	37 Weeks and Over Group III	Less than 37 Weeks Group IV	37 Weeks and Over Group V
Percent of all deliveries	1	2	2 to 4	2 to 4	90 ± 3
Neonatal mortality (%)	65	10	3 to 4	2	Less than 0.5
Appellations	Immature premature	Premature	"Small for dates" Dysmature Postmature Pseudopremature Fetal malnutrition Intrauterine growth retardation Chronic fetal distress	"Pseudoterm"	
Characteristics	Weight loss, 20 percent ± 10 percent Translucent and edematous skin Decreased tone Erratic extremity movement Periodic breathing Moderate jaundice Physiologic immaturity in enzymatic and functional development	Weight loss, 10 percent ± 5 percent	Minimal weight loss, less than 5 percent Malnutrition Dry and scaly skin Increased tone Restricted Moro reflex Increased oxygen consumption Minimal jaundice Cries for and has increased capacity for food Anxious, open-eyed appearance	Same as for Group II but less marked	Normal newborn infants
Complications	Respiratory distress syndrome common Susceptible to infection Asphyxial injury to capillaries, with hemorrhage	Respiratory distress syndrome common	Respiratory distress syndrome rare Hypoglycemia common Reduced skeletal growth Increase in congenital anomalies May have had chronic intrauterine asphyxia	Respiratory distress syndrome occasionally Often neglected because of the false reassurance of their size	
Special requirements	Incubator care		Early water, glucose, calories, and vitamins	Same as for Groups I and II	
Exceptions	Some immature infants who are also malnourished and undersized for their gestation, with some of the characteristics and nutritional requirements of Group III		Infants who are biologically small due to race, family pattern, or early growth arrest; usually not malnourished		Up to 10 percent of normal infants, who have had some degree of fetal malnutrition as in Group III, particularly when of postdate delivery

Source: Babson, S. G., and Benson, R. C.: Primer on Prematurity and High-risk Pregnancy. St. Louis, C. V. Mosby, 1966. (Modified from Yerushalmy, J., van den Berg, B. J., Erhardt, C. L., and Jacobziner, H.: Birth weight and gestation as indices of "immaturity." *Am. J. Dis. Child.* 109:43, 1965.

intrauterine growth have been determined for Caucasian infants, and serve as a guide for identification of appropriate birth weight for an infant's gestational age (Fig. 28-1 and Table 28-1).

Infants may now be categorized as *appropriate in weight for gestational age, small for gestational age* (also referred to as small-for-dates), and *large for gestational age*. In addition, the length of gestation can be determined, either by history of the mother's last menstrual period or by physical and neurological evaluation of the newborn (Chapter 27), and the infant categorized as *preterm* (less than 37 weeks gestation), *term* (37 to 42 weeks gestation), and *postterm* (more than 42 weeks gestation).[1] Weight serves as an assessment of growth, and gestational age as an assessment of maturity. An infant born at 40 weeks gestation and weighing less than 2,500 Gm. would be mature but undergrown, a condition generally referred to as *intrauterine growth retardation*. Similarly, an infant born at 35 weeks gestation and weighing more than 2,500 Gm. would be immature but overgrown, the most common example of this being the fat, edematous but underdeveloped baby of a diabetic mother. The term *premature* seems most appropriate for the *preterm*, immature infant regardless of birth weight. Preterm infants may also be small for gestational age, implying that at least two factors are involved: that causing the early delivery and that retarding the growth rate in utero.

Etiology

Preterm or premature

Premature or preterm infants are born before the thirty-seventh week of gestation, regardless of birth weight. Most babies who weigh less than 2,500 Gm. at birth are premature, as are almost all those weighing less than 1,500 Gm. The majority of these preterm infants are of appropriate weight for gestational age, but some are small-for-dates. The causes of early delivery in most of these infants who are appropriately sized remain obscure. Most studies of the factors associated with prematurity were based upon birth weight as the sole criterion; thus their data are clouded. However, some conditions have been clearly related to premature labor, including chronic hypertensive disease, toxemia, placenta previa, abruptio placentae, and cervical incompetence. Other socioeconomic and environmental factors are harder to evaluate, and often several related factors are inseparable and generally associated with poverty. Mortality rates are highest among premature infants and increase as birth weight decreases.[2]

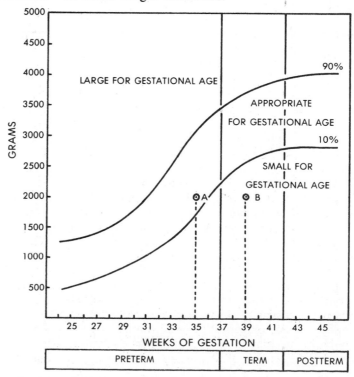

Figure 28-1. The birth weights of liveborn singleton caucasian infants at gestational ages from 24 to 42 weeks.

Small for gestational age

Infants whose weight falls below the tenth percentile for their gestational age have experienced impairment of the normal growth process during the prenatal period. This condition may occur at any gestational age, but the majority of small-for-dates infants are born at or close to term, and weigh less than 2,500 Gm. Under the old classification, these would have been called "premature," although their period of intrauterine life was not significantly shortened. Although small, these infants are mature and have needs and problems different from those of true preterm babies.

There are two different types of growth retardation, and these may occur separately or simultaneously. Fetal growth involves both an increase in the number of cells (hyperplasia) and an increase in the size of cells (hypertrophy). Embryonic growth largely involves rapid increase in the number of cells as the organs and body structures are formed, and later in pregnancy these cells increase in size. If an insult to the fetus occurs early in gestation, mitosis is impaired and fewer new cells are formed, resulting in small organs of subnormal weight. The cells, however, will be of normal size. If interference with growth occurs later, the cells will be normal in number but smaller in size, again resulting in smaller organs but in this instance due to reduced amounts of cytoplasm. An intrauterine insult throughout both phases of growth results in cells that are fewer in number and smaller in size. The classic example of the latter condition is the infant with the rubella syndrome. Fetal malnutrition and toxemia, which tend to be more prominent during later pregnancy, create the second type of growth retardation in which cell numbers are normal, but their size is reduced.

MALNUTRITION. Inadequate nutrition has long been suspect as a cause of impaired fetal growth, and animal studies show a direct causal relationship. Because human gestation is prolonged, effects of nutrition are harder to assess. In a study of near starvation conditions among pregnant women during World War II, it appeared that no significant undergrowth of infants occurred in utero unless the food shortage was present during the last weeks of pregnancy.[3] Poor placental growth in nutritionally deprived pregnant women has been demonstrated, supporting the concept of nutritional inadequacy as a cause of growth retardation.[4] The consistent positive association between poverty and low birth weight is also suggestive of a nutritional factor, but this relationship has not yet been satisfactorily explained. In the twin transfusion or parabiosis syndrome, when blood is transferred from one twin to the other through a placental shunt, the donor twin is anemic with smaller length, head size, weight, and size of organs than the recipient twin.

INFECTION. Certain intrauterine infections are known to cause decreased growth of the baby, most notably cytomegalic inclusion disease and rubella. Congenital syphilis does not seem to cause growth retardation, although it has previously been identified as a cause of prematurity. Intrauterine bacterial infections usually occur just prior to or during labor, but are not associated with the problem of growth retardation.

GENETIC FACTORS. With the separation of true premature from small-for-dates infants, it became apparent that most congenital malformations occur in undergrown infants. The smaller for gestational age, the greater the frequency of congenital anomalies. Additionally, the highest incidence of severe malformations was found to occur in small-for-dates infants with the longest gestation. Congenital malformations occur 10 to 20 times more frequently in small-for-gestational-age infants than in appropriate for gestational age infants.[5] Congenital disorders such as dwarfism often occur in infants who are small-for-dates, and in some families there are repeated births of infants who are small for age without associated abnormalities except mental retardation.

PLACENTAL INSUFFICIENCY. Impaired exchange between the mother and fetus, especially reduction of nutrients and hormones, has been conceptually defined as placental insufficiency and utilized to explain some instances of fetal malnutrition. There are some well-defined pathologic lesions of the placenta which are associated with inefficient placental functioning, but these occur in only a few instances. Included among these lesions are extensive fibrosis, occlusion of fetal vessels in the villi, large hemangiomas, and early separation of the placenta. Diabetes and toxemia also seem associated with placental insufficiency, but in most cases there are no apparent maternal disorders or morphologic abnormalities of the placenta. It seems logical that retarded fetal growth could be an end result of insufficient functioning of the placenta, but more study of this concept is needed.

OTHER FACTORS. Various other circumstances or conditions are associated with retarded intra-uterine growth. Infants born of multiple pregnancies are usually small-for-dates if born after 35 weeks gestation, presumably because the placenta can no longer supply the needs of the growing fetuses. Smoking is a significant statistical correlate to small-for-gestational-age babies, with moderate smokers having double the incidence of small birth weight babies and heavy smokers three times the incidence which occurs in nonsmokers. Mothers who smoke more than twenty cigarettes per day give birth to growth-retarded infants two to three times more often than mothers who do not smoke. Living at higher altitudes tends to be related to lower birth weight for the duration of pregnancy, but the reason for this is not known. Certain noxious agents such as x-ray, aminopterin and other antimetabolites result in growth impairment, malformations of the brain and cranial vault, and other anomalies depending upon timing of exposure. Infants of drug addicts, notably heroin addicts, are often small-for-dates.

Identification of the high-risk neonate

Although the causes of prematurity and growth retardation are not all well understood, several associated factors have been identified which alert nurses and physicians to the possibility of these problems. Early recognition of mothers with high-risk pregnancies and careful prenatal care can often contribute to a better outcome for the infant and the parents.

Prenatal factors

Characteristics of the mother
Age at conception under 16 or over 40;
Weight before conception under 100 pounds or over 200 pounds;
Alcohol or narcotics addict;
Poor socioeconomic status;
Mental retardation;
Cigarette smoker.

Previous pregnancy history
Grand multiparity (more than six pregnancies);
Surgical or complicated delivery, complications of pregnancy;
Prolonged labor (over 24 hours);
Fetal loss or infant death;
Premature or small-for-dates infant;
Infant with abnormalities;
Multiple pregnancy;
Infant over nine pounds;
Infertility;
Rh sensitization;
Abortion.

Health history
Hypertension;
Renal disease;
Diabetes;
Cardiovascular disease;
Thyroid disease;
Neurologic disease;
Major psychoses;
Anemia;
Tuberculosis;
Cancer;
Lupus erythematosus.

Present pregnancy
Toxemia;
Diabetes;
Bleeding after 12 weeks gestation;
Multiple pregnancy;
Hydramnios;
Rubella infection;
Exposure to noxious substances;
Urinary tract infection or persistent albuminuria;
Obesity or excessive weight gain;
Infectious diseases (syphilis, herpes, cytomegalovirus, toxoplasmosis);
Anemia;
Fundal height small-for-dates.

Intrapartal factors

Complications of labor and delivery
Labor longer than 24 hours in primigravida;
Labor longer than 12 hours in multigravida;
Second stage longer than 2 hours;
Ruptured membranes more than 24 hours;
Abnormal presentation or position;
Heavy sedation or injudicious anesthesia;
Maternal fever or infection;
Placenta previa or abruptio placentae;
Cesarean section;
Meconium-stained amniotic fluid;
Fetal distress by monitoring or scalp blood sampling;
Prolapsed cord;

High or midforceps delivery, difficult or operative delivery;
Premature labor.

Immediate problems of infant
Depressed, resuscitation required;
Low Apgar score;
Malformation or other significant abnormality;
Birth injury;
Failure to begin spontaneous respiration.

Neonatal factors

Characteristics of infant
Preterm or premature;
Small or large for gestational age;
Birth weight under 5½ pounds or over 9 pounds;
Low-set ears;
Enlargement of one or both kidneys;
Single palmar crease;
Single umbilical artery;
Small head size.

Clinical problems
Sucks and takes food poorly;
Anemia;
Hyperbilirubinemia;
Failure to maintain temperature;
Respiratory distress;
Hypoglycemia;
Polycythemia;
Infections;
Rh or ABO incompatibilities.

Assessment of gestational age

Accurate assessment of an infant's gestational age is of immediate and critical importance in the proper management of problems or anticipation of needs for care. The clinical course, outcome and problems are quite different for the preterm, immature infant and the small-for-gestational-age infant. In the first group, hyaline membrane disease, hyperbilirubinemia, apnea, and feeding problems are more common. In the second, frequent problems include hypoglycemia, congenital malformations, aspiration, pneumothorax, pulmonary hemorrhage, and polycythemia.

If concern develops during pregnancy because the fetus does not seem to be growing properly, a high-risk condition of the mother exists, or premature labor threatens, there are several procedures available for estimation of fetal age and well-being. The mother's last menstrual period is still a good index if she is reasonably certain about dates; however, these are sometimes confusing because of irregular periods, bleeding in the first trimester, or rapid succession of pregnancies.

Prenatal assessment
Reduced excretion of *urinary estriols* by the mother during pregnancy indicate defective placental function. Serial determinations are most helpful, for a sudden drop or disappearance of urinary estriol previously present is an ominous sign for the fetus, associated with hypoxia. Amniotic fluid obtained by amniocentesis during pregnancy provides several methods for assessing fetal status. Rising concentrations of *creatinine* during gestation are correlated with fetal gestational age, as creatinine concentrations less than 1.8 mg. per 100 ml. occur prior to the 36th week and greater than 1.8 mg. after the thirty-sixth week. A low level or absence of *bilirubin* probably indicates fetal maturity, although this is less reliable than creatinine. Pulmonary maturity is indicated by the sudden increase in the ratio of *lecithin to sphingomyelin* (also called the L/S ratio) which occurs in the amniotic fluid at 35 to 36 weeks gestation. Saturated lecithins and related phospholipids arise principally from the fetal lung and are produced in greater amounts as the lungs near maturity. If the L/S ratio is 2.0 or more, hyaline membrane disease is unlikely to occur. Fetal cells probably originating from sebaceous glands can be obtained from amniotic fluid and stained with *Nile blue sulfate.* The viable, more mature cells stain orange, the immature ones stain blue. Before 34 weeks gestation, the number of orange-stained cells is less than 1 percent; between 34 and 38 weeks, 1 to 10 percent; between 38 and 40 weeks, 10 to 50 percent; and beyond 40 weeks, over 50 percent.

Ultrasonic scanning can be used during pregnancy to measure the biparietal diameter of the fetal skull, permitting estimation of fetal maturity and serial assessment of the rate of fetal growth. This technique is proving to be quite accurate and its use is growing as it offers the additional benefit of posing no danger to the fetus. *X-ray examination* of the fetus for ossification centers in distal femoral and proximal tibial epiphyses has been used to assess fetal growth, but the dangers of radiation appear to

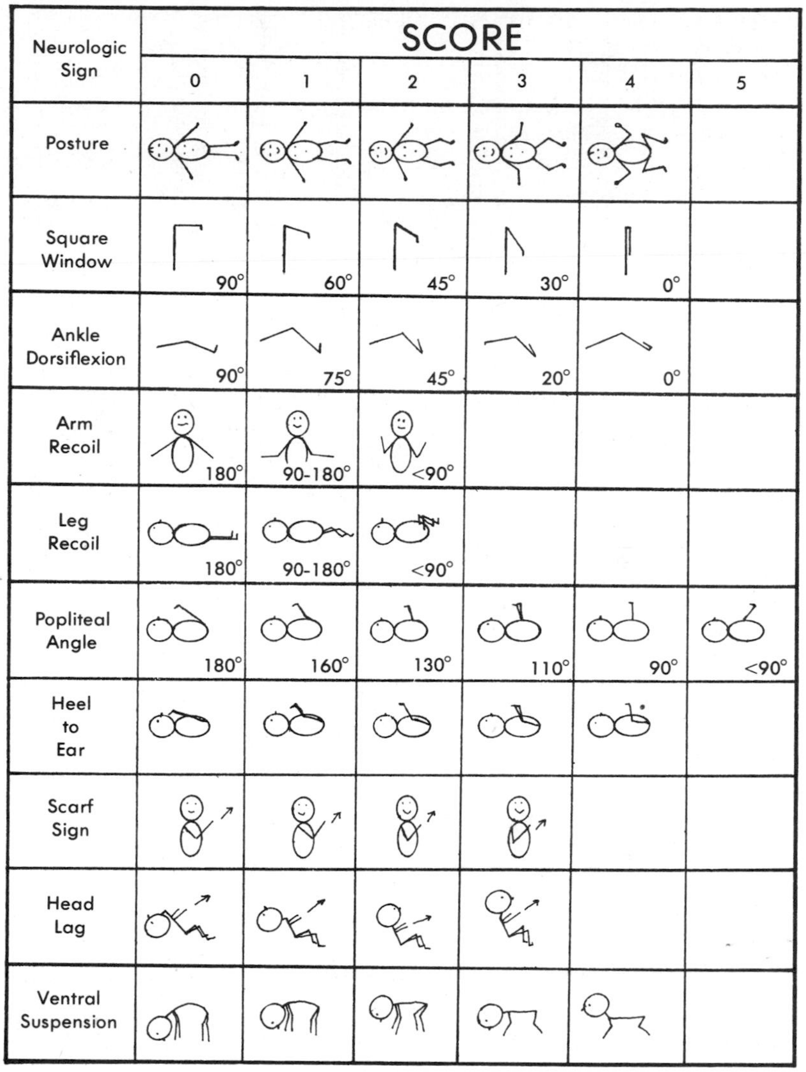

Neurologic Sign	SCORE					
	0	1	2	3	4	5
Posture						
Square Window	90°	60°	45°	30°	0°	
Ankle Dorsiflexion	90°	75°	45°	20°	0°	
Arm Recoil	180°	90-180°	<90°			
Leg Recoil	180°	90-180°	<90°			
Popliteal Angle	180°	160°	130°	110°	90°	<90°
Heel to Ear						
Scarf Sign						
Head Lag						
Ventral Suspension						

Figure 28-2. The scoring of neurologic findings.

outweigh the benefits. The femoral epiphysis is usually seen at 36 weeks gestation and the tibial at 38 weeks. However, gestational age can be predicted accurately only to within a range of about seven weeks, and infants with intrauterine growth retardation may have absent or markedly smaller epiphyses. A recent technique is injection of *radiopaque iodized lipid* into the amniotic fluid which dissolves in the vernix, thus outlining the fetal skin on x-ray. Based on the natural history of the vernix, almost all the fetal figure would be seen prior to 38 weeks gestation, limbs and abdomen patchily outlined between 38 and 40 weeks gestation, and only the back and head visible after 40 weeks.[6]

Postnatal assessment

After the infant's birth, a number of external physical characteristics and neurologic signs can be used to assess maturity. Standardized methods using these parameters have been developed over the past 15 years, and charts and scoring systems are available to make the procedures quicker and more accurate. Nurses as well as physicians involved in the care of high-risk infants need to be familiar with these physical characteristics and neurologic responses.

EXTERNAL PHYSICAL CHARACTERISTICS. During gestation, certain external physical characteristics develop and progress in an orderly fashion according to the age of the fetus. After

Table 28-2 Scoring System of External Physical Characteristics

External Sign	Score* 0	1	2	3	4
Edema	Obvious edema of hands and feet; pitting over tibia	No obvious edema of hands and feet; pitting over tibia	No edema		
Skin texture	Very thin, gelatinous	Thin and smooth	Smooth; medium thickness. Rash or superficial peeling	Slight thickening. Superficial cracking and peeling, especially of hands and feet	Thick and parchment-like; superficial or deep cracking
Skin color	Dark red	Uniformly pink	Pale pink; variable over body	Pale; only pink over ears, lips, palms, or soles	
Skin opacity (trunk)	Numerous veins and venules clearly seen, especially over abdomen	Veins and tributaries seen	A few large vessels seen over abdomen	A few large vessels seen indistinctly over abdomen	No blood vessels seen
Lanugo (over back)	No lanugo	Abundant; long and thick over whole back	Hair thinning especially over lower back	Small amount of lanugo and bald areas	At least ½ of back devoid of lanugo
Plantar creases	No skin creases	Faint red marks over anterior half of sole	Definite red marks over > anterior ½; indentations over < anterior ⅓	Indentations over > anterior ⅓	Definite deep indentations over > anterior ⅓
Nipple formation	Nipple barely visible; no areola	Nipple well defined; areola smooth and flat, diameter < 0.75 cm.	Areola stippled, edge not raised, diameter < 0.75 cm.	Areola stippled, edge raised, diameter > 0.75 cm.	
Breast size	No breast tissue palpable	Breast tissue on one or both sides, < 0.5 cm. diameter	Breast tissue both sides; one or both 0.5 to 1.0 cm.	Breast tissue both sides; one or both > 1 cm.	
Ear form	Pinna flat and shapeless, little or no incurving of edge	Incurving of part of edge of pinna	Partial incurving whole of upper pinna	Well-defined incurving whole of upper pinna	
Ear firmness	Pinna soft, easily folded, no recoil	Pinna soft, easily folded, slow recoil	Cartilage to edge of pinna, but soft in places, ready recoil	Pinna firm, cartilage to edge; instant recoil	
Genitals: Male	Neither testis in scrotum	At least one testis high in scrotum	At least one testis right down		
Genitals: Female (with hips ½ abducted)	Labia majora widely separated, labia minora protruding	Labia majora almost cover labia minora	Labia majora completely cover labia minora		

Source: Adapted by Dubowitz et al.: Clinical assessment of gestational age in the newborn infant. J. Pediat. 77:1, 1970. From Farr et al.: The definition of some external characteristics used in the assessment of gestational age of the newborn infant. Develop. Med. Child. Neurol. 8:507, 1966.

* If score differs on two sides, take the mean.

birth, the gestational age can be determined by presence or absence of a number of these characteristics. Scoring systems have been developed in which each physical characteristic is weighted increasingly as it changes with gestation. The scores obtained are added, and the total score is equated with the duration of pregnancy (Table 28-2).

NEUROLOGIC EXAMINATION. Gestational age may be assessed according to a number of neuromuscular responses of the newborn infant within the first few days of life. The infant's posture, the passive range of motion of certain parts, righting reactions, and various reflexes are evaluated and scored using a weighted scale in a method similar to that for assessing external physical characteristics. The neurologic examination requires the infant be in a quiet, rested state; this may not be possible immedi-

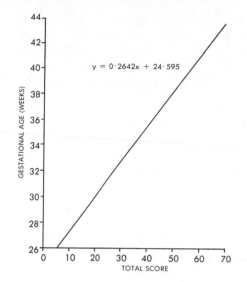

$$y = 0 \cdot 2642x + 24 \cdot 595$$

Figure 28-3. Graph for ascertaining gestational age from the total score of physical and neurologic development.

Table 28-3   Techniques of Neurologic Assessment

Posture

With the infant supine and quiet, score as follows:

arms and legs extended	= 0
slight or moderate flexion of hips and knees	= 1
moderate to strong flexion of hips and knees	= 2
legs flexed and abducted, arms slightly flexed	= 3
full flexion of arms and legs	= 4

Square Window

Flex the hand at the wrist. Exert pressure sufficient to get as much flexion as possible. The angle between the hypothenar emenence and the anterior aspect of the forearm is measured and scored according to Fig. 28-2. Do not rotate the wrist.

Ankle Dorsiflection

Flex the foot at the ankle with sufficient pressure to get maximum change. The angle between the dorsum of the foot and the anterior aspect of the leg is measured and scored as in Fig. 28-2.

Arm Recoil

With the infant supine, fully flex the forearm for five seconds, then fully extend by pulling the hands and release. Score the reaction according to:

remain extended or random movements	= 0
incomplete or partial flexion	= 1
brisk return to full flexion	= 2

Leg Recoil

With the infant supine, the hips and knees are fully flexed for five seconds, then extended by traction on the feet and released. Score the reaction according to:

no response or slight flexion	= 0
partial flexion	= 1
full flexion (less than 90° at knees and hips)	= 2

Popliteal Angle

With the infant supine and the pelvis flat on the examining surface, the leg is flexed on the thigh and the thigh fully flexed with the use of one hand. With the other hand the leg is then extended and the angle attained scored as in Fig. 28-2.

Heel to Ear Maneuver

With the infant supine, hold the infant's foot with one hand and move it as near to the head as possible without forcing it. Keep the pelvis flat on the examining surface. Score as in Fig. 28-2.

Scarf Sign

With the infant supine, take the infant's hand and draw it across the neck and as far across the opposite shoulder as possible. Assistance to the elbow is permissible by lifting it across the body. Score according to the location of the elbow:

elbow reaches the opposite anterior axillary line	= 0
elbow between opposite anterior axillary line and midline of thorax	= 1
elbow at midline of thorax	= 2
elbow does not reach midline of thorax	= 3

Head Lag

With the infant supine, grasp each forearm just proximal to the wrist and pull gently so as to bring the infant to a sitting position. Score according to the relationship of the head to the trunk during the maneuver:

no evidence of head support	= 0
some evidence of head support	= 1
maintains head in the same anteroposterior plane as the body	= 2
tends to hold the head forward	= 3

Ventral Suspension

With the infant prone and the chest resting on the examiner's palm, lift the infant off the examining surface and score according to the posture shown in Fig. 28-2.

Source: According to Dubowitz *et al.* from Amiel-Tison, C.: Neurological evaluation of the maturity of newborn infants. *Arch. Dis. Child.* 43:89, 1968. To be used in conjunction with Fig. 28-2.

ately after delivery. Most infants can be examined during the latter part of the first day of life, but others are not ready until the second or third day. The score obtained on the neurologic examination is totaled according to the scale indicated (Fig. 28-2 and Table 28-3). The neurologic examination score and the external physical characteristics score are added, and if used properly will provide a quite accurate assessment of gestational age when applied to the accompanying graph for interpretation (Fig. 28-3).

Characteristics and physiology of small-for-gestational-age infants

Appearance at birth

Small-for-dates infants appear thin and wasted, with skin that is loose, often dry, and frequently scaling. Meconium staining, involving the nails, skin and umbilical cord, is common. Such infants have very little subcutaneous tissue, and the trunk and extremities do not appear to have as much musculature as would be expected. Their faces appear wizened and are not full and round, with generally sparse hair on the head. Although their weight is low, length is often normal, as is head size. Shortly after birth these infants are usually alert, active, and hungry. They frequently do not urinate during the first several hours of life, and may go as long as 24 hours without voiding if fluids are withheld. The umbilical cord tends to dry more rapidly than that of normal infants. Some small-for-dates infants appear proportionately small without wasting, meconium staining, and the other characteristics described. These babies appear old for their size and seem to have been undergrown for a long time; it is in this group that anomalies tend to occur.

Physiologic problems

In adaptation to extrauterine life, the problems encountered by the small-for-gestational-age infant are different from those of the appropriate-for-gestational-age, preterm (premature) infant. If the problem of poor growth in utero has been detected during pregnancy, nurses and physicians skilled in resuscitation should be present at delivery.

ASPHYXIA. Small-for-dates babies tend to have increased incidences of neonatal asphyxia, particularly those who are markedly under-nourished. They may need immediate metabolic and ventilatory resuscitation, so delivery personnel must be skilled in techniques of intubation and resuscitation, and have appropriate equipment on hand. Temperature control is another common problem, and these infants must be carefully watched for significant drops in temperature. Aspiration of amniotic fluid leading to aspiration pneumonia and pneumothorax occurs more frequently in small-for-dates babies, while hyaline membrane disease is the primary pulmonary problem of premature infants.

HYPOGLYCEMIA. Neonatal hypoglycemia, or blood glucose concentration of less than 20 mg. per 100 ml., is more frequent in males and predominantly small-for-gestational-age infants. It occurs in 50 percent of these infants who are below the third percentile for gestational age, and who are markedly wasted. Although hypoglycemia usually occurs during the first 12 hours of life, it may appear as late as 48 hours. Blood sugars of these infants must be carefully monitored and early feeding instituted.

THERMAL REGULATION. Lacking subcutaneous tissue and fat, small-for-dates babies have difficulty maintaining body temperature. In addition to body composition, basal metabolic rates differ from normal newborns. The temperature setting on the incubator should be determined by closely monitoring the infant's temperature, with the goal of maintaining abdominal skin temperature between 36.0 and 36.5 degrees C.

POLYCYTHEMIA. Infants with intrauterine growth retardation have been found to have increased red blood cell volume, elevated erythropoietin levels, and a central hematocrit often greater than 60 percent. The cause of this polycythemia is unknown, but hypoxia in utero has been suggested. Although the condition is usually asymptomatic, when hematocrit values reach 70 percent, blood viscosity rises precipitously and may lead to such signs as tachypnea, intercostal retraction, grunting, nasal flaring, tachycardia, pleural effusion, scrotal edema, priapism, and convulsions. It is not unusual for hyperbilirubinemia to be present also. The treatment for polycythemia consists of removing small quantities of blood followed by serial hematocrits until a value of 50 to 60 percent is obtained. Often plasma is used to replace the volume of blood withdrawn.[7]

Characteristics and physiology of the premature infant

General description at birth

As there are many degrees of prematurity, there are also various stages of anatomic and physiologic development. Many of the symptoms described below may vary in infants of approximately the same fetal age, depending on the factors associated with prematurity and the physical condition of the mother and the infant.

At birth the premature baby lacks the subcutaneous fat which is deposited during the last two months of intrauterine development. This gives the skin a transparent appearance with the blood vessels easily seen through the skin, which often is of a deep red color, sometimes with a cyanotic hue. These premature babies are prone likewise to develop icteric skin changes. Lanugo is usually abundant all over the skin surface but disappears within a few weeks.

The external ears and the nose are very soft, due to the underdeveloped cartilage. The ears lie very close to the head. The skull is round, in contrast with the long anteroposterior skull diameter of the full-term infant. The fontanels are large, and the sutures prominent. The fingernails and toenails may be immature, often not reaching the ends of the fingers and the toes.

The infant may be puny and small or may approximate full-term weight; yet the internal organs may be imperfectly developed, and these babies appear to be reluctant to assume the responsibility to live. The respiration is shallow and irregular, due to the lack of lung expansion and proper gaseous exchange. There are often periods of apnea. Due to the irregular respiration and the poorly developed function of swallowing, there is danger of aspiration of milk or vomitus, causing cyanosis and predisposing to pulmonary infections. The premature baby regurgitates food readily, because the stomach is tubular in form, and the sphincters are poorly developed. The urine is usually scanty.

The walls of the blood vessels are weak, and the tendency to hemorrhage is great. Since the central nervous system is not fully developed, the premature infant is sluggish and must be wakened to be fed, and the muscular movements are feeble. The temperature is usually subnormal and fluctuating, due to the underdeveloped heat-regulating center. The cry is monotonous, whining, "kittenlike" and effortless, showing a lack of energy. All these symptoms are evidenced in varying degrees, according to the degree of immaturity.

Physiologic considerations

As we have seen in Chapter 21, the newly born infant must make certain adaptations to extrauterine life. While the various stages or steps have not been delineated for the premature baby as they have for the normal newborn, it is apparent that his adaptations will be even greater and more difficult due to his anatomic and physiologic deficits.

RESPIRATORY SYSTEM. The development of the lungs will depend upon the degree of maturity. For instance, the lungs of an infant weighing 2 pounds (900 Gm.) or less show small alveoli lined with cuboidal epithelium and surrounded by a meager supply of capillaries (which prevent efficient gaseous exchange); the lungs of an infant weighing 6 pounds (2,730 Gm.), on the other hand, show large alveoli, the walls of which are virtually formed by bare capillaries. There is a great increase in the capillary network between the twenty-sixth week and the thirty-sixth week of intrauterine life, and for this reason the ability of the lungs to sustain extrauterine life increases with each week of intrauterine existence. The more immature the infant, the less blood flow there is through the lungs, the remainder being shunted through the ductus arteriosus.

As we have seen with the mature newborn, the most critical event in the adjustment to extrauterine life is the establishment of ventilation by the previously unused lungs. The unexpanded lungs of any fetus are not just crumpled air sacs waiting to be filled; rather they are fluid-filled organs requiring a great deal of negative intrapleural pressure (up to 60 cm. water has been used experimentally) for expansion. This great effort is necessary because of the viscosity of the fluid in the lungs, surface tension effects, and tissue resistance. The premature baby is often not capable of this enormous task because of the previously mentioned inadequacy in the capillary anatomy which impedes appropriate gaseous exchange, and because the respiratory centers of the brain which regulate depth and rate of respiration are not fully developed. In addition, these infants are hampered by weak respiratory muscles, a yielding thoracic cage, a decreased amount of pulmonary lipoprotein which reduces surface tension in the lungs, and a deficient amount of fibrinolysins; hence primary and secondary atelectasis is common to these infants. The nasal passages are extremely narrow and the mucous membrane easily injured. The cough reflex is poorly developed or absent, making the danger of inhalation of regurgitated fluids very real.

In general then, an unstable respiratory system is a result of these deficits. Respiration tends to be irregular in rhythm and depth; there are periods of apnea during which cyanosis may develop. The infant utilizes his diaphragm more than his chest in his breathing, and if there is much atelectasis, the thoracic cage is dragged down with each inspiration. In severe cases, the sternum is sucked back toward the spine with inspiration, and expiration is accompanied by a short feeble grunt. It is important to remember that with these infants, respirations must be counted for at least a minute if any accurate respiratory rate is to be determined (Fig. 28-4).

CARDIOVASCULAR SYSTEM. *The heart* is relatively large at birth and often its action is slow and feeble. Extrasystoles occur and murmurs may be present at birth or soon after, which may later disappear as the fetal openings gradually close. As previously stated there is a decrease in the density of available capillaries in vital organs to take up sufficient oxygen in babies under about 1,000 Gm. The extreme capillary fragility, especially of the intracranial vessels, together with the low plasma prothrombin level leads to a bleeding tendency in these infants. This tendency is evidenced by the frequency of ecchymosis of the skin as well as intraventricular hemorrhage and other internal bleeding.

The *systolic blood pressure* at birth is lower than that of the mature infant, and decreases with the birth weight. Infants weighing between 2 to 4 pounds (900 to 2,270 Gm.) generally have a systolic pressure of 45 to 60 mm. of mercury as compared with the 80 mm. of mercury for term infants. The level rises with the age of the child, by about 20 mm. by the end of the second week, and an additional 5 mm. by the age of two months.

The *pulse rate* ranges between 100 and 160, with the average around 140. Because of the tendency to arrhythmia, the pulse rate is most accurately obtained (as with the term infant) with a stethoscope, counting the apical beat for a minute.

As with the mature infant, the premature has a relatively high *hemoglobin concentration* at birth which decreases to around 7 Gm. per 100 ml. of blood at four to eight weeks of age. This is due to the premature's inadequacy in manufacturing hemoglobin, together with his relatively rapid rate of growth. After this time, the rate gradually increases until about four

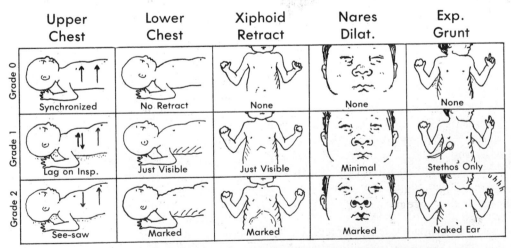

OBSERVATION OF RETRACTIONS

Figure 28-4. An index of respiratory distress is determined by grading each of five arbitrary criteria; grade 0 indicates no difficulty, grade 1 moderate difficulty, and grade 2 maximum respiratory difficulty. The "retraction score" is the sum of these values; a total score of 0 indicates no dyspnea, whereas a total score of ten denotes maximal respiratory distress.

months, when there is a second fall, characterized by hypochromia of the red cells. If a severe enough anemia develops in the first phase of hemoglobin decline, it may be treated with iron therapy. Some investigators have found for some unknown reason that *parenteral* (but not *oral*) administration of iron is useful in prevention of the first phase of anemia. However, the later phase responds well to oral iron therapy and thus it has become customary to institute the oral form of therapy from the third week onward.

WHITE BLOOD CELLS. The white blood cell count at birth is lower than that usually found in the term infant (see Chapter 21). There is a predominance of polymorphonuclear cells, as with the mature infant, and the same decrease occurs in the total white cell count during the first week of life. However, the change to lymphocytic predominance may occur slightly later for the mature infant.

JAUNDICE IN THE PREMATURE. The majority of premature infants become jaundiced around the second or third day of life. As is the case with term infants, the jaundice intensifies from the fourth to the sixth day and generally disappears by the second week. As far as we know, the mechanism responsible for this condition is approximately the same as that described for mature infants (see Chapter 21). Weight and degree of development appear to be related to the serum bilirubin value. The smaller the infant, the higher the peak of bilirubin value; 13 mg. per 100 ml. of blood is beyond the physiologic limit. In the very small premature, a value of 15 to 20 mg. per 100 ml. is often found, because of the inability of the premature's immature liver to dispose of the bilirubin which is liberated by the breakdown of the red blood cells.

When hyperbilirubinemia occurs (serum bilirubin in excess of 18 to 20 mg. per 100 ml. of blood), kernicterus may occur, and when the infant is particularly stressed (e.g., respiratory distress, difficult delivery) even lower concentrations of bilirubin are required to produce kernicterus. Other conditions which predispose to this condition before the second day of life are 1) erythroblastosis, concomitant with the immature liver function and 2) early gestational age of the infant.

TEMPERATURE REGULATION. Even more so than the normal newborn, the premature infant's temperature regulating mechanism is poorly developed at birth. Since his peripheral circu-

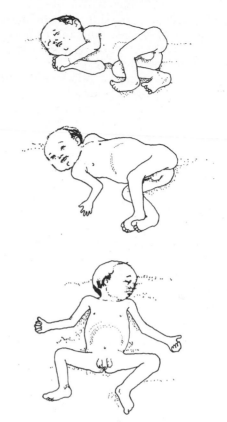

Figure 28-5. Posture of premature infant: (Top) Immediately after birth, (center) several hours later, and (bottom) after several days.

lation is also poor, his peripheral responses to heat and cold (i.e., sweating and shivering) are inadequate. Heat production is low and heat loss high because of the relatively greater body surface (in proportion to the weight) and the lack of subcutaneous fat.

NEUROLOGIC SYSTEM. The stage of development of the nervous system at birth will depend upon the degree of maturity. As with the normal newborn, all the premature's neurons are present, but they are not as fully developed and remain so for months and sometimes years. The least mature infants tend to lie quietly unless disturbed, waking only at intervals for feeding. External stimulation results in weak purposeless jerky movements and perhaps a feeble cry. As the infant matures, his movements tend to occur in little bursts of activity which can be quite vigorous, resulting in his wiggling from one end of the incubator to the other. At first the less mature infant will lie on his side in the "fetal position"; later he uncurls and after several days he lies on his back with his head rolled to one side, his hips flexed and abducted, and his knees and ankles flexed (frog position) (Fig. 28-5). The less mature the infant, the worse his muscle tone.

The vital centers controlling respiration and temperature are poorly developed, as are the centers controlling such important reflexes as coughing, swallowing and sucking. The Moro and tonic neck reflexes are present in normal infants of both low birth weight and early gestational age, as are the Chvostek and Babinski signs. Tendon reflexes are variable in all immature infants.

GASTROINTESTINAL SYSTEM. Larger prematures may have fairly good sucking and swallowing ability. The less mature infants, however, generally have feeble reflexes which, in the very immature, may be absent altogether. Because of the poorly developed mechanism for closure of the cardia and the relatively strong pyloric sphincter, regurgitation is common.

Again the powers of digestion depend upon the degree of prematurity, being rudimentary in infants of 26 to 28 weeks gestation but becoming more efficient as maturity increases. The stomach of a 2-pound (900-Gm.) infant at birth shows little folding of the mucosal surface (which reduces the surface area for absorption) and poor development of the secretory glands and muscle layers, as compared with that of a term baby with his deeply folded mucosal layer and relatively well-developed glands and muscle tissue. The premature infant appears to digest and absorb carbohydrates easily, proteins less well and fats badly, even though fat-splitting enzymes are present at birth. This inability to manage fat leads to the often seen greasy and foul-smelling steatorrheic stools. When the newborn premature uses his glycogen stores he depends as usual on his body fat for energy; when food becomes available, he uses more calories from the carbohydrates and less from the fats than the term baby; thus, he resembles the fetus more in this respect since the fetus also depends on carbohydrates for its main source of energy.

The musculature of the bowel is weak and easily distended, so that there may be a tendency to constipation. Because of the thin abdominal wall, gastric peristalsis is seen; if distention is present, intestinal peristalsis also becomes visible.

URINARY SYSTEM. In comparison to the normal newborn, the premature's renal function is impaired. Since the kidney tubules continue to be formed until term, the premature's kidneys are poorly developed. Thus, he cannot concentrate his urine well (which becomes important when he suffers from conditions involving an excessive water loss such as diarrhea or vomiting) and he is unable to excrete sodium and chloride well with resultant early water retention and edema. It is believed by many that the tendency to a more marked and prolonged acidosis in the newly born premature and his inability to excrete many drugs is probably due to the relatively poor development of the kidneys. Low pH levels (normal is 7.42) are regularly found in apparently healthy immature infants, and are not considered dangerous unless accompanied by conditions such as respiratory distress, vomiting or diarrhea.

Urination is scanty and infrequent for a few days after birth, due to the small amount of fluid that is usually administered. Urates are commonly present in some excess, thus giving a false positive for albumin by heat, acetic acid or trichloracetic acid tests.

HEPATIC SYSTEM. The liver is relatively large but its function is poorly developed in smaller infants. This immaturity of the liver predisposes to jaundice (see p. 565) because of the inability of the liver to conjugate and excrete bilirubin. It has also been suggested that the low blood sugar found in the premature is hepatogenic, due to small liver glycogen stores. Lower serum protein levels, deficiency of blood clotting factors, and the deficient conjugation and detoxification of certain drugs are all attributed to liver immaturity.

Physical care of the infant

Often, the first hours of the small-for-gestational-age or premature infant's life will determine the outcome. These babies need warmth, meticulous physical care, gentle handling, precise and careful feeding and protection from infection. Born either before the body systems have had enough time to develop and mature appropriately, or of a suboptimal uterine environment which has caused growth retardation, these infants must fight against almost insurmountable odds to make a viable adjustment to extrauterine life. The nurse is a key person in assisting these babies to maximize their resources in the struggle to live and grow, and in preventing the development of external complications which would further jeopardize their chances.

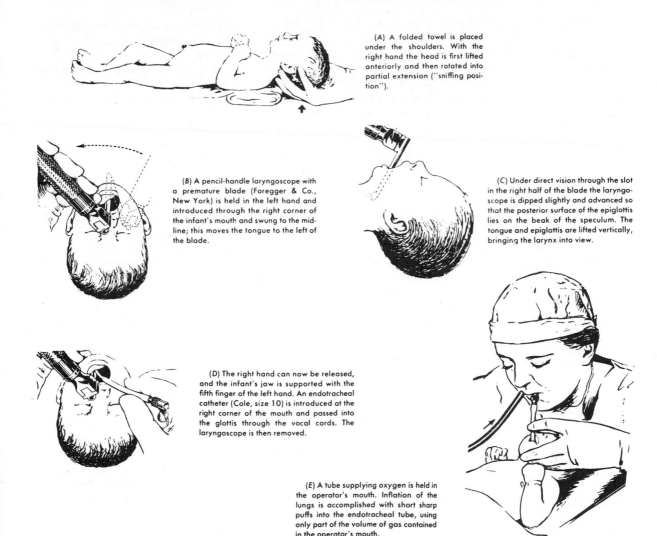

(A) A folded towel is placed under the shoulders. With the right hand the head is first lifted anteriorly and then rotated into partial extension ("sniffing position").

(B) A pencil-handle laryngoscope with a premature blade (Foregger & Co., New York) is held in the left hand and introduced through the right corner of the infant's mouth and swung to the midline; this moves the tongue to the left of the blade.

(C) Under direct vision through the slot in the right half of the blade the laryngoscope is dipped slightly and advanced so that the posterior surface of the epiglottis lies on the beak of the speculum. The tongue and epiglottis are lifted vertically, bringing the larynx into view.

(D) The right hand can now be released, and the infant's jaw is supported with the fifth finger of the left hand. An endotracheal catheter (Cole, size 10) is introduced at the right corner of the mouth and passed into the glottis through the vocal cords. The laryngoscope is then removed.

(E) A tube supplying oxygen is held in the operator's mouth. Inflation of the lungs is accomplished with short sharp puffs into the endotracheal tube, using only part of the volume of gas contained in the operator's mouth.

Figure 28-6. Technique of mouth-to-tube resuscitation. (Silverman, W. A.: Dunham's Premature Infants, p. 97, New York, Harper & Row, 1961)

Immediate care

Since these infants come into the world "before their time," and under adverse conditions, it is often the nurse's duty to assist with the delivery and/or the care immediately after the delivery. Even if the delivery has been effected under aseptic conditions, the care given a premature or small-for-dates infant may differ from that given to the full-size baby, depending on his condition. For the very small and feeble premature baby, the urgency of providing immediate warmth, humidity and oxygen as indicated may precede the care of the eyes and completion of the care of the cord. Moreover, the premature is often one of a multiple birth; also, his birth is often accompanied by pre-mature separation of the placenta, hemorrhage and other disorders; thus his delivery complicates the mother's safety as well as his own. Teamwork, that is, the combined efforts and skill of the obstetrician, pediatrician, anesthesiologist and nurse, is essential.

Whenever possible, the doctor will wait until the cord pulsation weakens before clamping it, so that the baby will benefit from the placental blood. The cord will be clamped or tied with special care because of the softness of the tissue, and often left longer to facilitate umbilical infusion. The cord should be inspected at frequent intervals for bleeding, because of the increased incidence of secondary hemorrhage. If a high-risk birth is anticipated, the pediatrician and anesthesiologist are usually notified to assist in their special areas. In almost all of these deliveries general anesthesia is contra-indicated because high-risk infants are so easily depressed by anesthetic and analgesic drugs. Therefore, the more specialized talents of the anesthesiologist are often required, and he will also attend to any resuscitation needs of the infant, leaving the obstetrician free to attend the mother. Direct laryngoscopy, tracheal aspiration, intubation and mouth to tube insufflation have all been used. If there is any rule of thumb, it is "do only what has to be done" since the more manipulation, instruments, etc. that are introduced, the more danger there is with respect to injury and infection. In flaccid infants the tongue may lie against the pharyngeal wall and obstruct the airway. After the airway is cleared of foreign material, the head is extended and a small-sized pharyngeal airway is inserted which often corrects the obstruction. If spontaneous respiration does not immediately occur, the lungs are inflated (Fig. 28-6). If the mouth-to-tube technique has been used, then antibiotics are generally instituted to guard against infection. Care must be exerted to prevent injury of small premature infants during resuscitation. Injudicious squeezing of the chest and abdomen (see Chapter 29) may result in multiple rib fractures or subcapsular hemorrhage of the liver. Various types of drugs have been used to aid in establishing and/or maintaining respiration. The opiate antagonists (N-allylnormorphine) have been effective when given to mothers who have had large doses of opiates. There was a significant reduction in the time required to establish respiration and in the need for resuscitation in the babies. Some physicians inject N-allylnormorphine in an isotonic saline solution directly into the umbilical vein of the depressed infant with satisfactory results. It is stressed, however, that depression may be deepened if the apnea is due to other causes; therefore, great caution is used with these drugs. Various respiratory stimulants including nikethamide, alphalobeline, picrotoxin, and even caffeine sodium benzoate have been found to exert little or no significant effect on alleviating depression. Some physicians give sodium bicarbonate to depressed infants who have not responded to initial oxygen therapy. This is to alkalize the probable acidotic condition engendered by depression of respiration; heart action and blood flow through the lungs are thereby improved. The nurse will be responsible for collecting all materials and equipment and assisting the physicians in any manipulations of them (or the infant) that are required. She or he will also be responsible for notifying the various physicians and units of the high-risk infant's impending arrival. Critical observation of the infant before, during and after any procedures is especially important at this time. The completion of necessary recording is to be accomplished quickly since early transfer of the infant is usually requested.

Since high-risk babies are more susceptible to infections, asepsis is imperative. However, if the infant's condition is very labile and/or critical, the installation of prophylactic eyedrops may have to be deferred until his condition stabilizes; in these cases, the eyes can be wiped with moist sterile gauze. These infants are usually placed in the supine position with the shoulders elevated so that the abdomen is lower than the thorax. This is accomplished by placing a folded towel under the shoulders and back. It is thought that this position prevents the voluminous liver from being forced back by gravity to impinge upon the dome of the diaphragm, thus reducing respiratory capacity (Fig. 28-7).

The maintenance of body temperature is essential. The high-risk infant's temperature tends to fall even more precipitously than the normal infant's at birth, because of his poor heat-regulating ability. Therefore the baby should be wrapped in a warmed blanket and placed in a warm environment (90 to 92° F.) or under radiant overhead heat. This attention to warmth must be continued even while resuscitation is being performed. After any immediate resuscitation efforts are concluded, the infant is generally transferred as quickly as possible to the high-risk unit to insure a proper environment. The usual weighing, temperature taking, thorough physical examination, and eye prophylaxis are generally delayed until the infant is transferred to the nursery. Obvious congenital anomalies can be noted before the infant is transferred.

Continuing care

Because of the magnitude of the high-risk problem, special nurseries and referral centers have developed for these infants in many urban areas. Space is usually allotted in the hospital separate from the term newborn nursery. In some cities, there is a large neonatal intensive care nursery (NICN) located in a medical cen-

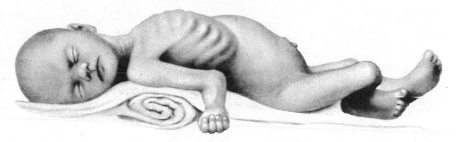

Figure 28-7. The position for premature infants recommended by Rossier. With the infant supine, a folded towel is placed under the back so that the abdomen is at a lower level than the thorax. In this position the neck is in slightly hyperextension.

ter. When these infants must be moved from a hospital to a center or from a rural area to a hospital, effort is made whenever possible for safe transport to and from the hospital. A special transport incubator designed to maintain temperature and administer oxygen is generally used. It is strongly advised that the nurse who accompanies the infant be trained in resuscitative techniques.

As with initial care, continuing care revolves around maintaining temperature, preventing infection, and maintaining respiration and nutrition of the infant.

NEONATAL INTENSIVE CARE NURSERY. These special nurseries, developed to provide highly skilled nursing and medical care to high-risk and sick neonates, require extensive and complicated equipment. Such life-support devices include reverse-isolation type incubators, radiant heaters, ECG-respiration-blood pressure monitors, head hoods, oxygen/air ratio controllers, oxygen analyzers, mechanical ventilators, heated nebulizers, infusion pumps, phototherapy units, and amplifying stethoscopes. The care and management of these machines present as great a problem as the treatment of the patients. It is necessary to have technicians who can maintain this "hardware" in the intensive care nursery as well as other special units throughout the hospital. Nurses should be free from the need to "nurse the equipment" because the critical condition of their tiny patients requires constant attention and full utilization of their special skills and knowledge.[8]

TEMPERATURE MAINTENANCE. Many babies have subnormal temperatures, sometimes as low as 90° F., when they arrive at the intensive care nursery. Bringing their temperature to normal and maintaining it is extremely important, as high-risk infants whose temperatures are kept between 97 and 98° F. from birth have significantly higher survival rates.

It is important to remember that these infants increase their heat production in cooler environments; this requires more oxygen, which places an added and at times an impossible burden on the already immature and often diseased lungs.

The high-risk infant's body temperature as well as his respiration is maintained in the artificial environment of the incubator, or as it is sometimes called, the Isolette. The modern air-conditioned Isolette is a miniature room in which the infant can live and be cared for under ideal conditions (i.e., desirable levels of heat, humidity and oxygen). As the infant matures, he will have less need for all three of the above in such exacting measured quantities; finally he will progress to a crib. There are several kinds of incubators currently in use, but the principle is the same, the differences being in the special construction details developed by various manufacturers. The nurse will want to familiarize herself with them since she will have a major responsibility in checking and maintaining the previously mentioned levels.

Modern incubators have controls on the outside of the unit to regulate the environment accurately and to adjust the bed from the horizontal to the tilted positions (Trendelenburg and reverse-Trendelenburg positions) to facilitate treatments and care. Some have the "Servo-Control" to automatically adjust to needed temperature and humidity settings by means of an automatic sensing device (thermistor) attached to the infant's skin. Special oxygen inlets provide adjustable oxygen concentrations (30 to 40 percent is the usual recommended "maintenance" flow). Regardless of these built-in sensors, the nurse will want to check and record the oxygen concentration with a reliable oximeter (oxygen analyzer) placed at the level of the infant's nose; a similar device can be used to ascertain the humidity level. When oxygen therapy is no longer required, the incubator can be ventilated with fresh air from the

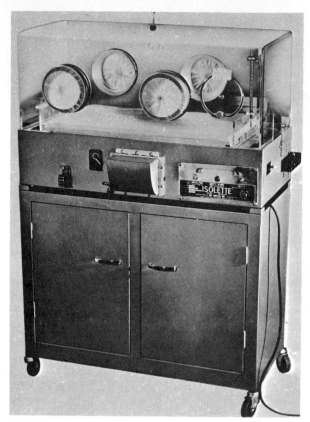

Figure 28-8. The Isolette incubator. (Air-Shields Inc., Hatboro, Pennsylvania)

room through a large, replaceable air filter or through an outside air attachment. Humidity can be controlled, and, by means of a nebulizer, supersaturated atmosphere can be created. Constant temperatures within the incubator can be regulated and maintained with a double-thermoswitch-controlled, sealed heating unit. Other features which are nonetheless important to the nurse are that these incubators are so designed that the infant can be observed from all sides through transparent windows. Moreover, hand holes with air-tight doors and self-adjusting "sleeves" permit the nurses and the physicians to care for the infant without disturbing the atmospheric conditions. The incubators are made of stainless steel and plastic and constructed for easy removal of all essential parts, without tools, to permit proper cleansing and sterilizing (Fig. 28-8).

The unit is usually preset at a skin temperature of 97° F. (98.6° F. rectally). As the baby's temperature rises, that of the Isolette decreases. When skin temperature of the infant reaches 97° F., the Isolette temperature is maintained at this setting. The baby's extremities may be wrapped with 4 x 4 gauze and Kerlix bandages for retention of body heat.

PREVENTION OF INFECTION. Even though the Isolette provides a more or less ideal environment, solicitous care must still be taken. The maintenance of asepsis in every detail must be maintained for these fragile babies. Scrupulous hand washing and gowning technique is to be observed. Personnel are also cautioned to avoid contact with sources of infection which might be transferred to the babies. There are usually special nursery gowns which will be worn when one is assuming care of these infants. The gowning procedure will vary from institution to institution but the underlying principle will be to keep as clean as possible anything that comes in contact with the high-risk infant. Masks are infrequently used in modern care as they have been found to harbor a rich source of contamination since moisture and bacteria from the nasopharynx collect in the mask folds, and even ordinary conversation distributes the infectious contents throughout the environment.

Ancillary personnel assume the task of cleaning incubators, respirators and suction equipment. All equipment is to be cultured after cleaning. Incubators that are in use are often cultured once a week and changed immediately if any bacterial growth is present. For long-term patients, it is well to change incubators once a week. For additional prophylaxis, a culture plate can be placed in each Isolette unit for two hours per day, and if any growth occurs the baby can be transferred to clean equipment.

MAINTAINING RESPIRATION. As previously stated, the establishment and maintenance of respiration is one of most critical import for these infants, and it is the nurse's responsibility to make careful, frequent observations and precise verbal and written recordings. It has been demonstrated that the first five minutes of life are crucial for the later successful outcome of the infant with respect to respiratory depression. Infants with unimproved respiratory function after these five minutes have a four times greater chance of dying in the first days than those infants whose condition improves or is good during this time. A majority of premature infants must receive oxygen initially because of respiratory depression or cyanosis or concurrent pathologic conditions such as hemorrhage or erythroblastosis. Oxygen therapy is often a life-saving measure for the infant, but it must be used judiciously and is to be administered at the lowest concentration compatible with life, since the oxygen requirements for these infants will vary according to weight, maturity and general condition of morbidity. If an incubator is not immediately available at birth (and respiratory difficulties are present) after necessary suctioning, the infant may be given oxygen by mask which is placed over the nose and mouth. This is to be considered a temporary emergency measure, and is to be removed promptly when the crisis is over and/or an incubator becomes available. The flow of oxygen can be set at a *maximum* of 3 liters when this method is used. When the premature infant is in an incubator, the lowest oxygen *concentration* to relieve the respiratory symptoms is to be employed; oxygen should not be ordered by liter flow when the incubator is utilized. Occasionally, higher concentrations (near 100 percent) may have to be employed to relieve general cyanosis or other conditions, but hourly reductions in the oxygen concentration must be carried out after these needs are met, to decrease any overoxygenation in the arterial blood of the infant.

Treatment of Respiratory Distress. If an infant is experiencing respiratory distress upon arrival at the intensive care nursery, he is placed in an Isolette and immediate assistance in breathing is given by means of "bagging." In this technique, a special plastic bag inflated with moist warm oxygen is placed over the infant's head and tied around his neck. A small roll can be placed under the shoulders to hyperextend the neck and provide a more efficient airway. Under constant surveillance, an umbilical catheter is inserted by the physician to obtain arterial blood for gas studies. Intra-arterial fluids may be administered via infusion pump, and periodic blood gas studies are done to determine the oxygen pressure (Po_2). Oxygen administered to the infant is adjusted according to arterial oxygen pressures. The pH and bicarbonate levels are also determined, and sodium bicarbonate may be used to correct acidosis.

The infant's extremities must be restrained during these procedures, and while the umbilical arterial catheter is in place. If the catheter should be displaced, severe hemorrhage may result. Respiratory and cardiac monitors are connected to these babies, with hourly recording of vital signs, temperature of bag oxygen and incubator, and oxygen concentration. If the infant cannot maintain respirations after a reasonable amount of bagging, he may be placed on a respirator. This is usually a grave sign, for most infants placed on the respirator do not survive. Antibiotics are started when the umbilical catheter is inserted and continued for two days after its removal. The dosage is determined according to the infant's weight.[9]

Retrolental fibroplasia is one of the inherent dangers of high arterial concentrations of oxygen (see Chapter 29). It has been demonstrated that there is a relationship between the prolonged use of relatively high concentrations (40 percent or more) of oxygen and the occurrence of this disease, which causes blindness in the premature infant (but not in the term infant). The high concentrations of oxygen cause arterial spasm of the fragile, still developing retinal vessels of the infant. The spasm is followed by obliteration and later by neovascularization, hemorrhage and retinal detachment. These processes produce the dense, fibrous tissue from which the disease takes its name. The premature (and not the term) infant is so susceptible to high oxygen concentrations because of the immaturity of his retinal development. By 24 weeks gestational age, the retinal vessels have grown about 6 mm. from the optic nerve. Between 24 and 30 weeks no further growth occurs ("immature" fundus); after this time, however, growth again begins ("transitional" fundus). By about 34 weeks (weight 4 lbs. 6 oz. or 2,000 Gm.) the fundus is usually mature. During the "immature" and "transitional" developmental stages of the fundus, infants are liable to become victims of the disease, when injudicious concentrations of oxygen are employed which initiate the above pathologic process; hence the preponderance of this disease among the very early gestational age and very low birth weight infants. Again, the nurse is responsible for seeing that the appropriate concentration is maintained.

Respiratory Patterns. The most common respiratory rhythm of a quiet, larger healthy premature is the steady cogwheel type, with no pause between inspiration and expiration; the next most common is the so-called adult rhythm with its inspiration, expiration pause. Other patterns such as inspiration-pause-expiration also occur. Sighs that interrupt the regular pattern are common and a sigh is often followed by an apneic pause. Periodic breathing, consisting of two or more periods of breathing per minute separated by an apneic pause of three seconds or more is more common among the small infants. Many authorities consider that anything that increases the minute volume of respiration reduces the incidence of this type of respiration.

"Normal" respiratory rates are difficult to determine since it is difficult to define the "normal" premature and the "normal" conditions under which they prevail. Two patterns have been associated with a low mortality rate and have thus been described as "normal." In the first pattern about 40 respirations per minute occur from birth onward without any significant fluctuations. In the second pattern rates over 60 respirations per minute occur in the first hour, with no significant increase, and subsequently decline. A significant increase is 15 or more respirations per minute above the average rate obtained in the first hour after birth.

The following patterns are always abnormal in the healthy term infant; so too in the premature but they are more expected because of the premature's developmental deficits. Simple retraction may be seen, in which the chest and abdomen rise together, with a slight indentation over the sternal area. When this occurs, the nurse knows that observations must be increased and sharpened. This pattern is a warning sign and the physician may want to be alerted. Paradoxical breathing is considered a critical condition; the abdomen rises while the chest sinks. There is a marked chin lag and an audible respiratory grunt, indicating respiratory distress. The nurse will want to alert the physician, and keep him informed of any progress in the condition. This will mean exacting observation and frequent reporting.

Prolonged apnea (which is different from the periodic apnea discussed above) often occurs in cases of respiratory distress syndrome (see Chapter 29), as well as other pathologic conditions such as infection, pneumonia and central nervous system injuries. Treatment usually consists of positive pressure oxygen therapy, and it goes without saying that these babies must have continuous observation since these spells are often repeated.

The nurse will also want to regulate other procedures such as bathing and weighing, to conserve the infant's strength and prevent apnea from sheer exhaustion. She will also want to position the infant in a lateral Sims's position or the supine position previously recommended to prevent mucus from reaching and remaining in the lungs. Changing position every two to three hours also aids in ventilating the lungs.

MAINTAINING NUTRITION. There is increasing evidence that delaying food and water in low birth weight infants lessens their chances for normal growth and development. Early feeding of these infants is associated with a reduced incidence of hyperbilirubinemia and symptomatic hypoglycemia. The nutritional requirements of low birth weight infants are higher in calories per unit of body weight than normal infants, because their growth is more comparable to that of a fetus. During the first few days, most of these babies will need intravenous infusion of a 10 percent glucose solution with appropriate electrolytes. Caloric requirements range from 110 to 140 calories per kg. of body weight per day, depending upon maturity of the infant. Protein intake should be about 3 to 4 Gm. per kg. per day, and 40 percent of the calories should be supplied by carbohydrates.

Extremely immature infants are usually given intravenous feedings. If the infant is somewhat more mature and healthy, oral feeding may start 6 to 12 hours after birth. A bottle with a soft nipple can be used if the infant is able to suck efficiently; if not intermittent gavage is recommended. Breast-feeding may be tried for infants of 36 weeks gestational age or when a similar level of maturity is reached.[10]

In planning the feeding schedule for the premature and low birth weight infant, it is important to establish a food tolerance, since the intestinal tract (as well as other organs) is underdeveloped. The caloric needs of the low birth weight baby are estimated according to the body weight. At first, the feeding should be in small amounts and then increased gradually to the amount that will produce a consistent gain, since vomiting and consequent aspiration, distention and diarrhea may be due to overfeeding. Early and more nearly optimal feeding in the case of the larger infant will contribute to lessen mortality and morbidity by preventing nutritive depletion and maintaining biochemical homeostasis.

Those infants in good condition (these are usually but not always the larger infants) with active peristalsis may be started on oral 5 to 10 percent glucose water 6 to 12 hours after birth. For the infant in poor condition, no matter what the cause, oral feedings are usually withheld for several days if necessary and

| | | Volume Ranges | | | |
| | | ml./kg./day | | ml./lb./day | |
Formula	Age (in days)	Immature*	Undergrown*	Immature	Undergrown
10% glucose	0	20	30	9	14
Half, 10% glucose and half, full-strength	1	30	45	14	20
	2	40	60	18	26
	3	50	75	22	32
	4	60	90	26	40
	5	70	105	30	48
Full-strength formula (24 cal. per 30 ml.)	6	80	120	35	55
	7	90	135	40	60
	8	100	150	45	70
	9				
	10	110	160	50	75
	12	120	160	55	75
	15	130	160	60	75
	20	140	160	65	75

1. The volume ranges allow a choice of feeding amounts. Most premature infants are more safely fed in the lower ranges. *Supplemental parenteral fluids will be necessary if dehydration, lethargy, or excessive weight loss occurs.*
2. Multiply infant's weight (kg. or lb.) by volume to be given for that day and divide by twelve (number of feedings) for amount to be fed at 2-hour intervals.
3. Infants on reaching 1.5 kg. (3 lb. 5 oz.) should be placed gradually on a 3-hour feeding schedule (total volume given, divided by eight feedings).
4. Infants on the bottle and on reaching 1.8 to 2 kg. (4 to 4½ lb.) may be fed on a modified demand basis and at increased feeding intervals.
5. Volume taken may range *above* 200 ml. per kg. (90 ml. per lb.).

Exceptions:
1. Infants in poor condition *for any reason* require a delay in oral feedings and the institution of parenteral fluids *from the first few hours of life.*
2. Any baby with distention, cyanotic or apneic attacks, or vomiting should have his feedings stopped and condition evaluated.
3. A stomach residual (at the time of the next gavage feeding) of over 1 ml. indicates a delay in emptying time. Feedings should be reduced and the event reported to physician for evaluation.
4. Malnourished infants require glucose and water soon after birth to support brain metabolism, due to deficient glycogen stores in liver.

* *Immature* refers to the very small, weak, and hypotonic premature infant. *Undergrown* infants are those who are small for their gestational age, with a greater need for calories.
Source: Babson, S. G., and Benson, R. C.: Primer on Prematurity and High-risk Pregnancy. St. Louis, Mosby, 1966.

parenteral fluids instituted. If the infant is fed orally some physicians begin the infant on a trial of plain water; if it is retained, then glucose water or dilute modified cow's milk formula is instituted at two-hour intervals. Some physicians begin with 5 to 10 percent glucose water. Thus, there is a gradual replacement of water feedings by milk feedings, and a gradual increase in the amounts of milk and water at each feeding until caloric and fluid requirements are met. If an infant is taking about 180 ml. of full-strength modified cow's milk formula per kilogram of body weight per day, then he is getting about 120 calories per kilogram per day which ensures an adequate weight gain (Table 28-4).

Some physicians still prefer breast milk as the feeding of choice; unless the infant is vigorous, it is difficult to manage him on this type of feeding since there are very few mother's milk banks in this country, and it is often difficult for the mother to manually express enough milk for her baby's needs. A modified cow's milk formula has been found most effective as an all-around diet to supply nutritional requirements in the form and proportions that the premature can readily handle.

Prematures who weigh 3 pounds or less may be fed every two or three hours. Infants who weigh over 3½ pounds may be placed on a four-hour feeding schedule. In addition to the feedings, the diets usually include vitamin and iron preparations. These additions are introduced when the feeding and schedule are fairly

the high-risk infant: low birth weight and premature   573

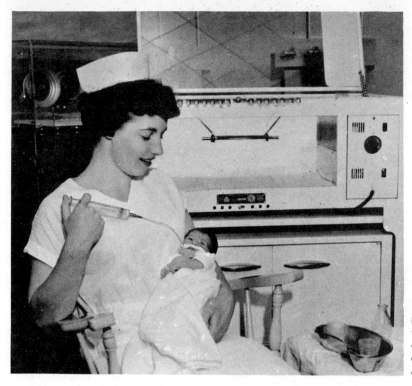

Figure 28-9. Gavage feeding. When the premature infant does not require oxygen, the nurse can take him out of the incubator and hold him as she feeds him. (Babies and Childrens Hospital, The University Hospitals of Cleveland, Cleveland, Ohio)

well established, and the infant is able to tolerate them. The stomach of the premature baby needs rest between feedings as much as that of the full-term baby; therefore, the interval should be regulated accordingly. The schedule should be as near that of a normal infant as is compatible with his progress.

When a very small and weak infant is on a two- to three-hour feeding schedule, gavage feeding is usually indicated (Fig. 28-9). More recently, the indwelling catheters have not been recommended because mucus is produced which can block the airway in the weak premature; also, purulent rhinitis and conjunctivitis may develop even with frequent tube changing; finally, the tube partially obstructs the airway. In addition, dropper feeding is not recommended because the swallowing reflex may be weak and easily fatigued, with a chance of overflow and aspiration. Also considerable skill is required in controlling the volume and speed of release of feedings.

Feeding responsibilities are the nurse's, and often she must pass the nasogastric tube as well. When gavage feeding is instituted, a French catheter no. 8 is introduced through the mouth; the distance is measured from the nose to the xiphoid process and is marked on the catheter. The infant is observed for any choking or gasping, which indicates the possibility of tracheal entry. The open end of the gavage tube can be inserted into a container of sterile water and if bubbles appear, then it is certain that the tube is in the trachea. The tube then must be removed and inserted properly. When the catheter is correctly placed, the tube is aspirated gently with a syringe; if a feeding residual of up to 1 ml. is returned, then the amount of the feeding is decreased by that amount. The residual need not be discarded; it can be fed as part of the new feeding. The nurse reports a residual of 1 ml. or more and skips that feeding. After checking the formula to determine correct temperature (tepid), the nurse will pour the formula through the barrel of the syringe; the milk is allowed to run slowly, with no pressure and minimal elevation of the syringe. During the feeding the infant is supported in a semireclining position. If the infant requires oxygen, he will be fed in the incubator. After the feeding, the infant is replaced in the incubator, and positioned with his head and shoulders slightly elevated, unless the physician prefers, and so specifies, another position. The larger infants may be placed on the abdomen or on the right side to facilitate emptying of the stomach. These positions guard against regurgitation and aspiration.

Bottle-feeding requires that the infant have a good sucking and swallowing reflex which may take days or weeks to develop. The baby will indicate his readiness for the bottle by consistently sucking on the gavage tubing. When bottle feeding is instituted, the time of feeding is not to exceed 15 minutes as this will tire the baby too much. A soft, average sized nipple with an adequate opening is used. The nurse can help the infant open his mouth to accept the nipple by applying gentle pressure on the infant's chin and touching his lips with the nipple. Again, the infant is held in the semierect position to facilitate "burping" and nursing. After the feeding he is positioned as described above. There are several precautions that the nurse will want to be aware of. The infant is not to be urged to accept more formula than is easily taken. Moreover, the bottle should be removed if the infant appears to be getting the milk too fast; in this case the infant will usually gasp, choke, or swallow so quickly as to interfere with his respirations. Any infant who shows reluctance to eat on two successive occasions will need critical reassessment. Feedings are to be discontinued if the baby vomits, becomes cyanotic, overdistends or develops frequent or diarrhea stools. Feedings should also be discontinued if there is 1 ml. or more of residual; again, the infant needs reevaluation. Finally, the bottle of the premature is never to be propped. Any change of feeding habits in these infants is critical and *may be the first sign of illness.*

The other necessary care of the infant such as temperature taking, weighing, bathing, and dressing (if required) is usually done in conjunction with the feeding periods so that the infant may rest without interference at the other times. The nurse will want to gather any materials needed and plan care carefully. Frequently entering the incubator is not in the interests of good aseptic technique and, of course, is very tiring to the infant.

The skin is extremely delicate and tender; and if diapers are used, they should be changed as soon as they become wet or soiled. Sometimes only a small pad is placed under the baby. Indeed, no clothing is really needed because of the controlled environment of the incubator.

Each institution will have its particular procedures for routine care in the intensive care nursery, but the principles are the same as those involved in attending the normal newborn.

Care of the mother and father

The parents of high-risk newborns often have adaptational needs or problems which necessitate sensitive and thoughtful nursing care. Not only are they making the transition to new parenthood with all its requirements, but they must cope with the unusual situation of a small, different and often sick baby. The importance of the early postpartum period for establishment of bonds between parents and the newborn, and for laying the groundwork for healthy attitudes toward future relationships with the child, must not be underestimated.

Maternal-infant attachment

The process of attachment, or bonding, between mothers and their babies has received considerable attention in the last several years. Behavioral studies in humans and animals indicate that the events immediately before and following delivery probably have a great influence on later maternal interaction with the young. Animal studies have shown species-specific maternal behavior patterns preceding and following birth which are essential for normal mothering to occur. If these patterns are interrupted, there is often severe distortion of mothering to such an extent that the offspring may not survive. Anthropological research among numerous human cultures found that every society exhibited some regularized manner of dealing with the entry of a new member, usually by secluding mother and infant and relieving the mother of other duties for a certain period of time. In light of this data, it is of particular interest that the routine complete separation of mother and infant in the first days after delivery occurs only in the high-risk and neonatal intensive care nurseries of the Western world.[11]

PRENATAL AND INTRAPARTAL PERIOD. A woman's own childhood experiences, how she herself was mothered, and a myriad of complex factors undoubtedly have significant influence upon how pregnancy is approached and the meanings of impending motherhood. Pregnancy is considered as a maturational process, with a series of adaptive tasks, each dependent upon completion of the preceding one. Although many women are initially upset and may experience grief and anger when they first become pregnant, these feelings usually resolve by the end of the first trimester, and pregnancy is accepted. During this stage, the mother identifies the growing fetus as an integral part of herself. The next stage arises when fetal movement initiates a process of thinking of the fetus as a separate individual, and the woman begins to fantasize about what the baby will be like and attributes to it certain physical and personality characteristics. Now there is further acceptance of the pregnancy, and usually anticipation of caretaking by making plans for the infant, selecting a name, purchasing clothes or a crib, or arranging a place in the home.[12] The steps in attachment, all of which are felt to be essential for healthy mother-infant bonding to occur, have been identified as follows: [13]

Planning the pregnancy;
Confirming the pregnancy;
Accepting the pregnancy;
Positive response to fetal movement;
Accepting the fetus as an individual;
Birth experience;
Seeing the baby;
Touching the baby;
Caretaking.

Although little data are available on the impact of the labor and delivery process upon monther-infant bonding, it has been suggested that certain experiences during labor, such as the nature and extent of touching the mother receives, are important to her subsequent ability to touch and care for her baby. While unconsciousness during delivery does not seem to result in rejection of the infant, mothers who are relaxed, have good rapport with attendants and receive support during labor tend to be more pleased with their infants on first sight.

EARLY POSTPARTUM PERIOD. During initial contacts with their babies after delivery, human mothers appear to have a routine behavior pattern, as do other animal species. When presented with their nude, full-term infant, mothers begin with fingertip touching of the infant's extremities and within a few minutes proceed to massaging, encompassing palm contact of the infant's trunk. Mothers of premature infants also follow this sequence, although they proceed more slowly. The "en face" position, in which the mother seeks eye-to-eye contact with the infant by moving her head so her eyes and those of the infant meet fully in the same horizontal plane, occurs during early contact among mothers of both full-term and premature babies. It has been suggested that eye-to-eye contact may initiate or release maternal caretaking responses. Interestingly, the time the mother seeks this eye contact coincides with the early functional development of the infant's visual pathways. In the newborn period, those maternal affectional ties which have developed during pregnancy and immediately postpartum can be easily disturbed by such minor problems as poor feeding and mild respiratory distress, and perhaps affected permanently.[14]

Interactional Deprivation. Prolonged mother-infant separation, such as is routine practice in most premature and high-risk nurseries, is currently under investigation for its effects on attachment. Shortly after the infant's birth, the mothers in the early contact group are admitted into the nursery and encouraged to touch and to perform such caretaking duties as the infant's condition allows. Mothers in the late contact group are not permitted into the nursery until after their infants reach almost one month of age. Results to date reveal detectable differences in mothering performance between these two groups. In one study, high contact mothers had higher scores on an attachment interview, maternal performance, "en face" feeding and the amount of fondling of infants when tested one month after delivery.[15] In another study comparing late and early contact mothers one month after discharge of the infants, and after 200 feedings at home, the late contact mothers held their babies differently, changed positions and burped less, and were not as skillful in feeding.[16] Some mothers who were barred from interaction with their babies in the nursery resumed prior interests when then returned home, and the babies had to compete with these interests when they were discharged. The possible implications of such studies suggest that prolonged separation may adversely affect commitment or attachment between mother and infant, reduce confidence in mothering abilities, and detract from the mother's ability to develop an efficient routine of care. When mothers were allowed into the high-risk nursery for early and frequent contact and caretaking of their infants, there was no increase in nursery infections or disruption of nursery routine.[17]

Modifying hospital routine to allow mothers early contact with their high-risk infants appears to alter later maternal behavior positively. This lends support to the concept of a sensitive time for bonding to occur between the human mother and her infant. This time is probably within the first several hours of delivery. Greater maternal attentiveness and better caretaking seem related to later exploratory behavior in infants; thus, removing barriers to maternal attachment during the sensitive period may have a potent influence on the later development of these babies.

Paternal-infant attachment

Fathers have been observed to go through the same series of behaviors when first touching and handling their newborn infants as previously described for mothers. In one study, when fathers had access to infants or saw the child first, their affection for the baby was initially stronger than the mother's, although her affection increased when she was later allowed to provide care.[18] The nature of the man's tie to his child is little understood and less studied. Paternal motivations for procreation have variously been described as ranging from a desire for immortality to a reaffirmation of masculinity, but these fail to explain the caring or affectional bond which develops. Among humans, with their long-term pairing and relatively permanent relationships, there is, no doubt, some species-specific process by which father-infant attachment takes place. This is an area requiring much more investigation.

Parental reactions and psychologic tasks

The birth of a premature or high-risk infant is often experienced as an acute emotional crisis by the family. This causes a certain amount of disorganization in the parents before they are able to master their feelings and come to accept the event. Since the baby may be born before term, parents often are deprived of the last six to eight weeks in which the final psychologic (and sometimes material) preparation for the birth is made. Few of the physical and emotional signs of approaching labor (enumerated in Chapter 18) may happen. These are helpful to the mother in alerting her to the near approach of another new phase in the childbearing process, and this awareness in turn assists her in achieving psychologic preparation. The result, then may be a rather abrupt arrival of the infant, and the event may be surrounded by several anxiety-provoking features: an unattended delivery, a longer hospital stay for her baby and perhaps herself, separation of the infant and herself, and most heartrending

of all, a delicate infant who may be in danger of death.

Guilt feelings and a certain amount of grieving (see Chapter 29) in both parents are an invariable accompaniment. The parents ask themselves time and again such questions as: "What went wrong? What did we do? What made it happen? Can I really carry babies?" These guilt feelings and grief may be manifested in a variety of ways: general anger with the whole situation, self-deprecation, numerous complaints, blaming the spouse and/or attendants, insistent bids for reassurance and attention, profuse crying, or extreme quiet and immobilization. Loneliness is also a problem, for the mother may have no opportunity to see, hold, feed and examine her child as the other mothers have. We are all familiar with the wistful figure at the nursery window, gazing longingly through the glass, while the other mothers are occupied with feeding, changing and cuddling their infants. The loneliness continues when the parents go home without their infant, and because of the continued separation, the task of integrating the new member into the household is delayed. In addition, most mothers are concerned about whether they will be able to take adequate care of their babies when they do bring them home. The mother may still carry a picture of the frail infant surrounded by all the nursery paraphernalia and not realize that her baby will be reasonably mature when he is discharged from the hospital.

To cope with this concern, she may ask many questions while she is in the hospital and demand reassurance about the baby's condition; on the other hand, she may be quiet and uncommunicative, quite overwhelmed with the anticipated enormous responsibility. The economic drain on the finances cannot be overlooked, either; with medical and hospitalization expenses what they are today, the cost is considerable. Even for those who have adequate medical insurance, the maternity benefits are usually distressingly low. This, of course, adds to the general anxiety and strain of the situation.

The psychologic processes the parents generally go through after the birth of a premature or high-risk infant include:

Shock, disbelief and denial;
Anger and searching self and others for causes;
Grieving over loss of perfect fantasized infant;
Grieving over own inability to produce perfect infant;

Anticipatory worrying over loss of infant;
Initiation of contact with infant;
Belief and desire that infant will live;
Readiness to establish caretaking relationship.

SUPPORTIVE CARE. Although there is much that is specialized in the physical care activities for the premature infant, the mother's physical care remains generally the same as that for any normal postpartal course. Thus, the emphasis on care for these mothers is two-fold: 1) they need help to facilitate their emotional adjustment (this holds true for the father as well) and 2) they need help in preparing for the care of the infant when they bring him home.

The nurse can do much to strengthen the mother's ego by helping her work through her guilt feelings and grief and thus reinforce her concept of herself as an adequate, worthy person. To do this, the nurse must provide opportunities for the mother to ventilate her feelings and to question the situation. It is often difficult for the nurse to answer all the questions the mother and father ask her, especially if the prognosis for the baby is guarded. Yet, to avoid the questions or problems is to deprive the parents of a valuable avenue of coping with the problem. The fears and the fantasies engendered by not knowing are often worse than the facts, even though the facts are unfortunate. As the nurse listens to the mother and the father and reflects their concerns, they are helped to arrive at a clearer notion of the reality of the situation; thus they are able to separate fact from fancy and to work through to a more positive acceptance of their situation. The nurse can expect some negative feelings to be expressed, and the patient may go through a period of self-pity. An accepting, nonjudgmental attitude will help the patient to move to a more positive frame of mind.

Keeping the lines of communication open between the nursery staff and the patient is another useful supportive measure; the nurse on the postpartal unit can be prepared with the latest reports regarding the baby's condition, so that this information can be given to the parents. Especially when the mother cannot be taken to see her baby in the premature nursery, it is very helpful if the nurse in the premature unit can make regular visits to the mother on the ward to inform her of her infant's progress. If circumstances within the unit prevent this, contact with the mother by telephone may be substituted. This two-way communication between the floor and the nursery helps the patient to feel that everyone is "tuned in" on her situation and concerned about her. It also gives her the opportunity to know the personnel who are responsible for the care of her baby, and this is reassuring in itself.

When the mother is able, she can be allowed to visit the nursery at least to observe her baby for a time. Some mothers find this difficult at first, especially if the infant is very small and/or ill. It is a wise nurse who allows the mother to indicate her readiness for such visits and gives appropriate encouragement as the mother is able to face the situation and take more responsibility.

Before the mother comes to the nursery, it is best to describe all the equipment surrounding the infant, and what the baby will look like. The nurse's presence beside the mother when she first sees her baby permits answering any questions which might arise and provides support during this difficult period. If the infant is under the bilirubin light, it is important to remove the eye patches so the mother can see the baby's eyes.

All avenues of support are to be explored with the parents. If the mother seems to benefit from visitors or visiting with the other patients, then there need be no restriction of visiting privileges. There is no reason to isolate a mother in a room by herself (even if there has been a fetal demise) without ascertaining whether the mother needs to be alone for a time. If possible, the same nurse should be assigned to her care, for if the mother is to work through her feelings, she must have time to build a trust relationship, and this takes at least several encounters. Other personnel, such as the social worker, may be helpful if aid is needed financially, or strict budgeting is necessary. Another source of help that can prove invaluable is the public health or visiting nurse. The need for a referral for these patients and their infants should never be overlooked. Most patients are delighted to have someone to rely on during the first difficult days when they bring the baby home. Furthermore, some patients cannot make much progress during their short hospital stay in expressing their feelings and in working through the problem. Thus, they need a competent person when they return home to help them in this, as well as in making necessary arrangements in preparation for the baby's homecoming.

Some hospitals encourage mothers to return to the nursery to feed and care for their babies until such time as the infant's condition permits discharge. Of particular help would be a counseling program on feeding and psychologic aspects of care, which incorporates anticipatory guidance concerning the condition and the needs of the infant on arrival home. Coping with sibling rivalry also may be included. This approach is very helpful, for it alleviates some of the separation and loneliness between mother and child and later fosters self-reliance and confidence in the mother at home.

In implementing care, the nurse will want to remember that the advent of a high-risk birth is a crisis in itself; however, the parents may have to adjust to various related crises (e.g., a sudden, downward turn in the baby's condition, financial embarrassment, unexpected developments regarding other children and relatives, etc.). Nurses must be prepared to help the parents to deal with these as they arise, and to seek appropriate resources for them if the matter lies beyond their competence. Knowledge of the principles of communication and supportive care will be utilized here as they would be in any other crisis. Willingness and ability to allow the parents to ventilate and work through their feelings about the situation is of prime importance. The nurse is one of the key persons in the care of high-risk infants and their parents.

Growth and development

Growth and development of the premature are primarily dependent upon the degree of immaturity at birth. Much will depend on the ability of the infant to meet the conditions attendant at birth and to adjust to the changes in his new environment. The majority (about 65 percent) of prematures weigh between 2,000 and 2,500 Gm. Outcomes for these infants are good barring complications. An additional 20 percent weigh between 1,500 to 2,000 Gm. and if prompt good care is provided, they also have a chance of a good outcome. As birth weight decreases, chances of satisfactory growth and development also decrease, even though "survival" rates may be good. In general, infants who react well to prompt treatment and care make their adjustment usually by the end of the first year. Others may require several years to match the "normal" child at that age, and some, unfortunately, really never "catch up" in

various respects. Nearly all longitudinal studies indicate a continued difference in height and weight as compared with standard populations. Caution must be used in interpreting these findings, since these data may be confounded by the inclusion of children who show reduced growth as a result of central nervous system damage or deficiency, poor nutrition, or low birth weight with intrauterine growth retardation. When these children are excluded, few significant differences are found.

Recently attention has focused upon the effects of malnutrition on the growth of the brain. Although the issue is far from resolved, evidence suggests that malnutrition during the period of most rapid brain growth may be associated with permanent reduction in the total number of cells. Among humans, the critical period probably occurs during the last few months of pregnancy and the first few months after birth. Continuous malnutrition extending through pregnancy and the first several postnatal months could thus reduce the quantity of brain cells irrevocably and permanently impair intellectual functioning, if the above holds true.

This has special significance for the small-for-gestational-age infant whose intrauterine environment has obviously been impaired. Retardation of brain development in small-for-dates infants and the inability to catch up after birth because of postnatal malnutrition form the combination most likely to result in permanent brain impairment. Not all studies of undergrown infants reveal reduction in intelligence or mental retardation, however. Small-for-dates infants born into high socioeconomic group families were reported to have intellectual functioning as good as or better than their peers at ages 10 to 12 years, while small-for-dates infants of lower socioeconomic groups functioned below their matched peers.[19]

The implications of this suggestive data that malnutrition is a pervasive cause of subnormal mentality are profound. If malnutrition is accepted as being socially remediable, it is contingent upon societies and governments to take the necessary action to ensure adequate nutrition.

The integrity and functioning of the infant's nervous system and continued appropriate growth and development are of primary concern to parents, nurse and physician. In the absence of congenital abnormalities, the incidence of retardation and neurologic conditions such as cerebral palsy appears to be declining among infants discharged from neonatal intensive care nurseries. Nervous system disorders which may leave permanent sequelae are often secondary to metabolic, physical, infectious or environmental conditions. With increased knowledge in the field of neonatology and techniques and equipment to intervene effectively in these problems, early recognition and careful management can significantly reduce the number of permanent neurologic deficits.

The nurse is often asked by the parents if their premature or low birth weight baby will ever develop as well and become as strong and sturdy as a normal sized newborn. As we have seen, depending upon birth weight, the infant has a good chance of doing so. Although he may be slower in regaining his birth weight, he is likely to gain approximately the same amount of weight (i.e., an average gain of 13 to 15 pounds) as the full term infant during the first year. Individual variations occur, of course, but the developmental level achieved by the small premature infant during his first year generally will be lower than that expected for his chronologic age. For this reason, parents are encouraged to think of premature babies in terms of actual age since conception, which gives more realistic expectations for developmental level.

Parents of premature or low birth weight infants invariably need special guidance and support to help them develop confidence in their ability to care for their baby, particularly in anticipation of taking him home from the hospital. The nurse has a real responsibility to help them so that they are adequately prepared for the baby's homecoming.

Bibliography

1. Klaus, M. H., and Fanaroff, A. A.: *Care of the High-Risk Neonate.* Philadelphia, W. B. Saunders, 1973, pp. 37, 40, 26-27, 50, 98-102.
2. Korones, S. B.: *High-Risk Newborn Infants: The Basis for Intensive Nursing Care.* St. Louis: Mosby, 1972, p. 87.
3. Smith, C.: Prenatal and neonatal nutrition. *Pediatrics* 30:145, 1962.
4. Winick, M.: Cellular growth in intrauterine malnutrition. *Ped. Clin. North Am.* 17:69, 1970.
5. Klaus and Fanaroff, *op. cit.*
6. *Ibid.*
7. *Ibid.*
8. Silverman, W. A.: Intensive care of low birth weight and other at-risk infants. *Clin. Ob. and Gyn.* 13:87-106, Mar. 1970.
9. DeMarco, J. P., and Reed, R.: Care of the high-risk infant in the intensive care unit. *Nurs. Clin. North Am.* 5:375-386, Sept. 1970.
10. Babson, S. G.: Feeding the low birth weight infant. *Pediatrics* 79:694-701, Oct. 1971.
11. Klaus, M. H., and Kennell, J. H.: Mothers separated from their newborn infants. *Ped. Clin. North Am.* 17:1015-1037, Nov. 1970.
12. Bibring, G.: Some considerations of the psychological processes in pregnancy. *Psychoanal. Stud. Child* 14:113, 1959.
13. Kennel, J. H., and Klaus, M. H.: Care of the mother of the high-risk infant. *Clin. Ob. and Gyn.* 14:926, 1971.
14. *Ibid.*
15. Klaus, M. H., *et al:* Maternal attachment: Importance of the first postpartum days. *New Eng. J. Med.* 286:460, 1972.
16. Klaus and Kennell, *op. cit.*
17. Barnett, C., *et al:* Neonatal separation: The maternal side of interactional deprivation. *Pediatrics* 45:197, 1970.
18. *Ibid.*
19. Drillien, C.: The small-for-dates infant: Etiology and prognosis. *Ped. Clin. North Am.* 17:9, 1970.

Suggested Reading

Babson, S. G., and Benson, R. C.: *Primer on Prematurity and High-Risk Pregnancy.* St. Louis, Mosby, 1966.
Gunders, S., and Whiting, J. W. M.: Mother-infant separation and physical growth. *Ethnology* 7:196-206, Apr. 1968.
Kaplan, D. M., and Mason, E. A.: Maternal reactions to premature births viewed as an acute emotional disorder. *Am. J. Orthopsychiat.* 30:539, July 1960.
Scarr-Salapatek, S., and Williams, M. L.: A stimulation program for low birth weight infants. *Am. J. Pub. Health* 62:662-667, May 1972.
Powell, L. F.: The effect of extra stimulation and maternal involvement on the development of low birth weight infants and on maternal behavior. *Child Devel.* 45:106-113, Mar. 1974.
Warrick, L. H.: Family-centered care in the premature nursery. *Am. J. Nurs.* 71:2134-2138, Nov. 1971.
Wiener, G., and Milton, T.: Demographic correlates of low birth weight. *Am. J. Epidem.* 91:260-272, 1970.

the high-risk infant: disorders of the newborn

29

Parental and Staff Reactions to Defects and Disorders / Neonatal Respiratory Distress / Injuries / Infections / Malformations / Inborn Errors of Metabolism / Miscellaneous Disorders

The care of the newborn infant and the developing relationship between the mother and her infant have been discussed previously. The focus in this chapter will be on certain disorders of the neonate that are encountered at times in the maternity unit. Fortunately for all concerned, these usually are not seen frequently; yet their appearance, however infrequent, is traumatic for both parents and staff. The principles of supportive care which were delineated in Chapters 21, 25 and 28 are appropriate here. At times modification will be needed, especially when separation of mother and infant is necessary, or when parental response makes the acceptance of the infant difficult. As the various disorders are discussed, the particular aspects, modifications, and the like, which are peculiar to the condition will be described. It is important to remember that the parents of babies with disorders have all the usual tasks of adjusting to the coming of a new infant. In addition they must cope with all the restrictions, limitations, and complications that the disorder imposes.

Parental and staff reactions to defects and disorders

There are certain characteristics inherent in the maternity unit that tend to give rise to and intensify certain interactional elements of the physician-patient-nurse relationship. First, the maternity patient usually comes to the hospital to be assured of a safe delivery for herself and her infant. This means, among other things, freedom from infection. Hence, the primary orientation of the unit is toward the control and prevention of infection. To this end the ward is restricted, that is, it may be actually physically set apart from the other units of the hospital; only obstetric patients are admitted to the unit; personnel (and often patients) are specially gowned, scrubbed and cleansed in a particular manner; visitors and traffic are restricted. All of this protocol tends to make patients and staff feel isolated. Second, the maternity unit is set apart from other units by the rather unique service it offers. In our culture, the childbirth process is considered part of the normal reproductive function of a woman. This normality as a life process, together with the predictability of events, leads to a set of expectations with consequent standardization and routinization of the technical and organizational aspects of the units. Third, the overall expectation is that a healthy patient arrives in anticipation of a happy outcome. Usually *two* healthy persons are returned to the community instead of only the one who entered, and the maternity staff often derives from this tangible production a sense of achievement and satisfaction so highly valued in our society.

It could be hypothesized, then, that the social interaction will be influenced by the interrelatedness of the above characteristics. When a traumatic event occurs, such as the birth of a defective child, both parents and staff will be affected in different ways and degrees.

Working through a crisis

As stated previously, many parents think of labor and delivery as the end of something rather than the beginning of a whole new phase in the family cycle. Probably the enormous responsibilities involved in being parents are responsible in part for this psychologic adaptation. It can be said with certainty, however, that becoming a parent is a turning point in life, and it is particularly so for the parents of a child who has a disorder. They can emerge from this crisis less mentally and emotionally healthy than they were, or they can move on to increased maturity. If they utilize maladaptive coping mechanisms to deal with the crisis, the former no doubt will occur; if they can be helped to work through positively, this experience will stand them in good stead for future stressful situations.

It is the responsibility of the members of the health team to help them cope with this situation adequately. However, staff members, too, are only human, and at times they are hampered by their own anxieties, feelings, and fantasies. Thus, it is especially important for the staff to understand the psychodynamics that are occurring in both the parents and themselves so that they may choose a therapeutic course of action to help the parents.

During pregnancy, all women wish for and fantasize a perfect child, and they also fear that their babies might be abnormal. Their fantasies of the expected child are a composite of the images of the people who are important to or admired by them. Thus, when the infant devi-

ates drastically from the anticipated child, the simultaneous occurrence of the sudden loss of the idealized child and the necessity of accepting a deviant child can be overwhelming. The greater the deviation from normal, the greater can be the impact of the experience.

It is important to remember that the parents have to grieve for the lost "perfect" child before they can form an attachment to the imperfect one. The process of grief, as will be shown, involves anger which can be directed toward anyone involved in the situation—including the infant. Mourning also impairs the capacity to recognize, evaluate, and adapt to reality appropriately. Thus, whenever possible, *long-range* planning for the infant should be delayed until the parents, particularly the mother, can participate in them; otherwise the mourning and depression may persist for an undue amount of time.

Anxiety is another dominant reaction. It is thought that the sources of the most serious anxiety are the threats to the parents' sense of adequacy, self-esteem, and social status. One of the earliest questions expressed, "What caused this?" is charged with feelings of biologic inadequacy. Indeed, what the parents are really asking is, "What's the matter with us as progenitors of children?" Particularly for the mother, her failure to produce what she has so long prepared herself to create may well be a threat not only to her femininity, but to her whole unique personhood as well. Moreover, these feelings hold true even for those who have not consciously "planned" the child or who have had several children. Procreating a defective child strikes at the very core of the woman's being. This is very understandable since the child just born is still, in effect, an extension of the mother, and a defect in him is tantamount to a defect in herself. The degree of the mother's anxiety is also related to a deep narcissistic wound, since the psychologic work during pregnancy includes an increase in narcissism—the need to "take in." Hence, feelings of shame and embarrassment are the general accompaniment of personal feelings of inadequacy. The nurse will remember that these feelings may be heightened by any reserve, avoidance, rejection, and the like that the parents encounter from their families and the professionals with whom they have contact.[1]

The culture and the society in which the parents live will influence the kind and the intensity of their feelings toward their defective and/or ill child. Our culture sets rigid standards with respect to appearance and intellectual capacity and functioning. Perfectly formed and good looking persons represent the societal ideal; thus, any visible physical defect or intellectual impairment represents a basis for class and caste distinctions. It is important to remember also that, since in our culture, one of the greatest threats is loss of standing in one's particular community, the anxiety about the child's birth is directly related to the parents' ego status. Thus, they seek a security-producing answer to support themselves in a situation in which they are vulnerable to devaluation by family and friends.

In spite of our sophisticated and "scientific" society, defects and deformities are still closely identified in much of the public mind with varying degrees of disqualification. For instance, for some, there still lurks the unspoken verdict that congenital conditions have a "sinful" or stigmatized basis. Hence, the parents may feel that the child's condition is retributive—that is, it happened as punishment for some sin of commission or omission. They may search themselves for some prior misdeed and immediately or at a later time attribute the defect to some act or occurrence in their lives. If the pregnancy was originally unwanted, the feelings of punishment may be particularly pronounced.

Some of the variables affecting the parents' coping behaviors include past experiences the parents have had in their own growing-up period. If their childhood experiences have fulfilled their needs for mastery, they will have gained trust, security in human relationships, feelings of optimism and the ability to cope, and freedom from crippling guilt and fear. They will also have learned tolerance for frustration. All of these will be of great help to them in their present crisis. Positive experiences with other handicapped or retarded adults and children can also affect the degree of concern and attitude the parents will have. On the other hand, if they remember hostility directed toward the defective person, or if they (or others) responded to him with guilt, pity, repugnance, or overprotectiveness, these feelings may become reactivated when they are confronted with the abnormality of their own child.

Another variable which may influence the response of the parents to their stress is the degree of energy they have at their disposal at the time of the crisis. The mother who has had a long, physically exhausting labor will have less energy for coping with stress than will the mother who has had a rapid, nonexhausting one. The father who has been at the mother's side coaching her during labor and delivery will have less reserve than one who has not performed the physical and emotional effort which accompanies coaching. In addition, having to attend to other-related life situations, such as making emergency preparations for the care of other children, making arrangements for job-related problems, and the like, also takes valuable energy away that is needed for coping.

Many other variables also may influence the responses of the parents. For example, differences in class, economic background, the physical and emotional maturity of the parents, the birth order of the child, all may have important bearing on the immediate significance which the event will have for them.[2]

AVOIDING NEGATIVE COMMUNICATION. In the delivery room, the physician, patient, and nurse are intensely involved with one another as noted in Chapter 18. The patient needs guidance, coaching, and explanation at this time. Since the time in the delivery room is short, and the events that occur very important, tensions rise with the imminence of birth. Therefore, the interactions are characterized by intense alertness to behavioral cues. Moreover the mother is encouraged verbally by the staff that she is "doing well" and that everything is going along "well." Whenever a disorder is apparent at birth, especially if it is of any magnitude or of a long-term nature (an anomaly, acute respiratory distress, and the like), the tension may be prolonged and intensified instead of being released in the more customary ways. The physician and the nurse will know about the disorder immediately or shortly thereafter. Both their verbal and nonverbal behavior are apt to convey their shock and disappointment to the mother. Their posture may become rigid or they may use their bodies to shield the baby from the mother; their conversation may dwindle or cease; or if an emergency ensues, their actions quicken and conversation is directed to each other and away from the mother and is of a technical nature. If the mother is conscious, she may sense this heightened tension and become increasingly aware and terrified that all is not well. As was stated, it is not always possible for the staff to stop their activities and to respond to the mother's questions; not only are their efforts often going into lifesaving measures for the infant, but they are having to cope with their own emotional reactions. For instance, it is not unnatural for the staff (and the parents later) to have, and perhaps to express, death wishes for a severely defective child. They feel frustrated and resentful toward a situation that they can neither control nor in many cases change. It may be an extremely difficult time for the physician, for it may seem to him that he has "failed" somehow, since he cannot heal the patient. The mother, in turn, may sense the attendants' frustration and misinterpret it as hostility or resentment toward her—that she also has "failed." This negative communication only intensifies the trauma that is experienced by all concerned. In addition, the new mother feels sadness, a completely different emotion than the joy she had anticipated; furthermore, it comes at a time when she may be physically and emotionally exhausted (see Chapter 18).

FORMING A RELATIONSHIP OF TRUST. The total response of the mother will depend on the type and the severity of the disorder and on her past experiences with stress and life in general as stated previously. During this immediate period when the disorder or defect may become apparent, the nurse can be a key person in easing the concern. She should utilize the relationship with the patient that hopefully she has established in the labor room, for it is vitally important that a trust relationship be formed with the patient if she and her partner are to weather this hardship. She can try to communicate her concern and empathy in any way that seems acceptable to the patient. This may be by just staying with the patient and/or holding her hand. Certainly allowing and encouraging the mother to express her feelings, either verbally or by crying, or by letting her be silent, are constructive measures on the part of the nurse. The nurse should never underestimate the importance of her mere presence; she is someone to share the mother's burden. However, she sometimes has to cope with her own inclinations to flee or to avoid the topic.

The situation may be a challenge to those working with the parents, since the birth of a defective and/or sick infant deeply affects them also. They, too, are products of their culture and are influenced by their previous learning experiences and their knowledge of what the experience means to the parents. As stated above, nurses, as well as physicians and other staff, may feel helpless, anxious, and angry. More-

over, they may also feel threatened and uncomfortable and not know what to say, with the result that the parents may misinterpret again and perceive the staff as matter-of-fact, uninterested, casual, and detached. Unfortunately, when nurses retreat, leaving the parents to bear their anxiety alone, the flight only adds to the feelings of worthlessness and inadequacy which parents are feeling. In addition, the nurse's anxiety is transmitted to the parents and contributes to a loss of confidence in her when the parents need her the most.

TELLING THE PARENTS. Many physicians agree that the mother and father should be informed as soon as possible (preferably immediately) of the disorder. However, research has indicated that many physicians tend to seek or develop strategies for delaying the announcement of "bad" news (see Suggested Reading). If this occurs, it can mean significant and far-reaching consequences for the mother and father. Since the mother has the expectation that she will see or at the very least be told about her infant, if this does not happen, she will become suspicious and alarmed and eventually mistrustful. The important immediate establishment of a "trust" relationship will be impeded. Moreover, there will be implications for the attainment of the future goals of the professional services and for the parents' image of professional workers in general.

Sometimes, however, the abnormality makes the condition of the infant so critical that he must be transferred immediately to more suitable facilities. Thus, for entirely different reasons, the mother may not receive a glimpse of her baby. Therefore, *what* the parents are told about the condition and *how* they are told become critical issues. All too often one hears parents complain bitterly about the "bluntness," "coldness," and "unconcern" that the staff demonstrated. Worse still is the "conspiracy of silence" that tortures the already overwrought pair, in which each professional avoids saying anything, pretending or assuming that the other will handle the matter, or that it is better left alone. It is important to recognize that the so-called coldness, avoidance, and so on, are not really manifestations of the staff members' true feelings, but rather are unsuccessful coping mechanisms on their part to allay their feelings of helplessness, anxiety, and inadequacy. However, it is part of the nurse's professional responsibility to explore her feelings in these matters and to develop more effective ways of handling them.

Most physicians want to tell the parents of the disorder themselves; on rare occasions the telling may be delegated to the nurse. In any case it is imperative for her to confer with the physician, so that each can be aware of what is being told to the parents, thus fostering effective communication.

It is imperative that the nurse make herself available to the parents at the time when the diagnosis of the abnormality or illness is communicated. If she can understand that the anger which may be directed at the health personnel is not personal, and if she is able to stay near the parents, support them, and help them in their mourning, she will be making a tremendous contribution to both the parents and the infant. She will also be able to get cues regarding the best type of intervention by observing the parents' behavior at this time. The nurse will want to remember that the mother cannot invest feeling in the defective child until she can feel and talk about her disappointment, sense of failure, helplessness, and/or fears regarding the infant's health and future. The process of grieving is facilitated through repeated discussions before reality can be faced. Interpretations of the baby's condition must be synchronized with this mourning process so that the parents can assimilate facts and reality as they move through the process. When anger or guilt is not expressed, tremendous energy is utilized to contain it, and this energy can be better used in forming a viable relationship later with the child. Moreover, the lack of opportunity to discuss their feelings will hinder the parents' ability to test reality. Therefore, it is necessary that each fear be clarified as the parents are able to bring it into consciousness. In this way, distortions of thinking, feeling, and perception are reduced.

To accomplish this, nurses and other professional personnel will want to encourage parents to react as fully as they desire in an emotional climate and physical environment where they are assured their behavior and feelings are accepted. An attitude of warmth and acceptance which is communicated by actions (physical care, comfort measures, simply sitting with the couple), as well as words, help the couple regain self-esteem. It may be difficult for the professional personnel, since our culture frowns on frank expression of deep feeling. Yet, it is much easier for the parents to accept their own feelings if they are accepted by the professionals around them. A mother will feel understood if the nurse conveys that her feelings and behavior are natural.[3]

The nurse will want to be particularly cognizant about maintaining communication regarding the parents' responses to their situation, the condition of the infant, and any other factors that have bearing on the situation. In this way, a coordinated effort can be made by all members of the health team for comprehensive care.

Realistic Appraisal and Reassurance. In order to give the parents a realistic appraisal of the situation, many authorities feel that the parents should be informed immediately of the disorder and the prognosis, especially if repair or long-term care is involved. This information, of course, must be explained in terms that the couple can understand, and reinforcement over the days probably will be necessary.

Whatever specifics are told, it is important that two aspects of realistic reassurance be given the mother and father: first, that they and their child are acceptable, and second, that the hospital and personnel are there to render any assistance possible. Particularly in the cases of some defects and deformities (e.g., phocomelia or myelomeningocele) the parents must understand that although their child may not be made whole, he usually may be helped to some degree. This kind of reassurance demonstrates an attitude of understanding and sharing of the parents' feelings of hurt and loss, and at the same time it does not minimize the gravity of the situation.

ACCEPTANCE OF THE INFANT BY THE STAFF. It is generally the physician who determines when the parents, and especially the mother, will see and care for her infant. The parents' first encounter with their infant is another crucial time. Particularly in cases in which there is an obvious anomaly, it is vitally important that the physician or the nurse who is showing the baby demonstrate an attitude of warmth and acceptance of the infant; if revulsion or rejection is manifested, the parents' own feelings of despair and ostracism will be intensified.

One way the staff can demonstrate to the parents that their child is valuable and important is to hold him close, cuddle him, and call him by name. At this time, if it seems to be indicated, the positive points in the prognosis can be reiterated or reinforced. This may be a difficult time for all concerned, since staff members are also trying to cope with their own possible feelings of rejection. Therefore, an attempt should be made to avoid a common type of destructive behavior that tends to be demonstrated unconsciously, that of isolating the patient under the guise of "protecting" the mother. In this kind of destructive behavior the mother may not be allowed to see her infant at all (or very infrequently) until she is "stronger"; no one talks to her of her child's handicap or death, because it will "upset" her, visitors are often restricted, and so on. The baby, in turn, is isolated and often overtreated (i.e., time- and energy-consuming procedures are employed which lead to very little change in the infant's condition). All this only emphasizes the enormity of the problem for the parents and hinders them in attaining a successful resolution of the problem.

GRIEVING. Grief can be considered a response to loss. It is most often known to us as a response to a loss through death or separation of a loved person, but it can occur following the loss of anything, tangible or intangible, which is highly valued. This may be such things as a material possession, a highly valued expectation (such as a well, whole infant), a position of status, a prized faculty, or even a place one is forced to leave. The ability to experience grief is gradually formed in the course of normal development and the capacity for grieving is closely related to the person's capacity to develop meaningful object relationships. Therefore, those who are able to form relationships at all become attached even to situations and places which are less than optimal and grieve for them (however briefly), even when moving to better conditions. Grief, then, is a universal, normal, developmentally evolved adaptive process. It progresses through three general predictable phases, and this progress enables the individual to deal adaptively with the disturbance of his psychologic equilibrium which is inevitably caused by object loss. Fortunately it is self-limiting if not allowed to deteriorate into deep-seated depression, and gradually diminishes over a period of about a year. Only the very early, acute phase is actually incapacitating, and even this phase, with appropriate professional help, may not grossly interfere with the person's normal functioning in many areas of his life. The staff can expect the parents to show signs of grieving when a substantial defect (or death) occurs. The couple must come to terms with a difficult and perhaps unex-

pected situation, one in which the prognosis may be poor. Both parents will demonstrate grief, and the father's needs should not be forgotten. He is particularly vulnerable, since it is on him that the early decisions, making arrangements, and so on, usually fall, and he often does not have the time or the privacy to express his own sorrow.

Several phases are encountered in the grief reaction, and how intensely the parents experience these will vary according to the nature and the gravity of the disorder and their capacity for grieving.[4]

In the first phase are shock and disbelief; this phase may be manifested by a refusal to accept or to comprehend the fact of the disorder or the loss. The person may appear stunned, immobilized, or may try to carry on ordinary activities; intermittent flashes of anguish and despair occur as reality penetrates. Occasionally, there is an overtly intellectual response to the reality of the situation: the mother or father may try to comfort the other, make any necessary arrangements, and the like. This type of response takes place only if the full emotional impact is not allowed to reach the consciousness. The loss is recognized, but its painful character is muted. This phase may last from minutes to days; the longings for a "perfect child" may be recalled, felt intensely, and discharged gradually. This process serves to free the parents' feelings so that they may proceed to the next phase. The nurse's presence is beneficial at this time, for it helps the parents to feel that they are not entirely alone.

The nurse may notice that, at this time, the parents may withdraw initially. This is a strategy to escape the painful reality of the situation; hence, at times they want only silence and solitude. It is important not to label this behavior as "rejection of the child," for if criticism of this kind is manifested or implied, the parents' anger may be directed toward the child so that they continue to not wish to see him. These parents are experiencing great psychic pain and their concerns naturally center on their own feelings. They are trying to sort out what this defect or illness means to them personally. Nurses can be of great assistance, if they can respond to withdrawal with understanding and a great deal of giving, even in the face of seeming disinterest and apathy. This demonstration of giving will help relieve the mother's feelings of guilt about her lack of motherliness if the nurse helps her to understand that such feelings always develop gradually as a mother cares for and handles her child. As the nurse "gives" to the mother, she is presenting a role model for the mother to follow. As grieving is gradually resolved, the mother will follow the nurse's example and "give" to her infant. If the guilt is not resolved, anger again may be directed toward the child, which will arouse more guilt and form the basis for subsequent pathologic overprotectiveness.[5]

On the other hand, however, if the mother appears to indicate an *initial* overprotectiveness toward the infant, this behavior should also be respected since it is a defense against the mother's anxiety and disorganization. Self-pity may become displaced as pity for the child and, if the nurse is critical of this attitude, the defense will only be deepened. Thus, the mother is not to be made to feel that others are trying to intrude between her and her infant. Those appropriate aspects of nurturance and care that she attempts to give can be reinforced and praised and gradually she can be helped to realize the limits of her assistance.

The second phase, that of developing awareness, involves a *feeling* of loss and disappointment, accompanied at times by affective and physical symptoms (i.e., emptiness in the epigastric or chest regions, sadness, and the like). Now the painful feelings are allowed to become conscious. The parents (particularly the mother) may cry, express anger toward a variety of persons and things, talk about the situation, or be unable to express any verbal emotions, although they want to. A relationship between the nurse and the parents that is based on helping is most effective at this time; the nurse's approach should be dictated by the parents' reactions. When she is accepting and encourages the expression of feelings (and provides privacy for their expression), she is helping to prepare the way for the next phase. Developing awareness may take a long time—days or months. The nurse in the hospital usually will see its beginning, but very infrequently will she see its termination.

During the grieving process, the mother needs more physical rest than the usual postpartum patient since she needs increased energy to cope with the tragedy. Regression is natural at this time and dependency needs are increased in the presence of anxiety. When the nurse lets the parents depend on her, she helps in preventing further frustrations for the couple. When she accepts the mother's increased need for personal care, she demonstrates that she is accepting both the mother and the child who deviates in some degree from normality.

As mentioned previously, the nurse, by taking meticulous care of the baby and showing affection and interest for him, demonstrates a realistic investment in him. This reassures the mother that the child is worthwhile and others can love and accept him—this allays her feelings of inadequacy over time. The nurse will want to be alert to the times that the mother shows signs of wanting to learn to care for the infant. Fortunately, now, mothers are given more opportunities to care for and feed their infants, even when the infants may be in a special nursery.

The feeding experience is extremely significant for the mother. When she can feed her infant and sense some response in him, she will begin to have some tangible, positive reinforcement that she can perform a crucial nurturing activity for her baby. Thus, her self-esteem is increased. It must be remembered, however, that every time the mother does feed (or performs any other care-giving activity for) her infant, she must face the baby's defect or illness, and her initial feelings of anxiety, frustration, and guilt are apt to be reactivated. Over time, these initial feelings gradually diminish with successful trials of feeding or care giving. However, if the mother refuses to feed her infant or prefers to "skip" one or two feedings, it is wise to be unblaming, since nothing is to be gained by pushing the mother into prematurely caring for the infant. As the mother learns to feed her infant and do other specific activities for the infant, she channels some of her own dependency feelings into the activities and gradually gains confidence in her competence as a mother. When caring for these mothers and infants, it is most important that the nurse be extremely observant of the infant and his cues for care. Because of the grieving, the mothers may not be able to be as observant and/or receptive as mothers of normal infants to their infants' cues. Moreover, any equipment attached to the baby—special incubators, and so on—all distract the mother from her baby's actual behavior (see Chapter 25). Thus, she needs all of the extra observational skills that the nurse can give her.

The nurse must remember that the birth of a defective child may have grave implications for the marital bond. After the immediate shock of the birth, the parents, in this second stage of grieving, begin to reflect on the many problems facing them because of the defect. Often one of them becomes very concerned about imparting information about the deviation to the other, and sometimes to close family or friends as well. This concern will be especially evident if the parent feels responsible in some way because of a family history of congenital defects, irresponsibility, or the like. This concern is manifested irrespective of whether the marriage is stable or not. Submergence of one's own feelings in deference to the partner's may occur in more stable unions, while blame may be attributed in less happy marriages. This latter response, particularly, only adds another source of stress. If either partner was afraid of what the birth of the baby might do to their relationship, the fears will only be intensified with the birth of a defective or ill child.

Fathers who have become aware of the emotional changes which accompany pregnancy, labor, and delivery, and who realize the mothers' vulnerability at this time, will be in a better position to give appropriate support to their partners than those who are not aware of the mothers' needs and who are withdrawn into their own grief. The arrival of a defective or ill child makes great demands on the father, and this fact is often overlooked, since attention is more frequently directed toward the mother since she is hospitalized. Often the father's responsibilities are so overwhelming that he cannot perceive or provide the support his partner so earnestly needs. Unless he too receives assistance in coping with his feelings about the birth, the parents' relationship may suffer a severe setback. He needs to know that his feelings are important also—that he is being considered as a person, not just as an expeditor or errand boy. As he realizes that his grief is acceptable and the professionals care about what he is experiencing, he will be able to cope with his feelings better and be able to offer more support to the mother.

The third and final phase of grieving involves restitution and resolving of the experience. During restitution mourning occurs, in which mutual grief and loss are expressed by the parents and sympathetic friends and relatives. At this stage religious beliefs and rituals are helpful, for they help to clarify the ambiguity about suffering, eternity, and death. In this,

the final phase of grief, resolution of the problem gradually occurs; this phase may take from six months to a year. Here memories and expectations are intensely experienced by repeated questioning, ruminating, and recalling the experience to mind. The wise nurse will listen empathetically in this phase, reflect what is being said, and gently probe to help the parents arrive at reality.* As already implied, the nurse in the community health agency will be in the best position to do this, and enlisting her help will entail appropriate referral on the part of the hospital staff.

Occasionally, grief is not resolved adequately, and the nurse will see in long-term situations what has been described as pathologic grieving or morbid grief.[6] These symptoms are not to be confused with a high degree of mourning or grieving that is seen in the acute phases of grieving. Time appears to be the crucial factor here—grief that is not resolved after a year or more can be considered pathologic or morbid. This includes the following symptoms: overacting without a sense of loss; acquisition of symptoms belonging to the last illness of the deceased; psychosomatic reactions such as ulcerative colitis, asthma, or rheumatoid arthritis; alterations of affectional ties in relation to friends and relatives; furious hostility against specific persons; repression of hostility, leading to a wooden and formal manner resembling schizophrenic behavior; lasting loss of patterns of social interaction; adoption of activities detrimental to one's social and economic existence; and finally, agitated depressions.

The interdisciplinary team

Many institutions are now employing an interdisciplinary team when the disorder is grave and/or of a long-term nature. In the case of a child who is born with a cleft palate, a pediatrician, plastic surgeon, otologist, orthodontist, psychologist, maternity nurses, and community health nurses may all be involved in the care. Since the parents easily can become lost in a maze of appointments, it is wise to have one central person (e.g., the private physician or a social worker) to be the mother's

* The articles in Suggested Reading that deal with grief, stillbirth, deformities, and the like, will help the student gain more explicit insight into the process of grief and the types of effective communication and intervention that are necessary in these cases.

liaison with the other members of the team. The nurse can be instrumental in helping to arrange this.

Stillbirth or neonatal death

Occasionally, parents and staff will be faced with the unfortunate circumstance of a still-birth or a neonatal death. All of the responses of both personnel and parents that have just been described may be apparent in these cases. Grief and mourning will be noted particularly, and it will become the nurse's responsibility to provide an environment in which the mother and father can express their feelings. Nursing care is essentially the same as that just described.

Recent research has postulated that the length and intensity of mourning after the death of an infant is proportionate to the close-ness of the relationship prior to death.[7] More-over, it has been found that caring for an infant who subsequently dies or touching or fondling a dead infant is not unduly upsetting to an emo-tionally healthy mother (one who does not have a history of psychiatric problems). All too often the reason given for not allowing the mother and father contact with their dying or dead infant is that it will be "too upsetting." Fortunately, it is now known that affectional bonding is enhanced (as with all babies) with tactile stim-ulation and caretaking and that this type of contact does not result in pathologic grieving. It appears that affectional bonding is necessary in order that the parents may relinquish the dead child and work through the symbiotic relationship that was extant before birth. Thus, a high degree of mourning appears to be a nor-mal phenomenon of the grieving process and should not be considered pathologic or abnor-mal. The student is referred to the Suggested Reading for further specific examples of cur-rent research, nursing approaches regarding this phenomenon.

One of the most frequent complaints of par-ents, and especially mothers, is that the staff, including nurses, do not "know what to do with me." That is, the mothers are treated as if nothing had happened and no mention is made of the tragedy; this is part of the "con-spiracy of silence" that we mentioned previ-ously. It is difficult to outline specific measures for the nurse since her ability and depth in interaction will depend to a great extent on her own feelings about death (and deformities) and her experience in dealing with death and dying. Schuman has outlined some approaches that she has found to be helpful in the initial encoun-ters. She suggests that the nurse sit down as close as possible to the mother and try to ap-pear relaxed and unhurried. Eye contact should be established and the nurse should introduce herself by name and job classification. This latter point gives the mother a frame of refer-ence so that she perceives more fully to whom she is speaking and what help she may expect. After these preliminaries, it is suggested that the nurse state gently *but clearly* that she is sorry that the *tragedy* had to happen to the mother. This may start the mother crying, but this emotional demonstration need not be feared. The nurse can then put her arms around the mother and encourage her to con-tinue, assuring her that this and other grieving behavior is acceptable. If the mother continues to cry, the nurse can gently reassure her. If the mother begins to talk about the tragedy, the nurse will be able to pick up cues which may call for further reassurance that she was not "guilty" of anything or perhaps the need for factual information. It may be that, initially, the nurse will only be able to say that she is sorry and to ask if the mother would like to talk to her about it. The general goal is to meet the parents' spoken and unspoken cries for compassion, understanding, and factual in-formation.[8]

Decisions will be difficult for the parents, and whenever possible, especially in everyday mundane matters concerning hospital routine, the nurse should try to structure the situation so that the mother is not overburdened with choices. It is often easier for the mother to respond to "I thought you would like your bed made now," than to "Would you like to shower now, or should I make your bed?" One other point needs special consideration. The nurse must be careful not to offer the mother unhelp-ful platitudes, such as, "Please don't feel so bad. You have such lovely children at home." Or "You can always have another baby." State-ments of this kind are not only unhelpful but are detrimental to the situation, since they con-vey to the patient the nurse's great lack of understanding and/or her disinterest in the situation. The parents will trust the nurse to the degree that they perceive her understand-ing and empathetic perception of their problem, and to this same degree will they trust her and permit her to help them arrive at a positive solution of their problem.

Getting help from instructors and supervisors

All of the responses that have been described (both for parents and staff) are related to emotionally charged areas (e.g., disappointment, loss, and death). As previously implied, these topics often are not discussed easily, and the nurse may encounter resistance on the patient's part in the form of hostility when she attempts to speak of these subjects. It is one thing to *talk* about letting patients express their feelings; it is quite another to permit them to *do* this. At times the inexperienced nurse may become very uncomfortable if a response of resistance is not anticipated. Since the student must have consistent and supportive help to plan effective care (and to manage her feelings and responses adequately) in these cases, she should turn to her instructors and other supervisory personnel for help in this regard. Faculty and supervisors who make themselves readily available as "supportive listeners" to students and anticipate the need for this role can be key persons in helping all concerned to resolve the trauma associated with a disorder or a loss.

In the foregoing section some general aspects related to parental and staff reactions as well as nursing care have been described. In the following pages the specific disorders and principles of care related to them will be discussed. The student may benefit from review of this section as she proceeds with the specific disorders.

Neonatal respiratory distress

Asphyxia of the newborn

The three causes of intrauterine injury of the central nervous system—narcosis, hypoxia, and brain hemorrhage—all produce a similar clinical picture, characterized by apnea as its prime objective manifestation. Formerly, this condition was known as *asphyxia neonatorum*. The course and prognosis of this syndrome vary with the degree of hypoxia, the location and extent of the hemorrhage, and the degree of asphyxia. This latter term describes the condition of the infant's arterial blood and connotes hypoxia plus hypercapnia and acidosis. This acidotic asphyxial state is more injurious and difficult to correct than hypoxia alone.

The normal oxygen saturation of the arterial blood of the fetus at birth is approximately 60 percent, but in severe cases may drop as low as 12 percent. In addition, the blood of these infants has a high concentration of lactic acid and a very low pH. In addition to apnea, babies suffering from asphyxia often exhibit other evidence of injury in the color of their skin, their muscle tonus, and their heart rate. Thus, the Apgar score provides a better assessment of the newborn infant than any single observation, such as the breathing or crying time. In milder cases, the infant's skin is bluish (formerly called *asphyxia livida*), but when shock is superimposed the skin is white (*asphyxia pallida*). In the presence of any significant degree of hypoxia, the muscle tone is weak, and in severe cases the infants are completely limp. A very slow heartbeat is characteristic, with the rate often dropping below 50 beats per minute. The bradycardia usually responds dramatically to oxygen, even in cases where the ultimate outcome is unfavorable. Since hypoxia may cause the rectal sphincter to relax, it is not unusual for these babies to be covered with meconium.[9]

Prevention of asphyxia of the newborn

Preventive treatment is very important and is the responsibility of the health team. It begins with the first antepartal visit when the pelvis is measured to make sure that it is large enough to allow passage of the infant's head without compression. Good diet and hygiene contribute greatly to the health of the infant at birth. During labor, the physician can do much to prevent asphyxia of the infant by care in the use of analgesic and anesthetic drugs and by avoiding as much as possible the more difficult types of operative delivery. Moreover, by monitoring the fetal heart tones, the attendant may detect early signs of impending fetal distress (slow and/or irregular rate), and, with this warning, it may be possible for the physician to deliver the infant before serious trouble develops. The passage of meconium-stained amniotic fluid is another sign of fetal distress, but is of no value in breech presentations, since the passage of meconium—ordinarily pure meconium—is the rule in breech cases.

In the past, many physicians believed that the administration of vitamin K to the mother late in pregnancy and during labor tended to prevent cerebral hemorrhage in the newborn by improving the clotting power of the fetal blood. This antihemorrhagic vitamin passes readily through the placenta and raises the prothrombin concentration of the fetal plasma, which ordinarily is low. Recent studies indicate, however, that hyperbilirubinemia is associated with the parenteral administration of a vitamin K analogue antepartally; this is particularly true in the case of premature infants. Therefore, the prophylactic administration of this drug to the mother during labor should be viewed with caution. Current practice is to administer a small dose (1.0 mg.) of water-soluble vitamin K to the infant immediately after birth as a prophylaxis against the coagulation defect related to vitamin K deficiency.

Treatment of asphyxia of the newborn

It has been recommended that all members of the delivery room team be trained in methods of resuscitation for mother and baby since both may have difficulty at the same time. Indecisive or ineffective therapy may lose precious moments in which the infant's life can be saved. All equipment necessary for resuscitation should be checked before each delivery and should include a suction apparatus, a plastic oropharyngeal airway, a laryngoscope equipped with a premature blade (and working batteries), and a Cole plastic endotracheal tube with a stilet (Fig. 29-1). In addition, oxygen should be available.

Generally, the anesthesiologist will assume responsibility for the maintenance of the resuscitation equipment per se. Since he is usually responsible for the immediate measures of resuscitation, it will fall to the nurse to assist him in any way that she can. Moreover, it is the nurse's function to keep the delivery room prepared for adequate and prompt treatment of asphyxia (as well as other emergencies), whether it is expected or not. Therefore, she should have supplies and equipment in readiness. These may include the resuscitator, warm blankets, oxygen, and the aforementioned equipment. She is to be prepared to position the infant during the procedures, if necessary, and to make and to report accurate observations. Her skill and competence in assisting the physician in caring for the infant and the mother will go far in giving the mother the reassurance and the support that she needs at this time.

Any infant who has an Apgar score (see Chapter 15) of 0, 1, or 2 is severely depressed and deserving of immediate treatment. In treat-

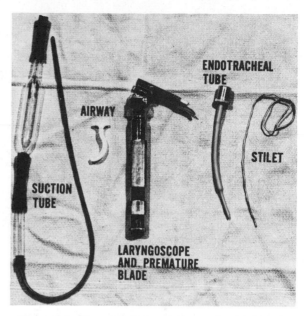

Figure 29-1. Tray-resuscitation apparatus. (Special Committee on Infant Mortality of the Medical Society of the County of New York: Resuscitation of the Newborn, rev. ed., p. 5, Fig. 4, Philadelphia, Smith Kline & French Laboratories, 1963)

ing an infant who does not breathe at birth, there are five main principles to keep in mind.

GENTLENESS. These infants are often in a state of shock, and rough attempts to resuscitate them—as by vigorous spanking or other overvigorous methods of external stimulation—do more harm than good. Methods of physical stimulation should be limited to gentle rubbing of the back and, at the most, to light patting of the buttocks. When anoxia is present, oxygen is necessary to overcome it, and the use of measures which act as external irritants will not oxygenate the tissues.

WARMTH. Heated cribs and other means of maintaining body warmth, such as radiant lights and warm blankets, must be in readiness. This is particularly important to remember, because the measures employed to resuscitate infants, unless care is taken, tend to expose their completely naked bodies (accustomed to the temperature in utero) to room temperature; and this may aggravate the state of shock. The body of the infant should be kept covered as much as possible.

POSTURE. Some obstetricians hold the infant up by the feet momentarily after birth in order to expedite drainage of mucus from the trachea, the larynx, and the posterior pharynx. Others cradle the baby in the arm with the hand sup-

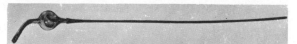

Figure 29-2. Catheter and glass bulb with a trap, for aspirating mucus in the treatment of asphyxia. (Chicago Lying-in Hospital)

porting the head, which is held down. The baby is then placed on his back in a slight Trendelenburg position (head turned aside, lower than buttocks), also to favor gravity drainage of mucus.

REMOVAL OF MUCUS. Cleansing the air passages of mucus and fluid is essential, since effective respiration cannot be accomplished through obstructed air passages. The head-down position will promote drainage of mucus and fluid from the respiratory passages, but postural drainage alone is often not adequate for this purpose, and suction of one type or another is frequently necessary. An ordinary catheter is used, size 12 to 14 French; in premature infants a smaller size (8 to 10) is advisable. A glass trap (Fry) is inserted into the catheter to arrest mucus which otherwise might be drawn into the operator's mouth (Fig. 29-2). Milking the trachea upward will help bring mucus and fluid into the posterior pharynx, where it may be aspirated by the catheter. Gentleness is essential, since the mucous membrane of the infant's mouth is delicate. Although the physician occasionally does so, the nurse should not introduce the catheter farther than the posterior pharynx. Mechanical suction devices are provided with most of the modern machines for infant resuscitation and are very convenient.

RESUSCITATION. Moderately depressed infants (Apgar score 4 to 6) are limp, cyanotic, or dusky and dyspneic. Respirations may be shallow, irregular, or gasping. The heart rate is normal, however, and there is at least a fair response to flicking the sole of the foot. Management entails the same regimen described for normal infants during the first minute after birth (see Chapters 15 and 18). If, however, effective spontaneous respiration is not established thereafter, ventilatory support is essential, especially in the presence of continued cyanosis and flaccidity. Initially, a laryngoscope is inserted. With the larynx visualized, suction is applied through a catheter attached to a De Lee trap. The trap may be operated by suction from the operator's mouth. This will as-

sure removal of any blood clots, large-sized particles of meconium, vernix, or thick mucus. The suction catheter is then removed and a curved plastic airway is inserted between the tongue and palate to prevent the base of the tongue from falling backward over the glottic opening into the larynx. Oxygen is administered through a tightly fitting face mask attached to a hand-operated bag that receives 100 percent oxygen and delivers it to the infant in high concentrations. The chest of the baby will rise with each squeeze if the oxygen is delivered adequately. If this procedure is effective, spontaneous respirations should begin within one minute and cyanosis and hypotonicity should disappear. Oxygen should still be supplied by mask, however, until the infant is stable. If color and respirations have not improved after one minute or the heart rate falls below 100 beats per minute at any time, endotracheal intubation is urgently indicated.

If the infant is severely depressed (Apgar 0 to 3), "gentle swiftness" is the essence of resuscitation. These infants are usually blue or pale, limp, and make little or no effort to breathe. The heart rate, if present at all, is under 100 beats per minute, and the preliminary resuscitation efforts are of no avail. Suction and endotracheal intubation under direct visualization with a laryngoscope are the only procedures that can save an infant in this condition. Generally, once the lungs are oxygenated, the response is gratifying. Immediate improvement may be noted, although intubation for ten minutes or longer is recommended. With the return of effective cardiac function, the baby becomes pink and some muscle activity can be noted. If heart activity is absent after three or four bag insufflations, external cardiac massage is mandatory. It is important to remember that *only after cardiovascular function is restored*, intravenous administration of sodium bicarbonate and dextrose is essential since the hypoxia causes metabolic acidosis and may produce hypoglycemia as a result of rapid depletion of glycogen stores.

EXTERNAL CARDIAC MASSAGE. As stated previously, if the heartbeat has not returned after three or four insufflations, external cardiac massage is instituted immediately. It should be performed by an assistant, leaving the primary operator free to manage ventilation. With the application of downward pressure at the left margin of the lower sternum, the heart is compressed (systole) and by releasing the pressure, the heart is dilated (diastole). The index and middle fingers are placed on the midthorax at the level of the sternum and the area is pressed downward and released. The total downward displacement of the chest wall should not exceed one inch. Excessive vigor may cause a laceration of the liver with severe blood loss (Fig. 29-3).

It is imperative to maintain both the cardiac massage and the ventilation. This can be accomplished by alternating the two maneuvers. The heart is compressed two or three times (approximately 120 times per minute) after which a breath of oxygen is given. The two procedures must not be performed simultaneously because the pressure applied during cardiac massage may rupture a lung that has just been inflated by the ventilation. If the procedure is effective, the femoral or temporal artery pulses are palpable in synchrony with depression of the sternum. The procedure is to be discontinued periodically to determine the presence of spontaneous cardiac activity. When the latter occurs, cardiac compression may be discontinued.[10]

No drugs have been found to be effective as respiratory stimulants for the infant. However, if the infant's respiratory depression is related to maternal narcosis from opiates, then the physician may administer levallorphan (Lorfan, 0.25 mg.) or nalorphine (N-allylnormorphine: Nalline, 0.1 mg. per kilogram of body weight) into the umbilical vein. Respiration may be improved. These drugs should be used only when a specific opiate has been used for the mother, as they otherwise will act as respiratory depressants for the baby (see Suggested Reading).

CONTINUED OBSERVATION. It is important that close observation be continued after resuscitation methods have ceased. Generally, the baby's condition will improve; occasionally, however, it will worsen, especially if the difficulty is due to mucous obstruction or to drugs administered to the mother. The Apgar method of infant evaluation, as well as the other observations described in Chapter 15, can be utilized in these cases. The continuing observations that should be made when the infant is transferred to the nursery are described in Chapter 18.

Aspiration syndromes

Among the multiple causes of neonatal respiratory distress is a range of abnormalities that are presumably caused by aspiration of

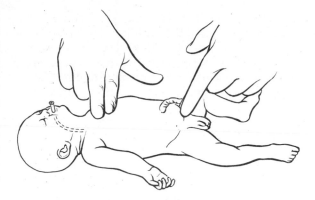

Figure 29-3. Closed-chest cardiac massage in the newborn infant. *Note:* The infant is placed on a flat surface which is tilted so that his head is on a lower level than his body, facilitating drainage of his airway. In addition, the infant's neck is extended; thus, his natural air passage is straightened.

amniotic fluid and its contents into the respiratory tract or retention of fetal lung fluid. Thus, in both of these instances, the flow of air is obstructed in varying degrees by the presence of fluid and/or particulate matter in the respiratory tract. The spectrum of abnormalities is composed at one end by diffuse emphysema of both lungs without collapse and at the other end by collapse of large areas of the lungs (*atelectasis*).

The clinical entity in which emphysema predominates has been called *transient tachypnea* of the newborn, *respiratory distress syndrome, Type II*, or *obstructive emphysema* of the newborn. It may affect infants born prematurely or at term. Respiratory distress begins at birth or shortly thereafter, and is characterized by tachypnea, retractions, flaring of the nostrils, and expiratory grunt. Generally, there has been no difficulty with the onset of breathing. There are no rales, but cyanosis in room air may be noted which usually clears with the administration of small increments of oxygen. Grunting and retractions may resolve within 24 to 48 hours and the clinical course is usually about four days. The prognosis is good for these infants. Treatment consists of oxygen and initial pH correction with sodium bicarbonate. In spite of the respiratory dysfunction, these infants seem to manage their alveolar gas exchange sufficiently well to maintain normal blood gas tensions. Supportive care and careful feeding to avoid choking is also indicated.

The clinical condition in which occlusion and collapse of the lungs are more prominent is *meconium aspiration*, or the *massive aspira-*

tion syndrome. In these cases, meconium has been passed into the amniotic fluid and the fetus aspirates particles of meconium, which, during the first few breaths, may be inspired more deeply into the alveoli. In contrast to transient tachypnea, affected infants often have difficulty establishing respirations. The subsequent signs of their respiratory distress are similar to those described for transient tachypnea except that rales are often present.

Respiratory abnormalities generally subside in 48 hours, although they may be apparent for as long as six or seven days. The prognosis is better than for hyaline membrane disease, although pneumothorax and pneumomediastinum may complicate the course.

Care is aimed at supporting the infant and correcting the varying degrees of mixed respiratory and metabolic acidosis. Thus, alkali therapy and oxygen administration may be necessary for severely ill babies for several days as well as intravenous or gavage feeding.[11]

Pneumonia

This condition is the largest pulmonary cause of death in infants dying after 48 hours and is noted in as many as 20 percent of all newborn autopsies. The incidence is usually bimodal, that is, two peaks occur. One is in the first 12 hours of life and is usually secondary to maternal infection. The second peak comes after 48 hours of life, and is probably acquired in the nursery.

Infection that has been acquired in utero (*congenital pneumonia*) is usually associated with obstetric abnormalities such as early rupture of the membranes, prolonged duration of labor, maternal infection, and uncomplicated premature delivery. The bacteria most frequently involved are *Escherichia coli* and other enteric organisms, *staphylococci* and group *B streptococci.* Symptoms may be evident at birth or within 48 hours thereafter. When these babies are affected at birth, they are flaccid, pale, or cyanotic. Resuscitation is often necessary. Once respirations are established, they tend to be rapid and shallow with some slight retractions. When the infection is severe, repeated apneic episodes occur and these infants must be observed carefully. Temperature elevation is more likely in term, full-sized infants; the premature infants often have subnormal temperatures.

Postnatally acquired pneumonia is generally caused by *Pseudomonas aeruginosa,* penicillin-resistant staphylococci, and enteric organisms. With this infection, clinical signs usually appear after 48 hours of life. The most common presenting signs are rapid respiration, poor feeding, or aspiration during feeding. Vomiting and aspiration sometimes occur during feeding because previously unsuspected pneumonia is already present. In these instances, the chest film reveals densities that cannot be attributed with certainty to effects of aspirated formula or to preexisting pneumonia. Recovery from postnatal pneumonia is more frequent than from congenital pneumonia.

Antibiotic therapy, oxygen, and supportive care, together with close observation, are the treatments of choice for these conditions. It is wise to place these infants on their abdomens or sides after feeding to avoid aspiration if regurgitation occurs.[12]

Since many newborn nursery units transfer a baby to a pediatric unit if the infant is born with or develops a serious disorder or infection, separation from her infant may be a problem for the mother. The principles regarding this aspect of nursing care will be essentially the same as those described in Chapter 25.

Idiopathic respiratory distress syndrome (hyaline membrane disease)

Hyaline membrane disease is a syndrome of neonatal respiratory distress in which the alveoli and the alveolar ducts are filled with a sticky exudate, a hyaline material, which prevents aeration. Although it is known that the hyaline material is a protein, the cause of hyaline membrane formation is not definitely known. Three main theories are now under study. The first proposes an alteration in the fibrinolytic enzyme system in the lung or blood which leads to the proliferation of the protein (fibrin) exudate. The second suggests an absence or alterations of the pulmonary surfactant which reduces alveolar ventilation and promotes atelectasis. The third indicates pulmonary hypofusion rather than surfactant deficiency. This hypofusion begins with intrauterine asphyxia and also results in reduced alveolar ventilation and atelectasis. Whatever the exact causes and mechanisms, surfactant activity is indeed deficient, and, as a result, there is incomplete expansion of the lung and failure to establish normal functional residual capacity (absence of alveolar stability). Thus, the lungs are atelectatic, and this is a hallmark of the disease.

Pulmonary compliance, or the capacity of the lung to increase in volume in response to a given amount of applied pressure during inspiration, is diminished in this syndrome. The stiffness of the lungs and their limited distensibility contributes significantly to the work of breathing in these sick babies. *Pulmonary vasoconstriction* is another injurious factor of major importance. This vasoconstriction results in increased resistance within the pulmonary circuit and causes hypofusion of alveolar capillaries, and, hence, the lungs are ischemic as well as atelectatic. Thus, the fetal circulatory state persists in varying degrees and this becomes life-threatening to the neonate. After a few breaths, continued impairment of gas exchange enhances hypoxia, hypercapnia, and acidosis. This, in turn, increases the pulmonary vasoconstriction and ischemia; surfactant activity is further diminished and atelectasis becomes more extensive. Pulmonary compliance decreases and the energy required for the simple act of breathing increases intolerably. All this leads to further impairment of gas exchange and a vicious cycle is established which soon becomes incompatible with life without intensive treatment.

The greatest incidence occurs in preterm infants weighing between 1,000 and 1,500 Gm., and it is observed in about 10 percent of all premature infants. It also occurs in about 50 percent of all infants of diabetic mothers and also in infants whose mothers experienced antepartal vaginal bleeding. The condition has also been noted in infants born by cesarean section; however, cesarean section in otherwise *uncomplicated* full-term deliveries is probably not associated with any increased incidence of the disease. This disease is not found in stillborn infants.

It was formerly believed that a free interval existed after birth before the onset of symptoms. However, when infants are observed closely and examined carefully, symptoms can be noted immediately after birth. A chest x-ray usually confirms the diagnosis and rules out congenital cardiovascular disease. Expiratory grunting or whining (observable when the infant is not crying), sternal and subcostal retractions, nasal flaring, rapid respirations (more than 60 per minute), and low body temperatures are seen early and are diagnostic clues. Grunting, which is the most important and useful clinical sign, may be the only and earliest indication of the disease. Conversely,

cessation of grunting is often the first sign of improvement. The infant may be cyanotic in room air. Infants who are badly affected may be cyanotic even with oxygen therapy yet paradoxically exhibit a normal respiratory rate. Auscultation of the chest reveals poor air entry, decreased breath sounds, and at times, fine rales. Bowel sounds are often absent in the early hours of the illness and the urine output is low during the first two or three days of life. If the disease progresses, respiratory rate increases, chest retractions become more marked, and see-saw respirations ensue (see Fig. 28-4, p. 564). Peripheral edema increases, and muscle tone decreases. With the increase in cyanosis, the body temperature tends to drop and short periods of apnea are noted. The heart rate is often fixed except for periods of bradycardia accompanied by severe cyanosis and grunting. Many symptoms are related to asphyxia which depresses the respiratory center and causes apneic episodes as well as changes in the blood distribution throughout the body. This latter fact accounts for the pale gray skin color of the severely affected infant. In addition the rate of heat production is also decreased. If treatment is instituted promptly, modern care has resulted in about a 50 to 70 percent salvage rate for these infants. If treatment is not prompt and/or the infant is small or does not respond to treatment, death may occur within 48 hours.

It is important that the nurse make meticulous observations and recordings about the respiratory signs and symptoms, especially of infants who are born prematurely or who are delivered by cesarean section. The outcome for the premature is usually poorer and depends a great deal on his birth weight: the smaller he is, the graver is the prognosis. For example, infants who weigh 1,000 Gm. or less generally succumb, since their lungs are not developed enough to make the adjustment to extrauterine life.

TREATMENT. Since the cause and complete pathophysiology of this entity are not understood, the principles of management center around alleviation of the clinical manifestations. Thus, approaches to treatment are made both directly, by treating the infant with oxygen and alkali, and indirectly, through influencing oxygen need and acid production by regulating the infant's body temperature, water balance, and caloric requirements. Treatment therefore involves 1) regulation of body tem-

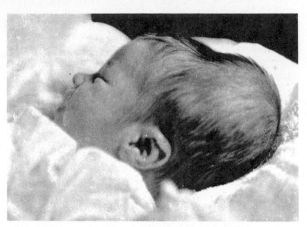

Figure 29-4. Caput succedaneum. (MacDonald House, University Hospitals of Cleveland)

perature, 2) intravenous feeding and base therapy, 3) oxygen therapy, and 4) assisted ventilation, if necessary.

The nurse is a key figure in all of these modalities. Accurate recording and reporting of all the data from the monitoring devices—skin, cardiac, apenia, and telethermometer—is necessary. The sites of these attachments must be watched carefully for abrasions or skin breakdown. Adequate oxygenation of the infant is imperative. Different criteria are used at different institutions and they are not universally agreed upon. In some institutions, oxygen is given the infant to assure an arterial oxygen tension (Po_2) of 50 to 60 mm. Hg, an arterial hemoglobin oxygen saturation of 85 to 90 percent, or a skin color devoid of cyanosis. The first two criteria are preferred if an arterial catheter has been inserted in the infant so that arterial blood sampling can be obtained. If an arterial catheter is not present, the third criterion can be used. Cyanosis usually will not be present until the arterial Po_2 is below 50 to 60 mm. Hg. It is well to remember that the smallest concentration of incubator oxygen necessary to achieve these criteria is used. Accurate reporting, recording, and observations of these levels is an important nursing responsibility. If the infant is receiving intravenous fluids (and he most likely will if very ill) scrupulous attention is to be given to the site to prevent and/or detect dislodgement or infection. One method used to protect the site is to take a plastic medicine glass and snip it in half lengthwise. Bind the edges with tape and apply over the IV site, securing with paper tape. This prevents direct contact with the needle by all persons coming in contact with the infant. Careful monitoring of the amount and flow of the infusion is also indicated. A urine bag is often taped in place when exact output is required. The presence of glucose in the urine can be detected in the absence of a bag by pressing a prepared glucose stick against the moistened diaper and comparing it with a standard chart. Glucose spillage in the urine calls for reduction of the amount of glucose being administered.

If an umbilical catheter is inserted, the umbilical site and the connecting points along the tubing are to be inspected frequently to prevent an undesired loss of blood. If the umbilical dressing and the connecting points along the tubing are exposed, bleeding can be readily ascertained. Any leakage should be reported to the physician immediately and direct pressure with sterile gauze sponges to the umbilical stump should be instituted.[13]

By 72 hours, infants with this condition will usually show either marked improvement or definite deterioration. When the infant remains stable for 12 to 24 hours in terms of acid-base and clinical status, small feedings of clear fluids may be instituted and the intravenous feedings discontinued if the oral feedings are retained.

Since infants delivered by cesarean section who have had a stormy labor are prone to develop this complication, many physicians prescribe that they be placed in an incubator with oxygen and high humidity immediately on delivery as a prophylactic measure. The stomach contents may be aspirated, and the oropharyngeal suctioning is done to remove mucus and fluid from the nose and the mouth.

Injuries

Caput succedaneum

Prolonged pressure on the head during a protracted first stage of labor, when the membranes rupture before the cervix is fully dilated, causes an edematous swelling of the soft tissues of the scalp over the area where it is encircled by the cervix (Fig. 29-4). This condition is called *caput succedaneum,* and in its milder forms is very common—so common that it may be regarded as normal.

It is due to an extravasation of serum into the tissues of the scalp at the portion surrounded by the cervix. The term is not confined to vertex cases; the corresponding swelling which forms on any presenting part is also, for the sake of uniformity, known as caput succedaneum. The condition always disappears within a few days without treatment. A prompt and simple explanation should be given to the parents, since this condition, although benign, can be somewhat disfiguring. Once the parents know that the caput will disappear of its own accord, they usually are reassured and will not press for "treatment."

Cephalhematoma

Cephalhematoma is another swelling of the scalp which resembles caput succedaneum in certain respects. It is caused by an effusion of blood between the bone and the periosteum (Fig. 29-5). This explains why the swelling appears directly over the bone. It is most common over the parietal bones. It is seldom visible when the infant is born and may not be noticed for several hours or more after delivery, since subperiosteal bleeding occurs slowly. The cephalhematoma increases gradually in size until about the seventh day after labor, when it remains stationary for a time and then begins to disappear. The infant usually recovers without treatment. It may be due to pressure in normal labor, or by forceps; but it is also seen occasionally in breech cases in which no instruments were used or prolonged pressure exerted on the aftercoming head. Such cases, however, are not common. Sometimes an x-ray will reveal a linear skull fracture beneath the hematoma. However, there are no known pathologic sequelae, even in the presence of a fracture. Occasionally, especially if the condition is bilateral, hyperbilirubinemia may result from the breakdown of the accumulated blood. Again, the parents should receive assurance regarding the temporary nature of this condition and its spontaneous disappearance.

Intracranial hemorrhage (cerebral hemorrhage, subdural hematoma)

In contradistinction to the two conditions just described, *intracranial hemorrhage* is one of the gravest complications encountered in the newborn. It may occur any place in the cranial vault, but is particularly likely to take place as the result of tears in the tentorium cerebelli with bleeding into the cerebellum, the pons, and the medulla oblongata. Since these structures contain many important centers (respiratory center, and so on), hemorrhage in these areas is very often fatal.

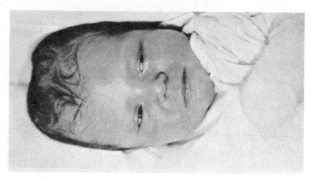

Figure 29-5. Cephalhematoma. (MacDonald House, University Hospitals of Cleveland)

Intracranial hemorrhage occurs most often after prolonged labor, especially in primiparae, and is particularly likely to take place in difficult forceps deliveries and in version and extractions. It is also seen more commonly in precipitate deliveries as the result of the rapid propulsion of the infant's head through the birth canal. It is due primarily to excessive or unduly prolonged pressure on the fetal skull. This causes excessive molding of the head and such overriding of the cranial bones that the delicate supporting structures of the brain (tentorium cerebelli, falx cerebri, and so on) are torn, with consequent rupture of blood vessels.

The development of symptoms in cerebral hemorrhage may be sudden or gradual. If the hemorrhage is severe, the infant is usually stillborn; if less marked, apnea of the newborn may result, often with fatal outcome. Many infants who are resuscitated with difficulty at birth succumb later from brain hemorrhage. On the other hand, the infant may appear normal after delivery and develop the first signs of intracranial hemorrhage several hours or several days later.

The nurse should be familiar with the common signs of cerebral hemorrhage, which are described as follows. Any such signs should be reported immediately.

CONVULSIONS. Convulsions may vary from mild, localized twitchings to severe spasms of the whole body. Twitching of the lower jaw is characteristic, particularly when associated with salivation.

CYANOSIS. Cyanosis may be persistent but is more likely to occur in repeated attacks.

ABNORMAL RESPIRATION. Grunting respiration is characteristic; or it may be irregular, of Cheyne-Stokes type, very rapid and shallow, or very slow. Very slow breathing, usually associated with cyanosis, suggests respiratory paralysis due to pressure on the medulla oblongata and is a grave sign.

A SHARP, SHRILL, WEAK CRY. This cry is similar to that seen in meningitis.

FLACCIDITY OR SPASTICITY. If this condition is present, it usually portends a fatal outcome. Somnolence also may be present. In other cases there may be generalized spasticity with backward arching of the head and neck and extension of the legs (*opisthotonos*).

TREATMENT. Prevention is most important and is largely the responsibility of the physician. It consists in protecting the infant from trauma, particularly in difficult operative delivery. As stated previously, many obstetricians believe that the administration of vitamin K to the mother before delivery decreases the likelihood of cerebral bleeding. This is done less frequently now due to the possibility of hyperbilirubinemia. A small dose of water-soluble vitamin K_1 (1.0 mg.) may be given the infant after birth, however (see p. 591).

Curative treatment can be effective if damage is not too extensive.

Complete rest with the very minimum amount of handling is imperative. Infants suspected of having a cerebral hemorrhage are placed in intensive care. All supportive measures of maintaining heat, oxygenation, and vital signs monitoring are employed. Intravenous feeding or gavage are employed. If a subdural hematoma is suspected, a spinal tap will be done for diagnostic purposes and excess subdural bloody fluid may be removed as a therapeutic measure. Usually the physician will order some form of sedative for convulsions. Vitamin C and water-soluble vitamin K may be used to control the hemorrhage, and antibiotics may be given prophylactically. The head of the infant is kept a few inches above the level of the hips, because this position is believed to lower intracranial pressure. Moreover, the infant should *not* be placed in Trendelenburg position after delivery.

The parents, of course, will need and deserve adequate explanation and reassurance. Since it is difficult to prognosticate in this condition (as well as in several of the other disorders) until the extent and the severity of the injury can be determined, personnel will not want to give the parents false hopes nor yet seem to be unduly pessimistic. The physician and nurse, however, as they report to the parents, can always add an expression like today or at this time to their explanations, even if the news seems to be unfortunate (e.g., "The baby is responding satisfactorily to the medicines today." "He is progressing at this time."). This will give the parents a more realistic reassurance and yet subtly alert them to the fluidity of the situation.

Facial paralysis

Pressure by forceps on the facial nerve may cause temporary paralysis of the muscles of one side of the face so that the mouth is drawn to the other side. This will be particularly noticeable when the infant cries. The condition is usually transitory and disappears in a few days, often in a few hours. Since the infant can look grotesque, the parents will need an explanation concerning the temporary nature of this affliction. If the mother is allowed to feed the baby, the nurse will want to be with her more consistently during the first feedings to help her as necessary. Sucking may be difficult for the infant, and the mother will need to develop patience and skill in the feeding of her baby. If one eye remains open because of the affected muscles, the physician will prescribe such treatment as is appropriate. Any necessary instruction regarding this continuing care after discharge should be given the mother before she leaves the hospital. Very often parents are afraid to handle their infants when disorders occur for fear of hurting the child; this may happen even if the condition is short-term and fairly innocuous. Thus, parents should be encouraged to hold and cuddle their infants whenever the condition permits.

Arm paralysis (Erb-Duchenne's paralysis, brachial palsy)

This condition results from excessive stretching of the nerve fibers that run from the neck through the shoulder and down toward the arm (brachial plexus). It is a result of forcible pulling of the shoulder away from the head during delivery, usually during a breech extraction. Generally, only the muscles of the upper arm are involved, and the infant holds his arm at the side with the elbow extended and the hand rotated inward. The hand and fingers may not be involved. If the nerves are merely stretched, recovery occurs in several weeks; if they are broken within their sheaths, healing will not be complete for several months. If healing fails to occur within that time, surgery is indicated; the outcome for recovery in these cases is guarded. To reduce tension on the brachial plexus, the physician usually will place the arm in a splint or cast in an elevated, neutral position. While the arm is healing, the physician will order gentle manipulation and massage of the muscles to prevent contractures. The mother is to be instructed in these procedures so that she may continue the care.

Fractures and dislocations

Fracture of a long bone or dislocation of an extremity may be the result of a version; or it may occur following a breech delivery in which the arms were extended above the head and were brought down into the vagina. Fractures of the clavicle or of the jaw, or dislocation of either of these bones, may follow forcible efforts to extract the aftercoming head in cases of breech presentation. Fracture or dislocation of the cervical spine, usually accompanied by damage to the spinal cord may also be the consequence of a difficult breech extraction. The vertebrae most usually affected are C5 and C6. If the cord is not completely severed, surgical repair is often effected. These babies will have a flaccid paralysis of the trunk and extremities and breathe abdominally, since the diaphragm is innervated by the nerves which have been injured in the dislocation or fracture.

Fractures in the newborn baby, particularly in the long bones usually heal rapidly, but it is often difficult to keep the parts in good alignment during repair. Immobilization of the part often can be achieved by swaddling and positioning the infant on his side. Splints, slings, and other apparatus are useful. However, these often make handling the infant difficult and cumbersome; hence parents tend to avoid touching the infant for fear of "hurting" him. Care should be taken by the staff to encourage the parents to give their infant adequate love and attention if these apparatuses are used. This will mean that the parents will have to be shown how to manipulate the apparatus effectively so that they will not traumatize the injury. Dislocation should be reduced at once, or there will be great danger of permanent deformity in the joint. Follow-up supervision is necessary in order to prevent permanent deformity. Physiotherapy under orthopedic direction is important.

Infections

Most institutions have an area designated as an isolation nursery where any infant who has or is suspected of having an infection is placed immediately. Once the infant has been transferred to the isolation nursery, he should not be returned to the newborn nursery even though the infection has been treated and/or cured. Strict aseptic technique is used in the care of these babies, and therefore the principles of infectious disease nursing must be understood and carried out by all personnel coming in contact with the infants. Separation of the mother and the infant may be necessary, depending on the type and the severity of the infection. This may require consequent nursing action that has been discussed in Chapter 15.

Ophthalmia of the newborn (gonorrheal conjunctivitis)

This is a serious condition which may result in total blindness, but if suitable treatment is adopted at the very outset of the disease and intelligently carried out, usually the sight can be saved. The entire treatment is, of course, under the direct supervision of the physician.

Fortunately, state laws making the use of an antibacterial prophylaxis compulsory for all infants at birth have reduced the incidence of this infection immeasurably. Before eye prophylaxis became mandatory, however, 25 to 30 percent of all children in schools for the blind suffered impaired sight as the result of the infection. This condition is of gonorrheal origin and is characterized by a profuse, purulent discharge in the eyes due to infection, generally from the genital canal at the time of birth. However, the causative organism, *Neisseria gonorrheae*, can be transmitted also on the hands of personnel working with infected mothers and by articles (e.g., towels, tissues, and so on) that come in contact with the infection. Thus, the importance of proper hygiene for those working with infected persons cannot be stressed enough. Prompt diagnosis and treatment of those suspected of having the disease is also vital, since the mother may reinfect her infant as she handles him.

The most common reason for delay in the diagnosis is the assumption by inexperienced persons that all conjunctivitis in the first few days of life is a consequence of the prophylactic silver nitrate (or the antibiotic ointment). A degree of conjunctival inflammation with catarrhal discharge may occur with silver nitrate and to a lesser degree with the various antibiotic preparations. However, the nurse should give primary consideration to infection in the presence of purulent exudate during the first days of life or catarrhal conjunctivitis persisting longer than three days. It is well to remember also that the widely used procedure of phototherapy for neonatal hyperbilirubinemia necessitates shielding the infant's eyes during the procedure and may result in obscuring this disease—thus, the pads should be removed regularly and the eyes examined.

If the infection occurs at the time of birth, the disease appears within two or three days; but as the septic discharge may be introduced into the eye at a later period by neglect of the proper care of the infant, the onset may be later. Both eyes are usually affected; and at first they are suffused with a watery discharge and considerable inflammation of the eyelids. Within 24 hours, the lids become very much swollen, and a thick, creamy, greenish pus is discharged. Later, unless treatment has been instituted early, the swelling becomes so marked that the eyes cannot be opened, opacities of the cornea occur, the conjunctiva is ulcerated and then perforated, and the eye collapses and finally atrophies.

The preventive treatment consists of the use of an antibacterial agent, usually 1 percent silver nitrate, or penicillin ophthalmic ointment, which is instilled immediately after birth. However, if infection does occur, penicillin intramuscular injections may be given. If the infection persists, intensive penicillin administration should be carried out. Thanks to this drug, gonorrheal ophthalmia, which used to be one of the most stubborn and grave afflictions and demanded the utmost in elaborate and prolonged nursing and medical care, is now cured within 12 to 24 hours. The swelling and the pus usually disappear in even less time than this. It must be remembered, however, that success depends on prompt diagnosis and treatment. Moreover, with the increased high incidence and prevalence of gonorrhea in the general population, this infection has come back into prominence and staff need to be alert to its importance.

Ophthalmia of the newborn is a distinctly infectious disease, and there is extreme danger of conveying it to others. This applies not only to other infants' eyes but to the genital tract of other mothers. Even the eyes of the nurse herself may become infected, unless she is most conscientious in her methods. The infant should be isolated, and all articles used should be sterilized.

Staphylococcus of resistant types occasionally cause purulent discharge; all such cases require the care of a physician until recovery.

Bacterial skin infections of the newborn

There continues to be concern about the spread of staphylococcal infection in hospitals and its increasing resistance to antibiotic therapy. The newborn nursery is one of the most vulnerable areas because of the infants' low tolerance to infections.

In studies of staphylococcal infection of the newborn, strains of the organism have been found not only in skin lesions of the infected infants, but also in the nasopharynx of a high percentage of apparently well infants. Nurseries at this time must be considered potential epidemic centers. Many factors contribute to the large numbers of infants found to harbor these organisms. *Crowding* of infants in a nursery has always been a serious problem and a contributing factor in any epidemic disease outbreak. The usually recommended minimum of 25 square feet of space per infant may actually not be adequate to prevent spread of infection. *Hospital personnel* have been found to be carriers of staphylococcus coagulase-positive organisms. These organisms are highly resistant to most antibiotics in current use, and when they are transmitted to infants, they may result in such manifestations as skin lesions, pneumonia, septicemia, conjunctivitis, omphalitis, osteomyelitis, and other forms of infection from mild infections to those of extremely serious nature. In many studies, there appears to be a direct transmission of the offending organisms from hospital personnel to infant, from infant to infant, from infant to mother and to the family at home, and even into the community (see Chapter 23). Hospital sanitation must be critically appraised, since these organisms may be air-borne and can exist in many contaminated or unclean surfaces of the nurseries, wards and other hospital areas. The type of walls, floors and equipment used must be of materials which can be easily and satisfactorily cleaned. Housekeeping personnel, their equipment and methods are to be constantly evaluated and supervised. There is no substitute for cleanliness, aseptic technique and isolation of infected patients and staff in controlling the spread of infection.

Manifestations of staphylococcal infection of the newborn frequently appear as pyoderma, stuffy noses, pneumonia, and conjunctivitis. Few infants develop serious staphylococcal disease without preceding or accompanying pyoderma. Treatment usually consists of antimicrobial drugs given parenterally.

Pyoderma of the skin may occur in epidemic form in the nursery. This was formerly called "impetigo contagiosa" and the term gives some hint of its infectiousness. The condition manifests itself by the eruption of small, semi-globular vesicles or pustules. Although these may appear on any part of the body, they are most frequently encountered on moist opposing surfaces, such as the folds of the neck, the axilla and the groin. Thence they may spread rapidly by autoinoculation to any part of the body. The lesion is small and varies from the size of a pinhead to a diameter of half an inch. It contains yellow pus. The bacterium involved is usually the staphylococcus or the streptococcus.

TREATMENT. The treatment is essentially preventive, and outbreaks rarely occur if the nursery techniques have been meticulous. *Failure to wash hands properly between handling of different infants is undoubtedly the principal mode of spread of infection by any organism. Nothing is more fundamental and important to proper nursery hygiene than handwashing.* This fact is restated here to reinforce its importance. Each hospital will have its particular scrub and handwashing procedures which hopefully are derived from the Center for Disease Control (Atlanta) and/or the local health department's recommended procedures. Another source for details of nursery techniques and measures for the management of nursery epidemics is presented in the *Standards and Recommendations for Hospital Care of Newborn Infants* (1971) published by the American Academy of Pediatrics.

Treatment consists of prompt isolation and local treatment of the lesions. Bathing infants with hexachlorophene detergent is well documented for its effectiveness in minimizing the rate of staphylococcal colonization and the incidence of disease. However, there is some evidence that, by reducing staph colonization with hexachlorophene, the prevalence of gram-negative rods is increased (see Suggested Reading).

In December 1972, the Food and Drug Administration and American Academy of Pediatrics recommended that routine total body bathing of infants, using hexachlorophene, be discontinued since there was some evidence in nonhuman subjects that this detergent produced cystic lesions in the brain (in doses far exceeding those used in humans). Moreover, blood levels of hexachlorophene in human newborns (primarily prematures) had been demonstrated, presumably absorbed from the skin. Several weeks after these reports, the Center for Disease Control reported outbreaks of staphylococcal disease throughout the nation, and this has continued in institutions that have discontinued the use of the detergent. Thus, the original statements of the Food and Drug Administration and the American Academy of Pediatrics were subsequently modified to recommend that hexachlorophene bathing be utilized in the presence of a staphylococcal outbreak. Many institutions have adopted modified routine procedures: diluting the detergent and/or giving only an admission and discharge bath. Systemic antibiotic therapy may be required in severe outbreaks. A high nutritional level must be maintained and scratching should be controlled. If the lesion is a bleb, the fluid in it is infectious and all materials coming in contact with it are to be taken care of according to isolation procedures.[14] (See Herrmann article in Suggested Reading for specifics regarding infection control in the nursery.)

Thrush

Thrush is an infection of the mouth caused by the organism *Candida albicans*, the organism which causes monilial vaginitis in the mother (see Chapter 18). The infant may acquire the infection as it passes through the birth canal of a mother so infected. However, the infection may be transferred from infant to infant on the hands of attendants and is favored by lack of cleanliness in feeding, in the care of the mother's nipples, or in the care of the bottles and the nipples. It is most likely to occur in weak, undernourished babies and in those receiving antibiotic therapy, since the use of certain antibiotics alters the oral flora making it more susceptible to this opportunistic organism.

The condition appears as small white patches (due to the fungus growth) on the tongue and in the mouth. These white plaques may be mistaken at first for small curds of milk. The infant's mouth must be kept clean, but great gentleness is required to avoid further injury to the delicate epithelium, and any attempt to wipe away the plaques will usually cause bleeding.

Some physicians advise painting the spots with an aqueous solution of 1 percent gentian violet, in which case the spots are touched gently with a sterile, soft cotton swab saturated with the medication. This is an effective treatment, but is temporarily disfiguring and stains clothing and bed linen (stains can be removed with a paste of sodium bicarbonate). Care should be taken to avoid applying an excess of this solution since it may be irritating when swallowed. The infant can be placed face down after the application so that saliva containing the drug can drain out more easily. Another more simple and as effective a drug is nystatin. This drug is given as an oral instillation (100,000 units per ml.), 1 ml. four times a day at intervals of six hours. The solution is slowly and gently instilled so that there is an opportunity for it to be widely distributed throughout the oral cavity before it is swallowed.

Special care must be taken with the bottles and nipples used for infants who have thrush. These bottles and nipples must be kept separated from the others used in the nursery. It is preferred that disposable bottles and nipples be used for these infants. If this is impossible, both the bottles and nipples are soaked in an antiseptic solution, washed thoroughly, and sterilized before they are cared for in the routine way with bottles and nipples of other infants.

Diarrhea of the newborn

Several bacterial agents can produce primary diarrhea. The most common and important is the enteropathic *Escherichia coli*. Serologic techniques have identified 140 groups of *E. coli*. and over a dozen have been implicated in nursery epidemics of diarrhea. Other bacteria —salmonella, shigella, and staphylococci—are infrequent causes.

Whatever the etiology, a pattern of signs and symptoms of the infection develops: there is refusal to feed, weight loss (as much as a pound a day), and hypoactivity. These may precede the diarrhea itself by a day or two. Blood and pus in the stool are rare, except in shigellosis. As diarrhea continues, the infant becomes toxic, dehydrated, and acidotic (meta-

bolic acidosis). These symptoms may appear somewhat abruptly during the early phase of explosive diarrhea. Dehydration is even more rapid if vomiting is also present. An ashen gray color or pallor is indicative of impending vasomotor collapse and death. Rapid correction of the metabolic acidosis and dehydration are therefore crucial. Milder forms of the disease are not uncommon; in these cases, there may be fewer stools, but the diarrhea is protracted and there is failure to feed.[15]

Two of the most important predisposing factors in these outbreaks are overcrowding and faulty nursery techniques—that is, failure to scrub properly before entering the nursery, *failure to wash hands before touching a baby*, failure to maintain proper cleanliness in equipment, clothing, supplies, and so on, that come in contact with the infant. The guiding principle involved is that everything coming in contact with the baby's mouth and nose should be in a surgically aseptic condition. All nursing and medical techniques are to be planned accordingly. Various health departments have set up helpful guidelines and regulations in the hope of preventing epidemics.

TREATMENT AND PREVENTION. When a case is discovered, immediate and absolute isolation is necessary; therefore, the infant is transferred from the newborn nursery. A culture of the stools is done to find out the causative organism. This is done so that specific therapy can be instituted as soon as possible. Neomycin or polymycin given orally have been found to be most effective against the *E. coli* organism and are instituted even before the results of the cultures are in. Often the cultures do not show either a bacterial or viral agent and to date these situations defy explanation. These drugs may be given prophylactically to exposed but uninfected infants until their discharge. Penicillin is sometimes administered to prevent or control the secondary infection that might occur in the debilitated infants. Supportive fluid therapy by the intravenous route also may be utilized. Oral fluids—water, 5 percent glucose in water, or commercially prepared electrolyte fluid replacement for oral use—are given in small amounts. Whole blood is given by transfusion if indicated.

If necessary, the nursery is closed to new admissions until the epidemic clears up. These nurseries are washed and disinfected before being opened again for new admissions. In the prevention of this disease there seems to be nothing more effective than strict aseptic nursery technique. Hand washing with surgical soap preparation or bacteriocidal and water after changing diapers, before feeding the infant and after handling the infant or any of its equipment is a rigid rule that should be stressed.

If an outbreak occurs, there should be a follow-up of all infants discharged in the preceding two weeks, and any infants needing treatment are readmitted to the pediatric service of the hospital. All infants exposed at the time of an outbreak are given prophylactic therapy. Complete control of this disease, which formerly led to closing of the nursery, can be gained by prompt reporting, rigid techniques, and immediate treatment.

Because of the "explosive" and virulent character of this disease and the startling debilitation of the infant, the parents usually become very anxious about their baby and with good reason. The baby is usually not allowed to go out to the mother, as a measure to prevent the spread of the infection and to guard against secondary infection of the infant. Thus, breast-feeding is interrupted for a time at least. The nurse can be helpful in keeping the mother and father informed about the status of the infant and helping the mother to work through her anxiety and grief positively. If it appears that breast-feeding can be resumed shortly, then the nurse can also show the mother how to empty her breast by manual expression to keep the milk supply available until nursing is resumed.

Syphilis

Even with the rise in the rate of this disease in the general population in recent years, syphilis in the newborn can be prevented when antepartal care is adequate. It has decreased greatly in the 42 states where serologic tests on the blood of all pregnant women are required. This condition shows lesions only if the infant has early prenatal syphilis. They may be present at birth or may appear from a few days up to four months of age, predominantly on the face, the buttocks, the palms, and the soles. Mucous patches occur in the mouth, and condylomata about the anus. These lesions are highly infectious. The eruption is usually maculopapular and not quite so generalized as in acquired syphilis. Bullae may appear on the palms and the soles, a type of lesion never found in acquired syphilis. The palms and the soles may desquamate as a result of the lesions. Less frequently seen are papular lesions or purely macular or, very rarely, vesicular or somewhat pustular ones. The nails may be deformed, and alopecia may be present. In such cases the blood test for syphilis is usually strongly positive. In addition to the cutaneous manifestations of syphilis, other signs and symptoms may arouse suspicion of the presence of the disease. The infant becomes restless, develops rhinitis (snuffles), and a hoarse voice. The baby does not gain weight as it should. The lymph nodes are enlarged, especially the epitrochlear nodes. The liver and the spleen are enlarged, as are also the ends of the long bones.

In the treatment of syphilis of the newborn, the physicians will rely chiefly on penicillin. The broad-spectrum antibiotics may be used if sensitivity makes the use of penicillin inadvisable. Usually additional therapy is unnecessary; however, most of these infants are kept under surveillance for one or two years after treatment.

Babies born to mothers who have been treated early in the antepartal period for syphilis are seldom born with the disease.

Malformations (intrauterine growth deviations)

There are approximately 250,000 babies born each year who have abnormalities that cause a significant alteration in the structure or function of their bodies. The incidence of these disorders has not changed greatly over the decades; however, the techniques of prenatal diagnosis, repair and correction have improved immensely, thus offering a great deal of hope and consolation to the parents and the children who are afflicted with these conditions. Indeed, there is increasing specialization in *teratology* —the study of the relationship of genetic and environmental factors in the production of congenital abnormalities.

The etiology of birth defects is not completely understood, but a multifactor etiology is generally accepted and it is recognized that most of these defects have an environmental component in their causes. Malformations may arise from 1) genetic factors such as change in the chromosome number, mutation, or structural abnormalities, and 2) environmental factors, such as irradiation, infection, and drugs. It should be emphasized that the most frequent of the genetically influenced malformations are multifactorial in nature. Thus, these defects result from interactions among multiple genetic and environmental factors. In addition, it is estimated that about 65 percent are due to unknown factors.[16]

Congenital deformities may range from minor abnormalities, such as supernumerary digits to grave malformations incompatible with life, which include *anencephalia* (absence of the brain), *hydrocephalus* (excessive amount of fluid in the cerebral ventricles with tremendous enlargement of the head), and *various heart abnormalities*. These grave defects are second only to accidents as a cause of death in childhood. Moreover, these youngsters represent a serious community health problem when one considers the numerous sequential surgical procedures with the attendant expense these families must undergo. In addition, the special rehabilitation and education that many require plus the drain on the parents' time and emotional and physical reserves, can have a grave social impact.

Since these conditions are so numerous and varied, this section will present selected disorders—those more commonly seen that are apparent at birth or soon thereafter and/or those with which the maternity nurse will have to deal. As indicated on pages 581 to 589, the care of these infants and their parents presents a great challenge to the nurse. She must give competent and, at times, complex nursing care to the babies, and she must help the parents to convert their feelings of disappointment and, often, despair to constructive efforts of habilitation of the infant. In addition, the negative feelings that are aroused in the nurse must be handled. The young student will find that discussing these feelings with her instructor or supervisors will help her to cope with them.

Congenital heart disease

At the time of birth and for weeks thereafter, there are great changes in the circulation of the newborn. When the cord is clamped and expansion of the lungs occurs, the pulmonary circulation increases in volume. The foramen ovale, the ductus arteriosus, and the ductus venosus are no longer needed and therefore close gradually over a period of several months. Usually the foramen ovale is closed by the third month of life and the ductus by the second; during the period of closure, signs or symptoms of patency rarely occur. When they do, they may be an indication of defects in these structures or other parts of the heart. Congenital heart disease has an incidence of about 3 percent per 1,000 at birth and 1 percent per 1,000 at the age of 10. Cardiovascular malformations account for approximately 50 percent of the deaths from congenital defects in the first year of life. The role of heredity as an etiologic agent is not as yet well understood. Congenital lesions may be recorded in as many as three generations and siblings seem to manifest the disease more often than in the preceding or succeeding generations. *Maternal disease during pregnancy influences the bodily structures of the developing fetus,* yet the etiology and dynamics of cardiovascular lesion are not known definitively. However, there is a higher incidence of other congenital defects among infants with congenital heart disease. Thus, the infant may suffer from multiple disorders.

Distress from congenital heart disease is often hard to distinguish from the distress that is secondary to pulmonary disease, such as respiratory distress syndrome. Yet accurate diagnosis is essential so that effective cardiac surgery can be instituted when indicated. The physical signs of both the normal and the abnormal newborn infant, such as right ventricular overactivity, behavior of the second heart sound, and color, are governed largely by the pulmonary artery pressure level, the rate of constriction of the ductus arteriosus, and the amount of placental transfusion. These are important and can mask the signs of congenital heart disease. The most severe of these diseases which occur in early infancy are not associated with loud murmurs, and many which eventually are associated with loud murmurs most often are not manifested immediately after birth.

Loud, abnormal heart sounds, however, together with a rapid rate, may constitute the first sign of serious illness. A gallop rhythm is an extremely helpful sign which indicates the presence of congestive heart failure. The presence of a single heart sound after the first 12 hours of life is almost always abnormal and should stimulate further search for cardiopulmonary disease. An ejection click is normally noted only during the first few hours of life, when it may accompany the normal hypertension which characterizes the transitional pulmonary circulation. After that time, the presence of a loud click may denote a large aorta (found in pulmonary atresia), a large pulmonary artery (found in the hypoplastic left heart syndrome), or a large single vessel (found in truncus arteriosus).

It must be remembered that peripheral cyanosis occurs a great deal in the newborn period; arterial blood oxygen tensions are significantly lower shortly after birth than they will be several days later. Thus, cardiac malformations which are associated with severe arterial oxygen desaturation later in the neonatal period may be present in a relatively acyanotic form owing to the good mix of oxygenated and unoxygenated blood that results temporarily from continued patency of the ductus arteriosus or foramen ovale.

Reduced amplitude of arterial pulses is always an important sign in this time and implies reduced cardiac output into the aorta. Bounding pulses usually imply a large aortic run-off such as is seen with patent ductus arteriosus or truncus arteriosus. Tachypnea is another useful sign. A respiratory rate in excess of 50 beats per minute usually means that a cardiopulmonary disorder is present. Congestive heart disease is characterized by tachypnea without much respiratory effort. In severe pulmonary disturbances, obvious labored respiration is a striking feature.[17]

Close nursing observations may disclose other signs which are indicative. These include ready tiring, reluctance to feed, constant or sporadic respiratory embarrassment of varying degrees, shallow "panting" respirations, sudden periods of distress accompanied by crying suggestive of pain, changes in color characterized by pallor, grayishness, or intense cyanosis. The older infant may exhibit a failure to thrive syndrome. These symptoms can occur in any combination at any time after birth.

Diagnosis is established from the history, physical findings, roentgenographic and electrocardiographic examinations. If doubt still exists, cardiac catheterization, angiocardiography, and aortography usually supply the needed confirmatory data. These latter procedures are strenuous, and, if the child is severely distressed or in danger of circulatory failure, they may very well threaten his life. Therefore, great effort is made to utilize astute observation, history findings, and the roentgen and electrocardiograph findings.

Nursing care of these infants is directed to offset those factors observed to aggravate symptoms. Severely affected infants may be transferred directly to the pediatric facility; however, less distressed infants may remain on the maternity unit especially during the time a diagnosis is being established.

The following nursing goals will be kept in mind: reduction of the work of the heart, maintenance of nutrition, reduction of respiratory distress, prevention of respiratory and other infection, reduction of the parents' anxiety, and their support and teaching.

Every precaution is taken to keep the infant from exposure to infection. The principles discussed in the care of the immature infant apply here. In addition, unnecessary disturbance is to be kept at a minimum as startling, or physical effort often distresses these babies. When the infant shows signs of severe respiratory embarrassment, relief is sometimes achieved by raising the head and shoulders. When these episodes are accompanied by crying which is suggestive of pain, the baby is sometimes eased if a warm hand is applied over his abdomen and he is very gently inclined over the upper margin of the supporting hand. In the case of severe distress, the baby may lie with his head loosely retracted; this should not be corrected as the infant assumes a position most suitable for aeration. Restlessness is often apparent, and, hence, clothes and positioning should allow for maximum freedom of movement. Profuse diaphoresis is often seen and sponge baths with tepid water can supplement the daily bath. Oxygen is to be ready at all times for these babies, and the physician may want to prescribe digitalis if heart failure appears imminent. Feedings are usually given more frequently and in less amounts than to the healthy term infant. The aim, of course, is to avoid undesirable pressure of a distended stomach on the diaphragm and heart. If the infant can suck without distress, a bottle is the feeding method of choice. If bottle feeding does result in cyanosis or impaired respiration, a spoon or gavage tube may have to be utilized. Breast-feeding is almost always discouraged because of the suddenness and capriciousness of the respiratory difficulties.

Supportive care is necessary for the parents of these babies; keeping lines of communication open between the parents and the staff (i.e., obstetrician, pediatrician, heart surgeon, nursery nurses, pediatric nurses) will do much to help alleviate anxiety and help in the adjustment. As with infants with other types of defects or the immature infant, there is no contraindication for the parents to "visit" their infant. He usually is viewed through a window to prevent exposure to infection. When the parents indicate a desire for a visit the nurse can arrange for it.

Cleft lip and cleft palate

These deformities, which may occur separately or in combination, result from the failure of the soft and/or bony tissues of the palate and the upper jaw to unite during the fifth to tenth weeks of gestation. The defect may be unilateral or bilateral (Fig. 29-6). Only the lip may be involved, or the disunion may extend into the upper jaw or into the nasal cavity.

Each year about one in 700 white infants and one in 2,000 black infants are born with a cleft lip and/or cleft palate; thus, this condition is one of the most common of the birth defects. More males than females appear to be affected by the combination cleft lip and palate disorder.

A clear-cut etiologic pattern for these deformities remains obscure. Variables found to be associated with them include genetic variables, drugs, radiation, obstruction in utero, maternal illness during pregnancy, and dietary influences. Recently, the hypothesis has been put forward that palatolabial defects may be due to sex-modified multifactorial inheritance.[18]

TREATMENT. The plan of treatment and outcome will depend on the severity of the condition. If only the lip is involved, the surgery may take place within the first few days, although some physicians prefer to wait until the child is eight to twelve weeks of age because they feel that there is more tissue available at that time to facilitate operative precision. When the palate is involved, the repair is usually done when the child is 18 to 24 months or when he reaches a weight of 20 to 22 pounds. Time is not the only salient variable; a child that is free from infection and who is nutritionally sound is perhaps even more important.[19]

When surgery is performed later a prosthetic speech device usually is fitted so that speech development may not be hindered. Cleft palates usually involve other difficulties, frequent respiratory infections, orthodontia and speech problems, and so on; therefore, the care of these children involves the coordinated activities of the pediatrician, plastic surgeon, orthodontist, hospital and community health nurses, speech therapists and, very often, the social worker. Fortunately, modern treatment is so effective that this defect becomes a relatively minor handicap.

Nevertheless, the parents require a great deal of supportive help initially, as mentioned earlier, especially since this disorder is so disfiguring. In our culture a high value is put on physical attractiveness and beauty; and when this condition occurs, particularly if the baby is a girl, it may come as a tremendous shock and burden to the parents. However, repair is generally successful, and it is very helpful if the parents know and understand this. One institution has one or two members of the team involved in the reconstruction process visit the mother after a comprehensive assessment of the infant has been made. The purpose of this visit is to assure the mother that the defect is correctable. Color transparencies are shown to

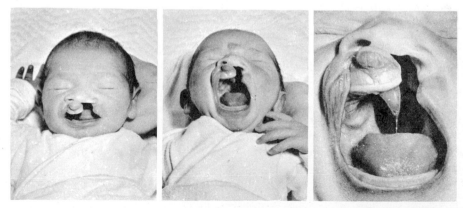

Figure 29-6. Cleft lip and complete cleft palate. In this case surgical closure of the harelip was performed less than 18 hours following birth, with excellent results. (MacDonald House, University Hospitals of Cleveland)

her of an infant with a similar defect and the results of the surgery. This visual reassurance has been found to be more effective than any verbal explanation. This initial visit has been found not only to placate the parents' fears, but also to restore their confidence that their baby will become a useful member of society and will be socially acceptable. No rejection of infants has been observed in the eight years this practice has been in operation. In addition, the pattern of treatment is explained to the mother so that she can know and begin to participate in the feeding and care of her child.[20]

More frequently now, the infant is sent home with the mother to become older and well-nourished enough to withstand the various procedures. Unless the baby reaches a state of adequate nutrition, the outlook for successful management by any specialty is diminished. Thus, caloric, fluid, and chemical balance is best realized through the baby's regular oral intake of a normal diet.

Feeding is usually one of the most immediate and difficult problems in the daily care of the infant. It can best be accomplished by placing the infant in an upright position and directing the flow of milk against the side of the mouth. This will decrease the possibility of aspiration as well as the amount of air swallowed during feeding. Since sucking strengthens and develops the muscles needed for speech, a nipple is used for feeding whenever possible. A variety of nipples may be tried, including a regular nipple with enlarged holes, a soft rubber nipple, a cleft palate nipple, or a duck bill nipple. The last two are more expensive and should be used only after the others have been tried. Specific instructions are necessary with their use. If the infant cannot use any of the nipples, then a spoon or a rubber-tipped medicine dropper may be tried. The flow of milk will have to be adjusted to the infant's swallowing and should not be released until the infant attempts to suck. The feedings are given at a pace which will neither cause the infant to become unduly tired nor result in aspiration of the liquid. Since these infants tend to swallow a large amount of air, they should be bubbled at frequent intervals, and the mother will need to be instructed in this technique. The nurse will want to help the mother to attain ease in feeding her baby and should arrange to stay with her during at least several of the sessions. She then can ascertain by demonstration and observation how well the mother is progressing. Gavage feeding usually is unnecessary and should be used only when the other methods fail, since it does not stimulate the sucking and swallowing reflexes and promotes aspiration.

One author has suggested that the feeding procedure and equipment needed for the cleft babies are to be considered essentially the same as for the normal newborn. A plastic nursing bottle with a presoftened "preemie" nipple is recommended. The nipple can be attached to the bottle by a circular collar which allows for some head movement and also eliminates vacuum formation in the bottle. The plastic bottle can be squeezed gently to assist the infant, thus decreasing his effort and lessening the time needed for feeding. Cross-cut nipples have also been found to be very helpful. They stay closed until the baby, with minimal pressure, opens it as he chews and swallows, establishing a nursing rhythm.[21]

The mother may want to breast-feed her infant, and there is no contraindication as long as the milk can be given in a way that the baby can take it. This may mean that the mother may have to express her milk and offer it in a bottle.

Frenulum linguae

The frenulum of the tongue is a sharp, thin ridge of tissue that arises in the midline from the base of the tongue and attaches to its under surface for varying distances toward the top. When the attachment extends far forward, a concavity or groove is apparent at the tip of the tongue on its upper surface. This has been called tongue-tie. It never interferes with feeding nor does it produce a speech impediment as formerly thought. Therefore, incising the frenulum is not indicated, since it provides a portal of entry for infection and there is danger of severing the large vein in the area of the frenulum.

Hypospadias and epispadias

In *hypospadias*, the urethra opens on the under surface of the penis proximal to the usual site. Minor degrees of this condition are quite common, and no surgical intervention is necessary. If the opening is at the base of the penis or far back on the shaft, plastic surgical repair will be necessary. In *epispadias*, the urethral opening is on the dorsal surface of the penis. If the defect is pronounced, it also will require repair. Surgical correction is usually made by two years of age. Definitive urethroplasty should be performed before the boy enters school so that it will be possible for him to urinate in the standing position. Since the foreskin is used in the repair, boys with hypospadias are not to be circumcised.

Spina bifida

Spina bifida is a rather common malformation and is due to the congenital absence of one or more vertebral arches, usually at the lower part of the spine. When the membranes covering the spinal cord bulge through the opening, the condition is known as *meningocele*. It forms a soft, fluctuating tumor filled with cerebrospinal fluid. The tumor can be diminished by pressure and enlarges when the baby cries. The extrusion of the cord along with the coverings is known as *meningomyelocele*. When the tumor is very small and shows no signs of increasing in size, it may merely be protected from injury and infection by carefully applied dressings; but the more severe cases must be treated surgically. When the repair is massive, the outlook can be discouraging. Hydrocephalus may occur if not already present. However, new techniques have been developed to relieve this latter condition. The situation and prognosis for the infant may be guarded, and the parents will need a good deal of support and instruction about the continuing care of their infant (see Suggested Reading). The physician will prescribe regarding the care that is to be given at home.

Umbilical hernia

Umbilical hernia, or rupture at the umbilicus, may appear during the first few weeks of life. The associated protrusion of intestinal contents may be made to disappear entirely on pressure, but it reappears when the pressure is removed, or when the baby cries. This is due to a weakness or an imperfect closure of the umbilical ring and is often associated with nonunion of the recti muscles. The condition usually disappears spontaneously by age one. There is a great deal of controversy regarding the utility of strapping the abdomen to reduce the hernia. Most authorities feel that the strapping technique is useless and some feel that it may be deleterious. Surgery is usually avoided unless the hernia persists until the age of three to five years, causes symptoms, becomes strangulated or enlarges. Some mothers may need to be discouraged from placing a coin or button beneath a home fashioned umbilical dressing; this practice was used for many years as a "home remedy." It has no value and prohibits adequate approximation of the margins of the abdomen.

Obstructions of the alimentary tract

ATRESIA OF THE ESOPHAGUS. This condition, although less common than some which have been mentioned, is quite serious, and immediate steps must be taken to prevent aspiration. The defect, which occurs during embryonic development, results in the esophagus ending in a blind pouch rather than a continuous tube to the stomach. A fistula usually occurs into the trachea near the bifurcation of the esophagus and the trachea. When the baby attempts to swallow liquids or even normal secretions, there is an overflow into the trachea from the blind pouch. This malformation should be suspected whenever the infant demonstrates excessive drooling, coughing, gagging, or cyanosis during feeding. The nurse must report these symptoms immediately; unless necessary surgery to correct the defect is prompt, the baby will contract bronchitis or pneumonia from repeated aspiration of milk and secretions. The infant is placed in the supine position, with his head elevated 30° or more to prevent any gastric secretions from rising into the trachea through the fistula. The baby usually is placed in a heated, humidified incubator after surgery. This atmosphere is needed to liquefy the tenacious mucus that collects. Nasopharyngeal suction is necessary, and the nurse should watch carefully for any cyanosis or labored respiration that indicates the need for this. Blood, plasma, parenteral fluids, and antibiotics are also given. The extent of the repair and the condition of the baby determine when oral feeding will be begun.

PYLORIC STENOSIS. This is a congenital anomaly and usually manifests its symptoms from the first week to the second or third week by the onset of vomiting which becomes projectile in character and occurs within 30 minutes after every feeding. The infant loses weight, the bowel elimination lessens, highly colored urine becomes scanty, and the symptoms of dehydration appear. Upon examination, gastric peristalsis is found to be present, and the pyloric "acornlike" tumor may be palpated. Surgery is the treatment of choice. Since it is not usually an emergency operation, there is sufficient time for supportive treatment to prepare the infant for surgery to correct any dehydration or electrolyte imbalance. If the hemoglobin is below 70 percent, transfusion is indicated. Gastric lavage, from one to two hours before operation, should be done until returns are clear. Maintaining body heat before and after the operation is essential. Transfusion should be given if indicated. Four ml. of 5 percent glucose in saline is given postoperatively for four feedings. If no vomiting develops, 8 ml. are given hourly for the next four feedings, then 16 ml. hourly for four feedings. If these feedings are retained, 1 ounce of formula is given an hour after the last feeding of clear fluid and repeated two hours later. By this stepwise increment, the amount of feedings and the interval between them are increased until a full feeding program is reinstituted in about 48 hours.

OBSTRUCTION OF THE DUODENUM AND THE SMALL INTESTINE. These conditions are relatively easy to diagnose. Vomiting occurs with the first feeding, and no meconium is eliminated. The vomitus may or may not be bile-stained, depending on whether the obstruction is high or low in the intestinal tract. If the obstruction is low, usually there is marked distention. A roentgenogram is used to confirm the diagnosis, and immediate surgery is indicated. However, the newborn infant should be allowed at least 12 hours for the respiration and kidney function to become stabilized. The operation is usually accompanied by continuous parenteral fluids, and blood should be available if needed. Postoperative care includes maintaining body temperature, intravenous fluids until peristalsis is established (about a week), followed by feedings as given in pyloric stenosis. If distention occurs, nasoduodenal suction may be necessary. If the distention is severe, the infant is placed in an oxygen tent.

IMPERFORATE ANUS. This abnormality consists of atresia of the anus, with the rectum ending in a blind pouch. Careful examination of the infant in the delivery room usually reveals the condition. Surgical treatment is, of course, imperative.

Chromosomal abnormalities

In the past decade, several striking chromosomal abnormalities have been found. When a particular chromosome is in triplicate rather than the usual duplicate (pair) it is called trisomy. Three such trisomies have been identified in man—trisomy 13 to 15, trisomy 17 to 18, and trisomy 21 to 22 (Down's syndrome). The clinical pictures of these conditions are so distinct that they can be recognized in the delivery room or the nursery and hence are included here for consideration by the maternity nurse.

As we have seen in Chapter 7, in the normal person, there are 46 chromosomes which are found in 23 pairs: one pair of sex-determining chromosomes and 22 pairs of autosomes. It is not yet possible to distinguish which chromosome is present in triplicate in a specific trisomy; thus, the numerical designations of suspect pairs are included in each particular trisomy aberration. Nor has the mechanism by which the offending chromosome produces its particular abnormality been determined. However, three distinct clinical patterns appear at birth. The extra chromosome found in trisomy results from nondisjunction (see Chapter 7) which can occur at any time in a cell's lifetime. Two different cytologic pictures emerge in trisomic cells. In the first, there is a free extra chromosome giving 47 chromosomes. In the second, the extra chromosome is translocated, that is, attached to another chromosome. The total number is 46, but one of the chromosomes is the size of two chromosomes put together. There is an increased incidence of all three types of trisomy with advanced maternal age. This phenomenon is thought to be related to the long storage of oocytes in the mother. These germ cells are laid down during the mother's own fetal life; they wait, however, until the time of their individual ovulation to complete their meiotic divisions. Thus, it appears that nondisjunction tends to occur in older oocytes.

TRISOMY 13, OR D. This trisomy is characterized by an extra chromosome in the D group which includes pairs 13 through 15 (see Chapter 7). Infants with this abnormality frequently have difficulty establishing and maintaining respiration. One of the most striking features is the abnormal cranial development. The cranium is usually small with a sloping forehead. The ears may be malformed and low set and the eyes usually have some defect (cataracts, iris defects, unusual smallness) often bilaterally. Cleft palate and lip are commonly present. In addition, the hands and feet are often grossly deformed. Extra digits are common on both hands and feet. The thumbs may be retroflexible (double jointed) and the foot frequently has a posterior prominence of the heel sometimes accompanied by a convex sole known as "rocker bottom" foot. Other defects may include a bulbous nose, umbilical and diaphragmatic hernias, abnormal genitalia, scalp defects, and extensive capillary hemangiomata far in excess of what is usually found in the normal newborn. Neurologic examination reveals these infants to have a weak or absent Moro reflex and little or no response to loud noises; hence they appear to be deaf. They are prone to develop myoclonic seizures and all suffer from apneic spells of unknown origin. Autopsy often reveals the complete absence of olfactory nerves and tracts. All of these infants are mentally retarded and the majority have severe cardiac defects (dextroposition of the heart, ventricular septal defects) which are the major contributors to death in these infants. The average life span for these youngsters is less than a year, although several have lived to the age of five years.

TRISOMY 18, OR E. This trisomy is characterized by an extra chromosome in the E group, which includes pairs 17 and 18 (see Chapter 7). These babies are usually born at term but are small, averaging about 5 pounds. Their placentas are often very small. The head is small with a prominent occiput but in proportion to the body size. The eyes are usually normal but the ears are generally malformed and low-set. The mouth appears small because of the short upper lip and the mandible is small giving a receding chin. The hands of these babies are always malformed but in a different way from the trisomy 13, and they give the best diagnostic clue to the condition. These babies keep their fists clenched most of the time, with the index finger overlying the third finger. Profuse lanugo covers the forehead, back and extremities, and the skin usually has a mottled appearance. The sternum is very short, hence the abdomen appears long. The pelvis is small with limited abduction of the hips. There also may be abnormal genitalia. Inguinal and umbilical hernias are frequent; diaphragmatic eventration (elevation of a thinned portion of the diaphragm) rather than frank hernia occurs more often in these patients. Neurologic examination reveals abnormal muscle tone; these babies progress from a hypertonic state to frank opisthotonus. Since the sucking reflex is poor, gavage feeding is often instituted. Unlike trisomy 13, no gross brain abnormalities can be demonstrated, although cardiac abnormalities are common and either these or aspiration account for the de-

mise of these babies. Their survival rate is less than six months on the average. During this time they become progressively undernourished and present a failure to thrive syndrome. As with trisomy 13, some infants have survived to childhood, so that death in infancy cannot be predicted.

TRISOMY 21, OR DOWN'S SYNDROME. In this condition an extra chromosome belonging to either pair 21 or 22 or a translocation of 15/21 is found (see Chapter 7). Although these babies are apt to have congenital defects and are more susceptible to infection, they can be expected to live much longer and have less severe mental retardation (although it can be very severe) than the other trisomies. The reader may be more familiar with the term "mongolism" used in reference to this syndrome, but recently this has lost favor, because it bears a connotation which is not only unfortunate but incorrect.

For many years the term "mongolism" has been given to the condition of infants who present a definite clinical picture, the configuration of their faces resembling that of a Mongol or an Oriental. Their eyes are set close together, are slanting, and the palpebral fissures are narrow. The nose is flat. The tongue is large, fissured, and usually is very obvious as it protrudes from the open mouth. The head is small, and posteriorly the occiput appears flat above the broad, pudgy neck. The hands are short and thick, especially the fingers (the little finger is curved), with simian creases apparent on the palmar surfaces. In addition to having defective mentality and the deformities mentioned above, these infants have underdeveloped muscles, loose joints, heart and alimentary tract abnormalities. Although these infants sometimes live past the age of puberty, the majority succumb earlier to some infection.

INCIDENCE AND ETIOLOGY. The incidence of Down's syndrome has been estimated at 1.5 in 1,000 births. Advanced maternal age has been known to play a very important role in the etiology of this condition, over a third of these children being born to mothers who are 40 years of age or older. Several decades ago it was suggested that this condition might be associated with a chromosomal aberration, but it was not demonstrated until recently that the etiologic factor in Down's syndrome is the result of one of the three chromosomal abnormalities.

TYPES. The most common chromosomal defect of the ovum in Down's syndrome is trisomy of the chromosome 21 or 22, resulting in a total chromosomal count of 47 instead of the normal number of 46. This type, commonly referred to as standard trisomy, usually occurs in infants born to older women and is rarely familial. The incidence of standard trisomy is 1 in 600 births. The second type of abnormality results from a 15/21 translocation; in this type the actual chromosomal count is 46. The translocation type of Down's syndrome usually occurs in infants born to younger parents, is the familial type and is rare. The third type of the disorder, mosaicism, is very rare. A unique factor in mosaicism is that one individual may have cells with different chromosomal counts. Laboratory tests may demonstrate that the affected person's blood cells, for example, have 47 chromosomes, whereas his skin cells may show 46 chromosomes. This is not a familial type of Down's syndrome, and, moreover, the abnormalities may be less.

The usual causes of death in these babies are heart defects and infectious illnesses. The average survival rate with effective antibiotic treatment has been extended to beyond nine years. Children with Down's syndrome are essentially retarded but have been found to be far more educatable than was previously thought. Thus the decision to institutionalize the child is an exceedingly difficult one and should not be forced on the parents by well-meaning professionals.

The key approach to trisomy conditions lies in prevention since treatment does not alter the long range prognosis. With respect to prevention, education of the public regarding the effect of maternal age is the key issue. We have seen the incidence of all three trisomies goes up with increased maternal age. The later *thirties* and *forties* are less safe for childbearing (from many points of view), and elective childbearing is better done when the mother is younger. Genetic counseling is another aspect of public education (see Chapter 27). Parents who have had a trisomic child (or if trisomy has appeared among their siblings) would do well to talk to their physician concerning the risk of producing more of these children. In some families, trisomies are not the result of nondisjunction and hence have an appreciable chance of recurring, depending on the interaction of the variables of family history, maternal age, and chromosomal arrangement. For instance, if a couple produced a trisomy infant in their twenties, the child may have received a translocated chromosome from one of them. If they continue to produce children, these children would stand a high chance of also inheriting the translocated chromosome. Parents clearly deserve to be told the facts of the matter so that they may be in a better position to make valid decisions regarding future childbearing. A young patient who has had a translocation (hereditary type) child is a candidate for amniocentesis with cell culture and karyotyping in a subsequent pregnancy. This may be done as early as 14 weeks and thereby provide the option of therapeutic abortion, should the abnormality be present again. This approach of antenatal diagnosis can now be applied to an ever increasing number of chromosomal abnormalities as well as biochemical disorders.[22]

Immediate care will be supportive for the infant. Warmth, prevention of infection, fluid and electrolyte balance, and often oxygen therapy will be under the supervision of the physician. Nursing therapy will be aimed primarily at support of the parents and helping them to work through their grief. This latter aspect is particularly important because of the grave prognosis for these babies. It is often helpful to institute community health and/or visiting nurse referrals since the parents may need technical help upon arriving home with the infant. If a fetal demise occurs, supportive help from a public health nurse is also helpful.

Phocomelia

In 1961-1962 many thousands of newborns in Germany were afflicted with an extremely pitiful type of malformation characterized either by total absence of the arms and the legs or by such stunting of the extremities that they were mere nubbins. The deformity is known as *phocomelia*. Investigation revealed that practically all the mothers who gave birth to such infants had taken a certain sedative drug, *thalidomide*, during the first part of pregnancy, and that this drug was undoubtedly the cause of the malformations.

Largely as the result of the thalidomide tragedy, the United States Food and Drug Administration, a federal agency authorized to approve new drugs, greatly tightened the regulations concerning new drug approval. But from the viewpoint of nurses and physicians, the most important lesson to be drawn from this sad experience is that *no pregnant woman should take any drug whatsoever* unless, in the opinion of her physician, it is urgently necessary for her health (see Chapters 10 and 20).

This rule does not apply to the routine administration of vitamins and iron, nor to the use of laxatives when indicated, but it does apply very strongly to most other drugs, particularly those often employed in the treatment of insomnia, nausea, and anxiety.

The child with deformed or missing limbs has special rehabilitation problems that do not occur in the treatment of adults who undergo a loss of a limb (see Suggested Reading). His physical characteristics and contours are different from those of an adult, and they are constantly changing as he grows. This complicates fitting an adequate prosthesis. Furthermore, his psychosocial adjustment demands continued attention, for he does not have the chance to make his adjustment to society as a whole person, and he therefore is likely to have some feelings of inadequacy and devaluation in a culture geared to the nonhandicapped. Fortunately, there are about 15 child amputee clinics throughout this country. They are located in Alabama, California, Connecticut, Florida, Georgia, Illinois, Maryland, Michigan, New York, North Carolina, Oklahoma, Pennsylvania, and Washington. These clinics are invaluable in helping parents to learn that their child can be fitted with a functional prosthesis and achieve satisfaction in its use. Even when the deformity is multiple, the child can achieve at least limited function with proper training. Since much of the success of the plan of treatment depends on the parents, it is particularly important that they be informed and reassured of these positive aspects in the situation. It has been demonstrated that the sooner the parents receive this knowledge, the more chance there is of an effective prosthetics program.

The newborn infant with a congenital amputation will be discussed here since nurses in the maternity unit will have initial contact with these infants and will need to instruct parents on various aspects of daily care. (For a thorough, interesting discussion of amputations in children of all ages, see the Steele article in the Suggested Reading.)

The usual sleeping position for the newborn is prone with the pelvis raised and the knees tucked under the abdomen. When the lower extremities are missing, the infant is unable to assume this position and, in addition, will not be able to indulge in the kicking behavior which appears to give a good deal of gratification. The baby with missing upper extremities presents other problems. Prior to feeding, the infant is usually occupied with a good deal of hand to mouth contact and this of course, will be altered. If both hands are missing the infant will be deprived of one of his major sources of sucking gratification. It is known that the need for sucking and the need for feeding often do not coincide, and, hence, the normal infant uses his fingers to complete the gratification of this need. Therefore the nurse will want to offer a pacifier to these infants. Clinging behavior in the human infant is not clearly understood, but it is observed that as the infant matures he tends to grasp things and bring them to his mouth possibly for further identification. In the absence of both upper limbs, this behavior also will be altered. The nurse will also want to instruct the parents that, when the infant is older, he may not be able to lift his head up (while in the prone position) since he can not raise up on his elbows to look around. A wedge-shaped pillow or thick folded blanket placed under the infant's chest will correct this handicap a great deal.

The development of body image begins in infancy and will play an increasingly important role in the development of these youngsters. The normally developed infant first perceives his moving arms (and legs) as part of the outside world; as he grows, he incorporates them into his body image and, hence, his self-concept. The infant amputee may not be aware that his body is different from others, but as he matures, he begins to compare himself with others and his concept about himself changes as he slowly integrates his defect into his existing body image. Obviously, the more positive attitudes he encounters with respect to his defect, the more positive his concept of himself can become. It is important for the nurse to remember that while the defect may seem rather minor to her (in comparison to some of the life-threatening conditions recently discussed), in the parents' eyes, it may be catastrophic. The principles of care, as given at the beginning of the chapter, especially with regard to how the nurse actually handles the baby are especially germane here. Guilt may be present, especially if the defect is thought to be the result of taking drugs or from contact with viral diseases. Denial also may be apparent, with the parents actually refusing to look at or admit, the defect. The nurse's warm, accepting attitude in this case is very helpful since the parents' denial is often related to their apprehension regarding how others will view their infant. Fortunately, these infants are usually in apparent good health in other respects and will thrive if given the chance. They do not seem to be handicapped by multiple abnormalities as is the case with some of the other disorders. Calling attention to the positive aspects of the baby's growth, development and general features will help the parents place the amputation in its proper perspective after the initial shock and grief have been worked through.

Inborn errors of metabolism

Numerous metabolic disorders, so-called inborn errors of metabolism, are now known to originate from mutations in the genes which alter the genetic constitution of an individual to the extent that normal function is disrupted. These biochemical disorders arise because of the disturbance (mutation) in a *molecule of the gene* itself. They *do not* stem from some mishap or alteration during the embryonic development of tissue or organs. The mode of transmission of these inborn errors usually is recessive; that is, a child must receive a pair of defective genes (one from his mother and one from his father) to be affected. The mother and the father in these cases would be carriers of the defective genes but would not be affected by the resulting disorder per se. Fortunately, defective genes are found rather infrequently in the general population, and the chance of their joining is even rarer; hence, the diseases they produce are commensurately rare. Some of the more familiar hereditary metabolic disorders and resulting conditions include:

1. Defects in metabolism and transport of amino acids
   A. Phenylketonuria
   B. Maple sugar urine disease
2. Defects in protein metabolism
   A. Agammaglobulinemia
3. Defects in metabolism and transport of carbohydrates
   A. Diabetes mellitus
   B. Gargoylism (Hurler's disease)
   C. Galactosemia
   D. Arachnodactyly (Marfan's syndrome)
4. Defects in metabolism and transport of lipids
   A. Cerebroside lipidosis (Gaucher's disease)
   B. Ganglioside lipidosis (Tay-Sachs disease)
   C. Sphingomyelin lipidosis (Niemann-Pick disease)

It is important to remember that these inborn errors of metabolism *do not produce symptoms* that are apparent at birth. Therefore, the maternity nurse rarely will see evidence of these disorders. However, two conditions do concern us here. The one directly because nursery personnel play an important role in the early detection of the condition; this disorder is phenylketonuria. The other is more indirect since it is the babies of mothers with the condition that we must attend; this latter condition is diabetes mellitus.

Phenylketonuria

This disease, commonly known as PKU, is an inborn error of metabolism of the essential amino acid phenylalanine, characterized by a deficiency in the liver enzyme phenylalanine hydroxylase, which is essential in phenylalanine metabolism. High blood levels of phenylalanine occur, and phenylketone bodies are excreted in the urine. Phenylalanine makes up 5 percent of the protein factor of all foods. Normally, phenylalanine is converted to tyrosine in the liver and then is further metabolized. The phenylketonuric child is able to digest protein and to absorb the resulting amino acids. However, there is a block in the normal metabolic pathway at this point, and the excess dietary phenylalanine, unable to be converted to tyrosine, builds up in the tissues (blood levels of this amino acid reach as high as 60 mg. per 100 ml., as compared with the normal 1 to 3 mg. per 100 ml.) and spills into the urine in the form of phenylpyruvic acid, excess phenylalanine, phenylacetic acid, and orthohydroxyphenylacetic acid. These components, excreted in the urine and the perspiration, give the child a characteristic musty odor.

Without treatment, the condition usually results in mental retardation, although the rest of the clinical picture will vary. Typically, the child with PKU is hyperactive and demonstrates unpredictable erratic behavior. Usually he does not relate well in interpersonal contacts, either within the family or with strangers, and he appears very immature and overly dependent. The three R's, routine, relaxation, and repetition (as used with other mentally retarded youngsters), are effective in helping him make a more satisfactory social adjustment. The main foci of management, however, is early detection of the condition and dietary management restricting the phenylalanine intake. If treatment is initiated before six months of age, the child probably will fall into the borderline-to-normal range of intelligence (70 to 100 IQ).

DIAGNOSIS. This disorder may be diagnosed from both blood and urine tests. The former are more advantageous, since they can be done before the infant leaves the hospital, and they give a low rate of false positive reactions. One of the easiest and most efficient to perform is the microbiological assay (MIA), more commonly known as the Guthrie method. In this test 1 or 2 drops of blood are secured from the infant's heel from the second day to the day of discharge and are placed immediately on filter paper. The laboratory then uses a bacterial inhibition assay method on the serum phenylalanine to determine the phenylalanine level. A result of 8 mg. percent or above is considered to be diagnostic of PKU. The nurse may be asked to collect the specimen for this test and/or to prepare the infants for the physician. Usually several babies will be tested at one time, therefore, she can facilitate matters by placing the infants in the prone position, which makes the heels easily accessible. The babies then can be covered loosely with a blanket so that they will remain accessible but will not be unduly exposed. After the heel has been wiped with a disinfectant solution, pricked (usually with a disposable blood lancet), and the specimen obtained, the infant should be observed for bleeding from the heel. In addition, the infant is to have a formula feeding prior to the test to insure appropriate blood levels of nutrients. Other blood tests have been developed which require more blood. They are as reliable as the Guthrie method and with proper laboratory facilities are often utilized.

The urine tests utilize ferric chloride as the testing agent; this solution is dropped on a freshly saturated diaper. A green reaction indicates probable phenylketonuria. The urine tests are effective only after the infant is six weeks old; they are useful in screening large populations of infants and are most often done in well-baby clinics. Since early diagnosis is imperative, the blood tests are the tests of choice.

TREATMENT. Restriction of phenylalanine intake is the basis of treatment, and yet enough protein must be available for growth and de-velopment; hence the child's diet becomes all-important. Commercial products (e.g., Lofenalac, a special food which is mixed with water) are available that provide adequate protein for growth with minimal phenylalanine content. The plan of dietary treatment should be reviewed carefully with both parents, so that they have an understanding of how to prepare the formula, use the meal guides and food exchange lists (see Suggested Reading) and prepare menus from them.

Requesting the parents to review their understanding of the problem, diet, and so on, often will elicit the areas that need clarification. The parents must be supported until they feel comfortable in discussing the problem; until this happens, they cannot be receptive to further teaching. Since this is a long-term condition and requires consistent counseling and follow-up, the need for a referral to the public health nurse becomes evident.

Care should be taken so that the parents of an affected child are not led to believe that all babies treated will have the usual pattern of growth and development (intellectual development may be slow, for instance). This cannot be guaranteed. *Early detection* and *prompt treatment* prevent mental retardation. The control of this condition demands consistent and disciplined supervision and follow-through on the part of the parents.

The infant of the diabetic mother

The successful control of diabetes with insulin has led to the survival and fertility of an increasing number of diabetic women (see Chapter 21). However, despite recent advances in the management of the diabetic mother, intrauterine surveillance of the fetus and therapy during delivery and the first days of life, the infant of the diabetic mother still runs a high risk of dying. Most institutions where expert care is given report a mortality rate between 15 and 25 percent. Where special care is not available, the mortality may be as high as 50 percent.

Most of these infants have a distinctive appearance. They have been called "a colossus on feet of clay."[23] They are usually large, often 10 pounds or over, and present a cushingoid appearance. Their tremendous weight is not due primarily to an excess of extracellular fluid as was formerly believed, but rather to an excess of fat. The obesity is a result of fetal hyperinsulinism, originating from transformation of carbohydrates to triglycerides.[24] These infants appear bloated and tend to be "jumpy" and tremulous after the first 24 hours of life. They are also subject to cyanotic attacks, respiratory distress syndrome, hypoglycemia, hypocalcemia, and hyperbilirubinemia.

Among the many causes of these babies' deaths and morbidity are the higher incidences of congenital anomalies and early delivery with the resulting prematurity, respiratory distress, hypocalcemia, and hypoglycemia. Many of these problems in turn are brought about by inadequate control of the maternal diabetes. Meticulous control of maternal blood sugar, therefore, may lead to fewer problems and lower infant mortality.

Traditionally, concern has been directed toward the effect on the fetus of maternal hypoglycemia. Severe prolonged hypoglycemia will damage the fetus. However, it has been pointed out that the newborn can tolerate a blood sugar level of as little as 20 percent with no damage and perhaps the fetus can also. Thus, loosely controlling the maternal diabetes (with one insulin injection per day and little dietary control) in an effort to provide the fetus with adequate blood sugar can instead lead to fetal death or to hypoglycemia in the newborn. The more current belief is that maternal hyperglycemia leads to the same condition in the fetus since glucose is rapidly transferred across the placenta. The fetal pancreas hypertrophies in response to repeated high "doses" of sugar and produces large amounts of insulin in an attempt to control the fetus' blood sugar and indirectly the mother's. However, since insulin is not transferred across the placenta, the fetus cannot help the mother. The excess sugar that pours across the placenta lodges in the fetal liver and other tissues, either as glycogen or fat, and produces the characteristic large, puffy infant of the diabetic mother.

It is felt that fetal hyperglycemia probably contributes to the death in utero of the thirty-sixth to thirty-seventh week fetus. To combat this, most physicians wish to deliver the infant at 35 to 36 weeks. However, early delivery subjects the baby to all of the hazards associated with prematurity. If the fetus can remain in utero until 37 or 38 weeks or longer, its outlook is improved. With the newer techniques of intrauterine assessment, some of the guesswork regarding the baby's maturity and ability to withstand an extrauterine environment has been diminished.

When the infant is delivered and the umbilical cord cut, he faces yet another problem. His external supply of glucose is now cut off, yet his hypertrophied pancreas continues producing large amounts of insulin, and this cannot be readily stopped.[25] Thus, the infant rapidly becomes severely hypoglycemic and can suffer brain damage and death. Care must be taken in the administration of glucose for this condition since the hypertrophied pancreas is highly sensitized to glucose and even small quantities will trigger rebound hypoglycemia.

MANAGEMENT. In general, these infants are to be treated as premature infants, although their size may be deceiving. Hence, all the vital signs and blood chemistry monitoring devices are appropriate for them. Adequate temperature control and an aseptic environment are to be provided. The baby's electrolyte balance is maintained with intravenous fluids until the eating pattern and sucking reflex normalize. An infusion pump should be used to insure that fluids are given at a constant rate so that the pancreas is not stimulated to produce excess insulin in receiving more glucose one hour and less the next. Treatment by large quantities of glucose by vein for the maintenance of glucose levels has been found ineffective for the above reason; however, this treatment for immediate *seizures* has had some effect when used in a 20-percent concentration. The use of glucagon to mobilize liver glycogen is also limited by the fact that it also stimulates insulin release and rebound hypoglycemia. Hypoglycemia can be detected by means of Dextrostix. If the infant can take fluids orally and if the blood sugar by Dextrostix is less than 45 mg. per 100 ml., the baby can be given 10-percent glucose water to bring levels to normal.

Epinephrine 1:1,000 intramuscularly can be used to decrease the amount of insulin released since it appears to inhibit the release of insulin from the pancreas. It also stimulates the liver and muscles to release glucose, and the fat tissue to release fatty acids for glucose production. The sudden death of these infants from heart failure can be caused either directly or indirectly by a deficiency of epinephrine. Indirectly, a deficiency of this substance leads to a lack of free fatty acids, a vital part of the heart's fuel supply. Without epinephrine and fuel, the heart is overtaxed and thus cannot handle the increased stress after delivery.

The nurse will also want to be watchful of the development of hypocalcemia (serum calcium below 7 mg. per 100 ml. or 3.5 mEq. per 1), which can occur with or without hypoglycemia. Symptoms are usually imperceptible and nonspecific. They include irritability, coarse tremors, twitches, and convulsions. Two peaks of incidence occur, the first during the first 48 hours and characterized by apnea, cyanotic episodes, edema, high-pitched cry, and abdominal distention but no neuromuscular involvement. It must be noted that these manifestations have not been proved to be solely of hypocalcemic origin. The second form occurs between the fifth and tenth days of life and is sometimes called *neonatal tetany*. It occurs when the infant is fed milk formulas (especially evaporated milk) which causes a hyperphosphatemia and depresses the activity of the parathyroid gland which, in turn, diminishes serum calcium. Here the symptoms include the neuromuscular signs—jitters, twitching, and focal or generalized convulsions. The preventive treatment is to feed the infant a milk formula that simulates the calcium phosphorus ratio of human milk. Actual treatment of the acute stage is intravenous instillation of 10 percent calcium gluconate 1 to 1.5 ml. per kg. of body weight, given slowly over a period of five minutes to prevent bradycardia. The heart rate is monitored constantly during the infusion and, if it drops below 100 beats per minute, the infusion is discontinued immediately. It may be restarted after the heart rate has been normal for 30 minutes.

The nurse will also have the responsibility to monitor the infant's blood oxygen level and neurologic function. He may be lethargic, so frequent position change is important. Respiratory distress is managed as in any premature. If the baby is having respiratory difficulties, he can be positioned on his chest and neck in as straight a line as possible to reduce interference with his air passages. His shoulders can be slightly elevated and his body tilted slightly backward.

Hydration is also of extreme importance. It is advisable to use a urine bag connected to straight drainage to collect and measure urinary output. If the bag can be attached so that it can stay in place for 24 to 48 hours, there is less of a chance of the skin becoming excoriated from frequent bag changes. As the infant responds to treatment during the first 24 to 48 hours, oral feedings can be started. However, care must be taken to see that the baby does not aspirate formula since these infants are usually poor feeders and their size makes easy handling difficult. It is difficult to hold up the head of such a large infant when he is in an Isolette, therefore he can be placed on his side for feeding and be bubbled by placing him on his abdomen or rotating him from side to side.[26]

The infant can be placed in an open crib when his respirations, reflexes, and body temperature are stabilized and within normal ranges. However, he is still to be watched carefully since reversals can occur. Recurrence of hypoglycemia and hypocalcemia is possible and hyperbilirubinemia often occurs. Neurologically, these babies reflect their gestational age, so swallowing and evacuation may be a problem for some weeks. Parents can be taught to handle their baby as if he were premature until he is on his way to stability.

Prenatally, supportive measures for the mother with diabetes should be planned with two objectives: the delivery of a normal baby and a minimum of maternal swings in blood sugar. This requires careful control of maternal blood sugar, which implies meticulous medical and nursing supervision and cooperation by the mother.

Postpartally, the parents, as part of their health education, will be alerted to the possibility that their infant may be prediabetic. If the hyperinsulinism that results from the stimulation of the fetal pancreas by maternal glucose is too prolonged or too severe, pancreatic exhaustion may ensue. This, along with genetic makeup, may lead to diabetes in the child either in the neonatal period or months or years later. Thus, parents need to receive adequate instruction about the nutritional needs of the child as well as a review of the signs and symptoms of diabetes. Parents can be encouraged to follow their child carefully following periods of stress, such as illness, injury, growth spurts, and so on. If any such symptoms occur, medical attention is indicated. Since the birth process is often traumatic for these parents and they have much to accomplish psychologically as for any trauma, a community health referral is indicated to assure follow-through on the teaching.[27]

Hyperbilirubinemia of the newborn

Hyperbilirubinemia, as previously stated, is present beyond physiologic bounds when the total serum bilirubin levels reach 18 to 20 mg. per 100 ml. of blood. This may occur particularly in premature infants as an exaggeration of physiologic jaundice or as a consequence of excessive hemolysis, such as severe hemolytic disease of the newborn. Occasionally, this condition is found in term infants who have no blood group incompatibilities. Therefore some authorities suggest that this term, "hyperbilirubinemia of the newborn," be applied only to those infants whose primary problem is a deficiency or inactivity of bilirubin transference rather than an excessive load of bilirubin for excretion. Certain conditions of the mother (e.g., diabetes, as well as neonatal conditions arising from the use of certain drugs, bacteremia and prolonged cyanosis) appear to be implicated in causing this condition. Occasionally this disorder appears among breast-fed infants during the second week of life. For some reason the mother manufactures a substance in her milk that inhibits the conjugation of bilirubin. If breast-feeding is discontinued, serum bilirubin levels return to normal within five days, and apparently no lasting damage is done to the infant. The significance of hyperbilirubinemia, of course, lies in the high incidence of kernicterus associated with it, which, as previously explained, can be lethal to the baby.

The use of intense fluorescent light to reduce serum bilirubin gained acceptance in the United States after a decade of use abroad. Blue light decomposes bilirubin by photooxidation, which appears to take place in the skin. The chemical nature of the products formed in the breakdown of bilirubin has not been precisely determined, nor have long-term outcomes been evaluated as well as the theoretic effects of intense light upon a wide spectrum of biologic processes. For these reasons, there are some reservations about the unqualified use of this treatment for all jaundiced babies.

Phototherapy is applied by exposing the nude infant to fluorescent daylight bulbs that supply 200 to 400 foot-candles on the skin surface. Optimal intensity or duration of therapy have not been determined. The infant's eyes are shielded from the light by means of patches. The nurse will want to be sure that the lids are closed when the blindfold is applied. The bandages are to be removed at least once each shift to inspect the eyes for conjunctivitis.[28]

Miscellaneous disorders

Hemorrhage from cord

Hemorrhage from the cord may be of two types: 1) primary, due to the slipping or loosening of the umbilical clamp, and 2) secondary, coming from the base of the cord when it separates from the body of the baby. In the first instance, the bleeding is from the end of the cord and not from its base and can be controlled by the proper application of a fresh clamp. The secondary hemorrhage, from the base of the cord, occurs at about the fifth to the eighth day when separation takes place. It is often preceded by a slight jaundice; it is not an actual flow of blood but a persistent oozing which frequently resists treatment. This variety of hemorrhage, which is a rare occurrence, is usually due to one of two causes: 1) the baby may be syphilitic, or 2) the peculiar condition known as hemorrhagic diathesis may be present. In this condition, the baby's blood shows no disposition to coagulate, and bleeding from any denuded surface is persistent and often profuse.

The nurse's responsibility in the treatment of secondary hemorrhage from the cord consists in applying a sterile dressing to the bleeding surface. The physician should be notified promptly; and if, by the time he arrives, the use of the dressing has not effectually controlled the oozing, he will doubtless clamp the base of the umbilicus. When this form of bleeding is at all severe and persistent, recovery is doubtful; and even if the umbilical hemorrhage is controlled, bleeding may appear in the nose, the mouth, the stomach, the intestines, or the abdominal cavity; or purpuric spots may develop on various parts of the body. The prompt administration of vitamin K has greatly improved the prognosis in these cases.

Retrolental fibroplasia

Retrolental fibroplasia is an acquired disease, associated with prematurity, in which retinal pathology occurs in those infants receiving continuous oxygen therapy in high concentration. The incidence of the condition depends on 1) the concentration of oxygen given, and 2) the degree of immaturity of the eyes at the time when oxygen is given (see Chapter 25). The disease is characterized by spasm, then obliteration, of the developing retinal vessels which is followed by neovascularization, hemorrhage, and retinal detachment. The disease has both an acute and a cicatricial phase; both eyes are affected, although different stages may be present in the two eyes; spontaneous arrest may occur at any stage.

The onset of the acute stage is usually between the ages of three weeks and three months and the smaller the birth weight, the *later* the onset. Dilatation and tortuosity of the retinal blood vessels occur, with the fundus becoming pale. Hemorrhages appear adjacent to the vessels and spread into the vitreous; separation of the retina follows. After several weeks, the acute stage passes into the cicatricial stage, characterized by formation of the retrolental membrane. The anterior chamber becomes shallow and impairment of vision may be accompanied by squint, photophobia, and nystagmus. In severe cases, microphthalmia and secondary glaucoma may be sequelae. Because most of the damage is mechanical, one cannot determine the extent of detachment that will occur. When the condition is detected early, and proper measures are instituted promptly (i.e., reduction in concentration of oxygen administered) the condition in the infant may regress at any stage of the disease, or, on the other hand, partial or complete blindness may result.

Extensive research, carried on during the years since retrolental fibroplasia was first described, has established the cause and the means of prevention of the disease. It is now a fact that almost all cases of retrolental fibroplasia in the premature infant are the result of intensive oxygen therapy. Today oxygen is administered to an infant in the lowest concentration compatible with life and is discontinued as soon as feasible. The maximum oxygen concentration of the incubator housing the premature infant is kept at less than 40 percent whenever possible, and this is done only for as long as it is *absolutely* necessary (see Oxygen Therapy.

Drug addiction in the newborn

This condition is being seen more frequently with the rise of drug addiction in the general population. Furthermore, it is the nurse who may be the first to discover this condition. The symptoms of the infant are due to withdrawal rather than narcosis; they may appear almost immediately after birth, or they may be delayed for several hours, depending on the time of the mother's last injection of narcotic, the dose, and the interval between the administration of the narcotic and the delivery. The infant may manifest restlessness, tremors, shrill crying, convulsions, or twitchings of the extremities and/or face. The Moro reflex may be incomplete, and the deep tendon reflexes may be increased. Diarrhea, vomiting, anorexia, yawning, sneezing, and excessive mucus also may be present. These symptoms parallel somewhat those found in the adult undergoing withdrawal symptoms from narcotics. If the signs of withdrawal are unrecognized, the baby may die; if the infant is treated (hydration, supportive measures, and diminishing doses of sedatives), recovery and permanent cure are assured since the infant does not have a psychic dependence on narcotics. However, some physicians believe that the infant should be removed from the mother's environment if it carries a threat of readdiction. This possibility will present a problem that will require a multidisciplinary approach, and the nurse can be helpful in beginning the process through appropriate and accurate reporting and recording. There is some evidence to support the theory that withdrawal symptoms can be lessened in the newborn if the mother can be treated with methadone therapy antepartally. The use of this substitution therapy has caused controversy, but its proponents maintain that the results for the infant as well as the mother warrant its use.[29] Another drug problem, perhaps of a more indirect but nevertheless important nature, concerns abuse in the use of the drug lysergic acid (LSD-25). This drug, a consciousness expander, was developed for research use and was never intended for indiscriminate use by the general population. Recent research has documented that LSD-25, when taken by mothers during pregnancy results in a significant increase in chromosomal abnormalities in their babies. This fact is also true, but to a lesser degree, of children of mothers *who took the drug before, but not during pregnancy.* How and in what manner any malformations will be manifested as a result of these chromosomal abnormalities is as yet uncertain. However, it is recommended that any agent capable of inflicting chromosomal damage should be treated with extreme caution until all the genetic implications are understood. Antenatal chromosomal analysis might also be of help in this group of patients.

Bibliography

1. Waechter, E. H.: The birth of an exceptional child. *Nurs. Forum* 9:202-205, 1970.
2. *Ibid.*, pp. 205-207.
3. *Ibid.*, pp. 207-208.
4. Engel, G. L.: Grief and grieving. *Am. J. Nurs.* 64:93-98, Sept. 1964.
5. Lindemann, E.: Symptomatology and management of acute grief. *Am. J. Psychiat.* 101:141-418, 1944.
6. Kennell, J. H., *et al*: The mourning response of parents to the death of a newborn infant. *New Eng. J. Med.* 283:344-349, Aug. 13, 1970.
7. *Ibid.*
8. Schuman, H.: Thoughts and comment. *JOGN Nursing* 48-49, May/June 1974.
9. Hellman, L. M., and Pritchard, J. A.: *Williams Obstetrics*, ed. 14. New York, Appleton-Century Crofts, 1971.
10. Korones, S. B., *et al*: *High-Risk Newborn Infants, The Basis for Intensive Nursing Care*. St. Louis, Mosby, 1972, p. 495.
11. *Ibid.*, pp. 140-143.
12. *Ibid.*, pp. 198-199.
13. Kumpe, M., *et al*: Care of the infant with the respiratory distress syndrome. *Nurs. Clin. North Am.* 6:25-37, Mar. 1971.
14. Korones, *op. cit.*, p. 200.
15. *Ibid.*, pp. 201-202.
16. Persaud, T. V. N., and Moore, K. L.: Causes and prenatal diagnosis of congenital abnormalities. *JOGN Nursing* 50-55, July/Aug. 1974.
17. Rowe, R. D.: Serious congenital heart disease in the newborn infant: Diagnosis and management. *Pediatrics Clin. North Am.* 17:969-971, Nov. 1970.
18. Walton, R. L.: A study of etiological variables in palatolabial malformations. *J. Kansas Med. Soc.* 73:370-377, Aug. 1972.
19. Shapiro, C. S., *et al*: Nursing care of the cleft lip/cleft palate child. *RN* 36:46-48, Aug. 1973.
20. Wood, B. G.: Pre-surgical correction of the deformed maxillary arch. *Nurs. Times* 66:1420-1425, Nov. 1970.
21. Kelley, E. E.: Feeding cleft palate babies—today's babies, today's methods. *Cleft Palate J.* 8:61-64, Jan. 1971.
22. Hall, J., and Hercht, E.: Autosomal trisomies. *Am. J. Nurs.* 64:87-91, Nov. 1964.
23. Picaud, F. J., *et al*: The newborn of diabetic mothers *Biol. Neonate* 24:1-30, 1974.
24. *Ibid.*, p. 3.
25. Guthrie, D. W., and Guthrie, R. A.: The infant of the diabetic mother. *Am. J. Nurs.* 11:2008-2009, Nov. 1974.
26. Leifer, G.: *Principles and Techniques of Pediatric Nursing*. Philadelphia, W. B. Saunders, 1972, pp. 42-50.
27. *Ibid.*
28. Korones, S. B., *op. cit.*, pp. 176-177.
29. Addicted babies. *Briefs* 38:86-90, Summer 1974.

Suggested Reading

ARGRAFIOTIS, P. C.: Teaching parents about the Pierre Robin syndrome. *Am. J. Nurs.* 72:2040-2041, Nov. 1972.

ASCARI, W. Q., *et al*: Incidence of maternal Rh immunization by ABO compatible and incompatible pregnancies. *Brit. Med. J.* 1:399-401, Feb. 15, 1969.

BARNETT, C. R., *et al*: Neonatal separation: The maternal side of interactional deprivation. *Pediatrics* 45:197-205, Feb. 1970.

BARSON, C., *et al*: Neonatal diabetes. *Nurs. Mirror* 138:81-82, Mar. 29, 1974.

BRANEY, M. L.: The child with hydrocephalus. *Am. J. Nurs.* 73:828-831, May 1973.

BRAVERMAN, S. J.: Death of a monster. *Am. J. Nurs.* 69:1682-1683, Aug. 1969.

COHEN, M. M., *et al*: The effect of LSD-25 on the chromosomes of children exposed in utero. *Pediatrics Research* 2:486-492, Nov. 1968.

CUNNINGHAM, G. C.: Two years of PKU testing in California. *Calif. Med.* 110:11-16, Jan. 1969.

DIONNA, T.; *et al*: Acute subdural hematoma in the newborn: A case report and review of the literature. *Neuropaediatrica* 10:181-190, May 1974.

DONNELLY, E.: The real of her. *JOGN Nursing* 48-53, May/June 1974.

EASTMAN, N. J., AND HELLMAN, L. M.: *Williams Obstetrics.* ed. 14. New York, Appleton-Century Crofts, 1971.

ENGLE, G. L.: Grief and grieving. *Am. J. Nurs.* 64:93-98, Sept. 1964.

FINAL REPORT OF THE COMMITTEE ON PHOTOTHERAPY IN THE NEWBORN. Washington, D.C., *National Research Council, National Academy of Sciences*, 1974.

FIRM TO MAKE LIVE VACCINE FOR MEASLES. *Los Angeles Times* 88, No. 189: Part I, p. 5, June 10, 1969.

FLEMING, J. W.: Recognizing the newborn addict. *Am. J. Nurs.* 65:83, Jan. 1965.

FOGERTY, S.: The nurse and the high-risk infant. *Nurs. Clin. North Am.* 8:533-547, Sept. 1973.

FOX, H. P., AND ROBERTSON, W. O.: Closing the information gap. *Northwest Med.* 68:124-125, Feb. 1969.

GARDAM, J. W.: Diarrheal diseases. *J. Med. Soc. New Jersey* 66:27-30, Jan. 1969.

GLASER, B. G., AND STRAUSS, A.: The social loss of dying patients. *Am. J. Nurs.* 64:119-121, June 1964.

GUTHRIE, R., AND STEWART, W.: Phenylketonuria. Children's Bureau Publication No. 41. Washington, D.C., U.S. Government Printing Office, 1964.

HALL, J. G., AND HEICHT, F.: Autosomal trisomies, *Am. J. Nurs.* 64:87-91, Nov. 1964.

HARDGROVE, C., AND WARRICK, L. H.: How shall we tell the children? *Am. J. Nurs.* 74:448-450, Mar. 1974.

HERRMANN, J., *et al*: Infection control in the newborn nursery. *Nurs. Clin. North Am.* 6:55-65, Mar. 1971.

HEY, D. J., *et al*: Neonatal infections caused by group B streptococci. *Am. J. Ob-Gyn.* 116:43-47, May 1973.

INGLES, T.: Maria, the hungry baby. *Nurs. Forum* 5, 2:36-47, 1966.

JOHNSON, J. M.: Stillbirth—a personal experience. *Am. J. Nurs.* 72:1595-1596, Sept. 1972.

KASLOW, R. A., *et al*: Staphylococcal disease related to hospital nursery bathing practices: A nationwide epidemiologic investigation. *Pediatrics* 51:608-615, April 1973.

KENNEDY, J. C.: The high-risk maternal-infant acquaintance process. *Nurs. Clin. North Am.* 8:549-557, Sept. 1973.

KLAUS, M. H., *et al*: Mothers separated from their newborn infants. *Pediatrics Clin. North Am.* 17:1015-1037, Nov. 1970.

McDONAGH, B. J.: Congenital atrial flutter. *Arch. Dis. Child.* 43:731-733, Dec. 1968.

MERCER, R. T.: Mothers' responses to their infants with defects. *Nurs. Research* 23:133-137, Mar./April 1974.

NEW YORK STATE DEPT. OF HEALTH: PKU in expectant mothers. *Health News* 45, No. 8:i, 1968.

OSTWALD, F. F., AND PELTZMAN, P.: The cry of the human infant. *Sci. Am.* 230:94-100, Mar. 1974.

PARMELEE, A. H., AND HAVER, AUDREY: Who is the high risk infant? *Clin. Ob. and Gyn.* 16:376-387, Mar. 1973.

PEEPLES, E. H., AND FRANCIS, G. M.: Social-psychological obstacles to effective health team practice. *Nurs. Forum* 7, 1:28-37, 1968.

PIDGEON, V.: The infant with congenital heart disease. *Am. J. Nurs.* 67:290-293, Feb. 1967.

QUESTIONS AND ANSWERS ON RUBELLA. National Communicable Disease Center, Health Services and Mental Health Administration, Public Health Service. Washington, D.C., U.S. Dept. Health, Education and Welfare, Atlanta, Georgia.

RAVITCH, M. M., AND ROWE, M. I.: Surgical emergencies in the neonate. *Am. J. Ob-Gyn.* 103:1034-1057, April 1, 1969.

ROWE, R. D.: Serious congenital heart disease in the newborn infant: diagnosis and management. *Pediatrics Clin. North Am.* 17:967-982, Nov. 1970.

STEELE, S.: Children with amputations. *Nurs. Forum* 7, No. 4:411-423, 1968.

TAYLOR, A.: Autosomal trisomy syndromes: A detailed study of 27 cases of Edwards Syndrome and 27 cases of Patoy's Syndrome. *J. Med. Genetics* 5:227-252, Sept. 1968.

UJHELY, G. B.: Grief and depression—implications for preventive and therapeutic nursing care. *Nurs. Forum* 5, No. 2:23-35, 1966.

VAN LEEUWEN, G.: The nurse in prevention and intervention in the neonatal period. *Nurs. Clin. North Am.* 8:509-520, Sept. 1973.

VAUGHN, V. C., III, MCKAY, R. J., AND NELSON, W. E. (EDS.): *Nelson Textbook of Pediatrics*. Philadelphia, W. B. Saunders, 1975.

WHICH WOMEN CAN SAFELY RECEIVE THE RUBELLA VACCINES? *JAMA* 207:1804-1805, Mar. 10, 1969.

WOOD, B. G., *et al*: Nursing care of babies with cleft lip and palate: The Pierre Robin syndrome. *Nurs. Times* 66:1385-1389, Oct. 1970.

———: Pre-surgical correction of the deformed maxillary arch. *Nurs. Times* 66:1420-1425, Nov. 1970.

———: The immediate pre- and post-operative nursing care. *Nurs. Times* 66:1490-1493, Nov. 1970.

WRIGHT, D. I., *et al*: Acute bacterial infections in the newborn. *Mississippi Med. Assn.* 11:493-500, Sept. 1970.

YASUNAGA, S., *et al*: Cephalhematoma in the newborn. *Clin. Pediatrics* (Philadelphia) 13:256-260, Mar. 1974.

YATES, S. A.: Stillbirth—what staff can do. *Am. J. Nurs.* 72:1592-1594, Sept. 1972.

ZACHMAN, R. D., *et al*: A neonatal intensive care unit: A four-year summary. *Am. J. Diseases of Child.* 128:165-170, Aug. 1974.

ZAHOUREK, R.: Grieving and the loss of the newborn. *Am. J. Nurs.* 73:836-839, May 1973.

ZANGER, N. W., *et al*: Ophthalmia neonatorum is still with us. *J. Med. Soc. New Jersey* 69:674-681, Aug. 1972.

Conference Material

1. In your own hospital setting, evaluate the facilities for and the care of the newborn infants in relation to the prevention of infection.

2. A mother's firstborn infant has a cleft lip and cleft palate. The infant is apparently normal otherwise. The distraught mother can see only "my poor deformed baby girl" and blames herself for this "tragedy," because she did not follow her physician's instructions during pregnancy, particularly in relation to good nutrition. How might the nurse handle the nursing problems in this situation?

3. How do you account for the high infant mortality during the neonatal period?

4. What community agencies in your city render services for handicapped children? What is the procedure for making the referral to such agencies? How can the public health nurse function most effectively in such cases?

5. What legislation in your city or state has contributed to reducing the incidence of congenital syphilis?

6. What methods are used by your hospital, well-baby clinics, and/or other community agencies for the detection of phenylketonuria?

1. Which of the following signs and symptoms should the nurse anticipate when a pregnant patient has a history of heart disease?
   A. Dyspnea
   B. Slow pulse rate
   C. Decrease in blood pressure
   D. Hemorrhage

   Select the number corresponding to the correct letter or letters.
   1. A only
   2. B only
   3. A, C and D
   4. All of them   _____

2. Which of the following factors influence the answer which you have given in Question 1?
   A. Increased need for oxygen intake
   B. Increased blood volume
   C. Toxic damage to the heart
   D. Failure of kidneys to excrete

   Select the number corresponding to the correct letters.
   1. A and B
   2. A and C
   3. B, C and D
   4. All of them   _____

3. Which of the following signs and symptoms would the patient with a ruptured fallopian tube manifest?
   A. Hegar's sign
   B. Intense pain
   C. Profound shock
   D. Irregular fetal heart tones
   E. Vaginal bleeding

   Select the number corresponding to the correct letters.
   1. A and B
   2. A, C and D
   3. B, C and E
   4. B, D and E   _____

4. Which of the following factors must exist before an erythroblastotic infant can be produced?
   A. Rh-negative mother
   B. Rh-positive father
   C. Rh-positive fetus
   D. Rh-positive substance from the fetus must find its way into the mother's bloodstream to build up antibodies.
   E. Mother must have had a previous Rh-positive pregnancy or transfusion.

   Select the number corresponding to the correct letters.
   1. A and D
   2. A, C and D
   3. B, C and E
   4. All of them   _____

5. Which of the following statements concerning diabetes complicated by pregnancy are correct?
   A. The size of the placenta tends to be in direct relationship to the size of the infant.
   B. Toxemia occurs more frequently than in nondiabetic pregnancies.
   C. Deliveries are always performed by cesarean section, usually two weeks prior to term.
   D. The fetus tends to be large.
   E. Hypoglycemia occurs in the infant following delivery.

   Select the number corresponding to the correct letters.
   1. A and B
   2. B, D and E
   3. B, C, D and E
   4. All of them   _____

6. Which of the following are causes of bleeding in the first and second trimesters of pregnancy?
   A. Menstruation
   B. Abortion
   C. Abruptio placentae
   D. Placenta previa
   E. Ectopic pregnancy

   Select the number corresponding to the correct letters.
   1. A and B
   2. A, B and D
   3. A, B and E
   4. B, C, D and E   _____

7. How is inevitable abortion distinguished from threatened abortion?
   A. Dilatation of the cervical canal
   B. Rupture of the membranes
   C. Pain
   D. Bleeding

   Select the number corresponding to the correct letter or letters.
   1. A only
   2. B only
   3. A, B and D
   4. All of them   _____

8. What is the effect of tetanic contractions on the pregnant uterus?
   A. Descent and rotation are hastened.
   B. Ruptured uterus is imminent.
   C. Fetal distress may occur.
   D. Uterine inertia may follow.
   E. Perineal lacerations may occur.

   Select the number corresponding to the correct letter or letters.
   1. A only
   2. B only
   3. A, C and D
   4. B, C and E   _____

9. Insofar as the toxemias are concerned, which of the following symptoms during labor should be reported to the physician promptly?
   A. Hard, painful uterine contractions
   B. Epigastric pain
   C. Dimness of vision
   D. Headache
   E. Decrease in urinary excretion

   Select the number corresponding to the correct letters.
   1. A, C and D
   2. A, C and E
   3. B, C and D
   4. B, C, D and E   _____

10. Which of the following conditions contribute to postpartal hemorrhage?
    A. Toxemias of pregnancy
    B. Overdistention of the uterus due to twins or hydramnios
    C. Unwise management of the third stage of labor
    D. Involution
    E. Retained placental fragments

    Select the number corresponding to the correct letters.
    1. A and C
    2. A, B and D
    3. B, C and E
    4. All of them   _____

11. A patient in the first stage of labor develops hypotonic dysfunctional labor. Which of the following are important in the treatment of this condition?
    A. Pitocin
    B. Sedation
    C. Fluids
    D. Bed rest
    E. Ambulation

    Select the number corresponding to the correct letters.
    1. A, B and D
    2. A, C and E
    3. B, C and D
    4. B, C and E   _____

12. To which of the following causes may urinary tract infections during the puerperium be attributed?
    A. Poor hygiene
    B. Urinary retention
    C. Uterine inertia
    D. Subinvolution
    E. Trauma sustained during delivery

    Select the number corresponding to the correct letters.
    1. A and B
    2. A, B and E
    3. B, D and E
    4. All of them   _____

13. Which of the following are the chief dangers from sore, cracked nipples?
    A. Infection of the infant from nursing
    B. Invasion of bacteria resulting in abscess of the nipple
    C. Invasion of bacteria through the nipple into the breast tissue
    D. Formation of scar tissue which will prevent normal nursing thereafter
    E. Formation of a permanent fissure in the nipple

    Select the number corresponding to the correct letters.
    1. A and C
    2. B and C
    3. B, D and E
    4. B, C, D and E
    _____

14. Which of the following veins is likely to be involved in puerperal thrombophlebitis?
    A. Splenic vein
    B. Popliteal vein
    C. Renal vein
    D. Ovarian vein
    E. Saphenous vein

    Select the number corresponding to the correct letters.
    1. A, B and D
    2. B, C and E
    3. B, D and E
    4. All of them
    _____

15. The nurse sometimes observes swelling of the newborn infant's scalp which may be due to caput succedaneum or cephalhematoma. Which of the following statements are true concerning cephalhematoma?
    A. It is due to an extravasation of serum into the tissues of the scalp.
    B. It is seldom visible when the infant is born and may not be noticed for several hours or more after delivery.
    C. The infant usually recovers without treatment.
    D. It always disappears within a few days.
    E. It gradually increases in size until about a week after the infant's birth, when it remains stationary for a time and then begins to disappear.

    Select the number corresponding to the correct letters.
    1. A and B
    2. A, C and D
    3. B, C and D
    4. B, C and E
    _____

16. What are some of the signs of cerebral hemorrhage which may be observed by the nurse caring for infants in the newborn nursery?
    A. Convulsions
    B. Slow, deep, rhythmic respiration
    C. Twitching of extremities
    D. Flushed face with circumoral pallor
    E. Weak, whining cry

    Select the number corresponding to the correct letter or letters.
    1. A only
    2. A and C
    3. B, C and E
    4. All of them
    _____

17. A newborn infant develops respiratory distress after birth, and the diagnosis of hyaline membrane disease is made. Which of the following statements have bearing on this condition?
   A. The infant was born prematurely.
   B. The infant is cyanotic and dyspneic.
   C. Progressive respiratory difficulty is evidenced by increased cyanosis and marked sternal retractions.
   D. Treatment primarily consists of the administration of oxygen and maintenance of high humidity.
   E. A protein material is obstructing the flow of air and the exchange of oxygen and carbon dioxide in the lungs.

   Select the number corresponding to the correct letters.
   1. A, B and C
   2. B, D and E
   3. C, D and E
   4. All of them   _____

18. Which of the following conditions are congenital disorders?
   A. Phimosis
   B. Chloasma
   C. Umbilical hernia
   D. Retrolental fibroplasia
   E. Seborrhea capitis

   Select the number corresponding to the correct letters.
   1. A and C
   2. B, C and D
   3. B, D and E
   4. All of them   _____

19. The most effective treatment of erythroblastosis is accomplished by blood transfusion. Which one of the following is the best method to use?
   A. Exchange transfusion with Rh-negative blood
   B. Exchange transfusion with Rh-positive blood
   C. Exchange transfusion with blood plasma
   D. Repeated small transfusions with Rh-negative blood
   E. Repeated small transfusions with Rh-positive blood
   F. Repeated small transfusions with blood plasma   _____

20. Hemolytic disease of the newborn may be produced by the union of parents with which of the following blood types?
   A. Rh-positive mother with Rh-negative father
   B. Rh-negative mother with Rh-negative father
   C. Rh-negative mother with Rh-positive father
   D. Type O mother with Type A father
   E. Type A mother with Type B father

   Select the number corresponding to the correct letters.
   1. A and C
   2. B and D
   3. C and D
   4. All of them   _____

21. Which one of the following infectious diseases, when contracted by the mother during the first trimester of pregnancy, will most often produce congenital anomalies in the infant?
    A. Scarlet fever
    B. Rubella
    C. Diphtheria
    D. Rubeola
    E. Typhoid fever
    _____

22. Some disorders which affect the infant in the neonatal period are manifestations of inborn errors of metabolism. Which of the following conditions would this include?
    A. Phenylketonuria
    B. Icterus neonatorum
    C. Galactosemia
    D. Down's syndrome
    E. Erythroblastosis fetalis

    Select the number corresponding to the correct letter or letters.
    1. A only
    2. A and C
    3. B, C and D
    4. B, D and E
    _____

23. What has recently become the best method to prevent erythroblastosis fetalis?
    A. Injection of the mother soon after delivery with Rh immune globulin to prevent maternal sensitization.
    B. Transfusing the mother during pregnancy.
    C. Transfusing all Rh-negative fathers.
    D. Transfusing all Rh-negative babies.
    E. Repeated small transfusions of Rh-positive blood to the mother.

    Select the number corresponding to the correct letter or letters.
    1. A only
    2. A and B
    3. B, C and D
    4. C, D and E
    _____

24. Which of the following features are characteristic of the preterm infant and distinguish him from the full-size infant?
    A. The infant is usually puny and weighs less than 2,000 Gm.
    B. The infant's head is proportionately large, his skull is round or ovoid in shape, and his facial features are small and angular.
    C. The skin is soft, transparent and may be covered with lanugo.
    D. These infants whimper and cry rather constantly, although the cry is weak.
    E. The body temperature is unstable and thus responds rather readily to changes in the temperature of the environment.

    Select the number corresponding to the correct letters.
    1. A and B
    2. B, C and D
    3. B, C and E
    4. All of them
    _____

25. When the mother learned that her preterm infant was receiving gavage feedings she asked the nurse why this was being done. Which of the following reasons may be correct for the nurse to reply?

   A. "This method of feeding your baby was indicated because he became exhausted when he tried to swallow."

   B. "Feeding your baby this way prevents him from vomiting and thus eliminates the danger of his aspirating formula into his lungs."

   C. "Feeding your baby this way conserves his strength and permits him to receive food into his stomach when sucking or swallowing may be difficult."

   D. "He can be given his formula quickly this way and so he does not have to be handled as much."

   E. "A tiny baby's resistance to infection is poor, so gavage feeding is really a protective measure against such infections as thrush, which he might acquire if he were bottle-fed."

   Select the number corresponding to the correct letter or letters.
   1. A only
   2. C only
   3. B, C and D
   4. B, D and E

26. In caring for preterm infants, which of the following precautions should be taken against retrolental fibroplasia?

   A. The administration of oxygen should be discontinued as soon as feasible.

   B. The concentration of oxygen in the incubator housing the infant should be tested periodically and kept at less than 30 percent when possible.

   C. Daily determinations of the serum bilirubin level should be done when there is any indication of proliferation of the retinal capillaries.

   D. High humidity should be maintained in the incubator constantly.

   E. The infant's eyes should be protected from bright lights.

   Select the number corresponding to the correct letters.
   1. A and B
   2. A, C and D
   3. B, D and E
   4. All of them

27. How can the community health nurse assist the family in the care and the supervision of the preterm and low birth weight infants?

   A. Visit the home before the infant leaves the hospital to evaluate the home situation and give anticipatory guidance to the parents as necessary.

   B. Help the family to understand that the infant is still premature and must have the same kind of skillful, protective care in a sheltered environment similar to that in the hospital premature nursery.

   C. Make daily visits to the home to bathe the infant, prepare the formula and, in general, give suggestions and guidance to the mother about her infant's care.

   D. Visit the home again after the infant is discharged from the hospital to give the family guidance and assistance as necessary.

   E. Help the family to understand that this infant requires a great amount of undisturbed rest and thus should not be held or cuddled as much as the full-size infant.

   Select the number corresponding to the correct letters.
   1. A and D
   2. A, C and E
   3. B, C and E
   4. All of them

28. The premature infant has difficulty in regulating his body temperature because heat regulation is one of the least developed functions of his body. Which of the following conditions are responsible for this?

A. The surface area of the premature infant is relatively smaller than that of a normal full-term infant in proportion to body size.

B. Lack of subcutaneous fat which would furnish a measure of insulation

C. Limited ability to produce body proteins

D. Poor reflex control of skin capillaries

E. Frequent episodes of diaphoresis causing loss of body heat

Select the number corresponding to the correct letters.

1. A and C
2. B and D
3. B, C and E
4. All of them

_____

special considerations in maternity nursing

Home Delivery
Obstetrics During Emergency
History of Maternity Care

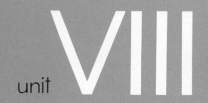

unit VIII

home delivery

30

The Home Birth Movement / Nurse-Midwifery / Approach to Home Delivery by Nurse-Midwife and Physician Teams

Childbirth in the home, once the predominant mode for almost all deliveries, has come to be viewed as an anachronism by the professional community. Significant strides were made in reduction of maternal and infant mortality by utilization of the hospital for deliveries over the last half century. Hospital asepsis led to control of puerperal infection, while surgical intervention and availability of blood transfusions reduced death from hemorrhage. Complex technical equipment and procedures for infant resuscitation and treatment of neonatal illness enabled reduction in infant deaths. Prenatal care instituted early in pregnancy correlated with positive outcomes for mother and baby.

With the obvious benefits of technological progress, the steadily growing incidence of childbirth in the home puzzles and bemuses many health professionals. To understand this movement, we must examine the cost in terms of the quality of the human experience that is exacted by hospital delivery. Health care institutions and professionals must also consider whether the acute hospital as we know it today is really the appropriate place for normal, uncomplicated labor and delivery to occur. There are many considerations on each side of the

home delivery issue, and these will be discussed in this chapter.

Nurse-midwives are often associated in the minds of many lay and professional people with home births. This association is not uniformly accepted by nurse-midwives themselves, as their professional organization and leaders have repeatedly emphasized that the nurse-midwife ideally functions within a team including an obstetrician, and provides care within established health care institutions. Although nurse-midwives are undoubtedly the best prepared professionals to participate in home deliveries, the tendency is to minimize this aspect of their functions and emphasize provision of the full range of maternity care to underserved populations in collaboration with the physician.

The home birth movement

Although accurate statistics are difficult to obtain, there is a recognized and growing trend among certain segments of the U.S. population to elect to deliver in the home, whether attended or unattended by professionals. In the Seattle-King County area the number of home births increased from 1.5 per 1,000 births in 1966 to 2.0 in 1969, with evidence that the number was doubling for 1971.[1] In California in 1971 the overall incidence of out-of-hospital births was 0.6 percent, but certain counties had incidences as high as 2.6 to 4.8 percent. Marin County, just north of San Francisco, reported out-of-hospital births at 6.1 percent in 1972.[2] Many of these home births are unattended, an estimated 100 per month in the San Francisco Bay area.[3]

Nurses and physicians have been reluctant to address the issue of home births, although those involved in prepared childbirth programs and county health departments receive many questions from interested parents. Not uncommonly, the parents are dismissed with curt replies or threats of numerous dangers for mother and baby, thus left on their own to seek information and prepare as best they are able. The implications of this rejection of traditional methods of prenatal and delivery care deserve professional attention, for although the numbers are now small, this group may represent the more radical expression of a widespread discontent with the status quo in maternity care.

Why couples elect home delivery

Many types of people arrive at the decision to deliver their babies at home, ranging from professionals disillusioned with the cold and dehumanizing hospital experience to counterculture and communal residents who seek oneness with nature and return to the spiritualism of birth. Childbirth is a physiologic, emotional, and for some an extremely spiritual experience, a truly unique peak happening in the lives of the involved people. Impersonal, anesthetic, detached, and restrictive environments such as that of the modern acute hospital markedly interfere with the freedom of the childbearing couple and significant others to feel and act as they deem important.

One reason for rejecting hospital delivery has to do with the nature of prenatal and intrapartal services provided by the health system. Rules are made by physicians and nurses and imposed upon the childbearing couple. Frequently they do not understand the reasons for certain expectations or restrictions. If they question the rules, they are often regarded as "problem patients" and told in subtle or obvious ways that they are bad parents and endangering the expected baby. Mature people expect to gather information and make decisions for themselves based upon their understanding and interpretation of the data. Relinquishing all decision making to the expert professionals places a person in the dependent-child position, which signifies immaturity. It is not difficult to understand why thinking people reject the paternalistic health professional's approach.

When the couple has sought a program to prepare them for childbirth, and developed a plan of action to cope with labor, or identified certain components of the labor-delivery experience which are important to them, health professionals often present barriers to these. Instead of asking why and examining the validity of the numerous rules and traditions surrounding the delivery area, doctors and nurses tend to engage in power struggles with the couple and demand conformity as the price for their services. The alienating effects of such actions need little elaboration. Some parents consider hospital treatment as disrespectful and dehumanizing, as one laywoman who assists at births has stated:

> Today women giving birth in hospitals are frequently forced to endure outrageous insults to body and intellect . . . the baby is detached from the sounds, smells, and closeness that are his birthright . . . Where is there room for love?[4]

Although soaring hospital costs have been cited as reasons for having a home delivery, many parents deny saving expenses as a significant motivation. What seems more important is avoiding the negative things which are imposed by hospital deliveries, such as enemas, artificial rupture of the amniotic sac, episiotomies, fundal pressure, traction on the umbilical cord for delivery of the placenta, intravenous infusions, pain medication, and in some cases use of oxytocin. These women generally want to either squat or lie on their sides for delivery, not maintain a strapped lithotomy position. They want to nurse their babies immediately after delivery or shortly after the cord is cut. They want to allow the perineum to iron out rather than have a hastened delivery with episiotomy and forceps. As such mothers will breastfeed, they do not want glucose water given to their babies as is the nearly universal nursery practice, and want the babies with them continuously. Few hospitals will agree to most of these practices.[5]

Continuity with a natural lifestyle is another reason why couples opt for home births. There is considerable reaction against society's present artificial and plastic nature and against practices of additives or substitutes for natural products as well as encroachment upon nature's rhythms and cycles. Many people of various persuasions object to these, as the growth of the natural foods industry and increased interest in mysticism and parapsychology attest. There is a spectrum in people's movement back toward a more natural existence; some simply change their diet while others move physically away from congested centers of population and establish communes or smaller group residences in isolated and remote areas. Such groups also move psychologically very far away from accepted social values and standards of behavior, seeking an ecological style of living in which mind, body and the natural elements are in harmony. Free expression of the full range of human feelings without social restraints is possible in this setting. Again, there are many degrees of this more natural and free lifestyle, and its proponents may be found in cities as well as rural areas.

Childbirth in the home is a reflection of the values associated with this lifestyle. It is a joyful and spiritual experience in which all "family" members share both risks and accomplishments. The rituals and ceremonies which used to surround childbirth are reconstituted, and it assumes once again great significance for the social group. The mother delivers her child rather than is delivered by the expert, with those people who are important to her close by, providing support and assistance. Self-sufficiency, total community involvement, complete sharing, and growth through accomplishment are the values which this process expresses. An experience of such magnitude will not easily be given up, despite risks and efforts by health professionals to discourage parents.

Many couples planning home births seek prenatal care, when it is available to them. They may or may not inform their physician, depending upon his attitude and their relationship with him. In some instances, the physician agrees to attend the birth or stand by, but the number of physicians who will do this is extremely small. Nurses or nurse-midwives may also be involved, but more commonly a lay-midwife or experienced friend attends the laboring woman. It is not uncommon for couples to attend prepared childbirth classes, as they appreciate the importance of learning about the process of labor and delivery and want tools enabling them to cope with the experience.

These couples are usually aware of the risks for mother and baby, but have decided that physical safety is secondary to obtaining the most meaningful experience possible during childbirth. Realistic planning for home delivery also includes options in case of complications or emergency.

Conduct of home delivery

Equipment for home delivery can be purchased in many drugstores, and generally includes bulb syringe, cord ties, scissors to be soaked in isopropyl alcohol, padding for the bad, a rubber sheet to protect the mattress, perineal pads, plastic pail and liners, a large bowl for catching the placenta, and newspapers to spread on the floor. Cord ties are generally new, unopened dental floss or shoestrings. Pads to put under the woman's buttocks during labor can be made from newspaper covered with soft muslin or cotton, but many women say these are crackly and uncomfortable. Old towels and rags that have been laundered, dried in a dryer and stuffed in a clean pillow case are preferred. For eye prophylaxis against gonorrhea in the newborn, an antibiotic ophthalmic ointment such as Bacitracin is frequently used.

After labor begins, women walk about much longer than hospitalized patients do. They eat nourishing snacks but restrict solids after labor becomes active. For pain relief, certain teas, such as raspberry tea, are prized, or marijuana in small amounts may be used. Ethyl alcohol and calcium are also sometimes recommended. As the second stage nears, most women recline in bed or assume a semiupright position. Breathing and distraction techniques learned in prepared childbirth classes are utilized, and the father and friends administer comfort measures. Delivery may occur in varying positions, such as squatting with knees moderately spread apart, sitting up and holding the knees apart, or standing with support on either side. The hands and knees position is also commonly used, and is favored for breech births. When the perineum begins to bulge and the head to crown, the father or attendant supports it with two fingers and waits for extension of the head. The perineum is given the opportunity to iron out, and the attendant tries to ease it around the head without laceration. At birth, the bulb syringe may be used to suction mucus from the

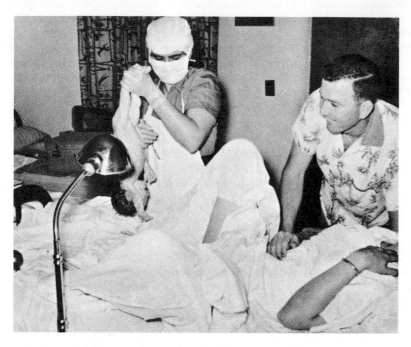

Figure 30-1. The certified nurse-midwife conducting a home delivery. The father at the bedside encourages his wife and simultaneously derives considerable satisfaction from his participation in the birth of their baby. (Catholic Maternity Institute, Sante Fe, New Mexico)

baby's nose and mouth, although recent techniques indicate that this probably is not necessary routinely. Cord tying is delayed until the cord is flaccid, so the baby may benefit from placental transfusion. Usually the baby is put to breast immediately, as soon as the cord is long enough. When the cord is tied and cut, attendants usually wash their hands thoroughly, and some may use gloves. The placenta is stored for about 24 hours in case of complications (Fig. 30-1).

After the delivery is complete, the mother's perineum is cleansed or she takes a shower, and she has a meal. Then she and the baby usually go to sleep together. If there has been a perineal laceration, or if bleeding is excessive, the mother usually goes to the emergency room, bringing the placenta when medical assistance is sought. Most physicians will only suture perineal lacerations within the first six hours postpartum. The second and third stages of labor in home births tend to be longer than health professionals might consider safe. Some women consider delivery of the placenta a voluntary act, in which they decide when to "release" it. If labor is prolonged, or other complications such as fever or heavy bleeding occur, the woman is usually taken to the emergency room. Vaginal examinations during labor at home are minimized or avoided because of the risk of infection. In some areas, pedia-tricians will agree to care for or do initial examinations on babies born at home, but parents must usually bring the baby to the emergency room or office.[6]

Risks of home delivery

When discussing the topic of home births, most professionals will note that when labor and delivery go well, it is a beautiful and natural process which really does not require any intervention by experts. However, when it goes badly it can be disastrous and even life threatening. In a certain proportion of cases, difficulty can be predicted. Women with cardiac or kidney disease, diabetes, Rh negative women, those with previous premature delivery, pre-eclampsia, successively larger babies, prolonged labors, or who are under 20 or over 35 years of age have a higher incidence of complications. But among other women, it is almost impossible to predict whether or when problems will arise. Many problems are accidents of labor or delivery and constitute emergency situations, such as prolapse of the cord, hemorrhage, and neonatal asphyxia. Others develop more slowly but have equally grave implications, such as amnionitis, failure to progress in labor, dysfunctional labor, and maternal exhaustion. The need for immediate medical intervention when serious complications arise is the major reason for professional reservations about home births.

Proponents of home births point out the low incidence of such serious complications. Professionals argue that in the individual case, when technologic services can prevent death or damage, this low incidence means nothing. Thus the issue of safety versus quality of the experience is crystallized, and individual choices must be made as to which takes precedence.

There are also differing professional opinions on the non-life-threatening practices, such as episiotomy. Ironing out the perineum to avoid episiotomy can be overdone, because in this process there is marked separation of the pelvic floor muscles whether or not a tear occurs. This separation of deep muscles can lead to pelvic relaxation and cystorectocele in later life, just as can extensive tears with inadequate repair. Tears into the anal sphincter when improperly repaired can lead to rectovaginal fistulas. Thus episiotomy may be indicated even after a certain amount of ironing out of the perineum, because there is not adequate elasticity of the tissues to prevent laceration or deep muscle rupture.

Although an obstetrician is certainly not needed for most deliveries, this medical presence represents a form of insurance against unforeseen complications. If parents shop around among physicians and hospitals, they can frequently find those who are willing to cooperate with parental desires regarding conduct of labor and delivery. In this way, the couple could experience most of the things they consider important yet have the safety of expert attendance and modern facilities in case of complications.

The health care system and the
human experience

The question is often raised whether the health care system can change its environment and practices enough that parents could obtain the warm, human experience which they desire from childbearing. Home deliveries are viewed as a symptom of failure in society and the health care system in that health professionals have not demonstrated enough caring about people and have disregarded their wants and needs. It has become necessary for growing numbers of parents to reject the health care system in order to obtain the human experience. There are many changes which could improve the quality of service provided by physicians, nurses and hospitals. Parents could be included as equal partners in the health care team, fully informed and involved in every decision. Their ideas could be elicited and discussed openly and nonjudgmentally. Professionals could be more willing to examine their biases and consider alternate approaches according to the true merits of the practice, rather than perpetuating traditional approaches just because these are widely used.

Efficiency of operation and cost would have to be considered for certain major changes. Could the hospital provide room space for an extended family group to attend labor and delivery? Could hospital rooms be made more homelike, warm and comfortable? Could the place and manner of delivery be changed from the surgical delivery room and still maintain standards of safety? Perhaps many hospital and public health codes would need to be amended. Would administrators and public officials agree with this? In considering the numerous small differences in conduct of labor and delivery which the parents favoring home birth desire, could nurses and physicians forego some of what they consider technological progress in favor of a more natural process? Can those in the nursery set aside concerns over heat regulation and infection control to permit continuous family-baby contact? Can feeding regimens for babies be completely optional?

A new approach within the health care system is presently in its earliest stage of development. The concept of a lying-in cottage is being revived, in which parents would conduct most of the labor, the delivery, and a short postpartum recovery period in a special institution organized just for this service. Emergency equipment would be on hand, as would arrangements for transfer to an acute hospital should a serious complication develop. Two such institutions are being planned, one in connection with the Maternity Center Association in New York and one by a group in Oregon. Nurse-midwives and physicians will collaborate in provision of prenatal, intrapartal and postpartum care for a group of patients who plan to use the lying-in cottage for delivery. Practices surrounding conduct of labor and delivery will be flexible and geared to parent preferences.

Another sign of change within health care institutions is the growing professional interest in the work of French obstetrician Frederick LeBoyer. This approach is intended to minimize the trauma associated with birth for the infant. After a prepared labor with parent participation, delivery is conducted in a warm,

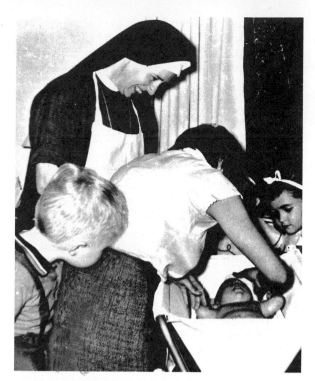

Figure 30-2. Postpartal care and teaching in the home provided by the certified nurse-midwife. (Catholic Maternity Institute, Sante Fe, New Mexico)

dark and very quiet room. Frightening stimuli such as bright delivery lights, cold environment, and harsh loud noises are eliminated. Delivery is slow and controlled, with gentle easing out of the baby. No suction with bulb syringe or catheter is employed, as it has been found that mucus drains naturally out of nasal and oral passages from gravity and pressure upon the thorax still in the birth canal. If delivery was hastened, there might not be enough time for this natural process to adequately drain mucus. Small amounts left in the respiratory passages are absorbed. When birth is complete the infant, still attached to the cord, is placed upon the mother's abdomen. She may enfold or nurse the baby. After the cord is cut, the baby's body is submerged in a tub of warm water which approximates the intrauterine existence with which the baby is familiar. All talk is conducted in whispers. During this process babies have been noted to open their eyes and apparently look around, to smile and emit small grunts, but they do not generally cry. The sounds the baby makes are interpreted as expressions of pleasure or comfort, rather than the terrified screaming of the baby with a

shocking and painful birth experience. LeBoyer has studied children born by the nontraumatic approach, and believes that they are better adjusted, less fearful, more open, stable children than the general population. The modifications necessary for this new approach to delivery are minimal, and can readily be accommodated by most standard delivery rooms.[7]

Despite the adoption of changes which humanize the health delivery system, some parents will still reject institutionalized labor and delivery. They explain that no matter what is done within the hospital, it is still not the same as the home environment. The sense of familiarity, the comfort, the freedom to do what one wants, the ability to have significant others totally involved with home delivery— these advantages simply cannot be matched by an institution. For this group, modifications in labor and delivery practices and hospital environments will not really make any difference. For a much larger group, however, such modifications will be enthusiastically welcomed, and may mean the difference between choosing a home or a hospital delivery. Maternity nurses and other health care professionals have an obligation to respond to a public which is providing sober testimony to the quality of services currently being provided.

Nurse-midwifery

The preponderance of maternity care throughout the world is provided by the nurse-midwife. In this country, nurse-midwives are registered nurses who have completed a recognized program of study and clinical experience leading to a certificate in nurse-midwifery. In other countries they may be specialized groups of nurses who have received the major part of their training in the area of maternity care. U.S. nurse-midwives consider theirs an extended nursing role, with equal emphasis on all phases of the maternity cycle. They are prepared to give comprehensive care to childbearing couples, including both physical management and educational-counseling aspects. Nurse-midwives are prepared to assume primary responsibility for prenatal, intrapartal, and postpartal care of women having normal pregnanices (Fig. 30-2).

History of nurse-midwifery in the U.S.

FRONTIER NURSING SERVICE. The history of the trained nurse-midwife in this country began in 1925, when an organization was established in the mountains of eastern Kentucky to handle the maternity problem in the rural and isolated areas of that territory—the now famous Frontier Nursing Service. This organization was founded by the late Mrs. Mary Breckinridge at Wendover, Ky., the headquarters of the public health nurse-midwifery service. Today, FNS is organized with Hayden Hospital, which has a full-time Medical Director (an M.D.), and five outpost clinics, each staffed with nurse-midwives. These nurses often travel by horseback from the outposts to serve families in the even more remote areas, but along the highways and roads they travel by jeep or station wagon. This organization has demonstrated clearly that graduate nurses prepared in midwifery can help to lower mortality rates in a large population in rural and isolated areas.

Frontier Nursing Service gives a wide range of medical care to 10,000 patients annually. In the last decade and a half, during which more than 5,000 mothers have been safely delivered by these nurse-midwives, there have been no maternal deaths. In the fall of 1939, the Frontier Nursing Service inaugurated the Frontier Graduate School of Midwifery in Hayden, Ky.

THE MATERNITY CENTER ASSOCIATION was founded in New York in 1918, and in 1932 the Center established its school of nurse-midwifery for graduate nurses. The Lobenstine Midwifery Clinic was established to provide a field service for this school. It trained about 12 students a year in a six-month course which provided obstetric theory and supervised practice by an obstetrician and by graduate nurse-midwives. In 1935, the Maternity Center Association and the Lobenstine Midwifery Clinic applied to the State of New York to consolidate under the name of Maternity Center Association. The progress achieved in this endeavor included certification of 413 nurse-midwives in a 30-year period, use of nurse-midwives in municipal hospitals by the New York City Department of Health, and development of closer relationships with the American College of Obstetricians and Gynecologists. In 1970 the Maternity Center Association received a grant to establish a series of regional refresher courses for nurse-midwives, to double the number of schools and programs of nurse-midwifery, and to expand the enrollment of existing schools.

THE AMERICAN COLLEGE OF NURSE-MIDWIFERY was established in 1955 as an organization of nurse-midwives to study and evaluate the activities of nurse-midwives, to plan and develop

educational programs meeting the requirements of the profession, and to perform other related functions. In 1957, the College became a member of the International Confederation of Midwives, a midwifery organization with members from some 31 countries throughout the world.

At the annual meeting of the College in May, 1962, the definitions of the nurse-midwife and nurse-midwifery were accepted by the membership and stated as follows:

> The Nurse-Midwife is a Registered Nurse who by virtue of added knowledge and skill gained through an organized program of study and clinical experience recognized by the American College of Nurse-Midwifery, has extended the limits (legal limits in jurisdictions where they obtain) of her practice into the area of management of care of mothers and babies throughout the maternity cycle so long as progress meets criteria accepted as normal.

THE AMERICAN COLLEGE OF NURSE-MIDWIVES had its inception in 1969 when the American College of Nurse-Midwifery amended its Articles of Incorporation.[8]

The objectives of the American College of Nurse-Midwives are as follows:

1. To enable nurse-midwives to concentrate their efforts in the improvement of services to mothers and newborn babies in cooperation with other allied groups.
2. To identify the area of nurse-midwifery practices as they relate to the total service and educational aspects of maternal and newborn care.
3. To study and evaluate the activities of the nurse-midwife in order that qualifications for these activities may be established.
4. To plan and develop with the assistance of allied educational groups educational programs in nurse-midwifery that will meet the qualifications of the profession.
5. To establish channels for communication and interpretation of midwifery to allied professional and nonprofessional groups on a regional, national, and international basis.
6. To sponsor research and develop literature in the field of nurse-midwifery.

Medical association endorsement of nurse-midwives

Physicians had long opposed any widespread use of nurse-midwives in the delivery of maternity care in the U.S. Many barriers had been raised to the practice of midwifery, including restrictive legislation and refusal of hospital privileges. Midwifery was even illegal in some states. In 1970, however, the American College of Obstetricians and Gynecologists took a positive stance toward nurse-midwives, issuing a joint statement with the Nurses Association of ACOG and the American College of Nurse-Midwives:

> The American College of Obstetricians and Gynecologists, the Nurses Association of the American College of Obstetricians and Gynecologists and the American College of Nurse-Midwives recognize the increasing needs for general health care and, more specifically, the deficits in availability and quality of maternity care. The latter, which are not confined to any social class, can best be corrected by the cooperative efforts of teams of physicians, nurse-midwives, obstetric registered nurses and other health personnel. The composition of such teams will vary and be determined by local needs and circumstances. The functions and responsibilities of team members should be clearly defined according to the education and training of the individuals concerned.
>
> To achieve the aims of providing optimal maternity care for all women the following recommendations are made:
> 1. The health team organized to provide maternity care will be directed by a qualified obstetrician-gynecologist.
> 2. In such medically directed teams, qualified nurse-midwives may assume responsibility for the complete care of uncomplicated maternity patients.
> 3. In such medically directed teams, obstetric registered nurses may assume responsibility for patient care according to their education, training and experience.
> 4. In such medically-directed teams, other health personnel who have been trained in specific areas of maternity care may participate in the team functions according to their abilities and within the definitions of responsibility established by the team.
> 5. Written policies describing the specific functions of each of the team members should be prepared. They should be reviewed and revised periodically according to changing needs.[9]

This joint statement recognized the common goal among nurses, nurse-midwives and physicians to improve and expand health services provided to women. It is expected to encourage preparation of more nurse-midwives and greater utilization of their services. Many nurse-midwives are in educational or administrative positions rather than providing direct care to patients, largely because their practice has been so restricted. Hopefully more will move into the practice settings as physicians become willing to cooperate and affiliate with nurse-midwives.

Issues in nurse-midwifery

The relationship of nurse-midwifery to nursing has long been a matter of some dissension. Early in the development of midwifery, the reluctance on the part of the professional nursing organizations to incorporate this "splinter group" led to formation of a separate organization for nurse-midwives. The American College of Nurse-Midwives approves nurse-midwifery programs and administers the certifying examination to graduates. Although not licensed separately from registered nurses, nurse-midwives must have this certificate to practice as well as meet other requirements which states may set. For instance, New York, Ohio, New Mexico and California have separate laws pertaining to nurse-midwifery, and in New York City the health code defines nurse-midwifery practice.[10]

Nurses may think of nurse-midwives as delivery technicians, but the comprehensive approach to maternity care most midwives provide is far from this. Nurse-midwives have been accused of being physician-dominated or essentially physician's assistants. Midwives contend that this is simply not true, that theirs has been a separate profession for over 40 years under the control and direction of nurse-midwives. Most of their education, licensing and certifying activities are conducted by nurse-midwives, not physicians. While they readily enter colleague relationships with physicians, practices are complementary. Nurse-midwives do not give up their integrity; rather, they share in the provision of care. Nurse-midwives believe that the care they provide to women with uncomplicated pregnancies is qualitatively different from obstetrical care, and more extensive because of its educational component.

Differences between nurse-midwives and maternity nurses or maternity clinical specialists are often questioned. Some nurses feel that nurse-midwifery merely adds "baby-catching" to maternity nursing. Although some of the differences may be more apparent than real, probably the one area of significant difference in nurse-midwifery practice is assumption of responsibility for complete management of the woman and baby during normal childbearing. Nurse-midwives are more mobile and provide care during all phases of childbearing, while nurses or clinical specialists tend to concentrate on one phase, such as prenatal or postpartal. The new nurse-practitioner role closely approximates nurse-midwife functions, with the exception of the intrapartal phase. Both are responsible for management of physical and emotional aspects of maternity care in uncomplicated cases. In all likelihood nurse-practitioner preparation will extend to the intrapartal phase in the coming years, which might lead to an eventual merging of nurse-midwifery and maternity nurse-practitioner roles.

A common misconception about nurse-midwives involves their functioning mainly in rural areas where there are no physicians. The saga of the Frontier Nursing Service with its nurse-midwives on horseback no doubt contributed to this image. Before the American College of Obstetricians and Gynecologists recognized the place of the nurse-midwife on the obstetrical team in 1970, it is true that most nurse-midwives functioned in areas where there was a lack of medical care, whether in rural or urban settings. However, since that time nurse-midwives have been increasingly incorporated into teams providing care to women of all social groups in locations representing a great range of population densities. Nurse-midwives reiterate that they are not substitutes for physician care to the poor, but are extenders of both quantity and quality of maternity care to all segments of the population.[11]

The role of the nurse-midwife in home deliveries is another issue of contention. Because of historic associations, nurse-midwives are closely connected with home births. Their preparation equips them well to deal with conduct of normal labor outside of institutional settings. Their philosophy of practice values minimal interference with normal labor processes and supports concepts of family involvement and participation. Many nurse-midwives are sympathetic to parents who opt out of the institutional health care system and choose to deliver at home, and no doubt many have formally and informally been involved in attending home deliveries. However, there are concerns about provision of safety when deliveries are conducted in the home which keep nurse-midwives from openly endorsing this practice. They feel that an adequate emergency support system is not generally available to administer care on the spot or transfer the patient to the hospital rapidly enough. One may perceive a slightly more positive stance, however, in reading literature by nurse-midwives about home deliveries in the last few years. Counterforces no doubt exert an important influence upon nurse-midwife attitudes, as manifest by the position of most obstetricians of strong opposition to home deliveries. Dr. Louis Hellman, renowned obstetrician and long-time supporter of physician/nurse-midwife teams, delivered a typical admonition in an address to a section of the American College of Obstetricians and Gynecologists:

> The nurse-midwife will have profound impact on maternity care, not by her influence on practice, but because she will increase the access to a health service and because she will facilitate the continuity of care . . . (but if nurse-midwifery) continues to press for a return to the naturalism of the past with the zealotry that seems to be its present penchant, much progress may be lost and a true team approach may become difficult.[12]

Approach to home delivery by nurse-midwife and physician teams

Even though at the present time the vast majority of mothers in this country are delivered in hospitals, there is still a small percentage of deliveries attended by physicians and qualified midwives at home, the majority of which take place in rural areas. When a home delivery is preferred, such factors as the normality of the patient, accessibility of the obstetrician, facilities at home and available care are important considerations.

Preparations for home delivery should be begun early in pregnancy to enable the family to make adequate preparations. Today in many areas the public health nurse visits the patient in her home routinely during the antepartal period and assists the physician in the management and care of the mother. When there is a home delivery service, these nurses may attend the delivery with the physician. The nurse can be most helpful with preparations for delivery because of special knowledge and expertise.

Many obstetricians give their patients a list of supplies that they will need for delivery at home, but where the matter is left to the parents and the nurse, the following suggestions may be helpful.

Supplies provided by the mother will necessarily vary in the individual situation. The following list contains supplies which will be needed:

Sheets and pillowcases (4)

Bath towels and washcloths (4)

Waterproof material—large enough to protect the mattress (about 1½ yards square). Rubber sheeting, plastic or white table oilcloth are preferable, although heavy brown paper can be used.

Receiving blanket for the infant

Delivery pads (4 to 6). These bed pads are made from 12 thicknesses of newspaper opened to full size (sewed together at the edges) and covered with freshly laundered old or new muslin. Quilted pads or large-size paper diapers may also be purchased for this purpose. Or, old towels and rags may be cleaned and used to make pads.

Newspapers. A supply of clean newspapers should be saved for the many uses to which they can be put at this time.

Small enamel wash basins (2 or 3) for solutions and sponges used in cleansing the patient's genitals, to receive the placenta, and a hand basin.

Large pail with cover

Covered kettles or stew pans (2), one for cooled boiled water and one for boiling water

Ladle or dipper

Enema can with tubing and rectal tip

Board for placing under mattress of delivery bed (table leaf or ironing board without legs may be used)

Hot-water bottle and cover

Bedpan

Nightgowns or pajama tops (3 or 4)

Brassieres (3 or 4) (may be improvised from straight binders, 10 in. wide, or large smooth cotton towels)

Sanitary pads (2 to 3 doz.). If they cannot be purchased, they may be made from freshly laundered, soft, absorbent material, folded and ironed ready for use.

Sanitary belts or T-binders (3 or 4)

Safety pins: 1 doz. small and 1 doz. large

Pitcher or Mason jar with cover

Sterile absorbent cotton (1 lb.) in original package, unopened

Sterile gauze squares 4″ x 4″ (1 doz.)

Mineral oil

Plain white petroleum jelly (tube)

Soap

New nail brush and orangewood stick

Umbilical tape or bobbin tape (narrow cotton) for tying cord (1 yd.)

Scissors

Roll of toilet tissue, unopened

In preparing supplies, such as sheets, drapes, towels and bed pads to be used during delivery, these articles are to be washed with soap and water and dried in the sun if possible, ironed and folded so that the ironed surfaces are folded upon each other. The ironed surface should be used for the field of delivery. These articles should be put away in a pillowcase or wrapped in a piece of ironed paper. The other articles needed at the time of delivery should be laid aside ready for use. Packages of absorbent cotton, gauze squares, sanitary pads and toilet tissue should be put away unopened.

Packages of sterile delivery supplies may be available from a local health agency, or it may be possible to have a package, assembled at home, autoclaved at a local hospital. Although autoclaving is most desirable, it is possible to sterilize dressings, etc., in the oven at home. The simplest method is to place the materials in small muslin bags, or bags of some other heavy white cotton material, and then place these bags in an old pillowcase and pin it shut (double wrapped). This package should be baked on the top shelf in a moderate oven, 325° for 1 hour. If an oven thermometer is not available, place a large white potato (washed and scrubbed) in the oven, and when it is done, the supplies in the pillowcase should be sterilized. The pillowcase should not be opened until the time of delivery, and if it has not been used within a month, it must be resterilized.

The more simple and careful the preparations are, the more efficient will be the results. The important factor to be achieved in a home delivery is cleanliness. Soap and water, sunshine and a hot iron have proved to be effective. On the whole, only a few articles must be sterile.

The room chosen for delivery should be the room in which the patient will be most comfortable. Many mothers during this period have to assume certain responsibilities for the management of the household, so it means much to be where the household affairs can be directed with the least exertion.

Ideally, it should be a room that is light, airy, quiet, cheerful and comfortable, conveniently near a bathroom. The room furnishings should be simple, so that they are easy to keep clean, as cleanliness is one of the first essentials of good obstetric care. The bed should be so placed that it can be approached from either side, and so that the light is convenient either day or night. Ample light is a necessity.

The nurse must make sure that the room has not been occupied recently by a patient suffering from any contagious, infectious or suppurative disease. The instructions set forth in the manual *The Control of Communicable Disease in Man*, American Public Health Association, regulate the isolation, quarantine and disinfection practiced in the care of the patient with communicable disease. In case of such disease, adaptation of procedures to facilities in the home is made as necessary.

In any event, the room must be cleaned thoroughly, and all unnecessary furniture removed, only enough being left to make the room comfortable and cheerful. The obstetrician will need a plain table or a substitute. The nurse will need a table or chair for supplies, unless perhaps the top of the bureau may be used. A card table may be very practical.

The delivery bedsprings should be in good condition, and the mattress firm and level. A single bed is preferable to the wider or double bed, because it is easier for the obstetrician and the nurse to care for the mother. If the bed is low, it may be raised to a more convenient height by using blocks. The bed should be so arranged that after the labor the mother may be made clean and comfortable without too much disturbance. The best way to accomplish this is first to prepare the bed as it is to be used after delivery and then to add the necessary preparations on top for the labor and the delivery.

The mattress may be supported by means of boards placed between it and the springs, so that it will be perfectly firm and level and not sag. Table leaves, a flat ironing board or plain board may be used for this purpose. Such supports should lie crosswise under the mattress at a point directly under the mother's buttocks and should be removed at the conclusion of the

delivery. A firm, flat mattress helps to prevent the patient's hips from sinking into the bed.

The mattress should be covered with a piece of waterproof material, if available; if not, heavy brown paper, newspaper or water-repellent paper may be used. Over this covering, a white cotton sheet should be placed and tucked in securely along the edges. The top sheet, the blanket and the spread may be fanfolded to the foot of the bed, where they will be convenient to cover the mother immediately after the delivery. Covered newspaper or moistureproof pads afford excellent protection and are so arranged that they protect the bed at the time of delivery, and a fresh pad is left under the mother after delivery.

Special equipment for the physician or nurse-midwife might include:

Box of medicines:
    Syntocinon (2 amp.)
    Methergine (2 amp.)
    Ergotrate tablets (50)
    Silver nitrate 1 per cent (2 wax amp.)
    Vitamin K_1 (2 amp.)
    File
    Chromic catgut #2 (2 tubes)
Sterile gloves:
    Size 7 (2 pairs)
    Size 7½ (2 pairs)
Sterile pack containing:
    Hand towel (1)
    Doctor's gown (1)
    Leggings (2) with towel clips (2)
    Towels (6)
    Gauze squares 3″ x 3″ (12)
    Cord dressings (2) with cord ties (4)
    Perineal pads (package)
    Towels for pelvic examination (package of 5)
Case of instruments:
    1-2 cc. syringe with No. 25 needles (2)
    Mayo scissors (1)
    Metal box with needles
    Sponge holder (1)
    Kelly clamps (2)
Muslin case with scales, tape measure, bottle of cord tape, 3″ x 3″ gauze squares (2 pkgs.)
Large basins (2)
Liter cup (1)
Bag of cotton (to be placed in cup)
Enamel covered container

Muslin case containing:
  Applicators, tongue depressors, razor and box of blades, and finger cots
  No. 14 catheters (2):
  1 for bladder catheterization
  1 for suctioning the infant
  No. 28 rectal tube with glass connecting tip (1)
  Rubber bulb syringe (1)
Muslin case containing enema equipment
Muslin case containing:
  Aprons (2)
  Caps (2)
  Masks (4)
Box containing:
  Mouth thermometer
  Rectal thermometer
  K. Y. jelly
  Alcohol 70%
  Green soap
  Bottle of antiseptic No. 3
  Mercury cyanide
  Brush and orangewood stick
  Paper napkins (12)
  Paper towels (12)
  Aromatic spirits of ammonia
Folder containing:
  Labor and delivery procedure
  Standing orders
  Procedure for care of premature infants
  Birth certificate book
  Labor and delivery records (12)
  Infant records (6)
  Baby's care (6)

Delivery procedure

During the antepartal period the patient and her partner will have prepared the needed supplies and been instructed concerning the symptoms of labor and when to call the physician and the nurse. Many physicians wish to be with the mother from the onset of labor; or they may wait for the nurse-midwife's call that delivery is imminent.

A few preparations cannot be made until labor begins, such as boiling the two kettles of water (for 20 minutes) in covered vessels and setting one aside to cool. It is a good idea also to boil a ladle or dipper in the kettle that is set aside to cool. The bed and the crib can be prepared and the delivery supplies arranged (Fig. 30-3).

The underlying principles for the care of the mother being delivered at home are the same as those for hospital delivery (see Chapter 18), although procedures will necessarily have to be modified because of the home situation.

According to the physician's specific orders, a low soapsuds enema may be given to empty the lower intestine in order to make more room for the descending head and to prevent fecal discharge during the delivery. The vulva may be shaved and the external genitalia cleansed with aseptic technique. The mother may need an explanation that the former practice of keeping a perineal pad on while in labor has been largely discarded because of the danger of carrying infection, notably the colon bacillus, to the parturient canal from the anal region.

During the first stage of labor the mother is usually allowed to be up and about until labor becomes very active, or the membranes rupture. The physician may suggest liquids to be given freely and that light nourishment be offered, such as tea and toast or crackers, if delivery is not imminent. As labor progresses, careful explanation will provide comfort and reassurance.

The nursing care of the mother in labor at home is essentially the same as in the hospital. Observations of the mother's temperature, pulse, respirations, blood pressure, intake and output and the progress of labor are made consistently. The fetal heart tones are checked routinely, and the mother is watched closely for any complication which might develop. If membranes rupture in the first stage of labor, the danger of prolapse of the cord must be kept in mind. In addition, if the physician is not present, he must be notified immediately, as would be the case if complications developed. If the physician needs to be called for this reason, it should be done without alarming the mother, especially if this is her first labor. From the beginning of true labor, the mother should use a commode or bedpan and be encouraged to empty her bladder at fairly frequent intervals to avoid bladder distention, as well as to keep her more comfortable.

As soon as it is apparent that the mother is nearing the second stage of labor, she should be put to bed, if she has not been already. The nurse should now have everything in readiness for delivery, if possible. On the arrival of the physician, he will, in all probability, want to do a rectal or a vaginal examination at once to determine the amount of dilatation of the cervix and the progress the mother has made.

All instruments required for the delivery are usually provided by the physician and are brought to the home in sterile packages. However, if such equipment as catheters, hypodermic syringes and needles and the various instruments are not sterile, these are boiled in a tightly covered container for 20 minutes. Sterile packages must not be laid open, or sterile equipment laid out, until just before they are to be used for the delivery.

In certain cases the nurse or nurse-midwife will find it necessary to manage the entire labor, either because of precipitate delivery or through delay in securing the services of a physician.

It is needless to say that labor in such cases progresses rapidly, and that almost before anything else can be done, the contractions are recurring with such frequency and severity that the mother must be put to bed and be given the undivided attention of the nurse. If time permits, much can be done for the comfort of the mother while preparations are made for delivery. Undoubtedly, the calmness of the nurse at the bedside will be transferred to the mother.

It seldom happens that the nurse and the patient are entirely alone; usually the father, a relative, or a friend in the home can be called upon to assist and bring the necessary things to the bedside. In an emergency, when there has been no previous preparation, an ordinary pair of scissors and pieces of clean, soft, white cord or tape may be boiled and used for tying and cutting the cord. As there is usually never any special hurry about tying and cutting the umbilical cord, there is time for scissors and tape to be boiled. Time may be saved by using only enough water to cover the instruments, but it must be sufficient to allow for evaporation. Also, anything which will float, such as the tape, should be weighted down with the scissors. The pan may be covered with a second pan, thus sterilizing both. (See the section on Emergency Delivery by the Nurse in Chapter 18.)

Bibliography

1. Disbrow, M. A., and Horn, B. M.: The impact of individual differences on maternity care. In J. P. Clauson, *et al* (eds.): *Maternity Nursing Today.* New York, McGraw-Hill Book Company, 1973, p. 148.
2. State of California, Department of Health. Birth Records 11/26/73.
3. Edwards, M. E.: Unattended home birth. *Am. J. Nurs.* 73:1332-1335, Aug. 1973.
4. Lang, R.: *Birth Book.* Ben Lomand, Ga., Genesis Press, 1972.
5. Home delivery—advance or retreat? *Briefs.* Maternity Center Association, Publication Office, New Jersey, Sept. 1973, pp. 104-108.
6. Edwards, *op. cit.*
7. LeBoyer, F.: *Birth Without Violence.* New York, Alfred A. Knopf, 1975.
8. American College of Nurse-Midwives: Articles of incorporation of American College of Nurse-Midwives. Amended April, 1969, New York, N.Y.
9. American College of Obstetricians and Gynecologists: Joint statement on maternity care. Approved by liaison group, October 2, 1970.
10. Bean, M. A.: The nurse-midwife at work. *Am. J. Nurs.* 71:949-952, May 1971.
11. Lubic, R. W.: Myths about nurse-midwifery. *Am. J. Nurs.* 74:268-269, Feb. 1974.
12. Crucial questions on nurse midwifery. *Family Practice News.* Dec. 1, 1973, p. 30.

Suggested Reading

BURNETT, J. E.: A physician-sponsored community nurse-midwife program. *Am. J. Ob-Gyn.* 40:719-723, Nov. 1972.

GOLDSMITH, S. B.: Obstetricians' attitudes towards nurse-midwives. *Am. J. Ob-Gyn.* 111:111-117, Sept. 1971.

HELLMAN, L. M.: Nurse-midwifery. *Annals New York Acad. Sci.* 156:896-902, Dec. 1969.

MAECK, J. V. S.: Obstetrician-midwife partnership in obstetric care. *Am. J. Ob-Gyn.* 37:314-319, Feb. 1971.

OBRIG, A. M.: A nurse-midwife in practice. *Am. J. Nurs.* 71:953-957, May 1971.

PETTY, C.: No more home deliveries! *RN* 35:42-55, Oct. 1972.

obstetrics during emergency

Commonalities of Disaster Situations /
Emergency Nursing in the Hospital /
Disaster Protection for Mothers and
Infants / Psychologic Reactions in
Emergency Situations

When any large-scale emergency arises, it is usually sudden and calls for immediate action, whether it is caused by hurricane, flood, fire or war. In the event of such catastrophe, babies are likely to be born rapidly, and many women may abort. When organized rescue work is hampered, it may fall to those who are in the immediate area to manage as best they can. The nurses in the area need to be able to assist with measures for the safety and the welfare of maternity patients and their newborn infants.

All nurses who have completed the basic course in maternity nursing are familiar with antepartal care, the conduct of labor and the immediate care of the newborn infant, but their preparation has been carried out, for the most part, in an organized environment (such as a hospital) where supplies, equipment and medical direction are available. It requires considerable imagination on the part of the nurse to conceive of an emergency situation in which she might be required to work without the availability of these facilities. Yet in any large-scale disaster, whole communities may be isolated and left to their own resources when telephone and radio communications are wrecked; roads may become impassable if they are inundated by water and blocked by debris, and an area may be without safe water, means of power and light and medical supplies.

Commonalities of disaster situations

It has been established that all disaster emergencies have certain similarities and differ only in scope, intensity, and effect. It has also been demonstrated that there are usually two kinds of people remaining, those who *need* help and those who *are able* to help. It is safe to assume that in any extreme, large-scale emergency, the medical-health requirements of the surviving population will lead to an unprecedented need for hospital space (improvised if necessary) and for skilled professionals to care for the ill and injured and to keep the well well.

In extreme disaster conditions nursing care is usually administered on an austere basis, but, whenever possible, in accordance with established medical principles designed to save life, prevent the spread of disease, alleviate suffering and promote recovery. If the emergency is dire but confined to an area, the resources and manpower of the unaffected regions can be brought to bear upon the situation, thus allowing all health care to proceed along the above lines. In the case of a thermonuclear holocaust involving a whole nation, then survival will depend upon self- and buddy-help, with only life-sustaining care provided by the necessarily limited resources which must be conserved for a prolonged period.

Every responsible practitioner will want to familiarize herself with basic emergency and disaster nursing techniques (see Suggested Reading). It is well to remember, however, that the required knowledge and skills for nursing under these conditions are essentially the same as those required in daily patient care; *only the priorities change*. Thus, treatment will be based on available personnel, drugs, supplies and equipment.

The organization of emergency nursing services in the hospital environment

Disaster strikes with little if any warning, and a hospital's emergency department must be prepared to face almost any situation. Definitions of disaster vary. Some disaster authorities define a major accident as having occurred when there are 50 or more living casualties. From a hospital's point of view, a disaster or emergency occurs when, with no warning, more casualties of varying severity arrive than the hospital is prepared or staffed to handle at that particular time.

With all the attendant noise, confusion, horror and tragedy of a disaster, there is no time to plan the management of mass casualties. Thus, planning must have been carried out beforehand and viable plans must be in readiness.

The following paragraphs provide an outline of one suggested plan that has proven successful.

The alert

When such facilities are available, the emergency or accident service usually has the responsibility for alerting the rest of the hospital; the message can be conveyed to the hospital telephone operator by some person designated as the alerting or casualty officer. Hospitals that do not have specific emergency room facilities per se can set aside some room that might serve this purpose. If the physical plant is such that this is impossible, these hospitals might act as "overflow" facilities for those casualties who are not so badly injured.

When the various wards of the hospital are alerted, the following information about the disaster needs to be given: the type of disaster, where and when it took place, the number of casualties involved and the nature of the injuries. The hospital's preparation for multiple injury cases from a plane crash, for instance, will differ from that required for a large number of burned patients or casualties suffering from smoke inhalation or exposure to cold.

The phased response

The casualty officer (person designated to give the alert) is responsible for deciding the level of response initially required by the hospital to cope with the disaster. For instance, a Phase 1 response might be designed to cope with an internal disaster affecting the hospital itself, such as fire, explosion, or bomb threat. A Phase 2 response might cope with a small number of casualties involving just the emergency room facilities. Finally, a Phase 3 response would alert and mobilize the entire hospital to deal with a classic disaster.[1]

The disaster chest

Once a disaster has been declared, the nurse or other health personnel in charge (and there should be a special person so designated) goes to the "disaster chest" which is easily identifiable and contains all the necessary documents and equipment for organizing the emergency service. Some item of identification, an armband, badge, and the like, must be available for the disaster officer to wear—this is appropriate also for any of her deputies—since many bottlenecks and disorganization is created by not being able to identify appropriate personnel in charge of activities. In addition to the identifying material, each box ought to contain a number of "action" cards which incorporate written information, advice and instruction for members of the nursing staff. Standard 5″ x 8″ cards can be used for basic instructions; for more complicated diagrams, larger cards may be necessary. These instructions need to be clear, short and unambiguous.[2]

The contents of the disaster chest are described below.[3] These chests and their contents are also suitable for transfer to the scene of a disaster (with suitable action cards) if it is advisable to give emergency treatment at the scene. Hospital and civil disaster officials caution against including drugs (particularly narcotics) in the disaster chest, even when it is to be used exclusively in the hospital, because they are subject to theft and deterioration. Arrangements can be made to assure that local physicians, hospitals, police and ambulance/rescue teams provide drugs at the disaster scene if the chest is to be transported there.

Basic Contents of a Disaster Chest

Applicator sticks	Matches, safety
Armbands, medical	Muslin, uncut
Bandages:	Pencils:
Adhesive	Indelible
Gauze roller,	Skin-marking,
Head	red and white
Muslin roller,	Pitchers, 2-quart
Triangular	Safety pins
Basins, emesis	Salt, table
Bedpans	Sanitary pads, binders
Blankets, disposable	or belts
(fireproof and	Scissors
waterproof)	Soaps:
Cotton, absorbent	Hand
Cups, paper	Tincture of green
Dressings:	soap
Tubular gauze	Soda, baking
4″ x 4″s and other	Splints, basswood
sizes	Swabs, alcohol
Eyepads, adult and	Tags, medical
child sizes	Tape, adhesive
Instrument sets	Tongue depressors
(4 hemostats,	Tourniquets
1 tissue forceps,	Toweling, paper
1 scissors)	Twine, balls of

Triage or casualty sorting

The process of casualty sorting in the saving of lives bears repeating here. The aim of this endeavor is to identify those casualties whose lives can be saved by the early application of medical skills and resuscitation procedures and to concentrate available medical and nursing resources on these people. An experienced physician is appointed as triage officer and as each casualty is brought in, he is rapidly assessed and assigned one of the following priorities: Priority 1: these individuals can easily die and may need blood transfusions, plasma infusions for burns or surgery soon to close cavity wounds. Laboring women, especially if wounded, are assigned to this category and the delivery as well as treatment of injuries is given first priority. Priority 2: these casualties are unlikely to die immediately or soon from the injuries sustained. Pregnant women who are not in labor may be given this priority unless they are wounded or some complication is anticipated. Priority 3: these persons are obviously dying from the injuries sustained.

It has been suggested that Priority 2 patients be given first aid, and then be left in the care of first aiders until more help can be given. After Priority 1 casualties have been attended to and when resources permit, attention can then be redirected to those with a 2 classification. Those who are dying need to be offered comfort and compassion by auxiliary personnel but not by medical and nursing personnel, whose efforts need to be directed toward saving the lives of those who can be helped.[4]

Primary treatment areas

Several kinds of facilities are needed; they may have to be improvised. The *resuscitation rooms* must be close to the ambulance entrance and suitably equipped so that hemorrhage can be controlled, airways established by tracheostomy if necessary and fractures supported and stabilized. Once the patient has been resuscitated, he can be reassessed and moved to another treatment area as quickly as possible.

In the *urgent treatment area*, wounds are covered, splints applied, shock treated and patients prepared for later care. Operation priorities are made before the patients leave this area. In the *nonurgent treatment area* which may include the *ambulatory casualty area*, patients are received for care of minor wounds, burns and simple fractures. Special provision is made for those with minimal or no injuries who are suffering from the effects of emotional shock. If a woman is near term and/or having any cramping or spotting or appears to be in labor, she may be held in the ambulatory area until further assessment can be made.

It is recommended that two registered nurses staff each of these areas, one of whom has some experience with disaster nursing. In addition, two nurses need to help the triage officer, while the casualty officer supervises the total operation. Nursing auxiliary personnel and/or volunteers can escort patients to other parts of the hospital.[5]

Some communities have instituted a mobile Disaster Nurse Corps whose members go to the scene of a disaster and carry out most of the procedures described above. Working with physicians and other paramedical personnel, they are able to render life-saving care to many victims whose injuries would have been compounded by improper handling.[6]

Disaster protection for mothers and infants

Insuring the lives and health of pregnant women and their newborn during national or extensive local disasters requires planning for this purpose predicated on the belief that plans and preparations prior to these events are essential and imperative.

In planning for the safeguarding of mothers and newborn infants prior to a disaster, certain assumptions can be made and specific factors considered:

Pregnant women will be subject to all of the risks and injuries to which men and nonpregnant women will be exposed. Their general care needs to be in accordance with provisions made for the population at large. However, their obstetric care does require additional planning and facilities, for it should be separate from hospital and emergency facilities for casualties if possible. Two lives are at stake, lives of particular import to the future of the country. The need for care of the pregnant woman is predictable, since sooner or later she must inevitably be delivered, and in the process will need medical attention to a greater or lesser extent. In the vast majority of instances, probably in 90 percent of all cases, the birth process, whether it results in a viable infant or abortion, will be essentially uncomplicated. The most formidable complications to be encountered with any frequency will be hemorrhage, obstructed or prolonged labor, infection, mild and severe toxemias of pregnancy with convulsions and miscellaneous medical and surgical conditions accompanying pregnancy.

It is estimated that at any given time approximately 2 percent of the total population will consist of women in various stages of pregnancy. In applying this prevalence rate to a given geographic area, allowance must be made for the character of the area, since the rate will, of course, be affected by the presence of large industrial plants and offices employing large numbers of males.

If the foregoing concepts are accepted and remain valid in disaster planning, what then should be the planning for minimal essential care for mothers and newborn infants in disaster situations? To the extent that it is possible, the facilities which are normally available for pregnant women during the antepartal, delivery and postpartal periods should be available.

However, we have learned from experience that in the event of large-scale catastrophes such as tornados, hurricanes, floods, or bombing, these facilities may not be functioning. Therefore adequate preparation for the care of mothers and babies during a disaster, particularly a large-scale one, requires that thought be given and plans made for the training of families for their own protection and survival. This is especially true for the pregnant woman and her family. Thus, a large percentage of the population needs to be trained to carry out minimal essentials of care (buddy system) to save the lives of other people.

As we have said, it can be assumed that in any major disaster, physicians, nurses and other specially trained professional personnel will be almost completely absorbed in the task of caring for casualties; normal women in labor at such times will have to rely largely on nonprofessional personnel for their needs. Just who will these nonprofessional people be? They will have to be other women who have received instruction in the procedures described. In other words, each community must contain a corps of laywomen who understand the basic concepts contained in this brief review and have been given at least minimal training in providing this type of care. Preparation for disaster is a family affair. Every citizen and every family need to have the information necessary to protect the individual, the family, and the community well in advance of a disaster or an enemy attack. Those responsible for planning and implementing disaster plans have the unique responsibility for making this information available to individuals in communities in a way which they can understand and accept.

The only hope we have for the saving of lives of mothers and newborn infants depends on the family's ability to carry out the plans made with and for them.

Every expectant mother needs to know her physician's expectation of the kind of delivery she will have, so that if she needs any special facilities, she will be able to go where these are available. She needs to understand the care she and her baby will need during delivery and immediately afterward.

There are differences of opinion about how much information pregnant women should have about their own condition and the conduct and the outcome of the delivery. It is assumed that in the event of large-scale disasters, women will have to carry much of the responsibility for their own safety. Therefore, adequate information about what to do, where to go and what constitutes essential equipment will be comforting to them rather than alarming.

Essential equipment is quite minimal and is available to almost every woman in her own home. A package should be made up and kept accessible with other emergency supplies if the area is disaster prone. Contents include a clean sheet, towels, washcloth and soap; blankets, clothing, a nipple and a bottle for the baby; a pair of blunt scissors; 2 pieces of clean linen tape, 6 inches long and ¼ inch wide, wrapped separately from the other articles, and a package of powdered milk for the mother. A can of powdered infant formula is also good insurance in the event that the establishment of lactation is delayed.

Those who are giving care to pregnant women need to understand that the pregnant woman's normal dependent needs may be greatly enhanced by separation from and concern for her husband and family and by increased fear for herself and her baby. Understanding in meeting this exaggerated need for mothering and providing a warm accepting environment will increase the confidence of the pregnant woman in her ability to have her baby and will comfort her and relieve some of her fear and apprehension. Every effort needs to be made to have someone with the patient throughout labor. The emotional support which patients in labor (who have had some preparation) derive from each other should be utilized.

There are certain preparations for impending labor and/or abortion that can be made in the immediate period of evacuation. As quickly as possible after a shelter, Field Aid Point or First Aid Station is occupied, all pregnant women should be registered and the expected date of birth recorded. As we stated previously, the nurse may be the only health professional on the scene; in that event she may want to delegate this activity to someone who appears able to carry through this activity *accurately*. The pregnant women who will be of special concern are 1) those who are in labor or expecting at any time, 2) those who are expecting within a week or two, and 3) those who have had difficulty with previous confinements and/or who have reason to expect difficulty by reason of disease or abnormalities. *They should be apprised of these facts by their physician.*

The nurse can assign someone to assist the laboring mother. In all probability, the nurse will be too occupied with other activities to assist herself if she is the only health professional. The attendant is to be informed of the expected date of birth and any information which the mother may have learned during her prenatal care. In addition, the nurse will need to instruct the attendant in the course of labor and the activities necessary at the time of birth. A delivery area can be selected away from the general living or gathering area if space permits. It should be prepared with respect to quiet, warmth (or coolness), cleanliness, available supplies and equipment. The mother will need a clean surface to lie on for the actual delivery. Clean plastic material and/or paper can be used for padding the actual delivery bed. The mother will need clean towels or a clean garment or sheet. A warmer covering such as a sweater, jacket or blanket is also desirable. Hopefully, she will have brought these articles for the baby with her. The infant's crib can be improvised from a carton and lined with any suitable material (paper or a blanket) available. It goes without saying that the mother's confidence may be temporarily shattered; her courage may not be, however. If the nurse can convey that while conditions may be very austere, labor and delivery can progress normally, she will do much toward helping the mother mobilize her resources to proceed through labor. The nurse will instruct the mother or attendant to report the first evidence of the onset of labor. This will usually give enough time to make the immediate preparations for delivery.

Essentials of care during the first stage of labor include the maintenance of physical and emotional reserves, the interpretation of the progress of labor to the patient and the family, the provision of rest and fluids, the maintenance of cleanliness, and the preparation for the second stage of labor, including frequent emptying of the bladder.

There needs to be constant review of progress and observation of signs of complications. As the patient approaches the completion of the first stage of labor, she will need special care and encouragement and should not be left alone.

During the second stage of labor, constant observation, encouragement and interpretation are all-important. A clean delivery area needs to be maintained, and there should be continual observation of the patient's general condition for signs of exhaustion and other complications. The maternal pulse rate and the quality should be observed.

A progress report to the supervising physician or nurse can be made by the person giving the care. In the absence of the physician during the delivery, the nurse, the nurse-midwife or the attendant who is helping the patient can teach her that when the baby's head is in sight to take a deep breath at the beginning of each contraction, to hold her breath and exert downward pressure, while the infant's head is controlled. As soon as the contraction is over, the patient can be encouraged to relax completely and wait for the next contraction.

Supportive care is especially important. The back can be rubbed for low back pain and the legs stretched for muscle cramps. The explanation of the progress of labor often provides the encouragement which the patient needs to complete the second stage of labor with minimal emotional stress.

When the head crowns, the perineum should be supported and protected with a clean towel if a sterile towel is not available. If there is no clean material for this purpose, it is important that the attendant be instructed *not to touch the birth canal or surrounding area of the perineum. Moreover, the mother must be instructed to keep her hands away from these areas also.* If clean material is available and the *attendant has had some professional training,* then gentle pressure can be applied against the head as it emerges to prevent too rapid delivery of the head. If the attendant is not skilled and/or seems to be rather overwhelmed by events, it is wiser to allow the infant's head to deliver spontaneously and simply support it as it is born.

Immediate removal of the membranes from around the baby's head is important. If the umbilical cord is around the neck, it is slipped over the head whenever this can be done easily. The mucus should be wiped from the baby's mouth and nose. Occasionally, spontaneous rotation of the head to one side or the other will not take place within a reasonable period of time. Under such circumstances, gentle rotation of the head in the direction toward which it tends to go more easily will suffice to bring one shoulder anteriorly behind the symphysis.

If the nurse is delivering the infant, she can next deliver the anterior shoulder by gently grasping the head in both hands, and exerting gentle but steady pressure toward the floor. With this maneuver, the anterior shoulder slips under the symphysis pubis, and the upper portion of the arm can be seen. Then the direction of traction is reversed upward in order to deliver the posterior shoulder over the perineum. These maneuvers are to be carried out *slowly and carefully*; there is no need to hurry.

The baby's body is supported as it is born and is wrapped in a warm sterile towel or clean cloth and placed on the mother's abdomen with the head lower so that the mucus will drain out. Pulling on the cord is avoided. The mother will want to know about the baby and see it as soon as it is born. If the baby does not cry immediately, or if there is mucus, the nose and the mouth should be cleared and postural drainage instituted. Gentle rubbing of the back helps to stimulate the baby's breathing. When the cord stops pulsating, it is tied in two places and cut between the two ties. After the cord is cut, the baby is warmly wrapped and placed in the mother's arms.

During the delivery of the baby and the beginning of the third stage of labor there should be constant observation of the mother's general condition and of signs indicating the separation of the placenta. If the attendant assisting with the delivery places her hand on the mother's fundus, she can report the changes to the person conducting the delivery. When the uterus rises upward in the abdomen and becomes globular and firm, and the umbilical cord extends 3 or 4 inches out of the vagina and there is a gush of blood, the patient can be asked to bear down with the next contraction. This pressure is usually sufficient to expel the placenta, which is received in a clean receptacle. In order to express the placenta, it may be necessary occasionally to apply gentle pressure on the fundus of the uterus when it is well contracted. The direction of pressure should be toward the vaginal outlet. Following the expulsion of the placenta, if the uterus tends to become soft, and bleeding occurs, the uterus should be massaged vigorously with the fingertips to promote uterine contraction, and the baby put to the breast.

The placenta and membranes should be examined to determine whether there are any missing portions.

If the uterus remains small and firm, nothing need be done other than to keep the hand on the fundus for one hour following the delivery of the baby. The patient is made comfortable, given nourishment, encouraged to void and allowed to rest.

The attendant rewashes her hands before beginning care of the infant. When it is apparent that the mother can be left safely, the baby is to be identified according to the method established by the particular health department. If the usual identification tapes or bands are not available, some method is to be improvised. The infant need not be washed for 24 hours, and can wait even longer if water is in short supply. The vernix caseosa may seem unpleasant but will protect the infant much more than unclean "cleansing" materials. Baby oil can be used as a substitute for water and mild soap after 24 hours. The cord stump is to be kept clean and, if at all possible, a sterile dressing is to be applied and left in place until the cord dries. The infant is to be examined for injuries and malformations.

Essentials of nursing care for the baby include gentle handling, observation of breathing, color, appearance, activity, skin and body temperature, stools, weight (if possible), and umbilical cord for bleeding and healing; provision needs to be made for warmth, proper food and protection from infection.

Mother and newborn baby can be considered an inseparable unit. If a mother cannot take care of her baby, full-time mothering care must be provided to enhance the baby's chances of survival and promote his well-being. Irregularities in breathing, mucus in air passages, weak sucking reflex, skin irritation and unstable temperature-regulating mechanism point to the importance of constant observation and an environment adapted to meet the needs of the individual infant.

Breast-feeding is preferable. The infant may be put to breast immediately after birth and at two- to four-hour intervals for three- to five-minute periods until the milk supply is established. If this regime tires the mother, the intervals between nursing periods can be lengthened. Once the milk supply is sufficient to satisfy the baby, feedings can be given as often as necessary to meet the need. Artificial feedings may be necessary until the mother's milk supply is adequate or in instances in which the mother is unable to nurse. Formula may be prepared from powdered infant formula or dried skim milk immediately prior to feeding since there will be no refrigeration facilities. Diluted canned evaporated milk is also a suitable formula. (One part milk to two parts water, boiled if possible.) If a bottle and nipple are unavailable, the baby can suck on a teaspoon placed on his lower lip, or milk can be dropped on the inside of the cheek with a medicine dropper. The formula does not have to be heated. Disposable diapers are preferred, but sheets substitute nicely. Of course, any absorbent material can be used if these are not available.

The newborn is particularly susceptible to infection. Anyone with any evidence of infection, such as rash, diarrhea or upper respiratory infection, should not give infant care.

When the infant is found to be premature and in need of special care, or to have congenital malformations, the emergency facilities which have been developed for such conditions can be utilized.

When the mother and infant are to be discharged from the place where care has been given during labor and delivery, it is important for arrangements to be made with the family and others for the mother to be relieved of responsibilities except the care of her baby and herself, if possible. The mother, the family and the attendant should know where and whom to call if she or the baby have any conditions or symptoms needing medical care.

To increase the number of people with some training in the care of pregnant women and newborn infants, the existing educational programs need to be expanded. These include mother and baby care classes, such as those given by the Red Cross and other health agencies, parent education groups, home nursing classes, first-aid training, classes for baby sitters and junior and senior high school students, and midwifery training programs. Planning for training and the achievement of the training of persons who carry this responsibility in a disaster are not easy.

During a disaster, it is assumed that it will be the responsibility of nurses, certified nurse-midwives and licensed nonprofessional midwives to carry on an intensive program of on-the-job training of whoever is available to help and to supervise the care of mothers and babies.[7]

Psychologic reactions in emergency situations

It has been found that human behavior in disaster, like human behavior in other life situations, falls into fairly predictable patterns. Since the nurse's role is so vital in the event of disaster, she will need to prepare herself with knowledge of these reactions, since coping with large numbers of persons suffering massive emotional shock will become every bit as important as rendering help for physical trauma and illness. Moreover, it will help the nurse to better understand her own responses to the catastrophe.

Periods of a disaster

For purposes of our analysis disaster can be said to have various periods. These may include a prodromal or warning period, an impact period, an immediate reaction period, and finally, a delayed response period. During these segments there are characteristic modes of behavior that people may exhibit.

In the *prodromal or warning period* certain persons tend to demonstrate disorganized and/or destructive behavior. They mill around, disobey instructions, break things or lash out at anyone getting in their way. Some others, however, are able to function in the face of even grave personal danger incredibly effectively; still others become immobilized and, for all practical purposes, helpless.

Some of the above individuals may respond to the warning signals as if the catastrophe had already occurred and demonstrate a penchant for ineffective action. These persons fall into two general groups. The first are those who have been through a similar experience before in which they were helpless and have developed a subsequent fear and/or helpless response to disaster or its warnings. The second group comprises those who always become helpless in any dangerous or frightening situation. These persons often present a difficult problem for helping personnel since, if left to themselves, these people often precipitate wild panic in others because of their own panicky behavior. They need to be taken aside and given definite tasks to do, no matter how simple. Clear, brief instructions and frequent reassurance help these people to regain control of their emotions.

At the *impact period*, almost everyone will experience many frightening feelings, no matter how adequate the training or drilling; thus, there will be at least some period of confusion. This is especially true in the case of an emergency in which there is no warning, such as a dam breaking, a sudden explosion or an electrical storm. Many respond with physical signs and symptoms. They may exhibit shortness of breath, rapid pulse and respiration, trembling, sweating, and so on. Adequate anticipatory training and drilling have been found to shorten the period of this uncontrolled activity, thus reducing the confusion period.

The *immediate reaction period* after impact is most crucial. Noneffective behavior at this point exacts a heavy toll in terms of the lives and well-being of the survivors. On the other hand, effective action will save lives, diminish disability, reduce abnormal behavior, and decrease the confusion immeasurably. It is imperative that normal behavior be resumed as quickly as possible, not only for each individual's personal safety but also to assure help for those unable to act because of an injury.

Immediately following impact, especially in a disaster of any magnitude, almost all persons will be unable to think, move or express concern, although given a reasonable length of time, most will make a tremendous effort to adjust. Some will manage this more quickly than others, and they will have to help their slower brethren in their adjustments. Help usually will be available from the relatively uninjured since professionals are often not available as we have stressed. Thus, it is wise for the less able to team with those who appear more able —the buddy system is more effective and often invaluable.

The *delayed response period* begins when the immediate danger has passed. Groups often unite for mutual protection and it is at this period that the less acutely affected psychologic casualties can be salvaged. It is important to remember that minimal attention may be all that is needed, but it *must be given* and *given early* in this period. Those afflicted are often highly suggestible, and will follow almost any advice or take cues for action from the behavior of others. This can be a double-edged sword, for while they respond well to instructions and reassurance, they also tend to become infected easily with anxiety and panic, and will, in turn, precipitate panic reactions in others if not carefully watched. It is important at this time for all to realize that the menace has passed; thus, verbal reinforcement and reiteration are important. Valuable information can also be conveyed by signs and facial expressions to aid individuals in achieving some measure of security.

Types of behavior

We have spoken of the different periods in a disaster and of some of the general behavior that might be exhibited. It would be well at this point to expand on the various types of behavior that can be demonstrated in response to danger or threat in general.

Under the heading of "normal reactions" comes apparent calmness, at least for a time. More usually seen, however, are physical or bodily manifestations such as sweating, trembling, weakness or rapid pulse. Included here also are nausea, vomiting and diarrhea of a temporary nature. Confusion, crying and immobilization of a short duration are not uncommon and can still be classified as "normal." The ability and the length of time required to collect oneself with or without help seem to be the most likely criteria for classification in the "normal" category.

When the above reactions become prolonged and/or incapacitating, the individual condition is thought of as more serious. "Conversion hysteria" can occur in which the person unconsciously converts his massive fear into a belief that some part of his body has ceased to function. And in fact, the organ does not function in spite of the fact that no organic damage can be demonstrated. These people cannot be treated as malingerers or "fakers." Since the disability is at the level of the unconscious, the person is as truly disabled as if he had had physical injury to the limb or organ. Nausea and vomiting arising from emotional origins are also seen in prolonged and incapacitating cases. Difficulty arises in diagnosis since these symptoms are indicative of radiation sickness also. Moreover, the person may interpret his symptoms as due to radiation exposure. Problems of isolation and decontamination multiply. These cases tax both the diagnostic astuteness and the emotional reserve of those dealing with them.

Somewhere between the normal reactions and the gross abnormal reactions fall panic and depressed and overactive responses. Panic is not expressed as frequently as one might expect, but its danger lies in its contagiousness. It can spread and cause a mass headlong flight of a crowd. Driven by a compulsion to flee, persons in the grip of this phenomenon often crush and trample one another. Purposeless uncontrolled motor behavior is indicative of a panic stage; it is evidenced by such behavior as uncontrolled weeping and running around. Sheer horror (the sight of family maimed) or the belief that avenues of escape are being blocked are the two most frequent precipitating conditions. Helping to move individuals and a crowd away from the presenting danger *in an orderly fashion* is the best preventive for this phenomenon.

Depressed reactions are characterized by a general slowing down of motor and mental processes. Persons sit and stare; they seem numb and confused. They do not respond when spoken to or if they do, it is with monosyllables. These individuals cannot initiate action even to escape threat. Fortunately they can be salvaged if help can be given to get them moving before too long a period. Other victims respond with a flurry of overactive responses. They will chatter ceaselessly about inappropriate topics, they run back and forth and are avid rumor spreaders. If given a task, they are soon off doing something else, although to their minds, they have completed it to perfection. An unreal confidence in their abilities is their hallmark. This causes them to assume more responsibility than they can possibly discharge and to become very intolerant of other ideas or plans. They are especially troublesome to those who are demonstrating effective leadership.

It is not possible to present a blueprint for dealing with these situations and behavior. There are some principles of behavior, however, that the nurse can utilize and which can be conveyed easily to those who will help her. First of all, she should try to accept *each person's right to his own feelings*. A quick appraisal of one's own feelings at this time makes one realize how difficult it is to make a conscious choice of one's deeper feelings. An ability to make a conscious choice depends upon what we do about our feelings to relieve the tensions they create within us. Nothing is gained by trying to deny the existence of the distressed feelings in ourselves or others, simply because they appear different from what we would ordinarily expect or experience in everyday life. If we can help someone to take appropriate action, the distressed feelings may change, either quickly or gradually. Each person brings to the disaster a varied experiential background which contributes greatly to his coping with the effects of the disaster. Letting a person know that you understand *how he feels at the moment* will be the first step toward helping him. As with any patient, pity will overwhelm him; if the nurse can convey by gesture or short conversation that she is trying to see the events through his eyes, she will be helping him to find constructive outlets for his feelings and thereby aid him in rehabilitation.

A second principle involves *accepting a person's limitations*. If a person is obviously physically shattered, one does not expect him to carry on as usual. Yet, when the nurse finds herself tired, frustrated and trying to maintain her own emotional equilibrium, she is apt to resent enormously the vague "unseen" disabilities of others. This is, perhaps an understatement, for the feeling of irritability will be enhanced because others will seem to have "pulled themselves together" considering the circumstances. Again these patients, for they are patients, need understanding and patience —not resentment—because they too are laboring under a great load.

A third principle involves the *ability to assess accurately and quickly the capabilities of others*. A very upset person can easily cause the nurse to forget that he can be of real assistance; therefore it is wise to be on the lookout for skills and other assets that might be revived and utilized. The nurse can begin to help the patient reorganize his world by inquiring into what has happened to him and letting him reply in his own way. Allowing him to talk of his experiences (without letting him ramble on and/or become more upset) will greatly relieve some of his feelings of despair and helplessness. The nurse can explore briefly his concern about his family and friends, giving him an honest estimate regarding the possibility of his reestablishing contact with his dear ones. If he is too depressed to talk freely, she can talk to him about what may have happened to him and to them. This may increase his confidence in the nurse to the point where he can make conversation. Brief questions regarding his occupation will give clues to his interests and basic capabilities. The nurse can then draw conclusions as to how he can best be utilized. While this may sound exploitive, keeping someone gainfully occupied is a genuine therapeutic coup. Treating someone as a potentially valued member of the disaster team will increase his effectiveness immeasurably.

Finally, the last but perhaps the most important principle: try to *accept your own limitations in the relief role*. We have stressed the responsibility of the nurse's role to herself and others, perhaps to the detriment of the real limitations in herself that the nurse will encounter. There will be much that the nurse will want to do in a disaster; some things,

however, will be beyond her strength and skill. Thus, the nurse will need to establish a set of priorities, not only with respect to what she must do for patient care but what she must undertake in the realm of responsibility generally. The first priority is to whatever emergency job that she has been assigned (or has volunteered for). In practice this job may well be more than full-time; therefore the nurse must select those activities which will be worth trying and those which would be a waste of time. While she will be pushing herself to the limits of her capacity, it is imperative that she not extend herself beyond those limits lest she become as ill as those whom she treats. If pushing herself beyond endurance is a personality characteristic, then it is wise that she acknowledge it early and pace herself accordingly. A reasonable candid self-appraisal is an important prerequisite for anyone attempting psychologic first aid! If one is to deal effectively with others, then one's own concerns must be dealt with *first and promptly*. If they are, the nurse will be less likely to become bogged down when she is trying to aid others. No matter how thorough the nurse's training has been, it is important that she recognize that she will not be immune to all personal disturbance if her community is torn apart by a terrible tragedy. Her first psychologic job then is to look to her own defense. If she understands herself reasonably well, she may justifiably hope to endure and control her own anxieties in the midst of a community-wide disaster and render excellent assistance to those who need her.[8]

Reactions of nurses to disaster situations

Research has indicated that while nurses may experience a great deal of anxiety and stress in a disaster while ministering to patients, this does not apparently interfere with effective performance.[9,10] Causes of greatest stress for the nurse appear to be the excessive physical demands made on her and concern for her own safety. Next most stressful is concern about supplies—either because supplies are inadequate or because they cannot be replenished. Other concerns include worry about one's own family, disorganization, and concern for those who have lost their home and all their possessions.

Excerpts from interviews are instructive.

PHYSICAL DEMANDS:

We had to walk up several flights of stairs, back and forth, up and down, for anything we needed (no elevators because of power loss). We carried water up the stairs. We helped carry trays up.

The hardest thing was having to move all the patients out into the halls, from both sides of the hall. It was hard physical work because we had all the windows shut and there was no air-conditioning and it was very hot.

Evacuating the patients from the top floors was the hardest. We couldn't use the elevator, just had to carry them down the stairs, two and three flights.[11]

CONCERN FOR SAFETY:

I think, trying to safeguard the patients during the worst part of the hurricane, when it just looked like the walls were going to come down.

I heard that all the windows had blown in and I tried so desperately to get over there. Some men forced open the hall door so I could go down the stairwell and I was kind of sorry after I got in the stairwell, because I was in there by myself and I have never felt such pressure in my life. I felt as though my ears would burst.

I was worried and concerned because I had a patient on a Stryker frame that I couldn't take down the stairs. Finally, the engineers took her down the elevator by hand-pulling the ropes. Seemed like it was 30 minutes just to come down from the sixth to the third floor.

Safety of the patients and myself. I was really frightened. Of course, I tried to control my feelings. I couldn't let the patients see that I was frightened and really think I would have been more frightened if I had not had so much to do. In trying to see to the patients' care and trying to keep them calm and protected from the flying debris, the flying gravel, rocks, and glass, and protect them from the slamming doors, I just didn't have time to be as afraid as possibly I should have because it was real, real bad.[12]

OTHER CONCERNS:

I didn't know what was happening to my family; well, that was the most stressful thing. I didn't know until three o'clock the next day, except I knew they weren't dead because there weren't that many people killed. I felt like they weren't.

I was mainly concerned about the children. So many were hurt by broken glass.

I think what really got me most was the people with large families that had small children. Small children that didn't even have a place to lie down or rest, and not a change of clothes, and no food. One lady with six or eight children came in and I asked her what I could do for her. She said, "Oh, I'm not too concerned about myself right now; I am more concerned about my children, and if I could just get a bottle of water for my children and for my baby."[13]

These quotes illustrate that the nurse is, indeed, human and vulnerable. As we have said previously, however, if she understands herself reasonably well, she will be able to cope when a disaster occurs and render excellent assistance to those who are in need of her services.

Bibliography

1. Hirst, W., and Savage, P.: Disaster planning. *Nurs. Times* 70:186-189, Feb. 1974.
2. *Ibid.*
3. Zanotelli, P.: Civil disasters? These nurses are ready. *RN* 34:50-52, September 1971.
4. ———: Major disasters and plans to deal with them. *Nurs. Mirror* 130:40-41, June 28, 1974.
5. Hirst, and Savage, *op. cit.*
6. Zanotelli, *op. cit.*
7. Fetter, S. E., *et al: Bull. Mat. Welfare* 49:9, 1957.
8. ———: The psychology of disaster. *Nurs. Clin. North Am.* 2:349-358, June 1967.
9. Rayner, J.: How do nurses behave in disaster? *Nurs. Outlook* 6:572-576, Oct. 1956.
10. Laub, J.: Psychological reactions of nurses in disaster. *Nurs. Research* 22:343-347, Jul./Aug. 1973.
11. *Ibid.*, p. 345.
12. *Ibid.*
13. *Ibid.*

Suggested Reading

ARANOW, S., *et al: The Fallen Sky, Medical Consequences of Thermonuclear War.* New York, Hill and Wang, 1963.

BLAKELY, J.: *The Care of Radiation Casualties.* London, William Heinemann Medical Books, 1968.

EDE, L., *et al: Emergency care and the nurse. *Nurs. Care* 6:23-27, Sept. 1973.

———: Major disasters and plans to deal with them. *Nurs. Mirror* 130:40-41, June 28, 1974.

EICHERLY, E. E.: Nursing in thermonuclear disaster. *Nurs. Clin. North Am.* 2:325-335, June 1967.

EMERGENCY HEALTH PROGRAMS. *J. S. Carolina Med. Assoc.* 65:23-24, Jan. 1969.

MELBER, R.: The nurse's role in obstetrical emergencies in the hospital setting. *Nurs. Clin. North Am.* 2:261-269, June 1967.

PSYCHOLOGY OF DISASTER. *Nurs. Clin. North Am.* 2:349-358, June 1967.

history of maternity nursing

32

Obstetrics Over the Centuries /
Background and Development of Maternal
and Infant Care in the United States /
The Emergence and Development of
Maternity Nursing / Future Possibilities

Obstetrics over the centuries

The bearing of children is an event of enormous social significance, and has certain symbolic meanings for all peoples. Traditions, rites, and practices have been developed surrounding this event to encourage positive outcomes for the individual and society. Roles for attendants during the reproductive process are formalized in one way or another, and differ greatly among cultures. Involvement of the sciences in childbearing grew gradually through the ages, but continued to be interwoven with folk beliefs and customs. Even today, alternate approaches to childbearing are practiced by certain groups in highly scientific, Western cultures. In the less developed countries, ancient folk practices continue to prevail in the care provided during pregnancy, delivery, and postpartum.

This account of the history of obstetrics is a brief outline of the major stages in the development of medical involvement in care during the reproductive process. The student may obtain more complete information from sources listed in Suggested Reading.

Obstetrics among primitive peoples

We know little about obstetrics among the primitive races, but from careful study of the customs of the aboriginal American Indians and the African peoples, we are able to learn some of the customs which were part of the obstetric practice of the ancients. Childbirth in primitive times was a relatively simple process. The mother retired to a place apart from the tribe and there gave birth to her child without great difficulty. It is known that intertribal marriages were relatively rare; therefore, there was not the conglomeration of mingled races which exists today. A realization of this fact alone makes possible an understanding of the relative simplicity of childbirth under these circumstances. The fetal head and body were accommodated satisfactorily within the anatomic range of the maternal pelvis. The lack of mixed marriages prevented the resultant disproportion between passenger and pelvic passages. It became customary for women who had attended other women in labor to be asked to assist or accompany more of them, and they became the primitive counterpart of our latter-day midwife. The only real danger a primitive mother faced was that of abnormal presentation, which usually terminated fatally for both mother and child. Toxemias and other complications are largely the products of more advanced civilization and were rarely if ever met among primitive peoples.

Egyptian obstetrics

In Egypt a highly organized state of society existed, and with it there arose a more complicated, if not more advanced, type of obstetrics. The priesthood in Egypt was interested in all the activities of society, and obstetrics was not neglected. They had a supervisory interest in it and took an active part in the care of abnormal or operative cases. They are known to have had obstetric forceps, to have performed cesarean sections on dead mothers, and podalic version was a part of their art.

Oriental obstetrics

Hindu medicine was probably the first authentic system of medicine to be given to the world. Among the earliest Hindus of whom there is written record was Susrata, one of the most prolific of Hindu writers. The exact date of his existence is still a matter of dispute, but he is variously stated to have worked and written between 600 B.C. and A.D. 500, more probably about the latter date. His knowledge of menstruation and gestation was quite modern. He knew and described intelligently the management of normal and abnormal labor. He described the use of forceps and cesarean section upon dead mothers to remove living children, and gave excellent antepartal and postpartal advice. He advised cleanliness on the part of the obstetrician; cutting the beard, the hair, and the nails closely; the wearing of clean gowns; and thorough disinfection of the operating rooms prior to operation or delivery. His surgical antiseptic technique seems remarkable to modern students.

Chinese obstetrics was largely of a legendary nature until the publication of a Chinese household manual of obstetrics, *Ta Sheng P'Ien*, which, according to the author's own statement, "is correct and needs no change or addition of prescription." There were monographs on obstetrics prior to this, but none so complete. Many of his statements are unfounded; in fact, the knowledge is scanty or incorrect, but the author had the saving grace of objecting to unnecessary interference and counseled patience in the treatment of labor. He had a poor opinion of midwives in general, stating that "the majority of them are fools." The reviews of Chinese obstetrics and obstetric drugs by Maxwell are excellent and give a detailed account of an interesting phase of obstetrics, which for lack of space we are forced to dispense with in this account.

Grecian obstetrics

Prior to Hippocrates, the Asclepiads, or followers of Aesculapius, the father of medicine, had a slight and largely supervisory interest in obstetrics. Abortions were not illegal. There is little definite knowledge concerning this period, but it seems probable that obstetric treatment was of a primitive nature.

The Hippocratic Period. During this age normal obstetric cases were handled by midwives under the supervision of the physicians. Abnormal labor was entirely in the hands of the medical profession. To Hippocrates is accredited the Hippocratic oath, which is still a part of the exercises for all students graduating from medical school. Treatises upon obstetrics attributed to Hippocrates are the oldest records available of the Western world's obstetric methods.

Greco-Roman Obstetrics. This period was one of progress, which was due largely to the work of Celsus, Aëtius, and Soranus (second century). The last reintroduced podalic version and is responsible for the first authentic records of its use in the delivery of living children. He gave an excellent technical description of the procedure and the indications for its use.

Byzantine, Mohammedan, Jewish and medieval periods

These periods may be said to have been characterized by a complete absence of progress, and as a corollary, a retrogression and loss of previously known practice resulted. This was due in large part to the general failure of science in the medieval period, but the interference of the Roman Church in secular matters, particularly those of a scientific nature, must be held responsible for a large share of it. The paucity of operative treatment in difficult labor may be judged from the recommendations contained in the only textbook of the day on obstetrics and gynecology, which read as follows: "Place the patient in a sheet held at the corners by four strong men, with her head somewhat elevated. Have them shake the sheet vigorously by pulling on the opposite corners, and with God's aid she will give birth." However, hospitals and nursing services were organized in this age.

Although the ancient Jews gave very little assistance to the woman during labor and delivery, they were interested in the hygiene of pregnancy and cleanliness at the time of childbirth. Hygiene and sanitation were apparently a part of their religion. At the time of difficult deliveries, the women "were comforted until they died." The stool or obstetric chair was used at this time and continued to be used until about the 19th century A.D. Reference is made to this chair in the Bible, in the first chapter of Exodus, "when you do the office of the midwife to the Hebrew women, and see them upon the stools. . . ."

The renaissance period

The Renaissance was characterized by advances in medicine and obstetrics commensurate with those in other fields. During this time appeared the first English text on obstetrics, the *Byrthe of Mankynde*, published by Raynalde. Both it and its German counterpart by Roesslin are copies of Soranus, and with their publication podalic version was reintroduced to obstetric practice. Many famous men were responsible for the progress in obstetrics—among them Leonardo da Vinci (who made the first accurate sketches of the fetus in utero) and Vesalius (who accurately described the pelvis for the first time).

To Ambrose Paré, the dean of French surgeons and obstetricians, must go the chief credit for making podalic version a useful and practicable procedure. Due to his skill, he preferred its use to cesarean section in difficult labor. By his careful studies of its indications and technique, he made possible the removal of obstetrics from the hands of the midwives, where it had rested since the fall of the Roman Empire, and its establishment as an independent branch of medicine. Regulations were enacted for the practice of midwives, and schools were established during this period for their training. Paré's work on version and his discouragement of cesarean section were opportune.

Sections had been practiced since antiquity upon dead mothers, but the first authentic section performed upon a living mother is credited to Trautman, of Wittenberg, in 1610. This was done upon a woman with a large ventral hernia which contained the uterus. Prior to this, Nufer, a sow gelder, is reputed to have performed the operation on his wife, after obstetricians and midwives had failed to deliver her. It has been stated that Jane Seymour was delivered by a section done by Frère, a noted surgeon of the time, at the request of Henry VIII. That she died a few days after the birth of Edward VI adds credence to the story, but no absolute confirmation is available. Due to the frightful mortality from hemorrhage, sepsis, and so on, it did not become popular in spite of the advocacy of the Church. Through the following centuries it was done occasionally, but not until the advent of uterine sutures and aseptic technique did it become a practical procedure.

The origin of its name has been ascribed to Julius Caesar, but, as his mother lived many years after his birth, this seems improbable—considering the high mortality of all abdominal operations before the time of Lister. A more accurate explanation is that Numa Pompilius, one of the earlier Roman kings, passed a law making it compulsory to perform the operation upon all mothers who died while pregnant in order that the mother and the child might be buried separately. This was known as the "Lex Regis" and with the advent of the Caesars as the "Lex Caesaris"—and subsequently "cesarean section." The name has been attributed to *cedere*, the Latin verb meaning to cut, but the former explanation seems to be more reasonable.

The 17th century was notable for many famous obstetricians. Mauriceau, of Paris, was the first to correct the view that the pelvic bones separated in normal labor. He was also the first man to refer to epidemic puerperal fever. His description of an obstetrician, or rather of the qualities an obstetrician should possess, is both interesting and amusing. He stated:

> He must be healthful, strong and robust; because this is the most laborious of all the Operations of Chirurgery; for it will make one sometimes sweat, so he shall not have a dry Thread, tho' it were the coldest Day in Winter. . . . He ought to be well shaped, at least to outward appearance, but above all, to have small hands for the easier Introduction of them into the Womb when necessary; yet strong, with the Fingers long, especially the Fore-finger, the better to reach and touch the inner orifice. He must have no Rings on his Fingers, and his Nails well pared, when he goeth about the Work, for fear of hurting the Womb. He ought to have a pleasant Countenance, and to be as neat in his Clothes as in his person, that the poor women who have need of him be not affrighted at him. Some are of the opinion, that a Practitioner of this Art ought on the contrary to be slovenly, at least very careless, wearing a great Beard, to prevent the Occa-

sion of the Husband's Jealousy that sends for him. Truly some believe this Policy augments their Practice but 'tis fit they should be disabused; for such a Posture and Dress resembles more a Butcher than a Chirurgeon, whom the woman apprehends already too much, that he needs not such as Disguise. Above all he must be sober, no Tipler, that he may at all times have his Wits about him. . . .

Van Deventer, of Holland, has been called the father of modern obstetrics and is credited with the first accurate description of the pelvis, its deformities and their effect on parturition. He also shares with Ould, of Dublin, the first description of the mechanism of labor. As time passed, customs changed, and the term "accoucheur" replaced the objectionable "midman" and "man-midwife." Obstetric forceps were invented, probably about 1580, by Peter Chamberlen but were kept as a family secret until 1813 in an effort of the Chamberlens to monopolize the field. When the Chamberlen forceps were finally revealed to the profession, their need had been met by other men, and the Chamberlens were thus justly punished for the discredit they had brought upon their calling.

This century witnessed severe population dessication due to plagues, wars, and the like. In England, William Pelty realized that controlling communicable diseases and saving infant lives would prevent continued diminution of the population. To this end he recommended isolation for plague patients and maternity hospitals for unmarried pregnant women. Such ideas were too far in advance of the time, however, and hence had no immediate consequences.

The eighteenth century

Population continued to be a great general concern to the governments of the world. Those who were concerned with general matters of health felt that governments ought to take a more active role in overseeing health matters. Between 1779 and 1817, Johan Peter Frank in Germany wrote several volumes entitled *System einer vollstandigen medicinischen Polezey*. This work is even today considered a landmark in the history of thought on the social relations of health and disease. His recommendations concerning childbirth were many and as with Pelty, farsighted for his time. He insisted that all childbirth be attended by trained persons, and further urged that a midwife be consulted prior to the expected date of confinement. In addition, he proposed legislation to enforce a reasonable period of bed rest during the puerperium and to free the mother for several weeks from any work in or outside the house which might prevent her from giving the necessary attention to her infant. When necessary, he felt that the state should support parturients for the first six weeks after delivery. He then expanded upon the above and outlined a detailed child welfare program. Acceptance of his work and ideas spread to all countries in close cultural contact with Germany.

The eighteenth century was also marked by a succession of other famous men connected with obstetrics such as Palfyne, the Hunters, Smellie, White, and others. Palfyne is credited with the invention of obstetric forceps, as he presented a copy in 1770 to the Academy of Medicine of Paris.

Smellie taught obstetrics with a manikin and made improvements on the obstetric forceps in use at that time, adding a steel lock and curved blades. He also laid down the first principles for their use and differentiated by measurement between contracted and normal pelves.

William Hunter, though a pupil of Smellie, was opposed to the use of forceps, and frequently exhibited his rusted blades as evidence of their uselessness. In conjunction with his brother he laid the foundation of modern knowledge of placental anatomy.

Charles White published an obstetric thesis advocating the scrubbing of the hands and general cleanliness on the part of the accoucheur; he was the pioneer in aseptic midwifery. John Harvie, 90 years before Credé, advocated external manual expression of the placenta, and it is known that a similar procedure was in use in Dublin at that time. One of the most active and famous English obstetricians of the time, John Clarke, had his fame commemorated in this epitaph:

> Beneath this stone, shut up in the dark
> Lies a learned man-midwife y'clep'd
>   Dr. Clarke.
> On earth while he lived by attending men's
>   wives,
> He increased population some thousands of
>   lives;
> Thus a gain to the nation was gain to himself,
> An enlarged population, enlargement of pelf.
> So he toiled late and early, from morning
>   to night,
> The squalling of children his greatest delight;

Then worn out with labours, he died skin
and bone
And his ladies he left all to Mansfield and
Stone.

There were many famous obstetricians on
the Continent in this period, chief among them
being Baudelocque, who invented the pelvimeter and named and described positions and
presentations. In America, prejudices against
men in midwifery were carried over from
Europe; as late as 1857 a demonstration before
the graduating class at Buffalo roused such a
storm of criticism that the American Medical
Association had to intervene. Their judgment
was that any physician who could not conduct
labor by touch alone should not undertake
midwifery.

The 18th century produced such men as
Moultrie, Lloyd, and Shippen. The last was a
pupil of Smellie and Hunter; in 1762, he opened
a school for midwifery in Philadelphia, and,
since he provided convenient lodgings for the
accommodation of poor women during confinement, he may be said to have established the
first lying-in hospital in America. With Morgan,
he founded the School of Medicine of the University of Pennsylvania, becoming its first Professor of Anatomy, Surgery, and Midwifery.

The nineteenth and the
twentieth centuries

The increased knowledge, interest and ability which physicians brought to obstetrics were
largely offset by the increased mortality due
to puerperal fever. During the 17th, the 18th,
and the 19th centuries it became a pestilence,
at times wiping out whole communities of puerperal women. The mortality rates varied in the
best European clinics at Paris and Vienna from
10 to 20 percent. The origin and the spread of
the disease were little understood or studied.
Obstetricians wasted futile hours on a study of
minor alterations in instruments or technique
and ignored the vast loss of life from puerperal
fever. Oliver Wendell Holmes, of Harvard, first
presented his views on the contagiousness of
puerperal fever in 1843, and in 1855 he reiterated them in a monograph on *Puerperal
Fever as a Private Pestilence*. This was, and
still remains, a medical classic on the subject.
His statements aroused great controversy in
America, and he received a great deal of abuse
and criticism from Meigs and Hodge, two of
the foremost American obstetricians of the
day. One of them stated that it was ridiculous

to conceive of any gentleman carrying contamination on his hands from patient to patient.

While Holmes first conceived the correct
idea of the nature of the disease, it is to Ignaz
Philipp Semmelweiss that the glory must go of
finally proving without question the nature
of its source and transmission. He was an
assistant in the Viennese clinic for women,
and while his associates fussed with unimportant details of technique, he was studying and
mourning the tremendous death rate among
puerperal women in the clinic. He observed
that the death rate in Clinic I, where women
were delivered by medical students or physicians, was always higher than that of Clinic II,
where midwives officiated or received instruction. After fruitless study and manifold changes
in technique in order to follow more closely
that of Clinic II, the cause of the disease was
brought home to him in a desperate and
startling fashion. His friend, Kalletschka, an
assistant in pathology, died after performing
an autopsy upon a victim of puerperal fever,
during which Kalletschka had sustained a
slight cut on his finger.

At postmortem the findings were identical
with those of puerperal sepsis, and Semmelweiss concluded that the disease was transmitted from the dead, by contact from the
physicians and the students, who often went
directly from the postmortem room to deliveries. Accordingly, he immediately instituted
and enforced a ruling which made it obligatory
that all physicians and students wash their
hands in a solution of chloride of lime after
attending autopsies and before examining or
delivering mothers. In seven months he had
reduced the mortality in Clinic I from 12 to
3 percent, and in the subsequent year had a
mortality lower than Clinic II, a hitherto un-
heard-of feat. Subsequently, he observed that
puerperal sepsis could be transmitted from
patient to patient by contact of contaminated
material, or attendants, as well as from the
postmortem room, and in 1861 he published his
immortal work on *The Cause, Concept and
Prophylaxis of Puerperal Fever*.

Medicine provides pitiful figures in profu-
sion, but none, it seems, met such a cruel reception and ultimate fate as Semmelweiss. His
colleagues (for the most part, but with a few
notable and loyal exceptions) distorted and
criticized his teachings. Had they stopped there,
it might have been bad enough, but they carried
their distaste for his views to the stage of per-

secution. He was forced to leave Vienna and go to Budapest, where a similar attitude—if possible a more malignant one—awaited him. A disappointed man, he died in 1865 from a brain abscess which may have originated in an infection similar to that of his friend Kalletschka. To the tragedy of his life, his death added satire. His work, however, has lived on; Pasteur and Lister added to it; and with a more modern and tolerant age his worth has been recognized.

The organisms causing puerperal fever probably were seen by several early workers beginning with Mayrhofer, who, in 1863, described "cylindrical vibrios" or "strings of pearls" in the lochia of puerperal sepsis. In 1864, 310 deaths occurred in the 1,350 confinement cases in the Maternité hospital in Paris, and that "Vestibule of Death" had to be closed in 1865.

Pasteur, in 1879, saw "cocci in chain" in cases of puerperal sepsis and contributed definitely to our knowledge of the causal streptococci, demonstrating to doctors the "presence of the invisible foe" in a drop of blood obtained by a "simple pin-prick on the finger tip of the unhappy woman doomed to die the next day" and recommending methods of aseptic technique for their control.

The 19th and the 20th centuries were largely notable for their utilization of drugs to alleviate the pains of childbirth. The use of ether as an anesthetic was first discovered in America, but it was first utilized for childbirth by Simpson in Great Britain. He brought back the lost art of version by making it a safer procedure and eventually substituted chloroform for ether. As with almost every advance in medicine, it was opposed bitterly. The opposition was loudest and most vehement from the clergy, but, in 1853, Queen Victoria accepted it for delivery and by her action silenced most of the criticism. Nitrous oxide had been used in 1880 and has continued to be popular ever since that time.

Obstetric analgesia and anesthesia have made great strides during the 20th century (see Chapter 17, Analgesia and Anesthesia in Labor).

The present century will be remembered largely for the development of antepartal clinics and the more concentrated care of the expectant mothers that came with them. The application of advances in general medicine, metabolism and public health to obstetrics has led to a marked decrease in mortality and morbidity from cardiac, pulmonic, metabolic, venereal and associated medical conditions complicating pregnancy. The consideration of adequate vitamin, mineral, and caloric contents in connection with the diet of pregnant and puerperal women not only has decreased the morbidity but also has enhanced the health of all mothers and children who receive adequate obstetric care.

Many other contributions have been made and are being added constantly to the science of obstetrics, not the least of which is more intensive training and study in this specialty demanded by the public as well as the medical profession. The advent of routine external expression of the placenta, anti-bacterial prophylaxis in the eyes of the newborn, purified ergot and pituitary preparations in hemorrhage control and prevention are but a few of the methods and medications which have marked the early 20th century.

The morphologic and anthropologic studies of Naegele, Roberts, Williams, Goodwin, Caldwell, Moloy, and others have done much to improve our understanding of the various types of pelves and some of their importance in labor. Roentgenologic pelvimetry, cephalometry, and tokodynamometry have greatly advanced our knowledge of the probable course of labor and delivery; Thoms, Caldwell and Moloy, Hanson, Jarcho, and countless others have contributed to our advances in this field (see Chapter 5).

In a necessarily brief and incomplete fashion, an endeavor has been made to touch upon some of the more interesting phases of the history of obstetrics—a fascinating subject.

Background and development of maternal and infant care in the United States

As we know it today, maternal and child care developed into its present status through various avenues of investigation and many by-paths of interrelated activity and work. Individuals, both from the profession and the laity, as well as private and municipal organizations, contributed time, money and interest until, at last, government action was obtained.

1866. A story was written which concerned cruelty to a child. Some thoughtful person referred the case to *The Society for the Prevention of Cruelty to Animals.* Henry Bergh, a former diplomat to Russia, was the founder and director of this association and was influential in having the judgment pronounced on the ground that a child was a human animal. This incident stimulated interest in the general treatment of children.

1873. *The New York Diet Kitchen Association*, the oldest public health organization in America, was opened at the request of doctors from "de Milt Dispensary" on the lower East Side of New York City. It was first organized as a soup kitchen, and milk, gruel, beef tea, and cooked rice were taken to the sick in their homes, with the idea of restoring health. In 1892, they began to make formulas for sick babies and still later dispensed free milk or sold it at 3 cents a quart. Maria L. Daniels was the first nurse director and contributed much for many years to public health progress. In 1926, this group was organized as *The Children's Health Service of New York*. The organization grew with the times, changing its program from curing the sick to preventive work—keeping well babies well. Although the organization devoted its major effort to work with babies and preschool children, it also included antepartal care in its program.

1876. The beginning of child-welfare legislation in the United States was the act passed by the New York State Legislature, granting to *The Society for the Prevention of Cruelty to Children* a charter that gave it wide power with regard to the protection of child life. The inception of this legislation was based on the incident of the "child as a human animal" (1866).

1893. The first *Infant Milk Station* in the United States was established in New York City by Nathan Strauss. Through his persistence, milk was finally made "safe" through pasteurization; and many such stations were set up.

1900. *The United States Census Bureau* was made a permanent organization. Up to this time, *vital statistics* were considered to be of so little importance in the United States that, as soon as the population was tabulated and classified, the bureau was disbanded, to be re-established and reorganized every ten years.

1906. *The United States Census Bureau* published mortality statistics which drew attention to the appalling loss of life among babies and children. Up to this time, very little thought had been given to maternity and infant protection.

1907. Due to the growing interest, Mr. George H. F. Schrader was stimulated to give money to *The Association for Improving Condi-tions of the Poor* (now the *Community Service Society*) for the salaries of two nurses to do antepartal work. This was the first consistent effort to prevent deaths of babies by caring for the mothers *before* the babies were born. Two reasons were given as to why antepartal care would be of value: 1) nurses in convalescent homes for postpartal mothers thought that if patients had better care during pregnancy, the health of mothers would be improved; 2) social workers going into the homes felt that they were not adequately prepared to advise pregnant mothers.

1907. *The New York Milk Committee* was organized. Its object was the reduction of infant mortality through the improvement of the city's milk supply. It established milk depots which proved beyond question their great value in the reduction of infant mortality by dispensing clean pasteurized milk and by educating mothers.

1908. In this year the *Division of Child Hygiene* was established in New York City, the first in the United States, and it was important enough to be recognized nationally. Josephine Baker, M.D., was appointed chief. This was a pioneer achievement, and the methods that were evolved had no precedent.

1909 to 1914. At approximately this time, Mrs. William Lowell Putnam, of Boston, promoted a demonstration of organized antepartal care. It was called *The Prenatal Care Committee* of the Women's Municipal League. The members of this committee worked in cooperation with the Boston Lying-In Hospital through Robert L. DeNormandie, M.D., of Harvard Medical School, Dr. Ruggles, of the then Homeopathic Hospital, and the Instructive District Nurses Association. The committee functioned long enough to establish the fact that good obstetric care was not possible without antepartal care.

1909. In this year *The American Association for the Study and Prevention of Infant Mortality* was organized and held its first meeting in New Haven, Connecticut. This committee was composed of both professional and lay members and devoted itself entirely to problems connected with child life, particularly to studying and trying to correct the high mortality rate. At this time there were no records of births or deaths, and the causes of deaths were unknown. The education of physicians and nurses was shamefully unsatisfactory; there was no public health in the schools, and practically no activity on the part of municipal, state, or the federal government to prevent infant mortality. The first president of this association was J. H. Mason Knox, M.D., and Gertrude B. Kipp was the first secretary. The committee consisted of the Honorable Herbert Hoover, Livingston Ferrand, M.D., L. Emmet Holt, M.D., Richard Bolt, M.D., and Philip Van Ingen, M.D. The work of this organization was of profound significance. In 1918, its expanding activities caused it to change its name to *The American Child Hygiene Association*, and in 1923 the name was changed to *The American Child Health Association*. In 1935, after having contributed to every angle of this pioneer work, the association was disbanded.

1909. *The First White House Conference*, on "The Dependent Child," was called by President Theodore Roosevelt. These investigations resulted in the establishment of the U.S. Children's Bureau in 1912. According to some authorities, this conference was called through the influence of a public health nurse.

1910. *The Census Bureau* published another report, this time on the mortality of infants under one year of age and at "special ages." As a result of this report maternity hospitals made an effort to improve the care given to infants.

1911. In New York City *the first strictly municipal baby-health stations* were organized under the jurisdiction of the Department of Health, and the full cost of the work was borne by the municipality. Soon the dispensing of milk was of minor importance, and emphasis was placed on prevention. They are now called *Child-Health Stations*.

1911. *The New York Milk Committee* (1907) made an investigation at the baby-health stations and found that 40 percent of all infant deaths (112 per 1,000) occurred within the first month of life before the mothers registered their babies at the health stations. This indicated the necessity for care *before* birth. The committee then decided to carry on an experiment in antepartal work. (See 1917.) They were convinced that much could be hoped for as a result of organized antepartal care.

1912. *The Babies' Welfare Association* (formerly *The Association of Infant Milk Stations* [1893]) represents the first comprehensive and successful attempt to coordinate the various child-welfare agencies in any community. All of the organizations of this type agreed to coordinate their activities by preventing dupli-

cation and overlapping without interfering with the organizations. In 1922, the name was changed to the *Children's Welfare Federation* of New York City. It continued to act as a clearing house and, among its other activities, managed the *Mother's Milk Bureau*.

1912. The *U.S. Children's Bureau* was established. It began in the Department of Commerce and Labor; in 1913 it was made a part of the Department of Labor and, in 1946, was transferred to the Federal Security Agency. This was created by Congress through a federal act (government sanction). This bureau was to set up special machinery to study and protect the child and to study all matters pertaining to the welfare of children and child life among all classes of our people, to assemble and accumulate factual information and to disseminate this information throughout the country. Miss Julia Lathrop was chosen as chief. Much of the success of this bureau is credited to Miss Lathrop's vision. Fortunately, her successor, Miss Grace Abbott, continued the work with equal zeal.

1915. *The Birth Registration Area* was established as a federal act. The information is compiled in a uniform manner, giving the birth and the death statistics on which are based our information on mortality rates.

1915. Dr. Haven Emerson, Health Commissioner of New York City, appointed a special committee (Ralph W. Lobenstine, M.D., Clifton Edgar, M.D., and Philip Van Ingen, M.D.), in cooperation with the New York Milk Committee, to make an analysis of the facilities for maternity care in the city. The result of the survey showed that there was little antepartal work and no uniformity, and that only a very small number of pregnant mothers were receiving care. It showed also that hospitals took care of 30 percent of the deliveries, midwives delivered 30 percent, general practitioners delivered 30 percent, and private physicians, who might be classified as obstetricians, delivered 10 percent. Previous to this time little or nothing had been done to regulate or control the midwives.

1916. *The National Society for the Prevention of Blindness* was created after much pioneer work and investigation, locally and throughout the states, by Carolyn Van Blarcom, R.N. She was chosen to be the executive secretary. Through these investigations it was learned that by far the greatest cause of blindness was ophthalmia of the newborn. These findings led to the passing of a law compelling all physicians and midwives to use prophylaxis in newborn babies' eyes. Also, as a direct result of Miss Van Blarcom's surveys, a school for lay midwives was started, Belleview School for Midwives (no longer in existence). Miss Van Blarcom took out a midwife's license and was the first nurse in the United States so to register. The first obstetrical nursing textbook to be written by a nurse is to Miss Van Blarcom's credit. Her later contribution to the better care of mothers and babies was to secure for Johns Hopkins Hospital the E. Bayard Halsted Fund for medical research.

1917. The Women's City Club of New York City and the New York Milk Committee opened three antepartal centers. The one sponsored by the Women's City Club was organized as the *Maternity Service Association* and, with Frances Perkins as the first executive secretary and Miss Mabel Choate as president, provided stimulating leadership. Dr. Ralph W. Lobenstine, a famous obstetrician, gave much time, labor, authority and direction as chairman of the medical board. In 1918, this organization was incorporated as the *Maternity Center Association* and carried out the first extensive piece of organized antepartal work in the United States. Miss Anne Stevens was director. Miss Annie W. Goodrich's wise counsel, as a member of the nursing committee, gave impetus to the organization's accomplishments. Louis I. Dublin, Ph.D., associated with this movement from the beginning, made an analysis of the first 4,000 records collected by the association. This revealed the startling fact that, through antepartal care, 50 percent of the lives of mothers might be saved and 60 percent of the lives of babies. Antepartal training and experience were extended to nurses throughout the world. This piece of intensive antepartal work fired increased interest in the care of mothers and babies. In 1929, the Maternity Center Association opened a school for the training of nurse midwives.

1919. *The Second White House Conference* was called by President Woodrow Wilson as a result of the activities of the U.S. Children's Bureau. It was organized in five sections. Each section was interested in a different phase of maternity and child care.

1919. *The American Committee on Maternal Welfare* was founded. The object of the committee was to stimulate interest of the medical profession in cooperating with public and private agencies to protect the lives and health of mothers and infants, and to teach principles and practice of personal hygiene and health to parents, physicians, nurses, and others dealing with the problems of maternity. The Committee was incorporated as a nonprofit organization in 1934 for the purpose of studying the maternal mortality rate in the United States and the management of obstetric problems generally. For more recent progress, see 1957 and 1964.

This organization publishes the magazine *The Bulletin of Maternal and Child Health*. It also promoted the American Congress of Obstetrics and Gynecology, which was held every three years.

1921. *The Sheppard-Towner Bill* was passed by Congress, an act for the promotion of the welfare and hygiene of maternity and infancy, to be administered by the U.S. Children's Bureau. This bill was introduced in the 65th Congress by Congresswoman Jeanette Rankin of New Jersey. It was reported out of committee favorably but failed to pass. A second bill was introduced in the 66th Congress. It passed in the Senate but, through delays, was not considered by the House. In the first session of the 67th Congress the bill was again introduced by Senator Sheppard and Congressman Towner and, after much agitation, finally passed—an epoch in child-welfare legislation. An appropriation of $1,240,000 per year was granted for five years. The Cooper Bill, passed in 1927, extended it for two more years. This law was accepted by all of the states except three. This legislation gave a tremendous impetus to the education not only of laity but also of physicians. Because of this legislation there was created at once, in the states which did not already have them, departments which now are quite uniformly labeled Divisions or Bureaus of Maternity and Child Health. In 1935, the Social Security Act was passed, following the plan of the Sheppard-Towner Bill. This Act appropriated $3,800,000. In 1939, the Social Security Act was amended, increasing the appropriation to $5,820,000. The amount has been increased gradually, and by 1952 (82nd Congress), $30,000,000 was appropriated for Maternal and Child Health, Crippled Children and other Child Health Services.

1923. *The National Committee for Maternal Health* was formed with Robert L. Dickinson, M.D., as secretary and later as president. This was a clearing house and a center of information on certain medical aspects of human fertility. The object was to gather and analyze material, to stimulate research, to issue reports to the medical profession and to persuade it to take a leading part in the scientific investigations of these problems in preventive medicine. No other group existed for this purpose. It was dissolved in 1950.

1923. *The Margaret Sanger Research Bureau* came into being, an affiliation of the Planned Parenthood Federation of America, Inc., for research in the field of infertility, contraception and marriage counseling.

1923. Mary Breckinridge began her investigations in Kentucky, which led to the organization of the *Frontier Nursing Service*. With this concentrated effort of all phases of maternity and infant care, the striking results proved the value of prenatal care. Through her vision, determination and unfaltering energy, Mary Breckinridge has made this organization one of worldwide renown. In 1936, the Frontier Nursing Service opened a school for the training of nurse midwives.

1925. *The Joint Committee on Maternal Welfare* was formed. This consisted of the American Gynecological Society, the American Association of Obstetrics and Gynecology and Abdominal Surgeons and the American Child Health Association (1909). Later the section of Obstetrics, Gynecology and Abdominal Surgeons of the American Medical Association was represented. The Committee issued a pamphlet entitled *An Outline of Delivery Care*. This stimulated the Children's Bureau to publish a concise pamphlet, *Standards of Prenatal Care* (1925), an outline for the use of physicians, which did much to standardize routine procedures.

1930. *The Third White House Conference* was called by President Herbert Hoover. Mr. Hoover's interest in child welfare was very evident. The conference was very comprehensive and far-reaching and was devoted to all aspects of maternity and child care. The Children's Charter was adopted and became a federal act. The 45,000,000 children were analyzed in chart form to show the paramount importance of care during pregnancy and the early years.

1938. *The Conference on Better Care for Mothers and Babies* was called by the Children's Bureau. This was the first time that representatives from the states, private and public organizations, both lay and professional people, met to pool ideas.

1939. *The Maternity Consultation Service* in New York City was organized to further antepartal education and care.

1940. *The Fourth White House Conference* on Children in a Democracy was called by President Franklin D. Roosevelt. It considered the aims of American civilization for the children in whose hands its future lies; how children can best be helped to grow into the kind of citizens who will know best how to preserve and protect our democracy. By 1940, the 48 states, the District of Columbia, Puerto Rico, Alaska, and Hawaii (then Territories) were cooperating with the Children's Bureau in its administration of child-welfare services.

1940. *The Cleveland Health Museum* was opened to the public—the first health museum in the Western hemisphere. It is significant in the maternity field because, in its workshops, it is reproducing the *Dickinson-Belskie models*, acquired in 1945. Dr. Bruno Gebhard, Director, says that, in his belief, the use of this sculptural series in professional and lay education will advance knowledge on this all-important subject more quickly and more accurately than any other visual means thus far available.

1943. *The Emergency Maternity and Infancy Care Program* was launched to care for the wives and the babies of enlisted men in the armed forces. From $17,000,000 to $45,000,000 per year was appropriated. This act also furthered interest in prenatal and child care.

1944. *The Public Health Service Act* was signed on July 3, 1944 and brought together all existing laws affecting the public health service. In addition, the act also revised existing laws, provided authority for grants and authorized expansion of the federal-state cooperative public health programs which had bearing on maternal and child health programs. This act was to exert a great indirect impact on the care of mothers and infants because of its provisions funding research and education of personnel needed in these areas.

1946. The *World Health Organization*—an agency of the United Nations—became a reality. At the first meeting in Paris, 64 nations signed the constitution. The membership as of 1965 totaled 117 countries. The object of the organization is "the attainment of the highest possible level of health of all the peoples." So far, much has been accomplished toward that end.

1950. *The Fifth White House Conference*, with emphasis on children and youth, was called by President Harry S Truman.

1950. *The Fred Lyman Adair Foundation* of the American Committee on Maternal Welfare was established. Its purpose is to collect funds from charitable sources to underwrite research and educational projects in this field.

1955. *The American College of Nurse-Midwifery* was established as an organization of nurse-midwives to study and evaluate the activities of nurse-midwives, to plan and develop educational programs meeting the requirements of the profession and to perform other related functions. In 1957, the College became a member of the International Confederation of Midwives, a midwifery organization with members from some 30 countries throughout the world.

1957. *The American Association for Maternal and Infant Health* (formerly the American Committee on Maternal Welfare) was activated at the Seventh American Congress held in July. Prompted by the spectacular improvements and advances in maternity care which have taken place since its founding, the board of directors of the committee voted unanimously to change the name, the role and the character of the organization. The new American Association for Maternal and Infant Health provides close integration of the various disciplines which participate in providing modern maternity care, and will serve as a forum for their mutual problems related to maternal and infant health.

1960. *The Sixth White House Conference,* concerned with the nation's children and youth, was called by President Dwight D. Eisenhower. The theme of this "Golden Anniversary" Conference was "Opportunities for Children and Youth to Realize Their Full Potential for Creative Life in Freedom and Dignity."

1962. *The Conference on Maternal and Child Health Teaching in Graduate Schools of Public Health* was convened in response to the dire reports of the lack of qualified personnel with any public health background in the area of maternal and child health. The conference recommended that an MCH career development program be established to offset the existing and predicted shortages of personnel. Such a program was established at the University of California at Berkeley with financial aid from the federal government (U.S. Children's Bureau) in 1965. The objectives of early recruitment of qualified physicians and the provision of specialized training in obstetrics or pediatrics with general community health maternal and child health content has been realized.

In the same year *The National Institute of Child Health and Human Development* was authorized. The goals of this Institute were support of research and training in special health problems and needs of mothers and children. This Institute also now conducts and supports research in the basic sciences relating to the processes of human growth and development, including prenatal development. Five conferences were held in 1967, which sought to find the problems involved in maternal and infant mortality and morbidity and to establish guidelines for change towards more optimal care.

1963. *The Maternal and Child Health and Mental Retardation Planning Amendments of 1963* was enacted. This law will make it possible for the Children's Bureau to carry out some of the major recommendations of the President's panel.

1964. *The American Association for Maternal and Child Health* (formerly the American Association for Maternal and Infant Health), as a multidisciplinary organization, is one of the most potentially valuable groups interested in matters concerning infant, child and maternal health. The board of directors of the Association altered the official title of the organization, not to imply any change in its proposed program but to present a more accurate definition of the organization in terms of its aims and objectives.

1964. *The Nurse Training Act,* one of the amendments of the Public Health Act, was an indirect aid to maternal and infant care. This act authorized grants for the expansion and improvement of nurse training, assistance to nursing students, scholarship grants to schools of nursing, and the establishment of a National Advisory Council on Nurse Training.

1965. *Amendments to the Social Security Act* provided for a new five-year program of special project grants for comprehensive health care and services for school and preschool children, particularly in low income family areas. These amendments also increased the authorization for money to support maternal and child health service programs. There are now 54 such projects in existence due to this legislation.

1965. *PKU Testing* became mandatory for all infants in the states of Illinois and Michigan, thus setting a precedent for other states.

1966. *The Department of Health, Education, and Welfare* issued a policy statement on birth control which stated that the Department would support, on request, health programs making family planning information and services available. Due to this unique statement, federally supported family planning programs have since slowly begun to evolve.

The Federal Food, Drug and Cosmetic Act was instituted on June 14, 1966. This legislation required labelling of ingredients of food represented for special dietary use. Infant foods, particularly, were specified.

The Child Protection Act of 1966 banned the sale of toys and children's articles containing hazardous substances, regardless of labelling.

1967. *The Public Health Law 89-749* is considered by health authorities to be one of the most significant health measures passed by Congress since it provides for increasing flexibility at state and regional levels to attack special health problems which have regional or local impact.

1967. *Medicaid* programs were increasing among the states (30 in 1967) to provide health care for low-income families. Care during pregnancy and child care were included.

1968. *Head Start* programs provided educational opportunities for underprivileged children of preschool age, often associated with nutritional and health screening programs.

1968. The second report of the *President's Committee on Mental Retardation* noted that three-fourths of the country's mental retardation was found in isolated and impoverished urban and rural areas, and cited evidence of a close relationship between diet and mental and nervous disorders. It recommended federal action to improve manpower shortages and develop facilities for care of the mentally retarded.

1968. The *Citizens' Board of Inquiry into Hunger and Malnutrition in the United States* issued its report "Hunger—U.S.A." which supported the presence of widespread hunger among millions of U.S. citizens.

1969. A live virus vaccine for *rubella* (German measles) was released and the U.S. Public Health Service began immunization programs.

1969. The *National Center for Family Planning* was established under the Health Services and Mental Health Administration, Department of Health, Education and Welfare (DHEW), to serve as a clearinghouse for information about contraception.

1969. *Neighborhood Health Centers* pilot projects began in many Southern states and Northern urban slums to provide medical care to the poor.

1969. *Pediatric Assistants* consisting of nurses and physician's assistants were being trained in several university pediatrics departments.

1969. *Amniocentesis* was used to diagnose hereditary disease in the fetus.

1969. *The White House Conference on Food, Nutrition and Health* was charged to formulate a national nutritional program, based upon reports of malnutrition among lower income population and the consequences of nutritional deficiency for the growth and development of infants.

1970. A nationwide drive was spearheaded by the *Center for Disease Control* in Atlanta, Georgia, to vaccinate children against rubella.

1970. *The Seventh White House Conference on Children and Youth* met, and recommended the establishment of a child advocacy agency by the federal government with full ethnic, cultural, racial, and sexual representation.

1969-1970. The *Office of Child Development* was established within DHEW to administer child development programs (Head Start, day care) and coordinate activities of governmental and private agencies involved in programs for children and youth.

1970. New York state liberalized its *abortion law* to leave the decision up to the woman during the first 24 weeks of pregnancy, permitting abortion after that time only to save the woman's life.

1971. *National Commission for the Study of Nursing and Nursing Education*, Jerome Lysaught, director, reported study of nursing roles and recommended nursing roles be expanded, educational systems repatterned, and more nursing input into health care.

1971. *National Health Insurance* was debated in Congress but no bills passed.

1971. The American Nurses Association and American Academy of Pediatrics jointly developed guidelines for *training pediatric nurse associates*, and held a national conference to implement these. The ANA and American College of Obstetricians and Gynecologists also met to draw up guidelines for training clinical nurse specialists in obstetrics-gynecology.

1971. Funds were awarded to six innovative *child advocacy demonstration projects* by two agencies of DHEW.

1972. *Home Start* programs were inaugurated to help disadvantaged parents provide child development services in their own homes, and be the primary educators of their own children.

1972. The *Office of Child Development* sponsored programs to help teenagers learn how to become good parents, and in coordinated efforts with Head Start and Community Mental Health Centers strove to improve the quality of mental health care including prevention, diagnosis and treatment for Head Start children and their families.

1972. *The Committee to Study Extended Roles for Nurses* reported to the secretary of DHEW that functions of nurses "need to be broadened" so they can "assume broader responsibility in primary care, acute care, and long-term care." The new "nurse practitioner" was functioning in expanded nursing roles in many areas including obstetrics, pediatrics, psychiatry, and medical-surgical nursing.

1972. *Professional Standards Review Organizations (PSRO)* were required by an amendment to the Social Security Act to be set up to oversee care given by physicians to Medicare and Medicaid patients in hospitals.

1973. The *U.S. Supreme Court* struck down almost all state statutes prohibiting or restricting *abortion*, leaving the abortion decision to the woman and her physician during the first three months of pregnancy, and that afterwards the state could only regulate abortion procedures in the interest of maternal health. Essentially the decision to abort became the right of the individual woman, with the state unable to interfere in her choice except to assure that the abortion be performed under safe conditions.

1973. The *Child and Family Resource Program* began as an experimental project designed to strengthen the role of the family by providing or making available prenatal health and nutritional education, after-school tutoring for primary grade children, and mental health services to parents about child development.

1973. Data showed that immunization of women with *anti-Rh antibodies* shortly after delivery was highly effective in preventing Rh sensitization in the Rh negative mother (Rhogam).

1973. *The National Commission for the Study of Nursing and Nursing Education*, directed by Jerome Lysaught, reported on the implementation phase of the study. To encourage the expansion of nursing practice, it conducted educational and informational activities aimed at nursing and the public, developed a national joint practice commission between medicine and nursing with state counterparts, and developed statewide planning committees to generate changes in patterns of education and practice.

1973. Several pilot projects to test the feasibility of *institutional licensure* were instituted in certain states, with considerable opposition from nursing organizations.

1973. *National Center on Child Abuse and Neglect* was established in DHEW's Office of Child Development to act as clearinghouse on information about the problem, a *National Commission* formed to study the role of the federal government in this area and the adequacy of state laws, and funds made available to regional child abuse prevention and treatment demonstration programs.

1974. *Guidelines on Short-Term Education Modules for the Obstetric-Gynecologic Nurse Practitioner* were drawn up by the Interorganizational Committee of Obstetric-Gynecologic Health Personnel.

1974. Federal *child health screening program* strengthened (Public Law 92-603), states required to inform Medicaid families about availability of child health screening services and provide these when requested.

1974. Funds made available to study *Sudden Infant Death Syndrome* from the National Institute of Child Health and Human Development.

1975. The Division on Maternal and Child Health Nursing Practice of the American Nurses' Association issued a *guide for short-term continuing education* programs for nurse clinicians in neonatal and maternal-fetal care, an outgrowth of a joint effort among several organizations.

1975. The ANA Commission on Nursing Education offered *accreditation for nondegree granting nurse practitioner programs*, including the OB-GYN nurse practitioners.

1974-1975. Several states revised their *nurse practice acts* to broaden the definition of nursing practice and include the functions of extended role nursing. Nurse practitioners are considered included under these revised acts, although methods of regulation, certification and supervision related to the extension of practice into medical areas remain to be established.

1974-1975. The issue of mandatory *continuing education* in nursing was debated, and a law passed in California requiring this after 1977. Nurses were also increasingly recognizing the need for *collective bargaining* to influence wages and working conditions, as federal funds for nursing programs and educational assistance were cut.

The emergence and development of maternity nursing

From time immemorial women have taken care of other women during pregnancy and childbirth; most cultures, both primitive and modern, have a well-developed "motherlore" which keeps alive instructions and practices to be used during the childbearing period.

Midwifery

In every primitive society, there seems to have been someone present to care for the mother and the infant. Usually this task fell to women, who in essence were the ancient forerunners of maternity nurses. These women might be female relatives or others who had borne children, or in some societies were the equivalent of a nurse-midwife. Midwives no doubt have existed for centuries untold, and Homer made reference to a nurse-midwife in the *Iliad*. They continued to attend the majority of deliveries in Roman and Medieval times, although the role of physicians was enlarging. During the 18th century maternity cases began to receive more attention, as many lying-in charities were formed and midwives were included in training programs in London and Paris.

As midwifery assumed a more scientific status, special lying-in hospitals increased, and the last 50 years of the eighteenth century saw a remarkable decrease in maternal and infant deaths in these hospitals due to better techniques of nursing management. The male physicians remained mostly uninvolved in parturient care unless needed for special procedures in difficult labors.[1] It was not until the 19th century that physicians participated extensively in obstetrics, and much opposition had to be overcome from both physicians and public before the "he-midwives" were widely accepted. In the United States, a school for midwifery was started in 1762 by a physician from Philadelphia. Both nurse-midwives and physician-midwives practiced during the eighteenth and nineteenth centuries, though the nurse-midwives predominated.

Emergence of professional maternity nursing

A variety of factors, cultural, social, and technological, have had important roles in shaping the growth and development of maternity nursing. One of the most important and direct of these factors was the shift from home to hospital delivery. At the turn of the century, almost all women were delivered at home by a midwife or physician. At the present time, more than 90 percent of mothers deliver in the hospital. Two other factors, in turn, brought about this change to hospital delivery and helped shape the kind of care received there. An increase in the understanding of asepsis made physicians much more attentive to this aspect of care, particularly for maternity patients. A growing conviction developed that delivery in a hospital was mandatory. As more women began delivering in hospitals, provision had to be made for quick, efficient, aseptic care and certain time-saving devices and work simplification procedures were borrowed from industry. "Assembly-line care" soon flourished. Compliance with "time-saving" techniques, performance of the somewhat ritualistic procedures called for to maintain asepsis, and the increasingly overall bureaucratic structure generated by the complex modernizing hospital all went into defining and shaping the very essence of maternity care. Hence there arose the ritualistic, rigid adherence to rules and procedures (with rather little thought to the patient) that characterizes so much of maternity care even today. It was during these early times that antepartal care was conceived and developed as an aspect of preventive medicine. Thus, women increasingly had longer contact with their physicians during the childbearing time and this, together with the still prevalent Victorian notion of dependency, served to cement the obstetric relationship. In order to do justice to this relationship, physicians even more strongly began to insist on hospital deliveries.

Maternity nursing developed as obstetrics developed and not surprisingly, was based on the medical model of obstetrics in which pathology was the main focus. Thus, the nursing student's experiences were oriented to the physical care of her patients, with emphasis on technical competence. Moreover, a good deal of the student's "patient experiences" was in reality service to the hospital. The early hospitals were, in fact, staffed largely by students.

This type of service-to-the-institution, technical competence orientation produced a nurse who was efficient in organizing care for many patients. However, because of the great numbers, no in-depth nursing therapy was either attempted or possible. Little or no public health experience was offered and the nurse gradually became more "institution (i.e., hospital) oriented" and the physician's veritable right arm.

NURSING ROLES AND WOMEN'S STATUS. Undoubtedly part of the reason why nursing was so subjugated by medicine was due to the powerless status of women, and the distaste with which working women were viewed. It is unfortunate that maternity nursing split so completely with nurse-midwifery so that two different fields were eventually formed. Midwives were also suppressed by medicine, however, to the point that their practice became illegal in some states, and was generally discredited and maligned. Maternity nurses have conducted, with more or less vigor, the long struggle toward more responsibility and autonomy that parallels the women's movement for full and equal status.

COMPARTMENTALIZATION AND ROUTINIZATION. In the third and fourth decades of this century, hospitals themselves became larger and more complex and the nurse gradually had to assume more and more administrative and organizational duties. Similarly, medical science enlarged and with the new knowledge and progress, more functions, formerly in the province of the physician, were delegated to the nurse. These factors together with the acute hospital personnel shortage precipitated by World War II, combined to develop and promote impersonal routinized care for the mother and her infant.

As more became known about the transmission and control of pathogenic organisms, various subunits were designated for the use of the mother, the well newborn, the sick newborn, and the premature infant. Thus, restrictions and compartmentalization of nursing function (nursery nurse, postpartum nurse, and so on) proliferated in the name of "better technique" but at the expense of unity in the mother-infant relationship. Perhaps even worse was the compartmentalization of thinking and communication that also evolved. The postpartum nurse knew and cared about the progress of the particular mothers in her charge while they were on the ward. She rarely knew how they responded to their pregnancy in general. She might know something about how they had withstood their labors, but only in the physical sense, and then only in relation to their immediate postpartum course. The nursery nurse knew about the babies in her nursery, but very little about the parents who would take them home or the environment into which they would go.

The experience of childbearing, once common to all members of the social group and centered in the home with involvement of most family members, had now become a disjointed, technical, and alien process about which parents were generally ignorant. Complex and mystical, childbirth had become the province of physicians and specialized nurses, to be enacted in a strange, threatening institution in which the parents were the most powerless members. It is not hard to understand why there was widespread dissatisfaction with this state of affairs, leading to the many far-reaching and sometimes radical changes which occurred over the last twenty years.

RECENT DEVELOPMENTS. The concept of *family-centered maternity care* began to gain support among nursing circles during the 1960s. This approach advocated consideration of other members of the family, particularly the fathers, during pre- and postdelivery care. The pregnant woman, who had been viewed largely in isolation as a medical problem, was recognized as having social and emotional needs which deserved the nurse's attention as did physical care. It seems strange now that nurses had to be reminded that pregnant women had families, with psychologic needs for some involvement in this most momentous event, as well as very real practical problems and social concerns which often could be helped by nursing attention. But, this indeed had been the outcome of years of emphasis on efficiency and routinization on the one hand and influence of the medical model on the other.

The *participant childbirth* movement brought about significant changes in the practice of obstetrics through consumer pressure. Its purposes closely paralleled the family-centered approach, but even greater involvement of the father was advocated. As the ideas and techniques of Dick-Read, Lamaze, and Bradley caught on in the United States, childbearing women and their partners began to seek knowledge and demand choice in the conduct of their own pregnancies, labors, and deliveries. Women wanted to be aware and awake, to feel a central part of the process, to become equipped to cope with the stress of labor without heavy medication, and to have their partners by their side to share the experience. Prepared childbirth usually involved education about the processes of parturition and instruction in techniques to reduce pain perception and enhance the sense of control over the process (see Chapter 16). Fathers frequently served as labor coaches, and through this type of involvement pressure was brought to bear on hospitals to allow their presence in the labor room, an area previously off limits. *Fathers in the delivery room* was soon to follow, as the ludicrousness of allowing them to assist their partners all during labor, only to be dismissed just at the climax of the entire process brought economic and logical pressures on physicians, nurses and hospital administration. This gain was not achieved easily, and took a period of some years before reluctant physicians and nurses accepted the fact that prepared fathers were not going to faint or become irate over necessary procedures or during unexpected complications.

Interest in a more natural and less regimented *style of parenting* developed during the late 1960s and early 1970s. Piaget's theories of childhood learning processes and Dr. Spock's widely-read approaches to childrearing brought recognition of infants and children as individuals with unique needs and characteristics. The *back-to-nature* movement which was an expected reaction to the increasing use of artificial substances and chemical additives in a wide variety of materials and products served as an impetus to rediscovery of *breast-feeding*. Organizations were formed to assist mothers relearn the art of breast-feeding and encourage success through information and support, such as LaLeche League. More parents became interested in modifying table foods for infants rather than using canned and preserved commercial baby foods. In response to maternal need, postpartum nurses began themselves learning about breast-feeding and how to help mothers initiate satisfactory breast-feeding patterns during their first days of nursing their babies in the hospital.

The impact of changing *abortion laws* in the United States was considerable for many nurses involved in the care of pregnant women.

Abortion was permitted only to save the life of the mother until the mid-1960s, when statutes in some states began to be liberalized. Following the lead of New York, more than half of the states considered or revised their abortion laws in 1967 to legalize the procedure if the mother's mental or physical health was threatened, if there was danger of fetal deformity, or if the pregnancy resulted from rape, incest or other felonious intercourse. In January, 1973, the U.S. Supreme Court made its landmark ruling that during the first three months of pregnancy the abortion decision was a matter between the woman and her physician, that during the second trimester the state could regulate the abortion procedure in ways reasonably related to maternal health, and that after the fetus had developed enough for survival on its own, abortion could be regulated or proscribed except to preserve the life or health of the mother. For many nurses in labor areas and postpartum units, these laws created problematic situations because religious or personal convictions prevented them from participating in abortions. The situation improved with the development of *outpatient abortions* and *abortion clinics* for pregnancies prior to 12 weeks gestation. Midtrimester abortions are still performed in hospitals, however, and continue to present a difficult situation for many health workers. The generally accepted practice now is that nurses or physicians can refuse to participate in care directly related to the abortion for these hospitalized patients. For many women, the liberalization of abortion laws has allowed them the freedom of choice they regard as their right in control of their reproductive facilities. The majority of the U.S. population seems to support the concept of abortion as a woman's right, although there are attempts currently underway to restrict or repeal the present laws.

Family planning services have been greatly increased in the last two decades, with the federal government encouraging that contraception be available to all who desire it, and providing monies to make this possible. Free or low cost clinics are widely dispersed throughout the states, and counseling the couple in contraceptive methods has become a standard part of maternity nursing practice. This is in marked contrast to several years ago when sex and birth control were never mentioned, and were treated as taboo subjects. The area of *sexuality and sex education* has received much attention since the early 1970s, as both the literature and available counseling resources have increased rapidly. Sexual problems are voiced by clients and help is sought from health professionals, as human sexuality develops into a new specialty in health care. Nurses involved in maternity care are recognizing that sexuality is an integral part of this field also, for many problems develop or are recognized during the prenatal and postpartal periods. The level of sexual therapy which consists of education about sexuality and sexual response, reinforcement and validation of sexual practices, and some interpersonal counseling falls within the scope of practice of maternity nursing. Increasingly, nurses are becoming prepared to undertake such practice through extending their own education in the field of sexuality.[2]

Following increased concern about family involvement in the childbearing process, *mother-baby couple care* was instituted in many postpartum units to facilitate development of the early mother-infant relationship. The forerunner of this practice was *rooming-in*, when mothers who elected to do so, and could afford a private room or could be placed with a roommate who also wanted rooming-in, would have their babies placed in the mothers' room during the duration of hospitalization. Rooming-in had a varying course over the years, with persistent professional resistance which mothers had to overcome, often only to be left largely on their own with their new babies. Mother-baby couple care represents a commitment on the part of the postpartum and nursery staff to restructure the hospital units so mothers and babies may be together the greater part of the day and night. Usually satellite nurseries are developed to serve each wing of the maternity unit, and postpartum and nursery nurses move back-and-forth within the wing or area. Babies are out with their mothers except for specified times back in the nursery for physical examinations, tests or procedures, or if mother or baby are temporarily sick. Although the logistics of mother-baby couple care require some working out, and nurses need some retraining in the area of their lesser experience, the benefits of each mother-baby couple having the same nurse responsible for their care are enormous. In this way, the same nurse knows the condition and needs of both mother and baby, enhancing the development of the mother-infant relationship through intimacy and close contact, immediate response to

needs or problems, and elimination of the communication gap.

When the birth is complicated or high risk, or the infant is seriously ill, *neonatal intensive care nurseries* have been developed recently to respond to special needs for complex care (see Chapter 29). These special nurseries utilize the latest advanced equipment and procedures for treating neonatal problems. As the body of knowledge in this area enlarges, and modalities for treatment are expanded, a new specialty has emerged called *neonatology*. Both physician and nurse neonatologists receive advanced preparation to provide the complex care needed by infants with life-threatening problems in this intensive care setting (see Chapter 29).

Another new specialty to emerge within the last decade is the *maternity clinical specialist*. These clinicians undergo advanced study of maternity nursing at the graduate level, and are able to provide in-depth intervention for many of the adaptational and physiologic problems encountered in maternity care. Frequently clinical specialists have an area of expertise within the specialty field, such as a maternity clinical specialist with special expertise in the care of pregnant diabetics, breast-feeding mothers, parents experiencing neonatal death or abnormalities, Rh sensitized mothers, and so on. These nurses with Masters degrees also serve as consultants to other maternity nursing staff, assisting them to plan care for difficult problems or special situations encountered on the unit. Although clinical specialists may also be involved in staff education, their primary function is direct patient services utilizing a high degree of knowledge, skill, and competence in their area of specialty.[3]

The latest new role to emerge on the nursing scene is that of the *nurse practitioner*. Beginning in about 1965, physicians and nurses started working together in several settings to "broaden the role" of the nurse in provision of care to patients in ambulatory and out-patient settings. Impetus for such changes was provided by the health manpower crisis and disillusionment of the American public with its health care nonsystem which erupted during the mid-sixties. With an undersupply of physicians that was predicted to get worse, and underutilization of the knowledge and skills of hundreds of thousands of registered nurses, many voices cried out for an extension of the scope of nursing practice to help meet the health needs of the nation. Some nurses had previously been identifying health problems and providing limited treatment, notably in public health and private office settings, but their effectiveness was reduced by lack of a systematic approach and a body of knowledge to enable them to carry out treatment. As the nurse practitioner role evolved, it encompassed additional skills in the techniques of physical diagnosis which were formerly in the realm of medicine, as well as the knowledge base to diagnose and treat common problems and minor illness. Health prevention and maintenance, including examination, testing and education, as well as management of stabilized chronic illness are also included in nurse practitioner functions. The nurse practitioner combines the nurse's sensitivity to emotional needs and focus on adaptation and social aspects of patient care with the techniques and knowledge of medicine to diagnose and treat pathophysiologic problems. These nurses usually practice in a primary care setting, defined as the first contact in any given episode of illness with the health care system, and responsibility for continuance of care including maintenance of health, evaluation and management of symptoms, and appropriate referrals.[4,5]

The maternity nurse practitioner, or OB-GYN nurse practitioner, provides prenatal care for uncomplicated pregnancies with a physician consultant available. The nurse takes a health and pregnancy history, performs the physical and obstetrical examination, orders, and interprets laboratory and other diagnostic studies, plans for necessary treatments and medications in conjunction with the physician, and assesses family relationships and psychosocial needs. Throughout the pregnancy the nurse practitioner sees the woman on antepartal visits, sometimes alternating with the physician, and evaluates the progress of the pregnancy as well as manages minor physical problems. Information and counseling related to pregnancy and childbirth and assessment of the couple's adjustments and family problems are also part of the nurse practitioner's role. Referrals to community agencies, prepared childbirth classes, and other medical specialties may also be done. Most maternity nurse practitioners are skilled in provision of contraception, and can select appropriate methods for the patient including oral contraceptives, insertion of intrauterine devices, fitting for diaphragms, and teaching about the other methods.

Family nurse practitioners also provide care during pregnancy, as they are generalists who care for all family members similarly to family practice physicians. In addition to the functions described above for maternity nurse practitioners, family practitioners provide post-delivery care for the mother and newborn care. They are also able to care for the baby as it grows, thus providing continuity during the reproductive process except for the intrapartal phase.

Future possibilities

In speculating about the future of maternity nursing, several significant recent developments in health care and social patterns must be taken into consideration. Perhaps the most far-reaching is the declining birthrate in the United States, with its associated slowing of the rate of population increase. In the decade from 1940 to 1950 U.S. population increased 14.5 percent, and from 1950 to 1960, 18.5 percent. This led to predictions of even greater population increases for the following decade, with anticipation of the need for much greater numbers of health personnel in maternal and child care. During the 1960s, however, concern over the burgeoning world population and changing attitudes toward birth control led to widespread conviction of the need to limit population growth. Awareness of the world's ecological balance and finiteness of its resources also contributed to this, and a declining increase of population was seen after 1965. From 1960 to 1965 there was a 3.3 percent decrease in the rate of population growth, from 1965 to 1970 a 1.7 percent decrease, and from 1970 to 1973, an 11 percent decrease. Although the absolute number of people in the United States continued to increase every year, the rate of this increase slowed markedly. This is reflected in the declining birthrate, in which there were 3.73 million births in 1970, 3.26 million in 1972, and 3.14 million in 1973. While the U.S. population grew from 204.9 million in 1970 to 210.4 million in 1973, fewer babies were being born each year.

The most overt manifestation of the decrease in birthrate was the closing of maternity units in many small to moderate sized hospitals in this country. It became economically impossible to maintain these units because of a falling census, so consolidation of obstetrical services in a few designated hospitals became common. In some of the larger cities with higher concentrations of physicians, some obstetricians and pediatricians were hard-pressed to find enough business. However, the maldistribution of health care services continued as before, with lower income and inner city or outlying rural populations still left with inadequate services. With Zero Population Growth the watchword, some went so far as to say maternity nursing would soon be obsolete.

But, as we all know, women will continue to get pregnant and babies continue to be born, even though in decreased numbers. Maternity nursing will no doubt continue, but may need to expand its scope or change its focus. The desires of the consumers of maternity care also signify a growing need for changes, as the routinized and standardized care organized in settings most convenient for the providers rather than consumers of care are less and less acceptable. Parents are asking for full participation in all phases of childbearing, the right to be involved in decisions affecting their bodies and health, and the right to institute practices which they believe are important for the happiness and well-being of parents and baby. A growing body of literature and research is reaffirming the importance of early and continued close contact between mother and baby, a situation many of our modern hospital practices have made impossible to attain. The importance of natural practices, such as breast-feeding and avoidance of highly processed and chemically preserved foods suggests that health professionals support rather than discourage parents who wish to follow these practices. Question is being raised as to the appropriateness of routine delivery of normal, uncomplicated maternity patients in the acute hospital with its focus on disease and illness. New data about the importance of immediate, active intervention in delivery of high-risk pregnancies and the postdelivery care of depressed, sick or anoxic infants reinforce the need for highly trained personnel and well-equipped delivery rooms and intensive care nurseries, however. The situation appears paradoxical, and answers will not be easy. It is safe to say that what have come to be accepted as routine practices in the care of maternity and newborn patients are being seriously questioned by both experts and public.

Maternity nursing must enlarge its scope if it is to remain a viable entity. Narrow concentration on the processes of childbearing and newborn care limit the services the maternity nurse can offer the patient and family. Because reproduction is basically a sexual event, both physiologically and in terms of role and identity, the most obvious areas for extension of maternity are into sexuality and contraception. To some extent, this is now occurring. Abortion care is another natural extension, as it is a variation within the process of reproduction. Increasing expertise in early childhood development, and being familiar with the normal growth and development of children equips the nurse to provide much-needed assistance to families beyond the immediate childbearing period. Skill in counseling families and knowledge of family dynamics permit the nurse to be of service when problems or needs arise not only in integrating the new baby, but also with relationships between parents and other children and relatives. Another area with potential for involvement of maternity nurses is that of women's search for a satisfying identity and sense of productivity and self-realization, generally thought of as the "women's movement." With an inquisitive mind and open attitudes, and a willingness to question personal and social tenets, perhaps both nurse and patient could attain more satisfying levels of existence.

It is hard to predict where the nurse practitioner role will go, for this certainly embodies an enlargement of the scope of maternity and other nursing practice. One possibility is an eventual merging of maternity nurse practitioner with the nurse-midwife, resulting in provision of the full range of childbearing services by such nurses to uncomplicated cases. Should this occur, relationships with the medical profession would have to be altered, as physicians would primarily provide care to high-risk and complicated cases, perform gynecologic surgery, and serve as consultants to the nurses providing care during normal childbearing. Or, perhaps maternity nursing will split off into two separate specialties, one the nurse practitioner type involved in prenatal and postpartal followup, the other the acute hospital nurse involved in intrapartal and immediate postdelivery care. Nurse-midwifery undoubtedly will increase as restrictive laws change and programs develop to more equitably distribute care to all the American population.

Whatever the future portends, its hallmark will be change. Health care, medical care, and nursing care are all undergoing major upheavals as the decade of the seventies draws to a close. The issues of national health insurance, the role of third-party payers, problems with malpractice insurance, federal controls and peer review organizations, changing practice laws of nursing and medicine, the exorbitant costs of health care and the increasingly vociferous consumer advocacy movement, the development of health maintenance organizations and community health networks, all signify that health care in this country is experiencing radical changes. Maternity nursing must read the winds of change, and nursing leaders take initiative in shaping the new form this specialty will take in the years to come to serve the best interests and needs of families during all phases of childbearing.

Bibliography

1. Bullough, V. L., and Bullough, B.: *The Emergence of Modern Nursing.* Toronto, The Macmillan Co., Collier-Macmillan Canada, Ltd., 1969, pp. 4, 17, 28-29, 76-78.
2. Tanner, L. M.: The maternity nurse as counselor in human sexuality. In E. H. Anderson (ed.): *Current Concepts in Clinical Nursing.* St. Louis, Mosby, 1973, pp. 169-178.
3. Riehl, J. P., and McVay, J. W.: *The Clinical Nurse Specialist: Interpretations.* New York, Appleton-Century Crofts, 1973.
4. National Commission for the Study of Nursing and Nursing Education. Jerome Lysaught, Director. *An Abstract for Action.* New York, McGraw-Hill, 1970.
5. *Extending the Scope of Nursing Practice.* A Report of the Secretary's Committee to Study Extended Roles for Nurses. Washington, D.C., Department of Health, Education and Welfare, Nov. 1971.

Suggested Reading

ANDERSON, E. M., LEONARD, B. J., AND YATES, J. A.: Epigenesis of the nurse practitioner role. *Am. J. Nurs.* 74:1812-1816, Oct. 1974.

BARRETT, J.: The nurse specialist practitioner: A study. *Nurs. Outlook* 20:524-527, Aug. 1972.

CHANGING PATTERNS OF OBSTETRIC CARE. *Am. J. Nurs.* 73:1723-1727, Oct. 1973.

CONTEMPORARY NURSING SERIES: Maternal and newborn care: Nursing interventions. Compiled by M. H. Browning and E. P. Lewis. *Am. J. Nurs.* New York, 1973.

FOWLER, M. M.: The maternity nurse clinician in practice. In E. H. Anderson (ed.): *Current Concepts in Clinical Nursing.* St. Louis, Mosby, 1973, pp. 210-215.

GORDON, M.: The clinical specialist as change agent. *Nurs. Outlook* 17:37-39, Mar. 1969.

HEATON, C. E.: Obstetrics and gynecology in America. *N. Carolina Med. J.* 8:35, 1947.

———: Fifty years of progress in obstetrics and gynecology. *New York J. Med.* 51:83, 1951.

HELLMAN, L. M.: Nurse-midwifery in the United States. *Ob-Gyn.* 30:883-888, Dec. 1967.

HILLIARD, M. E.: The changing role of the maternity nurse. *Nurs. Clin. North Am.* 3:277-288, June 1968.

LUBIC, R. W.: Myths about nurse-midwifery. *Am. J. Nurs.* 74:268-269, Feb. 1974.

LYNAUGH, J. E., AND BATES, B.: Physical diagnosis: A skill for all nurses? *Am. J. Nurs.* 74:58-59, Jan. 1974.

MARTIN, L. M.: "I like being an FNP". *Am. J. Nurs.* 75:826-828, May 1975.

McCORMACK, G. B.: The visiting nurse becomes a nurse practitioner. *Nurs. Outlook* 22:119-123, Feb. 1974.

MERENESS, D.: Recent trends in expanding roles of the nurse. *Nurs. Outlook* 18:30-33, May 1970.

OZIMEK, D., AND YURA, H.: Who is the nurse practitioner? Dept. Bacc. and Higher Degree Prog., National League for Nursing, New York, Pub. No. 15-1555, 1975.

REED, D. E., AND ROGHMANN, K. J.: Acceptability of an expanded nurse role to nurses and physicians. *Med. Care* 9:372-377, July/Aug. 1971.

SMITH, M. R., et al: The RN obstetric assistant: A clinical trial. *Am. J. Ob-Gyn.* 38:308-312, Aug. 1971.

SPEERT, H.: Obstetrics and Gynecologic Milestones. New York, Macmillan, 1958.

THE NURSE PRACTITIONER QUESTION. Round table discussion. *Am. J. Nurs.* 74:2188-2191, Dec. 1974.

appendix

Answer Key for Study Questions
Glossary
Conversion Table for Weights of Newborn
Aid for Visualization of Cervical Dilatation

answer key

for Study Questions

UNIT II

1. A: Diagonal Conjugate
   B: Obstetrical Conjugate
   C: Tuberischii Diameter
2. A: B
   B: A
   C: C
3. C
4. A: 4
   B: 3
   C: 1
   D: 2
5. C
6. B
7. B
8. A: 2
   B: 3
   C: 3
9. B

10. A
11. C
12. A
13. C
14. B
15. B
16. B
17. A
18. 2
19. A
20. 4
21. D
22. B
23. A
24. A
25. B
26. B

UNIT III

1. 2
2. A, 3
   B, 3
3. B
4. B
5. F
6. C
7. C

8. A, 2
   B, 3
9. A: 1
   B: 3
   C: 3
10. A, 3
    B, 1
11. B

12. D
13. A
14. D
15. 1
16. 2
17. D

UNIT IV

1. A: Full Dilatations
   B: Effacement
   C: Amnisic
   D: Uterine Atony
   E: Episiotomy
   F: Lightening
2. Situation No. 1: 3
   Situation No. 2: 2
   Situation No. 3: 2
3. A, 2
   B, 3
   C, 2
4. 1

5. 3
6. C
7. B
8. 4
9. 2
10. 1
11. 3
12. A, 3
    B, 2
13. A, 3
    B, 1
    C, 4
    D, 4

UNIT V

1. 3
2. 2
3. 1: G
   2: D
   3: B
   4: C
   5: G
   6: G

7: D
8: G
4. 4
5. 2
6. 1
7. 3
8. 1
9. 1

10. 2
11. D
12. E
13. B
14. C
15. C
16. 2
17. 3

UNIT VI

1. 3
2. 2

3. 2
4. 1

5. 3
6. 1

UNIT VII

1. 1
2. 1
3. 3
4. 4
5. 2
6. 3
7. 1
8. 2
9. 4
10. 3

11. 3
12. 2
13. 2
14. 3
15. 4
16. 2
17. 4
18. 1
19. A
20. 3

21. B
22. 2
23. 1
24. 3
25. 2
26. 1
27. 1
28. 2

glossary

Note: The pronunciations indicated below follow Webster's Second International Dictionary.

āle, chȧotic, câre, ădd, ăccount, ärm, ȧsk, sofȧ; ēve, hẹre, êvent, ĕnd, silĕnt, makēr; īce, ĭll, charĭty; ōld, ȯbey, ôrb, ŏdd, soft, cŏnnect; fōͦd, fŏͦt; out; oil, cūbe, ûnite, ûrn, ŭp, circŭs, menü; chair; go; sing; then, thin; natûre; verdûre; k = ch in German ich or ach; bon; yet zh = z in azure

abdominal (ăb-dŏm'ĭ-năl). Belonging to or relating to the abdomen.

a. delivery. Delivery of the child by abdominal section. See *cesarean section.*

a. gestation. Ectopic pregnancy occurring in the cavity of the abdomen.

a. pregnancy. See *gestation* above.

ablatio placentae. See *abruptio placentae.*

abortion. The termination of pregnancy at any time before the fetus has attained a stage of viability, i.e., before it is capable of extrauterine existence.

abruptio placentae (ăb-rŭp'shĭ-ŏ plȧ-sen'tē). Premature separation of normally implanted placenta.

acromion (ȧ-krō'mĭ-ŏn). An outward extension of the spine of the scapula, used to explain presentation of the fetus.

adnexa (ăd-nĕk'sȧ). Appendages.

a., uterine (ū'tĕr-ĭn). The fallopian tubes and ovaries.

afibrinogenemia (ȧ-fī"brin-ō-jen-ē'mē-ă). Lack of fibrinogen in the blood.

afterbirth (ȧf'tĕr-bûrth"). The structures cast off after the expulsion of the fetus, including the membranes and the placenta with the attached umbilical cord; the secundines.

afterpains (ȧf'tĕr-pāns"). Those pains, more or less severe, after expulsion of the afterbirth, which result from the contractile efforts of the uterus to return to its normal condition.

agalactia (ăg'ȧ-lăk'shĭ-ȧ). Absence *or* failure of the secretion of milk.

allantois (ȧ-lăn'tȯ-ĭs). A tubular diverticulum of the posterior part of the yolk sac of the embryo; it passes into the body stalk through which it is accompanied by the allantoic (umbilical) blood vessel, thus taking part in the formation of the umbilical cord; and later, fusing with the chorion, it helps to form the placenta.

amenorrhea (ā-mĕn"ŏ-rē'ȧ). Absence or suppression of the menstrual discharge.

amnesia (ăm-nē'zhĭ-ȧ). Loss of memory.

amnion (ăm'nĭ-ŏn). The most internal of the fetal membranes, containing the waters which surround the fetus in utero.

amniotic (ăm"nĭ-ŏt-ĭk). Pertaining to the amnion.

a. sac. The "bag of membranes" containing the fetus before delivery.

analgesia (ăn"-ăl-jē'zī-a). Drug which relieves pain, used during labor.

androgen (ăn'drȯ-jĕn). Any substance which possesses masculinizing activities, such as the testis hormone.

android (ăn'droid). The term adopted for the male type of pelvis.

anencephalia (ăn-ĕn"sĕ-fā'lĭ-ȧ). Form of monstrosity with absence of a brain.

anovular (ăn-ōv'ŭ-lēr). Not accompanied with the discharge of an ovum; said of cyclic uterine bleeding.

anoxia (an-ox'e-ah). Oxygen deficiency; any condition of absence of tissue oxidation.

antenatal (ăn-tē-nā'tăl). Occurring or formed before birth.

antepartal (ăn"tĕ-pär'tal). Before labor and delivery or childbirth; prenatal.

areola (ȧ-rē'ȯ-lȧ). The ring of pigment surrounding the nipple.

secondary a. A circle of faint color sometimes seen just outside the original areola about the fifth month of pregnancy.

articulation (är-tĭk"ŭ-lā'shŭn). The fastening together of the various bones of the skeleton in their natural situation; a joint. The articulations of the bones of the body are divided into two principal groups—*synarthroses,* immovable articulations, and *diarthroses,* movable articulations.

Aschheim-Zondek test (ăsh"hīm-tsŏn'dĕk). A test for the diagnosis of pregnancy. Repeated injections of small quantities of urine voided during the first weeks of pregnancy produce in infantile mice, within 100 hours, 1) minute intrafollicular ovarian hemorrhage and 2) the development of lutein cells.

asphyxia (ăs-fĭk'sĭ-ȧ). Suspended animation; anoxia and carbon dioxide retention resulting from failure of respiration.

a. neonatorum (nē"ȯ-nȧ-tō'rŭm). "Asphyxia of the newborn," deficient respiration in newborn babies.

attitude (ăt'ĭ-tūd). A posture or position of the body. In obstetrics, the relation of the fetal members to each other in the uterus; the position of the fetus in the uterus.

axis (ăk′sĭs). A line about which any revolving body turns.

pelvic a. The curved line which passes through the centers of all the anteroposterior diameters of the pelvis.

bag of waters. The membranes which enclose the liquor amnii of the fetus.

ballottement (bă-lŏt′mĕnt). Literally means tossing. A term used in examination when the fetus can be pushed about in the pregnant uterus.

Bandl's ring (Bän′dls). A groove on the uterus at the upper level of the fully developed lower uterine segment; visible on the abdomen after hard labor as a transverse or slightly slanting depression between the umbilicus and the pubis. Shows overstretching of lower uterine segment. Resembles a full bladder.

Bartholin's glands (Bär′tô-lĭn). Glands situated one on each side of the vaginal canal opening into the groove between the hymen and the labia minora.

bicornate uterus (bī-kôr′nāt). Having two horns which, in the embryo, failed to attain complete fusion.

bimanual (bī-măn′ū-ăl). Performed with or relating to both hands.

b. palpation. Examination of the pelvic organs of a woman by placing one hand on the abdomen and the fingers of the other in the vagina.

blastoderm (blăs′tô-dûrm). Delicate germinal membrane of the ovum.

b. vesicle. Hollow space within the morula formed by the rearrangement of cells, and by proliferation.

Braxton Hicks sign. Painless uterine contractions occurring periodically throughout pregnancy, thereby enlarging the uterus to accommodate the growing fetus.

B.H. version. One of the types of operation designed to turn the baby from an undesirable position to a desirable one.

breech (brēch). Nates or buttocks.

b. delivery. Labor and delivery marked by breech presentations.

bregma (brĕg′mă). The point on the surface of the skull at the junction of the coronal and sagittal sutures.

brim (brĭm). The edge of the superior strait or inlet of the pelvis.

caked breast. See *engorgement*.

caput (kā′pŭt). 1. The head, consisting of the cranium, or skull, and the face. 2. Any prominent object, such as the head.

c. succedaneum (sŭk″sē-dā′nĕ-ŭm). A dropsical swelling which sometimes appears on the presenting head of the fetus during labor.

catamenia (kăt-ă-mē′nĭ-ă). See *menses*.

caudal (kô′dăl). The term applied to analgesia or anesthesia resulting from the introduction of the suitable analgesic or anesthetic solution into the caudal canal (nonclosure of the laminae of the last sacral vertebra).

caul (kôl). A portion of the amniotic sac which occasionally envelops the child's head at birth.

cephalhematoma (sĕf″ăl-hē″mă-tō′mă). A tumor or swelling between the bone and the periosteum caused by an effusion of blood.

cephalic (sĕ-făl′ĭk). Belonging to the head.

c. presentation. Presentation of any part of the fetal head in labor.

cervix (sûr′vĭks). Neckline part; the lower and narrow end of the uterus, between the os and the body of the organ.

cesarean section (sĕ-zâ′rĕ-ăn). Delivery of the fetus by an incision through the abdominal wall and the wall of the uterus.

Chadwick's sign (tshăd′wĭks). The violet color on the mucous membrane of the vagina just below the urethral orifice, seen after the fourth week of pregnancy.

change of life. See *climacteric*.

chloasma (klô-ăz′mă). Pl. *chloasmata*. A cutaneous affection exhibiting spots and patches of a yellowish-brown color. The term chloasma is a vague one and is applied to various kinds of pigmentary discoloration of the skin.

c. gravidarum, c. uterinum. Chloasma occurring during pregnancy.

chorioepithelioma (kō′rĭ-ō-ĕp-ĭ-thē-lĭ-ō′mă). Chorionic carcinoma; a tumor formed by malignant proliferation of the epithelium of the chorionic villi.

chorion (kō′rĭ-ŏn). The outermost membrane of the growing zygote, or fertilized ovum, which serves as a protective and nutritive covering.

chromosome (krō′mo-sōm). One of several small, dark-staining and more or less rod-shaped bodies which appear in the nucleus of the cell at the time of cell division and particularly in mitosis.

circumcision (sûr″kŭm-sĭzh′ŭn). The removal of all or part of the prepuce, or foreskin of the penis.

cleft palate (klĕft păl′ĭt). Congenital fissure of the palate and the roof of the mouth.

climacteric (klī-măk-tēr′ĭk). A particular epoch of the ordinary term of life at which the body undergoes a considerable change; especially, the menopause or "change of life."

clitoris (klī′tô-rĭs). A small, elongated, erectile body, situated at the anterior part of the vulva. An organ of the female homologous with the penis of the male.

coitus (kō′ĭt-ŭs). Sexual intercourse; copulation.

colostrum (kô-lŏs′trŭm). A substance in the first milk after delivery, giving to it a yellowish color.

c. corpuscles. Large granular cells found in colostrum.

colporrhaphy (kŏl-pōr′ă-fē). 1. The operation of suturing the vagina. 2. The operation of denuding and suturing the vaginal wall for the purpose of narrowing the vagina.

colpotomy (kŏl-pŏt′o-mē). Any surgical cutting operation upon the vagina.

conception (kŏn-sĕp′shŭn). The impregnation of the female ovum by the spermatozoon of the male, whence results a new being.

condyloma (con-dil-o′mah). Pl. *condylomata*. A wartlike excrescence near the anus or the vulva; the flat, moist papule of secondary syphilis.

confinement (kŏn-fīn′mĕnt). Term applied to childbirth and the lying-in period.

congenital (kŏn-jĕn′ĭ-tĕl). Born with a person; existing from or from before birth, as, for example, congenital disease, a disease originating in the fetus before birth.

conjugate (kŏn′jōō-gåt). The anteroposterior diameter of the pelvic inlet.

contraception (kŏn″trå-sĕp′shŭn). The prevention of conception or impregnation.

coronal (kŏr′ŏ-nål). Belonging to, or relating to, the crown of the head.

c. suture. The suture formed by the union of the frontal bone with the two parietal bones.

corpus luteum (kôr′pŭs lū′tē-ŭm). The yellow mass found in the graafian follicle after the ovum has been expelled.

cotyledon (kŏt″ĭ-lē′dŭn). Any one of the subdivisions of the uterine surface of the placenta.

cul-de-sac (kōōl′dē-săk′) **of Douglas.** A pouch between the anterior wall of the rectum and the uterus.

cyesis (sī-ē′sĭs). Pregnancy.

decrement (dĕk′rē-mĕnt). Decrease; also the stage of decline.

delivery (dē-lĭv′ĕr-ĭ). [French, *délivrer*, to free, to deliver.] 1. The expulsion of a child by the mother, or its extraction by the obstetric practitioner. 2. The removal of a part from the body; as *delivery* of the placenta.

dizygotic (dī″zī-gŏt′ĭk). Pertaining to or proceeding from two zygotes (ova).

Döderlein's bacillus (ded′er-līnz). The large gram-positive bacterium occurring in the normal vaginal secretion.

Douglas' cul-de-sac (kōōl′dē-săk′). A sac or recess formed by a fold of the peritoneum dipping down between the rectum and the uterus. Also called *pouch of Douglas* and *rectouterine pouch*.

ductus (dŭk′tŭs). A duct.

d. arteriosus (är-tē″rĭ-ō′sŭs). "Arterial duct," a blood vessel peculiar to the fetus, communicating directly between the pulmonary artery and the aorta.

d. venosus (vĕ-nō′sŭs). "Venous duct," a blood vessel peculiar to the fetus, establishing a direct communication between the umbilical vein and the inferior vena cava.

Duncan (dŭng′kăn) **mechanism.** The position of the placenta, with the maternal surface outermost; to be born edgewise.

dystocia (dĭs-tō′shĭ-å). Difficult, slow or painful birth or delivery. It is distinguished as *maternal* or *fetal* according as the difficulty is due to some deformity on the part of the mother or on the part of the child.

d., placental. Difficulty in delivering the placenta.

eclampsia (ĕk-lămp′sĭ-å). Acute "toxemia of pregnancy" characterized by convulsions and coma which may occur during pregnancy, labor or the puerperium.

ectoderm (ĕk′tō-dûrm). The outer layer of cells of the primitive embryo.

ectopic (ĕk-tŏp′ĭk). Out of place.

e. gestation. Gestation in which the fetus is out of its normal place in the cavity of the uterus. It includes gestations in the interstitial portion of the tube, in a rudimentary horn of the uterus (cornual pregnancy) and cervical pregnancy as well as tubal, abdominal and ovarian pregnancies. See also *extrauterine pregnancy*.

e. pregnancy. Same as *ectopic gestation*.

effacement (ĕ-fās′mĕnt). Obliteration. In obstetrics, refers to thinning and shortening of the cervix.

ejaculation (ĕ-jăk″ū-lā′shŭn). A sudden act of expulsion, as of semen.

embryo (ĕm′brĭ-ō). The product of conception in utero from the third through the fifth week of gestation; after that length of time it is called the fetus.

emphathy (ĕm′på-thĭ). The projection of one's own consciousness into that of another. Empathy may be distinguished from sympathy in that the former state includes relative freedom from emotional involvement.

endocervical (ĕn′dŏ-sûr′vĭ-kăl). Pertaining to the interior of the cervix of the uterus.

endometrium (ĕn″dŏ-mē′trĭ-ŭm). The mucous membrane which lines the uterus.

engagement (ĕn-gāj′mĕnt). In obstetrics, applies to the entrance of the presenting part into the superior pelvic strait and the beginning of the descent through the pelvic canal.

engorgement (ĕn-gôrj′mĕnt). Hyperemia; local congestion; excessive fullness of any organ or passage. In obstetrics, refers to an exaggeration of normal venous and lymph stasis of the breasts which occurs in relation to lactation.

entoderm (ĕn′tō-dûrm). The innermost layer of cells of the primitive embryo.

enzygotic (ĕn-zī-gŏt′ĭk). Developed from the same fertilized ovum.

episiotomy (ĕp″ĭs-ĭ-ot′ŏ-mĭ). Surgical incision of the vulvar orifice for obstetric purposes.

Erb's paralysis. Partial paralysis of the brachial plexus, affecting various muscles of the arm and the chest wall.

ergot (ûr′gŏt). A drug having the remarkable property of exciting powerfully the contractile force of the uterus, and chiefly used for this purpose, but its long-continued use is highly dangerous. Usually given in the fluid extract.

erythroblastosis fetalis (ĕ-rĭth″rŏ-blăs-tō′sĭs). A severe hemolytic disease of the newborn usually due to Rh incompatibility.

estrogen (ĕs′trŏ-jĕn). A hormone secreted by the ovary and the placenta.

extraperitoneal (ĕks″trȧ-pĕr-ĭ-tŏ-nē′ăl). Situated or occurring outside the peritoneal cavity.

extrauterine (ĕks″trȧ-ū′tĕr-ĭn). Outside of the uterus.

   e. pregnancy. Pregnancy in which the fetus is contained in some organ outside of the uterus, i.e., tubal, abdominal and ovarian pregnancies.

fallopian (fă-lō′pĭ-ăn). [Relating to G. *Fallopius,* a celebrated Italian anatomist of the 16th century.]

   f. tubes. The oviducts—two canals extending from the sides of the fundus uteri.

fecundation (fē″kŭn-dā′shŭn). The act of impregnating or the state of being impregnated; the fertilization of the ovum by means of the male seminal element.

fertility (fĕr-tĭl′ĭ-tĭ). The ability to produce offspring; power of reproduction.

fertilization (fûr-tĭ-lĭ-zā′shŭn). The fusion of the spermatozoon with the ovum; it marks the beginning of pregnancy.

fetus (fē′tŭs). The baby in utero from the end of the fifth week of gestation until birth.

fimbria (fĭm′brĭ-ȧ). A fringe; especially the fringe-like end of the fallopian tube.

fontanel (fŏn″tȧ-nĕl′). The diamond-shaped space between the frontal and two parietal bones in very young infants. This is called the *anterior f.* and is the familiar "soft spot" just above a baby's forehead. A small, triangular one (*posterior f.*) is between the occipital and parietal bones.

foramen (fŏ-rā′mĕn). A hole, opening, aperture or orifice—especially one through a bone.

   f. ovale (ŏ-vā′lē). An opening situated in the partition which separates the right and left auricles of the heart in the fetus.

foreskin (fōr′skĭn). The prepuce—the fold of skin covering the glans penis.

fornix (fôr′nĭks). Pl. *fornices* (fôr′nĭ-sēz). An arch; any vaulted surface.

   f. of the vagina. The angle of reflection of the vaginal mucous membrane onto the cervix uteri.

fourchette (fŏŏr-shĕt′). [French, "fork."] The posterior angle or commissure of the labia majora.

frenum (frē′nŭm). Lingual fold of integument or of mucous membrane that checks, curbs, or limits the movements of the tongue (ankyloglossia). Congenital shortening.

Friedman's test (frēd′măn). A modification of the Aschheim-Zondek test for pregnancy; the urine of early pregnancy is injected in 4-ml. doses intravenously twice daily for two days into an unmated mature rabbit. If, at the end of this time, the ovaries of the rabbit contain fresh corpora lutea or hemorrhagic corpora, the test is positive.

FSH. Abbreviation for follicle-stimulating hormone.

fundus (fŭn′dŭs). The upper rounded portion of the uterus between the points of insertion of the fallopian tubes.

funic souffle (fū′nĭc sŏŏ′f′l). A soft, blowing sound, synchronous with the fetal heart sounds and supposed to be produced in the umbilical cord.

funis (fū′nĭs). A cord—especially the umbilical cord.

galactagogue (gȧ-lăk′tȧ-gŏg). 1. Causing the flow of milk. 2. Any drug which causes the flow of milk to increase.

galactorrhea (gă-lak-tō-re′ȧ). Excessive flow of milk.

gamete (găm′ēt). A sexual cell; a mature germ cell, as an unfertilized egg or a mature sperm cell.

gastrula (găs′trŏŏ-lȧ). The early embryonic stage which follows the blastula.

gene (jēn). An hereditary germinal factor in the chromosome which carries on an hereditary transmissible character.

genitalia (jĕn-ĭtăl′ĭ-ȧ). The reproductive organs.

gestation (jĕs-tā-shŭn). The condition of pregnancy; pregnancy; gravidity.

gonad (gŏn′ăd). A gamete-producing gland; an ovary or testis.

gonadotropin (gŏn″ăd-ŏ-trō′pĭn). A substance having an affinity for or a stimulating effect on the gonads.

Goodell's sign (gŏŏd′elz). Softening of the cervix, a presumptive sign of pregnancy.

graafian follices or **vesicles** (grăf′ĭ-ăn). Small spherical bodies in the ovaries, each containing an ovum.

gravida (grăv′ĭd-ä). A pregnant woman.

habitus (hăb′ĭt-ŭs). Attitude, disposition or tendency; to act in a certain way; position acquired by frequent repetition.

Hegar's sign (hā′gärz). Softening of the lower uterine segment; a sign of pregnancy.

homologous (hŏ-mŏl′ŏ-gŭs). Corresponding in structure or origin; derived from the same source.

hormone (hôr′mōn). A chemical substance produced in an organ, which, being carried to an associated organ by the blood stream, excites in the latter organ a functional activity.

hydatidiform (hi″dah-tid′ĭ-form) **mole.** Cystic proliferation of chorionic villi, resembling a bunch of grapes.

hydramnios (hī-drăm′nĭ-ŏs). An excessive amount of amniotic fluid.

hymen (hī′mĕn). A membranous fold which partially or wholly occludes the external orifice of the vagina, especially in the virgin.

hypofibrinogenemia (hī″pŏ-fī-brĭn″ō-jen-ē′mē-ȧ). Deficiency of fibrinogen in the blood.

hypogalactia (hī″pŏ-gă-lăk′she-a). Deficiency in the secretion of milk.

hypoxia (hī-pŏks′ĭ-a). Insufficient oxygen to support normal metabolic requirements.

iliopectineal line (ĭl″ĭ-ŏ-pĕk-tĭn′ē-ăl). The linea terminalis.

impregnation (ĭm″prĕg-nā′shŭn). See *fertilization.*

increment (ĭn′krĕ-mĕnt). That by which anything is increased.

inertia (in-ûr′shĭ-a). Inactivity; inability to move spontaneously. Sluggishness of uterine contractions during labor.

infant (ĭn′fănt). A baby; a child under two years of age.

infertility (ĭn-fûr-tĭl′ĭ-tĭ). The condition of being unfruitful or barren; sterility.

inlet (ĭn′lĕt). The upper limit of the pelvic cavity (brim).

introitis (ĭn-trō′ĭ-tŭs). A term applied to the opening of the vagina.

in utero. Inside the uterus.

inversion (ĭn-vûr′shŭn). A turning upside down, inside out, or end for end.
  i. of the uterus. The state of the womb being turned inside out, caused by violently drawing away the placenta before it is detached by the natural process of labor.

involution (ĭn″vō-lū′shŭn). 1. A rolling or pushing inward. 2. A retrograde process of change which is the reverse of evolution: particularly applied to the return of the uterus to its normal size and condition after parturition.

ischium (ĭs′kĭ-ŭm). The posterior and inferior bone of the pelvis, distinct and separate in the fetus or the infant, or the corresponding part of the innominate bone in the adult.

jelly (jĕl′ĭ). A soft substance which is coherent, tremulous, and more or less transparent.
  j. of Wharton. The soft, pulpy, connective tissue that constitutes the matrix of the umbilical cord.

labia (lā′bĭ-a). The nominative plural of *labium.* Lips or liplike structures.
  l. majora (ma-jō′ra). The folds of skin containing fat and covered with hair which form each side of the vulva.
  l. minora (mĭ-nō′ra). The nymphae, or folds of delicate skin inside of the labia majora.

labor (lā′bēr). Parturition; the series of processes by which the products of conception are expelled from the mother's body.

lactation (lăk-tā′shŭn). The act or period of giving milk; the secretion of milk; the time or period of secreting milk.

lambdoid (lăm′doid). Having the shape of the Greek letter λ (lambda).
  l. suture. The suture between the occipital and two parietal bones.

lanugo (la-nū′gō). The fine hair on the body of the fetus. The fine, downy hair found on nearly all parts of the body except the palms of the hands and the soles of the feet.

leukorrhea (lū″kŏ-rē′a). A whitish discharge from the female genital organs.

LH. Abbreviation for luteinizing hormone.

lightening (līt′n-ĭng). The sensation of decreased abdominal distention produced by the descent of the uterus into the pelvic cavity, which occurs from 2 to 3 weeks before the onset of labor.

linea (lĭn′ē-a). Pl. *lineae* (lĭn′ē-ē). A line or thread.
  l. alba (ăl′ba). The central tendinous line extending from the pubic bone to the ensiform cartilage.
  l. nigra (nī′grä). A dark line appearing on the abdomen and extending from the pubis toward the umbilicus—considered one of the signs of pregnancy.
  l. terminalis. The oblique ridge on the inner surface of the ilium, continued on the pubis, which separates the true from the false pelvis. Formerly called the iliopectineal line.

lingua (lĭng′gwĭ). Tongue.
  l. frenum. Tonguetie.

liquor (lĭk′ēr). A liquid.
  l. amnii (lĭ′kwôr ăm′nĭ-ī). The fluid contained within the amnion in which the fetus floats.

lochia (lō′kĭ-a). The discharge from the genital canal during several days subsequent to delivery.

mask (máski) of pregnancy. See *chloasma.*

maturation (măt″ŭ-rā′shŭn). In biology, a process of cell division during which the number of chromosomes in the germ cells is reduced to one half the number characteristic of the species.

meatus (mĕ-ā′tŭs). A passage; an opening leading to a canal, duct or cavity.
  m. urinarius (ū″-rĭ-nā′rĭ-ŭs). The external orifice of the urethra.

mechanism (mĕk′a-niz′m). The manner of combinations which subserve a common function. In obstetrics refers to labor and delivery.

meconium (mĕ-kō′nĭ-ŭm). The dark-green or black substance found in the large intestine of the fetus or newly born infant.

menarche (mĕ-när′kĕ). The establishment or the beginning of the menstrual function.

menopause (mĕn′ō-pŏz). The period at which menstruation ceases; the "change of life."

menorrhagia (mĕn″ō-rā′jĭ-a). An abnormally profuse menstrual flow.

menses (mĕn′sēz). [Pl. of Latin *mensis,* month.] The periodic monthly discharge of blood from the uterus; the catamenia.

menstruation (mĕn″strōo-ā′shŭn). The cyclic, physiologic uterine bleeding which normally recurs at approximately four-week intervals, in the absence of pregnancy, during the reproductive period.

mentum (mĕn′tŭm). The chin.

mesoderm (mĕs′ŏ-dûrm). The middle layer of cells derived from the primitive embryo.

metrorrhagia (mē-trŏ-rā′jĭ-à). Abnormal uterine bleeding.

migration (mī-grā′shŭn). In obstetrics refers to the passage of the ovum from the ovary to the uterus.

milia (mĭl′ē-ă). Plural of *milium*.

milium (mĭl′ē-ŭm). A small white nodule of the skin, usually caused by clogged sebaceous glands or hair follicles.

milk-leg. See *phlegmasia alba dolens.*

miscarriage (mĭs-kăr′ĭj). Abortion.

molding (mōld′ĭng). The shaping of the baby's head so as to adjust itself to the size and shape of the birth canal.

monozygotic (mŏn″ŏ-zī-gŏ′tĭk). Pertaining to or derived from one zygote.

  m. twins (mŏn″ŏ-zī-gŏ′tĭk). Pertaining to or derived from one zygote.

mons veneris (mŏnz vĕn′ĕ-rĭs). The eminence in the upper and anterior part of the pubes of women.

Montgomery's tubercles (mŭnt-gŭm′ĕr-ĭz). Small, nodular follicles or glands on the areolae around the nipples.

multigravida (mŭl″tĭ-grăv′ĭ-dà). A woman who has been pregnant several times, or many times.

multipara (mŭl-tĭp′à-rà). A woman who has borne several, or many, children.

navel (nāv′ĕl). The umbilicus.

neonatal (nē″ŏ-nā′tăl). Pertaining to the newborn, usually considered the first four weeks of life.

nevus (nē′vŭs). A natural mark or blemish; a mole, a circumscribed deposit of pigmentary matter in the skin present at birth (birthmark).

nidation (nĭ-dā′shŭn). The implantation of the fertilized ovum in the endometrium of the pregnant uterus.

nullipara (nŭ-lĭp′à-rà). A woman who has not borne children.

occipitobregmatic (ŏk-sĭp″ĭt-ŏ-brĕg-măt′-ik). Pertaining to the occiput (the back part of the head) and the bregma (junction of the coronal and sagittal sutures).

oligohydramnios (ŏl″ĭ-gŏ-hī-drăm′nĭ-ŏs). Deficiency of amniotic fluid.

omphalic (ŏm-făl′ĭk). Pertaining to the umbilicus.

oocyesis (ō′ŏ-sī-ē′sĭs). Ovarian pregnancy.

ophthalmia neonatorum (ŏf-thăl′mĭ-à). Acute purulent conjunctivitis of the newborn usually due to gonorrheal infection.

os (ŏs). Pl. *ora* (ō′rà). Mouth.

  o. externum (*external os*). The external opening of the canal of the cervix.

  o. internum (*internal os*). Internal opening of canal of cervix.

  o. uteri. "Mouth of the uterus."

ova. Plural of ovum.

ovary (ō′và-rĭ). The sexual gland of the female in which the ova are developed. There are two ovaries, one at each side of the pelvis.

ovulation (ō-vŭ-lā′shŭn). The growth and discharge of an unimpregnated ovum, usually coincident with the menstrual period.

ovum (ō′vŭm). The female reproductive cell. The human ovum is a round cell about 1⁄120 of an inch in diameter, developed in the ovary.

oxytocic (ŏk″sĭ-tō′sĭk). 1. Accelerating parturition. 2. A medicine which accelerates parturition.

oxytocin (ŏk-sĭ-tō-sĭn). One of the two hormones secreted by the posterior pituitary.

palsy (pôl′zĭ). A synonym for paralysis, used in connection with certain special forms.

  Bell's p. Peripheral facial paralysis due to lesion of the facial nerve, resulting characteristic distortion of the face.

  Erb's p. The upper-arm type of brachial birth palsy.

para (păr′à). The term used to refer to past pregnancies which have produced an infant which has been viable, whether or not the infant is dead or alive at birth.

parametrium (păr-à-mē′trĭ-ŭm). The fibrous subserous coat of the supravaginal portion of the uterus, extending laterally between the layers of the broad ligaments.

parity (păr′ĭ-tĭ). The condition of a woman with respect to her having borne children.

parovarian (păr-ŏ-vâr′ĭ-ăn). Pertaining to the residual structure in the broad ligament between the ovary and the fallopian tube.

parturient (păr-tū′rĭ-ĕnt). Bringing forth; pertaining to childbearing. A woman in childbirth.

parturition (păr″tŭ-rĭsh′ŭn). The act or process of giving birth to a child.

patulous (păt′ŭ-lŭs). Spreading somewhat widely apart; open.

pelvimeter (pĕl-vĭm′ē-tēr). An instrument for measuring the diameters and capacity of the pelvis.

pelvimetry (pĕl-vĭm′ē-trĭ). The measurement of the dimensions and capacity of the pelvis.

penis (pē′nĭs). The male organ of copulation.

perineorrhaphy (pĕr″ĭ-nē-ŏr′à-fĭ). Suture of the perineum; the operation for the repair of lacerations of the perineum.

perineotomy (pĕr′ĭ-nē-ŏt′ō-mĭ). A surgical incision through the perineum.

perineum (pĕr″ĭ-nē′ŭm). The area between the vagina and the rectum.

peritoneum (pĕr″ĭ-tŏ-nē′ŭm). A strong serous membrane investing the inner surface of the abdominal walls and the viscera of the abdomen.

phimosis (fī-mō′sĭs). Tightness of the foreskin.

phlegmasia alba dolens (flĕg-mā'zhĭ'a ăl'ba dō'lĕnz). Phlebitis of the femoral vein, occasionally following delivery.

Pitocin (pī-tŏ'sĭn). A proprietary solution of oxytocin.

placenta (pla-sĕn'ta). The circular flat, vascular structure in the impregnated uterus forming the principal medium of communication between the mother and the fetus.

   ablatio p. See *abruptio placentae.*

   abruptio p. Premature separation of the normally implanted placenta.

   previa p. A placenta which is implanted in the lower uterine segment so that it adjoins or covers the internal os of the cervix.

polygalactia (pŏl″ē-ga-lăk'shē-a). Excessive secretion of milk.

polyhydramnios (pŏl″ĭ-hī-drăm'nĭ-ŏs). Hydramnios.

position (pô-zĭsh'ŭn). The situation of the fetus in the pelvis; determined by the relation of some arbitrarily chosen portion of the fetus to the right or the left side of the mother's pelvis.

postnatal (pōst-nā'tăl). Occurring after birth.

postpartal (pōst-pär'tal). After delivery or childbirth.

preeclampsia (prē-ĕk-lămp'sĭ-a). A disorder encountered during pregnancy or early in the puerperium, characterized by hypertension, edema and albuminuria.

pregnancy (prĕg'năn-sĭ). [Latin, *praeg'nans,* literally "previous to bringing forth."] The state of being with young or with child. The normal duration of pregnancy in the human female is 280 days, or 10 lunar months, or 9 calendar months.

premature infant. An infant which weighs 2,500 Gm. or less at birth.

prepuce (prē'pūs). The fold of skin which covers the glans penis in the male.

   p. of the clitoris. The fold of mucous membrane which covers the glans clitoris.

presentation (prĕ″zĕn-tā'shŭn). Term used to designate that part of the fetus nearest the internal os; or that part which is felt by the physician's examining finger when introduced into the cervix.

primigravida (prī″mĭ-grăv'ĭ-da). Pl. *primigravidae* (prī″mĭ-grăv'ĭ-dē). A woman who is pregnant for the first time.

primipara (prī-mĭp'a-ra). Pl. *primiparae* (prī-mĭp'a-rē). A woman who has given birth to her first child.

primordial (prī-môr'dĭ-ăl). Original or primitive; of the simplest and most undeveloped character.

prodromal (prō-drō'măl). Premonitory; indicating the approach of a disease.

progesterone (prō-jĕs'tĕr-ōn). The pure hormone contained in the corpora lutea whose function is to prepare the endometrium for the reception and development of the fertilized ovum.

prolactin (prō-lăk'tĭn). A proteohormone from the anterior pituitary which stimulates lactation in the mammary glands.

prolan (prō'lăn). Zondek's term for the gonadotropic principle of human-pregnancy urine, responsible for the biologic pregnancy tests.

promontory (prŏm'ŭn-tō″rĭ). A small projection; a prominence.

   p. of the sacrum. The superior or projecting portion of the sacrum when in situ in the pelvis, at the junction of the sacrum and the last lumbar vertebra.

pseudocyesis (sū″dō-sī-ē'sĭs). An apparent condition of pregnancy; the woman really believes she is pregnant when, as a matter of fact, she is not.

puberty (pū'bĕr-tĭ). The age at which the generative organs become functionally active.

pubic (pū'bĭk). Belonging to the pubis.

pubiotomy (pū'bī-ŏt'ô-mĭ). The operation of cutting through the pubic bone lateral to the median line.

pubis (pū'bĭs). The os pubis or pubic bone forming the front of the pelvis.

pudendal (pū-dĕn'dăl). Relating to the pudenda.

pudendum (pū-dĕn'dŭm). [Latin, *pude're,* to have shame or modesty.] The external genital parts of either sex, but especially of the female.

puerperium (pū″ĕr-pē'rĭ-ŭm). The period elapsing between the termination of labor and the return of the uterus to its normal condition, about six weeks.

quickening (kwĭk'ĕn-ĭng). The mother's first perception of the movements of the fetus.

rabbit test. See *Friedman's test.*

Rh. Abbreviation for *Rhesus,* a type of monkey. This term is used for a property of human blood cells, because of its relationship to a similar property in the blood cells of *Rhesus* monkeys.

Rh factor. A term applied to an inherited antigen in the human blood.

Ritgen maneuver (rĭt'gĕn). Delivery of the infant's head by lifting the head upward and forward through the vulva, between contractions, by pressing with the tips of the fingers upon the perineum behind the anus.

Schultze's mechanism (shoŏlt'sĕz). The expulsion of the placenta with the fetal surfaces presenting.

secundine (sĕk'ŭn-dīn). The afterbirth; the placenta and membranes expelled after the birth of a child.

segmentation (sĕg″mĕn-tā'shŭn). The process of division by which the fertilized ovum multiplies before differentiation into layers occurs.

semen (sē'mĕn). 1. A seed. 2. The fluid secreted by the male reproductive organs.

show (shō). 1. Popularly, the blood-tinged mucus discharged from the vagina before or during labor.

Skene's gland. Two glands just within the meatus of the female urethra; regarded as homologues of the prostate gland in the male.

smegma. A thick cheesy secretion found under the prepuce and in the region of the clitoris and the labia minora.

souffle (soof'f'l). A soft, blowing auscultatory sound.

funic s. A hissing souffle synchronous with the fetal heart sounds and supposed to be produced in the umbilical cord.

placental s. A souffle supposed to be produced by the blood current in the placenta.

spermatozoon (spûr″ma-tô-zō'ŏn). Pl. *spermatozoa* (spûr″ma-tô-zō'a). The mobile microscopic sexual element of the male, resembling in shape an elongated tadpole. The male reproductive cell.

stillborn (stĭl'bôrn″). Born without life; born dead.

stria (strī'a). Pl. *striae* (strī'ē). A Latin word signifying a "groove," "furrow" or "crease."

striae gravidarum (grăv-ĭ-där'ŭm). Shining, reddish lines upon the abdomen, thighs and breasts during pregnancy.

subinvolution (sŭb'ĭn-vô-lū'shŭn). Failure of a part to return to its normal size and condition after enlargement from functional activity, as subinvolution of the uterus which exists when normal involution of the puerperal uterus is retarded.

succedaneum (sŭk'sĕ-dā'nĕ-ŭm). See *caput*.

superfecundation (sū'pēr-fē-kŭn-dā'shŭn). The fertilization at about the same time of two different ova by sperm from different males.

superfetation (sū'pēr-fĕ-tā'shŭn). The fecundation of a woman already pregnant.

symphysis (sĭm'fĭ-sĭs). The union of bones by means of an intervening substance; a variety of synarthrosis.

s. pubis (pū'bĭs). "Symphysis of the pubis," the pubic articulation or union of the pubic bones which are connected with each other by inter-articular cartilage.

synchondrosis (sĭng″kŏn-drō'sĭs). A union of bones by means of a fibrous or elastic cartilage.

testicle (tĕs'tĭ-k'l). One of the two glands contained in the male scrotum.

thrush. An infection caused by the fungus *Candida albicans,* characterized by whitish plaques in the mouth.

tonguetie. See *lingua frenum*.

toxemia (tŏks-ē'mĭ-a). The toxemias of pregnancy are disorders encountered during gestation, or early in the puerperium, which are characterized by one or more of the following signs: hypertension, edema, albuminuria, and in severe cases, convulsions and coma.

trichomonas (trĭk-ŏm'ô-năs). A genus of parasitic flagellate protozoa.

t. vaginalis. A species sometimes found in the vagina.

trophectoderm (trŏf-ĕk'tô-dûrm). The outer layer of cells of the early blastodermic vesicle; it develops the trophoderm—the feeding layer.

umbilical (ŭm-bĭl'ĭ-kăl). Pertaining to the umbilicus.

u. arteries. The arteries which accompany and form part of the umbilical cord.

u. cord [Latin, *funis umbilicalis*]. The cord connecting the placenta with the umbilicus of the fetus, and at the close of gestation principally made up of the two umbilical arteries and the umbilical vein, encased in a mass of gelatinous tissue called "Wharton's jelly."

u. hernia. Hernia at or near the umbilicus.

u. vein. Forms a part of the umbilical cord.

uterus (ū'tēr-ŭs). The hollow muscular organ in the female designed for the lodgement and nourishment of the fetus during its development until birth.

vagina (va-jī'na). [Latin, a sheath.] The canal in the female, extending from the vulva to the cervix of the uterus.

vernix caseosa (vûr'nĭks kā″sĕ-ō'sa). "Cheesy varnish." The layer of fatty matter which covers the skin of the fetus.

version (vûr'shŭn). The act of turning; specifically, a turning of the fetus in the uterus so as to change the presenting part and bring it into more favorable position for delivery.

vertex (vûr'tĕks). The summit or top of anything. In anatomy, the top or crown of the head.

v. presentation. Presentation of the vextex of the fetus in labor.

vestibule (vĕs'tĭ-būl). A triangular space between the labia minora; the urinary meatus and the vagina open into it.

viable (vī'a-b'l). A term in medical jurisprudence signifying "able or likely to live"; applied to the condition of the child at birth.

villus (vĭl'ŭs). A small vascular process or protrusion growing on a mucous surface, such as the chorionic villi seen in tufts on the chorion of the early embryo.

vulva (vŭl'va). The external genitals of the female.

Wharton's jelly (hwôr'tŭnz). [Thomas *Wharton,* English anatomist, died 1673.] The jellylike mucous tissue composing the bulk of the umbilical cord.

witches' milk (wĭch'ĕz). A milky fluid secreted from the breast of the newly born.

womb (woom). See *uterus*.

zona pellucida (zō'na pĕll-ū'sĭd-ä). A transparent belt; translucent or shining through.

zygote (zī'gōt). A cell resulting from the fusion of two gametes.

Conversion Table for Weights of Newborn

(Gram equivalents for pounds and ounces)

For example, to find weight in pounds and ounces of baby weighing 3315 grams, glance down columns to figure nearest 3315 = 3317. Refer to number at top of column for pounds and number to far left for ounces = 7 pounds, 5 ounces.

POUNDS→ OUNCES↓	3	4	5	6	7	8	9	10
0	1361	1814	2268	2722	3175	3629	4082	4536
1	1389	1843	2296	2750	3203	3657	4111	4564
2	1417	1871	2325	2778	3232	3685	4139	4593
3	1446	1899	2353	2807	3260	3714	4167	4621
4	1474	1928	2381	2835	3289	3742	4196	4649
5	1503	1956	2410	2863	3317	3770	4224	4678
6	1531	1984	2438	2892	3345	3799	4252	4706
7	1559	2013	2466	2920	3374	3827	4281	4734
8	1588	2041	2495	2948	3402	3856	4309	4763
9	1616	2070	2523	2977	3430	3884	4338	4791
10	1644	2098	2551	3005	3459	3912	4366	4819
11	1673	2126	2580	3033	3487	3941	4394	4848
12	1701	2155	2608	3062	3515	3969	4423	4876
13	1729	2183	2637	3090	3544	3997	4451	4904
14	1758	2211	2665	3118	3572	4026	4479	4933
15	1786	2240	2693	3147	3600	4054	4508	4961

Or, to convert grams into pounds and *decimals* of a pound, multiply weight in grams by .0022. Thus, 3317 × .0022 = 7.2974, i.e., 7.3 pounds, or 7 pounds, 5 ounces.

To convert pounds and ounces into grams, multiply the pounds by 453.6 and the ounces by 28.4 and add the two products. Thus, to convert 7 pounds, 5 ounces, 7 × 453.6 = 3175; 5 × 28.4 = 142; 3175 + 142 = 3317 grams.

Aid for Visualization

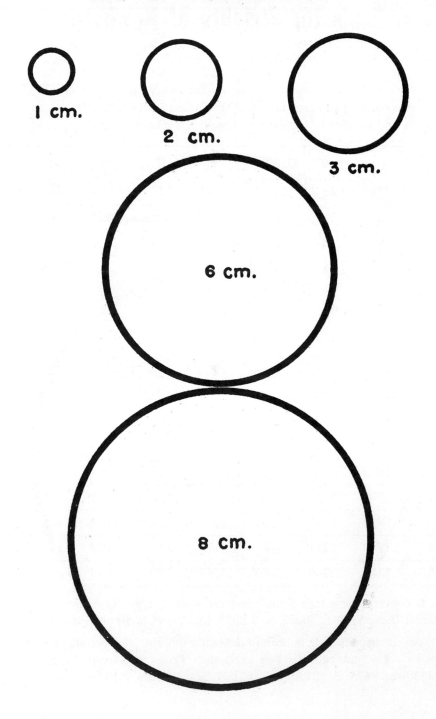

# of Cervical Dilatation

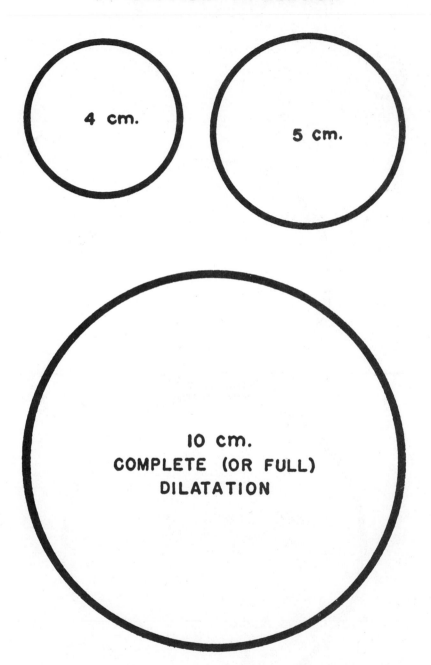

index

Page numbers in italics refer to tables.

Abdomen:
  changes in, during pregnancy, 147, 149, 155-56
  examination of, during labor, 310-11
  lifting of, 281-82
  postpartal involution, 361
  support garments for, 201
Abdominal pregnancy, 479
ABO hemolytic disease, 545-46
Abortion, 54, 474-77
  causes, 14, 475-76, 549, 550
  classification of, 474-75
  incomplete, 475
  inevitable, 474-75
  with intrauterine device, 125
  laws regarding, 129, 668, 669, 672
  and maternal mortality, 43, 131, 464
  prevention of, 90, 474
  procedures for, 129-31
  rate of, 14
  Rh factor in, 545
  risks of, 121
  therapeutic, indications for, 484, 549-50 (see also Genetic counseling)
  treatment of patient, 476-77
  tubal, 478
  United States Supreme Court ruling, 129, 475, 669, 672
Abruptio placentae, 481-82
  and hemorrhage, 508
  and hypertension, 549
Abscess of breast, 524-25
Acidosis, detection of, in fetus, 543-44
Adolescence, 119
Adoption:
  and conception, 136
  difficulty of, 121
After-pains, 362-63
Agalactia, 522
Age. See Gestational age; Maternal age
Albuminuria, 465, 466
Alcohol, and lactation, 391
Alimentary tract, congenital obstructions of, 608-9
Altitude, and infant size, 557
Ambulation, postpartal, 362, 365, 372-73, 518, 520
Amenorrhea, 91, 123-24
American Academy of Pediatrics, 199, 601, 668
American Association for Maternal and Child Health, 667

American Association for Maternal and Infant Health, 667
American Association for the Study and Prevention of Infant Mortality, 663-64
American Association of Obstetrics and Gynecology and Abdominal Surgeons, 666
American Child Health Association, 664, 666
American Child Hygiene Association, 664
American College of Nurse-Midwifery, 637, 667
American College of Nurse-Midwives, 637, 638
American College of Obstetricians and Gynecologists, 637, 638, 639, 668
American Committee of Maternal Welfare, 464-65, 665, 667
American Congress of Obstetrics and Gynecology, 665
American Gynecological Society, 666
American Institute of Family Relations, 225
American Medical Association, 188, 661, 666
American Nurses Association, 668, 669
American Public Health Association, 641
American Society for Prophylaxis in Obstetrics, 224
Amnesia, induction for labor, 291
Amniocentesis:
  to assess gestational age, 558
  to detect congenital abnormalities, 535, 536
  first use of, 668
  meconium in, 531
  procedure for, 538-39
  in prolonged pregnancy, 549
  and Rh disease, 547
  risks of, 538
  and trisomy, 611
Amniography, 529, 535
Amnion, 108
Amnioscopy, 534
Amniotic fluid:
  aspiration of, by newborn, 593
  embolism, 509-10
  and lungs of fetus, 398
  studies of, 531-32, 534, 535. See also Amniocentesis
  weight of, 148
Amniotomy, 457-58

Amputation, congenital, 612
Analgesia, for labor, 325. See also Anesthesia
Anatomy, reproductive, 65-84
Androgens, 376
Andrology, 132
Anemia:
  fetal, 534, 546-47
  physiologic neonatal, 400
  among poor, 57
  during pregnancy, 149, 485-86
  in premature infant, 565
Anencephaly, 535, 536, 604
Anesthesia, 289-98. See also types of anesthesia
  administration of, prior to delivery, 329
  for forceps delivery, 450-51
  general, 296-98
  history of, 662
  in premature births, 568
  and reaction to birth, 338-39
  regional, 291-96
  and special obstetrical problems, 298
  spinal, ambulation following, 372-73
  and urinary retention, 373
Anesthesiologist, 591
Anger, and pain, 266
Antepartal care, 161-215. See also Pregnancy
  for alternate lifestyle parents, 32-33
  in community setting, 177-78
  general hygiene counseling, 195-206, 516
  history of, 12, 663, 664, 665
  initial visit, 167-68, 174
  instructions to patients, 170, 172-74
  nutrition counseling, 179-95
  physical examination, 168, 174-77
  preparations for baby, 212-14
  preventive care, 162-65
  and social class, 46-47
  supervision of, 165-70
Anticoagulants, 518. See also Heparin
Anti-D globulin, 547-48
Antimicrobial therapy, 519-20
Anus, 81-82
  imperforate, 609
  puerperal cleansing, 377
Anxiety:
  regarding defective child, 582
  regarding electrical monitoring equipment, 323-24

Anxiety: (continued)
   during labor, 277, 280-81, 291
   regarding uterine massage, 505-6
Apgar scoring system, 343-44
   in neonatal respiratory distress, 590, 591, 592
Apnea. See Asphyxia neonatorum
Arms:
   congenital amputation, 612
   neonatal paralysis, 598-99
Artificial insemination, 132
Aschheim-Zondek test, 157
Ascorbic acid (vitamin C), 57, *191*, 193
Asepsis, in delivery room, 329
Asherman's syndrome, 135
Aspiration:
   due to general anesthesia, 296-97
   neonatal syndromes, 593-95
Asphyxia neonatorum, 590-93
   livida vs. pallida types, 590
   prevention of, 590-91
   transitory, 398
   treatment, 591
   in undersized infant, 562
Association for Improving the Conditions of the Poor, 12, 663
Association of Infant Milk Stations, 664
Atelectasis, 593-94
Atony, uterine, 296, 504
Atropine:
   and breast milk, 362
   and fetal heart rate, 323

Babies' Welfare Association, 664
Backache, during pregnancy, 67, 208
Back labor, 268, 282
Bacterial infections, neonatal, 594, 600-1, 602
Ballottement, 156
Baptism, 346-47
Barbiturates:
   for eclampsia, 471
   for hyperemesis gravidarum, 484
   for labor pain, 291
   for preeclampsia, 468
Bartholin's glands, 76
Basal metabolism of newborn, 400-1
Bathing:
   in early puerperium, 373
   during labor, 307
   during last weeks of pregnancy, 516
   of newborn, 418-20, 430
Belladonna alkaloid, 291, 325
Belleview School for Midwives, 665
Bilirubin:
   amniotic levels, and fetal evaluation, 532, 534, 547, 558
   excess. See Hyperbilirubinemia
   neonatal levels, 400
   in premature infants, 565
Birth certificate, 9-10, 346
Birth marks, 119-20

Birthrate:
   by mother's age and race, *8*
   decline in, 7, 9, 674
   defined, 8
   in 1974, 42, 44
   and number of births, 10-11
Birth Registration Area, 664
Birth weight:
   effect of mother's smoking on, 58
   and gestational age, 553-55
   and mother's age, 54, 55
   significance of, 14
   and socioeconomic status, 56
Blacks. See also Race
   family lifestyle, 35-36
   infant mortality among, 56
Bladder:
   catheterization, 332, 374
   description, 81
   monitoring of, during labor, 324-25
   puerperal complications, 372, 525-27
   and uterine fundus, 360
   voiding, after delivery, 373-74
Bleeding. See Hemorrhage
Blemishes of newborn, 119-20
Blindness, 571
Blinking reflex, 402
Blood:
   changes in, during pregnancy, 148-49
   of infant, white cells, 400, 465
   in puerperium, 362
   uterine supply, 79
Blood coagulation:
   with abruptio placentae, 482
   in newborn, 400
Blood group:
   and fetal problems, 545-48
   of laboring mother, 307
Blood pressure:
   in antepartal care, 168
   after delivery, 370, 372
   in eclampsia, 470
   high. See Hypertension
   monitoring, during normal labor, 324
   of newborn, 399-400
   in preeclampsia, 465-66
   in premature infant, 564
Blood studies:
   for fetal evaluation, 534, 544
   for phenylketonuria, 614
Blood transfusion:
   exchange-type, for newborn, 547
   for postpartal hemorrhage, 506
Blood volume of newborn, 399
Body temperature, and menstrual cycle, 91-93
Bottle-feeding. See also Formula
   to complement breast-feeding, 387-88
   decision regarding, 379
   for premature infants, 575
Bottles, for formula, 425-26
Bowel habits during pregnancy, 203

Brachial palsy, 598-99
Bradycardia, fetal, 317, 320
Brain damage:
   from malnutrition, 579
   and reflexes, 401-2
Brassiere, for nursing mother, 375, 377
Braxton-Hicks contractions:
   prior to labor, 302
   sign of pregnancy, 156
Breast-feeding, 375-92. See also Breast milk; Lactation
   advantages of, 421
   and after-pains, 362
   alternate massage, 383
   and breast care, 375
   with cleft lip and solidus or palate, 607
   in communes, 30
   and complemental feeding, 387-88
   contraindications, 379, 387, 490, 524, 605
   decision regarding, 379
   in disaster conditions, 651
   with endometritis, 518
   from engorged breast, 522
   group instruction, 227
   and hyperbilirubinemia, 617
   and infant stools, 420
   initiation of, 381-86
   interruption of, 603
   and laxative use, 375
   in maternal infection, 409
   maternal nutrition for, 372, 390-91
   and menstruation, 363
   and need for rest, 372
   and nipple care, 386-87
   orientation of infant to, 384-86
   positions for, 383-84
   and postpartal hemorrhage, 507
   with premature infant, 572
   scheduling, 387-88
   and uterine contraction, 521
   weaning, 391-92
Breast milk, 361-62. See also Breast-feeding; Lactation
   and breast engorgement, 381
   composition of, 423
   ejection reflex, 380
   expression of, 388-90, 409
   precursor of, 148
   for premature infants, 573
   secretion of, 380, 522-23
Breast pump, 389-90, 409, 522
Breast shield, 385-86
Breasts. See also Nipples
   abscess of, 524-25
   antepartal care, 200, 375
   "caked," 522
   changes in, after delivery, 361-62
   changes in, during pregnancy, 147-48, 149
   engorged, 361, 375-76, 380-81, 522
   exercises for, 392
   of newborn, 408, *560*
   puerperal care, 375-76

Breasts (*continued*)
  puerperal disorders, 521-25
  signs of pregnancy, 154-55
  structure of, 82
  support garments for, 201, 375, 377
Breathing exercises, 224-25, 230-33, 271, 315. *See also* Prepared childbirth
Breech presentation, 244, 246, 298, 498-501
Bromides, and breast milk, 362
Brow presentations, 501-2
Bubbling, 387, 403, 426
Bulletin of Maternal and Child Health, 665

Calcium, dietary, *190*, 193
Calories. *See also* Diet; Food; Infant feeding; Nutrition
  food values, 183
  for newborn, 401, 424
  supplied by milk, *423*
Cancer, cervical, 169
Candidiasis, 212
Caput succedaneum, 596-97
Carbohydrates:
  infant requirements, 424
  metabolism of, during pregnancy, 148
  for premature infant, 572
  supplied by milk, *423*
Cardiac. *See also* Heart
Cardiac disease, and pregnancy, 486-87
Cardiac massage, 592-93
Cardiovascular system:
  malformations of, 604-6
  of premature infant, 564-65
Cathartics, and breast milk, 362
Caudal anesthesia, 292-94, 295-96, 298
Caul, 257
Cellulitis, pelvic, 518
Center for Disease Control (Atlanta), 601, 668
Central nursery system, 410-11
Cephalhematoma, 597
Cephalic presentation, 244
Cephalopelvic disproportion, 502-3
Cerebral hemorrhage, 597-98
Cervical mucus:
  during pregnancy, 146
  and menstrual cycle, 91, 127
Cervix:
  cancer of, 169
  changes in, during pregnancy, 146, 156
  description, 78, 79
  effacement and dilatation, 252, 255-57
  incompetent os, 477-78
  laceration of, 504
  obliteration of, 257
  puerperal changes, 360, 516
  in rectal examination, 311
  and spermatazoa, 102
  taking up of, 257

Cesarean section, 452-56
  in abruptio placentae, 482
  anesthesia with, 296, 298
  and bathing, 373
  for breech presentation, 500
  for brow presentation, 502
  with contracted pelvis, 502
  for diabetic gravida, 488
  history of, 658, 659
  and hyaline membrane disease, 595, 596
  in placenta previa, 481
  postpartal instructions, 227
  with prolapsed cord, 509
  in prolonged pregnancy, 548-49
  for shoulder presentation, 501
  for syphilis prevention, 550
  for uterine dysfunction, 495, 496, 507
Chadwick's sign, 155
Change of life, 91, 93-94
Cheeks of newborn, 405-6
Child and Family Resource Program, 669
Childbearing:
  education for, 220-26. *See also* Prepared childbirth
  fear of, 495
  husband-coached, 219, 225. *See also* Father
  motivations for, 42-44
  natural childbirth. *See* Prepared childbirth
  pain, uniqueness of, 265-66, 276
  sociocultural factors affecting, 44-45
Childbed fever. *See* Puerperal infection
Childbirth Education Association, 290
Child care instructions, 226-28
Child health, 6-7
Child-Health Stations (New York), 664
Child Protection Act, 668
Children. *See also* Infant
  recommended daily dietary allowances, *180*
  role of, 22-23
Children's Bureau, 17
Children's Health Service of New York, 663
Child Study Association, 17
Child-welfare legislation, 663
Chills:
  after delivery, 337, 366
  with puerperal infection, 517, 519
Chimerism, 551
Chinese obstetrics, 658
Chloasma, 149
Chloroform, 297, 298
Cholera:
  danger of, 550
  vaccine, 199
Chorea, 538

Chorion, 105, 108-10
  neoplasm of, 479-80
  and twinning, 510-11
Chorionic somatotropin, 150
Chromosomes:
  abnormalities, 99, 535-36, 609-11
  and fertilization, 96-98, 104
Circulation:
  changes in, at birth, 118, *119*
  of fetus, 117-18, *119*
  of newborn, 399-400
Circumcision, 408
  care following, 416
  contraindication, 608
Clamps, obstetric, 333
Cleft lip, 606-7
Cleft palate, 588, 606-7
Climacteric, 91, 93-94
Clitoris, 75-76
Clothing, during pregnancy, 200-2
Cluster visits, pediatric, 228
Coitus. *See* Sexual intercourse
Coitus interruptus, 128
Colostrum, 148, 361, 381
Coma, in eclampsia, 469-70
Committee on Maternal Nutrition, 181
Common cold, 489
Commune families, 27-28, 30-31
Community health nurse, 177-78
Community Mental Health Centers, 669
Community Service Society, 663
Conceptus, 107
Conception:
  and adoption, 136
  and ovum development, 95-105
  prevention of. *See* Contraception
Condom, 126, 128
Conference on Better Care for Mothers and Babies, 666
Conference on Maternal and Child Health Teaching in Graduate Schools of Public Health, 667
Congenital amputation, 612
Congenital heart disease, 604-6
Congenital malformations, 603-13
  of alimentary tract, 608-9
  antenatal detection, 534-36
  atresia, 608
  due to diabetes, 548
  due to rubella, 549-50
  in undersized infants, 556
Congenital pneumonia, 594
Congenital syphilis, 556, 603
Congestive heart failure, and pregnancy, 486
Conjugate, obstetric, 72-73
Conjunctivitis, 599-600
Constipation:
  antepartal, 149, 203, 208
  after delivery, 363, 374-75
  prevention of, 372
Contraception, 121-28
  current fertility trends, 42-43
  oral. *See* Oral contraceptives

Contraception (*continued*)
  permanent. *See* Sterilization
  postpartal, 128
  rhythm method, 91, 122, 126-27
  in social contract families, 28
  for teenagers, 55
Contraceptive withdrawal, 128
Contractions. *See also* Labor; Labor
    pain
  Braxton-Hicks type, 156, 302
  dangerously long, 315
  after delivery, 362-63
  dysfunctional, 493, 494-98
  in first stage of labor, 313-15
  mechanism of, 254
  pain due to, 267-69
  in true vs. false labor, *303*
Convulsions, 469-70, 597. *See also*
    Eclampsia
Coombs test, 546, 548
Cooper Bill, 665
Corona radiata, 99, 103
Corpus luteum, 88, 89, 147
Cortical steroids, fetal, 253-54
Cortisol, metabolism during preg-
    nancy, 151
Cough reflex, 402
Cramps:
  during labor, 327
  during pregnancy, 211
Creams, contraceptive, 125, 126, 127
Creatinine, 531-32, 558
Crisis:
  of defective child, 582-88
  and disaster conditions, 645-55
Crying, 417-18
  evaluation of, 413
  with intracranial hemorrhage, 598
  mother's concerns regarding, 430
  of premature infant, 563
  and pulse rate, 399
  postpartal, of mother, 370
Cumulus oophorus, 99, 103
Curettage, suction method, 130
Cyanosis of newborn, 343, 399, 414
Cyclopropane, 297, 298
Cystitis, puerperal, 526
Cytology, 531
Cytomegalovirus, 550, 551

Dancing reflex, 402
Death:
  neonatal, 589-90. *See also* Infant
    mortality
  of mother. *See* Maternal mortality
Death wishes, 584
Decidua, 107-8, 359-60
Dehydration, 483
DeLee glass trap, 342
DeLee-Hillis stethoscope, 316
Delivery:
  anesthesia prior to, 329
  blood pressure following, 370, 372
  complications of, 557-58
  in disaster conditions, 650
  of drug addict, 59

Delivery: (*continued*)
  of defective child, 583-84
  of diabetic gravida, 548
  emergency, by nurse, 347-48
  with forceps, 449-51
  in home, 629-43
  in normal labor, 329-34
  pain due to, 268
  parents' goals regarding, 273-74
  of preeclampsic gravida, 468
Delivery room:
  preparation of, 328-29
  transfer to, 326-28, 329
Delivery table, exercises for, 233
Depression:
  postpartal, 370
  with thrombophlebitis, 519
Destructive operations, 456
Diabetes mellitus:
  fetal problems due to, 317, 548
  and incidence of hyaline mem-
    brane disease, 595
  infant characteristics, 614-16
  infant death due to, *464*
  postpartal instructions, 227
  during pregnancy, 148, 487-88
Diapering after circumcision, 416
Diaper rash, 419-20
Diapers, sterilization of, 420
Diaphragm method, 125-26
Diarrhea, neonatal, 602-3
Diazepam, 290, 468, 471
Dick-Read method, 176, 223, 269, 290,
    671
Diet. *See also* Nutrition
  after delivery, 368
  for diabetic gravida, 488
  during labor, 324
  for lactating mother, 390-91
  in preeclampsia, 467-68
Digestion:
  after delivery, 362
  in newborn, 403, 421
  during pregnancy, 149
Disaster chest, 646-47
Disaster Nurse Corps, 647
Disasters, obstetrics during, 645-55
Discharge instruction for new
    mother, 395
Dislocations, neonatal, 599
Diuretics, for preeclampsia, 467-68,
    472
Doppler signal, 318
Douching:
  and contraception, 126, 127
  contraindications, 395, 516, 517
  during pregnancy, 203-4
Down's syndrome:
  fetal detection, 535
  genetic counseling aspects, 537-38
  incidence, 610-11
  origin, 99, 609
Drug addiction:
  effect on pregnancy outcome, 59-60
  neonatal, 618

Drugs. *See also* names or classes of
    drugs
  for home delivery, 641
  transplacental, 551
  use, by lactating mother, 391
  during pregnancy, 611-12
Duchenne's muscular dystrophy, 536
Duodenum, congenital obstruction,
    609
Dysmenorrhea, 91
Dyspnea:
  during pregnancy, 208-9
  in newborn, 399, 414
Dystocia, 498-503

Ears of newborn, 405, *560*
Eclampsia, 469-73. *See also* Toxemias
    of pregnancy
  fetal problems due to, 317, 549
  and nutrition, 57
Ectopic pregnancy, 101, 478-79
EDC, 115-16
Edema:
  in eclampsia, 470
  neonatal, 401-2, *560*
  perineal, 378
  in preeclampsia, 465-66
  during pregnancy, 211
  of scalp, 596-97
Egyptian obstetrics, 658
Electrocardiogram, fetal, 540
Electronic monitoring equipment,
    317, 323-24
Embolism:
  amniotic, 509-10
  pulmonary, 362, 518, 520-21
Embryo, 107-8, 111-12, 119
Emergency conditions, obstetrics
    during, 645-55
Emergency delivery, 347-48
Emergency Maternity and Infancy
    Care Program, 666
Empathy, 304-5
Emphysema, neonatal, 593
Employment during pregnancy, 196-
    98
Endocrine studies, fetal, 531, 533-34
Endocrine system:
  changes in, during pregnancy, 150-
    51
  fetal, 253-54
Endometriosis, 133-34
Endometritis, 517-18
Endometrium:
  biopsy of, 133
  in early pregnancy, 107-8, 116
  healing of, after delivery, 359-60,
    516
  and menstrual cycle, 88, 89
Enema:
  after delivery, 375
  during labor, 307
England, history of obstetrics in,
    659, 660, 662
Epidural anesthesia, 294-96, 298

Epinephrine:
 with chloroform, 297
 and insulin production, 615
Episiotomy, 349-50, 449
 advantages of, 332, 635
 anesthesia for, 291, 297
 avoidance of, 274
 with forceps delivery, 451
 and perineal discomfort, 378
 preparation for, 310
 timing of, 268
Epispadias, 607-8
Erb-Duchenne's paralysis, 598-99
Ergonovine:
 for endometritis, 517-18
 to prevent uterine hemorrhage,
  335-36, 506, 521
Erythema toxicum, 407
Esophagus, congenital atresia, 608
Estriol, role in fetal evaluation, 531,
 533, 548, 558
Estrogen:
 changes due to pregnancy, 150, 151
 effect on fetus, 116-17, 533
 and menopause, 93, 94
 non-menstrual functions, 90-91
 in oral contraceptives, 123
 origin of, 89
 at puberty, 86
 role, in onset of labor, 253
 to suppress lactation, 376
Ether, 297, 298, 662
Ethnicity, and diet, *186*, 187
Exercises:
 for breasts, 392
 for breathing control, 230-33. *See
  also* Prepared childbirth
 during pregnancy, 196
 postpartal, 233-35, 394-95
Expected date of confinement
  (EDC), 115-16
Eye contact, maternal-infant, 576
Eyes. *See also* Vision
 of newborn, 404
 care of, 344-46, 415
 of premature infant, 568

Face presentation, 244, 246, 501
Facial paralysis, neonatal, 598
Fallopian tubes, 78
 and infertility, 133-35
 ligation of, 128-29
 pregnancy in, 478-79
 transport of ovum, 100-101
False labor, 494
False pelvis, 67-68
Family, 17-38. *See also* Parents
 antenatal counseling, 176-77
 black, 35-36
 communal, 27-28, 29-31
 defined, 24
 as focus of maternity care, 671-72
 forms of, in 1970s, 26-28
 interactional approach to, 24, 25-26
 Japanese-American, 37-38
 Mexican-American, 36-37

Family (*continued*)
 roles in, 20-23
 with single parent, 29
 social contract style, 28
 study of, 24-26
Family planning, 121-36
 services, 165, 672-73
Father. *See also* Parents
 of defective infant, 583, 586, 588
 in emergency delivery, 347-48
 during labor, 219, 223, 224, 266, 270,
  299-300, *308*, 313, 325
 nurse's relation to, 306
 of premature infant, 575-77
 during puerperium, 393, 394
 response to infant, 339
 role of, 21-22, 672
 and rooming-in, 412
 single, 29
Fatherliness, 21
Fatigue:
 avoidance of, 195-96. *See also* Sleep
  and rest
 as sign of pregnancy, 155
Fats, infant requirement, 424
Fear of childbirth, 265, 303, 495
Federal. *See also* United States
Federal Food, Drug and Cosmetic
  Act, 668
Federal Security Agent, 664
Feeding. *See* Infant feeding; Diet;
  Nutrition
Femoral thrombophlebitis, 518
Fertility:
 and body temperature, 92
 regulation of, 121-36. *See also* Contraception
Fertility rate:
 by mother's age and race, *8*
 decline in, 7, 9
 present trends, 42-43
Fertilization, 103-4
Fetal. *See also* Fetus
Fetal anemia, 534, 546-47
Fetal distress:
 causes, 544-45
 due to uterine dysfunction, 495-96
Fetal heart rate:
 abnormal patterns, 541-42, *543*
 monitoring, 316-24, 496, 540
 and pregnancy detection, 157-59
Fetal mortality. *See also* Stillbirth
 defined, 8, 13-14
 in eclampsia, 470
 and size of fetus, 502
Fetal position:
 abnormal, 498-502
 diagnosis of, 247-49
 types of, 244-47
 version, 451-52, 505, 658, 659
Fetal presentation:
 breech, 244, 246, 298, 498-501
 brow, 501-2
 cephalic, 244
 foot, 244
 shoulder, 244, 246, 501

Fetus, 529-52. *See also* Fetal
 age determination, 530-32
 chronic problems, 545-51
 circulation in, 117-18, *119*
 descent, 258-59
 development of, 108-20
 disproportional to birth canal,
  502-3
 enlarged, due to diabetes, 548
 evaluation of, 532-36, 539-44
 and genetic counseling, 536-39
 growth retardation in, 550-51
 habitus, 243
 head, during labor, 243-44
 heart sounds of. *See* Fetal heart
  rate
 hyperglycemia in, 615
 hypoxia in, 320, 322
 lungs in, 398, 550
 measurement of, 530
 movements of, 159, 302
 outline of, 156
 period of, 119
 physiology of, 116-18
 in prolonged pregnancy, 548
 quickening of, 155
 scalp blood sample, 543-44
 size of, 110-11
 treatment of, 551-52
 undersized, 550-51
Fever:
 in newborn, 401
 puerperal, 12, 661-62
Flaccidity of newborn, 598
Flatulence, 208
Fluids:
 during labor, 324
 for lactating women, 391
 for newborn, 401, 424
 role in diet, 193
Fluothane, 297, 298
Foams, contraceptive, 127
Folic acid deficiency, 486
Follicle-stimulating hormone (FSH),
  89, 90
 and twinning, 511
Fontanels, 243
 appearance, 405
 fallen, 37
Foot presentation, 244
Footprints of infant, 346
Forceps, 449-51, 660
 in breech presentation, 500
Foreskin, 416
Formula, 423-26. *See also* Bottle-
  feeding
 for premature infant, 572-73
 and stools, 420
Fractures, neonatal, 599
France, history of obstetrics, 659,
  662
Free clinics, 163-64
Frenulum linguae, 607
Friedman test, 157
Fright, 37
Frog test, 157

Frontier Graduate School of Midwifery, 637
Frontier Nursing Service, 636-37, 639, 666
Fruits, role in diet, 192-93
FSH, 89, 90, 511
Fundus, palpation of, 370-71
Funic souffle, 158
Funis. *See* Umbilical cord

Gag reflex, 402
Galactorrhea, 523
Gametes, 95, 98. *See also* Ovum; Spermatozoon
Gamper method, 269
Garters, 201-2
Gastrointestinal tract:
  changes at birth, 403
  function in newborn, 420-21
  in premature infants, 566
Gate control theory, 275-76, 282, 284
Genes, 98, 99
  and blood type, 546
  and size of infant, 556
General anesthesia, 296-98
Genetic counseling:
  after LSD use, 618
  nurse's role in, 536-39
  and trisomy, 611
Genitals, and gestational age, *560*
Gentian violet, 602
German measles. *See* Rubella
Gestational age. *See also* Prematurity
  assessment of, 558-62
  and birth weight, 553-55
  infant small for, 556-57
Glass trap, DeLee, 342
Glucocorticoid, 551-52
Glucose, indications for, 484, 596, 609, 615
Goiter, 488-89
Gonadotropins:
  and menstrual cycle, 89
  during pregnancy, 151
  at puberty, 86
  and twinning, 511
Gonorrhea:
  and neonatal ophthalmia, 345
  during pregnancy, 492
  sign of, 211
Gonorrheal conjuctivitis, 599-600
Gonorrheal salpingitis, 121, 133
Goodell's sign, 156
Graafian follicle, 87-88, 89, 99
Grasp reflex, 402
Gravida. *See also* Primigravida
  defined, 143
  high-risk, 529-30
Grief:
  regarding defective child, 582, 586-88
  regarding neonatal death, 589
Group instruction, 221-28
Grunting, cause of, 595

Guilt:
  regarding defective child, 586-87
  regarding prematurity, 577
Guthrie method, in diagnosis of phenylketonuria, 614

Haase's rule, 110
Halothane, 297, 298
Harvard pump, 496
HCS, 531, 534
Head:
  of newborn, 404
  of premature infant, 563
Headache:
  in preeclampsia, 466
  due to spinal anesthesia, 296, 372-73
Head Start, 668, 669
Health grid, 6
Health Services Administration, 7
Hearing of newborn, 405
Heart. *See also* Cardiac
  changes in, during pregnancy, 149
  fetal sound, 157-59. *See also* Fetal heart rate
  of premature infant, 564
Heartburn, 207-8
Heart disease:
  congenital, 604-6
  and breast-feeding, 379
  and pregnancy, 486-87
Heat lamp, perineal, 378
Hegar's sign, 156
Hemangiomas, 406
Hematologic disorders, 485-86
Hematomas, 521
Hemoglobin concentration:
  of newborn, 400
  in premature infant, 564-65
Hemoglobinopathies:
  fetal detection, 536
  of pregnancy, 486
Hemolytic disease, 545-48
Hemorrhage:
  and abruptio placentae, 508
  maternal mortality rate, 12
  neonatal intracranial, 597-98
  postpartal, 335-36, 337, 374, 503-7
  during pregnancy, 473-82
  in premature infant, 563, 564
  in puerperal infection, 515
  vs. show, 482
  from umbilical cord, 617
Hemorrhoids:
  during pregnancy, 210-11
  after delivery, 363
Heparin, 518, 519, 521
Hepatic function:
  and choice of anesthetic, 297
  in newborn, 404
  in premature infant, 566
Hernia, umbilical, 608
Heroin addict:
  congenital, 618
  delivery of, 59
Hexachlorophene, 414, 601

High blood pressure. *See* Hypertension
High-level wellness, 5-6
HMG, 133
Hogben test, 157
Home delivery, 33-34, 629-43
  advantages, 632-33
  conduct of, 633-34
  equipment for, 633
  incidence of, 631-32
  risks of, 634-35
  vs. "sick role," 45
  supplies for, 640, 641-42
Home start programs, 668-69
Hormones, 88-91
Hospital:
  during emergency, 646-47
  number of births in, 13
Hospitalization, 13, 15
  admission and orientation to labor, 303, 306, 307
  for hyperemesis gravidarum, 483
  in preeclampsia, 467
  postpartal discharge, 373
  resistance to, 33-34
  shift to, 670
Hot flashes, 94
HPL, 531, 534
Human chorionic gonadotropin (HCG), 91, 105, 150, 157
  in fetal evaluation, 533-34
Human chorionic somatotropin (HCS), 531, 534
Human menopausal gonadotropin (HMG), 133
Human placental lactogen (HPL), 531, 534
Huntington's chorea, 538
Husband-Coached Childbirth, 269, 286. *See also* Fathers; Prepared childbirth
Hyaline membrane disease, 594-96
Hydatidiform mole, 479-80, 473
Hydramnios, 362, 504
Hydrocephalus, 503, 604
Hymen, 76
Hyperbilirubinemia:
  and breast-feeding, 617
  neonatal, 400, 616
  in premature infant, 565
  and vitamin K, 591
Hyperemesis gravidarum, 154, 482-84
Hyperglycemia, fetal, 615
Hypertension:
  and abruptio placentae, 549
  with eclampsia, 470
  effect of pregnancy on, 473
  fetal problems due to, 549
  and toxemia, 465
Hyperthyroidism, 488
Hypertonic saline abortion, 130-31
Hypertonic uterine dysfunction, 495-96
Hyperventilation:
  cause, during labor, 225, 271
  treatment, 283

Hypnosis, 225-26, 290
Hypnotics. *See* Barbiturates
Hypocalcemia, 616
Hypofibrinogenemia, 482, 509
Hypoglycemia, neonatal, 562, 625-16
Hypoprothrombinemia prophylaxis, 346
Hypospadias, 607-8
Hypotension, maternal, 295-96, 320
Hypothalamus, 89-90
Hypothyroidism, 489
Hypotonic uterine dysfunction, 496-98
Hypoxia, fetal, 320, 322
Hysterectomy:
    after abruptio placentae, 482
    with cesarean section, 454
    effects of, 94
    for uterine rupture, 507
Hysteria, in disaster, 652, 653
Hysterosalpingography, 134
Hysterotomy, 130-31

Icterus neonatorum, 407
Idiopathic respiratory distress syndrome, 594-96
Illegitimate births, rate of, *54*
Immunization, during pregnancy, 199, 490
Imperforate anus, 609
Incompetent os, 477-78
Incomplete abortion, 475
Incubator, 569-70
Induction of labor, 456-58, 548
Inevitable abortion, 474-75
Infancy, period of, 119
Infant, 397-440
    abnormalities in, 406-8, 581-618
    appraisal of, 342-43
    assessment of gestational age, 559-62. *See also* Gestational age
    baptism of, 346-47
    basal metabolism, 400-401
    behavior of, 413
    breast engorgement in, 408
    circulatory changes, at birth, 399-400
    daily cleansing of, 414, 418-20, 430
    drug-addicted, 59-60, 618
    after emergency delivery, 348
    environment of, 408-13, 427
    feeding of. *See* Breast-feeding; Bottle-feeding; Infant feeding; Nutrition
    full term vs. preterm, 474
    gastrointestinal changes, at birth, 403
    general appearance of, 404-6
    hepatic function, 404, 566
    high-risk, 557-58
    hypertonic, 418
    hypoglycemia in, 562, 625-26
    identification of, 346
    immature, 474
    immediate care of, 333, 338, 341-47
    infection in, 408-11, 594, 599-603. *See also* Infection

Infant (*continued*)
    injuries of, 596-99
    intensive care nursery, 569
    jaundiced. *See* Jaundice, neonatal
    kidney function, 403-4, 566
    malformed, 603-13. *See also* Congenital malformations
    menstruation in, 408
    mortality. *See* Infant mortality; Perinatal mortality; Stillbirth
    mother's bonding with, 575-77
    mother's concerns regarding, 430
    natal day observations, 333, 413-14
    newborn period, 119
    nursing care for, 413-20, 397-440
    physiological responses, 413-14
    physiology of, 397-404
    oversized, 502-3
    protection of, in disaster, 648-51
    postmature, 548-49
    premature. *See* Prematurity
    recommended daily nutritional allowances, *280*
    reflexes, 401-3
    respiratory changes, at birth, 398-99, 414
    respiratory distress, 590-96
    sucking behavior, 384-86
    suckling reflex, 382
    temperature changes, 400
    tetany in, 616
    types of care for, 410-13
    undersized, 556-57, 562
    urinary excretion, 403-4, 420
Infant feeding, 420-28. *See also* Bottle-feeding; Breast-feeding; Nutrition
    artificial, 423-26
    bubbling, 387, 403, 426
    of defective infant, 587, 607
    environment for, 427
    intravenous, 572
    mother's concerns regarding, 430
    of premature infant, 575
    schedule for, 387-88
    self-regulatory, 422-23
    and sucking behavior, 384-86
    weaning, 391-92
Infant Milk Station, 663
Infant mortality, 13-14. *See also* Perinatal mortality; Stillbirth
    in breech presentation, 499
    decline in, 7
    with diabetic mother, 614
    and diseases of mother, *464*
    first statistics, 664
    with hyaline membrane disease, 595
    and mother's age, 53
    and race, 55, 56
    rate, defined, 8
    in shoulder presentation, 501
Infection:
    of breast, 523-24
    fetal problems due to, 549-50
    and infant size, 556
    intrapartal, 495

Infection: (*continued*)
    neonatal, 408-11, 594, 599-603
    during pregnancy, 489-92
    puerperal. *See* Puerperal infection
    in premature infant, 570
    respiratory, 516
    of urinary tract. *See* Urinary system
    of uterus, 550
Infertility, 121, 131-36
Influenza, 490, 550
Injuries, neonatal, 596-99
Insemination, artificial, 132
Insufflation, uterine, 134
Insulin:
    fetal production, 615
    resistance to, 488
Intensive care nursery, 569, 576, 673
Intercourse. *See* Sexual intercourse
Internal version, 451-52
International Childbirth Education Association, 277
International Confederation of Midwives, 637, 667
Interorganizational Committee of Obstetric-Gynecologic Health Personnel, 669
Interstitial pregnancy, 479
Intestinal elimination:
    after delivery, 363
    of newborn, 420
    during puerperium, 374-75
Intestines of newborn, 403, 421
Intrapartal infection, 495
Intrauterine device (IUD), 124
    abortion with, 125
Intrauterine pressure (IUP), 318-19
Involution, 359-61
Iodides, and breast milk, 362
Iodine, role in diet, 195
Iron:
    function and sources, *190*, 194-95
    in neonatal period, 404
Iron deficiency anemia, in pregnancy, 149, 485-86
Irritability, reflex, 343
Ischium, 65-66
Isolette, 569-70
Isoniazid (INH), 490-91
IUD, 124, 125
IUP, 318-19
Ivac peristaltic pump, 496

Japanese-American families, 37-38
Jaundice, neonatal:
    physiologic, 400, 407
    in premature infant, 565
    due to Rh disease, 546
Jellies, contraceptive, 125, 126, 127
Jewish obstetrics, 658-59
Joint Committee on Maternal Welfare, 519, 666

Karyotype, 96-98
Kegal exercise, 235
Kelly clamps, 333

Kernicterús, 565. *See also* Jaundice, neonatal
Kidney disease:
  and breast-feeding, 379
  during pregnancy, 489
Kidneys:
  of newborn, 403-4
  of premature infant, 566
  during puerperium, 363

Labia:
  after delivery, 361
  description, 75
  cleansing of, 377
Labor, 299-350
  abnormal, signs of, 304
  analgesia during, 325
  anesthesia during, 289-98
  anxiety regarding, 219, 313-14
  back labor, 268, 282
  complications of, 493-512, 557-58
  concurrent discomforts, 272
  in disaster conditions, 649-50
  duration of, 254-56
  in eclampsia, 473
  enema administration, 307
  examinations during, 310-12
  false, 251, 272, *303*
  fear of, 303
  fetal well-being during, 539-44
  first stage, *308-9, 312-26*
  fourth stage, 336-41
  guidelines to mother's participation in, *308-9*
  in home birth, 633, 642-43
  hospital admission and orientation, 303, 306, 307
  under hypnosis, 225-26
  induction of, 456-58, 548
  informing mother of progress, 280-81
  latent vs. active phases, 255-56
  mechanism of, 258, 262
  onset of, 252-54, 302
  pain during. *See* Labor pain
  parents' goals and expectations of, 273-74
  phenomena of, 251-63
  positioning of mother, 270, 282
  premature, 254, 474, 550
  premonitory signs, 251-52, 302
  preparations for, 302
  presentation and position of fetus, 243-49. *See also* Fetal position; Fetal presentation
  reduction of noxious stimuli, 281-82
  after saline abortion, 130
  second stage, 325-34
  stages of, 256-63, *308-9*
  stimulation of, 151
  third stage, 334-36
Laboratory tests. *See also* names of tests
  antepartal, 168-69
  to detect pregnancy, 156-57
  on laboring mother, 307

Labor pain, 265-87
  and anxiety, 313-14
  assessment of, 268-75
  beliefs about, 265-66
  causes of, 267-68
  gate control theory, 275-76, 282, 284
  importance of control, 266
  relief measures, 280-85. *See also* Anesthesia
Lacerations:
  of birth canal, 348-49, 504
  repair of, anesthesia for, 291
Lactation. *See also* Breast-feeding; Breast milk
  and breast engorgement, 380-81
  and diet of mother, 390-91
  initiation of, 376
  mechanisms of, 379
  onset of, 361-62
  suppression of, 375-76
  variations in, 522-23
LaLeche League, 29, 672
Lamaze method, 223, 224-25, 269, 277, *278-79*, 282-83, 290
Lamp treatment:
  for diaper rash, 419
  of nipples, 386
  of perineum, 378
Lanugo:
  in assessment of gestational age, *560*
  in meconium, 420, 421
  neonatal appearance, 406
  of premature infant, 563
Laparoscopy, 129, 135
Laxatives:
  antepartal use, 203, 208
  and breast-feeding, 375
  after delivery, 375
Laws regarding abortion, 129, 668, 669, 672
Layette, 212-13
Learning concepts, 218
Lecithin/sphingomyelin ratio, 558
Leff fetal heart stethoscope, 316
Leopold maneuvers, 247-49
Lightening, 146, 251, 302
  effect on bladder, 150
Liley chart, 547
Linea negra, 149
Lips of newborn, 405-6
Liver. *See* Hepatic function
Lochia, 359-60
  in endometritis, 517-18
  observation of, 377
  with stilbestrol, 376
LSD-25, 618
L/S ratio, 558
Lumbar epidural anesthesia, 294-96, 298
Lungs:
  of fetus, 398
  neonatal problems, 590-96
  of premature infant, 563
Luteinizing hormone (LH), 89, 90
Lysergic acid, 618
Lysozyme, 375

Macrobiotic diet, 188
Magnesium sulfate:
  in eclampsia, 471
  in preeclampsia, 468
Malformations, congenital. *See* Congenital malformations
Malnutrition:
  and brain damage, 579
  and fetal growth, 556
Mammary grands. *See* Breasts
Mannitol, 472
Margaret Sanger Research Bureau, 666
Marijuana, 272
Marriage:
  common-law, 28
  effect on, of childrearing, 26
  group, 27, 30
  social contract, 28
Marriage rate, 8, 9
Mask of pregnancy, 149
Mask:
  indications for use, 410, 517
  contraindication, 570
Massage:
  alternate, in breast-feeding, 383
  cardiac, 592-93
  during labor, 284
Massive aspiration syndrome, 594-95
Mastitis, 523-24
Maternal age:
  effect on pregnancy outcome, 53-56
  and fertility, 8
  and genetic counseling, 537
  and maternal mortality, 11
  and use of antenatal services, 47
Maternal and Child Health and Mental Retardation Planning Amendments of 1963, 667
Maternal hypotension, 295-96, 320
Maternal and infant care projects (MIC), 49, 50
Maternal mortality:
  and abortion, 43, 129, 131, 475
  defined, 8
  with diabetes, 488
  with eclampsia, 470
  leading cause of, 297, 464
  and nutrition, 57
  with placenta previa, 480
  with puerperal infection, 515
  trends in, 11-13
  with uterine atony, 504
Maternal physiology, 85-94
Maternity care:
  current problems, 1-62
  family focus, 671-72
  for low-income groups, 49-52
  lying-in cottage concept, 635
  and prepared childbirth, 225, 269, 283
  role of communication in, 48-49
  school of nurse-midwifery, 637
  social factors, 41-52
  WHO definition, 4
Maternity Center Association, 17, 222, 665

Maternity clinical specialist, 673
Maternity Consultation Service (New York), 666
Maternity nursing. *See also* Nurse
  antepartal process, 170-78
  development of, 670-74
  during emergency, 645-55
  establishing nurse-patient relationship, 303-7
  future of, 674-76
  in home delivery, 629-43
  role of, 4-6
  teaching and counseling function, 217-35
Maternity Service Association, 665
Maternity services:
  factors in utilization of, 46-49
  trends in, 42-44
Maturity, period of, 119
Measles. *See* Rubella
Meat group, role in diet, 192
Meconium:
  in amniocentesis, 531
  in amnioscopy, 534
  and asphyxia, 590
  aspiration of, 593-94
  in breech presentation, 501
  and fetal distress, 544
  and newborn, 420
  passage of, significance, 316-17
Medicaid, 668, 669
Medical Letter on Drugs and Therapeutics, 199
Medical social worker, 178-79
Medicare, 669
Meiosis, 95, 96
Membranes, rupture of:
  artificial rupture, 457-58, 496
  in emergency delivery, 347-48
  and fetal heart rate, 317, 509
  in hypertonic uterine dysfunction, 495-96
  infection due to, 550
Menarche, 85, 86, 91
Meningomyelocele, 535, 536, 608
Menopause, 91, 93-94
Menstrual cycle, 88-91. *See also* Ovulation
  and body temperature, 91-93
  length of, 91
  and oral contraception, 123-24
  safe period, 91, 122, 126-27
Menstruation:
  after delivery, 363
  hormonal control of, 88-91
  in newborn, 408, 416
  and ovulation, 86-88
  and pregnancy, 88, 154
  suppression of, 154
Metabolism:
  changes during pregnancy, 148
  inborn errors, 613-17
Methadone:
  antepartal therapy, 618
  effect on fetus, 60
Methoxyflurane, 297
Mexican-American families, 36-37

MIC, 49, 50
Midwifery, 4, 670. *See also* Nurse-midwife
  Chinese attitude toward, 658
  Hebrew, 659
  history in U.S., 661, 670
  primitive, 657
  in Renaissance period, 659
Milia, 406, 407
Milk:
  composition, *423*
  and neonatal calcium metabolism, 616
  nutritional role, 189-90, 192
Milk-fever, 362
Milk leg, 518
Milk let-down, 151, 387
Milk of magnesia, 208
Minerals:
  infant requirements, 424
  nutritional role, *180*, 193-95
  in various types of milk, *423*
Miscarriage. *See* Abortion
Molding, 243
Momma League, 29
Mongolian spots, 406
Mongolism. *See* Down's syndrome
Mons veneris, 75
Mortality. *See* Fetal mortality; Infant mortality; Maternal mortality; Perinatal mortality; Stillbirth
Morula, 101, 104
Morning sickness, 154, 482
Moro reflex, 401-2
Morphine:
  in eclampsia, 471
  in preeclampsia, 468
  in pulmonary embolism, 520
  in uterine dysfunction, 495
Mosaicism, 611
Mother. *See also* Maternal; Maternity; Parents
  of defective child, 582
  disaster protection for, 648-51
  encouragement of, during labor, 304
  health of, 6-7
  high-risk, 164, 317, 557
  impressions of, 119-20
  of premature infant, 575-77
  problems and goals of, 427-28
  role of, 20-21
  single, 29
Motherliness, 20
Mouth of newborn, 405-6
Movements of newborn, 404
Mucus, cervical. *See* Cervical mucus
Multigravida:
  delivery of, 326
  fetal heart rate in, 316
  hospitalization of, 314
  lightening in, 302
  and rooming-in, 412
Multipara, defined, 143
Multiple births, 9
  after-pains, 362

Multiple births (*continued*)
  cause, 133
  effect on infant size, 557
  pregnancy, 510-12
Mumps, 199
Muscle control during pregnancy, 229
Muscle tone of newborn, 343
Muscular dystrophy, Duchenne's, 536
Myomectomy, 135

N-allylnormorphine, 568
Narcotics, for labor pain, 290
Nasopharynx, neonatal infection, 524
Natality, 9-10
National Academy of Sciences, 181
National Advisory Council on Nurse Training, 667
National Center for Family Planning, 668
National Center for Health Statistics, 8, 55
National Center on Child Abuse and Welfare, 669
National Commission for the Study of Nursing and Nursing Education, 668, 669
National Committee for Maternal Health, 665-66
National Health Insurance, 668
National Institute of Child Health and Human Development, 667, 669
National Institutes of Health, 56
National Natality Study, 46
National Office of Vital Statistics, 9, 10
National Research Council, 193, 390-91
Natural childbirth. *See* Prepared childbirth
National Society for the Prevention of Blindness, 664
Nausea, during pregnancy, 154, 207, 482
Neighborhood Health Centers, 668
Neonatal. *See* Infant
Neonatalogy, 673
Nesacaine, 292-93
Neurological system:
  and assessment of gestational age, 561-62
  changes in, at birth, 401-3
  of premature infant, 565-66
Neurosis, about pregnancy, 483
Newborn. *See* Infant
New York City:
  Child Health Stations, 664
  Children's Welfare Federation, 664
  Department of Health, 637
  Diet Kitchen Association, 663
  Division of Child Hygiene, 663
  Infant mortality, 14
  Milk Committee, 663, 664, 665
  Mother's Milk Bureau, 664

Niacin, function and sources, *191*
Nicotinic acid, dietary role, 193
Nipples. *See also* Breasts
　abnormalities of, 523
　artificial, 425, 607
　care of, 386-87
　inverted, 200
　of newborn, *560*
Nitrous oxide, 296, 297
　for breech presentation, 298
　first use of, 662
Nurse, 23-24, 48-49, 300-301
　in abortion cases, 477
　in antepartal care, 165-68, 170-78
　in cesarean section, 455-56
　in contraceptive counseling, 122-23
　with deformed child, 583-86
　in disasters, 654-55
　in eclampsia, 472-73
　in emergency delivery, 347-48
　in genetic counseling, 536-39
　in hypermesis gravidarum, 483-84
　in multiple births, 512
　in normal labor, 299-302, 304-6, 312-13
　in pain relief, 265-87
　in preeclampsia, 468-69
　in prevention of postpartal hemorrhage, 506
　with teenagers, 55-56
　in uterine dysfunction, 497-98
Nurse-midwife, 636-39. *See also* Midwifery
　first in U.S., 665
　history of, 636-37
　issues affecting, 638-39
　medical association endorsement, 637-38
　schools for, 665, 666
Nurse practitioner, 673-74
Nursery, 410-11
　equipment for, 213-14
　infections in, 600-601, 602-3
　intensive care, 569, 576, 673
Nurse Training Act, 667
Nurses Association of the American College of Obstetricians and Gynecologists, 638
Nutrition. *See also* Diet
　and age at menarche, 55
　and birth weight, 56-57
　of communal families, 30-31
　diet history and evaluation form, *184-85*
　of fetus, 116-17
　function and source of nutrients, *190-91*
　of newborn. *See* Infant feeding; Bottle-feeding; Breast-feeding
　during pregnancy, 34-35, 179-95
　and pregnancy outcome, 56-58
　in premature infant, 572-75
　psychological aspects, 188-89
　during puerperium, 372

Nutrition (*continued*)
　recommended daily allowances, *180*
　sample menus, *186*
　sources of information, 195

Obesity, 181, 182
Observation nursery, 411
Obstetric conjugate, 72-73
Obstetric examination, antenatal, 168
Obstetrics:
　defined, 3-4
　development of, in U.S., 662-70
　history of, 657-62
　largest problems of, 553
　operations, 449-58
　vs. pediatrics, 48
Office of Child Development, 669
Office of Economic Opportunity, 50
Ontario Perinatal Mortality Study, 58
Oophorectomy, 94
Ophthalmia neonatorum, 344-45, 599-600
Opiates, 362
　antagonists, 568, 593
Opisthotonos, 598
Oral contraceptives, 123-24
　and chloasma, 149
　and fertility trends, 42-43
　for nursing mother, 128
Oriental obstetrics, 658
Osmolarity, 532
Outpatient groups, postpartal, 227-28
Ovaries:
　description, 77-78
　and hormonal changes, 88, 91-93
　during pregnancy, 147, 151
　removal of, 94
Ovulation:
　and body temperature, 93
　and fertility, 104, 132-33
　hormonal aspects, 90
　and lactation, 363
　and menstruation, 86-88
　suppression of, 123-24
Ovum:
　description, 99-100
　and endometrium, 88
　in fallopian tube, 100-101
　fertilization of, 103-4
　implantation of, 104-5
　maturation of, 95-98
　number, 87
　penetration of, 103
　period of, 119
　release of, 99-100
Oxygen administration:
　in hyaline membrane disease, 596
　to incubator, 569-70
　during labor, 295-96, 320
　for newborn, 343-44, 592
　for premature infant, 570-71
　and retrolental fibroplasia, 617-18

Oxytocin:
　in abortion, 131, 477
　and breast-feeding, 362
　and cesarean section, 455, 456
　with chloroform, 297
　contraindications, 319, 320, 321, 322
　function, 151
　to induce labor, 456-58
　and lactation, 380, 381
　in multiple births, 512
　and onset of labor, 253
　to prevent postpartal hemorrhage, 335-36, 337, 504, 506
　for uterine dysfunction, 495, 496, 497
　and uterine rupture, 507
　source of, 90
Oxytocin challenge test, 534, 549

Pacifiers, 406
Pain. *See* Labor pain
Palmprints, 346
Palsy, 598-99
Panic:
　in disasters, 651
　during labor, 280
Panting, 233, 271. *See also* Breathing exercises; Prepared childbirth
Papanicolaou smear, 169, 175
Paracervical block, 292
Paralysis, neonatal, 598-99
Parametritis, 518
Para I, defined, 143
Parents. *See also* Father; Maternal; Maternity; Mother
　alternate life style, 32-33
　of defective child, 581-90
　goals and expectations about labor, 273-74, 285-87
　and home delivery, 632-33
　and infant feeding, 379
　other concerns of, during labor, 272-73
　and pain of labor, 266, *268*, 269-72, 274-75
　of premature infant, 575-79
　prepared childbirth classes. *See* Prepared childbirth
　role during puerperium, 392-95
　single, 29
Parents Without Partners, 29
Parity, 143. *See also* Multigravida; Primigravida
　and after-pain, 362
　and cervical os, 360
　and lochia quantity, 360
　and oxytocin use, 496
　and placenta previa, 480
　and postpartal hemorrhage, 505
　and pregnancy outcome, 53-54
　and shoulder presentation, 501
　and size of uterus, 360
　and uterine obstruction, 498
　and vaginal size, 361
Participant childbirth. *See* Prepared childbirth
Paternal-infant attachment, 577

Pediatric assistants, 668
Pediatric care, 227-28, 455
Pediatric cluster visits, 228
Pelvic cellulitis, 518
Pelvic examination, 175
Pelvic thrombophlebitis, 518, 519
Pelvimetry, 71-75
Pelvis, 65-75
    articulation and surfaces, 66-67
    contracted, 502
    divisions, 67-69
    false, 67-68
    healing of, after delivery, 360-61
    individual variations, 69-71
    measurements, 71-75
    organs related to, 81-82
    structure, 65-66
    true, 68
Penicillin:
    for general neonatal indications, 602, 603
    maternal indications, 491, 520
    for neonatal ophthalmia, 344-45, 600
Penis, 82, 84. See also Circumcision
    abnormalities of, 407-8, 607-8
Penthrane, 297
Pentothal, 298
Peridural anesthesia:
    caudal, 292-94
    lumbar, 294-96
Perinatal mortality, 8. See also Infant mortality
    and age of mother, 54
    with diabetic mother, 548
    in eclampsia, 549
    and mother's smoking, 58-59
    with prolapsed cord, 509
    and socioeconomic status, 56
Perineal heat lamp, 378
Perineum, 76-77
    anesthesia of, 291-92
    cleansing, during labor, 316
    at delivery, 268
    discomfort of, 378-79
    incision of. See Episiotomy
    lacerations of, 449, 504
    preparation for delivery, 310
    puerperal care, 376-79, 517
Peritoneoscopy, 134-35
Peritonitis, 519
Phenobarbital:
    in preeclampsia, 467
    for Rh disease, 547, 551
Phenylketonuria (PKU), 613-14, 667
Phimosis, 408-9
Phlegmasia alba dolens, 518
Phocomelia, 611-13
Phonocardiography, 318, 540
Phospholipids, 532
Phosphorus, dietary role, 193-94
Phototherapy, 617
Pill, "the." See Oral contraceptives
Pitocin. See Oxytocin
Pituitary gland:
    changes during pregnancy, 151
    role in menstruation, 89-90

PKU, 613-14, 667
Placenta:
    abruptio, 481-82
    and antithyroid drugs, 488
    birth of, 256, 261-62, 334-36
    description, 110
    effect on, of malnutrition, 556
    in emergency delivery, 348
    endocrine functions, 150, 151
    expression of, 335
    and fetal distress, 544
    function, 116, 117-18
    in home delivery, 634
    in hypertonic saline abortion, 130
    low-lying, 319
    manual delivery, 506
    in prolonged pregnancy, 548
    postpartal hemorrhage, 504, 508
    and Rh factor, 545
    separation of, 359-60
    and twinning, 510-11
    and undersized infant, 556-57
    weight of, 148
Placenta previa, 480-81, 505, 508
Planned Parenthood Federation of America, Inc., 666
Pneumonia, 550, 594
Poliomyelitis, 199, 491
Polycythemia, 562
Polygalactia, 523
Porro's operation, 454
Position of fetus. See Fetal position; Fetal presentation
Postmaturity, 548-49
Postpartal period. See also Puerperium
    after-pains, 262-63
    depression, 370
    exercises, 233-35, 394-95
    first hour, 262-63
    hemorrhage during, 507
    mother-child relationship, 219-20, 576-77
    physical examination, 363-64
    planning for, 214-15
    in preeclampsia, 468
    teaching, 226-28
Posture during pregnancy, 146, 228-29
Potassium, 467
Poverty, and maternal care, 46, 49-52
PPM. See Lamaze method
Preeclampsia. See also Toxemias of pregnancy
    blood study findings, 534
    fetal problems due to, 549
    signs and symptoms, 465-66
    treatment, 466-68
Pregnancy. See also Antepartal care
    abdominal, 479
    breast care during, 200, 375
    and breast-feeding, 379
    bowel habits during, 203
    coincidental diseases, 485-92
    comfort during, 228-29

Pregnancy (continued)
    complications of, 463-84, 557. See also Toxemias of pregnancy
    difficulty in achieving, 121, 131-36
    drug-taking during, 59-60, 611-12
    duration of, 114-16
    early loss, rate of, 107
    ectopic, 101, 478-79
    endocrine changes, 150-51
    hemorrhagic complications, 473-82
    interstitial, 479
    mask of, 149
    maternal impressions during, 119-20
    and menstruation, 88
    metabolic changes, 148
    minor discomforts of, 206-12
    multiple, 510-12
    normal, 143-51
    nutrition during, 179-95
    physiologic changes, 144-50
    positive signs of, 154, 157-59
    presumptive signs, 153, 154-55
    prevention of. See Contraception
    probable signs of, 153, 155-57
    prolonged, 548-49
    psychological effects, 150
    psychological tasks, 218-19
    risk factors, 53-62, 164-65
    social and cultural meanings, 42, 44-45
    teaching and counseling, 217-35
    in teenagers, 54-56
    termination of, 129-31, 471
    tests for, 156-57
    toxemias of. See Toxemias of pregnancy
Premature labor, 254, 474, 550
Prematurity, 553-80
    and birth weight, 553-55
    etiology, 555-57
    growth and development patterns, 579-80
    and hyaline membrane disease, 595
    physical care of infant, 566-75
    physiologic considerations, 563-66
    and retrolental fibroplasia, 617-18
    symptoms at birth, 563
Prenatal Care Committee, 663
Prenatal records, 168
Prepared childbirth:
    Dick-Read method, 176, 223, 269, 290, 671
    groups, 222-25, 283
    Lamaze method, 223, 224-25, 269, 277, 278-79, 282-83, 290
    nurse's role in, 313
    pain relief methods, 265-66, 269-72, 270-72, 277
Presentation. See Fetal position; Fetal presentation
President's Committee on Mental Retardation, 668
Preterm. See Prematurity

Primigravida. *See also* Gravida
  breech presentations in, 500
  defined, 143
  and eclampsia, 470
  episiotomy for, 350, 449
  and fetal heart rate, 316
  and forceps delivery, 450
  frequency of contractions, and hospitalization, 314
  lacerations in, 349
  lightening in, 251, 302
  perineal discomfort of, 378
  and preeclampsia, 465
  utilization of antenatal care, 46, 47
Primipara, defined, 143
Primitive obstetrics, 657
Professional Standards Review Organization, 669
Progesterone:
  assay, in fetal evaluation, 533
  and body temperature, 93
  in intrauterine device, 125
  and labor onset, 252-53
  non-menstrual functions, 90-91
  in oral contraceptives, 123
  origin of, 88, 89
  and ovulation, 133
  during pregnancy, 150, 151
Prostaglandins, 131, 254
Prosthetics, 612
Protein:
  for diabetic gravida, 488
  function and sources, *190*
  in hyaline membrane disease, 594
  infant requirement, 424
  lactation requirements, 391
  in preeclampsia, 467
  for premature infant, 572
  role in phenylketonuria, 614
Protestant Episcopal Church, infant baptism, 347
Psychoprophylactic method, 224-25. *See also* Lamaze method
Psychosexual method, 269
Ptyalism, 489
Public Health Service Act, 666, 667
Pudendal block, 291-92, 298, 450
Puerperal infection, 12, 515-20, 661-62
  history of, 661-62
  maternal mortality rate, 12
Puerperium. *See also* Postpartal period
  complications of, 515-27
  infant care during, 397-440
  nursing care during, 365-95
  physiology of, 358-64
  preparations for, 228, 233-35
  taking-hold phase, 368-70, 372
  taking-in phase, 367-68
Pulmonary embolus, 362, 518, 520-21
Pulse:
  after delivery, 371-72
  monitoring during labor, 324
  of newborn, 399, 417
  in premature infant, 564
  in puerperium, 362

Pump:
  Harvard, 496
  Ivac peristaltic, 496
  for milk expression, 389-90
Pyelitis, 525
Pyelonephritis, 489, 550
Pyloric stenosis, 608-9

Quadruplets, 510. *See also* Multiple births
Quickening, 155

Race:
  and antenatal care, 46
  and birthrate, 9
  and fertility, 8
  and incidence of cleft lip and/or palate, 606
  and infant mortality, 13, 55, 56
  and maternal mortality, 464
  statistical categories, 9
Rash of newborn, 407
Rectal examination during labor, 310
Red Cross, 221, 651
Reflexes of infant, 401, 566. *See also* names of reflexes
Reflex irritability, 343
Regional anesthesia, 291-96
Regurgitation, 403, 426
Relaxation:
  during labor, 270, 284-85
  during pregnancy, 229-30
Renal. *See* Kidneys
Reproduction:
  anatomy related to, 65-84
  clinical aspects, 121-36
  conception and ovum development, 95-105
  development and physiology of embryo and fetus, 107-20
  maternal physiology related to, 85-94
Respiration:
  changes in, during pregnancy, 149
  fetal, 398
  of infant, 343, 597-98
  initiation, in newborn, 398-99
  monitoring of, in normal labor, 324
  of premature infant, 563-64, 570-72
  during puerperium, 371-72
Respiratory distress, 590-96
Respiratory infection, 516
Rest and sleep. *See* sleep and rest
Resuscitation:
  disaster rooms, 647
  for newborn asphyxia, 591-93
Retrolental fibroplasia, 571, 617-18
Rh factor:
  antepartal tests, 169
  and fetal problems, 545-48, 552
  first immunization for, 669
  sensitization to, and uterine transfusion, 533
Rhogam, 547-48, 552
Rhythm method, 91, 122, 126-27
Riboflavin, 57, *191*, 193

Ritgen's maneuver, 332
Roentgenography:
  to assess gestational age, 558-59
  to detect pregnancy, 159
  to determine fetal position, 249
  pelvimetry, 73-75
Roman Catholic Church:
  and contraception, 122
  infant baptism, 346-47
  influence of, on obstetrics, 658, 659
Roman obstetrics, 4, 658, 659
Rooming-in, 411-12, 673
Rooting reflex, 402
Rubella:
  effect on fetus, 199, 490, 549-50
  immunization, 199, 668
  and infant death rate, *464*
Rupture:
  of membranes. *See* Membranes, rupture of uterus, 501, 507

Saddle block, 296
Salivary glands, 489
Salpingitis, 121, 133
Salpingotomy, 479
Salt:
  dietary role, in pregnancy, 182
  and preeclampsia, 466-67
Scopolamine, 291, 325
Scrotum, 82
Sebum, 375
Section, cesarean. *See* Cesarean section
Sedatives:
  for after-pains, 362-63
  after cesarean section, 456
  in eclampsia, 471
  in hyperemesis gravidarum, 484
  in preeclampsia, 468
Semen, 132
Septicemia, puerperal. *See* Puerperal infection
Sex:
  determination of, 96, 98-99
  fetal detection, 538
  and incidence of cleft lip and/or palate, 606
  and infant size, 502
Sex chromatin, 98-99
Sex hormones, 71
Sex-linked disorders, 536
Sexual intercourse:
  after delivery, 395
  before multiple births, 512
  during pregnancy, 204-6, 516
Sexual maturity, 85-88
"Shake test," 532
Shaking chills, after delivery, 337, 366
Sheppard-Towner Bill, 665
Shirodkar technique, 478
Shoes, during pregnancy, 202
Shoulder dystocia, 503
Shoulder presentation, 244, 246, 501
Show, 252, 315-16, 482

Shower, for laboring mother, 307
Sickle cell trait:
  and pregnancy, 486
  fetal detection, 536
Sign. *See* name of sign
Silver nitrate, 344-46, 599-600
Sims's position, 292
Skin, maternal:
    care of, during pregnancy, 199-200
    changes in, during pregnancy, 149-50, 155
    during puerperium, 363
  of newborn, 406, 414
    and assessment of gestational age, *560*
    bacterial infections, 600-601
    care of, 418-20
    of premature infant, 563, 575
Sleep and rest:
  after delivery, 366, 368
  of newborn, 399, 420
  during puerperium, 219, 372, 390
  simulation of, in labor, 270
Sleeplessness, 302
Small intestine, congenital obstruction, 609
Smallpox, 199, 490
Smegma, removal of, 310, 416
Smoking:
  and breast-feeding, 391
  and infant size, 557
  and pregnancy outcome, 58-59, 206
Sneeze reflex, 402
Socialization, steps in, 22-23
Social Security Act, 665, 667, 669
Socioeconomic status, and pregnancy outcomes, 56-58
Sodium chloride. *See* Salt
Souffle, 158-59
Spanish-American families, 51-52
Spasticity, 598
Spermacides, 127
  with diaphragm, 125, 126
Spermatozoon:
  in fallopian tube, 100, 101
  and fertility studies, 132
  maturation of, 95-98
  motion of, 101-3
  penetration of ovum, 103
  and vasectomy, 128
Spina bifida, 608
Spinal anesthesia, 296, 298
Stages of labor. *See* Labor
Standards and Recommendations for Hospital Care of Newborn Infants, 601
Standards for Maternity Care and Employment of Mothers, 197
Standards of Prenatal Care, 666
Startle reflex, 401-2
Starvation, 483
Stepping reflex, 402
Sterilization, 43, 128-29
Stethoscopes, 316

Stillbirth, 8, 589-90. *See also* Fetal mortality and diabetes test, 487
  due to intracranial hemorrhage, 597-98
  and mother's smoking, 58
  previous, and fetal monitoring, 317
  due to Rh disease, 545-46
  due to toxemias of pregnancy, 464
Stomach of newborn, 403, 421, 566
Stools of newborn, 403, 420
Stork bites, 406, 407
Streptococcus, in puerperal infection, 515
Stress:
  during pregnancy, 60-62
  during puerperium, 370
Striae gravidarum, 147, 149
Subdural hematoma, 597-98
Sucking, 406
Sucking pads, 403
Sucking reflex, 402, 421
Suctioning of newborn, 341, 342-43
Sudden infant death syndrome, 699
Superstitions:
  regarding birthmarks, 119-20
  regarding caul, 257
  regarding premature survival rate, 114
Supine hypotensive syndrome, 482
Support garments:
  abdominal, 201
  for breasts, 201, 375, 377
  stockings, 201-2
Suppositories, contraceptive, 127
Swallowing reflex, 402, 421
Sympathy, 304-5
Syntocinon. *See* Oxytocin
Syphilis:
  antepartal test for, 169
  and breast-feeding, 379
  congenital, 556, 603
  fetal problems due to, 550
  during pregnancy, 491

Tachycardia, fetal, 317, 319-20, 399
Tachypnea, neonatal, 593
Tarnier forceps, 450
Tay-Sachs disease, 535, 536, 538
Teenagers, pregnancy in, 54-56
Teeth, during pregnancy, 202
Temperature:
  infant's tolerance to, after delivery, 338, 341
  maintenance of, in infant resuscitation, 591
  maternal, during puerperium, 362, 371-72, 519
  monitoring, in normal labor, 324
  of newborn, 400, 414, 417, 419, 562
  and ovulation, 91-93, 126-27
  regulation of, for premature infant, 565, 568, 569-70
Ten-State National Nutrition Survey, 57
Teratology, 603
Testes, 84

Tetany, neonatal, 616
Thalassemia, fetal detection, 536
Thalidomide, 611
Therapeutic abortion, 484, 549-550
Thermography, 381
Thiamin, function and sources, *191*, 193
Thiopental sodium, 298
Thoms's pelvimeter, 73
Thrombophlebitis, 362, 372, 518-19
Thrush, 212, 601-2
Thyroid function during pregnancy, 151, 488-89
Tokodynamometer, 318
Tongue of newborn, 406
Tongue-tie, 607
Tonic neck reflex, 402
Toxemias of pregnancy, 464-73. *See also* Eclampsia; Preeclampsia
  classification, 464-65
  general examination during labor, 310
  and infant death, *464*
  maternal mortality rate, 12
  and nutrition, 57, 179-81
  use of anesthesia, 296
Toxoplasmosis, *464*, 550
Tranquilizers, 290-91
Transition phase, in labor, 268, 283, *309*
Transitory asphyxia, 398
Transverse lie, 244
Traveling during pregnancy, 198-99
Triage, 647
Trichlorethylene, 297
Trichomoniasis, 212
Trilene, 297
Triplets, 510. *See also* Multiple births
Trisomy. *See* Down's syndrome
Trophoblast, 104-5, 475
True pelvis, 68
Tubal ligation, 128-29, 473
Tubal pregnancy, 478-79
Tuberculosis:
  and breast-feeding, 379
  during pregnancy, 490-91
Tucker McLane forceps, 450
Twinning:
  causes, 511
  rate, 9
Twins. *See also* Multiple births
  delivery of, 512
  diagnosis, 511
  disproportionate development, 551, 556
  and eclampsia, 470
  and postpartal hemorrhage, 504
  types of, 510-11
Typhoid fever, 490, 550

Ultrasonic scanning:
  to assess gestational age, 530-31, 558
  to monitor fetus during labor, 318, 540

Umbilical cord:
  and bathing, 415-16
  care of, 344
  and circulation changes at birth, 118, *119*
  clamping, 333
  and congenital malformation, 344
  at delivery, 332-33
  description, 110
  in emergency delivery, 348
  and fetal distress, 544
  and neonatal hemorrhage, 617
  observation of, 414
  and placenta delivery, 335
  of premature infant, 567
  prolapsed, 322, 508-9
Umbilical hernia, 608
Umbilicus, during pregnancy, 147
United Nations. *See* World Health Organization
United States. *See also* Federal history of obstetrics, 661, 662-70
United States Census Bureau, 10, 663, 664
United States Children's Bureau:
  community health programs, 6
  establishment of, 664
  grants and publications, 666, 667
  MIC projects, 49, 50
  recommendations for expectant mothers, 197
  study of infant mortality, 53
  White House Conference on, 665
United States Department of Commerce and Labor, 664
United States Department of Health, Education, and Welfare, 464, 667-68, 669
United States Department of Labor, 664
United States Food and Drug Administration, 601, 611
United States Public Health Service, 8, 58, 668
United States Supreme Court, abortion ruling, 129, 475, 669, 672
Urinary system:
  changes in, during pregnancy, 150
  infection of, during pregnancy, 489
    due to sickle cell trait, 486
  of premature infant, 566
Urination:
  after delivery, 373-74
  of newborn, 403-4, 420
  during puerperium, 525-26
  during pregnancy, 154, 207
Urine:
  albumin in, 465, 466
  antepartal testing of, 168-69
  phenylketonuria test, 614
  and pregnancy tests, 157
  during puerperium, 363, 525-26

Uterine atony, 296, 504
Uterine dysfunction, 493, 494-98
Uterine souffle, 158-59
Uterotubal insufflation, 134
Uterus:
  after-pains, 362-63
  changes in, during pregnancy, 144-46
  contractions. *See* Contractions; Labor; Labor pain
  and decidua, 107-8
  description, 78-81
  in first hour after delivery, 370-71
  infection of, during pregnancy, 550
  and infertility, 135-36
  intrauterine device, 124-25
  inversion of, 508
  involution of, 359-60
  massage of, 505
  and ovum implantation, 104-5
  and placenta delivery, 334-35
  postpartal care, 337, 370-71
  relaxation of, agents for, 298
  removal of, 94, 454, 482, 507
  rupture of, 501, 507
  signs of pregnancy, 156
  and spermatozoa, 102
  subinvolution of, 521
  weight of, 360

Vaccinations, during pregnancy, 199
Vacuum aspiration, 130
Vacuum extraction, 451, 509
Vagina:
  description, 81
  examination via, 249, 311-12
  involution, 360-61
  lacerations of, 449, 504
  puerperal infection, 516-17
  signs of pregnancy, 155
Vaginal discharge. *See also* Lochia; Menstruation
  during pregnancy, 211-12
  prior to labor, 302
Valium, 290, 468, 471
Varicose veins, 209-10
Vasectomy, 128
Vegetables, dietary role, 193
Vegetarianism, 32, 34, 184, 187-88
Vernix caseosa, 406
  in amniocentesis, 531
  in assessing gestational age, 559
  after emergency delivery, 651
  first appearance of, 114
  in meconium, 421
Version, 451-52, 505
Vertex presentation, 244, 245, 246
Vision. *See also* Eyes
  blurred, 466
  of newborn, 405
Visiting Nurse Association, 222
Vital statistics, 7-9, 663

Vitamins. *See also* names of vitamins
  deficiencies, 57, 187, 483, 502
  function and sources, *191*
  lactation requirements, *180*, 391
  ointment form, 386
  recommended daily allowances, *180*, *181*
  role in diet, 193
  supplemental K for infants, 346, 400, 416, 590-91, 598
Vomiting:
  due to anesthesia, 296-97
  excessive, 154, 482-84
  morning sickness, 154, 482
  in newborn, 403
Vulva:
  description, 75-77
  puerperal lesions, 517
  shaving and washing, 307, 310
Vulvar hematoma, 521

Water. *See* Fluids
Weaning, 391-92
Weight:
  fetal, and viability, 474
  gain, during pregnancy, 148, 169-70, 181, 465-66
  of lactating mother, 391
  of newborn, 416-17. *See also* Birth weight
  puerperal loss, 363
  loss of, prior to labor, 302
Wellness, high-level, 5-6
White House Conferences on children, 664, 665, 666, 667, 668
White House Conference on Food, Nutrition and Health, 668
William's pelvimeter, 73
Witch's milk, 117
Withdrawal, contraceptive, 128
Women. *See also* Maternal; Maternity; Mothers
  economic role, 43
  liberation movement, 28, 29, 30
  status of, and nursing, 671
World Health Organization, 121-22, 666
  abortion terminology, 474
  Committee on Maternity Care, 4
  establishment, 666
  fetal death defined by, 13-14
  Manual of International Classification of Diseases, Injuries, and Causes of Death, 8
Wright method, 269

Yawn reflex, 402
Yellow fever, 199

Zona pellucida, 99, 103
Zygote, 95